THE AFRICAN TRYPANOSOMIASES

The African Trypanosomiases

EDITED BY

Colonel H. W. MULLIGAN

C.M.G., M.D., D.SC., I.M.S. (retd.)

Visiting Lecturer, Department of Biology, University of Salford
Formerly Director, Central Research Institute, Kasauli, India
Director, West African Institute for Trypanosomiasis Research, Kaduna, Nigeria
Director, Wellcome Research Laboratories, Beckenham, Kent

WITH THE HELP, FOR PART II, OF

W. H. POTTS

M.A. (Cantab.)

Commonwealth Institute of Entomology
Formerly, Chief Entomologist, East African Tsetse Research Organization
Shinyanga, Tanganyika

WITH A FOREWORD BY

PROFESSOR W. E. KERSHAW

V.R.D., M.D., D.SC.

Chairman, Trypanosomiasis Panel
Ministry of Overseas Development

London

GEORGE ALLEN AND UNWIN LTD

RUSKIN HOUSE MUSEUM STREET

FIRST PUBLISHED IN 1970

ISBN: 0 04 614001 8

PRINTED IN GREAT BRITAIN
in 10pt Times Roman type
AT THE PITMAN PRESS
BATH

Foreword by

W. E. KERSHAW

V.R.D., M.D., D.SC.

Chairman, Trypanosomiasis Advisory Panel and Chairman, Tsetse Attractants Committee
Ministry of Overseas Development
Professor of Biology, University of Salford
Formerly Professor of Parasitology and Entomology, Liverpool School of Tropical Medicine

The trypanosomiases of tropical Africa comprise a group of diseases of great social and economic importance. Sleeping sickness or trypanosomiasis in man has been responsible for serious mortality and much ill health; nagana or trypanosomiasis in livestock has directly contributed to the widespread malnutrition in Africa by decreasing the amount of protein food available to man. The World Health Organization, in delineating the ten major health problems facing mankind, placed the trypanosomiases of man and his domestic animals high on the list, along with malaria, cancer and heart disease.

The discovery of the aetiology of trypanosome disease and of its mode of transmission was made by British scientists over half a century ago and, during the years of British Colonial Administration in Africa, British investigators were responsible for acquiring much of the present-day knowledge of the trypanosomiases, although the important part played by French, Belgian and Portuguese workers must not be overlooked. Each colony had its own organization devoted to sleeping sickness control. It was established very early that the epidemiology and control of trypanosome infections in man and animals were closely related to the pattern of human and animal life; therefore, control was bound up with the use of land by man for settlement and the use of land by animals, both domestic and wild, for grazing. Medical and veterinary officers, entomologists and some distinguished amateurs were responsible for the conduct of control measures. Most of the observations made in the field could be regarded as naturalistic and ecological, and were not related to those made by workers in other vector-borne diseases such as malaria, filariasis or yellow fever, for it was the fashion to deal with each disease separately, both from an administrative and from a research point of view.

Even before the Second World War, a considerable body of knowledge had been established and was adequate in British, French, Belgian and Portuguese territories in Africa for sleeping sickness to be controlled quite successfully, in the relatively stable political conditions then obtaining, so that the day of the gigantic epidemic was regarded as over. So successful was the control of sleeping sickness that more attention was beginning to be directed to animal trypanosomiasis, the importance of which had long been recognized because of the urgent need for livestock to provide first class protein in the diet of African populations; the need to reorganize the traditional pattern of African agriculture, however, made this problem difficult to solve in the short term.

At the end of the Second World War, the British Colonial Office invited Professor P. A. Buxton, Professor T. H. Davey and Mr H. E. Hornby to examine and report upon the trypanosomiasis problem in the British Colonies in Africa. These experts advised that research on all aspects of the trypanosomiases should be integrated and organized on an interterritorial basis. Two major research institutes were established to serve the needs of East and West Africa, respectively. The East African Trypanosomiasis Research Organization was set up at Tororo in Uganda and the West African Institute for Trypanosomiasis Research at Vom and Kaduna in Nigeria. These two organizations did notable work for more than a decade. Control measures still remained in the hands of individual colonial administrations, apart from a brief period when the Institute in East Africa accepted responsibility for control as well as for research.

With the sometimes stormy advent of independence of the African territories in the 1950s and 60s, these control organizations became gradually less reliable for many reasons and the control of human trypanosomiases deteriorated until, in 1969, it was believed that there were up to a million cases of sleeping sickness in the Congo and that epidemics of vast proportions might well break out in other territories. Research, as well as control, in the field suffered from unstable political conditions.

Contemporaneously with this devolution, however, there was an enormous expansion of the biological sciences, dependent upon and arising from the pure sciences, which changed completely the role and place of research in trypanosomiasis; from being an offshoot of control carried out in Africa, research was already becoming part of the rapidly expanding development of fundamental research in pure science in the developed countries. The advances in molecular biology, the understanding of enzyme systems in microbiology, the development of immunology and immuno-chemistry, the advances in genetics, both of parasites and their vectors, together with enormous advances in organic chemistry and biochemistry, made it clear that fundamental work on the trypanosome and the tsetse fly should be instituted, not only for the obvious, urgent humanitarian reasons but for the advancement of knowledge. In 1960, Colonel H. W. Mulligan was Chairman of the Trypanosomiasis Advisory Panel of the Colonial Office and, on his initiative, a Working Party was established to advise the Panel on the kind of research to be promoted. Such research could obviously be done only in sophisticated laboratories which were part of large institutions devoted to fundamental research.

During the next ten years, therefore, the efforts of scientists in many disciplines have been supported by the Ministry of Overseas Development in institutions all over the British Isles as well as in Africa. The parasite and its vector are now understood far better than formerly and there has been, as a bonus, some fall out from this work into the general pool of scientific knowledge.

In other vector-borne infections such as malaria and filariasis, much has been done in the development of genetics, to the point where genetic manipulation of the vectors has quite sound prospects for use in control. Such work has only recently been started on the tsetse fly; the Ministry of Overseas Development has set up a new Committee, concerned with the promotion of fundamental work on tsetse behaviour and its understanding.

In the half century that has elapsed since the discovery of the aetiology and mode of transmission of the trypanosomiases, no comprehensive book has ever been published, for it would obviously be beyond the competence of any one man to encompass the whole subject. The late Patrick Buxton's classic book *The Natural History of Tsetse Flies* (1955) and A. Sicé's book *La Trypanosomiase humaine en Afrique Intertropicale* (published in 1937 but now out of print and out of date) represent the two most important publications in this field but they deal only with limited aspects of the subject. Two distinguished investigators, Drs A. J. Duggan and M. P. Hutchinson, of the Wellcome Museum of Medical Science in London, suggested to the Trypanosomiasis Advisory Panel of the Ministry of Overseas Development that the time was opportune for a standard reference work covering all aspects of the trypanosomiases and based on contributions from experts in the various disciplines involved. The Ministry agreed to sponsor such a work and were fortunate in securing the services of Colonel H. W. Mulligan as Editor. Colonel Mulligan, by reason of a long and distinguished career in tropical medicine, including research on medical and veterinary aspects of protozoal diseases, and his experience in the administration of, amongst other bodies, the West African Institute for Trypanosomiasis Research, is by qualification and temperament admirably fitted for the task, to which he has also brought his considerable experience and talents as an editor.

The twenty-seven contributors to the book are all men with intimate knowledge of the disciplines with which they deal and, where relevant, all have had extensive experience in tropical Africa.

The distillation of wisdom and experience in this book will, it is hoped, prove of value to many, particularly those in the former British, French and Belgian colonial territories and in the Portuguese colonies who are, sometimes alone and sometimes with the help of others, producing their own control organizations in difficult circumstances. Since many who are entering these control organizations will be new to the trypanosomiases, this book should give them a baseline from which to start their own investigations. It should also be informative to those pure scientists who, for divers reasons, wish to increase the range of possible application of their disciplines.

In the whole field of the African trypanosomiases, there have been so many devoted scientific workers that it is impossible, although it would be appropriate here, to pay them tribute by name. Let this book stand as their testimony.

The invisible contribution made by the Civil Servants of the British Colonial Office which became the Department of Technical Co-operation and is now the Ministry of Overseas Development must be acknowledged. As Chairman of the Trypanosomiasis Advisory Panel of the Ministry, I thank them for their administrative help, their whole-hearted co-operation in the promotion of research, their sense of responsibility towards the developing countries of Africa and for the manner in which they have made it possible for the scientists to get on with the job. Without their prompt and ready assistance, it is possible that this book would have remained a concept, instead of becoming a valuable work of reference for all those who, in Britain and in other countries, are working on this great African problem.

SEPTEMBER, 1969

List of Contributors

DR F. I. C. APTED

M.B., B.S., M.R.C.S., L.R.C.P., D.T.M. & H.

Director, Bureau of Hygiene & Tropical Diseases
Formerly Sleeping Sickness Specialist, Tanganyika

DR J. R. BAKER

Ph.D., D.Sc., F.I.Biol.

Reader in Parasitic Protozoology, London School of Hygiene and Tropical Medicine
Formerly Scientific Officer, East African Trypanosomiasis Research Organization, Tororo, Uganda

DR G. F. BURNETT

D.Sc.

Lecturer in Agricultural Zoology, University of Aberdeen
Formerly Deputy Director, Tropical Pesticides Research Institute, Arusha, Tanzania

PROFESSOR E. BURSELL

Ph.D., D.Sc.

Professor of Zoology and Chairman of the Division of Biological Sciences, University College of Rhodesia, Salisbury, Rhodesia

DR DAVID A. DAME

Ph.D.

Tsetse Fly Investigations Leader, Entomology Research Division, United States Department of Agriculture, Salisbury, Rhodesia

DR A. J. DUGGAN

M.D., D.T.M. & H.

Director, Wellcome Museum of Medical Science, London
Formerly Senior Medical Officer, Sleeping Sickness Service, Nigeria

R. N. FIENNES

M.A., M.R.C.V.S.

Head of Department of Pathology, Nuffield Institute of Comparative Medicine, The Zoological Society of London
Formerly Senior Veterinary Research Officer, Kenya, and Senior Lecturer (Veterinary Science), Department of Agriculture, University of the Gold Coast

J. FORD

M.A., B.Sc.

Wellcome Trust Study of the Role of Trypanosomiasis in Human Ecology
Formerly Director, East African Trypanosomiasis Research Organization Tororo, Uganda

DR J. P. GLASGOW

M.Sc., Ph.D.

St Mary Redcliffe and Temple School, Bristol
Formerly Chief Entomologist, Central Tsetse Research Laboratory, Shinyanga, Tanganyika

DR A. R. GRAY

M.A., Ph.D., Vet.M.B., M.R.C.V.S.

Senior Principal Research Officer, Nigerian Institute for Trypanosomiasis Research, Vom, Nigeria

DR C. A. HOARE

D.Sc., F.I.Biol., F.R.S.

Wellcome Research Fellow, Wellcome Museum of Medical Science, London
Formerly Head of Protozoology Department, Wellcome Laboratories of Tropical Medicine, London

DR A. M. JORDAN

B.Sc., Ph.D.

Tsetse Research Laboratory, School of Veterinary Science, University of Bristol
Formerly Principal Research Officer, West African Institute for Trypanosomiasis Research, Kaduna, Nigeria

K. J. R. MACLENNAN

O.B.E., B.Sc., M.R.C.V.S.

Chief Veterinary Tsetse Officer, Interim Common Services Agency, Kaduna, Nigeria

DR T. A. M. NASH

C.M.G., O.B.E., D.Sc.

Director, Tsetse Research Laboratory, School of Veterinary Science, University of Bristol
Formerly Director, West African Institute for Trypanosomiasis Research, Kaduna, Nigeria

DR W. E. ORMEROD

M.A., B.Sc., D.M.

Reader in Medical Protozoology, London School of Hygiene and Tropical Medicine

DR R. J. PHELPS

Ph.D.

Lecturer, Department of Zoology, University College of Rhodesia, Salisbury, Rhodesia
Formerly Entomologist, Tsetse Control Branch of the Federal Government of Rhodesia and Nyasaland

W. H. POTTS

M.A.

Commonwealth Institute of Entomology, London
Formerly Chief Entomologist, East African Tsetse Research Organization, Shinyanga, Tanganyika

DR D. S. SAUNDERS

B.Sc., Ph.D.

Lecturer, Department of Zoology, University of Edinburgh

LIST OF CONTRIBUTORS

DR D. SCOTT

O.B.E., M.A., M.D., D.P.H., D.T.M. & H.

Formerly Specialist Epidemiologist, Ministry of Health, Ghana, and in charge of Medical Field Units
Senior Lecturer, Department of Tropical Hygiene, Liverpool School of Tropical Medicine

PROFESSOR L. E. STEPHEN

D.V.M., D.A.P. & E., F.R.C.V.S.

Professor of Tropical Health and Protozoology and Chairman, Department of Tropical Health, School of Public Health, American University of Beirut, Lebanon
Formerly Officer-in-Charge, West African Institute for Trypanosomiasis Research, Vom, Nigeria

DR K. VICKERMAN

Ph.D.

Director, Nuffield Protozoological Research Unit and Reader in Zoology, University of Glasgow
Formerly Tropical Research Fellow of the Royal Society and Visiting Lecturer, University College, London

DR B. B. WADDY

D.M., D.P.H.

Formerly Reader in Tropical Hygiene, London School of Hygiene and Tropical Medicine. Specialist in Epidemiology and in charge of Medical Field Units, Ghana

DR P. J. WALKER

M.A., Ph.D.

Lecturer, Department of Zoology, University of Exeter
Formerly Scientific Staff of the Medical Research Council, Division of Chemotherapy and Parasitology

PROFESSOR B. G. F. WEITZ

O.B.E., D.Sc., M.R.C.V.S.

Director, National Institute for Research in Dairying, University of Reading
Formerly of the Lister Institute of Preventive Medicine, Elstree

J. R. WELCH

B.Sc., M.I.Biol.

Formerly Senior Tsetse Officer, Veterinary Division, Ministry of Agriculture and Cooperatives, Dar-es-Salaam, Tanzania

DR K. C. WILLETT

M.A., M.B., B.S., M.R.C.S., L.R.C.P.

Formerly Senior Medical Research Officer, East African Trypanosomiasis Research Organization, Tororo, Uganda. Director, West African Institute for Trypanosomiasis Research, Kaduna, Nigeria

DR J. WILLIAMSON

Ph.D.

National Institute for Medical Research, London
Formerly Biochemist, West African Institute for Trypanosomiasis Research Vom, Nigeria

Acknowledgements

My first and very pleasant duty is to acknowledge my indebtedness to the twenty-seven contributors to this book, not only for the high standard of their contributions but also for their unfailing courtesy and cooperation. I am particularly appreciative of the way in which each graciously accepted the editorial changes—often extensive—which were necessary to avoid unnecessary overlaps and to facilitate integration of the various disciplines with which the book deals.

I am particularly indebted to Mr W. H. Potts for his invaluable assistance in planning and editing Part II (Insect Vectors).

Helpful advice and encouragement were freely given by the Trypanosomiasis Panel of the Ministry of Overseas Development, especially by its Chairman, Professor W. E. Kershaw, and its Secretary, Mr P. G. Ottewill. I owe a special debt of gratitude to Professor Kershaw for contributing the Foreword and for providing excellent facilities for the editorial work in his Department at the University of Salford. Mr Ottewill handled the administrative aspects of the project with such skill and promptitude that no difficulties arose; he and his colleagues in the Ministry kindly supplied the information from which the list of names and former names of countries in Africa was compiled. For their help and courtesy on all occasions I offer my sincere thanks.

Grateful acknowledgements are made to all those—societies, editors of scientific publications, publishers and individuals—who have generously given permission to reproduce illustrative and other material from previously published work. Specific acknowledgements of the sources of this material are made, where appropriate, in the text of the book, usually in the legends accompanying the relevant figures.

Authorization to reproduce tables and figures has been given by the undermentioned Editors and Learned Societies:

Editor, *Annals of Tropical Medicine and Parasitology* (5 figures).
Editor, *Journal of Comparative Pathology* (3 figures).
Editor, *Nature* (2 figures).
Editor, *Revue d'Élevage et de Medicine véterinaire des Pays tropicales* (2 figures).
Editor, *Transactions of the Royal Society of Tropical Medicine and Hygiene* (2 figures).
Editor, *Veterinary Record* (3 figures).

The Commonwealth Animal Bureau
(*Veterinary Reviews and Annotations*, 1 figure).
The Commonwealth Institute of Entomology
(*Bulletin of Entomological Research*, 3 figures and 5 tables).
The Royal Entomological Society of London
(*Proceedings of*, 6 figures and 4 tables).
The Royal Society (*Proceedings of*, Series B, 1 figure and 1 table).
The Zoological Society of London (*Proceedings of*, 1 figure).

Various publishers have been equally generous in permitting the use, in this book, of previously published material. Messrs Baillière, Tindall and Cassel Limited, London, have kindly given permission to reproduce three figures from Hoare's *Handbook of Medical Protozoology* and one figure from Wenyon's *Protozoology*. Messrs H. K. Lewis and Co. Ltd., London (with the concurrence of the London School of Hygiene and Tropical Medicine) have generously authorized the reproduction of five figures from Buxton's *The Natural History of Tsetse Flies*. The Pergamon Press Ltd., Oxford, have graciously consented to the reproduction of three tables and five figures from Glasgow's *The Distribution and Abundance of Tsetse Flies* and to the quotation of several lengthy passages from the text. The Companhia de Diamentes de Angola, Lisbon, has kindly permitted the reproduction of four figures from Machado's *Revision systematique des Glossines de groupe* palpalis (*Diptera*). The Liverpool School of Tropical Medicine has most generously consented to the reprinting of twenty-nine figures from Newstead's *Guide to the Study of Tsetse Flies*.

In Chapter 6, the section on antigenic variation by Dr A. R. Gray is substantially a reprint of part of a prior publication by the same author (*Bulletin of the World Health Organization*, 37, pp. 177–93). The permission of the World Health Organization to use this material is gratefully acknowledged.

Special thanks are due to Dr C. E. Dyte for his generosity in making available still unpublished information on the genus *Thyridanthrax*, the systematics of which he is currently revising (*see* Chapter 25).

Individual contributors to this book have requested that acknowledgement be made of assistance they have received from various sources.

Dr F. I. C. Apted desires to record his thanks to all those—Ministries and individual workers—who have kindly supplied up-to-date information on the incidence and distribution of sleeping sickness in the countries of East and Central Africa (*see* Chapter 23).

Dr G. F. Burnett is grateful to many correspondents and in particular to Dr A. Challier, Dr G. F. Cockbill, Mr J. A. Gledhill, Mr C. W. Lee, Mr T. M. Leach, Mr J. G. Le Roux, Mr K. Riordan and Mr D. B. Turner, who provided unpublished information on current practice on insecticidal control measures in their departments.

Professor E. Bursell 'gratefully acknowledges the benefit of discussions with Dr R. J. Phelps, Dr D. A. Dame, Mr G. Vale and Mr A. Marks' in connection with his contribution on the dispersal of tsetse flies (Chapter 16).

Mr John Ford wishes to thank all those who have supplied information, or helped in other ways, in connection with his several contributions. He is particularly indebted to Dr A. de Barros Machado, Dr J. Itard, Mr D. B. Turner, Dr W. R. Wooff, Dr G. F. Cockbill, Mr A. G. Robertson and Professor B. W. Thompson. He also wishes to acknowledge the generous support of the Wellcome Trust.

Mr W. H. Potts wishes to express his indebtedness to Dr A. de Barros Machado for his valuable comments on Chapter 9, for his agreement to the reproduction of four figures from his previously published work, for making new information freely available and for permitting the citation of his as yet unpublished views.

Mr J. R. Welch wishes to thank Mr D. B. Turner, formerly Senior Tsetse

Officer, Tanzania, for making available many of the data on which the section on partial clearing in East Africa is based.

Dr K. C. Willett is greatly indebted to Mr J. G. le Roux, Chief Zoologist, Tsetse Survey and Control Unit, Kenya, to Dr W. R. Wooff, Chief Tsetse Control Officer, Uganda, and to Mr K. J. R. MacLennan, Officer in Charge of the Veterinary Tsetse and Trypanosomiasis Unit Northern Nigeria, for much of the detailed information given in Chapter 30. He also wishes to thank Dr P. E. Glover for permission to quote passages from unpublished work.

Many of the figures reproduced from earlier publications have been redrawn by Miss Tamsyn Trenaman and Mr J. J. Myles; their skill and care in the execution of this work is gratefully acknowledged.

My personal thanks are due to Mrs E. E. Robinson for the meticulous care and accuracy with which she has prepared all of the typescripts for the press and for help given in many other ways.

Finally, I wish to record my sincere thanks to the Publishers, Messrs George Allen and Unwin, Ltd., for their help and advice at all times.

EDITOR

Contents

METHODS

CONTROL OF POPULATIONS OF *GLOSSINA*

CONTENTS

Illustrations

FIGURE *page*

MAP

Illustrations

Names, Former Names and Political Status of Countries in Africa[1]

COUNTRIES WITH INDEPENDENT STATUS PRIOR TO 1956

Present Name	*Former Name*
Ethiopia	Abyssinia (1936–1941)
Liberia	Liberia
Libya	Libya
South Africa, Republic of	Union of South Africa
United Arab Republic	Egypt

COUNTRIES WHICH ACHIEVED INDEPENDENT STATUS SUBSEQUENT TO JANUARY 1, 1956

Present Name	*Former Name(s)*	*Former Administration*
Algeria	Algeria	France
Botswana	Bechuanaland	Great Britain
Burundi	Burundi	Belgium
Cameroon, Federal Republic of	French Cameroons (French Equatorial Africa)	France (UN trust)
	Southern Cameroons	Great Britain (UN trust)
Central Africa Republic	Ubangi-Shari (French Equatorial Africa)	France
Chad	Chad (French Equatorial Africa)	France
Congo (Brazzaville)	Middle Congo (French Equatorial Africa)	France
Congo (Kinshasa)	Belgian Congo	Belgium
Dahomey	Dahomey (French West Africa)	France
Equatorial Republic of Guinea	Fernando Po: Rio Muni	Spain
Gabon	Gaboon (French Equatorial Africa)	France

[1] Compiled from information obtained from *The Changing Map of Africa* prepared for British Information Services by the Central Office of Information, London, together with additional information kindly supplied by the Ministry of Overseas Development London.

Present Name	*Former Name(s)*	*Former Administration*
Gambia	Gambia	Great Britain
Ghana	Gold Coast	Great Britain
Guinea	French Guinea (French West Africa)	France
Ivory Coast	Ivory Coast (French West Africa)	France
Kenya	Kenya	Great Britain
Lesotho	Basutoland	Great Britain
Malagasy Republic	Madagascar	France
Malawi	Nyasaland	Great Britain
Mali	French Sudan (part) (French West Africa)	France
Mauritania	Mauritania (French West Africa)	France
Morocco	Morocco	France (protectorate) Spain (protectorate)
Niger	Niger (French West Africa)	France
Nigeria, Federal Republic of	Nigeria	Great Britain
Rhodesia[1]	Southern Rhodesia	Great Britain
Rwanda	Rwanda	Belgium
Senegal	Senegal (French West Africa)	France
Sierra Leone	Sierra Leone	Great Britain
Somali Republic	British Somaliland	Great Britain (protectorate)
	Italian Somaliland	Italy (UN trust)
Sudan	Sudan	Anglo-Egyptian Condominium
Swaziland	Swaziland	Great Britain (protectorate)
Tanzania, United Republic of	Tanganyika: Zanzibar	Great Britain
Togo	Togo (French West Africa)	France (UN trust)
Tunisia	Tunisia	France
Uganda	Uganda	Great Britain
Upper Volta	Upper Volta (French West Africa)	France
Zambia	Northern Rhodesia	Great Britain

[1] Independence declared in 1965 but not so far recognized by any other State.

Names, Former Names and Political Status

DEPENDENT TERRITORIES IN AFRICA

Present Name	*Former Name(s)*	*Present (1968) Administration*
Angola	Angola	Portugal
Ceuta and Melilla	Ceuta : Melilla	Spain
French Somaliland	French Somaliland	France
Ifni	Spanish West Africa	Spain
Mozambique	Mozambique	Portugal
Portuguese Guinea	Portuguese Guinea	Portugal
South West Africa	South West Africa	South Africa (UN trust)
Spanish Sahara	Spanish West Africa	Spain

General Introduction

This book, the first of its kind to be published, is designed to provide a comprehensive work of reference on the African trypanosomiases, a group of closely allied diseases of man and animals, caused by infection with species of the genus *Trypanosoma.* The main emphasis is placed on the pathogenic trypanosomes which are cyclically transmitted by species of the genus *Glossina* (tsetse flies) but others, not so transmitted, are also considered in less detail. The latter include the causative organism (*T. evansi*) of surra, a disease of camels and equines which is transmitted by blood-sucking flies other than tsetse, and the causative organism (*T. equiperdum*) of dourine, a disease of horses which is transmitted by direct contact during coitus.

The book is introduced by a review entitled 'An Historical Perspective' which, although concerned mainly with the disease in man, serves as a useful prelude to the subjects considered in detail in subsequent chapters. The relative paucity of precise information precludes the treatment of the animal trypanosomiases in a similar manner.

The remainder of the work is presented in four Parts. Aspects of the subject which have general application to the trypanosomiases as a group are considered in Parts I and II which deal, respectively, with the causative organisms and the insect vectors. Part III is devoted to human trypanosomiasis and is intended to meet the special needs of readers whose main interests lie in the medical field. Part IV deals specifically with the trypanosomiases of animals and is designed to satisfy the requirements of veterinarians and others responsible for the welfare of livestock.

Two main considerations led to the decision to prepare and publish this book at this time. Firstly, the voluminous literature on the subject is not always readily available to workers in areas where the trypanosomiases are endemic; secondly, the political emancipation of former African Colonies has been followed by the withdrawal from Africa of many recognized experts on different aspects of the trypanosomiases and it was obviously desirable to ensure that their unique knowledge and experience should be assimilated and recorded while still available. It has, however, been questioned whether the present is an opportune time to undertake this task, on the grounds that new knowledge of the subject is still being rapidly acquired. This contention is likely to be equally pertinent at any time and, indeed, hesitancy over appropriate timing may perhaps explain why no such work has been published hitherto.

The text of the book has been prepared by the twenty-seven contributors of whom details are given on pp. xi–xiii. The name of the contributor is given immediately following the title of the contribution for which he is responsible which, in most cases, comprises a separate chapter. Each contributor is a recognized authority on the particular discipline with which he deals and, with very few exceptions, each has had extensive first-hand experience of his subject in tropical Africa.

It is a notoriously difficult undertaking to produce an integrated and well-balanced textbook on the basis of multiple authorship but, in the case of the trypanosomiases, there is no alternative means of ensuring that each of the many disciplines involved is dealt with in an authoritative manner. The main difficulties in welding together the work of numerous contributors are to ensure complete coverage of the subject, to maintain reasonable continuity and uniformity in presentation and, particularly, to avoid unnecessary overlapping. If each discipline is to be developed by logical reasoning, some degree of repetition is inescapable. It has seemed preferable to accept a certain amount of repetition in the text rather than to deny the contributor the opportunity to develop his theme by logical argument or to subject the reader to the disturbing and time-consuming expedient of making frequent cross-references to other parts of the book. Care has, however, been taken to minimize repetition insofar as this is consistent with these aims. Wherever a particular topic has been exhaustively described in one contribution, only brief accounts of the relevant and salient points have been included in another. For example, a detailed review of the drugs available for the prevention and treatment of the trypanosomiases has been presented in Chapter 7, while the practical application of these drugs to the human disease has been considered in Chapters 36 and 37, and to the animal trypanosomiases in Chapters 42 and 43. Similarly, the nature of the contact between man and tsetse fly, a factor of prime importance in the transmission of Gambian sleeping sickness, has been fully described in Chapter 32 to provide background material for the description of the epidemiology of this disease which follows in Chapter 33.

In a book compiled from individual contributions from numerous authorities, some of them expert in the same or closely allied fields, it would indeed be remarkable if the views expressed on a particular subject were identical in all cases. The reader will discover some, usually slight, differences in the opinions of one contributor as compared with another but, where this occurs, it will be found that, in most cases, such differences in viewpoint relate to matters on which no final pronouncement can yet be made. It is hoped that variances of this kind will not give rise to confusion but that they will serve to indicate where further investigation is required. A good example is provided by the account of the dispersal of tsetse flies given in Chapter 16, in which the contributor offers explanations of observed facts which provide alternatives to those hitherto widely accepted and still held by some workers. This is calculated to stimulate the further investigation necessary before the true state of affairs can be declared with absolute conviction.

Editorial consistency has been sacrificed to practical expediency in respect of the systems of weights and measures used in different parts of the book. The increasingly used metric system has been adopted in those disciplines where it is already well established as, for example, in designating the dosage of drugs and in the specification of laboratory formulae. It is believed that the majority of readers will be familiar with, and accustomed to use, non-metrical systems in such other connections as the measurements of larger areas (square miles, acres, etc.), longer distances (miles, yards, etc.), heavier weights (avoirdupois) and larger volumes (gallons, etc.). For these reasons the systems of weights and measures adopted by individual contributors have been retained; these are the systems most likely to be followed by other workers in the same field, at least in English-speaking countries. Where this is not the case, the user will find it necessary to convert the weights and measures given to the system of his choice.

In the detailed treatment of the African mammalian trypanosomes (Chapters 1 and 2) the conclusion is reached that there are no sound taxonomic or other reasons for continuing to regard *T. brucei*, *T. gambiense* and *T. rhodesiense* as three separate species, as has long been the case, and that all should properly be regarded as belonging to the single species, *T. brucei*. At the same time it is recognized that confusion is likely to be caused by discarding the familiar and long-used names '*T. gambiense*' and '*T. rhodesiense*' which provide a convenient means of referring to recognized differences in the clinical manifestations of the disease in man. For this reason these names and the terms 'Gambian' and 'Rhodesian' sleeping sickness have been retained where appropriate.

The full scientific names of the various species of trypanosomes are used only in those sections of the book which deal with the systematics of the genus *Trypanosoma*. Elsewhere, the commonly recognized abbreviated forms have been used.

Similarly, to avoid what appears to be unnecessary pedantry, the full specific name of each species of the genus *Glossina* is given only in the list of species (Table 8.1) in Chapter 8, in Chapter 9 which deals with the systematics of the genus and on the occasion of the first use of the name in other chapters. Elsewhere abbreviated names are used unless there are special reasons to do otherwise.

It has been considered unnecessary to deal with the genus *Glossina* in minute detail because of the very detailed information available in Buxton's (1955) *The Natural History of Tsetse Flies*. In the present work, attention has been especially directed towards those aspects of the subject on which new knowledge has been acquired since Buxton's book was published, although, where necessary, earlier work has been cited in sufficient detail to permit the logical development of newer concepts.

The revision of the *palpalis* group assigns the name *Glossina fuscipes fuscipes* to the East African subspecies commonly known as *Glossina palpalis fuscipes*. This change in nomenclature is liable to cause confusion when considering earlier work in eastern Africa. To overcome this difficulty, references to *G. palpalis* in the original literature have been recorded as *G. palpalis* [*G. fuscipes*] where it is clear that reference is made to the form now considered to be a distinct species, *G. fuscipes*.

The vexed question of control of tsetse populations by destruction of the larger mammalian fauna is dispassionately considered in Chapter 28. While it is essential to record the facts concerning the use of this method of tsetse control it is not necessary to dwell upon the widely divergent views that have been expressed in the bitter controversy which the use of this method has aroused. It cannot be denied that, in certain circumstances, the complete, or even partial, elimination of game animals is an effective means of reducing or eradicating tsetse populations, but all reasonable people will agree that this distasteful method should be adopted only as a last resort. In this connection, it must be remembered that the continued presence of game animals in sufficient numbers to support tsetse populations is incompatible with a certain density of human settlement and the full and proper use of land. Game animals are themselves an important economic asset in some African countries and care is taken to ensure their preservation in extensive areas specially set aside for this purpose. Africa is a vast continent and it should not be beyond man's ingenuity to cater for the needs of the human population while at the same time ensuring the conservation of all other species of the mammalian fauna. If these simple truths were sufficiently recognized, a more rational attitude would be taken towards this method of tsetse control.

The various methods described for the control of tsetse fly populations are critically reviewed in Chapter 29. The administrative and organizational aspects of trypanosomiasis control programmes are considered in Chapter 30 which, for convenience, has been included at the end of Part II although it has relevance also to Part I.

Some discrepancies occur in the dates of the latest literature cited in different chapters. Each contributor accepted his task in addition to his regular duties and, in these circumstances, it is not surprising that an interval of almost two years separated the submission of the first and the last contribution. Consequently, the publication date of the latest literature available to individual contributors, at the time of writing, varied from 1968 to 1970.

The bibliography at the end of the book is extensive and representative but it is not claimed to be exhaustive. Many of the references cited in Chapter 7 are readily available in previous reviews and, for this reason, only those of special importance and those subsequent to 1961 have been included in the bibliography.

The emergence of new self-governing countries in Africa during comparatively recent years has, in many cases, resulted in a change of name. For the reader's convenience the former and present names of these territories are listed on pp. xxxiii–xxxv.

EDITOR

An Historical Perspective

A. J. DUGGAN

It is commonly believed that the trypanosomes which infect man in Africa have evolved from others which are morphologically similar or identical and which live as commensals in the bloodstream of antelope. In this respect, the paleogenesis of human trypanosomiasis has been given much thoughtful study, but it would be mistaken to assume that this evolution took place long ago as an event, or a series of events, which is now only of historic interest. The trypanosomes of man have neither abandoned their evolutionary cradle nor reached their ultimate parasitological destination; they still pursue the protracted odyssey which a parasite must follow during the hazardous traverse from an ancient host to a new one, and the consequences of human infection betray the insecurity of an undecided relationship. The less well adapted parasites with propensities still akin to those of their wild forerunners enjoy only the transient freedom of the peripheral blood in a patient whose days are numbered, while the older strains are destined to cripple their host during a final imprisonment within the nervous system. Neither of these is an ideal situation for an organism which depends for its survival upon the unlikelihood of ingestion by a bloodsucking fly of sylvatic disposition which, in a particular state of receptiveness, happens to feed on man. Unless the animal reservoirs had persisted throughout the prehistoric period and even up to the present time to provide a perennial source of trypanosomes for persistent evolutionary exploration, the phenomenon which we call sleeping sickness would have been lost, long ago, as a castaway amid the restless infinite sea of biological change.

The problem of African trypanosomiasis is therefore still dynamic and fluctuating; few, if any, aspects of it are comfortably predictable, and events which happen in one part of Africa are not necessarily explicable on the basis of experience elsewhere. As the whole phenomenon involves man, trypanosomes, tsetse flies, wild and domesticated animals and the various ecological situations within which they all subsist, it is hardly surprising that outbreaks of sleeping sickness have seldom been completely investigated. Measures have usually been taken to bring about an artificial change in the dynamics of transmission before the necessary team of experts, supposing such ever to have been available, could be brought to bear. Between times, new discoveries have been made by the investigation of isolated aspects and these have been applied, when possible, by those later confronted with the untoward effects of the entire complex. In this piecemeal fashion a large body of knowledge, scientific and empirical, has been established during this century. With care and discretion some of this can be used to illuminate past experiences and, if not to explain them in detail, at any rate to define, however vaguely, the fabric upon which the present pattern of the disease has been woven and to describe how the succession of events has gradually built up a recognizable design.

By the end of the nineteenth century a considerable amount of literature on sleeping sickness derived from observations in western Africa had become available. All of it was based upon clinical descriptions of patients with either enlarged glands or dramatic neurological symptomatology, and most accounts were tantalizingly deficient in other respects, particularly with regard to the precise geographical distribution of the disease. Nonetheless, retrospective enquiries from 1900 onwards revealed that in western Africa and in the basin of the Congo river, endemic foci of sleeping sickness had existed for so long that knowledge of the disease and, in some cases, its mode of transmission, had passed into tribal lore. Yet the existence of such ancient foci does not necessarily merit the belief that trypanosomiasis of man originated only in western Africa. Although to the east of the Rift Valley and in the Zambesi basin sleeping sickness has been observed only within the last sixty years and the African people of these regions have no traditional acquaintance with it, the acuteness of the symptomatology, the speed with which the ill-adapted parasite exerts its lethal effects and the fact that transmission occurs within a diffuse environment mitigate against a clear understanding of its nature as a distinct clinical entity by unsophisticated tribal observers. Even after the discovery of the aetiology of sleeping sickness it was some time before scientific workers became generally convinced that this neurological disease was, in reality, the late stage of a parasitaemic condition hitherto known as 'trypanosomal fever'.

The evolution of human trypanosomiasis occurred, and may still occur as a multifocal event. In western Africa the successful passage of trypanosomes from animals to man must have taken place long ago, and since then some strains of parasite have become more adapted to the human host by passage from man to man through riverine rather than woodland tsetse with the more restricted anthropological relationship which this implies. It is only to be expected that, even after a long period of time, this biological event has found certain geographical and ecological situations more favourable for its repetition than others, and this undoubtedly accounts for the focal nature of the endemic disease. But the chronicity of the clinical picture in long-established foci obscures the possibility that the original phenomenon of transference from animal to man may be repeated from time to time in those foci and in other places, although, as game becomes scarcer in the West African countryside, the frequency of such transference diminishes as the years go by. Acute trypanosomal infections have occasionally been detected in areas where the predominant strain of parasite was well-adapted to man, and these unusual cases serve as isolated reminders of the sporadic violence which accompanied the beginnings of the new host-parasite relationship. In eastern Africa, the adaptation of animal trypanosomes to man has proceeded much more slowly. Yet, although the circumstances of transmission are diffuse, even the acute ill-adapted infection characteristic of that part of Africa already tends to have a focal distribution in so far as some places have become more notorious than others as localities in which virulent sleeping sickness is likely to be contracted. Over the comparatively short time during which the disease has been observed in eastern Africa, there is no direct evidence that a predictably chronic form of sleeping sickness is emerging as a result of parasite adaptation, although individual cases are known in which the parasitaemia of an otherwise virulent infection has been accommodated for many months without serious harm. But the trypanosomes of animals are rejected by the majority of humans and this power of rejection may be conditioned by genetic factors. Possibly, the inborn nature of human stock in eastern Africa is such as to retard or even refute an evolutionary development that has succeeded in making progress among races elsewhere ever since ancient times.

The innate behaviour of the long-established foci in western Africa has had an enormous influence upon events. Old foci of chronic sleeping sickness wax and wane according to the propitiousness of the prevailing ecological circumstances at a particular time. When transmission by riverine tsetse becomes intensified in these places, sleeping sickness begins to spread into adjacent localities where normally it would never occur. Moreover, while the infection is thus advancing, the virulence of the trypanosome often appears to increase, so that the clinical and economic effects of the disease are far graver among the newly-invaded communities than among those who live in the area whence it sprang. The reason for this is completely unknown. By such means the original focus creates a sphere of influence in which new satellite foci are maintained until transmission in the primary focus dies down naturally or is eradicated by artificial means. Sometimes, however, a satellite becomes capable of an independent existence and this in its turn becomes a stable focus in its own right, contributing to the permanent endemicity within the region. Such localities tend to be intractable and, in nature, as Dutton and Todd observed in the Congo, 'no district in which sleeping sickness has once existed is known ever to become entirely free from the disease.'

Among the coastal forests of western Africa old foci undoubtedly exist in places such as Eket, but the disease is mild, and sudden acceleration of transmission is unusual. At the other extreme, towards the northern limits of tsetse distribution, in areas which we may call 'frontier zones' such as the northern savanna of the western Soudan, ancient foci tend to flare, and in some places such flares occur with a certain periodicity. Moreover, at such times the virulence of the infection seems to increase, giving rise to social disruption and economic devastation which does not normally occur in old trypanosomiasis foci in more afforested regions.

These ancient patterns are interwoven. In areas where man, woodland tsetse and game animals co-exist, the evolutionary transfer of animal trypanosomes to man is still possible. Endemicity is maintained by riverine tsetse in historic foci from which further spread takes place, sometimes with increased virulence. Lastly, no ancient focus in which the disease has settled down to a familiar pattern of clinical expression and epidemic rhythm is immune from the introduction of fresh trypanosome strains whose behaviour invalidates an otherwise predictable situation.

Until the end of the nineteenth century the dynamics of these phenomena were restrained by the relative stasis of human communities; even so, caravans arduously toiled their way for long distances, marauding warriors crossed wide tracts of land in search of booty, and even whole tribes migrated to improve their fortunes. Undoubtedly, these movements helped to arrange, however slowly, the biological dispositions which existed towards the end of the nineteenth century and which provided the libretto—and the cast—for the drama which was to be enacted during the next fifty years. If the cosmological view is taken, it appears that the things which happened were inevitable, but the rapid development of African territories, constantly accompanied by sociological changes, telescoped into half a century an inescapable evolutionary process that might otherwise have taken a thousand years.

The devastating forces inherent in these old, but restricted, endemic localities were first unleashed among the population of the Congo basin at the turn of the century. During the 1800s many observations were made upon the effects of sleeping sickness in 'Congolese' patients. This designation was used in a loose sense to describe not only the inhabitants of the Congo but also those of countries bordering the Gulf of Guinea, yet the work of Dutton and Todd in the early 1900s clearly defined the existence of a primary endemic focus along both banks of the Congo river for a distance of 100 miles upstream from its mouth. A number of smaller endemic areas, including at least one on the Ubangi tributary and others scattered upstream on the Congo itself over a distance of 400 miles inland had also come into existence in former times. It is convenient to regard all these Congolese foci as primordial, although any one may have arisen from any other as a permanent satellite. It has been argued that some of them may have originated from the Lake Chad basin through introductions by Hausa soldiers as late as the 1880s. In the present context such historical niceties may be set aside; the fundamental point is that the predominant trypanosome strain in these areas was comparatively well-adapted to man when confined in its ancient home, causing a chronic disease, and was conveyed by riverine tsetse.

In 1885 the Congo Free State came into existence. Within the next few years steamers were launched on the river and its tributaries, and regular traffic with inland areas became established. Soldiers and labourers from the endemic areas of the lower Congo became permanently employed on the upper reaches, and the exploitation of this vast waterway enabled the region to be effectively occupied to its uttermost headwaters. About ten years after these developments had begun, it became clear that sleeping sickness was spreading to places where hitherto it had been unknown. The endemic area at the mouth of the Congo expanded, and by 1905 a great region, stretching from the Lulua tributary eastwards for 250 miles to the shores of Lake Tanganyika had been invaded. It has been estimated that during this cataclysmic advance between 1896 and 1906, about half a million people died of sleeping sickness in the Congo basin.

As the spread continued, outbreaks occurred along the Sanga and Ubangi tributaries, carrying the disease further northwards through territory opened up by the French in 1890, towards the watershed in upper Ubangi which conceals the origins of the Shari river that flows to Lake Chad. Furthermore, dissemination of the disease took place from an endemic focus in the coastal district of

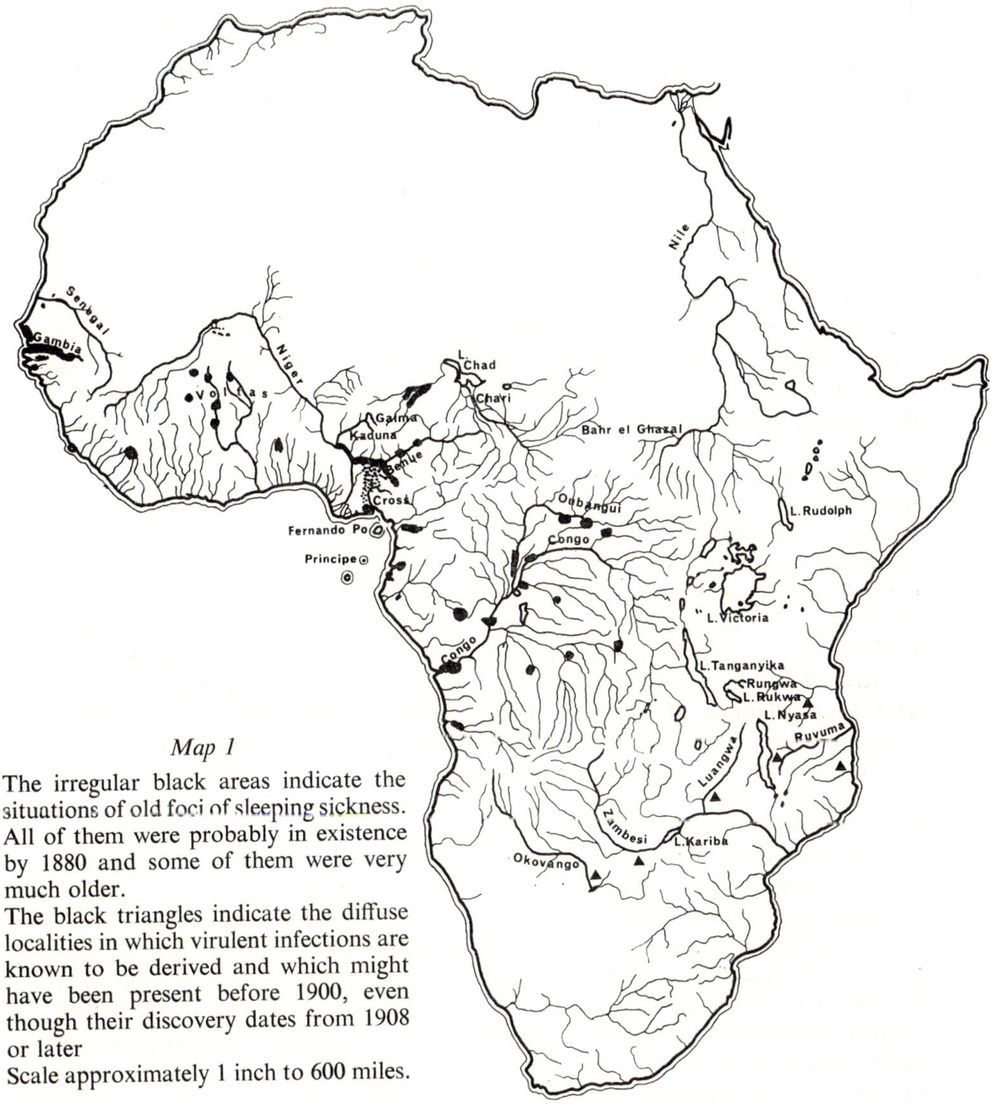

Map 1

The irregular black areas indicate the situations of old foci of sleeping sickness. All of them were probably in existence by 1880 and some of them were very much older.

The black triangles indicate the diffuse localities in which virulent infections are known to be derived and which might have been present before 1900, even though their discovery dates from 1908 or later

Scale approximately 1 inch to 600 miles.

Luanga from which porters, labourers and soldiers were recruited for employment in the western part of the French Congo.

During this time, another epidemic began in eastern Africa on the northern shores of Lake Victoria where the disease appeared in Busoga in 1896. Although this outbreak was discontinuous by some hundreds of miles from the nearest epidemic area in the Congo, it is generally believed to have been derived from that source by the immigration of infected Sudanese followers of Emin Pasha. Their arrival was followed by a heavy mortality among the indigenous people which, at the time, was attributed to a coincidental famine, but in 1901 the disease spread along the lake shore into districts in which food was plentiful and the true situation became manifest. By 1908, the population of this area, originally believed to be about 300,000, had been reduced to one-third. On the lake islands of Buvuma and Sesse the population fell from 79,000 to 22,000, and the survivors were evacuated in 1909.

By 1905 sleeping sickness was spreading from the Congo basin towards the Nile in a north-easterly direction. The Bahr-El-Ghazal was believed to be free from infection in 1907, but it had reached Raga by 1909. In the following year the Lado enclave, which had been leased to the Belgian Government, was redeemed, and an important focus of infection along the river Yei was disclosed. It is unlikely that the Yei focus had been in existence for many years before the transfer of political power, but whether the disease was introduced primarily from the French Congo to the west or from outbreaks to the south along the shores of Lake Albert or Lake Victoria is not known.

Elsewhere, to the south of the Congo basin an old focus of sleeping sickness existed in the valley of the Cuanza river, near the southern extremity of its distribution on the west coast of Africa. The first cases were clinically identified in 1871 and epidemics began in several localities near Cazendo during the construction of a railway line between Luanda and Mulanga during the 1880s. This focus claimed at least one notable satellite. According to Da Costa, sleeping sickness was introduced with tsetse flies into the island of Principe as a result of importing cattle from the west coast of Africa about 1825. Nevertheless, the disease remained very rare on the island and tsetse were regarded as harmless until 1877 when labour began to be introduced from Cazendo, whereupon the disease spread rapidly, and reached epidemic proportions by 1890. The population was virtually annihilated and the permanent inhabitants were reduced to no more than 350 by 1907.

Little information came to hand concerning the incidence of sleeping sickness in territories under Spanish influence along the river Muni and on the island of Fernando Po until 1909, when it appeared that the disease had been firmly entrenched in both places for a considerable time. A much later report, however, claims that the introduction of a new trypanosome strain in 1898 caused an epidemic which killed practically everyone at risk.

During the early part of this century the advance of the disease from its ancient home in the Congo basin was confined in the north by the highlands of the Cameroons and by the tracts of desert extending eastwards to the Bahr-El-Ghazal and the river Nile. Extensions eastwards from the Congo basin halted upon the eastern shores of Lake Victoria and Lake Tanganyika. To the south, new endemic areas came into existence in the southern part of the Congo basin and some of these became contiguous with other foci, both old and new, in Angola.

Meanwhile, westwards from the Cameroons, the governments of colonial territories along the coast of Africa as far as Senegal, which contains the northwest limit of tsetse distribution, began to show concern. Investigations made in these areas at this time revealed a number of primordial foci, and the authorities waited with apprehension for these latent sources of disaster to erupt. Yet nature was taking its time. Circumstances had not yet been made propitious, possibly for two reasons; in the first place the opening up of these countries was conducted more slowly than that of the Congo basin, and secondly the restricted navigability of rivers such as the Niger, the Benue and the Volta did not provide an internal communications system comparable to that of the Congo. Man and his trypanosomes waited for another twenty years before the development of roads and railways enabled them to fulfil their destiny.

By 1908 the turbulence in the Congo basin had involved a region as great in size as the Indian subcontinent, stretching from the mouth of the Congo to the eastern shores of Lake Tanganyika, and from the Bahr-El-Ghazal southwards to the Coanza valley. The sheer numbers of people involved and the obvious economic implication of the disease as a serious barrier to material progress led to widespread government-sponsored scientific enquiry by all the European nations whose interests were at stake. Each of them, by 1908, had put at least one Commission in the field; international agreements for the exchange of information and the control of the disease along interterritorial routes were negotiated; the most eminent medical scientists of the day, including Roubaud, Koch, Laveran and Manson were directing important lines of investigation. Before the twentieth century was four years old the discoveries of Dutton and Castellani had led men to understand the cause of the disease, and Bruce had shown that riverine tsetse was the vector. But as yet control measures were largely directed towards restricting the movement of persons known to be infected. This seemed an obvious line of approach and, given the conditions under which these territories were administered at that time, particularly in the Congo, it was also practicable; but in the light of later developments it was not the happiest of first principles to adopt. There was but one ray of positive hope, and it emanated from the genius of Paul Ehrlich. Efforts of others to find a means of curing sleeping sickness, ranging from inunctions of mercury to intrathecal lysol were reaching a stage almost of despair, when, after a long and precise chain of chemical deduction and biological experiment, he produced the pentavalent aromatic arsenical compound, Atoxyl, which began to be used about 1905. It was not a perfect weapon, but it offered a chance of life to the doomed, and encouraged medical men to continue the struggle. It lowered, if not abolished, parasitaemia, to the epidemiologists' relief. It was the first tangible success against African trypanosomiasis.

These great events concerned the transmission of well-adapted trypanosomes from man to man by riverine tsetse. It was thus ironical that the effects of the host-parasite complex were first discerned in relation to the far end of its evolutionary time-scale, as a chronic neurological affliction. But medical scientists were soon to make the acquaintance of this parasite in more savage and primeval form.

In 1908 an Englishman, by name William Armstrong, became infected with trypanosomes during a journey through the Luangwa valley of the Zambesi system, 200 miles south of Lake Tanganyika. The infection was of an extremely virulent kind and caused his death in little more than six months. His companion, Beith, soon afterwards shared the same fate. The virulence of the strain was expressed also in experimental animals in the blood of which a proportion of the organisms showed a tendency for their nucleus to take up a more posterior position than was the case with other trypanosomes that had been isolated from man at that time. Upon this evidence and certain other somewhat unstable characters the trypanosome was deemed to be of a different species from that which had caused the dramatic events far to the northwest. The award of separate specific status to this organism has probably led to more misunderstanding than any other single mistake in the history of African trypanosomiasis.

It is not proposed to describe the long and contentious scientific debates which have been pursued on this subject during the last fifty years, except to state that none of them can gainsay the evolutionary view of this phenomenon. Even the most radical theory, which maintains that these highly virulent trypanosomes have emerged only in recent times and that the majority of them have been derived from a single source, cannot obscure the evident appeal of the evolutionary standpoint. These virulent trypanosomes are now known to be harboured by animals and transmitted chiefly by tsetse flies of the woodland, and this association, combined with a specific identification of the trypanosome, gave rise for many years to the erroneous belief that while well-adapted trypanosomes were carried by riverine species, those more quickly lethal to man were transmitted only by woodland tsetse; only in comparatively recent times has this dual conception been refuted by clear cut field observations.

These virulent infections to which Armstrong was the first known victim, bear witness to the evolutionary embarkation of the African trypanosomes of man. It is, for the parasite, a difficult transition because the ecology of woodland tsetse itself depends upon the presence of no more than an attenuated human population which in any case plays but a minor role as a source of food for the fly. Moreover, the circumstances of transmission involve a further uncertainty since the majority of people have an inherent resistance to infection with most organisms of direct animal origin. Hence these infections are, in the main, sporadic, although clusters of cases are known to occur in localized areas where, occasionally, a human being becomes a carrier of virulent trypanosomes without succumbing to their pathogenic effects in the usual way.

It is difficult to maintain the view that this phenomenon has arisen only in recent times; it is significant that a high proportion of cases which first came to light were Europeans who were under much closer medical supervision than the indigenous population at that time. There is good reason for the absence of references to this disease in the folk lore of eastern Africa, for, as the Luangwa Sleeping Sickness Commission of 1911 pointed out, the duration of the disease is short, with little in the way of subjective symptomatology. No reasonable argument can assail the view that the transmission of virulent trypanosomes from game to man has sporadically occurred over a long period. The most cogent proposition is that of Lyndhurst Duke, who maintained that under normal conditions man (i.e. human society), is not seriously threatened by the polymorphic trypanosomes transmitted by woodland tsetse. The increasing numbers of cases of this kind of sleeping sickness which came to light after 1908 revealed 'nature taken unawares by the general upheaval of the old order of things that has attended the awakening of a continent'.

One such upheaval was provided by the cataclysm of the First World War. In the western half of Africa the effect of this disastrous epoch was to frustrate most of the plans for the civil development of colonies, except in so far as they were important for military operations. The eastern side of the continent, by contrast, was kept in turmoil by the marching and counter-marching of the German forces under Neumann in northern Tanganyika and more particularly under von Lettow to the south. After a long series of furtive engagements with Allied, largely British, troops, this commander, undefeated in the field, surrendered with the German capitulation of 1918. These operations unwittingly provided a unique experiment in the epidemiology of human trypanosomiasis in eastern Africa; large numbers of susceptibles, both African and European, were exposed for years on end to trypanosomal infection from woodland tsetse in country where game was abundant. Yet only nine European cases occurred in von Lettow's army, and eighteen cases, thirteen of them African, among the British force. Thus the rarity of this acute infection contrasts with the prevalence of riverine tsetse-borne disease in the Congo basin where, for example in one year, eight out of a handful of Europeans were infected on the Sangha tributary alone.

The interest of these infections among military personnel lay not only in their small numbers, but in that they were contracted in areas which, although diffuse by the standards of sleeping sickness foci in western Africa, were, nevertheless, fairly well defined geographically, the German cases having occurred in the vicinity of the Malanda river while the British troops became infected along a supply route known as the Port Amelia Line, running between Bandari and Anquabe. These localities were situated on either side of the Rovuma river, where the Portuguese had detected cases in 1909, or possibly even earlier.

One of the War's many futile consequences was practically to eliminate any further contribution by the Germans to the campaign against trypanosomiasis in the field. On the eastern shore of Lake Tanganyika they had established special camps to contend with the constant importation of sleeping sickness by travellers from the Congo. By 1908, over 1,500 patients were under treatment in these enclaves, and the supportive measures of bush clearance and restriction of movement were so energetically applied that by 1914 the disease had almost been eradicated from places in which it had established a foothold. In Togo on the west coast of Africa, even at this time, patients were treated with Atoxyl by a specially appointed medical officer in a fly-free camp at Hausberg. In the Cameroons, an old endemic focus on the Nyong river was located in 1910, and three others in the same vicinity were demarcated by 1912. By 1914, no fewer than fourteen doctors were working on sleeping sickness in that area under the direction of Kleine. The efficiency of the German response, even to such a comparatively small challenge, set an example which other nations were to follow, but not always with the same promptitude nor on the same scale.

In 1916 the French authorities in the Congo set up a special prophylactic service under Jamot, to undertake mass diagnostic and treatment campaigns by mobile teams, with one special medical officer for every 50,000 of the population. With these teams, in the Ubangui-Chari territory, Jamot found and treated 5,347 cases among 90,000 persons examined between July 1917 and August 1919. It seems that this was the first major field survey ever undertaken against trypanosomiasis by a fully equipped service with legislative support.

The Belgian authorities had instituted a special laboratory at Leopoldville in 1899 to study sleeping sickness, and in 1905 commissioned an expedition from the Liverpool School of Tropical Medicine to investigate and report upon the Congolese situation. Later efforts to control the disease by quarantine and compulsory isolation were disastrous, as the patients absconded and the populations of infected villages scattered and went into hiding. Likewise, the clearing of vegetation from river banks to eliminate tsetse failed for the lack of ecological studies; tall trees were cut down only to be replaced by low thicket which was more favourable for the breeding of fly. The resiting of villages often proved impossible because, except in certain districts of Katanga, there were few places which could be considered tsetse-free. In view of these setbacks, increasing reliance was placed upon the use of Atoxyl to eradicate trypanosomes from the blood of man. By 1913 the equivalent of £12,000 per year was being allocated for these therapeutic measures.

The exigencies of the War seriously retarded the progress of such campaigns, and undoubtedly cost many lives in areas where sleeping sickness was rampant. Elsewhere, particularly in the Cameroons, the grim fraternity of trypanosome and fly tightened its sinister hold in readiness for the days of peace.

In 1919 the victorious European powers in colonial Africa faced a situation in which numerous endemic foci had been located in the western territories, epidemic conditions were still extant in the Congo basin and sporadic cases of a virulent kind were being reported from Tanganyika, the Rhodesias and Portuguese East Africa. At this point the polices of English- and French-speaking nations diverged. The latter were confronted with an immediate and very serious problem in Congolese territories, and a committee under the leadership of Laveran recommended that the chief preventive measure should be to reduce the number of circulating trypanosomes in the human population by a method described as 'atoxylization of the sick'. To the members of this committee, tsetse eradication was little more than a dream, although it was appreciated that local clearing of bush at strategic points was a useful measure; if all failed, defeat would have to be acknowledged and the affected population moved. Hence in 1920 the Belgian authorities established a mobile anti-trypanosomiasis mission under Schwetz in the district of Kwango-Kasai, and between 1920 and 1923 this team carried out nearly 850,000 examinations; about 60,000 cases of sleeping sickness were found and treated with Atoxyl, sometimes combined with tartar emetic. Meanwhile, about 4,000 cases a year were being discovered by French workers in the 'prophylactic sectors' of the northern part of the Congo basin, and about 21,000 patients were finally treated.

The harsh breath of the ill wind which had threatened the west coast of Africa for so long, began to blow across the Cameroons. Transmission in the endemic foci along the Njong river had intensified during the years of neglect imposed by war, and Jamot undertook a survey of these areas in 1922 and 1923, disclosing over 30,000 cases. The situation was handled according to policy, by treatment brigades using Atoxyl, and by restricting the movement of patients to places outside the epidemic area. Before control was achieved in the Njong foci, sleeping sickness accounted for almost as many deaths as all other causes put together, and during the epidemic the general mortality was about twice as high as the birthrate. Jamot's campaign reduced the monthly death rate from 400 to less than 150 within a year. It was a dramatic forerunner of future events further to the west.

For the hard-line advocates of compulsory treatment and segregation such as Jamot and Schwetz, further help soon came to hand. Immediately the War was over, efforts were made to find a more satisfactory form of treatment than Atoxyl. With this drug, many patients needed long courses of injections which placed a considerable administrative burden upon treatment brigades and aggravated the frustrations of those whose liberty was curtailed. Success came in 1921 with the discovery of suramin, a colourless analogue of trypan red, following upon traditional German research into the biostatic properties of dyestuffs. This compound quickly eliminated trypanosomes from the peripheral blood, and in the early stages of the virulent trypanosomiasis of eastern Africa its curative effects were so predictable as to make possible the use of volunteers in experimental work. Moreover, in 1926 it was found to have protein-binding properties which delayed its excretion so that in certain circumstances it could be used as a prophylactic. The chief shortcoming of suramin was its inability to cure patients with neurological involvement. Yet this was made good by the almost simultaneous discovery of the pentavalent aromatic arsenical tryparsamide, which possessed this property in Congolese cases. The problem of curing virulent trypanosomiasis in eastern Africa after the nervous system had been invaded, remained intractable, but this was largely a concern of the British. Suramin and tryparsamide were a godsend to those who depended upon compulsory treatment as a means of control. Once the logistical problems were solved, the end of the epidemic era in the Congo basin could be foreseen.

To the British, the disaster on Lake Victoria was an isolated encounter and a thing of the past; in 1919 no serious sleeping sickness epidemic was affecting any of their territory and it seemed to them that trypanosomiasis of domestic stock was of far greater significance than the human disease. Their stake in the world had rested on the horse in war and the bullock-cart in peace, and in most of tropical Africa trypanosomiasis denied them both. On the majority of African farms there was hardly a quadruped to be seen, save for the ubiquitous goat. The problems were therefore approached in a more fundamental and objective way, and the Government asked the Imperial Bureau of Entomology to recommend lines of research with a view to controlling tsetse.

In eastern Africa the British were favourably placed for such investigations. The Royal Society Commission had begun work during the epidemic on Lake Victoria in 1902 and had remained in the field more or less continuously until 1914. The Commission made numerous researches into trypanosomiasis of man and animals in Uganda and Nyasaland during this time, and immediately after the War, Hale Carpenter returned to Lake Victoria under the auspices of the Commission for further observations on riverine tsetse. Moreover, Lyndhurst Duke, as an officer of the Uganda Medical Service, was working on trypanosomiasis in his laboratory at Entebbe, which later became the Human Trypanosomiasis Research Institute under his directorship in 1927. With no great difficulty it was therefore possible to build upon these traditions, and, partly owing to the good fortune of territorial contiguity, the academic influence of the research workers and the application of their discoveries finally held sway from the Nile almost to the Zambesi. Moreover British research in eastern Africa remained undistracted by sleeping sickness problems on a scale which might otherwise have diverted its manpower into overriding problems of field control. Under the continuing guidance of Swynnerton, Jackson and others, many problems concerning woodland tsetse were elucidated, and methods were promulgated of reclaiming land impoverished by the depredations of this fly upon domestic stock. In due course, research stations were established at Shinyanga and Tinde in Tanganyika, and long-term investigations were made into both tsetse flies and trypanosomes. For the space of a generation these institutions were to contribute enormously to the knowledge of the agents and vectors of trypanosomiasis in eastern Africa.

On the other side of the continent the recommendations of the Imperial Bureau materialized with the establishment of a Tsetse Investigation at Sherifuri in Northern Nigeria under Johnson and his deputy Lloyd, in July 1921. Sherifuri was situated at latitude 12°N in the Sudanese savanna zone of the Lake Chad basin whose rivers, flowing from the southwest as outspread fingers towards the palm of a hand, maintained vegetation sufficient to support both riverine and woodland tsetse. Moreover, at that time and by West African standards, the area was rich in game. The investigators settled down immediately to the comfortable study of tsetse ecology and mammalian trypanosomes. But the ill wind was not far away.

By this time the sleeping sickness situation in Nigeria had been fairly well defined by its Colonial Officers and by several special investigations such as those of Scott Macfie and Simpson. An ancient endemic focus had been located on the coast near Eket, and to the north of this an irregular pattern of isolated chronic infections could, and still can, be traced until the valley of the Cross River gives way to that of the Benue which flows westwards to find the Niger in the heart of the country. At around latitude 8°N the Niger-Benue valley sustains another well-defined focus of the disease, old beyond the span of African tradition. Shortly before Johnson took up his position at Sherifuri, northward extensions of sleeping sickness from this focus began to come about through road and railway communications with Kaduna and the great dynastic cities of Zaria and Kano. Originally, this focus occupied a strip no more than fifty miles deep along the north bank of the two rivers, but in 1916 an extension occurred for a short distance northwards to the garrison town of Wamba, forcing the troops to evacuate the place. Three years later the small village of Gimi established by a few hundred Christians near Zaria was quietly decimated by a northwards extension of over 200 miles, brought about by railway communication and the agronomic exploitation of the fertile watershed between the Kaduna and Galma rivers. But these isolated events were as raindrops before the tempest.

At about the latitude of Sherifuri, the northern limit of both woodland and riverine tsetse fly is contained by the arid inimical conditions of the outer Sahara frontiers. At these limits the fly is struggling for survival. Maximum temperatures are high, humidity is often very low, and relatively few flies, often limited in the range of their predatory excursions, feed on game and man. In the dry season, man, game and fly compete for the remnants of a desiccating land, and as the means of their existence become concentrated about the precious waterways, their contact becomes closer. Similar conditions are found 800 miles farther west at the same latitude in the region of the upper Voltas. It is now established by retrospection that both these 'frontier' zones were the scenes of violent and destructive sleeping sickness epidemics during similar periods in the nineteenth century, notably from about 1850 to 1870 and from 1886 to 1906. Significantly, perhaps, in these widely separated areas, history was now to be repeated.

In 1923 it became clear to Johnson that sleeping sickness was rapidly becoming more prevalent in riverine villages near Sherifuri. Although in that year only thirty-seven cases were reported from the usual medical sources throughout northern Nigeria, the research staff treated four times that number in the locality of their institute alone, including no fewer than six of their own workers. In the following year the situation became obscured by a heavy mortality from the pandemic of relapsing fever which had spread from the west along the southern marches of the desert. Moreover, suramin had been used for treating patients at Sherifuri, and in 1925 it was thought possible that the efficacy of this drug had stemmed a threatened sleeping sickness epidemic; but optimism was short-lived; the unpreparedness of Johnson's position was revealed by his having only sufficient suramin to treat 120 cases.

In 1927, over 400 cases were treated at Sherifuri and four special Sleeping Sickness Officers were appointed for curative work; in 1928 over 3,000 cases were treated by the extra staff, and their field excursions disclosed a great unbroken epidemic zone lying east of Kano. Under the guidance of the chief entomologist, strategic anti-tsetse clearances were made in the neighbourhood of highly infected villages, but in the absence of a proper organization to maintain them, they had but little permanent effect.

In 1928, Johnson visited the French Congo to acquaint himself with methods of mass diagnosis and treatment. On his return to Nigeria in the following year, two small mobile teams of African assistants were recruited and trained although treatment was voluntary and most patients absconded after two or three tryparsamide injections. In 1930 Paisley visited the French Cameroons to study its anti-trypanosomiasis organization which consisted of 10 medical officers, 20 sanitarians and 300 assistants working under Jamot. In 1931, the first Nigerian sleeping sickness team took the field. It was but a shadow of Jamot's brigade, but reserves were in training at the Investigation's new headquarters in Gadau, a few miles south of Sherifuri, which had been opened in 1929. In 1930 Johnson was succeeded by Lester who took command of both the Tsetse Investigation and the new Sleeping Sickness Service. It was a bold reorganization but it came too late. During the next five years about 18,000 cases were found and treated by Lester's teams in the Lake Chad basin, but the true scale of the epidemic will never be known. By 1935 it had died out; its disappearance from many areas was due to the voluntary movement of surviving settlements away from the rivers.

Eastwards of Sherifuri, also at 12°N, a new focus had been found in the region of Fort Lamy in the French Cameroons in 1923, and within three years nearly 2,000 cases had been diagnosed and treated in this area; by these energetic means an epidemic was snuffed out. It was a perfect contrast to the British situation. But in the Upper Volta, far to the west, the same mysterious epidemic synchronism began in 1925, and there, the French, too, were taken unawares.

The behaviour of the disease in the northern savanna of the western Sudan differs in several respects from that of classical sleeping sickness in other ancient foci and also from the sporadic virulent trypanosomal infections of eastern Africa. During epidemic periods the disease is acute by classical standards, usually causing death within two years. Trypanosomes are more easily found in the blood of patients than they are in classical zones and the response to treatment is less satisfactory, particularly after the nervous system has become involved. These properties give the epidemics their particularly destructive character. During the epidemic in the Lake Chad basin at least two trypanosome strains were isolated and found to be akin to the virulent trypanosomes of eastern Africa.

It has been proposed that the recurring epidemics along latitude 12°N are due to the propagation of a rather virulent trypanosome along the great trade route of the west African hinterland. Yet it is not easy to see how the perennial movement of caravans can be solely responsible for epidemics at fairly regular intervals of about thirty years. It is possible that between epidemics, sleeping sickness lurks in chronic form at low, even undetectable, levels of endemicity, breaking out with epidemic force under a climatological or other universal influence and behaving with increased virulence as it is known to do when it invades virgin territory. Neither is it possible to deny that in these regions, where life of all kinds congregates around the slender sinews of water, there exist circumstances under which the transference of trypanosomes from antelope to man can take place.

From 1930 onwards, extensions of sleeping sickness northwards from the Niger-Benue valley began to cause great concern. In 1926 an important administrative centre at Jemaa was abandoned, and from there the disease pursued its relentless course into the central province of Zaria. The watershed between the Kaduna river and its tributary, the Galma, became a permanent and strategic source of infection for a large area of countryside, extending northwards almost to Kano city, and eastwards to the ramparts of the Bauchi plateau. The development of tin mining, gold mining, and timber extraction in different parts of Northern Nigeria with their special occupational risks, intensified transmission, not only locally but among migrant labourers. In 1934 the headquarters of the Service moved from Gadau to Kaduna, the chief administrative centre of Northern Nigeria. In 1935, nearly 90,000 cases were diagnosed in the central provinces. Altogether, from 1930 to 1940, 300,000 patients with sleeping sickness were treated by mobile teams and at a number of strategically situated centres.

It is hardly surprising that the days of the Investigation as a research department were numbered, and although a skeleton staff remained at Gadau for some years after the headquarters had moved, the advent of World War II in 1939 made it impossible to carry on. By 1940 all that remained of the endeavour embarked upon so optimistically in 1921 were a permanent legacy of over 100 scientific publications and the continuing personal inquiries of medical officers and the chief entomologist, undertaken in such time as they could spare from the ever-present problems of field control.

Meanwhile, it became clear that the success of anti-trypanosomiasis campaigns depended not only upon medical skill and applied entomological knowledge but also upon the vital factor of political administration.

It is often overlooked that those whose duty it is to combat trypanosomiasis among the peoples of Africa and their domestic animals are indebted to administrators at all levels, from the high concourses of government to those less honoured in the field. The British Government, through the academic power of the Royal Society, gave great impetus to trypanosomiasis work from the earliest times. Sleeping sickness was being studied in London in 1891; in 1902 Mott's classic study of the neuropathology of the disease was carried out in Essex, and this was but one aspect of the work of the Royal Society Commission. In 1908 a Sleeping Sickness Bureau was established in London and, so immensely valuable were its services, that four years later it became a centre for the dissemination of information on tropical diseases in general, and still provides a continual flow of vital information on tropical medicine and hygiene throughout the world. High level meetings sponsored by governments followed in almost endless succession, from the International Sleeping Sickness Conference organized by the British Foreign Office in 1907 and the Anglo-German Agreement and Protocol of 1908, to the expert international organization set up by the League of Nations Health Committee in 1922, under the chairmanship of Balfour. The work of the League continued for six years and had the humane and sensible effect of restoring the authority of German scientists such as Kleine who lent his great experience to problems in the Congo and Tanganyika. Its major publications included another important contribution to the pathology of trypanosomiasis, by Peruzzi, and its timely and authoritative example concluded with the Second International Conference on Sleeping Sickness in Paris at the end of 1928.

Without the active intervention of governments, the special services for research and field control that had come into existence throughout Africa by the 1930s would never have been established. Even during times of stringent national economy, large grants were made for work in epidemic areas. In 1915, the German authorities made an allocation of one million marks for sleeping sickness control in the Cameroons. In 1921 the British Colonial Office provided no less than £50,000 for an investigation into a method of treating the disease by intrathecal salvarsanized serum. During the inter-war years, the greater part of the health budget in French West and Equatorial Africa was allocated to sleeping sickness work. These are but a few examples of the many subscriptions made by western governments for the campaign against African trypanosomiasis.

In the field, political administration, albeit at a less exalted level, remains of vital importance. The principle of eradicating trypanosomes from a human population by chemotherapy depends upon the examination of everyone at risk, the discovery of every case and the full treatment of every patient thus found. These methods, when first employed in French-speaking colonies, included the provision of medical passports to restrict the movement of patients and a legislative code which made attendance at surveys, and treatment, when indicated, a matter of compulsion. These obligations proved to be an embarrassment to the British who were given to a more indirect form of administration and in whose territories compulsory methods as applied to the practice of hygiene went somewhat against the political grain. Legislation was introduced, but usually enforced only under particularly dangerous circumstances such as existed in tin mines. The success of most campaigns depended upon the tactful persuasiveness exercised by administrative officers in dealing with reluctant and often uncomprehending native authorities.

It must be admitted that mass examination and treatment campaigns are cumbersome, lengthy, expensive and troublesome to all concerned. If not carried out efficiently, they are often worse than useless, simply prolonging epidemic conditions beyond their natural span and bringing the whole system into disrepute. It is a matter for admiration that in countless instances administrative officers played a vital part in bringing these operations to a successful conclusion.

Yet no man-made system is perfect. In such critical times as those of the early 1930s, serious situations can arise through administrative delay. Happily, such examples are not easy to find, but in the Upper Volta epidemic which began in 1925, momentary indecisiveness may, in retrospect have made all the difference to subsequent events. At this time the French authorities had a splendid record of anti-trypanosomiasis work in Equatorial Africa. The tenacity of Jamot had brought into being the famous Permanent Mission against sleeping sickness in 1926, and the special prophylactic service in 1927. In the French Cameroons the battle against human sleeping sickness had been virtually won by 1932. But the Upper Volta epidemic was confronted less promptly and when Jamot visited this region in 1934 he discovered nearly 32,000 cases, with serious epidemic conditions in the regions of Koudougou, Ouagadougou and Gaoua, involving many villages on tributaries of the Volta rivers. In the following year a special service on the lines of the Equatorial Mission was set up in French West Africa and a full-scale attack was finally launched. Nonetheless, this epidemic continued to spread and by 1939 an area of about 30,000 square miles had been invaded, reaching westwards to the Niger near Segou and involving nearly 80,000 patients.

In Dahomey, endemic sleeping sickness was discovered in 1926 around Djougou and Natitingou; in 1930 there was a sharp increase in prevalence and a special unit was set up to deal with the situation. Ultimately, about 6,000 cases were found in these areas and another 10,000 were discovered in 1934 in the neighbouring parts of Togoland; as a whole, this focus remained a formidable source of infection during the rest of the 1930s.

Farther to the west, the Gold Coast administration had long been aware that old foci existed in central Ashanti and parts of Brong-Ahafo. In 1909 to 1910 Kinghorn had found about a hundred cases in these areas, but there was little indication that epidemic conditions were likely to arise, as the infection was mild and maintained at a low endemic level. The first sign of misfortune was an increase in the numbers of cases diagnosed at medical institutions between 1929 and 1931, and in the following year it was realized that transmission was taking place in the east Mamprussi district in the north-east of the country. In 1934 a second epidemic area was located in the extreme north-west, and a treatment camp for sleeping sickness patients was opened near Lawra. In 1936 about 5,000 cases were diagnosed in the country; this was fifty times the number recorded in 1929.

In January 1937, a Trypanosomiasis Campaign was established to control the epidemic by mass examination of whole populations, immediate treatment of patients and protective anti-tsetse clearings at critical places in the worst affected villages. It seems that the epidemic reached its peak during the first two years of the Campaign; when the first mass surveys were performed, the prevalence of the disease was over 6 per cent in the north-east and nearly 3 per cent in the north-west. Over a ten-year period, more than 4,700 cases were treated in these areas.

Meanwhile, transmission had intensified in the central endemic areas of Ashanti and Brong-Ahafo where important lines of communication converged, bringing together peoples from all over the country. The prevalence in the strategic town of Ejura, for example, was 4·5 per cent. Fortunately the situation responded to the methods employed and in all areas the prevalence began to decline after the first mass treatment. By 1950, epidemic conditions had virtually disappeared.

Farther to the west, the old endemic foci in the coastal areas below latitude 8°N remained quiescent. From the accumulation of isolated records over the years it was known that places such as Tebo in the Ivory Coast, Bakratown in Liberia, and Sherbro Island of Sierra Leone were sources of chronic classical sleeping sickness at a low endemic level. The most difficult and elusive problem in this part of West Africa was found a little above 8°N in the hinterland of

Guinea where the frontiers of that country are shared with those of Liberia and Sierra Leone. Here, the epidemiology is associated with the habits and migrations of the Kissi tribe whose knowledge of the disease is traditional. They number nearly 300,000, two-thirds of whom live around Kissidougou and Gueckedou, in Guinea. Their population density is relatively high for this region, and as the political frontiers transect the whole ethnic group, movement between parties of the inter-related population from one country to another is considerable. The presence of trypanosomiasis among the Kissi was known as early as 1908, but no significant events took place until 1932 when an investigation into an unusually high number of recent deaths confirmed that they were due to this disease.

In 1934 over a thousand cases were found between Gueckedou and Kissidougou. During the next four years about 8,600 more cases were discovered in this area and more than two-thirds of these were from Gueckedou. The disease was taking a virulent form, and four main epidemic foci were located. By 1939 considerable spread had occurred and it had become established in the neighbouring areas of Sierra Leone, where, in 1940, the prevalence among Kissi had risen to about 20 per cent. In 1939 the Service de la Maladie du Sommeil was created by Muraz to deal with human trypanosomiasis in countries administered by the French in West Africa, and a long series of diagnostic and treatment surveys was put in hand.

Elsewhere in the French controlled colony of Guinea it had been known since 1906 that trypanosomiasis was endemic among tribes such as the Mandinga and the Soussous, and even as early as 1916 extensions of the disease from these tribal areas were thought possible. These anticipations were fulfilled in the early 1930s by an outbreak involving nearly 14,000 people around the important communication centre of Labe in the north of the territory.

Meanwhile farther west, in that part of Guinea administered by the Portuguese, sleeping sickness had been known to be endemic in the colony since 1855, about sixty-six cases having been reported during the nineteenth century. From 1900 until 1924, only twenty-six cases were diagnosed but, on the recommendation of the Sleeping Sickness Conference in London in 1925, a Mission was established under Barreto. As a result of his enquiries, it was believed that the disease did not constitute a serious threat to the population, but in 1932 twenty-eight cases were found by a Mission from the Lisbon School of Tropical Medicine and Hygiene under Fontoura de Sequeira. Sleeping sickness then became a preoccupation of the health authorities, and this resulted in the discovery of nearly 4,500 patients during the next twelve years. By 1944 sleeping sickness was considered to be the fourth most important communicable disease in the territory.

The disease had been known for many years among the tribes inhabiting the valley of the river Gambia which flows westwards parallel to the equator at approximately 10°30′N. This is the historic locality of the infection contracted by the European captain of a river steamer in 1902. He became the first patient in whose blood trypanosomes were unequivocally demonstrated. A year later Dutton and Todd showed that sleeping sickness extended upriver for 250 miles. In certain riverine villages the prevalence among small communities was thought to be as high as 5 per cent. Notwithstanding, little more was heard of the disease until 1925. Between 1925 and 1935 the number of cases reported annually increased from about twenty to over 1,000, and a survey in 1937 confirmed that sleeping sickness was widespread and that there had been a real increase in prevalence. This increase continued until 1940 since when the situation has remained relatively constant, with no major epidemics.

Senegal, a large territory surrounding the Gambia on all sides save to seaward, is at the north-western limit of tsetse distribution. The presence of sleeping sickness in this country was established by Corré in 1877, and old endemic centres exist in the delta of the Senegal river and southwards to Joal along the coastal strip. Ancient foci are also known along the tributaries of the Casamance river which traverses the Senegalese corridor between Gambia and Portuguese Guinea to the south. In anticipation of possible intensifications of transmission and spread from these areas, the twentieth-century history of this region became largely administrative. The passage of time was punctuated by a series of prophylactic activities including legislation, governmental proscriptions, treatment centres and other organizational projects. But apart from a small outbreak in 1915 which yielded 184 cases along the 'little coast' south of Dakar, no disturbing events took place. Perhaps eternal vigilance had been rewarded, or perhaps it was simply the nature of things.

Elsewhere, in 1935 and 1936 the epidemic in West Africa reached its zenith. Although in retrospect it is possible to define the main epidemic zones, the contemporary prospect was one of unrelieved danger and uncertainty. From most epidemic regions, cases were numbered by the thousand, if not by tens of thousands, and it is probable that during this epoch at least a quarter of a million infections were being contracted each year. At the same time the situation in the Congo basin had not come completely under control and its extensions were still causing anxiety. Only in the Cameroons and in Ubangi could it be said that control had been achieved.

Everywhere, governments were at work to overcome the threat or reality of disaster. By the end of the 1930s the French had 10 trained teams in the Upper Volta, 2 on the western border of the Ivory Coast, 3 in Dahomey, 1 in Senegal, and 2 in Guinea. The Belgians under Van Hoof were concentrating their medical effort upon rural districts and, according to their fashion, numerous organizations both official and unofficial were involved. Among the most distinguished of these was the specially endowed Foundation Reine Élisabeth pour l'Assistance Médicale aux Indigènes better known as Foréami, whose annual expenditure rose to over eleven million francs.

Notwithstanding these great national efforts it must be admitted that sleeping sickness epidemics are self-limiting, and it would be false to claim that the subsequent amelioration of the whole inter-territorial situation has been wholly attributable to human intervention. For many reasons not altogether purposeful, it is unlikely that there will ever be as much sleeping sickness in West Africa again as there was at that time. Yet times of great crisis in human history are apt to produce men of genius and unlimited energy who not only meet the seemingly impossible challenge but inspire others to expend themselves in what appears to be a cause without hope. The innumerable campaigns against sleeping sickness during and since that time have saved countless lives and even communities. For these, mankind must remain forever indebted to Jamot. Wearied by incessant toil, and contemplating the ever-increasing numbers of cases being reported in spite of every effort, he wrote in January 1935: 'Ces chiffres, qui ne représentent d'ailleurs qu'une faible partie du nombre total des malades, donnent une idée du tribut de vies humaines que l'Afrique occidentale paie sans arrêt, depuis un temps immémorial, à la maladie du sommeil.'

The behaviour of sleeping sickness in the Congo basin and in western Africa, with its variety of clinical expression, epidemiological rhythm and economic effects, contrasts with the predictability of its mood in the great river basin of the Zambesi. In African latitudes greater than 13°S, tsetse are represented almost exclusively by woodland species. These flies inhabit the land drained by this vast waterway in a series of discontinuous belts. The most easterly lies to the south of the river in Mozambique; on the north bank lies a smaller infested region extending westwards towards Chikoa. More centrally placed, the largest belt, over 600 miles long from north-east to south-west, embraces the whole Luangwa tributary of historic fame, crosses the Zambesi along a front 300 miles wide and terminates around latitude 18°S. A fourth great region, centred around the Busango swamp, lies to the west, and to the south-west of this in Ngamiland is another belt, sustained largely by the delta of the Okovango, whose waters are evaporated from the swamps of that name to such an extent that its link with the Zambesi is practically lost. This belt probably extends northwards into the Caprivi strip along the valley of the Kwando which flows into the Liambezi Lake. Farther to the north, on the Kwelo and Makondo rivers in Angola are the last, isolated domains of woodland tsetse. From these, westwards for hundreds of miles to Mossamedes and Benguella on the Atlantic coast, the continent purchases reprieve at the price of rain.

Within these belts, the behaviour of human trypanosomiasis has a number of common features. Although the disease has been scientifically located in these places only in the comparatively recent past, there is a general, if uncertain, belief that it has been known for a much longer period of time even though such knowledge may not have passed into traditional tribal lore. Infections occur chiefly within certain notorious localities within the belts and, generally speaking, a significantly high proportion of those infected are either persons of European stock or others who are not indigenous to the region. Sometimes, however, the traditional inhabitants contract the disease and although it often takes a virulent form in them, some appear to harbour trypanosomes in their blood without becoming seriously ill. Sometimes sporadic infections begin to become more frequent in any one locality and this frequency may build up to produce as many as a hundred cases or more in the course of a single year. When this occurs, it has been commonly described as an epidemic, although of course the prevalence hardly merits such a term by standards of the Congo and western Africa. This relatively high local incidence lingers on for several years, after which the outbreak subsides of its own accord.

Most of the evidence suggests that these events are related to the degree of contact between man and woodland tsetse in the presence of game. Infections are often derived during patrols, hunting expeditions and other excursions into thinly populated bush, but in contrast with the epidemiology of sleeping sickness carried by riverine tsetse, the movement of the fly belts themselves is a complicating factor which has made the interpretation of human trypanosomiasis in central and eastern Africa a matter of difficulty.

These movements of woodland tsetse have about them the inexorability which characterizes phenomena that are promoted by great natural forces, and some of the factors involved are still not fully understood. It is believed that the rinderpest epizootic of the late nineteenth century, possibly the greatest natural calamity ever recorded in Africa, caused the belts to contract owing to the elimination of the natural food hosts of the fly. Some of the extensions which have been noted in recent times may therefore indicate the recolonization of ancient fly belts consequent upon their repopulation by ungulate communities. If this is so, then there must have been a time when man, had he been more numerous, or resourceful, or had he followed a culture based upon social units greater than the household and an agrarian policy other than shifting cultivation, might have moved into those areas and made them his own. But the opportunity was lost, and it was the fly which finally prevailed again, adding further to the impoverishment and incapacity of the land and its peoples.

It is also probable that climatological cyles have an influence upon the degree of contact between man and fly and that periods of drought, occurring either locally or on a continental scale, cause man, game and fly to congregate about the more restricted waterbodies that persist during relatively dry periods.

There are many reasons why outbreaks of virulent sleeping sickness in these areas tend to be of transient duration and, even during so-called epidemic periods, the prevalence of the disease, overall, is relatively low. For one thing the life of the human host is so shortened by the infection that the statistical likelihood of further transmission from man to man is considerably reduced. Furthermore, the absence of riverine tsetse, with their greater affinity for man and their closer contact with village societies has, as it were, stultified the evolution of a parasite which is attempting to perpetuate itself through a process of adaptation to man.

There are many tsetse-infested areas in the Zambesi valley from which sleeping sickness has never been reported. The reason for this is not known, but it has been suggested that a certain immunity may be induced by continual inoculation of man with animal trypanosomes and that this may protect the inhabitants of such places against human trypanosomiasis. In these fly-belts therefore, we may witness the more obvious of the mysterious inter-related phenomena which are concerned with the evolution of sleeping sickness in its most primitive form.

In the easterly fly belt which lies in Mozambique from the valley of the Rio Save northwards to the Zambesi, sporadic infections have occurred along the railway which runs westwards from Beira, and have been numerous enough to warrant the localization of a diffuse endemic focus between Masaka and the Rhodesian frontier. In the second belt to the north of the Zambesi a better defined focus is found in the region of Tete, where the disease has been known since 1918 or even earlier. In this area sixty-three cases occurred in 1932 and 1933 and in 1941 a further sixty-six infected persons were discovered. In spite of treatment the case mortality rate was nearly 20 per cent.

Further to the east, in the great belt which extends into the Zambesi valley along the course of the Luangwa river, well-defined endemic foci have been located to the south of the river at Sebungwe, West Hartley, North Lomagundi and Kariba, and each series of sporadic infections has originated from at least one apparently healthy person with trypanosomes in the blood. In each of them the disease has prevailed during a well-defined period of time but never assuming epidemic form. Fewer than 200 cases have been reported from these foci in more than fifty years, and of these a significantly high proportion have been Europeans. The situation in the Luangwa valley was investigated under the auspices of the British-South African company before the First World War. Although occasional sporadic infections have been contracted along the length of this great tributary ever since, there has been no sudden increase in prevalence.

In the large tsetse belt to the north of Livingstone and west of Lusaka, the pattern of sporadic infection is similar, with a tendency for an increase in prevalence from time to time along certain parts of the Kafue system.

The discovery of human trypanosomiasis within the Ngamiland tsetse belt was also true to type. Two European constables became infected in 1934 while on patrol near the Chobe river. From one of them, as from Armstrong and Beith, historical distinction demanded the highest price. Further inquiries disclosed that the disease had been recognized by the local inhabitants for many years, and confirmed that woodland tsetse were distributed throughout parts of the Chobe district and to the south around the Okovango swamps. In 1938 four cases were diagnosed from this southern tsetse belt and investigation revealed a low prevalence of virulent sleeping sickness over a wide area. There is some disputed evidence that the disease increased between 1939 and 1942, involving a few hundred people. Thereafter infection continued at a low endemic level, yet cases occurred among the staff of the tsetse fly control organization among whom exposure to the bites of woodland tsetse is an occupational hazard. From 1958 onwards the number of cases reported from Ngamiland and Chobe has increased to about eighty per annum. Typically, an increased prevalence tends to occur in different localities at different times, and is not universal throughout the whole belt.

Hence the evolutionary character of the phenomena is clear, although the number of factors which influence the behaviour of tsetse, game and man in any given focus is large, and it is not always possible to unravel the inter-related causes of a sudden local outbreak. Although the individual effects of virulent trypanosomiasis as it occurs in uncomplicated fashion in the Zambesi valley may be lethal, communities as a whole do not suffer unduly, unless, by chance, infection is limited to those members whose productivity is vital to the welfare of everyone.

North-eastwards beyond the sphere of the Zambesi the African coastline bulges outwards to the city of Mozambique and is serrated by the mouths of numerous rivers which flow eastwards into the Indian Ocean. The greater part of the country between Lake Nyasa and the sea is occupied by woodland tsetse extending far to the north beyond Dar es Salaam. In this area the Portuguese have defined several endemic foci of virulent trypanosomiasis, notably in Mazimbwa and Mtengula on the Ruvuma river system as well as the focus inland from Port Amelia which the British have cause to remember. In Mazimbwa, near the mouth of the Ruvuma, an increase in the number of reported cases occurred between 1942 and 1947 involving over 600 people. In Mtengula, near the source of the river not far from Lake Nyasa, cases were found for the first time in 1946, but the focus has since declined in importance.

To the north-west, however, in the great belt of woodland tsetse east of Lake Tanganyika this now familiar epidemiological pattern suddenly becomes manifest with vicious intensity, as if the trypanosome, frustrated by the lack of a riverine vector to help its adaptation, were bent upon a human holocaust.

So efficient had been the German control of sleeping sickness on the shores of Lake Tanganyika, that immediately after the First World War few cases could be found except in a small persistent focus at the northern end of the lake near the Ruanda-Burundi frontier. Elsewhere, however, in the heart of the woodland, serious developments lay in store. From the early 1920s, outbreaks began to occur in various parts of this territory on a scale far greater than any experienced in the Zambesi valley, and the infection was more virulent than had ever been known.

Although several authorities have discerned in these Tanganyikan epidemics a directional force, impelling trypanosomiasis northwards from foci in the Luangwa and Ruvuma river basins, the dynamics are probably more complex. The first major outbreak, in Maswa district to the south-east of Lake Victoria, has been ascribed to trypanosomes introduced by Congolese soldiers during the First World War, but of this there is no definite proof. A major difficulty in taking an historical view of this epidemic is that unusually virulent trypanosomiasis transmitted by riverine tsetse was occasionally reported in the Congo basin when the classical epidemics were going on there. Indeed, it has been postulated that human trypanosomiasis in this crucial part of eastern Africa originated from a virulent Congolese trypanosome which was brought into the Zambesi basin as early as 1907 and travelled northwards from there. These theories depend upon the principle that new foci of virulent sleeping sickness in eastern Africa develop as a result of introductions by infected humans. However important this contention may be, more universal considerations should not be dismissed. The expansion of the tsetse belt which lies between Lake Tanganyika and Lake Victoria to the north-east should not be ignored, and neither should those circumstances which prevail in parts of this region whereby the transmission of trypanosomes from game to man can take place. Furthermore, the migration of game animals themselves can, in theory at least, bring this evolutionary phenomenon to operate in places where hitherto it could never have happened. To complicate the situation further the region is one upon which the vegetational characters of African forest and savanna converge and where the belts of woodland tsetse, typical of eastern Africa, impinge upon the realm of riverine fly.

The Maswa epidemic came to light in 1922 with the reporting of nearly 700 deaths, and had probably been incubating for several years, possibly since 1918. There was a serious shortage of field staff immediately after the War, and moreover the peoples of this area were seriously afflicted by influenza and famine at about this time. This, then, was another occasion in history when the beginnings of a sleeping sickness outbreak might have been obscured by the effects of coincident medical disaster. Once the situation was assessed, the population began to be withdrawn to a fly-free area and total calamity was averted. It seems clear that this was the first epidemic of its kind in Maswa district, but opinions still differ as to whether the chief reservoir of this virulent trypanosome was man or antelope.

Two years later, in 1924, these sombre events were repeated in the southern part of the tsetse belt in the woodland drained by the Rungwa river which flows into Lake Rukwa. Once deaths began to occur, people dispersed in panic and, possibly on this account, an epidemic of West African proportions developed, spreading as far north as Kahama and beyond. As many as 3,000 cases were notified from this area in a single year. By 1930, almost the whole of the western province of Tanganyika was involved, and in spite of control measures the disease finally spread to Mwanza and Ukerewe Island on Lake Victoria by 1939.

The extraordinary virulence of the trypanosome, which could cause death within three to eight months, has been ascribed to the effects of ever-accelerating passage through man as the epidemics built up. The case mortality rate was about 50%, and it has been estimated that of nearly 24,000 persons infected between 1922, when the Maswa epidemic broke, and 1946, at least 11,500 were doomed.

Among the early research workers in East Africa, Lyndhurst Duke was outstanding, and the results of his studies lent support to the theory that African trypanosomiasis originated as a zoonosis. As Director of the Human Trypanosomiasis Research Institute at Entebbe in Uganda from 1927 to 1936, he published papers which not only illuminated the relationships between the trypanosomes of man and animals, but had about them a certain prophetic quality which influenced lines of investigation elsewhere.

The experiments of Corson, for example, were of paramount importance. His object was to discover whether trypanosomes isolated from man and maintained by inoculation through a series of laboratory animals would lose their adaptation to the human host. By remarkable investigations, in which he played the dual role of scientist and experimental subject, he showed that infectivity to man was a stable property. This conclusion was confirmed by an experiment which he began at the Sleeping Sickness Research Station in Tinde and was continued by his successors. In this classic investigation a trypanosome strain was maintained in sheep for twenty-three years by cyclical transmission through woodland tsetse, without losing the power to cause human trypanosomiasis.

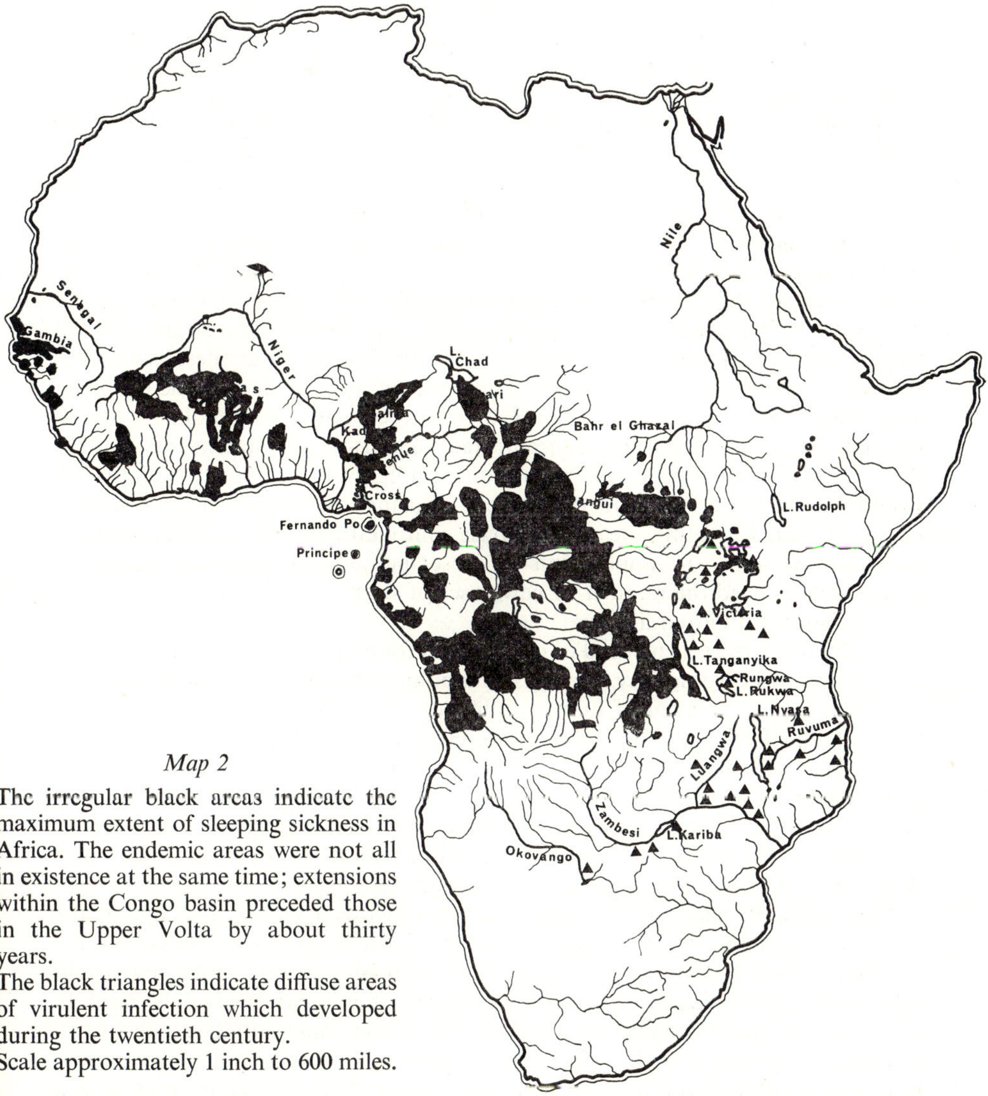

Map 2

The irregular black areas indicate the maximum extent of sleeping sickness in Africa. The endemic areas were not all in existence at the same time; extensions within the Congo basin preceded those in the Upper Volta by about thirty years.
The black triangles indicate diffuse areas of virulent infection which developed during the twentieth century.
Scale approximately 1 inch to 600 miles.

As time went on, field observations confirmed that man could derive infection on journeys through deserted woodland and on seasonal visits to fishing sites which at other times of the year were abandoned. Jackson noted that in a prohibited area south of Tabora, twenty-seven members of his staff contracted virulent sleeping sickness during the course of their field investigations.

The implication of these discoveries was far-reaching. The inference could be drawn that once a wild trypanosome overcomes the difficulties of adaptation to man, such propensity is not lost, but passed on to future generations. Furthermore, when man is not available, the strain can find harbourage as a commensal in its ancestral host without forfeiting its evolutionary advance.

More immediately, this information was vital to those in combat against the epidemic in Tanganyika. Hitherto, it had been anticipated that if an outbreak of sleeping sickness occurred, removal of the population could prevent further transmission, and it was believed that if human infection could then be eliminated, even by some simple holding operation for three years or so, the original area could be reoccupied with no more danger than existed before man-adapted trypanosomes had made their appearance in the locality. But these researches showed conclusively that temporary retreat was of no avail against the problem, and those at risk were therefore moved from their small households scattered through the woodland, and concentrated in permanent settlements with a population density of up to 100 to the square mile. In this way, woodland tsetse would be driven off by the consequent clearing of vegetation for farming purposes, thus liberating the society from continual exposure to trypanosomal infection. By 1936 the application of these methods by Maclean, Fairbairn and others reduced the number of new cases of sleeping sickness in Tanganyika to less than six hundred a year.

As time went by, this method of control was found to have certain limitations. As the newly-settled society grew, its inhabitants found a need for expansion; secondly, the withdrawal of human influence from wide areas gave woodland tsetse greater freedom to advance. It therefore became clear that the establishment of permanent settlements had to be combined with direct measures for the control and, if possible, the eradication, of tsetse. This problem was tackled largely by the Tsetse Research Department of Tanganyika Territory at Shinyanga under the direction of Swynnerton whose investigations were conducted with the skill and ingenuity of the born naturalist.

The wholesale clearing of bush was an obvious method, but unless the voluntary cooperation of a large number of adults could be obtained for reclamation work, the cost of making any impression upon the fly belt would have been prohibitive. Furthermore, in areas of comparatively low rainfall, such clearing could result in an adverse affect upon water supplies and lead to serious soil erosion. Lastly, if the clearings were not quickly utilized for cultivation, a type of vegetational regrowth could occur which is ideally suitable as a habitat for woodland tsetse. Hence part of the fly belt near Shinyanga was divided into blocks in which alternative methods were investigated. These included the proper organization of grass burning. Although this was practicable only in grassland of a suitable kind, it was later adopted in Uganda with encouraging results. In other experimental areas, fly and game barriers were formed by encouraging the growth of dense thicket. Fly traps were devised, and the advantages of protecting woodland from grass fires were also investigated on the principle that the vegetation thus spared ultimately becomes too dense for habitation by certain species of fly.

Much of this work was of relevance, not only to Tanganyika, but to every other country in eastern Africa. It completely justified the inclusion of professional entomological staff in every sleeping sickness control organization, and showed these workers to be indispensable for a complete understanding of the problems involved. Their scientific training and insight into the operations of nature in the field have often been the envy of their clinical colleagues. Moreover, as the problem of sleeping sickness is fundamentally one of applied biology, their objective outlook furnished a much-needed counterpoise to the anthropocentric views of medical personnel.

This is not to gainsay the part played by physicians. During the nineteenth century numerous clinical studies were made, from Winterbottom's observation of the glandular enlargements in the neck, a sign which has been acknowledged to him ever since, and the painstaking researches of Guerin who earned a doctorate in 1869 for a study of 148 cases among liberated Congolese on Martinique, to the careful analyses by Mackenzie and Manson in London. Soon afterwards, physicians such as the intrepid Christy of the Royal Society Commission, were suddenly confronted with complicated clinical problems of which they had no experience, little understanding and only elementary knowledge. It is true that their empiricism and mode of expression sometimes lacked scientific precision. Graf, for example, who gave his name to the primary skin lesion, referred to the 'sting' of the tsetse. Yet such inaccuracies need not detract from the merit due to those who in epidemic times worked at special risk, as the eponymous description of Kerandel's infection can testify. Later, medical men inoculated themselves with trypanosomes and were often among the first to take new compounds suggested for the prophylaxis and treatment of the disease.

One of the most remarkable aspects of East African research was its fruitful conduct during a time of the utmost financial stringency. That so much was done by relatively few with such primitive equipment under conditions of employment that would attract no scientist today, is an undeniable tribute to their vocational concern with the well-being of the inhabitants of eastern Africa.

In 1930, Duke published a warning that trypanosomiasis was again finding its way into Uganda. Almost at once, the economic recession necessitated a reduction of his staff at Entebbe, and at the end of 1935 his laboratory, from which exemplary scientific work had emanated for twenty-three years, was finally closed. By the time the trypanosome began its onslaught, the prophet had gone.

Meanwhile, in Northern Nigeria a resettlement scheme in connexion with sleeping sickness control was being undertaken for reasons which differed completely from those which were compelling men to retreat from tsetse in Tanganyika. In the countryside to the north of the Galma river, near the scene of the small but historic epidemic at Gimi in 1919, the disease had insidiously tightened its grip, and by 1934 about one-third of the population in a district called Anchau were infected, with serious loss of life.

By this time, entomological research had shown that riverine tsetse could be attacked by partial, as opposed to ruthless, clearing of riverine thicket. However, regeneration had to be eliminated by annual reslashing and, for this, communal labour had to be employed because the exploitation of cleared areas by farming was too irregular to guarantee permanent eradication. In Anchau, however, the population had become so attenuated that the available manpower was insufficient to maintain the necessary clearings by communal forces.

It was therefore planned to establish a tsetse-free corridor about 70 miles long and 10 miles wide containing about 60,000 inhabitants, and to increase the population density within it from 33 to 70 per square mile. For this purpose a grant of £95,000 over a ten-year period was made in 1936 from the Colonial Development Fund, on condition that the area was economically developed at the same time. The subsequent campaign placed a unique and formidable burden upon the Sleeping Sickness Service and the Administration.

In contrast to the foot-loose culture of the Tanganyikans, Anchau people lived in organized communities and their resettlement had to be reconciled with the intricate native laws of land tenure. Furthermore, the settlers had to be integrated with societies already living under stabilized local village administration. Apart from these difficulties, the campaign involved the building of a new town to house 600 people, chiefly from the decrepit slums of Anchau town itself.

The provision of water supplies entailed the sinking of over 120 wells which had the incidental, but much applauded, result of eliminating guinea worm which had plagued the inhabitants since time immemorial. Other prodigies of organization included road construction, the building of markets, health propaganda, education, the provision of shade trees and the introduction of crops such as soya bean, sugar cane, groundnuts and tobacco.

As woodland tsetse was absent, the eradication of riverine fly immediately conjured up the prospect of mixed farming. However, most of the cattle in the first imported herd were found already to have trypanosomiasis. The severity of the disease increased after anti-rinderpest inoculations, and within a year only two animals out of 140 survived. Notwithstanding this setback, further efforts were made and eventually about ninety head of cattle were established in the corridor. By this time, too, pig keeping had been introduced and the local breeds of donkey, chicken and goat had been improved.

In retrospect, Anchau was undoubtedly the most ambitious resettlement operation ever attempted by a sleeping sickness control organization, and its subsequent history has been as instructive as the lessons which were learned while the scheme was in progress. After 1939, as from all other colonial departments, the Second World War demanded its overriding tribute and the professional cadre of the Service became insufficient to train adequate numbers of Nigerians in the management of the technical problems involved. Yet this was not the only reason why the fortunes of this fly-free haven have declined.

In 1946, administration was virtually handed over to the native authority. As far as is known, the corridor has remained free of tsetse ever since, and the clearings are still regularly maintained, a task which becomes less burdensome as time goes by. But it is apparent that far too many social and economic innovations were attempted in too short a time. The peasantry in the corridor, having been denied by trypanosomiasis any tradition of animal husbandry, had never learned how to look after cattle and had little enthusiasm for doing so, manure or no manure, unless the effort resulted in immediate financial returns. Likewise, a decade of propaganda was hardly enough to overcome the prejudices and conservatism of the Anchau farmers who raised their pittance from the soil by methods that had not altered since the Iron Age. Furthermore, as sleeping sickness had been known in the district for not more than a generation, the inhabitants had, and probably still have, little understanding of the complicated scientific reasons for such an upheaval in their lives to eliminate a scourge which, to them, was simply one of countless inexplicable vicissitudes periodically suffered by West African societies since the birth of mankind.

So far, this elaborate scientific and social experiment had little in common with resettlement operations in Tanganyika. Yet the innate ability of woodland tsetse to take advantage of an ecological change can be discerned in the case of Anchau, as in eastern Africa. Towards the end of the 1940s it became clear that this fly was moving from a previously defined belt south of the corridor, northwards along its eastern limit in numbers and with a persistence that had never been recorded before. It therefore seems that the concentration of population within the corridor had created a vacuum into which woodland tsetse extended. To some extent, all tsetse-free islands, whether natural or artificial, tend towards ultimate imprisonment by this implacable invader.

By 1940 the epidemiological pattern of sleeping sickness in western Africa had begun to settle down. As Dutton and Todd had predicted, most of the primordial foci were still in existence and many of them had acquired permanent satellites. In these intractable places, the prevalence of the disease waxed and waned, although new extensions from them happily became less frequent. Trained African assistants enabled campaigns to be undertaken with fewer professional staff, and operations began to be conducted from permanent case-finding and treatment centres.

An epidemic still smouldered in Upper Volta, where, in February 1939, Muraz had taken over the campaign. The neighbouring parts of the Gold Coast near Lawra were involved, but following a campaign against riverine tsetse, sleeping sickness was virtually eliminated by 1945. Meanwhile Muraz, continuing Jamot's tradition, conducted about four million examinations and treated nearly four thousand patients in ten years, and also adopted measures against riverine fly in certain situations. Finally, under his constant pressure, the epidemic began to abate.

The Kissi focus was active during the War years. In Liberia from 1941 to 1943, 10,000 cases were discovered and in Sierra Leone, epidemic sleeping sickness occurred in the Kissi and Kono districts adjacent to the frontiers of Liberia and Guinea. In 1939 a campaign against sleeping sickness was launched, chiefly to contend with the Kissi influence in these eastern districts. During the next fifteen years over 12,000 cases were treated. In French Guinea, teams were working from 1934 onwards but even after ten years, village prevalences still ranged from 3 to 7 per cent.

During the 1940s it was seen that the control of sleeping sickness by mass diagnosis and treatment had not only an interminable future but was beginning to obey the law of diminishing returns. True, the method could reduce an epidemic situation to one of low endemicity, but for various reasons it could never achieve eradication of ancient West African foci on any significant scale. In the first place the source of infection in the riverine fly remained untouched. Secondly, it was impossible to undertake extensive surveys at frequent intervals, not only for economic reasons but because the lack of good rural communications often immobilized teams during the rains. The establishment of treatment centres at strategic places provided no answer to this problem as attendances were voluntary and few early cases reported. Most important of all, diagnostic methods had scarcely changed since gland puncture was advocated at the turn of the century and even when combined with blood examination, there was no guarantee, even in expert hands, of diagnosing every case even on repeated examination. In retrospect, this factor was probably responsible for more disappointments than any other shortcoming of the system. At this time it also became apparent, especially in certain areas of the Congo, that the curative effects of tryparsamide were declining, probably due to the emergence of strains of trypanosome which were resistant to arsenicals.

To contend with these problems, a few attempts had been made to use suramin as a prophylactic, but for various reasons this approach never became popular. However in 1940, the prophylactic effect of the aromatic diamidines was noted in experimental animals and Van Hoof lost no time in undertaking field trials of these substances in the Congo, and was soon followed by McLetchie, Lester's successor, in Nigeria. Subsequently, pentamidine, known to the French as Lomidine, was found to be the most efficacious and least toxic of these compounds. In French West Africa chemoprophylaxis with Lomidine was begun in 1946 and within the next eight years over $1\frac{1}{2}$ million doses had been given to people at risk in active foci. Notwithstanding the difficulties of contending with the widespread influences of the Kissi tribe, the disease in the Gueckedou and Kissidougou regions was finally brought under control. The method was also exploited in Belgian and Portuguese territories. In Nigeria, the drug was introduced in 1944, chiefly for the protection of labourers in tin mines and other persons at special occupational risk.

Yet, even to this day, well organized and skilful forces using mass survey methods, chemoprophylaxis and strategic anti-tsetse campaigns have seldom completely eliminated the old endemic areas that persist like the rocks of ages after the recession of the epidemic tide.

There are innumerable examples of the tenacity with which sleeping sickness persists in established foci. In the Sudan, the disease was fought with almost military efficiency after the establishment of a special Commission in 1905, which included Balfour within its ranks. Yet in spite of the meticulous application of control measures, including segregation of patients, seven intractable foci had developed by 1920, comprising the focus at Raga in the north-west, and six others associated with tributaries of the Bahr el Ghazal and the White Nile. By 1911 a small epidemic was going on at Yei, which had begun to develop into an agricultural centre. Situated on a trade route that traversed rivers and streams, the focus was clearly a menace to other areas and was tackled vigorously by segregation of cases and ruthless anti-tsetse clearing, as a result of which the disease died out by 1924. Similar measures at Raga had the same effect; control of another dangerous situation in Tembura district was attained by several methods including the establishment of a settlement for nearly 700 patients twenty-five miles away in 1920. The efficiency of this enterprise rivalled that of Anchau which it preceded by nearly twenty years in far more difficult terrain. In 1925 over 1,800 patients were undergoing treatment there.

Another endemic area at Yambio became the centre for the Zande resettlement and agricultural scheme in 1946. A low prevalence of sleeping sickness had obtained in this region since 1924, but after the development programme began, the reported cases increased to 64 in 1953 and 871 in 1957. The Yambio district of 2,000 square miles comprises a network of riverine vegetation infested with fly, making tsetse control or segregation practically impossible. The situation was therefore dealt with by mass pentamidine prophylaxis throughout a population of about 180,000. The prevalence rapidly diminished and transmission appeared to have ceased by 1961.

Meanwhile sleeping sickness was reintroduced into the Yei focus in 1943. For the next eleven years control measures kept the prevalence at a low level, but in 1954, owing to a sweeping political change, case-finding was given up and control work came to a standstill. By 1960 the number of reported cases had risen to 223 per annum, and pentamidine prophylaxis was put in hand. Thereafter the number of new infections rapidly declined. Although the position appears to be under control, there is no room for complacency. The area is strategically situated along lines of communication with other foci in the Congo basin and in Uganda. In 1962 a patient infected at Yei was found to have trypanosomiasis that was resistant to pentamidine in full curative doses. Thus, even after sixty years, and in spite of numerous campaigns, the threat of sleeping sickness lingers on.

A notable example of epidemic resurgence occurred in the Lake Chad basin of Northern Nigeria where Johnson's research team had been overrun by events in the 1920s. In 1948, transmission of sleeping sickness began again, and almost at once an experienced force began a widespread treatment campaign. The figures attained of 3¼ million examinations and 5,000 cases found were of West African proportions, but mass diagnosis and treatment could only contain, and not overcome, this outbreak. After five years the situation was still fluid and discriminative clearings were made against riverine tsetse in the flood valleys, but the immense cost of labour crippled this endeavour. From the economic point of view, times had changed since the first tree was felled in the Anchau corridor.

In this region the distribution of woodland tsetse coincides with that of riverine fly. By good fortune an insecticidal campaign against tsetse was being pursued in part of the riverine system by the Veterinary Department of Northern

Nigeria, using a technique that eliminated both kinds of fly. Hence in 1958, an insecticidal attack was launched against tsetse in the sleeping sickness areas, and within three years the situation was under control.

The use of mass diagnosis and treatment campaigns against epidemics in western Africa depends upon the principle that man is the only significant reservoir. Yet the cyclical epidemics around Sherifuri were never controlled by these methods; they ceased only when, either naturally or artificially, contact between man and fly was severed. In these and other respects they possess the overtones of a situation influenced by woodland tsetse and an animal reservoir.

Owing to the declining prevalence of infection in many countries during the 1940s, mobile services utilized solely for sleeping sickness work became polyvalent, and their experience and flexibility were used to combat other endemic and epidemic diseases. In the Congo, Foréami, originally designed for multipurpose campaigns, became committed to the control of many communicable diseases. In French West Africa the Service General d'Hygiene Mobile et de Prophylaxie (SCHMP), was formed, with its headquarters and a training school for medical auxiliaries at Bobo Dioulasso. The Nigerian Medical Field Units which began to be trained in 1946 were strengthened by workers with years of experience in the Sleeping Sickness Service. Similarly, the Portuguese, having created a special trypanosomiasis service in Guinea in 1945, turned it into a multi-purpose organization for endemic disease control eleven years later. All these organizations were destined to play important roles in campaigns against yaws, smallpox, yellow fever, and many other scourges of the West African peasantry. Yet notwithstanding the immense benefits thus derived, the intractability of ancient foci must still demand the retention of adequate expert staff to deal with the complicated and specialized problems of sleeping sickness control.

During the early 1940s, while in many parts of Africa human trypanosomiasis was entering upon a phase of biological repose, attention was alerted by reports from Uganda of another epidemic on the northern shore of Lake Victoria. The investigation of this outbreak by MacKichan of the Colonial Medical Service brought matters to light which were of far more than purely local concern.

The disastrous epidemic in this area at the beginning of the century was terminated by the wholesale evacuation of the population to a distance of up to fifteen miles. Most authorities agree that the disease was of West African type, the man-adapted trypanosomes behaving with unusual virulence in a virgin population weakened by coincidental famine. No one doubts that the vector was riverine tsetse. The handling of the situation has passed into the realms of historical controversy, illuminated by the writings of Sir Hesketh Bell, under whose administration the campaign was fought, and a later report by Fiske who anticipated further trouble in this area, although, as things turned out, not for the right reasons. By the time his report was written in 1926, remnants of the former population were moving back into the area in a somewhat irregular fashion.

Evidence began to accumulate during the 1930s that Uganda was at risk from the introduction of virulent trypanosomes from the south west, and in 1940 a handful of cases were found near Jinja. Immediate measures were taken to evacuate the lake shore between Kakira and Jinja to a depth of up to two miles, and efforts were directed towards isolating the township of Jinja, based upon the assumption that as in the distant past, the disease was being conveyed by riverine tsetse. Within a few months the clearings had apparently succeeded in controlling the outbreak, but shortly afterwards twenty cases were found, further to the east, among the inhabitants of a leper colony at Buluba. A month later infections occurring among forestry workers near Kiterera brought the total number of cases to eighty.

The population of the Busoga coastal area was then surveyed and protected by clearing and prophylactic suramin. It soon became clear however that the inland population to the north was also at risk, and in November 1941, a year after the first case had been discovered, others were found, at least twelve miles from the lake. Within the next two months the disease spread across the Sio river into Kenya. By March 1942 over 100 new patients were reporting each week, and in that year over 1,800 cases were treated. The disease was extremely virulent and many victims became moribund within six weeks of the onset of symptoms. Subsequently, the prevalence quickly declined; it seems that this regression was partly a natural phenomenon consequent upon the cessation of abnormally heavy rains. Problems of endemicity, however, have since persisted in this region.

The observations of MacKichan and, subsequently, Jackson pointed to the fact that this outbreak was conveyed, not by riverine tsetse, but by a woodland species, *Glossina pallidipes*. The incrimination of this particular fly as a vector of virulent trypanosomiasis not only explained a number of puzzling local features, but established a vital link in the evolutionary chain of transmission of trypanosomes from antelope to man. This tsetse fly is associated with certain types of thicket within the general landscape of East African woodland, and feeds upon bushbuck. The significance of the ecology of *G. pallidipes* and the enticing shade of its natural haunts now began to dawn, but one last fundamental discovery still had to be made.

The most widely held view is that the trypanosome responsible for this epidemic which involved nearly 2,500 people of whom 274 died in spite of treatment, was introduced from Tanganyika along the western shore of Lake Victoria. Its extraordinary virulence, however, suggests that it had not long forsaken the tranquillity of residence in the animal host, even though the focal nature of the ensuing outbreaks clearly indicated man-to-man transmission.

There is no more mysterious or beautiful region in Africa than the great rift which runs to the northeast from Lake Edward through the Semliki valley to Lake Albert which, abducting the waters of the Victoria Nile from the east, delivers its charge into the Albert Nile as far as Nimule. Here, as the waterway turns through an elbow, the White Nile is born and surges northwards, taking life to the Sudanese and Egyptian peoples. Immediately to the west, the basins of the Congo and the Nile struggle for dominion through mountain and valley, savanna and forest. These regions of immense complexity constitute the focal point of the continent's physical conformation, the biological labyrinth of Africa and the scene of man's own restless migrations.

At the end of the nineteenth century, sleeping sickness of West African type was introduced into the Nile basin, probably from epidemic areas on the Upper Ubangi of the Congo system. By 1904 several foci had become established along the Albert Nile from Nimule southwards to Wadelai. This stretch of river provides the eastern foreshore of the West Nile district of Uganda, and its political history bears witness to the turbulence of human activity so characteristic of this region. In 1876 much of this area was included in the Lado Enclave of Emin Pasha. In 1893 the Lado was leased to King Leopold of the Belgians, but on his death in 1909 it returned to Sudanese administration. In 1914, it became the Nile Province of Uganda, but the First World War then began and any preoccupation with sleeping sickness matters was postponed until the 1920s.

The early spread of sleeping sickness along the Albert Nile northwards and southwards from Wadelai resembled the insidious but remorseless advance of the disease in parts of West Africa. The Wadelai headquarters were abandoned on account of sleeping sickness in 1906 and moved to Koba about twenty-five miles to the south. There, too, the native people fished and hunted by the waterside within the ambit of riverine tsetse, and in 1910 about a thousand deaths were reported. Two years later the station was moved to Gulu over sixty miles to the northeast of Koba and many riverside people were evacuated. Yet the retreat was made only from one bank of the Albert Nile, and sleeping sickness was still smouldering in the valley in 1914.

By 1921 sleeping sickness was established among the Madi who occupied both banks of the Albert Nile near Nimule. It is possible that this area became involved by the movement of people from Kajo Kaji in the north, a small but important focus in the Sudan. Some evacuations were attempted, but the Madi were reluctant to move, and even those who left kept returning to their homes. Meanwhile, a serious famine befell them, and they began to migrate to the west in search of food. By 1927 the disease had become established at Aringa, and local epidemic conditions began. By the end of 1928, 700 cases had been diagnosed.

Control measures consisting of mass survey and treatment and strategic anti-tsetse clearings were put in hand. A special enclave for the segregation of patients was established in Aringa, and the Congolese system of restricting movement of peoples, legally enforced, with registration of the population in danger zones, was applied. As the Belgians had noted twenty years before, the imposition of such restrictions caused great confusion and led to further spread of the disease by surreptitious movements along unsupervised bush tracks in the wilderness. However, by 1930 the disease was on the decline in Aringa district although a new focus had arisen around the district headquarters of Arua. By the end of 1931 anti-tsetse clearings had achieved control in Arua and the prevalence in Aringa continued to fall. It is difficult to assess to what extent this decline was due to medical and administrative action, because the Madi famine came to an end in 1929 and the widespread peregrinations of starving people ceased. Communities became more settled, and now that the struggle for existence was less acute they became more favourably disposed towards inspection and treatment.

In 1933 it became apparent that epidemic conditions had again built up in Aringa and Terigo country and over a thousand cases were diagnosed throughout an area of 500 square miles on the western tributary systems of the Albert Nile. In spite of extensive and thorough control measures, by 1939 sleeping sickness was more or less endemic throughout West Nile except in the highlands. The disease was controlled by mass diagnosis and treatment at regular intervals, and by clearing. Since 1947 a low state of endemicity has prevailed, with local intensifications of transmission occurring at propitious times.

To the south of the Victoria Nile as it flows westwards in splendour to Lake Albert, is the Kingdom of Bunyoro. Sleeping sickness was discovered there in 1904 and in the following year it was reported that 200 deaths had occurred· During the next four years the disease extended to the mouth of the river and then spread southwards, decimating the fishing populations along the eastern shore of the lake. Hence in 1909 yet another retreat was sounded, and the shore was evacuated. The withdrawal was thorough, and in consequence much country along the Victoria Nile was invaded by woodland tsetse. Part of this area now contributes to the Murchison National Park, a reserve of great natural beauty obtained at the cost of a victory for trypanosomiasis.

By 1915 it seems that epidemic conditions on Lake Albert had died out, and after the First World War resettlement began along the north-eastern shore. The situation remained quiet until the late 1930s when trypanosomes were introduced from West Nile district, after which small local outbreaks occurred in Bunyoro for the next sixteen years. Of the cases diagnosed, about one third were unusually virulent infections and it is believed that this area may have been open not only to the influence of the endemic area of West Nile in the north, but also to that of an epidemic of virulent trypanosomiasis transmitted by woodland tsetse in Mengo district to the south. By 1951 organized hunting virtually eliminated this fly as far north as Masindi and consequent upon this achievement and the continuing low prevalence of the disease in West Nile, the situation along the eastern shore of Lake Albert has remained satisfactory, However, this region remains vulnerable as each year 25,000 migrant labourers make their way through the district in search of seasonal employment.

The great bastion of the Ruwenzori lies between Lakes Albert and Edward, looming across the waters of Lake George to the southeast and circumscribed on the west by the Semliki valley which falls within the political province of the Congo. The history of trypanosomiasis in this region is, like many another history, obscure, but it seems that the disease might have been present in the valley before its occupation by the Belgians in 1896, and that a notable epidemic occurred from 1915 to 1923 around the northern shore of Lake Edward.

To the south and east of the Ruwenzori mountains lies the district of Busongora, traversed by numerous rivers running from the great slopes into Lakes Edward and George. It seems that human trypanosomiasis was introduced into this area early in the present century, possibly by salt traders from the

Semliki valley in the west. By 1910 the disease prevailed among people living near Katwe on the northern shore of Lake Edward, with a heavy mortality among men engaged in canoe traffic. By 1913 it was spreading eastwards from Katwe along the Kazinga channel to the western shore of Lake George. In 1914 several lakeside communities were evacuated further into Busongora country, much of which, however, still lay within the domain of riverine tsetse.

The disease was of the insidious West African kind and, possibly for this reason, the situation attracted little further attention. However, by 1931, foci were still present in parts of the countryside, and imported cases were found among Congolese escaping from the sleeping sickness control regulations imposed by Belgian authorities in the Semliki valley. For a time, transmission in Busongora intensified and the disease tended to spread farther to the east. However, a programme of mass diagnosis and treatment combined with strategic anti-tsetse clearings was put in hand and, as is usual with outbreaks of classical sleeping sickness, the situation responded satisfactorily, leaving a few localized pockets of low endemicity.

In the vicinity of the great Rift, therefore, human trypanosomiasis behaved as it did in many places in western Africa. Serious local outbreaks occurred soon after its introduction and later these settled down into an overall endemic pattern of low prevalence and widespread distribution, with occasional flares in restricted localities under circumstances which, known or unknown, were temporarily propitious.

Close to the northern shore of Lake Victoria lies a chain of islands whose inhabitants, most of them fisherfolk, maintain contact with each other and with the peoples on the mainland by canoes of a kind which have plied smoothly and swiftly across the water ever since man himself learned to master wind and current with defiance and skill. The islands extend in a huge arc 150 miles long from the Sesse group, Bugala and Bukasa, in the west, through Kome, Damba, and Bugaia to Buvuma south of Jinja on the lakeshore, and beyond. Many of the islanders were smitten by the great epidemic at the dawn of this century, and the disease was carried eastwards into Kenya through Lolui, Mageta and Rusingwa, the stepping stones for its progression to the far side of the Kavirondo Gulf, where its appearance was recorded in 1902. The disease, transmitted by riverine fly, rapidly obtained a hold, particularly to the south of the Gulf, and within six years the lakeside populations of Nyanza had been seriously affected as far south as the border of Tanganyika. Camps established for the segregation of patients became unpopular as no treatment was given. Finally, of its own accord, the population moved away from dangerous areas and this self-inflicted retreat was followed by a decline in prevalence after 1910. The disease remained at a low endemic level for the next decade, but in the early 1920s a sharp outbreak occurred at the eastern extremity of the Gulf near Kisumu and on Mageta Island, to be followed in 1925 by a localized epidemic along the Miruwe river which flows into the Kavirondo Gulf from the southeast. The outbreak was controlled by clearing and by farming the reclaimed land and the valley has remained free of sleeping sickness for over forty years.

To the south of the Gulf the disease persisted with greater tenacity. In the 1930s further epidemics broke out in places on the Kuja-Migori river system and although the situation was tackled with mass treatment of patients, bush clearance and utilization of the reclaimed land, small outbreaks continued to occur for the next ten years. During the 1940s another epidemic spread up the headwaters of the Kuja river and an important focus of infection appeared on a tributary of the Nyando to the east of Kisumu. The most energetic and successful measures were eventually applied, at first by Wilson on the Nyando and later by Glover on the Kuja system, using insecticidal attack to exterminate riverine tsetse. Since these operations were completed in 1957 the chief influence in south Nyanza has been that of *G. pallidipes* whose depredations among new settlements in the Lambwe valley have resulted in a constant stream of virulent infections since 1960.

The history of sleeping sickness in Central Nyanza which embraces the lakeshore and its hinterland from the northern limit of the Kavirondo Gulf northwestwards to the Uganda border, is of great complexity, although in recent years the countryside has furnished the background for outstanding discoveries. Administratively this region is divided into a number of locations including Samia in the north, followed successively southeastwards by Yimbo (otherwise Kadimu), Sakwa and Uyoma along the lakeshore. Further from the lake, to the east of Yimbo, lies the Alego location. The peoples of this region have been exposed to incursions of classical sleeping sickness from Uganda since 1900; canoe traffic has provided the means of rapid spread, but the influence of the slower overland route, too, cannot be discounted. This pattern has been true to type, and epidemics have alternated with latent periods. The first serious outbreak occurred between 1902 and 1910 and the second began about 1920, prompting the League of Nations to dispatch the redoubtable van Hoof across the Lake from the Congo, taking treatment facilities with him. Finally the second epidemic began to die down, and after campaigns by MacLean and Southby the situation became quiescent.

A further outbreak was discovered in 1949 in the Yimbo and Alego locations to the south of the Yala swamp. This was countered by a campaign against riverine tsetse, and in 1950, of seven locations surveyed, sleeping sickness could be found in only three, Samia, Yimbo and Alego. By the end of 1954 the disease had virtually disappeared from these, but new infections were being discovered in Sakwa and Uyoma locations to the south.

It is now believed that complicated and significant biological events took place in and around Yimbo location after the mid-1940s. Comparative studies suggest that *G. pallidipes* greatly increased in range and numbers in this area during the next two decades. The inhabitants were no strangers to sleeping sickness, but the virulence of the trypanosomal infection which they derived after 1948 was of an order that they had never known before. To add to these disconcerting developments, hundreds of Yimbo cattle succumbed to a mysterious wasting disease a few months before the epidemic began. The first human infections were derived by farmers in a remote place known as Ulungu, the richest game area in Yimbo, at some distance from the lakeshore.

Until 1953 it was generally considered that most sleeping sickness in Central

Nyanza was due to well-adapted trypanosomes carried by riverine tsetse, even though it had been reported that the virulent form of the disease had entered Kenya during the epidemic in southeast Uganda which MacKichan had investigated more than a decade previously. By 1953 it had become clear that the disease was not responding satisfactorily to tryparsamide and in the following year a highly virulent strain was isolated from a patient in Uyoma. Sleeping sickness in Central Nyanza was going through a critical phase at this time and it now appears that the locations of Sakwa and Uyoma were harbouring a perennial endemic reservoir of virulent trypanosomes transmitted by *G. pallidipes*. In Samia there was a greater degree of contact between man and fly owing to the presence not only of *G. pallidipes* but to riverine tsetse as well, a circumstance which may have led to an increase in the number of reported cases of virulent trypanosomiasis in 1957 and in later years. In Yimbo itself, riverine tsetse were present with an increasing *G. pallidipes* population, bringing about another sharp outbreak in 1961. Thus it began to be discerned that riverine tsetse was supplementing woodland fly as a vector of ill-adapted trypanosomes, the number of infections being proportional to the degree of man-fly contact.

Meanwhile, in 1958 Heisch, McMahon and Manson-Bahr made a signal contribution by isolating a trypanosome of great virulence to man from the blood of a bushbuck shot in the Utonga forest south of Kadimu Bay. Although such a discovery had been anticipated for many years by Duke, Corson and others, their predictions do not detract from the scientific precision with which it was made nor from its profound significance in terms of human trypanosomiasis. The bushbuck, *Tragelaphus scriptus*, better known as the harnessed antelope, is distributed widely throughout Africa south of the Sahara and, in eastern Africa, serves as a food host for *G. pallidipes*, favouring the woodland thickets which are the usual haunts of this fly. The evolutionary chain of events was fast becoming clear, and in 1961 Lumsden forged yet another link by demonstrating virulent trypanosomes in *G. pallidipes* caught in the Uhaya forest. Thus in the space of a few years, nature was forced to yield secrets that had eluded medical scientists for over half a century, and then, as though not enough had been disclosed, an outbreak of human trypanosomiasis occurred in Alego in 1964.

The people of this location, unlike those of Yimbo, live in compounds known as *bomas*, enclosed by vegetation susceptible to colonization by a tsetse fly which, although closely related to the riverine species of West Africa, is able to breed in this peri-domestic environment, particularly when, as in this case, it is reinforced with *Lantana* thicket which has been rapidly multiplying in this part of Kenya for many years. It soon became clear that this vector alone was transmitting a virulent trypanosome which invaded the central nervous system within four months. Further important discoveries, by Onyango and Van Hoeve, demonstrated that, in Alego, trypanosomes from symptomless cattle were capable of producing a virulent infection in man and that such trypanosomes could be cyclically transmitted through woodland tsetse.

It can hardly be said that this remarkable succession of important discoveries has elucidated beyond doubt the complexity of the sleeping sickness situation in Central Nyanza; the numerous disclosures can be juxtaposed in so many ways that one could speculate almost endlessly upon the nature and origins of the outbreaks since 1949. However, the importance of all this evidence to a general theory of the history of trypanosomiasis is overwhelming; now, the whole succession of events, from the clandestine cycle between woodland fly and bushbuck to the uncertain harmonies of mild West African sleeping sickness in man, lies revealed.

It should not be assumed that the far-reaching discoveries made in so short a period by workers in Nyanza were dispensations of fortune; men of outstanding research ability did not happen by chance to be at the correct place at the right time with the appropriate facilities. Their enterprise resulted from the great surge of trypanosomiasis research which had begun, not only in East and West Africa, but in many other parts of the globe, after the end of the Second World War.

During this terrible collision of mighty powers, heavily depleted field control organizations managed, by Herculean efforts, to hold the position which had been attained during the late 1930s. The war years saw some, but relatively few, serious epidemics or new extensions of sleeping sickness; it has been alleged that others occurred, but remained undetected for the want of surveillance, yet this is unlikely. The territorial reports of that time may show evidence of over-strained services working hastily and untidily, but the ground was covered, and after 1946 no past evidence of serious oversight or neglect was found. From practically everywhere in Africa the number of reported cases was in decline.

Fundamental research, of course, suffered considerably and advances of a practical nature were restricted to the perfection of discriminative clearing techniques against fly and the emergence of a new group of therapeutic melaminyl arsenical compounds which began to be studied by Friedheim in 1939. After a protracted succession of syntheses and field trials a combination of Melarsen oxide and BAL was found to possess the long-sought properties of curing the virulent human trypanosomiasis of eastern Africa after the nervous system had been invaded and classical cases which were resistant to tryparsamide. The drug was toxic to a degree which is still in dispute but it remains an entirely justifiable form of therapy for late East African cases who were otherwise invariably doomed. In West Africa this agent, now known as Arsobal, is used in short courses for the treatment of early infections although some workers prefer to use longer courses of the less toxic Melarsen sodium. This was an exciting therapeutic departure by any standards, and, as in the case of previous anti-trypanosomal agents, physicans were guided to no small extent by impartial and meticulous scientific assessments made in the Chemotherapy Department of the Liverpool School of Tropical Medicine which had become world famous between the Wars under the direction of Warrington Yorke and his successor Lourie.

Even mankind's shameful epochs unaccountably bring their benefits. The Second World War accelerated the advance of modern technology, and after the conflict research workers in all fields of biology including trypanosomiasis found at hand revolutionary instruments and materials which had immediate application to many of their problems. The insecticide DDT, first used in a wartime typhus epidemic in Naples, was soon to be exploited against tsetse. In quite another sphere, the introduction of regular inter-continental air transport expedited collaboration between workers in western research centres and in Africa.

The British Government lost little time in putting trypanosomiasis research into full-scale activity. The Secretary of State, working through a reorganized Tsetse Fly and Trypanosomiasis Committee and advised by experts such as Davey and Buxton, whose masterwork on tsetse flies was then being compiled, established the West African Institute of Trypanosomiasis Research (WAITR) in northern Nigeria, at the formidable cost of £350,000. The work of this institution was to elucidate not only Nigerian problems but those of the other three West African territories under British administration. Important investigations were conducted into the epidemiological aspects of human sleeping sickness, of which the concise and detailed studies by Hutchinson in the Gambia and Sierra Leone were early examples. Further papers soon followed on protozoology, chemotherapy and chemoprophylaxis, especially in relation to animal trypanosomiasis, and emphasis was given to devising new techniques for the study of these aspects. The difficult task of maintaining the well-adapted trypanosomes of man was successfully overcome and one strain was maintained in animals by blood inoculation for at least ten years, its virulence fluctuating from time to time. In the entomological field, the ecology of riverine tsetse in western Africa was worked out with great precision.

The researches conducted on human and animal trypanosomiasis by the staff and visiting specialists at WAITR comprise much of the substance of this book, yet a discovery made there by Wijers in 1958 must be ranked as a milestone along the path of knowledge of trypanosomal behaviour. With great technical delicacy he showed that riverine tsetse become infected with trypanosomes very early in life, during the first or second blood meal. This at once illuminated phenomena, such as the low infection rate in wild flies, which had puzzled investigators for years, and enabled him to state the conditions which must be fulfilled if riverine tsetse were to become infected; the fly must feed upon a host with transmissible trypanosomes in the peripheral blood within twenty-four hours of emerging from its puparium, and must live for a further eighteen days before becoming a vector in the true sense. This work, in conjunction with entomological research at WAITR, incriminated the late dry season as the most dangerous time for the transmission of sleeping sickness by riverine tsetse in West Africa.

In East Africa research and tsetse reclamation were reorganized at the end of 1948 and it was decided to concentrate on experimental schemes of practical value. Among many important lines of research undertaken after the War, Fairbairn showed that the infectivity of virulent trypanosomes to man was seriously retarded by the presence in the same animal reservoir of other strains which had not begun their evolutionary journey. This discovery explained why virulent sleeping sickness was not of cosmopolitan distribution in the woodland tsetse belts of eastern Africa and why so many outbreaks of virulent trypanosomiasis depended upon introduction by man rather than by animals.

A few years later, Hornby's major assessment of animal trypanosomiasis appeared, and this work stimulated some new conceptions about the pattern of trypanosomiasis research in East Africa. Lumsden, appointed Director of the East African Trypanosomiasis Research Organization in 1957, soon put the necessary reorientation into effect. Until then, entomological control of trypanosomiasis had traditionally predominated over other disciplines whose research activities had been conducted on a more restricted scale. Moreover, difficulties had arisen because staff had been widely dispersed. It was therefore decided to close the famous field stations at Tinde and Shinyanga, and concentrate future activities upon the Institute at Tororo in Uganda, where work went ahead in the fields of immunology, protozoology and clinical medicine. Much of the highly successful research which followed in Nyanza was undertaken in collaboration with the Kenya Medical Department. As in the case of its counterpart in West Africa, the Institute continued to attract numbers of visiting scientists.

An early example of the part played by modern communications was provided by an investigation to discover the animal hosts on which different species of tsetse habitually feed. The necessity for such a study had been emphasized by the Health Organization of the League of Nations in 1928 and again by the East African Sub-Committee of the Tsetse Fly Committee in 1935. Yet it was not until 1949 that the problem began to yield to a sophisticated technique devised in East Africa and performed in England. This was made possible by the ease with which experimental material gathered in the field can now reach an investigator thousands of miles away. By this means light has been thrown upon many problems concerning the reservoirs of trypanosomiasis in man and domesticated animals.

Some support was given by these researches and by investigations carried out at WAITR, to an earlier proposition by van Hoof that the domestic pig may, if only temporarily, be capable of harbouring the well-adapted trypanosomes of man in western Africa.

Laborious ground-work undertaken in African research institutions enabled colonies of tsetse to be maintained almost anywhere in the world. Thanks to such ingenuity, trypanosomes and their vectors are now practically regarded as laboratory animals.

The trypanosomes of man have yielded their morphological secrets to the electron microscope in research centres all over the world. With this instrument, Vickerman in London concluded, at a few incisive strokes, a series of attacks made by British workers on the problem of so-called polymorphism. This had been studied by Fairbairn and Godfrey who related the lengths of trypanosomes to the virulence of the infection which they produced in domesticated animals and by Wijers and Ashcroft in respect of the variations of size and shape noted in the African trypanosomes which parasitize man. Vickerman was able to correlate these variations with the respiratory modifications that trypanosomes are compelled to make during their constant alternation between vertebrate and invertebrate hosts. He thus not only contributed to the solution of a complex morphological difficulty but revealed the immense adaptability of the parasite during the hazards of its evolutionary travail.

The preservation of trypanosomes at very low temperatures was exploited by both East and West African workers, permitting immunological studies to be conducted with trypanosomes of known pedigree as antigens. It had long been known that even though the sera of patients contained trypanosomal antibodies, they had but little effect in stemming the clinical course of sleeping sickness. In 1955 Soltys, Desowitz and other workers began to investigate the mechanisms involved using modern techniques, and set in motion a line of research which offers, perhaps, the brightest ultimate solution of all to the trypanosomiasis problem. They have revealed that trypanosomes possess a most complicated antigenic structure, and that a single strain of parasite can give rise to a significant number of antibody variants in the same host; meanwhile, during cyclical development in tsetse, the organism reverts to a standard antigenic constitution. It is not known how such variations occur but the problem may have to be solved before immunization procedures against human trypanosomiasis can be considered.

With so much research activity in view, the rapid exchange of information on an international scale was essential. At the end of February 1948 the most important trypanosomiasis conference ever held began at Brazzaville. It was attended by most of the leading research and field workers of the time, and strong and purposeful recommendations were made as to the directions in which research should be undertaken. As a result of this meeting, the Commission for Technical Co-operation South of the Sahara set up two important organizations. One of these, the International Scientific Committee for Trypanosomiasis Research, held its first conference in London in February 1949, and the immense task of consolidating the continental distribution of tsetse flies into a set of maps was projected. The Commission also set up the Permanent Inter-African Bureau for Tsetse and Trypanosomiasis in Leopoldville under Franco-Belgian technical direction, and in the same year this centre began to disseminate a steady stream of scientific information.

Thus a reformation was brought about, which justified the highest hopes. Until this period, as Pascal would have observed, circumstances and necessity had been the infallible masters; there had always been an awareness that man's decisions were dictated by the eternal magisterium of parasite and vector. At last it seemed to be broken, and the exponents of modern science were able to operate with freedom at one step removed from contingency.

In the field itself, control organizations, replenished with better trained staff than ever before, maintained their steady grip and in regions where sleeping sickness epidemics had formerly raged, prevalences were being calculated in fractions of a single percentage. Neujean, describing the situation in the Congo in 1959, stated that new infections were so few that no meaningful maps of regional endemicity could be drawn up and that the control of human trypanosomiasis had become a matter of logistics rather than research. A similar degree of control had been achieved in many other territories; statistics of the World Health Organization in 1949 recorded over 42,000 cases of sleeping sickness in twenty African countries. Ten years later, in spite of increasingly reliable case-finding machinery, patients in the same territories numbered little more than 6,000. Meanwhile, reclamation operations such as the Kano-Katsina-Zaria (KKZ) scheme in Nigeria and elaborate campaigns against woodland tsetse in eastern Africa promised a new era of agricultural prosperity.

At the end of the 1950s there might have been a moment when a trypanosomiasis worker in contemplative mood could have reflected with satisfaction upon the prospect, and caught, in his mind's eye, the figures of Jamot the warrior and Duke the prophet smiling on the scene. Almost within the instant, that vision would have been dispelled.

Just at this time, when many cherished hopes lay within reach, the modern political age dawned over Africa. By 1959 a few autonomous republics such as Ghana, Chad, Guinea and Sudan, had come into existence, but between 1960 and 1962 independence was adopted by at least 18 other nations whose frontiers contained endemic trypanosomiasis regions. It was not, of course, this widespread embrace of self-determination which caused the situation to become unstable, even though the replacement of a few extensive powers by a multitude of more restricted ones immediately led to problems of communication. The internal upheavals which accompanied the emergence of young African nations were of far greater significance.

Their effects quickly became apparent in the Congolese Republic. The Bureau at Leopoldville, ironically designated 'Permanent' only eleven years before, closed down in 1960, having disseminated nearly 3,000 medical and scientific communications, most of them in two languages. They had included numerous otherwise unobtainable reports, and monographs of unique reference value such as that which immortalized the clinical work of Saunders in Ghana.

In June 1962, a meeting of Ministers representing the West African territories formerly under British administration passed a resolution which deprived the West African Institute of Trypanosomiasis Research of its former legal basis, leaving the Institute in a state of doubt and uncertainty until an enlightened Nigerian Government assumed responsibility for it at the end of 1964.

The sleeping sickness situation became obscure in regions where permanent endemic foci still remained. The disruption of services gave rise to particular anxiety where control had been achieved by chemoprophylaxis alone, a measure which required legislative support and efficient administration and left the vector of the disease unchallenged. The system of survey and case-finding carried the overtones of colonial administration, and in many places the inevitable reaction caused attendances for examination and treatment to decline.

Often enough, social mobility in tropical Africa has been a factor in the spread of the disease, but the political changes after 1960 promoted the displacement of population on an unprecedented scale. At the beginning of 1967 it was estimated that there were nearly three quarters of a million refugees in Africa south of the Sahara, and that 300,000 of them were making their way to the Congo Republic from Angola and Sudan. Because some parts of the continent have been either under duress or held together by insecure administrative systems which impose restrictions upon communication, it is impossible to estimate the effect of these sad migrations. Indeed, of some places, one can only reiterate the words of Manson in 1898 that 'sleeping sickness lies between Senegal to the north and Loanda to the south and extends into the back country but how far, it is difficult to say'.

Nevertheless, epidemics do not seem to have occurred on any large scale. In 1965, twenty-four African states excluding the Congo Republic and Nigeria reported fewer than 3,000 cases and only 200 deaths from sleeping sickness. Although the movement of population helps the disease to progress from one place to another, the establishment of an endemic pattern of foci and satellites depends upon a certain degree of immobility to enable repeated personal contact between communities of man and tsetse to come about. The full significance of the turmoil in parts of Africa may thus emerge only after the return of stable conditions.

In many regions the transfer of political power was accomplished without exigency. In former French West African possessions, the loss of efficiency which followed the separation of interterritorial services was quickly recognized, and the Organization de Coordination pour la lutte contre les Grandes Endémies (OCCGE) was formed in 1960. This Organization has enabled institutions such as the École Jamot and the Centre Muraz at Bobo Dioulasso to function with financial aid not only from French sources but from other international bodies such as WHO and UNICEF. The activities of OCCGE, and the control that had been achieved by the French in the Cameroons and equatorial Africa have so far maintained a satisfactory situation.

In response to the difficulties of the early 1960s the World Health Organization exercised its great experience and resources upon the trypanosomiasis problem, bringing together experts on the disease and specialists in closely related disciplines. Its first Expert Committee on Trypanosomiasis was convened in June 1962 under the chairmanship of Vaucel, and the ensuing Report, together with an extensive series of articles in the Organization's *Bulletin* in the following year, provided an authoritative guide-line for those who were to work in Africa under the new political conditions. The Organization has since established a Trypanosomiasis Information Service and has arranged professional training courses for field workers at the Centre Muraz and in Kaduna. Specialists have been employed to investigate situations of particular concern in East and West Africa and the Congo Republic.

The Commission for Technical Co-operation continued its work undismayed by sponsoring investigations such as that conducted in the Kissi focus in 1964 and further meetings of the International Scientific Committee.

In retrospect, the 1960s has seen more international exchanges on African trypanosomiasis than any other period; many workers whose responsibilities in Africa were relinquished found an opportunity to contribute their experiences at conferences and meetings. Experts who had spent much of their lives in one region went to other places where the opportunities for research were still favourable. An outstanding example is to be found in the work of Morris who, already distinguished for tsetse control operations in Ghana, later undertook

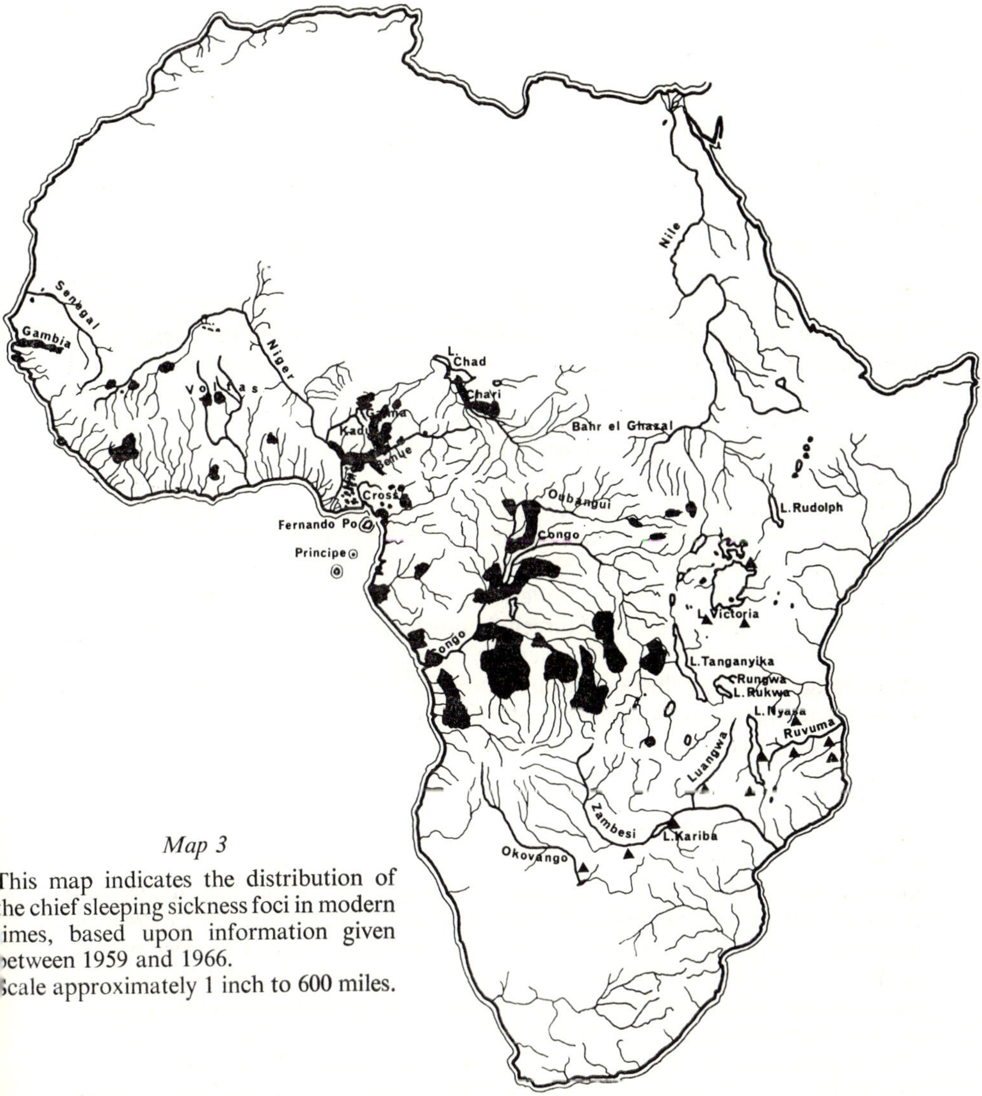

Map 3

This map indicates the distribution of the chief sleeping sickness foci in modern times, based upon information given between 1959 and 1966.
Scale approximately 1 inch to 600 miles.

research in Uganda and made numerous contributions to epidemiological knowledge in that part of Africa.

Throughout this period, British home-based research has continued unabated. The Government, working through its Trypanosomiasis Advisory Panel, has supported scores of projects, both fundamental and applied, on numerous aspects of trypanosomiasis in man and domesticated animals. Each year, investigators in colleges and research institutions throughout Great Britain meet at a seminar at which their work is fully discussed. Although many of their papers deal with experimental infections and are orientated towards animal trypanosomiasis, now recognized as one of the world's great biological problems, much of their work is applicable to human trypanosomiasis in the field.

From the clinical point of view, the two most desirable short-term objectives are a drug given by mouth which will cure sleeping sickness with the speed and certainty of a modern anti-malarial against Plasmodia, and a rapid and impeccable method of diagnosis. The first of these is made more urgent because the parasite, with its almost infinite resilience, can develop resistance to the melarsen group of drugs. If this should happen, according to the past predictions of Lourie's workers, the emerging strains may well prove resistant also to pentamidine and tryparsamide; this eventuality would precipitate a therapeutic predicament reminiscent of the early 1920s.

As to the second of these necessities, the shortcomings of definitive microscopical diagnosis still remain a great handicap to field workers, particularly in the detection of low endemic situations. The lack of accurate diagnosis invalidates statistics, and is one underlying reason for the persistence of endemic foci and the eventual failure of direct chemotherapeutic attack. The application of immunology's awakening power, by using methods for the detection of immunoglobulin and fluorescent antibody techniques, offers some hope of an eventual answer to this intractable problem.

As in the past, resourceful industries in the West continue to underwrite trypanosomiasis research. Much indebtedness is owed to pharmaceutical manufacturers, many of whose contributions to the therapy of the disease in man and animals belied the assertion that the profit motive is their only compelling purpose. Just as suramin bore for many years the alternative name of its German manufacturer, so Antrycide, the first great breakthrough in the treatment of animal trypanosomiasis, announced by Curd and Davey in 1949, had its origins in research sponsored by a great British industry. The titles of many an independent research fellow now engaged on trypanosomiasis work carry the names of industrial benefactors, not all of whom were originally concerned with medical science.

The unsatisfactory aspect of the present position lies in the ever-widening gap between rapid advances in fundamental knowledge and the administrative difficulties of applying them under field conditions for want of money, staff or receptive administration. It is, of course, only one recess in the great gulf between the pathways of societies in the forefront of science and of mankind elsewhere. Somehow it must be bridged ere man in Africa is left, harrowed by a host of biological contingencies of which trypanosomiasis is but one, while his fellows of the technological world, all heedless, throw their hands aloft to make a springboard of the lifeless moon.

Scientific discoveries and medical triumphs, like jewels, lose nothing by being set in the silver ring of time. Hence this story may help the reader of this book to perceive the reasons which prompted a great company of scientists, doctors and administrators to exert themselves, and to judge the merit and significance of their successes in contemporaneous terms.

But it is more difficult to convey the remorseless pressures, natural and contrived, which propel that cavalcade onwards to face new and greater difficulties with even more ingenuity and skill. It is clear that the problem of trypanosomiasis in domesticated animals is now of far greater concern than human infection to the health and prosperity of Africa. Its biological complexity is vast, its physical extent is only vaguely defined and its significance is almost immeasurable. The burden of sleeping sickness in the 1930s was but thistledown in comparison to the leaden weight of this gigantic load.

It may seem necessary to change the face of rural Africa before the scourge is eliminated, yet as Barzun reminds us, there is no use struggling to save a world in which one would find it hell to live when saved. An Africa without game, tsetse and trypanosomes could turn a noble ambition to dust, for they are the guardians of the land. Over-zealous guardians they may be, but their too peremptory dismissal from the scene could permit improvidence and exploitation on a ruinous scale.

If those who fought sleeping sickness to a standstill were blind to anything, it was the realization that in developing countries a balance must be kept between the improvement of communal health and the other processes of social and economic development. During centuries of exposure to a hazard, mankind adapts in order to survive, and after the sudden removal of the danger his adaptations, whether physiological, psychological or social, may recoil to his disadvantage. In our universal society whose history is documented largely in terms of slaughter, there can be fewer more creditable acts than that one man should save the life of another. But there is a difference between curing a patient of sleeping sickness and spraying a potent insecticide of unknown ultimate propensity throughout a swathe fifty miles long, and this distinction is as valid as that between the chemoprophylactic inoculation of an ox and the deliberate extermination of 25,000 head of game. As the scientific weapons at man's disposal increase in range and power, so the temptation towards total environmental interference at all costs will inevitably grow. Yet in the perspective of history, a less precarious alternative can be discerned.

The trypanosomes of man in Africa are clearly travelling towards commensalism. In the evolutionary time-scale they are now but an eye-blink from their destination; indeed, in some parts of West Africa, their goal has almost been attained. Long ago, Dutton and Todd in the Gambia described the strange longevity of their untreated patients; Scott Macfie at Eket was so impressed by the exquisite harmony between man and parasite as to suggest that the trypanosome involved was of a hitherto undescribed species; more recently, Lapeyssonnie announced his isolation of the innocuous Féo strain from a woman in northern Togo. Infections of this kind are commonplace enough, but the balance is too fragile, too unaccountable as yet, to slake the scientific thirst for predictability. The ideal situation would be for the inhabitants of tsetse-infested areas to harbour a commensal trypanosome which, in payment for eternal sanctuary, renders its host unassailable by its ill-adapted forbears.

Neither in Africa nor in other places has man the time to wait for such a dispensation, inevitable though it may be; a prompter solution surely lies somewhere within the compass of modern immunology and in the work of gifted men, proud, and yet humble enough, to toil in the footsteps and philosophy of Louis Pasteur. The biological complex of trypanosomiasis is in deep and mortal relationship with the life of Africa; to sever this relationship would be to change the bionomics of half a continent. It seems more commendable to leave the relationship alone, and simply to thwart the undesirable effects of its progression by methods which anticipate its own beneficent destiny.

Part I

THE CAUSATIVE ORGANISMS
THE GENUS *TRYPANOSOMA*

Chapter 1

The Mammalian Trypanosomes of Africa

C. A. HOARE

INTRODUCTION

Strictly speaking, the only mammalian trypanosomes that are confined to Africa are the tsetse-borne species, whose distribution normally coincides with that of their vectors, represented by flies of the purely African genus *Glossina*. These trypanosomes are also the most important parasites from the medical and veterinary points of view for they include the causative agents of human sleeping sickness (*Trypanosoma gambiense* and *T. rhodesiense*) and of trypano somiases affecting domestic mammals (*T. vivax*, *T. congolense*, *T. simiae*, *T. brucei*, *T. suis*), all of which are prevalent in the tropical zone of Africa. Among the pathogenic trypanosomes of mammals there are also two species, *T. evansi* and *T. equiperdum*, which—though not tsetse-borne—are closely related to *T. brucei* and have probably descended from the latter through the replacement of *Glossina* by mechanical inoculators (such as Tabanidae), in the case of *T. evansi*, or through the complete loss of a vector, in the case of *T. equiperdum*. The emancipation of these trypanosomes from the tropical tsetse flies as vectors has enabled the corresponding diseases, surra and dourine, to spread outside the 'fly belts' to the Mediterranean littoral of North Africa and even beyond this continent, to Europe, Asia and the Americas.

In addition to the tsetse-borne species and the allied forms, African mammals may harbour non-pathogenic trypanosomes, many of which have a cosmopolitan distribution. Thus, *T. theileri* and *T. ingens* are commonly found in domestic and wild ruminants, *T. lewisi* and allied forms in rodents and *T. vespertilionis* and *T. megadermae*-like trypanosomes in bats. Although these parasites are of no practical importance they cannot be entirely ignored for they are liable to be encountered in the course of surveys and it is essential that they should be differentiated from the pathogenic species.

PHYLOGENY

The relations between the diverse species of mammalian trypanosomes can be best appreciated against the background of their evolution which provides a basis for their classification on phylogenetic lines and which not only throws light on their affinities but serves also to unite species showing similarities in their physiology, antigenic constitution and host-parasite relations. These features in their turn have a direct bearing on the response of the trypanosomes to chemotherapy, on the immunological reaction of the host and on the clinical manifestations of the diseases caused by them.

Clues to the origin of mammalian trypanosomes are provided by the intestinal flagellates of insects of the family Trypanosomatidae which includes the genus *Trypanosoma*. While the insect flagellates are monogenetic, trypanosomes are digenetic parasites whose life cycle alternates between two hosts: one, an invertebrate representing the intermediate host or vector in which the flagellates develop primarily in the gut; the other, a vertebrate in which they inhabit the blood and/or tissues. In addition to *Trypanosoma*, digenetic flagellates are represented in vertebrates by *Leishmania* and *Endotrypanum*, and in plants by *Phytomonas*, but the last three genera need not concern us.

In accordance with recent revisions, based on electron microscopy and on taxonomic studies (Wallace, 1963; 1966), the monogenetic Trypanosomatidae are now divided into the following four genera, for the developmental stages of which a new terminology (Hoare & Wallace, 1966) was devised (Fig. 1.1).

1. Genus *Leptomonas*: comprises (a) promastigote (= leptomonad) stage, represented by elongated flagellates with an antenuclear kinetoplast situated in the anterior end of the body, where the flagellum emerges from a short reservoir; undulating membrane absent; and (b) amastigote (= leishmanial) stage (free and cysts) devoid of a free flagellum.

2. Genus *Herpetomonas*: comprises (a) typical promastigote stage (as in 1) and (b) opisthomastigote stage, represented by similar forms but with post-nuclear kinetoplast, situated at variable distances behind the nucleus; flagellum emerging at anterior end of the body from the bottom of a long reservoir which may extend as far back as the kinetoplast; undulating membrane absent; (c) amastigote stage (as in 1).

3. Genus *Blastocrithidia*: comprises (a) promastigote stage (as in 1, 2); (b) epimastigote (= crithidial) stage, represented by elongated flagellates with juxtanuclear kinetoplast; flagellum emerging at the side of the body out of a shallow reservoir and running along a short undulating membrane; (c) amastigote stage (as in 1, 2).

4. Genus *Crithidia* (syn. *Strigomonas*): comprises (a) choanomastigote stage, represented by short 'barleycorn'-like flagellates with truncated anterior end;

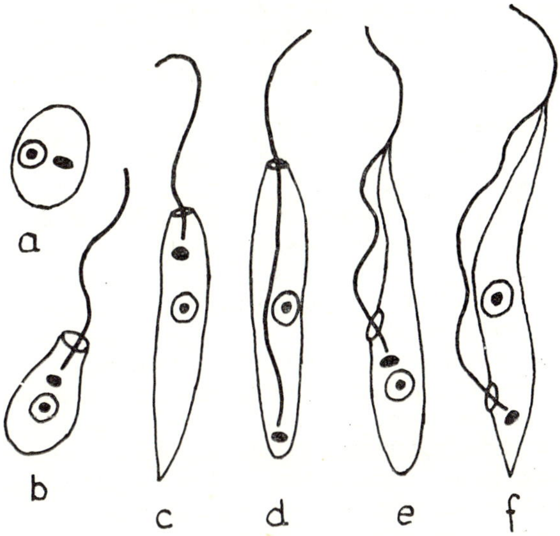

Fig. 1.1 Stages in Trypanosomatidae: a. Amastigote (= leishmanial); b. Choanomastigote (only in *Crithidia*); c. Promastigote (= leptomonad); d. Opisthomastigote (only in *Herpetomonas*); e. Epimastigote (= crithidial); f. Trypomastigote (= trypanosomal). (From Hoare & Wallace, 1966)

kinetoplast antenuclear; flagellum emerging from short funnel-shaped reservoir; undulating membrane absent; (b) amastigote stage (as in 1, 2).

In the foregoing four genera the rounded amastigote forms represent the infective stage; they are discharged with the droppings and are transmitted from donor-insect to recipient-insect when the latter ingests food polluted by the infected faeces, i.e. by the contaminative method.

5. The digenetic genus *Trypanosoma* is characterized by the appearance of a new stage, represented by the trypomastigote (= trypanosomal) forms. They are of the epimastigote type but their kinetoplast occupies a postnuclear position, while the flagellum likewise emerges from a shallow lateral reservoir to run along a lengthy undulating membrane. The other stages are as in (3) *Blastocrithidia*.

The hypotheses regarding the phylogeny of mammalian trypanosomes are based on the close resemblance of their stages of development in the insect-vector to the Trypanosomatid flagellates specific to insects, especially *Blastocrithidia*. The phylogenetic relations of trypanosomes were first considered by Léger (1904) who believed that they were descended from the monogenetic parasites of non-haematophagous insects which adapted themselves to life in vertebrate hosts when some of these insects acquired bloodsucking habits. On the other hand, Minchin (1908) advanced an opposite hypothesis according to which the ancestors of trypanosomes were originally parasitic in the intestine of vertebrates whence they passed into their blood and were eventually taken up by bloodsucking insects. However, this author soon abandoned his idea and accepted Léger's concept which was adopted by most subsequent authors, though a few still adhered to Minchin's original hypothesis (*see* Hoare, 1948; Baker, 1963).

Recently Hoare (1967) reviewed all the available evidence and found convincing support for Léger's hypothesis. The precursors of the intermediate hosts of mammalian trypanosomes, in common with other haematophagous insects, evolved from phytophagous and entomophagous ancestors while the forebears of the trypanosomes themselves are to be found among flagellates of the genus *Blastocrithidia* all stages of which are represented among the developmental forms of the trypanosomes in their vectors (Fig. 1.1, a,c,e,f). In these the flagellates may pass through the promastigote, epimastigote and amastigote stages which appear in different proportions and at various periods of the invertebrate cycle, according to the species of *Trypanosoma*.

As regards the trypomastigote (= trypanosomal) stage, it has no counterpart among the insect Trypanosomatids but first appears in the genus *Trypanosoma*, where it is represented in the mammalian host by the characteristic blood forms, and in the vector by the infective metacyclic forms or metatrypanosomes. In his electron microscopic studies Vickerman (1962, 1965) has shown that the stage assumed by them reflects the degree of development of the mitochondrial tubes arising from the kinetoplast which in turn is correlated with the respiratory metabolism of the flagellates. Thus, in the epimastigote forms an elaborate network of mitochondrial tubes is associated with a poor supply of respiratory substrate (glucose) in the insect gut, while the reduced mitochondrion of the trypomastigote forms indicates reduced mitochondrial activity and greater dependence of the blood forms on wasteful glycolytic respiration in a medium rich in glucose. The trypomastigote stage has therefore probably evolved from the ancestral insect flagellates when these first established themselves in mammalian hosts in which they underwent morphogenetic changes in response to the new environmental conditions in the blood. Conversely, when the blood trypanosomes are taken up by the vector, they revert to the epimastigote stage by proliferation of the mitochondrion. The close affinity between trypanosomes and the Trypanosomatid flagellates of insects is illustrated by historical examples when epimastigote flagellates discovered in the gut of bloodsucking insects were first mistaken for specific parasites of these insects, until it was proved that they were actually trypanosomes of vertebrates and the insects themselves were their vectors.

All species of *Trypanosoma* have a similar pattern of development in the vector: the trypanosomes ingested with the blood are earlier or later transformed into epimastigote forms which eventually give rise to the infective metatrypanosomes. The mammalian trypanosomes are divided into two major groups which differ in the site where the metatrypanosomes develop and in the mode of transmission of the infection (Wenyon, 1926; Hoare, 1949). In the great majority of species (e.g. *T. lewisi* of rodents, *T. theileri* of ruminants) the entire invertebrate cycle of development is confined to the alimentary tract of the vector, with the production of metatrypanosomes in the hindgut, whence they are voided with the droppings, to be transmitted to new individuals of the vertebrate host by faecal contamination. This course of development, terminating in the 'posterior station', is characteristic of trypanosomes belonging to section Stercoraria (*see* p. 17). However, in the tsetse-borne African trypanosomes with which we are mainly concerned only the initial stages of development take place in the gut of the vector while the final stages, terminating in the formation of metatrypanosomes, develop in the proboscis or salivary glands of the insect, i.e. in the 'anterior station'; in the case of *T. vivax* the entire development is restricted to the proboscis. Parasites with this life cycle belong to section Salivaria (*see* p. 18) and are transmitted to the mammalian host by the inoculative method, through the bite of the vector.

Of the two cycles the Stercorarian pattern is undoubtedly the more ancient and primitive type since it corresponds to that in the specific Trypanosomatid parasites of insects. Indirect evidence of the antiquity of the Stercoraria (*cf.* Hoare, 1967) is provided (a) by the perfect adaptation between these parasites and their vectors, up to 100% of which usually become infected; (b) by better adaptation to their mammalian hosts, to which they are as a rule not pathogenic, while the host-range is in most cases restricted; and (c) by a distinct pattern of metabolism (von Brand, 1956).

The origin of the Salivaria and their connection with insect-trypanosomatids is not clear since among the latter there are no examples of development in the anterior station. It is therefore evident that the course of evolution of the Salivaria differed from that of the Stercoraria. According to one hypothesis (Hoare, 1948; 1967), it is conceivable that the tsetse-borne mammalian trypanosomes were originally parasites of wild ruminants and that their development was completed in the posterior station of some other insect-vector which transmitted them by the contaminative method. It is further assumed that in addition to this cyclical transmission by their intermediate host, they were at the same time transmitted mechanically by tsetse flies. At first the trypanosomes merely survived in the proboscis of these flies but in the course of time they adapted themselves to *Glossina* so well that they began to develop cyclically in these insects, with the result that tsetse flies were transformed from purely mechanical inoculators into true intermediate hosts of the pathogenic trypanosomes, which were then transmitted by the inoculative method. The plausibility of this hypothesis is borne out by the existing species which appear to be relict groups whose evolution had come to a dead end and remained fixed at certain phases of their adaptation to tsetse flies. Thus, *T. vivax*, which undergoes its entire development in the proboscis and does not survive in the gut of the fly, illustrates the initial phase when the trypanosomes, instead of just surviving, began to develop in the mouth parts. The next phase is represented by *T. congolense*, the development of which already extended to the gut; and finally the last phase is exemplified by *T. brucei* and *T. gambiense* in which the development involved the salivary glands. However, it is not implied here that there is a phylogenetic succession between these species: they are merely landmarks on branches of the genealogical tree indicating the level of evolution reached by the trypanosomes in question. Presumptive evidence of the more recent emergence of the Salivaria, as compared with the Stercoraria, is provided (a) by their imperfect adaption to the tsetse vectors as reflected in their low infectivity for *Glossina* which diminishes in the order of the postulated evolution of the trypanosomes in question, as well as by the ease with which they lose their power to develop in tsetse flies; (b) by their virulence and correspondingly wide host-range; and (c) by their distinct metabolic activities.

An alternative hypothesis regarding the origin of tsetse-borne mammalian trypanosomes was proposed by Baker (1963) who suggested that the Salivaria and the trypanosomes of aquatic vertebrates transmitted by leeches have descended from parasites of the common ancestors of the annelids and arthropods, in which the flagellates completed their development in the anterior station. In the course of evolution, when these invertebrates eventually diverged, leeches became the vectors for the trypanosomes of aquatic vertebrates while tsetse flies became the vectors of trypanosomes of terrestrial vertebrates, including the pathogens of mammals. Although there can be no conclusive proof one way of the other, there is stronger circumstantial evidence to support Hoare's hypothesis which is moreover less speculative than Baker's.

In addition to the species of mammalian trypanosomes considered above that are separable on morphological grounds, there are groups of species as well as strains within the same species which are morphologically indistinguishable but differ from each other only in biological or physiological features. Such biological races had presumably evolved from homogeneous parental species by segregation of clones possessing new characters, the perpetuation of which was determined by favourable natural selection of those variants that were best adapted to a new hostal environment (Mayr, 1943; Hoare, 1943, 1955).

The Salivarian trypanosomes provide examples of this variation at various levels of the evolutionary process. They differ in the degree of isolation from each other and in stability, as well as in their bionomics which determine the extent of divergence reached by them and provide criteria for their differentiation. Thus, trypanosomes of the subgenus *Trypanozoon* (*T. gambiense*, *T. rhodesiense*, *T. brucei*, *T. evansi*, *T. equiperdum*) constitute a single complex of morphologically identical biological races whose stability and host-parasite relationship entitle them to a separate taxonomic status. On the other hand, some of these species comprise strains differing in minor serological, clinical or hostal features, which are comparable to 'types' among bacteria, the ultimate distinction between which in a given group is determined by differences in antigenic constitution. In view of the wide connotation of the word 'type' in biology, it has been proposed to use the term 'deme' for such variants (Gilmour and Heslop-Harrison, 1954; Hoare, 1955), while the nature of the differential criterion is indicated by an appropriate prefix.

Among the demes in Salivarian species the following can be recognized:

(a) plastodemes: strains characterized by extreme lability, determined by environmentally induced antigenic variations (e.g. 'relapse strains' in *T. brucei*);
(b) serodemes: stable, immunologically distinct strains exhibiting no cross-immunity (e.g. in *T. evansi*);
(c) xenodemes: strains differing in degree of host-restriction and range (e.g. hostal strains in *T. evansi*);

(d) clinodemes: strains showing a gradation in mensural characters of the parasite over the area of distribution of its host (e.g. in *T. vivax*, *T. congolense*, *T. evansi*); and

(e) nosodemes: strains differing in virulence and type of disease produced by them (e.g. in *T. congolense*, *T. gambiense-rhodesiense*).

Further details of the evolutionary trends in the different subgenera and species will be given in Chapter 2 (*see* also Hoare, 1967).

MORPHOLOGY

Until quite recently our knowledge of the morphology of trypanosomes was based entirely on stained preparations viewed by light microscopy which shows their general appearance as well as the essential internal structures. However, the revelation of the ultrastructure of the various constituents in the body of these parasites by phase contrast and especially by electron microscopy has necessitated a radical reappraisal of our former concepts regarding their cytology. Nevertheless, since in practice laboratory and field workers must continue to rely upon the conventional techniques, it is important that they should be familiar with the morphology of the trypanosomes as seen in dry-fixed blood films stained by one of the Romanovsky methods, provided their cytology is interpreted in the light of what is now known about their ultrastructure.

General Cytology

One of the first to describe the morphology of mammalian trypanosomes was Minchin (1909) but more detailed accounts were given in a number of text-books (e.g. Laveran & Mesnil, 1912; Wenyon, 1926; Hoare, 1949; Grassé,

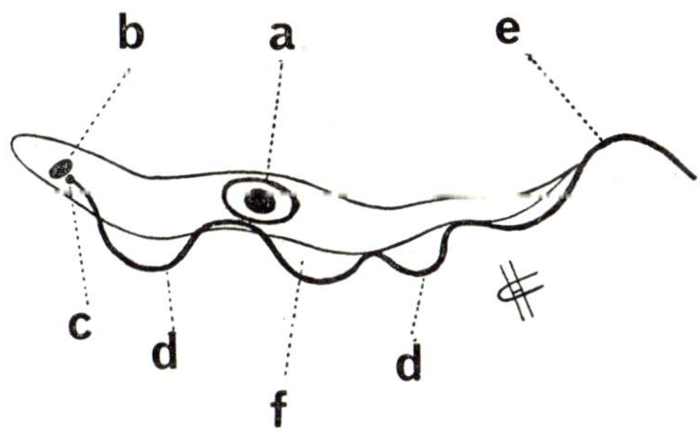

Fig. 1.2 Structure of Trypanosome: a. Nucleus; b. Kinetoplast; c. Basal body; d, e. Flagellum—marginal and free portions; f. Undulating membrane. (From Hoare, 1949)

1952). Mammalian trypanosomes typically have a more or less spindle-shaped flattened body (Fig. 1.2) which is usually curved, but its shape varies in different species. There is a single nucleus of the vesicular type containing a large achromatic karyosome and peripheral chromatin lining the membrane. However its exact structure is revealed only in preparations stained after 'wet' fixation, whereas in those fixed by the 'dry' method and stained by the Romanovsky technique the appearance of the nucleus is deceptive, for it shows no internal organization but appears to be filled with irregular granules produced by the deposition of the stain in the nucleus. The shape of the nucleus is typically round or elongated, according to the width of the body.

It is customary to describe that part of the body which is directed forward during locomotion as the anterior end. The organ of locomotion is represented by a single flagellum which starts behind the nucleus in the posterior part of the body, whence it emerges to run forwards along the outer margin of a frilled fold of the pellicle which extends throughout the length of the body and is known as the undulating membrane. When the flagellum reaches the anterior end it either becomes free (Fig. 2.2, a–f) or it terminates at the end of the membrane without a free portion (Fig. 2.3, a–d). The base of the flagellum is formed by the so-called 'basal body' (sometimes called the 'blepharoplast') which is usually inconspicuous but sometimes appears as a minute bulbous thickening. In close proximity to the basal body there is a characteristic dark-staining organoid known as the kinetoplast, which is disc-shaped but may appear to be rounded or rod-shaped according to its orientation in the body of the flagellate. The kinetoplast accompanies the base of the flagellum whenever the position of the latter shifts in the course of development but there is no obvious connection between these two elements, as was formerly assumed (e.g. Wenyon, 1926).

In addition to these major structural elements, trypanosomes may contain various cytoplasmic inclusions, especially different kinds of volutin granules, the number of which varies during the course of the infection and with the strain of the parasite and may be associated with the immune reaction of the host (Ormerod, 1958; 1961a; 1966).

The relatively simple organization of the trypanosomes described above is all that can be seen by light microscopy. Some new cytological features have been revealed with the aid of phase contrast microscopy by Clark (1959) who demonstrated the presence in trypanosomes of (a) a 'reservoir' representing an ectoplasmic invagination in the posterior end of the body; it encloses the sheathed flagellum which arises from its base and emerges from its 'mouth', and in some of them (b) a contractile vacuole lying at the side of the reservoir into which its contents are discharged. However, the cytology of trypanosomes revealed by electron microscopy has introduced the most revolutionary changes in our concept of their structure, throwing considerable light on the nature of the organoids. The ultrastructure of trypanosomes is described in Chapter 3.

Multiplication

There are two main modes of reproduction among the blood forms of mammalian trypanosomes: (a) by unequal binary or multiple division in the amastigote or epimastigote stages, and (b) by equal binary division in the trypomastigote stage. Among African species the former pattern is represented in *T. theileri* and *T. lewisi* (Fig. 1.3, b,d,f), while the latter is characteristic of the tsetse-borne pathogenic trypanosomes and allied forms (Fig. 1.3, g–l). It was previously thought that multiplication of a trypanosome is initiated by division of the

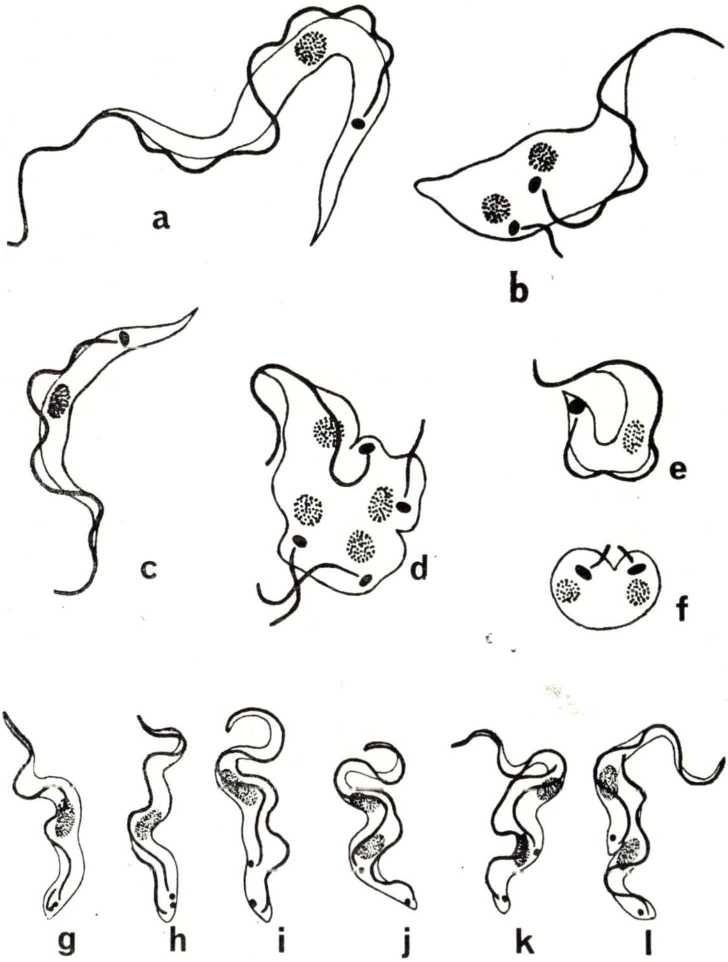

Fig. 1.3 Division of Trypanosomes (×2,000). a, b. *Trypanosoma theileri:* adult and dividing by unequal binary fission in epimastigote stage; c, d. *T. lewisi:* adult and dividing by multiple fission in epimastigote stage; e, f. *T. vespertilionis:* adult and dividing by binary fission in amastigote stage; g–l. *T. simiae* dividing by equal binary fission; g. Bipartition of kinetoplast, new flagellum arising near its posterior half; h, i. Kinetoplast divided and new flagellum growing parallel to old one; j, k. Nucleus divided, new flagellum fully developed; l. Division completed: daughter-individuals separating by cytoplasmic fission. (After Hoare, 1936, 1957)

'blepharoplast' into two but recent electron microscopic studies (Grimstone, 1961; Grassé, 1961) have demonstrated that in dividing flagellates the parental basal body 'induces' the neoformation of a second one in its proximity. In the meantime the kinetoplast undergoes bipartition, while the newly formed basal body gives rise to a daughter-flagellum and the nucleus divides in its turn. After the trypanosome has developed a double set of nuclei and other organoids (in the case of Salivarian species) the body itself undergoes longitudinal fission until finally the two daughter-individuals become separated (Fig. 1.3, 1). On the other hand, in the species reproducing by multiple division (*T. lewisi*) the various organoids continue to divide but fission of the cytoplasm is retarded until eventually it undergoes segmentation into several daughter-individuals (Fig. 1.3, d).

Nuclear division

It is generally agreed that the nucleus divides by a form of mitosis which has been studied more fully in the blood forms of *T. lewisi* (Wolcott, 1952) and in cultures of *T. theileri* and *T. cruzi* (Hartmann & Nöller, 1918; Noble *et al.*, 1953; Noble, 1955). At the beginning of mitosis (prophase) the peripheral chromatin migrates into the karyosome where it condenses and breaks up into three chromosomes during metaphase; these then divide giving rise in anaphase to two groups which separate in telophase to form two daughter-nuclei (Fig. 1.4).

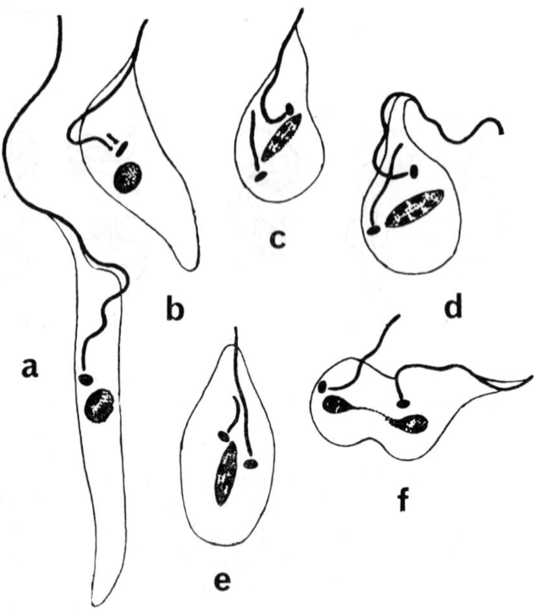

Fig. 1.4 Nuclear division in *T. theileri* culture (×2,000). a. Nucleus with 3 chromosomes in early prophase; b–e. Nuclei in late prophase and anaphase; f. Nucleus in telophase. (After Hartmann & Noeller, 1918)

Sexuality

Though from time to time there have appeared accounts of syngamy in trypanosomes, there is no evidence of nuclear changes to substantiate the existence of sexuality in these organisms. In fact, there is indirect evidence against it, for it was shown that genetical recombination resulting from sexual reproduction does not occur when trypanosome strains of the same species (e.g. *T. rhodesiense*, *T. equiperdum*) but resistant to different drugs are mixed in the same vertebrate or invertebrate host (Amrein & Fulton, 1959; Amrein, 1965).

LIFE CYCLE

In vertebrate host

The course of development of mammalian trypanosomes in the vertebrate host is relatively simple. It is initiated by the metatrypanosomes introduced into the mammal by the insect-vector, either passively by contamination of its mucous membranes or skin (in the case of Stercorarian species like *T. lewisi*) or actively by their inoculation through the bite (in the case of tsete-borne Salivarian species). The metatrypanosomes apparently find their way into the blood stream where they are transformed into trypanosomes with the characteristic structure of the species to which they belong.

The trypanosomes proceed to multiply in the blood (or, in the case of *T. cruzi*, in the tissues) by one of the methods described above. In the Stercorarian species, *T. lewisi* and *T. theileri*, multiplication is discontinuous being limited to a reproductive period at the beginning of the infection when as the result of repeated divisions 'adult' trypanosomes are produced which do not divide any more and constitute the established phase of the infection. However, in the Salivaria, to which the pathogenic African species belong, there is no special reproductive period but the trypanosomes multiply more or less continuously throughout the infection.

Further particulars of the development of trypanosomes in their mammalian hosts are given in Chapter 2.

In invertebrate host

When trypanosomes are ingested by their vectors together with the mammalian host's blood, they pass into the insect's gut. Except for species whose development is restricted to the proboscis (*T. vivax* and *T. uniforme*), the entire invertebrate cycle of development may be confined to the alimentary tract, as in the Stercoraria (e.g. *T. lewisi*), or it involves migration to the salivary medium of the anterior station (proboscis and/or salivary glands), as in the tsetse-borne Salivaria.

The main features of this cyle are similar in all the mammalian trypanosomes. They may assume any of the stages found in the insect-flagellates (e.g. *Blastocrithidia*), which appear in different proportions and at various periods of the invertebrate cycle, according to the species of trypanosome. Thus, in the parasites of African mongooses, *T. helogalei* and *T. ichneumoni*, promastigote forms predominate (Grewal, 1960; 1961), in *T. lewisi* chiefly epimastigote and trypomastigote forms are present (Minchin and Thomson, 1915), while in all the tsetse-borne species the intestinal stages are represented only by trypomastigote forms (Fig. 2.1). However, the most important and characteristic stage in the invertebrate cycle is the epimastigote form through which all the trypanosomes must pass before they are transformed into metatrypanosomes. The intermediate host is incapable of transmitting the infection to the mammalian host until this cycle (from blood trypanosome, through epimastigote stage, to metatrypanosome) is completed. This method of development is accordingly known as cyclical, to distinguish it from the mechanical mode of transmission when trypanosomes taken up with the blood merely survive for a short time in the mouth parts of the insect and are inoculated into a new mammalian host when the insect feeds again, without undergoing any development in the vector. This is the normal method of transmission of *T. evansi* by Tabanid flies.

In the Salivarian trypanosomes the invertebrate cycle of development is complicated by the anatomical peculiarities of the alimentary tract in tsetse flies, which are described below (p. 19).

DIAGNOSTIC CHARACTERS

The chief differential characters of mammalian trypanosomes are based on the appearance of the stained adult blood forms the morphology of which provides criteria upon which the diagnosis of species is based (*cf.* Wenyon, 1926; Hoare, 1966). Various species of trypanosomes may differ in size and shape of the body, in the position of the nucleus and kinetoplast, as well as in the degree of development of the undulating membrane and flagellum. A well-developed undulating membrane is convoluted and conspicuous whereas an undeveloped one is more or less flat and inconspicuous; the flagellum may or may not have a free portion of varying length. Mammalian trypanosomes differ also in the shape of the posterior end of the body which may be sharply pointed (*T. lewisi*), bluntly pointed (*T. brucei* and allied species), or rounded (*T. vivax*, *T. congolense*). The position and size of the kinetoplast are also of diagnostic value (Hoare, 1938; Schwetz, 1938). It may be far from the posterior end of the body (*T. theileri*), subterminal (*T. brucei*), marginal (*T. congolense*) or almost terminal (*T. vivax*), while among the Salivaria it is large in *T. vivax*, of medium size in *T. congolense* and small in the *T. brucei-gambiense* complex.

Mammalian trypanosomes are also distinguishable by their mensural characters (Fig. 1.5) comprising total length, including flagellum (L) distance from posterior end of the body to kinetoplast (PK) and to nucleus (PN), distance from kinetoplast to nucleus (KN), from latter to anterior end of the body (NA) and length of free flagellum (F). The length is measured by drawing with the aid of a camera lucida (say at $\times 2{,}000$) a line running through the middle of the body from the posterior extremity to the tip of the flagellum, and then measuring this line by means of a pair of fine compasses the points of which are separated 2 mm. ($= 1\mu$) (Bruce, 1909; Hoare & Broom, 1938). The other measurements are calculated by marking the appropriate positions (PK, KN, N, F) on the same line. Useful indices are available for indicating the position of the nucleus and kinetoplast. One of these, the nuclear index (NI), represents the ratio of the distance from the posterior end of the body to the nucleus to the distance from the latter to the anterior end (PN/NA) (Dias and Freitas, 1943). When NI = 1, the nucleus is in the middle of the body; when it is < 1, it is in the posterior part, and when it is > 1, it is in the anterior part. The other is the kinetoplastic index (KI), arrived at by dividing the distance from the posterior end to the nucleus by the distance from the kinetoplast to the nucleus (PN/KN). If KI is

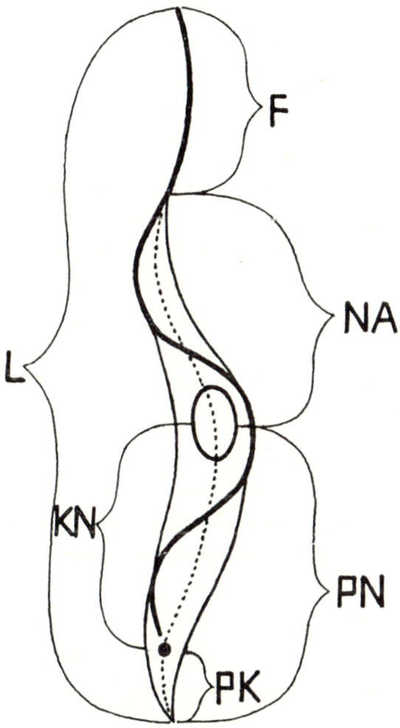

Fig. 1.5 Measurements of Trypanosomes. L = total length (including free flagellum); PK = distance from posterior end to kinetoplast; KN = from kinetoplast to middle of nucleus; PN = from posterior end to middle of nucleus; NA = from nucleus to anterior end; F = length of free flagellum. (Adapted from Dias & Freitas, 1943)

less than 2 the kinetoplast is nearer to the posterior end than to the nucleus; if it is 2 the kinetoplast is halfway between the two; if it is more than 2 the kinetoplast is closer to the nucleus (Keymer, 1967).

Statistical methods may be of value for the separation of related groups and for the study of variation in trypanosomes. As is shown in Chapter 2, biometry has been used successfully for the differentiation of species (*T. vivax*, *T. uniforme*), for the demonstration of polymorphism (*brucei*-complex, *T. simiae*) and for the study of strains varying in virulence (*T. vivax*, *T. congolense*, *T. evansi*). However, the application of biometry to the differentiation of trypanosomes may be misleading on account of the wide variation sometimes observed even within populations of the same strain (Davis, 1952; Hoare, 1956). Additional clues of taxonomic value are provided by biological characters such as the site and stages of development in the insect-vector, the virulence and host-range of the trypanosomes, and their immunological relations which are dealt with in other sections.

CLASSIFICATION

General

Since the genus *Trypanosoma* was created by Gruby in 1843 over a dozen different names of the genus-group have been proposed for trypanosomes. However all these generic and subgeneric names failed to gain general acceptance, leaving *Trypanosoma* as the only genus embracing all the known trypanosomes (for nomenclatural history, *see* Hoare, 1964).

The history of the systematics of the mammalian trypanosomes has passed through several phases. In the early days Laveran and Blanchard (1895) believed that the trypanosomes known at that time represented hostal varieties of the same species. Somewhat similar views were expressed by Alexeieff (1913) who maintained that all the mammalian forms were capable of being transformed one into another. The first serious attempt to differentiate these trypanosomes was made by Laveran and Mesnil (1912) who divided them arbitrarily into two groups according to whether they were pathogenic or not. This artificial classification was rectified independently by Duke (1913) and Roubaud (1913) who arranged the pathogenic African species into three groups on the basis of their mode of development in the tsetse vector, while Bruce (1914) amplified this classification by uniting with *T. brucei* the closely related *T. evansi* and *T. equiperdum*. It was extended by Knuth and Du Toit (1921) to the non-pathogenic trypanosomes and rationalized by Wenyon (1926) who separated the mammalian trypanosomes into two major divisions according to the site of their development in the vector. Further changes were introduced by Hoare (1957, 1964, 1966) who developed a natural classification of these parasites on phylogenetic lines based on both morphological and biological criteria.

The mammalian trypanosomes fall naturally into the two major divisions mentioned above which differ mainly in the course of development in their vectors: Section *A*, comprising species whose development is completed in the posterior station and transmission is contaminative, and Section *B*, comprising species whose development is completed in the anterior station and which are transmitted by the inoculative method. Until quite recently these sections were subdivided into groups and subgroups bearing the names of the typical species as follows: *A* containing the single I. *Lewisi* group, *B* containing three groups: II. *Vivax*, III. *Congolense*, and IV. *Brucei*, the latter consisting of subgroups *Suis*, *Brucei* and *Evansi*.

Although this scheme served its purpose well, it became too complicated owing to the progressive multiplication of subordinate groupings as knowledge advanced. This problem was solved (Hoare, 1964) by arranging related species of *Trypanosoma* into subgenera corresponding to the previous minor groupings while retaining the two major sections and designating them by the descriptive names Stercoraria (= Section *A*) and Salivaria (= Section *B*), which indicate the media (faecal and salivary, respectively) in which the flagellates complete the invertebrate developmental cycle.

The systematic position of *Trypanosoma* among the Protozoa and the revised classification of the mammalian trypanosomes (with special reference to African species) are as follows:

Phylum PROTOZOA Goldfuss, 1818; emend. Siebold, 1845.
Subphylum SARCOMASTIGOPHORA Honigberg & Balamuth, 1963.
Superclass MASTIGOPHORA Diesing, 1866.
Class ZOOMASTIGOPHOREA Calkins, 1909.
Order KINETOPLASTIDA Honigberg, 1963.
Suborder TRYPANOSOMATINA Kent, 1880.
Family TRYPANOSOMATIDAE Doflein, 1901; emend. Grobben, 1905.
Genus *Trypanosoma* Gruby, 1843.

A Section *Stercoraria*

Trypanosomes in which a free flagellum is always present; kinetoplast large and not terminal; posterior end of the body pointed. Multiplication in mammalian host discontinuous, typically taking place in the epimastigote or amastigote stages. Development in the vector is completed in the posterior station and transmission is contaminative. Trypanosomes typically not pathogenic.

1. Subgenus *Megatrypanum* Hoare, 1964

Large trypanosomes, with kinetoplast typically situated near the nucleus and far from the posterior end of the body.

African species: (a) *Trypanosoma* (*Megatrypanum*) *theileri* Laveran, 1902 (Fig. 1.3, a). Length up to 100 μ; reproduction by unequal binary fission in epimastigote stage. Hosts: bovines, antelopes. (b) *T.* (*M.*) *tragelaphi* Kinghorn *et al.*, 1913 (possibly = *T. ingens*). Length 53–73 μ; reproduction unknown. Hosts: antelopes. (c) *T.* (*M.*) *cephalophi* Bruce *et al.*, 1913 (possibly = *T. theileri*). Length 40–50 μ; reproduction unknown. Hosts: antelopes. (d). *T.* (*M.*) *ingens* Bruce *et al.*, 1910. Length 72–130 μ; reproduction unknown. Hosts: cattle, antelopes, chevrotains.

Megatrypanum also includes large trypanosomes of African (e) bats (e.g. *T. megadermae*, *T. heybergi*), (f) mongooses (*T. helogalei*, *T. ichneumoni*) and (g) primates (*T. irangiense*).

2. Subgenus *Herpetosoma* Doflein, 1901

Trypanosomes of medium size, with subterminal kinetoplast lying at some distance from the pointed posterior end of the body. Reproduction in mammalian host typically in the epimastigote stage.

African species: (a) *Trypanosoma* (*Herpetosoma*) *lewisi* (Kent, 1880) Laveran & Mesnil, 1901 (Fig. 1.3, c). Length 21–36 μ; reproduction by unequal multiple fission in epimastigote stage. Hosts: rats.

Herpetosoma also includes numerous other *lewisi*-like parasites from various African mammals: (b) rodents (about 10 species of trypanosomes), (c) shrews (*T. brodeni*) and (d) primates (*T. perodictici*, *T. primatum*).

3. Subgenus *Schizotrypanum* Chagas, 1909, emend. Nöller, 1931.

Trypanosomes relatively small and typically C-shaped; voluminous kinetoplast situated very near the short pointed posterior end of the body. Multiplication in mammalian host intracellular, typically in amastigote stage.

Type-species: *Trypanosoma* (*Schizotrypanum*) *cruzi* Chagas, 1909. Restricted to the New World; causative agent of Chagas' disease in man.

Only African species: *Trypanosoma* (*Schizotrypanum*) *vespertilionis* Battaglia, 1904 (Fig. 1.3, e,f). Mean lengths 15–24 μ. Hosts: bats.

B Section *Salivaria*

Trypanosomes in which a free flagellum may be present or absent; kinetoplast terminal or subterminal; posterior end of the body usually blunt. Multiplication in mammalian host continuous in trypomastigote stage. Development in the vector (*Glossina*) completed in the anterior station (except in mechanical vectors) and transmission inoculative (except in *T. equiperdum*). Trypanosomes pathogenic.

1. Subgenus *Duttonella* Chalmers, 1918

Trypanosomes of former *Vivax* group, represented by monomorphic forms in which a free flagellum is always present; posterior end of the body typically rounded; kinetoplast large and usually terminal. Development in *Glossina* takes place in proboscis exclusively.

Species: (a) *Trypanosoma* (*Duttonella*) *vivax* Ziemann, 1905. Long forms (means 21·0–25·4 μ). Hosts: ruminants, equines; (b) *T.* (*D.*) *uniforme* Bruce *et al.*, 1911. Short forms (means 14·6–16·5 μ). Hosts; ruminants.

2. Subgenus *Nannomonas* Hoare, 1964

Trypanosomes of former *Congolense* group, represented by small forms in which a free flagellum is absent; kinetoplast of medium size, typically marginal. Development in *Glossina* takes place in midgut and proboscis.

Species: (a) *Trypanosoma* (*Nannomonas*) *congolense* Broden, 1904. Monomorphic forms (means 12·2–17·6 μ). Hosts: ruminants, equines, pigs, dogs; (b) *T.* (*N.*) *simiae* Bruce *et al.*, 1911. Polymorphic forms (means 17·0–18·2 μ). Hosts: pigs, warthogs, camels.

3. Subgenus *Trypanozoon* Lühe, 1906

Trypanosomes of former *Brucei* group—*Brucei* and *Evansi* subgroups, represented by polymorphic forms, with or without free flagellum; kinetoplast small, subterminal. Development in *Glossina* takes place in midgut and salivary glands (except d,e).

Species: (a) *Trypanosoma* (*Trypanozoon*) *brucei* Plimmer & Bradford, 1899. Polymorphism constant. Mean lengths 17·0–20·0 μ. Hosts: domestic mammals, antelopes; (b) *T.* (*T.*) *rhodesiense* Stephens & Fantham, 1910. Polymorphism constant. Mean lengths 19·0–20·0 μ. Hosts: man, antelopes; (c) *T.* (*T.*) *gambiense* Dutton, 1902. Polymorphism constant. Mean length 20·0–21·0 μ. Host: man; (d) *T.* (*T.*) *evansi* (Steel, 1885). Polymorphism inconstant. Mechanical transmission by insects. Mean lengths 19·4–22·0 μ. Hosts: camels, equines, bovines, dogs, etc. (e) *T.* (*T.*) *equiperdum* Doflein, 1901. Polymorphism inconstant. Transmission by contact between vertebrate hosts (insect vector absent). Mean lengths 25·0–27·7 μ. Hosts: equines.

4. Subgenus *Pycnomonas* Hoare, 1964.

Trypanosomes of former *Brucei* group—*Suis* subgroup, represented by stout monomorphic forms with short free flagellum and small subterminal kinetoplast. Development in vector (*Glossina*) takes place in midgut and salivary glands. Monotypical: single representative: *Trypanosoma* (*Pycnomonas*) *suis* Ochmann, 1905. Hosts: pigs (wild and domestic).

Since the introduction of subgeneric names involves a complication in the citation of species, it should be noted that while the citation of genus and species is compulsory, the use of the subgeneric name is optional and it can be omitted. It must also be emphasized that a subgenus should not be cited without naming the genus. For example, both *Trypanosoma* (*Duttonella*) *vivax* and *Trypanosoma vivax* are legitimate citations but '*Duttonella vivax*' is not permissible. Those who prefer to ignore the subgeneric name can treat it as a new designation for the former group or subgroup to which the trypanosome in question belongs.

In a number of African mammalian trypanosomes the morphological characters separating the species intergrade while in others only biological differential characters are present. From the zoological point of view some of these groups could be classified as subspecies, e.g. (a) *Trypanosoma* (*Duttonella*) *vivax vivax* and *T.* (*D.*) *vivax uniforme* (Hoare & Broom, 1938); (b) *Typranosoma* (*Nannomonas*) *congolense congolense*, *T.* (*N.*) *congolense dimorphon* and *T.* (*N.*) *congolense simiae* (Hoare, 1959); (c) *Trypanosoma* (*Trypanozoon*) *brucei brucei*, *T.* (*T.*) *brucei gambiense*, *T.* (*T.*) *brucei rhodesiense*, *T.* (*T.*) *brucei evansi* and *T.* (*T.*) *brucei equiperdum* (Hoare, 1955). However, the adoption of a trinominal nomenclature would be too cumbersome for practical purposes.

Stages in tsetse fly

In the course of epidemiological studies of the tsetse-borne trypanosomes it is essential to recognize their developmental stages in *Glossina*. While exact criteria are available for the identification of the trypanosomes in the mammalian host, the differential diagnosis of the flagellates in the vector is uncertain, because the insect stages of species belonging to the same subgenus are practically indistinguishable even when there is a marked difference between their blood forms. Therefore, at the present state of knowledge it is possible to identify only the subgenus—but not species—to which the trypanosomes belong. Their differential diagnosis is based (a) on localization in the fly and (b) on their morphological characters. These are shown in Table 1.1 and illustrated in Fig. 1.6. The tsetse-borne trypanosomes include the crocodile-parasite *T. grayi* the developmental stages of which should be recognized and differentiated in order to avoid confusion with the mammalian parasites sharing the same vectors.

In order to understand the course of development of the tsetse-borne trypanosomes, it is necessary to describe the alimentary tract and its accessory

TABLE 1.1

Differential diagnosis of trypanosomes in* Glossina *(Modified after Hoare, 1966)

Subgenera	Species	Localization in fly				Characters
		Proboscis	Salivary glands	Midgut	Hindgut	
Duttonella	*T. vivax* *T. uniforme*	Trypomastigotes, epimastigotes and metatrypanosomes	No development	No development	No development	Kinetoplast large, free flagellum present in all stages
Nannomonas	*T. congolense* *T. simiae*	Trypomastigotes, epimastigotes and metatrypanosomes	No development	Trypomastigotes	No development	Kinetoplast medium, free flagellum absent in all stages
Trypanozoon	*T. brucei* *T. rhodesiense* *T. gambiense*	No development	Trypomastigotes, epimastigotes and metatrypanosomes	Trypomastigotes	No development	Kinetoplast small, free flagellum present in all stages except metatrypanosomes, in which it is typically absent
Pycnomonas	*T. suis*	No development	Trypomastigotes, epimastigotes and metatrypanosomes	Trypomastigotes	No development	Kinetoplast small, free flagellum present in all stages, including metatrypanosomes
Crocodile parasite	*T. grayi*	No development	No development	Epimastigotes (including filamental forms) and trypomastigotes	Epimastigotes and metatrypanosomes	Kinetoplast large, free flagellum present in all stages

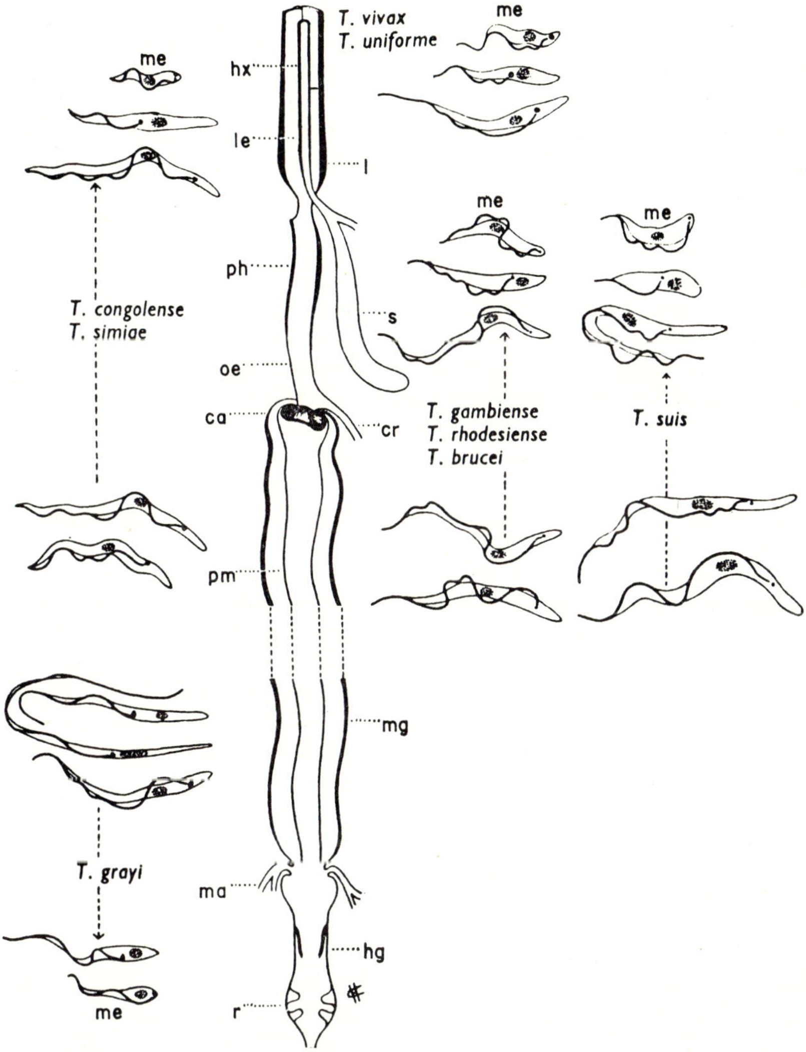

Fig. 1.6 Developmental patterns of trypanosomes in *Glossina*. ca. Cardia (= proventriculus); cr. Crop duct; hg. Hindgut; hx. Hypopharynx; l. Labium; le. Labrum-epipharynx (hx+l+le = proboscis); ma. Malpighian tubes; me. Metatrypanosomes; mg. Midgut; oe. Oesophagus; ph. Pharynx; pm. Peritrophic membrane; r. Rectum; s. Salivary glands (one cut off). Magnification of flagellates ca. ×1,500. (Adapted from Hoare, 1949)

parts of *Glossina* (Fig. 1.6) (Hoare, 1949). The tsetse fly pierces the skin of the mammalian host and ingests its blood by means of the proboscis consisting of two gutter-like pieces, the labium and labrum-epipharynx, which fit together to form the tubular food canal and enclose the long slender hypopharynx, whose anterior end is open, while the posterior end leads to the common salivary duct. The latter emerges into the body cavity where it divides into two ducts leading to two long convoluted salivary glands. The food canal leads to the pharynx and oesophagus, which opens into the midgut and gives off a duct leading to the crop.

The anterior end of the midgut forms a pyriform dilatation, the cardia (= proventriculus), while the rest of the midgut is coiled up in the abdominal cavity. The midgut is separated from the hindgut by a sphincter near which the two common ducts of the four Malpighian tubes open. The hindgut ends in a bulbar rectum which terminates in the anal aperture.

Within the midgut, starting from the cardia and extending as far as the hindgut is a peritrophic membrane which is a thin chitinous sleeve concentric with the alimentary canal. This membrane arises in the form of a circle of droplets secreted from glandular cells situated in the wall of the cardia near its junction with the oesophagus where there is an annular fold which is closely applied to the anterior wall of the cardia. As the secretion passes between this wall and the fold it is compressed and condensed, emerging into the lumen of the midgut in the form of a delicate cylindrical sleeve, the terminal part of which opens into the distal end of the midgut or the proximal end of the hindgut. When blood ingested by the fly passes into the midgut, it fills the lumen of the peritrophic membrane and is enclosed in the endoperitrophic space during the whole period of digestion. Since the trypanosomes ingested with the blood of the mammalian host are unable to pass through the tough peritrophic membrane, its presence has an important effect on the course of their development in *Glossina.*

The formation and function of the peritrophic membrane in tsetse flies were first described by Wigglesworth (1929) and recently amplified by Willett (1966). Its role in directing the development of trypanosomes was first elucidated in the case of the tsetse-borne crocodile-trypanosome, *T. grayi* (Hoare, 1931), and later confirmed for *T. gambiense*, *T. brucei*, *T. rhodesiense* and *T. congolense* (Taylor, 1932; Yorke *et al.*, 1933; Fairbairn, 1958; Gordon, 1957).

When ingested by the fly with the blood, the trypanosomes find themselves in the midgut within the endoperitrophic space where they continue to develop until they reach the open end of the peritrophic membrane or its ruptured wall in the hindgut. After escaping from the endoperitrophic space the flagellates invade the ectoperitrophic space; here they gradually advance forwards until they reach the cardia and find themselves in a *cul-de-sac.* The route by which the flagellates reach the anterior station to complete their development was demonstrated in *T. brucei*, *T. gambiense* and *T. congolense*, all of which pass from the ectoperitrophic space of the cardia into its endoperitrophic space by penetrating the least resistant portion of the membrane, namely through the fluid or semifluid part at or near the points where it is being secreted from the epithelial ridge. Having thus gained entrance into the inner lumen of the cardia the flagellates continue to migrate forwards, first into the oesophagus and pharynx and then into the proboscis. *T. congolense* completes its development here but *T. brucei*, *T. gambiense* and *T. suis*, enter the hypopharynx through its open anterior end after which they again turn back and find their way into the salivary ducts from which they invade the glands, where their development is completed. Since *T. vivax* is restricted to the proboscis its development is not affected by the peritrophic membrane.

The manner in which the flagellates surmount the obstacle presented by the peritrophic membrane in *Glossina* reveals their remarkable powers of adaptation. Although the membrane diverts the flagellates from their path this does not interfere with their development or ability to reach their ultimate destination by the shortest route through the series of manoeuvres described above.

The final stages of development of tsetse-borne trypanosomes take place in the proboscis (*T. congolense*) or salivary glands (*T. brucei* and allied species) where they assume the epimastigote stage before giving rise to the metatrypanosomes.

Chapter 2

Systematic Description of the Mammalian Trypanosomes of Africa

C. A. HOARE

SECTION A. STERCORARIA

Subgenus *Megatrypanum*

1 *Trypanosoma (Megatrypanum) theileri* Laveran, 1902.

Synonyms: *T. transvaaliense* Laveran, 1902; *T. tragelaphi* Kinghorn *et al.*, 1913 (*pro parte*); *T. cephalophi* Bruce *et al.*, 1915 (*pro parte*).

The only Stercorarian species of trypanosome that is of any economic interest is *Trypanosoma theileri* which is a common parasite of domestic and wild ruminants in Africa. This trypanosome was discovered in Transvaal in the blood of cattle suffering from gall sickness by Theiler (1903) who at first erroneously attributed the disease to this parasite but later recognized the causative agent as *Anaplasma*. *T. theileri* has a cosmopolitan distribution among domestic cattle throughout the world while in Africa it also occurs in various antelopes. As a rule the infection is cryptic and is usually detected by blood culture.

MORPHOLOGY AND LIFE CYCLE. *T. theileri* is one of the largest mammalian trypanosomes measuring on the average 60–70 μ, but sometimes upwards of 100 μ, in total length. The posterior end of the body is drawn out to a point; the large kinetoplast is typically near the nucleus, which occupies a more or less central position; the undulating membrane is well developed and there is a long free flagellum. Multiplication of *T. theileri* (Fig. 1.3, a,b) takes place in the blood by unequal binary fission in the epimastigote state (Reichenow, 1940).

In Europe the vectors of *T. theileri* are Tabanid flies, *Tabanus glaucopis* and *Haematopota pluvialis* (Nöller, 1925; Kraneveld, 1931), in which the development follows the typical Stercorarian pattern with the production of metatrypanosomes in the hindgut and contaminative transmission. Although similar flagellates were found in African horse-flies, *Tabanus secedens*, *Pangonia neavei* and *Haematopota vandenbrandeni* (Wallace, 1962), there is no experimental evidence that they belong to *T. theileri*.

HOST-PARASITE RELATIONS. Although *T. theileri* has been known for more than sixty years, there is still some controversy regarding its effect on the bovine host (*cf.* Herbert, 1964). According to the prevailing view, this parasite is completely harmless, but some veterinarians believe that it is potentially pathogenic, its dormant virulence being activated in the presence of some intercurrent disease. Thus, the infection in cattle is typically latent and produces no clinical manifestations in the host, but in infected animals suffering from certain concomitant diseases (e.g. piroplasmosis, rinderpest) parasitaemia may reach a high level. This phenomenon is particularly striking in the case of rinderpest and is usually observed in the course of immunization of cattle with living virus. Some authors (e.g. Curasson, 1925) believed that the course and symptoms of the concomitant disease were typical and were not aggravated by the presence of *T. theileri*, but others (e.g. Hornby & Bailey, 1929) maintained that the latter was responsible for some of the symptoms observed. However, there is no evidence of any specific pathological changes attributable to *T. theileri*. In this connection, it is significant that a flare-up of the trypanosome infection has never been reported in pure infections with this parasite.

SECTION B. SALIVARIA

Subgenus *Duttonella*

This subgenus is represented by monomorphic trypanosomes with a peculiar combination of characters distinguishing them clearly from the species in the

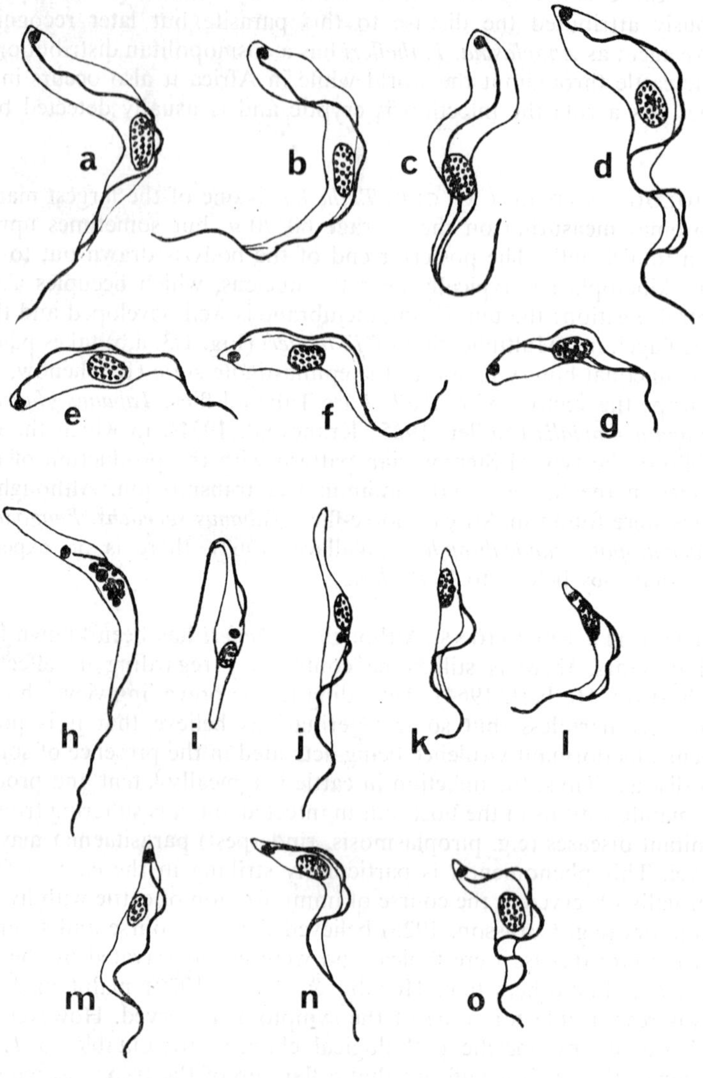

Fig. 2.1 Subgenus *Duttonella* (× 2,000). a–g. Blood forms: a, b, c. *Trypanosoma vivax*; d. "*T. caprae*"; e–g. *T. uniforme*. h–o. Developmental stages of *T. vivax* in proboscis of *Glossina*: h. Degenerating trypanosome in midgut; i, j. Epimastigote and k, l. Trypomastigote forms in food canal; m–o. Metatrypanosomes in hypopharynx. (After Bruce *et al.*, 1911, 1913; and Lloyd & Johnson, 1924)

other three subgenera of the Salivaria (Fig. 2.1). The body is somewhat club-shaped, being typically swollen and rounded at the posterior end and tapering towards the anterior end. The undulating membrane is usually slightly developed (except in Bruce's *T. caprae*) and there is a distinct free flagellum. The kinetoplast is typically terminal, but it may be subterminal, occupying a marginal position. The most remarkable feature of the kinetoplast is its large size, exceeding that in the other Salivarian species. This character is by itself of diagnostic value for it facilitates the identification of *Duttonella* even in imperfect preparations. Trypanosomes of this subgenus are parasitic chiefly in wild and domestic ruminants and do not readily infect laboratory rodents. The development of these trypanosomes in *Glossina* is confined to the proboscis.

Duttonella comprises two well-defined species, *Trypanosoma vivax* and *T. uniforme*, and one sub-species, *T. vivax ellipsiprymni*.

2 *Trypanosoma (Duttonella) vivax* Ziemann, 1905.

Synonyms: *Trypanosoma cazalboui* Laveran, 1906; *T. congolense* Broden & Rodhain, 1910; *T. bovis* Kleine, 1910; *T. caprae* Kleine, 1910; *T. viennei* Lavier, 1921.

RELATION TO DISEASE AND DISTRIBUTION. *T. vivax* is pathogenic to various domestic ungulates (cattle, sheep, goats, horses and camels). The disease, known as *souma* or *nagana* in Africa and *secadera* in South America, is characterized by fever. anaemia and cachexia, as well as paralysis of the hind-quarters.

T. vivax is widely distributed throughout tropical Africa wherever its tsetse-vectors are found. This species has also been introduced through human agency into distant countries outside Africa (Mauritius, West Indies, Central and South America).

HISTORY. *T. vivax* was first discovered and named by Ziemann (1905) who found this parasite in the blood of domestic ruminants in the then German Cameroons. A year later Laveran (1906) gave the name *T. cazalboui* to a similar trypanosome recorded from the Upper Niger region. There was some controversy as to whether these two species were identical but the demonstration by Bruce *et al.* (1911c) that they were morphologically indistinguishable settled the question in favour of Ziemann's name.

MORPHOLOGY (Fig. 2.1, a,c). According to Hall (1950: cited by Gordon and Willett, 1956), when sheep are inoculated with *T. vivax* through the bite of tsetse flies the trypanosomes are localized during the first forty-eight hours in the subcutaneous tissues, after which they invade the lymph glands and then appear in the blood. In addition to the general characteristics of *Duttonella* noted above, *T. vivax* is readily differentiated by its length which has a range from 18 μ to 31 μ (including free flagellum measuring 3–6 μ) with means from 21 μ to 25·4 μ, though over 90% of the measurements are between 20 μ and 26 μ (Hoare & Broom, 1938). However, Fairbairn (1953) found that the length distributions of *T. vivax* fall into two groups represented by (a) long forms

26–30 μ long (means 26–27 μ) and (b) short forms measuring 15–28 μ (means 21–24 μ). As will be shown below, the size of the trypanosomes in these strains is correlated with differences in their virulence. The mammalian host also appears to influence the mean lengths of the trypanosomes.

TRANSMISSION. Bruce *et al.* (1911a) were the first to demonstrate that *T. vivax* is transmitted by tsetse flies. All the species of *Glossina* that have been investigated appear to be capable of transmitting this trypanosome and the following species have been definitely incriminated as vectors (*vide* Buxton, 1955 and others): *G. morsitans* in Tanganyika, Rhodesia, Mozambique, Rwanda-Burundi and Nigeria; *G. palpalis* in Congo and Nigeria; *G. tachinoides* in Nigeria; *G. swynnertoni* in Tanganyika; *G. pallidipes* in Uganda, Tanzania and Zululand; *G. longipalpis* in Portuguese Guinea; *G. austeni* in Mozambique, and *G. vanhoofi* in Burundi (Berghe & Zaghi, 1963).

In general it would appear that *T. vivax* is better adapted to development in its vectors than the other Salivarian species for the infection rate of this trypanosome in 'wild' tsetse flies—though variable—reaches the highest level. Thus, in Nigeria, Lloyd and Johnson (1924) found *T. vivax* infections in about 19% of *Glossina morsitans*, in 7·6% of *G. tachinoides* and in 2·6% of *G. palpalis*. However, according to Buxton (1955), in the Congo about 10% of the last-named species were infected while in Rhodesia the infection rate in *G. morsitans* was 4·7%. On the other hand, in Tanganyika *T. vivax* was seen in only 2·1% of *G. swynnertoni* and *G. pallidipes*. The high infection rate is also evident from the fact that under experimental conditions about 20% of *G. palpalis* may become infected with *T. vivax* (Bruce *et al.*, 1911a).

In addition to tsetse flies which are the cyclical vectors of *T. vivax*, this species is readily transmitted by mechanical inoculators represented by other blood-sucking Diptera, especially Tabanid flies (*cf.* Hoare, 1947). Thus in Africa bovine infections with *T. vivax* occur in a number of areas free of tsetse flies, e.g. in Rwanda, Uganda, Mali, Eritrea and Sudan. Though in some of these cases the occasional introduction of infected *Glossina* cannot be ruled out, such contact is absent in Mauritius, West Indies and Central and South America, into which *T. vivax* had been introduced from Africa with infected cattle. In these countries trypanosomiasis caused by this species (known locally also as *T. viennei*) is transmitted chiefly by Tabanids. Moreover, in the course of their adaptation to mechanical transmission the New World trypanosome has lost its power to develop in *Glossina* (*cf.* Hoare, 1957a).

CYCLE IN VECTOR. The development of *T. vivax* in *Glossina* was first described by Bruce *et al.* (1911b) who established the fact that its cycle in the vector is confined to the proboscis. Further details of this development were given by Lloyd and Johnson (1924). When the trypanosomes are ingested with the blood, they attach themselves to the walls of the food canal between the labrum-epipharynx and the labium and also invade the hypopharynx. In this position the flagellates undergo their complete cycle of development, in the course of which the blood trypanosomes are transformed first into elongated trypomastigotes with the kinetoplast not far behind the nucleus and then into epimastigote forms which eventually give rise to metatrypanosomes (Figs. 1.6, 2.1 h–p, Table 1.1). The latter resemble the blood forms but are smaller (*ca.* 15 μ long). In all these stages the flagellates retain the free flagellum and the large kinetoplast characteristic of this species. Trypanosomes that find their way into the gut are detectable there only up to the fourth day; they rapidly degenerate or are simply digested together with the blood.

The duration of the complete cycle in tsetse flies varies and is probably influenced by the temperature at which they develop. Thus, Desowitz and Fairbairn (1955) have shown that in *G. palpalis* the development takes 12–13 days at 22°C and 5 days at 29°C.

T. vivax has not been cultivated in any of the conventional media but was grown in a medium containing tsetse-fly tissues (Trager, 1959).

HOST–PARASITE RELATIONS. As in the case of other pathogenic trypanosomes, the pathogenicity of *T. vivax* varies in different strains and mammalian hosts. It has already been mentioned that Fairbairn (1953) demonstrated the existence of two strains in which differences in dimensions are correlated with differences in virulence. Thus, the long trypanosomes are characteristic mainly of East African strains which cause chronic infections in bovines while the shorter trypanosomes are found chiefly in West African strains which cause acute infections though virulent strains have been recorded also from Kenya and Tanganyika. These strains correspond to clinodemes (see p. 9).

The course of infection in cattle also varies in different breeds. Thus, in tsetse-areas of Nigeria (Desowitz, 1959) Zebu cattle are highly susceptible to infection which tends to run a chronic course, while the Muturu and Ndama breeds are resistant, the infection in them being transient and terminating in recovery. But animals born and bred in tsetse-free localities are as susceptible as Zebu, the disease being acute in the case of Muturu and chronic in Ndama. In horses the infection is usually chronic and mild, with spontaneous recovery within one year, while in sheep, goats and camels the severity of the disease is variable but generally runs a mild course. On the other hand, pigs and dogs appear to be resistant to infection with *T. vivax* (Hornby, 1952).

T. vivax has been reported from a number of African antelopes (Wenyon, 1926; Silva & Silva, 1958) in which the infection is cryptic and symptomless. The innocuousness of this parasite to antelopes was demonstrated experimentally in animals challenged with infected tsetse flies (Desowitz, 1960). It is generally accepted that antelopes are the reservoir hosts of *T. vivax* from which the infection is transmissible to domestic ruminants.

Until recently most attempts to study *T. vivax* under laboratory conditions were unsuccessful owing to the resistance of rodents to experimental infection although in the past some success was obtained with rabbits. Ordinary inoculation either fails altogether to produce infection or the infection is transient and cannot be passaged. However, workers in West Africa (Desowitz & Watson, 1951, 1952; Unsworth & Nesbitt, 1952) succeeded in producing infection in rats and rabbits by inoculation of infected blood accompanied by sheep's serum. This strain of *T. vivax* was maintained in serial passages through rats at first with added serum, but later it adapted itself so well to rats, as well as mice, that it is now maintained in European laboratories by passages through these animals without supplementary sheep's serum.

T. vivax IN MAN. On two occasions human infections with *T. vivax*-like trypanosomes have been reported from Africa. In the first case (Macfie, 1917) from the Gold Coast (= Ghana) only forms identical with *T. vivax* were seen; in the second from Uganda (Lavier, 1927b) there was apparently a mixed infection of this species and *T. gambiense*. If these observations are correct, it is possible that in exceptional cases the enhanced virulence of a strain of *T. vivax* or a lowering of human resistance might have created conditions enabling this parasite to set up a temporary infection in man (Hoare, 1962).

3 *Trypanosoma (Duttonella) vivax ellipsiprymni* Keymer, 1970.

Synonyms: *T. caprae* (Bruce *et al.*, 1913); (nec *T. caprae* Kleine, 1910).

Working in Tanganyika (= Tanzania), Kleine (1910) found trypanosomes in goats which he named *T. caprae*. Later Bruce *et al.* (1913) described a caprine trypanosome from Nyasaland (= Malawi) which they identified with Kleine's *T. caprae*. However (as shown by Hoare & Broom, 1938), there are discrepancies between the accounts of *T. caprae* by Kleine (*loc. cit.*) and Kleine and Taute (1911) on the one hand, and by Bruce and his collaborators, on the other. In the description and illustrations given by the German authors the trypanosome is indistinguishable from typical *T. vivax*, and—like *T. bovis* (= *T. vivax*) from cattle described in the same papers—it evidently owes its name merely to the host in which it was found. However, the trypanosome described by the British authors (Fig. 2.1d), though having the same measurements as *T. vivax*, differs from this species—as well as from Kleine's *T. caprae*—in the possession of a well-developed undulating membrane and a broader body (*ca.* 3 μ). Kleine's trypanosome is therefore identical with *T. vivax* and since it is a synonym of this species, the name *T. caprae* is not available under the International Code of Zoological Nomenclature. Trypanosomes similar to Bruce's '*T. caprae*' have recently been described by Chardome and Peel (1967) from Rwanda-Burundi and by Keymer (1970) in waterbuck from Zambia, under the name *Trypanosoma vivax ellipsiprymni*. The type species accordingly becomes *T. v. vivax*.

As in *T. vivax*, the development of Bruce's '*T. caprae*' in tsetse flies (*Glossina morsitans* and *G. brevipalpis*) is restricted to the proboscis and it is infective to the same range of ruminants (Bruce *et al.*, 1915b).

4 *Trypanosoma (Duttonella) uniforme* Bruce *et al.*, 1911.

RELATION TO DISEASE AND DISTRIBUTION. Although the data regarding the pathological effects of *T. uniforme* are fragmentary, the available evidence indicates that the disease caused by it in domestic ruminants is manifested by a mild relapsing fever, but it may be occasionally fatal (Wilson, 1949; Hornby, 1952).

HISTORY. *T. uniforme* was first described and named by Bruce *et al.* (1911d) who found it in bovines from Uganda. It was later recorded from antelopes and buffalo in the same country, from bovines in Zululand and Congo (*cf.* Hoare & Broom, 1938) and possibly Ethiopia. It was also found in sheep and goats from Congo (van Hoof *et al.*, 1948), in cattle from Angola (Dias, 1946) and in giraffe from Tanzania (Baker *et al.*, 1967). The records of *T. uniforme* are thus scanty and its distribution restricted for it has been reported only within the region extending northwards up to the Equator in East and Central Africa and to about 15° Western longitude (Kinshasa & Luanda). However, the absence of records of *T. uniforme* from West Africa and its restricted distribution elsewhere are probably due not so much to its rarity as to failure on the part of observers to recognize and differentiate this species. Owing to these circumstances and because of its resemblance to *T. vivax*, there has been some scepticism regarding the independent status of *T. uniforme*, especially in view of its co-existence with the former species both geographically and in mixed infections in the same host. There was therefore a tendency to regard *T. uniforme* as a small variant of *T. vivax*.

MORPHOLOGY. The independence of *T. uniforme* was firmly established by a comparative biometrical study of this species and *T. vivax* (Hoare & Broom, 1938) the results of which were confirmed by Wilson (1949).

T. uniforme has all the general structural features of the subgenus *Dutonella* and closely resembles *T. vivax* from which it differs in its smaller size (Fig. 2.1, e–g). Its total length has a range from 12 μ to 20 μ (means 14·6 μ–16·5 μ), with over 90% measuring 13 μ–17 μ. Although the length distributions of *T. uniforme* and *T. vivax* slightly overlap between 18 μ and 21 μ, they can be readily differentiated by their mean measurement, viz. if it is less than 18 μ the infection is *T. uniforme*, if it is greater than 20 μ it is *T. vivax*. The independence of *T. uniforme* as a species is also evident from the fact that it retains its characteristic mensural characters, distinguishing it from *T. vivax*, both in pure infections and when accompanied by the latter in double infections.

TRANSMISSION AND CYCLE IN VECTOR. The range of vectors of *T. uniforme* is unknown for its development was studied only in experimentally infected *Glossina palpalis* (Fraser & Duke, 1912). As in the case of *T. vivax*, the infection in the vector is restricted entirely to the proboscis where stages of the flagellates similar to those of *T. vivax* are found free or attached in the food canal and in the hypopharynx (Figs. 1.6, 2.1 h–p, Table 1.1).

HOST-PARASITE RELATIONS. According to the available evidence, *T. uniforme* comprises strains varying in virulence to domestic ruminants. Thus, in cattle, goats and sheep, the infection may be transient and practically symptomless (Wilson, 1949) but the disease in cattle may be acute and fatal (Bruce *et al.*, 1911d), while severe outbreaks among these animals have been reported from Uganda and Angola. However, since strains of low virulence are more common, infections with *T. uniforme* are liable to be overlooked (Hornby, 1952). Symptomless infections were reported from some wild ruminants (buffalo, bushbuck, situtunga, waterbuck) which are presumably reservoir hosts of *T. uniforme*. Laboratory rodents are refractory to infection with this trypanosome.

Subgenus *Nannomonas*

The subgenus *Nannomonas* is represented by relatively small trypanosomes measuring between 8 μ and 24 μ in total length. They are typically devoid of a free flagellum and possess a medium-sized kinetoplast usually occupying a marginal position, while the undulating membrane is in most cases inconspicuous. One of the peculiarities of members of this subgenus is that the intracytoplasmic portion of the flagellum typically arises somewhat behind the kinetoplast before emerging from the opposite side of the body. The posterior end of the body is either rounded (in the smaller forms) or obtusely pointed (in the longer ones). The nucleus is situated near the middle of the body (Fig. 2.2, a–m). On the whole, *Nannomonas* exhibit a certain degree of polymorphism which is especially pronounced in *T. simiae*.

Although trypanosomes of this subgenus are the most important pathogenic parasites affecting domestic animals in Africa, there is still some uncertainty regarding the number of species belonging to this group. This is due mainly to the fact that certain forms, especially the short ones, are common to all the species. Since the proportion of such forms varies in different strains and populations, it is not always easy to identify the species in random samples. However, if we disregard those names which are undoubtedly synonyms (e.g. *T. nanum*, *T. pecorum*, *T. ignotum*, etc.), there remain two, *T. congolense* and *T. simiae*, which are generally regarded as valid species of *Nannomonas*. Nevertheless, among various strains attributed to *T. congolense* there are considerable morphological and biological differences on account of which some of them had been separated as independent species.

The development of these trypanosomes in tsetse flies takes place in the midgut and proboscis.

5 *Trypanosoma (Nannomonas) congolense* Broden, 1904.

Synonyms: *T. dimorphon* Laveran & Mesnil, 1904; *T. nanum* Laveran, 1905; *T. confusum* Montgomery & Kinghorn, 1909; *T. pecorum* Bruce *et al.*, 1910; *T. montgomeryi* Laveran, 1909 (*pro parte*).

RELATION TO DISEASE AND DISTRIBUTION. *T. congolense* is responsible for the most important form of African trypanosomiasis in domestic mammals such as bovines, equines, sheep, goats, camels and pigs, as well as dogs. The manifestations of the disease vary according to the strain and host of the parasite, being generally characterized by fever, anaemia and cachexia.

T. congolense occurs throughout the tropical regions of Africa wherever tsetse flies are present.

HISTORY. The name *T. congolense* was given by Broden (1904) to a small trypanosome discovered by him in domestic ungulates from Congo. Later in the same year Laveran and Mesnil (1904) created *T. dimorphon* for an apparently dimorphic trypanosome, while Laveran (1905) separated a strain of similar but smaller trypanosomes under the name *T. nanum*. With the mistaken idea of resolving the existing confusion, Bruce *et al.* (1910) proposed to unite all these

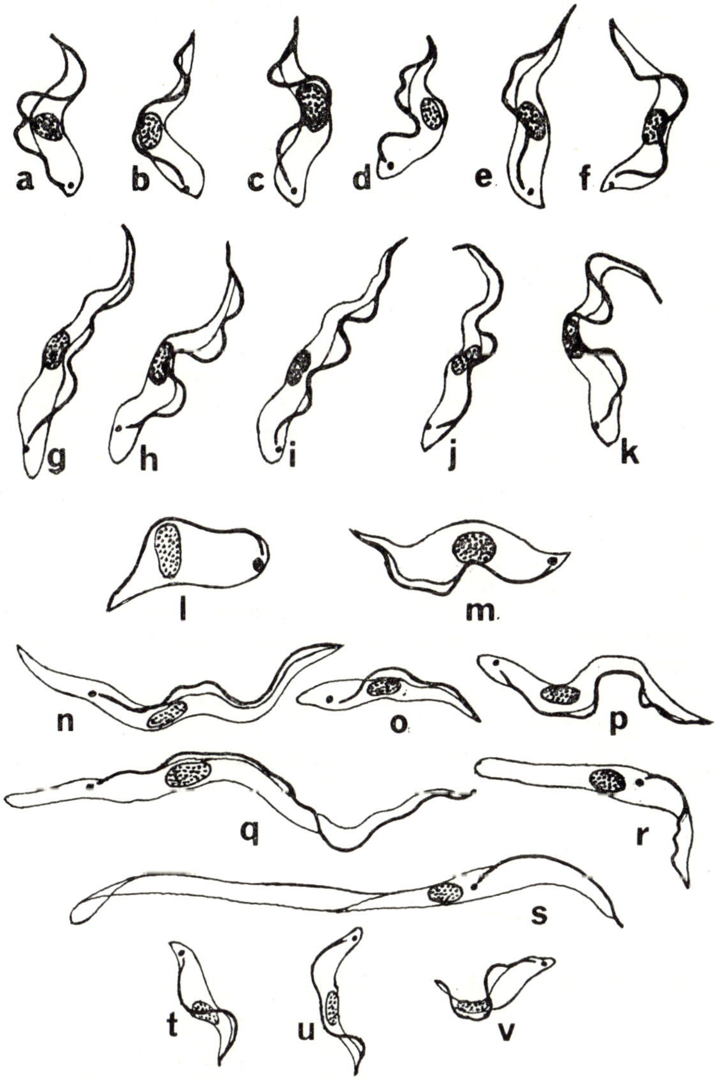

Fig. 2.2 Subgenus *Nannomonas* (×2,000). a–m. Blood forms: a–f. *Trypanosoma congolense*; g–k. *T. simiae;* l, m. "*T. montgomeryi*". n–v. Developmental stages of *T. congolense* in *Glossina*: n–p. Trypomastigote forms in midgut; q. Proventricular form in cardia; r, s. Epimastigote forms in food canal; t–v. Metatrypanosomes in hypopharynx. (After Bruce *et al.*, 1910, 1911, 1914; Kinghorn and Yorke, 1913; and Lloyd & Johnson, 1924)

species under a new name, *T. pecorum*. As shown below, there was some hesitation about the independence of *T. dimorphon* but at present all the above named species can be regarded as synonyms of *T. congolense*.

MORPHOLOGY. The blood forms of *T. congolense* are relatively small monomorphic forms with the general characteristics of *Nannomonas* (Fig. 2.2, a–f). According to recent biometrical studies, the overall total lengths of this trypanosome have a range from 8 μ to 24 μ with means 12·2–17·6 μ (Hoare, 1959) and 12·5–15·6 μ (Fairbairn, 1962). However, Laveran and Mesnil (1904) had separated from *T. congolense* an equine strain isolated in Gambia which they named *T. dimorphon*. It was said to be dimorphic, being characterized by the presence—in addition to the short forms—of long forms which are absent in typical *T. congolense*.

As *T. dimorphon* had not been adequately described its name was frequently misused and trypanosomes of both types were for many years cited indiscriminately as *T. congolense* and/or *T. dimorphon*. Owing to the resulting confusion, the latter gradually passed out of circulation and became a synonym of *T. congolense*. But in a revision of *T. dimorphon* based on the French authors' original material, Hoare (1959) demonstrated that this species could be differentiated from typical *T. congolense* on the basis of its length, which measured 11·3–24 μ (means 15·3–17·6 μ) as compared to 8–19·5 μ (means 12·2–14·4 μ) in the latter species. Since there was a definite gap between the highest mean of the shorter species (14·4 μ) and the lowest of the longer one (15·3 μ), there appeared to be justification for restoring *T. dimorphon* to its independent status.

However, in subsequent studies on *T. congolense* Godfrey (1960) revealed the existence in Nigeria of strains with intermediate mean lengths, viz. *ca.* 12·5–13·9 μ, while Fairbairn (1962) found similar strains in other parts of Africa with means *ca.* 14–15 μ. From these data it is evident that *T. dimorphon* cannot be regarded any longer as a distinct species and that *T. congolense* comprises at least three strains or races separable by their mean lengths, which are correlated with differences in their virulence (*see* below). These strains can be arranged according to their mean lengths (*M*) and percentages of short (*S*) and long (*L*) forms present as follows:

(i) *congolense*-type: M = (a) 11·2–13·8 μ,
(b) 12·5–13·8 μ, S = 29–57%
L = 0– 2%

(ii) intermediate-type: M = (a) *ca.* 13–14 μ
(b) 14–15 μ, S = 17–42%
L = 4–11%

(iii) *dimorphon*-type: M = (a) *ca.* 13·8–15·7 μ,
(b) *ca.* 14·9–15·6 μ, S = 4–16%
L = 20–36%

The variations in the means given by Godfrey (a) and Fairbairn (b) were attributed to the effect of different hosts upon the size of the trypanosomes.

TRANSMISSION. From the results of dissections of wild tsetse flies carried out in the course of surveys (*vide* Buxton, 1955 and others) it would appear that *T. congolense* can be transmitted by diverse species of *Glossina*. Thus infections with this parasite have been recorded from *G. palpalis* (Congo, Nigeria), *G. morsitans* (Tanganyika, Mozambique, Nigeria, Rwanda, Burundi, Kenya and Zambia), *G. austeni* (Tanganyika, Kenya, Zanzibar), *G. swynnertoni* (Tanganyika), *G. pallidipes* (Tanganyika, Kenya, Uganda, Zululand, Mozambique), *G. longipalpis* (Ghana, Portuguese Guinea), *G. tachinoides* (Nigeria), *G. brevipalpis* (Tanganyika, Burundi), and *G. vanhoofi* (Burundi).

The infectivity of *T. congolense* for tsetse flies is usually lower than that of *T. vivax* but higher than in species of the *brucei*-complex. Thus, in Nigeria this trypanosome was detected in 8·2% of *G. morsitans*, in about 2% of *G. tachinoides* but only in 0·6% of *G. palpalis* (Lloyd & Johnson, 1924) while the rate in experimentally infected *G. morsitans* from Nyasaland (= Malawi) was found to be 10% (Bruce *et al.*, 1915).

There is some evidence that *T. congolense* is transmissible also by mechanical vectors such as Tabanids and *Stomoxys* (*cf.* Hoare, 1947).

CYCLE IN VECTOR. The life cycle of *T. congolense* in *Glossina* was described by a number of authors (Duke, 1912; Robertson, 1913; Bruce *et al.*, 1915; Lloyd & Johnson, 1924; Roubaud, 1935; Gordon, 1957). The development of the trypanosomes ingested with the blood commences in the endoperitrophic space of the midgut (chiefly in its posterior third) where they assume an elongated trypomastigote form characterized by the position of the kinetoplast not far behind the nucleus (Figs. 1.6, 2.2 n–v, Table 1.1). In this stage the flagellates multiply for some days, and then escape through the open end of the membrane into the ectoperitrophic space, reaching the cardia by the twentieth day or earlier. Here they become longer and penetrate into the endoperitrophic space of the cardia, whence they migrate through the oesophagus to the proboscis, where they are transformed into epimastigote forms which attach themselves to the walls of the labrum and food canal. Finally they find their way into the hypopharynx in which the cycle is completed by transformation of the flagellates into metatrypanosomes measuring about 11 μ in length.

The developmental forms of *T. congolense* in the vector can be distinguished from those of all the other tsetse-borne Salivaria by the total absence of a free flagellum in all the stages. The entire cycle of development in *Glossina* may take from 19 to 53 days, after which the trypanosome becomes infective to the mammalian host.

T. congolense has been cultivated in modified Razgha's medium in which the flagellates correspond to the trypomastigote forms in the midgut of the vector, whereas the proboscis stages (epimastigotes and metatrypanosomes) do not develop *in vitro* (Reichenow, 1937; Hoare, 1949).

HOST-PARASITE RELATIONS. Practically all domestic mammals are susceptible to infection with *T. congolense*, the effects of which vary considerably according to the strain of the parasite and the physical condition of the host. Thus in most ungulates (bovines, sheep, goats, equines and camels), as well as in dogs, the disease may be acute, chronic or mild, while in pigs it usually runs a mild course (Hornby, 1949; Richardson & Kendall, 1957; Stephen, 1966a).

It has already been noted above that some strains of *T. congolense* are separable by their dimensions. Godfrey (1961) has shown that in Nigerian strains the mean lengths are correlated with the pathogenicity of the parasite for cattle, sheep, dogs and rats. Thus (i) the small *congolense* type is characterized by low infectivity, virulence and parasitaemia; (ii) in the intermediate type both infectivity and parasitaemia are high but virulence is low, while (iii) the long *dimorphon*-type is highly infective and virulent, with heavy parasitaemia. According to Fairbairn (1962), strains of the first two types occur over the breadth of the continent, from Zambia to Nigeria, while those of the third type are found in Sudan and Nigeria. Strains showing gradations of this type are comparable to clinodemes and nosodemes (*see* p. 9).

T. congolense is infective to practically all laboratory rodents which are therefore commonly used for the detection of infection in domestic animals. However, as in the case of natural infections, there is much variation in the virulence of different strains for laboratory animals. Thus Binns (1938), who inoculated rodents with diverse bovine strains of *T. congolense* from Malawi, demonstrated that some of them were infective but others were not; moreover, even the same strain when isolated from different individual bovines varied in its infectivity; and similarly there were differences in the susceptibility of individual rodents.

6 *Trypanosoma (Nannomonas) simiae* Bruce *et al.*, 1912.

Synonyms: *T. ignotum* Kinghorn & Yorke, 1912; *T. rodhaini* Walravens, 1924; *T. porci* Schwetz, 1932; *T. congolense porci* Schwetz, 1934; *T. montgomeryi* Laveran, 1909 (*pro parte*).

RELATION TO DISEASE AND DISTRIBUTION. *T. simiae* is a specific parasite of Suidae, being the only trypanosome that is highly pathogenic to domestic pigs in which it causes outbreaks of acute and fatal disease of very short duration.

About thirty years ago *T. simiae* was known only from East and Central Africa, viz. Tanganyika (Tanzania), Nyasaland (Malawi), Northern Rhodesia (Zambia), Southern Rhodesia and Congo. As there are no natural barriers to account for the absence of this parasite in West Africa, the lack of records was probably due to failure on the part of observers to identify it. And indeed, after its diagnostic characters had been firmly established (Hoare, 1936), it was discovered in pigs first in Ghana (Stewart, 1936) and subsequently in Portuguese Guinea, Guinea, Sierra Leone, Mali and Nigeria, as well as in new eastern and southern localities, viz. Kenya, Uganda, Burundi, Mozambique (Stephen, 1966a) and South Africa (Neitz: *in litteris*). It is now known that porcine trypanosomiasis of this type is common throughout most of tropical Africa.

In addition to pigs, which are the main hosts of *T. simiae*, it occurs in camels of Somalia (*cf.* Stephen, 1966a) while individual cases of infection were reported from a horse and an ox in Tanzania (Culwick & Fairbairn, 1947). Among wild mammals this parasite had been isolated only from warthogs and possibly bushpigs. The former, *Phacochoerus aethiopicus*, is regarded as the reservoir host of *T. simiae*.

HISTORY. *T. simiae* owes its inappropriate name to the fact that it was originally isolated by Bruce *et al.* (1912) in Nyasaland from a monkey challenged by infected wild tsetse flies. Somewhat later in the same year Kinghorn and Yorke (1912) similarly isolated the same trypanosome in Rhodesia and called it *T. ignotum*. After Bruce and his associates demonstrated that *T. simiae* was highly virulent for pigs and Belgian investigators in Congo recorded its natural occurrence in these animals, Schwetz (1932) proposed to rename this parasite *T. porci*, in spite of the priority of the original name. The problem of the nomenclature of the porcine trypanosome was discussed in detail by Hoare (1936) and Stephen (1966a).

MORPHOLOGY. *T. simiae* was described by Bruce *et al.* (1912, 1914) as a monomorphic species resembling *T. congolense* in general appearance. However, subsequent studies of *T. simiae* from infected pigs (*cf.* Hoare, 1936; Culwick & Fairbairn, 1947; Stephen, 1966a) established the fact that it was polymorphic and could be readily differentiated from *T. congolense*, especially when parasitaemia is high. Nevertheless, since certain morphological features are common to both species and because some populations of a given species do not contain all the characteristic forms, it may be difficult to identify this trypanosome in random samples.

The overall lengths of *T. simiae* and *T. congolense* are similar, viz. 8–24 μ (means 13·3 μ–19·2 μ) but, whereas the latter is monomorphic, *T. simiae* comprises three structural types or stages (Fig. 2.2, g–l): (i) standard type, represented by stout elongated trypanosomes measuring 14–24 μ (mean 18 μ), are the predominant forms (88·8–92·2%); they have a well-developed undulating membrane, the kinetoplast is subterminal and marginal, and the posterior end of the body is rounded or bluntly pointed; (ii) so-called *rodhaini*-type, represented by slender elongated forms with an inconspicuous undulating membrane but otherwise similar characters; they are 11–20 μ long (mean 15·8 μ) and are present in small numbers (5·2–7·8%); and (iii) *congolense*-type, represented by short forms (9–17 μ long, mean 13·3 μ) indistinguishable from typical *T. congolense*, but the proportion of these forms is very low (2–4·2%).

Among the longer trypanosomes (standard and *rodhaini* types) a few (0·8–3·9%) may appear to have a short free flagellum. However, owing to the extreme attenuation and delicacy of the undulating membrane in the anterior end of the body, it is easily obliterated and becomes invisible in old or defective preparations. In fact, as the writer has shown (Hoare, 1936a, b), the more recent and perfect the preparation the lower the proportion of forms in which a free flagellum appears to be present. It can therefore be assumed that—like *T. congolense*—*T. simiae* is typically devoid of a free flagellum in all its stages.

Since the standard forms of *T. simiae* show a superficial resemblance to the long forms of *T. brucei*, the absence of free flagellum and the marginal position of the kinetoplast are important differential characters (*inter alia*) separating the former from the latter.

TRANSMISSION. As in the case of other tsetse-borne trypanosomes, *T. simiae* can apparently be transmitted by diverse species of *Glossina*. *G. palpalis*, *G. fuscipes* and *G. morsitans* appear to be the most important vectors in East and West Africa, but *G. tachinoides*, *G. longipalpis*, *G. fusca*, *G. tabaniformis*, *G. brevipalpis*, *G. vanhoofi* and *G. austeni* have also been incriminated as vectors (Hoare, 1936; Stephen, 1966a; Berghe *et al.*, 1963).

In the case of epizootics of pig-trypanosomiasis tsetse flies apparently play a secondary role in the transmission of *T. simiae*. Most observers emphasize the paucity or absence of these flies in the immediate vicinity of the outbreaks. There is evidence that in these cases other blood-sucking flies, especially Tabanidae, which were in close contact with the pigs, were mainly responsible for the spread of the infection. It is therefore believed that in outbreaks of acute porcine trypanosomiasis *T. simiae* is first introduced from outside by a few tsetse flies, after which the infection is picked up by horse-flies and transmitted by them mechanically throughout the herd.

CYCLE IN VECTOR. The development of *T. simiae* in tsetse flies was first described by Bruce *et al.* (1914a) who used laboratory-bred *G. morsitans* in this study. They found that the cycle undergone by this species is similar to that of *T. congolense*, viz. it commences in the midgut in which the flagellates are represented by trypomastigote forms with a kinetoplast situated far from the posterior end of the body and near the nucleus. After migration to the proboscis the flagellates assume the epimastigote form and attach themselves to the walls of the food canal, and finally invade the hypopharynx where the metatrypanosomes are produced (Figs. 1.6, 2.2 n–v, Table 1.1). The latter measure 10–12 μ in length (Culwick & Fairbairn, 1947) and resemble the *congolense*-like blood forms. As in *T. congolense*, *T. simiae* is devoid of a free flagellum in all stages of its development in the vector.

The entire developmental cycle in *G. morsitans* and *G. brevipalpis* takes about twenty days (Bruce *et al.*, 1914a; Peel and Chardome, 1954d). As in the case of *T. congolense*, the infection rate of *T. simiae* in *Glossina* is fairly high, viz. up to 12·7% (*cf.* Stephen, 1966a).

T. simiae has been cultivated in modified Razgha's medium.

HOST-PARASITE RELATIONS. As already mentioned, *T. simiae* is essentially a porcine parasite. Bruce's graphic description of this trypanosome as 'the lightning destroyer of the domestic pig' is fully borne out by subsequent observations on its behaviour in outbreaks of the disease. According to Stephen (1966), who has brought together the data on pig trypanosomiasis, the infection may last on the average 3·6 days from the discovery of the trypanosomes in the blood and death of the host. In experimentally infected pigs the incubation period is about three days after inoculation with blood and 4–5 days after challenge by infected tsetse flies. Parasitaemia rises rapidly for 24 hours until the trypanosomes are swarming in the blood and the animal may be *in extremis* and dies soon afterwards.

The effect of *T. simiae* upon horses and cattle is unknown. Apparently this trypanosome causes a hyperacute disease in camels of Somalia. Under experimental conditions it is infective to sheep and goats producing in them disease that may last for some months. The only susceptible laboratory animals are *Cercopithecus* monkeys; rodents and dogs are refractory to infection. However, rabbits are sometimes susceptible: while in intact animals the course of infection is variable, in splenoctomized rabbits it is acute and fatal, with high parasitaemia (Desowitz & Watson, 1953). Among wild mammals examined, only warthogs proved to be infected with *T. simiae*. As they are frequently found in areas where infected tsetse flies and porcine trypanosomiasis are prevalent, these animals are undoubtedly the natural hosts and reservoirs of the infection in domestic pigs (*cf.* Hoare, 1936; Stephen, 1966a).

Status of *Trypanosoma montgomeryi*

The name *T. montgomeryi* was given by Laveran (1909) to a peculiar trypanosome recorded by Montgomery and Kinghorn (1909) from cattle in Northern Rhodesia (Zambia). Similar trypanosomes have been reported in various ruminants and dogs from different parts of Africa. The characteristics of *T. montgomeryi* described by some authors are as follows (Fig. 2.2, l,m): in general it resembles *T. congolense* but differs from it mainly in the great breadth of the body (up to 3·6 μ), while the kinetoplast is subterminal and marginal; there is occasionally a very short free flagellum (up to 1·7 μ long) and the body measures 10–20·8 μ in length (means 14·7–16 μ). In a critical revision of *T. montgomeryi*, Stephen (1963a, 1966a) has shown that although it may occasionally occur in pure infections, in most cases this trypanosome was associated either with *T. congolense* or *T. simiae*. Moreover, when passaged through susceptible animals this trypanosome never maintained its peculiar morphology. Stephen rightly concluded that *T. montgomeryi* is an atypical broad form found in species of *Nannomonas* and is therefore not a valid species. Some authors (e.g. Schwetz, 1934) believed that this form was characteristic of chronic infections with *T. congolense* while others (e.g. Gillain, 1937) regarded them as involution forms appearing during the terminal phase of the infection.

Subgenus *Trypanozoon*

The subgenus *Trypanozoon* is the most homogeneous group of Salivarian trypanosomes in that it contains a number of species which are morphologically indistinguishable but differ only in biological and nosological features. In Africa there are about five species, three of which (*T. brucei*, *T. rhodesiense* and *T. gambiense*) are tsetse-borne and develop in the midgut and salivary glands of the vector while the remaining two are transmitted directly, one (*T. evansi*) by mechanical inoculators (Tabanid flies) and the other (*T. equiperdum*) by contact between the mammalian hosts.

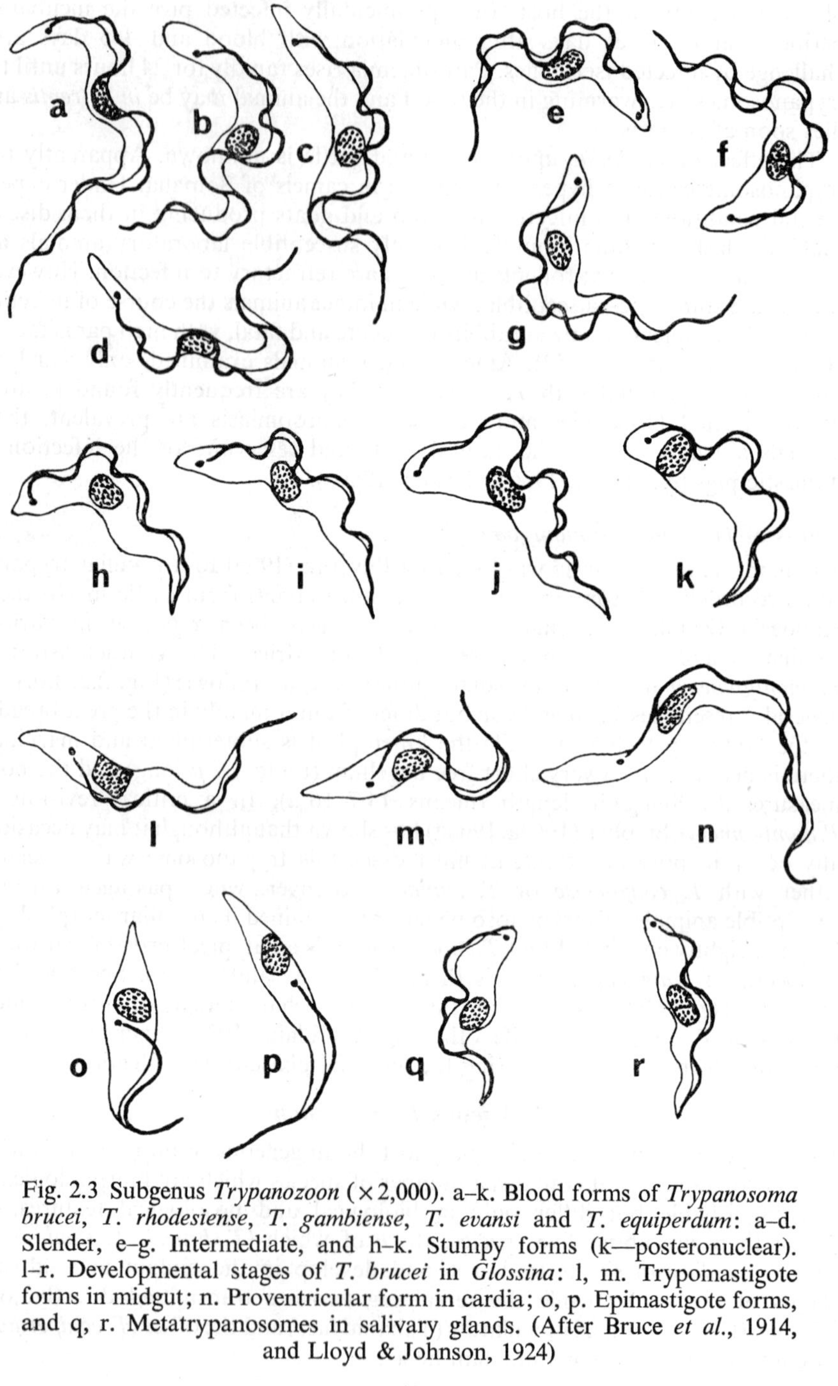

Fig. 2.3 Subgenus *Trypanozoon* (×2,000). a–k. Blood forms of *Trypanosoma brucei*, *T. rhodesiense*, *T. gambiense*, *T. evansi* and *T. equiperdum*: a–d. Slender, e–g. Intermediate, and h–k. Stumpy forms (k—posteronuclear). l–r. Developmental stages of *T. brucei* in *Glossina*: l, m. Trypomastigote forms in midgut; n. Proventricular form in cardia; o, p. Epimastigote forms, and q, r. Metatrypanosomes in salivary glands. (After Bruce *et al.*, 1914, and Lloyd & Johnson, 1924)

The blood forms of *Trypanozoon* (Fig. 2.3, a–k) measure from 11 μ to 42 μ in total length. They are typically polymorphic, being represented by three forms: (a) slender trypanosomes (mean lengths *ca.* 23 μ–30 μ) possessing a long free flagellum and a well-developed undulating membrane, elongated nucleus, subterminal kinetoplast and narrow posterior end drawn out to a blunt point or sometimes truncated; (b) stumpy trypanosomes (mean lengths *ca.* 17 μ–22 μ) which are stout and usually without a free flagellum, undulating membrane well developed, nucleus rounded (displaced to the posterior end in posteronuclear forms), kinetoplast near broadly rounded or obtusely pointed posterior end; and (c) intermediate forms (mean lengths *ca.* 20–25 μ) in which the flagellum is shorter, the posterior end blunter and the kinetoplast nearer to this extremity than in the slender forms. The kinetoplast in *Trypanozoon* is smaller than in any of the other Salivarian trypanosomes except *T. suis* (0·6–0·7 μ).

The polymorphism in members of the subgenus *Trypanozoon* is a variable character. The most characteristic forms are the slender ones, since they are always present in all the species, whereas the proportion of stumpy forms, which appear constantly in the tsetse-borne species (*T. brucei*, *T. rhodesiense* and *T. gambiense*), fluctuates in the course of the infection and they may disappear completely after prolonged mechanical passages. Thus laboratory strains maintained by blood inoculation eventually become monomorphic with only the slender forms present. These are also the only kind of trypanosomes in those species which are normally transmitted by the mechanical method, viz. in *T. evansi* and *T. equiperdum*. However, it has been demonstrated that stumpy forms comparable to those in the *brucei*-complex may occur sporadically in both these species. The morphological difference between the tsetse-borne and the mechanically transmitted species of *Trypanozoon* is therefore quantitative and resolves itself to the constancy of polymorphism in the former and its inconstancy in the latter (Hoare, 1956).

There has been considerable difference of opinion regarding the nature of polymorphism in the *brucei*-like trypanosomes. Recent investigations (Ashcroft, 1957; Wijers, 1959) indicate that the morphology of the trypanosomes is determined primarily by the degree of parasitaemia and antibody response of the host. When parasitaemia rises the slender forms proliferate and their numbers increase; when it falls stumpy forms are predominant, while the intermediate forms are transitional stages produced when the slender forms shrink to become stumpy forms and, *vice versa*, when the latter elongate to become slender again.

The close affinity between all the species of *Trypanozoon* finds further support in the possession by *T. brucei*, *T. evansi*, and *T. equiperdum* of common antigens, on account of which they cannot be differentiated by the complement fixation test (Robinson, 1926; Hoare, 1956; Richardson & Kendall, 1957).

7 *Trypanosoma (Trypanozoon) gambiense* Dutton, 1902.

Synonyms: *T. ugandense* Castellani, 1903; *T. castellanii* Kruse, 1903; *T. hominis* Manson, 1903; *T. fordii* Maxwell-Adams, 1903; *T. tullochii* Minchin, 1907; *T. rovumense* Beck & Weck, 1913; *T. nigeriense* Macfie, 1913.

8 *Trypanosoma (Trypanozoon) rhodesiense* Stephens & Fantham, 1910.

Synonym: *T. brucei* vel *rhodesiense* Bruce *et al.*, 1915.

RELATION TO DISEASE AND DISTRIBUTION. Both *T. gambiense* and *T. rhodesiense* are the causative agents of sleeping sickness or African human trypanosomiasis which is characterized in the initial stages by parasitaemia and polyadenitis, while in the later stages the nervous system becomes involved, eventually giving rise to meningo-encephalitis. The disease occurs in two main forms, the chronic Gambian and the acute Rhodesian, which are attributed to *T. gambiense* and *T. rhodesiense* respectively. However, the clinical manifestations associated with these trypanosomes are not clearly demarcated, for cases with symptoms of one type of sleeping sickness may occur in the area of distribution of the other type, while some of the other diagnostic characters differentiating the two types of the disease (virulence, vectors, response to drugs) are also of relative value (*cf.* Hoare, 1949).

Since *T. gambiense* and *T. rhodesiense* are morphologically indistinguishable, there can be no doubt that these two species are very closely related and probably identical, *T. rhodesiense* representing merely a virulent race of *T. gambiense* (Hoare, 1967). On account of this, they can be described collectively.

Sleeping sickness occurs exclusively in tropical Africa, where its distribution covers a wide belt, roughly between 15°N and 20°S of the Equator. The areas of distribution of the Gambian (*T. gambiense*) and Rhodesian (*T. rhodesiense*) forms of the disease are in most cases distinct though cases of one type may occur in localities where the other is prevalent. According to a recent review (Vaucel *et al.*, 1963), the Gambian disease is endemic throughout most of tropical Africa, viz. in Senegal, Guinea, Mali, Ivory Coast, Upper Volta, Togo, Dahomey, Niger, Cameroon, Gabon, Republics of Congo and Central Africa, Chad, Gambia, Portuguese Guinea, Sierra Leone, Liberia, Ghana, Nigeria, Spanish Equatorial region, Angola, Congo, Ruanda, Burundi, southern Sudan, Uganda and Kenya, while the Rhodesian disease is prevalent in Tanzania, Malawi, Zambia, Rhodesia and Mozambique as well as in the northern area of Lake Victoria lying in Kenya and Uganda. In the Zambezi basin and Botswana there is a third form of sleeping sickness occupying an intermediate position between the two classical types.

HISTORY. The causative organism of sleeping sickness discovered by Forde in 1901 in the blood of a patient from Gambia, was first recognized as a trypanosome by Dutton (1902) who named it *T. gambiense*. According to Davies (1962) this parasite was discovered independently by Castellani in 1902 in the cerebrospinal fluid of a patient in Uganda and named *T. ugandense*. The name *T. rhodesiense* was given by Stephens and Fantham (1910) to a strain isolated from a case of sleeping sickness from Rhodesia. It was differentiated from *T. gambiense* by the presence of posteronuclear forms and by its greater virulence for laboratory rodents.

MORPHOLOGY. The initial development of the sleeping sickness trypanosomes in cyclically infected susceptible mammals was studied in the case of

T. rhodesiense by Gordon and Willett (1956, 1958) and Fairbairn and Godfrey (1958). They demonstrated that in rodents the trypanosomes injected by the fly into the skin almost immediately invaded the blood stream, but in human volunteers the development of the trypanosomes during the first nine days was restricted to the primary nodule or 'chancre' which appears at the site of the bite, after which the trypanosomes invade the blood stream. The development of the metatrypanosomes into blood forms was observed *in vitro* at 37°C. After 12–20 minutes they were still unaltered but in the course of the next eight hours their body gradually elongated, a free flagellum developed, and the metatrypanosomes were transformed directly into slender blood forms. Similar forms were found in the chancre itself. There is reason to believe that man requires a minimum dose of 300–450 metatrypanosomes for infection with *T. rhodesiense* to be successfully established (Fairbairn & Burtt, 1946).

The morphology of *T. gambiense* and *T. rhodesiense* was studied by a number of authors (*cf.* Wenyon, 1926). In general it conforms to the polymorphic pattern of the subgenus *Trypanozoon* described above (Fig. 2.3, a–k). The comparative lengths of these trypanosomes given by various authors (*cf.* Hoare, 1956) are as follows:

	T. gambiense	*T. rhodesiense*
Range	12–35 μ	12–42 μ
Thin forms (slender and intermediate)	20–35 μ Mean *ca.* 27 μ	16–42 μ Means 28·4–29 μ
Stumpy forms	12–27 μ Mean *ca.* 20·5 μ	12–25 μ Means 17·5–19·4 μ

Since these measurements were based on various numbers from diverse hosts and at different periods of the infection, the slight differences between *T. gambiense* and *T. rhodesiense* are not significant and it can be assumed that these two species cannot be differentiated by their mensural characters.

The proportion of trypanosomes belonging to any of the three types (slender, intermediate and stumpy) is subject to wide fluctuation in the course of an infection but as a rule the flagellated thin forms are predominant. Although dividing trypanosomes occur among all the three forms, only the slender ones multiply in any appreciable numbers whereas the stumpy forms which are produced by shrinkage of the slender ones rarely divide. In addition to the three standard forms, there occurs in these trypanosomes a type in which the nucleus is displaced to the posterior end of the body near or even beyond the kinetoplast (Fig. 2.3, k). These posteronuclear forms are particularly common in *T. rhodesiense*, especially in experimentally infected laboratory animals. At one time it was thought that posteronuclear forms were peculiar to this species but they were subsequently recorded from Ugandan and Nigerian strains of *T. gambiense* (Lavier, 1927; Lester, 1933). It is generally agreed that the stumpy forms represent the infective stage capable of developing in tsetse flies (Wijers & Willett, 1960).

While cyclically transmitted strains retain their polymorphism, it is well known that laboratory strains maintained by blood passages lose the stumpy forms and become monomorphic. Thus in strains passaged through guinea-pigs the writer (Hoare, 1956) found that *T. gambiense* lost its polymorphism seven months after isolation from man while *T. rhodesiense* remained polymorphic for one year. In syringe-passaged strains some of the biological properties are also modified and they are therefore not comparable to cyclically transmitted strains. Thus their transmissibility by *Glossina* may be lost and their virulence for rodents increased with time (Duke, 1934, 1935). As regards their behaviour in man, it was shown (Fairbairn, 1956) that an old laboratory strain of *T. rhodesiense* lost its infectivity to man though a strain of *T. gambiense* was still infective to man after four years, when the strain was already monomorphic.

TRANSMISSION. It is well known that in the laboratory *T. gambiense* and *T. rhodesiense* are capable of developing in diverse species of *Glossina*, but under natural conditions their association with particular vectors is determined by the epidemiological peculiarities of the diseases caused by them, the Gambian type being essentially an anthroponosis, which is transmitted from man to man, while the Rhodesian type is an anthropozoonosis frequently transmitted by tsetse flies which had fed on infected wild mammals, especially antelopes. *T. gambiense* is normally transmitted by waterside flies of the *palpalis* group, represented by *G. palpalis* and *G. tachinoides* in West Africa and by *G. fuscipes* in East Africa. The zones occupied by these insects are characterized by scanty mammalian fauna but are usually situated near well populated places, the inhabitants of which frequently come in contact with the vectors whose food-hosts however are mainly crocodiles. The chief vectors of *T. rhodesiense* belong to the *morsitans* group, represented by *G. morsitans*, *G. swynnertoni* and *G. pallidipes*, which inhabit savanna-like woodland abundant in game animals (*cf.* Hoare, 1962). Among the wild mammals some, e.g. bushbuck (*Tragelaphus scriptus*), may harbour *T. rhodesiense* and serve as reservoir hosts of sleeping sickness (Heisch *et al.*, 1958).

However, the association between the two species of human trypanosomes with either of these groups of tsetse flies is not rigidly fixed for the suitability of a given species of *Glossina* as vector depends also upon the degree of contact between man and flies available locally. Thus, in north-eastern Uganda the vector of *T. rhodesiense* is a member of the *palpalis* group (*G. fuscipes*), while *T. gambiense* is transmissible cyclically through *G. morsitans* (Lester, 1933; Corson, 1938).

CYCLE IN VECTOR. Kleine (1909, 1909a) was the first to demonstrate that *T. brucei* underwent a definite cycle of development in *Glossina* before it became infective. This observation was soon confirmed for *T. gambiense* by Bruce *et al.* (1909) who described the stages of its development in *G. palpalis* but did not link them up into a definite life cycle. Later, Bruce *et al.* (1911) gave an account of the succession of stages of this trypanosome in the fly and proved that the metatrypanosomes in the salivary glands represented the infective stage. The complete life history of *T. gambiense* in its vector was elucidated by Muriel Robertson (1913) and amplified by others, while Bruce *et al.* (1914c, d) described the development of *T. rhodesiense* in *G. morsitans* and *G. brevipalpis.* More recent work on the behaviour of the human trypanosomes in tsetse flies was critically reviewed by Fairbairn and Culwick (1950).

Since the course of development of *T. gambiense* and *T. rhodesiense* (as well as of *T. brucei*) in *Glossina* is similar, it need not be described separately for each of these species. When these trypanosomes are ingested with the blood of the mammalian host, they find themselves in the endoperitrophic space of the midgut where they are transformed by the third or fourth day into a new trypomastigote form in which the undulating membrane is less pronounced than in the slender blood forms, the kinetoplast is situated about halfway between the posterior end of the body and the nucleus, and a free flagellum is always present (Figs. 1.6, 2.3, 1,m, Table 1.1). These flagellates, which may reach 35 μ in length, multiply intensely in the lumen of the gut for about ten days until large numbers extending to its posterior portion are present. As the flagellates reach the open end of the peritrophic membrane they enter the ectoperitrophic space of the midgut and gradually migrate forwards, reaching the cardia (= proventriculus) between the tenth and twentieth day. Here the trypomastigote flagellates become more slender and elongated and are known as the proventricular forms (Fig. 2.3, n) which now begin to penetrate into the endoperitrophic space of the cardia (*see* p. 22), whence they pass through the oesophagus and pharynx into the mouth parts. Here they enter the hypopharynx at its open anterior end and finally pass along the salivary ducts into the salivary glands, where they attach themselves to the walls and undergo the final stages of development. In the glands the proventricular forms are transformed into broad epimastigote forms (Fig. 2.3, o,p) which multiply and give rise to the metatrypanosomes (Fig. 2.3, g,r), represented by short forms measuring about 14·6 × 1·5 μ and resembling the stumpy blood forms. They are typically without a free flagellum though a very short one may occasionally be present; the kinetoplast lies near the posterior end and the nucleus is median. In the case of *T. rhodesiense* it was estimated (using the probing method) that the number of metatrypanosomes discharged by an infected *G. morsitans* may reach 40,000, the minimum infective dose being 300–450 metatrypanosomes (Fairbairn & Burtt, 1946; Harley *et al.*, 1966).

There is no agreement regarding the infection rate and the length of the life cycle of the sleeping sickness trypanosomes in *Glossina.* It is generally accepted (*cf.* Buxton, 1955) that under natural conditions the proportion of tsetse flies infected with *brucei*-type trypanosomes is the lowest among the Salivaria, viz. below 1%, while estimates of the time required to complete the development in the vector given by different observers vary from about 17 to 45 days and even longer. These discrepancies find a ready explanation in the light of experiments by Fairbairn and Culwick (1950) who showed that the fundamental factor governing the transmission of these trypanosomes is the temperature to which the tsetse flies are exposed during the development of the flagellates.

While it was already known that the infection rate can be increased by exposure of the flies to high temperatures (35°–37°C), these authors demonstrated in the case of *T. rhodesiense* and *G. morsitans* that both the infection rate and length of the cycle are determined primarily by the temperature at which the pupae had been kept but not upon the temperature at which the emerged adult insects were subsequently maintained, as shown below.

Maintenance temperatures		Infection rate	Average length of cycle
Pupae	Adult flies	(%)	(days)
Room t°	Room t°	2·7– 6·4	29
28°C	Room t°	2·8– 8·2	23
30°C	Room t°	10·8–17·5	12

It was concluded that the optimum conditions for the transmission of *T. rhodesiense* by *G. morsitans* obtained when the pupae were kept at 30°C and the adult flies at 28°C, with 80% relative humidity. The correctness of the data based on experimental conditions is borne out by field observations, indicating that fluctuations of the infection rates in tsetse flies from various localities are influenced by climate, especially temperature. Thus, according to Kinghorn and York (1912a), in Central Africa *G. morsitans* was more readily infected with *T. rhodesiense* in areas with a mean temperature of 27·6°C than in those where it was 17·9°C, while Fairbairn and Culwick (1950) observed the effect of seasonal variations of the temperature in Tanzania, where the incidence of sleeping sickness rises considerably at the end of the hot dry season. (For a review of this question *see* Ford and Leggate, 1961; Ford, 1965.)

It should be noted that the *brucei*-like trypanosomes do not always complete their cycle in the tsetse fly. In some cases the trypanosomes start developing in the gut but are unable to invade the salivary glands, in others they may disappear spontaneously from an infected fly (Duke, 1933; Hoare, 1940).

T. gambiense and *T. rhodesiense* have been grown *in vitro* in a number of blood-agar media, the most suitable of which are those devised by Tobie *et al.* (1950) and Weinman (1960). As in the case of other Salivaria, the flagellates in culture correspond to the trypomastigote forms in the gut of tsetse flies. Since the metatrypanosomes do not develop in these media, cultures of these trypanosomes are not infective to mammals.

HOST-PARASITE RELATIONS. It has already been noted that *T. gambiense* and *T. rhodesiense* typically produce two types of sleeping sickness, the clinical manifestations of which are not clearly demarcated, while in the Zambezi basin and in Botswana there occurs a third type (Ormerod, 1961b; Apted *et al.*, 1963) occupying an intermediate position between the classical forms of the disease. The general course of human infection is as follows (*cf.* Hoare, 1949).

In the earlier period there is intensive multiplication of the trypanosomes in the blood and in the lymph glands when they periodically appear in and disappear from the blood. Their disappearance (crisis) is due to destruction by trypanolytic antibodies aided by phagocytosis, leaving a certain percentage of resistant parasites to repopulate the blood stream thereby giving rise to relapse strains. As the infection progresses the trypanosomes are reduced in numbers and may be apparently absent from the blood for long periods, but can then usually be found in the lymph glands. They persist longer in the blood of patients infected with *T. rhodesiense*, in which blood examination usually reveals the parasites.

After a variable period—about one month in the Rhodesian disease and several months in the Gambian type—the trypanosomes invade the cerebrospinal fluid where they are usually found in small numbers. In later periods of the disease the central nervous system becomes involved, extending to the brain. In the cerebral tissues the trypanosomes are situated in the intercellular spaces but not in the cells themselves. After involvement of the central nervous system the disease may run a chronic course lasting up to several years in the Gambian type, or an acute course lasting only several months in the Rhodesian type, in both cases terminating fatally if untreated. However, symptomless carriers occur in infections with both *T. gambiense* and *T. rhodesiense*.

The course of sleeping sickness caused by these two species is a reflection of differences in their virulence to man, which is paralleled in their effect upon experimentally infected laboratory animals. As in the case of human infections, *T. rhodesiense* is more virulent to lower mammals than *T. gambiense*. Both these species produce heavy infections in monkeys (except baboons which are refractory) and are infective to laboratory rodents (e.g. rats) but, whereas *T. rhodesiense* succeeds in establishing itself in these animals directly, *T. gambiense* on first isolation from man does not readily infect them, although after passage through a monkey it becomes more virulent for the rodents. Other animals susceptible to infection with the human trypanosomes include dogs, cats, sheep, goats, cattle and pigs. In the blood of rats and mice the trypanosomes multiply rapidly, producing high parasitaemia which may kill the hosts in a few days. In guinea-pigs the infection is usually chronic, with a succession of crises and relapses, but ultimately terminates in the death of the animal.

Natural infections with *brucei*-like trypanosomes are quite common among wild African mammals including various antelopes, buffalo and warthog. In view of the absence of morphological differences between *T. gambiense*, *T. rhodesiense* and *T. brucei*, their identity in naturally infected hosts can be established with certainty only by experimental infection of susceptible animals, as well as of human volunteers, but in most cases the nature of the parasite is determined from circumstantial evidence provided by epidemiological data. Thus, trypanosomes found in animals from localities where the human disease is unknown are probably *T. brucei* while those occurring in endemic areas of the Rhodesian disease might be either *T. rhodesiense* or *T. brucei* according to whether or not the strain is infective to human beings. In endemic areas of the Gambian disease the differential diagnosis of *T. brucei* and *T. gambiense* is based on the relative virulence of the strain for laboratory rodents which are highly susceptible to infection with the former species but may be refractory to the latter.

In the past there was considerable circumstantial evidence that man may acquire Rhodesian sleeping sickness from wild ruminants (*cf.* Hoare, 1962). The correctness of the hypothesis that some of these animals are reservoir hosts of the human disease was confirmed by experimental infection of volunteers with trypanosomes isolated from bushbuck and from wild tsetse flies (Heisch *et al.*, 1958; Southon & Robertson, 1961), and there is convincing epidemiological evidence of the existence in Tanzania and in the Zambezi basin of enzootic foci of Rhodesian sleeping sickness (Apted *et al.*, 1963). Under natural conditions in the bush the infection circulates independently of man between donor-antelopes, their vectors and recipient-antelopes, while in endemic areas the circulation of the parasite involves man as well, with the result that he becomes both donor and recipient of the infection (Hoare, 1962). It is also possible that cattle may act as domestic reservoirs of *T. rhodesiense* (Onyango *et al.*, 1966). Although Gambian sleeping sickness is transmitted mainly from man to man, there is both experimental and epidemiological evidence that some domestic animals, such as pigs and goats, might serve as reservoir hosts of human infection (Duke, 1928; van Hoof, 1947; Fairbairn, 1954; Stephen, 1966a).

9 ***Trypanosoma (Trypanozoon) brucei*** **Plimmer & Bradford, 1899.**

Synonyms: *T. pecaudi* Laveran, 1907; *T. togolense* Mesnil & Brimont, 1909; *T. elephantis* Bruce *et al.*, 1909; *T. anceps* Bruce *et al.*, 1914; *T. ugandae* Stephens & Blacklock, 1913; *T. dukei* Knuth & du Toit, 1921.

RELATION TO DISEASE AND DISTRIBUTION. *T. brucei* is the causative organism of nagana affecting domestic animals; this disease is characterized by fever, anaemia, oedema, cachexia and frequently partial blindness and paralysis. The course of the infection varies according to the strain of parasite and host. It is usually acute in dogs, cats and horses; subacute in donkeys, sheep and goats; and chronic in pigs and cattle. Though morphologically indistinguishable from the human parasites, *T. gambiense* and *T. rhodesiense*, *T. brucei* is not infective to man.

T. brucei has the same geographical distribution as *T. congolense* (*see* p. 32) but the incidence of infection with this parasite is apparently lower. However, latent *T. brucei* infections are liable to be missed but can be revealed by inoculation of rats (Godfrey & Killick-Kendrick, 1961).

HISTORY. This trypanosome was first seen by David Bruce in 1894 in the blood of cattle suffering from nagana in Zululand and later was recognized by him (Bruce, 1895) as the causative agent of the disease. It was studied in England by Plimmer and Bradford (1899) who named it *T. brucei.* Since this strain was monomorphic while strains from Uganda proved to be polymorphic, Stephens and Blacklock (1913) regarded the latter as belonging to a distinct species and proposed for it the name *T. ugandae*. However, it was evident that the Zululand strain had lost its original polymorphism after maintenance in laboratory animals, therefore the valid name of this parasite is *T. brucei* (*cf.* Wenyon, 1926).

MORPHOLOGY. In the blood of its mammalian hosts *T. brucei* has all the characteristics of the polymorphic tsetse-borne trypanosomes of the subgenus *Trypanozoon* described above (p. 18). Like *T. gambiense* and *T. rhodesiense* it is represented by slender, intermediate and stumpy forms (Fig. 2.3, a,k), the lengths of which are as follows (Hoare, 1956).

Range 11–39 μ
Thin forms (slender and intermediate) 14–39 μ (mean 27 μ)
Stumpy forms 11–27 μ (means 16·6–20 μ).

For reasons already stated (p. 39), it is evident that *T. brucei* cannot be distinguished from the human trypanosomes by its mensural characters but it differs from *T. gambiense* in the common occurrence among the stumpy trypanosomes of posteronuclear forms, especially in infected laboratory rodents. In this respect *T. brucei* is indistinguishable from *T. rhodesiense*, on account of which some authors regarded the latter as merely a human strain of *T. brucei* (Bruce *et al.*, 1915b; Wenyon, 1926 and others). Like the human trypanosomes, *T. brucei* becomes monomorphic after prolonged passages through laboratory mammals. This phenomenon was first noted by Bruce (1914) while the writer (Hoare, 1956) found that this change can take place after thirty months.

For further particulars about *T. brucei* in the mammalian host the reader should consult the preceding section (p. 39).

TRANSMISSION. Like the other tsetse-borne Salivaria, *T. brucei* is capable of developing in any species of *Glossina*. Under natural conditions it is sometimes difficult to identify the specific vectors of *T. brucei* because in most surveys infections in the fly are recorded as belonging to the *brucei* group collectively. Therefore in the absence of tests for infectivity to laboratory mammals or (in the case of *T. rhodesiense*) to man the identification of the flagellates found in *Glossina* is determined from epidemiological evidence. According to the available data (Wenyon, 1926; Curasson, 1943; Buxton, 1955), the main vectors of *T. brucei* are species belonging to the *morsitans* group, viz. *G. morsitans* and *G. pallidipes*, but *G. brevipalpis* of the *fusca* group, as well as *G. tachinoides* and *G. palpalis* of the *palpalis* group have also been incriminated.

The transmission of *T. brucei* by tsetse flies was demonstrated by Bruce (1897) in the case of *G. pallidipes*, but Kleine (1909a) was the first to show that these trypanosomes went through a cycle of development in the fly before they became infective to mammals, while Bouet and Roubaud (1910) proved that *G. longipalpis*, *G. tachinoides* and *G. palpalis* were vectors of this trypanosome.

In addition to cyclical transmission by its intermediate hosts, *T. brucei* can be transmitted to mammals directly by mechanical inoculators, which are in some cases tsetse flies, in others Tabanid flies and/or *Stomoxys* (Duke *et al.*, 1934; Hornby, 1952; Buxton, 1955). The success of mechanical transmission depends upon the length of survival of the blood trypanosomes in the proboscis of the insect during the very short interval between interrupted feeds.

CYCLE IN VECTOR. The course of development of *T. brucei* was studied in *G. morsitans* by Bruce *et al.* (1914b, c). As it is similar to the cycle of *T. gambiense* and *T. rhodesiense* (Fig. 1.6, g, l–r; Table 1.1) and the factors affecting the infection rate and length of the invertebrate cycle are comparable to those in the human trypanosomes, the reader is referred to pp. 44 for a detailed account of the development of *T. brucei* in the vector. This trypanosome has been cultivated in the same media as the human trypanosomes.

HOST-PARASITE RELATIONS. From the medical point of view, the most important property of *T. brucei* is negative, viz. its inability under normal conditions to infect man, although in other respects this trypanosome is indistinguishable from the human parasites, especially *T. rhodesiense*. However, as shown below, there is circumstantial evidence that human infections derived from *T. brucei* might possibly occur in nature. In this connection it is interesting that man's closest anthropoid relation, the chimpanzee, proved to be susceptible to infection with both *T. rhodesiense* and *T. brucei* (Baker, 1962).

As the causative agent of nagana, *T. brucei* is of considerable veterinary importance for practically all domestic mammals are susceptible to infection. *T. brucei* is particularly virulent for horses and other equines and for sheep, goats and dogs, in which it may produce a severe and fatal disease (Hornby, 1952; Richardson & Kendall, 1957). Although pigs are readily infected with this trypanosome, its pathogenicity for this animal is usually low (Stephen, 1966a); cattle are relatively resistant. *T. brucei* is highly pathogenic to all laboratory rodents in which its virulence increases rapidly with passages until the animal succumbs within a few days. Like *T. rhodesiense*, *T. brucei* produces numerous posteronuclear forms in these animals.

Under natural conditions *T. brucei* has been recovered from many species of wild game and there can be no doubt that some of these mammals, especially antelopes, are reservoir hosts from which wild tsetse flies transmit the infection to domestic animals.

PHYLOGENETIC RELATIONS OF *brucei*-LIKE TRYPANOSOMES. It has already been shown that the three species, *T. gambiense*, *T. rhodesiense* and *T. brucei*, are morphologically indistinguishable both in their mammalian and insect hosts but they differ in biological properties manifested in their relationship to their mammalian hosts. They are all infective to diverse mammals but only *T. gambiense* and *T. rhodesiense* are capable of infecting man, producing chronic and acute sleeping sickness respectively, while laboratory rodents are highly susceptible to infection with *T. rhodesiense* and *T. brucei* but relatively refractory to *T. gambiense*. However, the Zambezi strain causes in man a chronic disease of the Gambian type but—like *T. rhodesiense*—is very virulent for laboratory mammals. There is thus no hard and fast line separating the Gambian and Rhodesian diseases which are linked by the Zambezian form.

Furthermore, except for its infectivity to man, *T. rhodesiense* is in every respect comparable to *T. brucei*, for both are extremely virulent for their mammalian hosts and are typical zoonoses, sharing the same vectors and depending upon big game as reservoirs of the diseases caused by them. *T. gambiense* is essentially a human parasite though some livestock may possibly be involved as reservoir hosts.

There can thus be no doubt that the tsetse-borne trypanosomes of the subgenus *Trypanozoon* are very closely allied but there is still some controversy regarding their phylogenetic relations.

While some authors (e.g. Willett, 1965) maintain that *T. rhodesiense* originated from a virulent strain of *T. gambiense*, others (e.g. Hoare, 1949, 1967; Lambrecht, 1964) believe that *T. gambiense* was derived from *T. rhodesiense* which in its turn descended from *T. brucei*. Lambrecht (1964) in attempting to trace the evolution of these trypanosomes suggested the following hypothesis. In prehistoric times, when early man first settled in the savanna zone of Africa, he was exposed to bites of tsetse of the *morsitans* group which harboured infection with *T. brucei* derived from naturally infected antelopes. Contemporary man, in similar situations, does not normally become infected but in those exceptional cases when this took place *T. brucei* probably caused in non-immune subjects an acute disease which has come to be ascribed to *T. rhodesiense*. In enzootic foci *T. rhodesiense* still retains its connections with the game tsetse as vectors and with antelopes as reservoirs of infection. In waterside zones, on the other hand, the trypanosomes became better adapted to man and produced a chronic form of the disease which has come to be ascribed to *T. gambiense*. The latter is transmitted by tsetse of the *palpalis* group which feed mainly on reptiles as opposed to wild mammals. According to this hypothesis *T. brucei* is the ancestral form from which *T. rhodesiense* evolved while the latter, in turn, gave rise to *T. gambiense*. Thus, the evolution of the diseases caused by trypanosomes of the *brucei* complex proceeded from a purely enzootic infection of wild ruminants (nagana) to an anthropozoonosis (Zambezian and Rhodesian disease in man) and ultimately to a pure anthroponosis (Gambian disease in man).

Since the biological characters of species of the *brucei-rhodesiense-gambiense* complex intergrade they can be regarded as subspecies of *T. brucei* and designated as *T. brucei brucei* and *T. brucei gambiense*, while *T. rhodesiense* is probably merely a virulent nosodeme of *T. gambiense*. Although *T. rhodesiense* is phylogenetically older than *T. gambiense*, the latter name must be retained on grounds of priority (Hoare, 1967).

10 *Trypanosoma (Trypanozoon) evansi* (Steel, 1885).

Synonyms: *T. evansi* var. *mborii* Laveran, 1903; *T. soudanense* Laveran, 1907; *T. soudanense* var. *berberum* Sergent *et al.*, 1912; *T. marocanum* Sergent *et al.*, 1915; *T. aegyptum* Nattan-Larrier & Noyer, 1932.

RELATION TO DISEASE AND DISTRIBUTION. *T. evansi* is the causative organism of the disease generally known as surra which affects diverse mammals and is characterized by fever and anaemia, followed by oedema and cachexia.

The symptoms of surra vary in severity according to the strain of parasite and species of host. Among domestic animals the disease assumes the most severe form in camels, horses and dogs (Curasson, 1943).

Surra is widely distributed in countries with hot and warm climates. On the Eurasian continent it is found in the Middle East and the south-eastern part of the Soviet Union, whence it passes into Soviet Middle Asia and extends eastwards through Iran, India, Indo-China and parts of southern China, as well as to islands of the Indian and Pacific oceans. Finally this trypanosome has found its way into Central and South America.

In Africa, the disease is known under various Arabic names, such as mbori, salaf, debab, tahaga, etc., and occurs along the Atlantic and Mediterranean littorals of North Africa where debab is prevalent in Morocco, Algeria, Tunisia, Libya and Egypt, whence it extends across Sahara into Senegal, Mali, Chad and parts of West Africa lying north of 15°–16°N, i.e. as far as the northern boundary of the distribution of tsetse flies. In the East the disease spreads further south to about 13°N in Sudan and almost up to the Equator in northern Kenya and Somalia (Barotte, 1925; Hoare, 1956). At the beginning of this century surra had been introduced with infected camels into South and South-West Africa but was soon stamped out there.

T. evansi has no true intermediate host, but is transmitted by mechanical inoculator represented chiefly by Tabanid flies.

HISTORY. Surra was known in India from time immemorial but its causative agent was first seen in 1880 by Evans in the blood of infected equines and camels. It was later found in Burma by Steel (1885), who named it *Spirochaete evansi*; its true nature was recognized by Crookshank (1886) and Steel's name was amended to *T. evansi* by Balbiani (1888). Subsequently the surra trypanosome was recovered from diverse mammalian hosts in different countries and in many cases distinct specific or varietal names were given to local strains (*see* synonyms above). However, *T. evansi* is now accepted as the only valid name for the parasite of surra (*cf.* Hoare, 1956).

MORPHOLOGY. In the blood of its mammalian hosts *T. evansi* (Fig. 2.3, a–g) is represented almost exclusively by the thin trypanosomes that are indistinguishable from the slender and intermediate forms of *T. brucei* and the allied human parasites (*see* p. 41) and need not be described separately. Although *T. evansi* is typically monomorphic, like the laboratory strains of *T. brucei*, some strains occasionally exhibit the same type and degree of polymorphism, including the presence of typical and posteronuclear stumpy forms, as *T. brucei* (Fig. 2.4). Such strains are indistinguishable from cyclically transmitted strains of the latter species but polymorphism in *T. evansi* appears only sporadically, in contrast to *T. brucei* in which it is a constant characteristic of normal strains. Although there is considerable variation in the dimensions of various strains and populations of typical *T. evansi*, its overall length distributions have a range from 15 μ to 34 μ (mean 24 μ), comparable to the measurements of the thin forms in the *brucei*-like trypanosomes (Hoare, 1956).

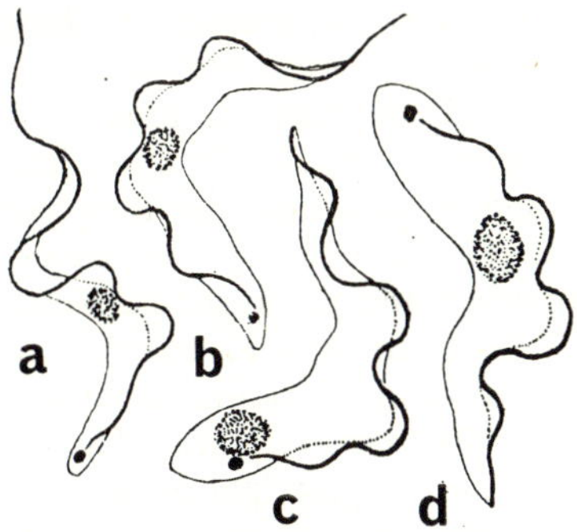

Fig. 2.4 *Trypanosoma evansi*, polymorphic strain (× 2,000). a. Slender, b. Intermediate, and c, d. Stumpy forms (c—posteronuclear). (From Hoare, 1952)

TRANSMISSION. There is abundant evidence that *T. evansi* does not undergo any cycle of development in an intermediate insect-host but is transmitted mechanically by bloodsucking Diptera other than *Glossina*. The most convincing experimental confirmation of the role of mechanical inoculators as vectors of *T. evansi* was provided by Nieschulz (1930) whose exhaustive researches on equine surra in Indonesia demonstrated that all the local species of *Tabanus* transmitted the infection during interrupted feeds with intervals up to one hour. However, stable-flies (*Stomoxys*) proved to be inefficient vectors. In Africa both horse-flies (*Tabanidae*) and stable-flies have been incriminated as transmitters of *T. evansi* (Barotte, 1925; Curasson, 1943). Apparently under field conditions the principal vectors are Tabanids, while in stables transmission is effected by *Stomoxys*. On the other hand, it was demonstrated experimentally (Hoare, 1940) that *T. evansi* is incapable of developing in *Glossina* for the trypanosomes ingested by the fly are killed in the gut within six hours and digested together with the blood. In the case of dogs, the infection can be transmitted by ingestion of meat from infected carcases.

HOST-PARASITE RELATIONS. *T. evansi* is pathogenic to all domestic animals, its effect upon the host depending upon (a) the virulence of the strain of parasite, and (b) the susceptibility of the host, but in various parts of Africa a given host-species may be affected in different ways (*cf.* Hoare, 1956, 1967). In those countries where camels are kept (North Africa, Egypt, Sudan, Somalia) these animals are highly susceptible to infection, the disease running an acute or chronic course and terminating fatally in untreated cases. Horses are similarly affected in North Africa whereas in Sudan and Somalia they are refractory to infection. In cattle and pigs the disease is mild and as a rule symptomless, but in dogs the course of infection is acute. *T. evansi* is thus represented by cameline, equine and bovine hostal strains or xenodemes which differ both in geographical distribution and in the degree of host-restriction (Hoare, 1955, 1956). *T. evansi* is pathogenic to all laboratory mammals which rapidly succumb to the infection.

PHYLOGENETIC RELATIONS OF *T. evansi*. As shown above, *T. evansi* has many features in common with *T. brucei* but—unlike the latter—it is typically monomorphic and occurs only outside the area of distribution of *Glossina*, where it is transmitted mechanically. On the other hand, laboratory strains of *T. brucei* also become monomorphic and lose their power to develop in tsetse flies. The parallelism between these two species leaves no doubt that they are phylogenetically closely related and the available facts provide strong evidence in favour of the origin of *T. evansi* from *T. brucei*. If this hypothesis is correct, the differentiation of *T. evansi* took place in mammalian hosts that had been in contact with tsetse flies infected with *T. brucei*. The clue to this supposition is provided by camels which are the principal hosts of *T. evansi* throughout the vast desert region of Africa lying beyond the northern boundary of the distribution of *Glossina*. Owing to the danger of tsetse-borne trypanosomiasis, camels are not usually taken south of this border but occasionally caravans do penetrate into the tsetse-belt or are attacked by these flies in isolated foci situated to the north of the boundary, thereby exposing the camels to infection with *T. brucei*. On the return of the caravans to tsetse-free areas (e.g. in North Africa and Sudan) the infection was spread among other camels by horse-flies. In the course of time *T. brucei* adapted itself to mechanical transmission, lost its transmissibility by *Glossina* and became monomorphic, i.e. assumed all the characteristics of typical *T. evansi*. From this point of view the occasional appearance of polymorphism in this species can be regarded as an atavistic trait. This problem is discussed in detail by Hoare (1940, 1947, 1956, 1957a, 1967).

11 *Trypanosoma (Trypanozoon) equiperdum* Doflein, 1901.

Synonyms: *T. rougeti* Laveran & Mesnil, 1901; *T. equi* Blacklock & Yorke, 1913.

RELATION TO DISEASE AND DISTRIBUTION. *T. equiperdum* causes dourine, a venereal disease of horses and donkeys, which is transmitted by direct contact during the sexual act. The first symptoms of the disease are associated with oedema of the genitalia but, at a later stage, plaques appear on the skin and the infection becomes generalized, with febrile and nervous symptoms. The disease usually terminates in death after several months or longer.

Formerly dourine was enzootic throughout most continents of the world but with improvement of control measures and the reduction of the equine population this disease is disappearing from more developed countries. The ease with which dourine was spread by imported horses is due to the fact that *T. equiperdum* is not affected by the territorial restrictions imposed upon cyclically transmitted trypanosomes by the climatic requirements of their insect-vectors (Curasson, 1943; Hornby, 1953).

In Africa *T. equiperdum* is prevalent mainly in countries bordering the Mediterranean Sea (Morocco, Algeria, Tunisia, etc.), which are probably the ancestral home of this parasite and in which it co-exists with *T. evansi*. It is conceivable that *T. equiperdum* actually originated from the latter by complete emancipation from the insect-vector (Hoare, 1967). Dourine is also present in South and South-West Africa, as well as Botswana, but it appears to be absent in West Africa (Curasson, 1943; Robinson, 1948a).

HISTORY. Dourine was known to Arabs and other horsemen of Asia and Africa for centuries but the causative organism was first recognized in 1894 by Rouget and named *T. rougeti* by Laveran and Mesnil (1901). However, they were anticipated by Doflein (1901) whose name *T. equiperdum* has a prior claim.

MORPHOLOGY. Though *T. equiperdum* is occasionally found in the blood of horses, it is essentially a tissue parasite which is normally confined to the lesions, and can be detected by examination of the fluid from the local oedemata of the genitalia or from the 'plaques'. In view of the scarcity of parasites in equine hosts, morphological studies on *T. equiperdum* have been carried out almost exclusively in infected laboratory rodents. In the mammalian host *T. equiperdum* (Fig. 2.3, a–g) is indistinguishable from *T. evansi* and from monomorphic laboratory strains of *T. brucei*. Like these species it is typically represented by slender and intermediate forms, measuring 15·5–36 μ (means 25·6–27·7 μ) in total length. However, as in the case of *T. evansi*, *T. equiperdum* occasionally becomes polymorphic, exhibiting typical and posteronuclear stumpy forms. Such a strain was described by Blacklock and Yorke (1913) who regarded it as a new species which they named *T. equi*. The presence of scanty stumpy forms in strains of typical *T. equiperdum* was also noted by Lavier (1933) while the writer had observed a laboratory strain in which a substantial number of such forms suddenly made their appearance.

TRANSMISSION. Dourine is transmitted exclusively by direct contact between stallion and mare during the sexual act, when the trypanosomes are transferred from the infected mucous membrane of the genitalia of the donor to that of the recipient into which they penetrate and thereby initiate the infection. Apparently foals can contract the infection through contamination of the conjunctival and nasal mucous membranes with the infected vaginal discharge of the mare (Robinson, 1948b).

HOST-PARASITE RELATIONS. The course of dourine depends upon the virulence of the trypanosome strain and the host-resistance. In some cases, e.g. in South Africa, the disease runs a prolonged but mild course (Parkin, 1948) while in others, e.g. in North Africa, it is chronic with local involvement of the genital organs and invasion of distant organs and tissues (Barotte, 1925; Curasson, 1943). In stallions the disease is invariably fatal but in mares its course is slower and the mortality lower. In laboratory animals the initial isolation of the trypanosomes from equines presents the greatest difficulty. In murines blood infection may be established only after hundreds of unsuccessful attempts or by first inoculating splenectomized animals. After the strain becomes adapted to these animals it can be passaged through rats and mice indefinitely like *T. evansi* and *T. brucei* (Watson, 1920; Haig & Lund, 1948). On the other hand, *T. equiperdum* can be maintained in rabbits only by inoculation into the testicles (Haig & Lund, 1948).

T. equiperdum is widely employed for various chemotherapeutic and immunological studies on trypanosomes in general. But, because of the difficulty of isolating this species, some of the existing laboratory strains have been in use from the beginning of this century. Since their origin and specific identity are now uncertain, it would be desirable to replace such doubtful strains by authenticated ones of recent isolation.

Subgenus *Pycnomonas*

The subgenus *Pycnomonas* is represented by a single species, *Trypanosoma suis*, which is characterized by stout monomorphic forms with a free flagellum and a small subterminal kinetoplast. It develops in *Glossina* like the tsetse-borne species of *Trypanozoon*, viz. in the midgut and salivary glands. Pigs are the only domestic mammalian hosts.

12 *Trypanosoma (Pycnomonas) suis* Ochmann, 1905.

RELATION TO DISEASE AND DISTRIBUTION. *T. suis* causes in domestic pigs a disease which runs a mild chronic course in adults but is highly pathogenic to young animals which die within two months. *T. suis* is the least known pathogenic trypanosome. The earliest record goes back to 1905 when it was found in a herd of sick pigs from north-eastern Tanzania; in 1912 this parasite was recovered from a warthog in western Tanzania. Nearly half a century had elapsed before *T. suis* was re-discovered, this time in Burundi. It is probable that further studies will reveal the presence of this species in other parts of tropical Africa. The vectors of *T. suis* are tsetse flies.

HISTORY. The history of the discovery of *T. suis* is very confusing. This name was given by Ochmann (1905) to a trypanosome found by him in East African pigs. A similar parasite was later recovered from a warthog by Geisler (1912) and adequately illustrated by Mayer (1912) who identified it with Ochmann's species. However, the early descriptions were inadequate to establish the identity and affinities of this trypanosome and various authors identified it as *T. congolense*, *T. simiae*, or *T. brucei* until Peel and Chardome (1954a) demonstrated conclusively that *T. suis* was a distinct species. Since its development is completed in the salivary glands of *Glossina*, it was referred to the former *brucei*-group as subgroup *Suis* which now constitutes the subgenus *Pycnomonas* (Hoare, 1956, 1966).

MORPHOLOGY. The structure of *T. suis* in the blood of the porcine host was fully described by Peel and Chardome (1954) and by Stephen (1963a). The appearance of this trypanosome is very characteristic and unusual (Fig. 2.5, a,b). Its body is very broad (*ca.* 3 μ) and short; the posterior end usually terminates in a short point, but sometimes it is rounded; a free flagellum (*ca.* 3 μ) is typically present. The small kinetoplast is usually situated near the posterior end and in the majority of cases occupies a marginal position, while the voluminous nucleus lies in the anterior part of the body and the undulating membrane is conspicuous. The total length of *T. suis* has a range from 13 μ to 19 μ (mean 16 μ) with a normal distribution, indicating that this species is monomorphic.

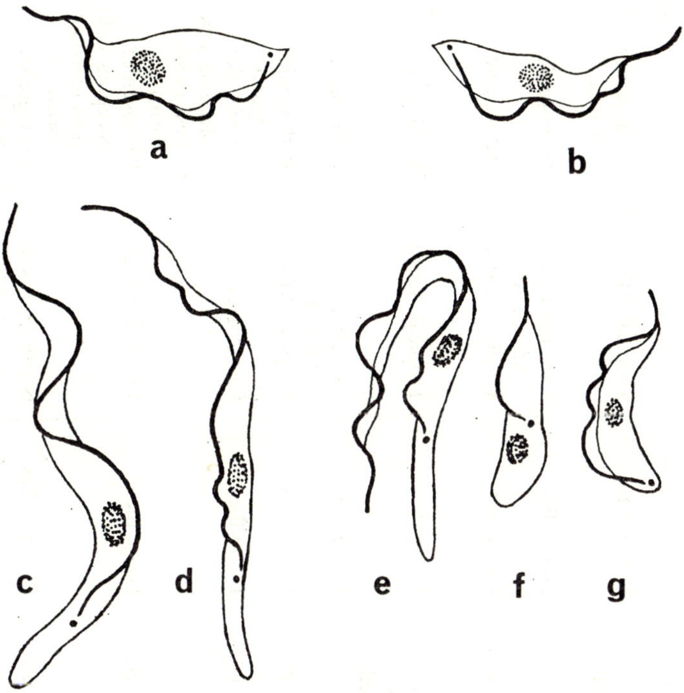

Fig. 2.5 Subgenus *Pycnomonas* (×2,000). *Trypanosoma suis:* a, b. Blood forms; c–g. Developmental stages in *Glossina*: c. Trypomastigote form in midgut; d, e. Proventricular forms in cardia; f. Epimastigote form in salivary gland; g. Metatrypanosome in hypopharynx. (After Peel and Chardome, 1954)

TRANSMISSION AND CYCLE IN VECTOR. Up to the present only two species of *Glossina* have been incriminated as vectors of *T. suis* in Burundi. In the eastern savanna area it is transmitted by *G. brevipalpis* while in the central rain forest this species is replaced by *G. vanhoofi* (van den Berghe *et al.*, 1963). The incidence of infection in wild flies of the former species varies from 1% to 2%, according to the season.

The cycle of *T. suis* in the tsetse fly (Peel & Chardome, 1954) is comparable to that of the *brucei*-like trypanosomes (Figs. 1.6; 2.5, c–g; Table 1.1). The Belgian authors did not define the stages of development but these can be recognized and pieced together from their illustrations. In the midgut and cardia the flagellates are in the trypomastigote stage, represented by long forms with the kinetoplast situated about halfway between the bluntly pointed posterior end and the nucleus. These flagellates are larger than the corresponding gut forms of the *brucei*-like trypanosomes, and—as in the latter—the proventricular forms are more slender than those in the midgut. The proventricular forms invade the salivary glands where they become stouter and shorter and assume the epimastigote stage, eventually giving rise to the metatrypanosomes which

TABLE 2.1

African trypanosomes of medical and veterinary interest

Parasite	Mammalian hosts	Susceptible laboratory animals	Vectors	Distribution	Effect upon host
1 *Trypanosoma (Duttonella) vivax*	Bovines, sheep, goats, equines, dogs, antelopes	Rodents (adapted)	Tsetse flies	Tropical Africa	Pathogenic: Souma
2 *T. (D.) uniforme*	Bovines, sheep, goats, antelopes	None	Tsetse flies	East and Central Africa, Angola	Pathogenic
3 *Trypanosoma (Nannomonas) congolense*	Bovines, sheep, goats, equines, pigs, dogs, antelopes	Rodents, etc.	Tsetse flies	Tropical Africa	Pathogenic
4 *T. (N.) simiae*	Pigs, warthogs possibly: bovines, equines, camels	Monkeys, rabbits (adapted)	Tsetse flies	Tropical Africa	Pathogenic
5 *Trypanosoma (Pycnomonas) suis*	Pigs, warthogs, bushpigs	None	Tsetse flies	Tanzania, Burundi	Pathogenic
6 *Trypanosoma (Trypanozoon) brucei*	All domestic mammals, antelopes	Rodents, etc.	Tsetse flies	Tropical Africa	Pathogenic: Nagana
7 *T. (T.) rhodesiense*	Man, bovines, antelopes	Rodents, etc.	Tsetse flies	East Africa	Pathogenic: Sleeping sickness (acute form)
8 *T. (T.) gambiense*	Man	Rodents, etc.	Tsetse flies	Tropical Africa	Pathogenic: Sleeping sickness (chronic form)
9 *T. (T.) evansi*	Bovines, equines, camels, dogs, etc.	Rodents, etc.	Tabanid flies	North and N.W. Africa, Sudan, Somalia	Pathogenic: Surra
10 *T. (T.) equiperdum*	Equines	Rabbits, rodents	None (transmission by coitus)	North, South, and S.W. Africa	Pathogenic: Dourine

show some resemblance to the blood forms of *T. suis*. Like these, they have a short free flagellum, which distinguishes them from the typical metatrypanosomes in *Trypanozoon* (Table 1.1). The metatrypanosomes migrate to the hypopharynx and may overflow into the food canal of the proboscis. The entire invertebrate cycle takes about twenty-eight days and the fly remains infective for the rest of its life.

HOST-PARASITE RELATIONS. *T. suis* is a specific parasite of the Suidae. Under natural conditions it occurs in wild animals, viz. warthogs (*Phacochoerus aethiopicus*), bushpigs (*Potamochoerus* sp.) and forest hogs (*Hylochoerus* sp.) which are presumably the reservoir hosts of this trypanosome (van den Berghe & Zaghi, 1963). Among livestock the only animal affected by *T. suis* is the domestic pig. Other mammals appear to be refractory to infection with this parasite, for all attempts to infect various laboratory rodents, domestic ruminants, donkeys, dogs and some primates were unsuccessful (Peel & Chardome, 1954).

The main characteristics of the pathogenic African trypanosomes are summarized in Table 2.1.

Chapter 3

Ultrastructure of *Trypanosoma* and Relation to Function

K. VICKERMAN

Our knowledge of trypanosome fine structure is based largely upon the study by electron microscopy of ultra-thin sections of fixed material embedded in an electron-transparent plastic supporting medium. Some information has also been gained by the examination of whole mounts of finely disintegrated organisms or surface replicas of such material. Living material cannot, as yet, be examined satisfactorily with the electron microscope. A more detailed account of trypanosome fine structure is given by Rudzinska and Vickerman (1968).

In an early study, bloodstream trypanosomes were disrupted in distilled water, leaving only the pellicle and flagellum intact. When such 'ghosts' were shadowed with a shower of metal atoms, their structure was thrown into relief, revealing in the pellicle longitudinal fibrils which run from one end of the body to the other (*see* Scanga, 1959). Sections of trypanosomes show that these fibrils are actually hollow (Fig. 3.1) and belong to a class of cytoplasmic organelles called microtubules (Schulz and MacClure, 1961). They underlie the membrane which limits the entire body of the animal. On analogy with other cells, it seems likely that in trypanosomes the microtubules constitute a deformable corset maintaining the elongated shape of the body.

Sections of the salivarian trypanosomes in their bloodstream phase show that the three-ply surface membrane (Fig. 3.1) is enveloped by a coat of amorphous material which is lost when the flagellate develops in culture or in the tsetse fly. In *T. rhodesiense* (and probably in others of the group) the coat is reacquired as the epimastigote forms transform into metacyclic trypanosomes. The variable antigens, detected in bloodstream trypanosomes by the agglutination reaction, must be located in this surface coat. The fact that different variants lose their antigenic identity and assume a common serotype when they are grown in the culture tube is explained by loss of the coat to reveal the naked surface membrane: the reversion of all strains to a basic antigen at the metacyclic stage corresponds to acquisition of the coat. The fact that the bloodstream and metacyclic forms are more positively charged than culture and fly midgut forms can be correlated with the presence of a coat in the former and absence of a coat in the latter.

One of the most striking features of the living trypanosome is the undulating membrane formed by the flagellum running along the pellicle. In flagellates which have been crudely disrupted in the manner described above the flagellum separates from the pellicle and in some electron micrographs can be seen to be composed of two parallel rod-like structures (Ray *et al.*, 1955), only one of which has its origin in the basal body. More details are revealed in transverse

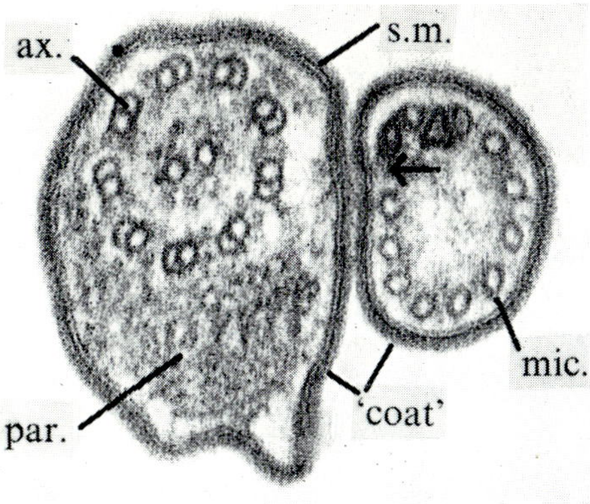

Fig. 3.1 Transverse section of anterior end of *T. rhodesiense* slender bloodstream form showing body (right) with attached flagellum (left). Both body and flagellum are limited by a 3-ply surface membrane (s.m.) which is covered by a coat of amorphous material. This surface coat may contain the variable antigens of the bloodstream trypanosome. Inside the flagellum note the axoneme (ax.) composed of nine double *plus* two single tubules, also the paraxial rod (par.). Within the body note the pellicular microtubules. The gap in these tubules (arrowed) corresponds to the row of stud-like structures which bind the flagellum to the pellicle; this section falls between 2 adjacent studs. (×92,000.)

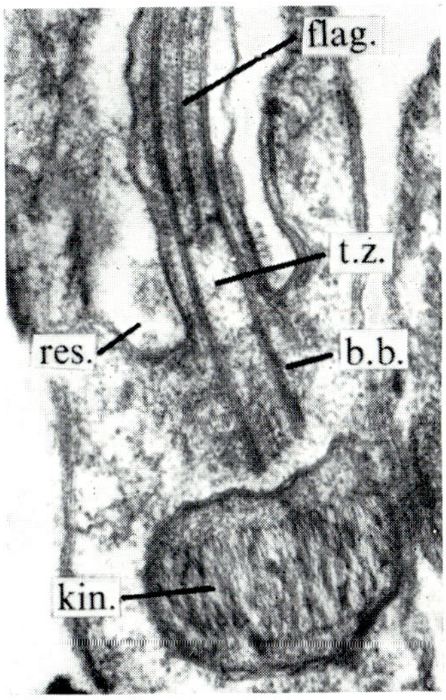

Fig. 3.2 *T. theileri*. Longitudinal section of the epimastigote form in the region of the flagellum base showing the basal body (b.b.), transitional zone (t.z.) and shaft (flag.) of the flagellum in relation to the flagellar pocket or reservoir (*res.*). The large fibrous kinetoplast (*kin.*) is surrounded by a double membranous mitochondrial envelope which shows no apparent connection to the basal body. (×35,000.)

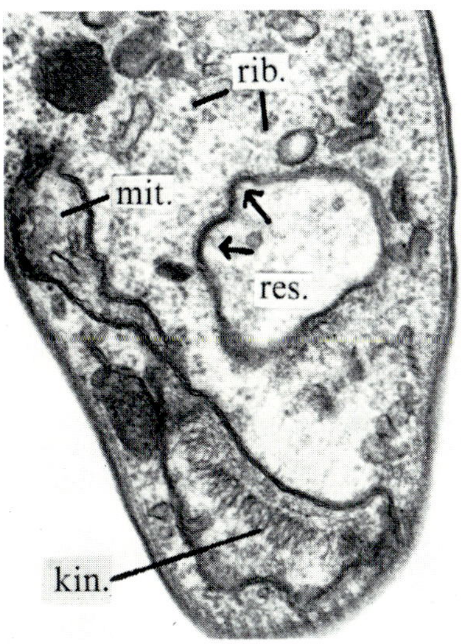

Fig. 3.3 *T. congolense*. Longitudinal section of bloodstream form showing kinetoplast (*kin.*) and part of the mitochondrial canal (*mit.*) with internal cristae. Ribosomes (rib.) abound in the surrounding cytoplasm. The reservoir (*res.*) shows bulges (arrowed) which may represent incipient pinocytosis. The basal body of the flagellum is out of the plane of this picture. (×38,000.)

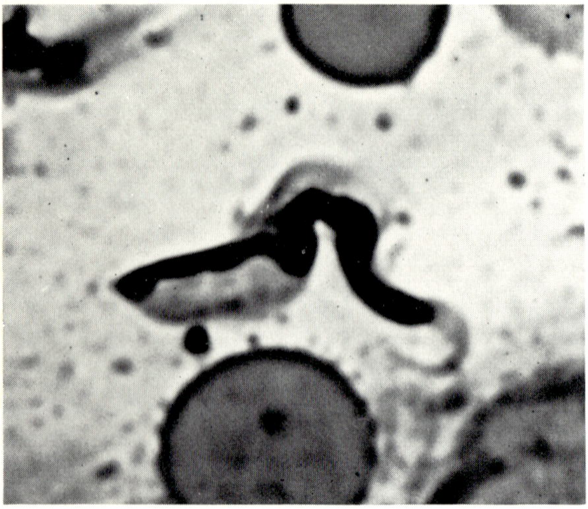

Fig. 3.4 *T. brucei*. Intermediate bloodstream form which has been stained for the mitochondrial enzyme NAD diaphorase so that the mitochondrion is revealed as a single canal running the length of the body. (×3,500.)

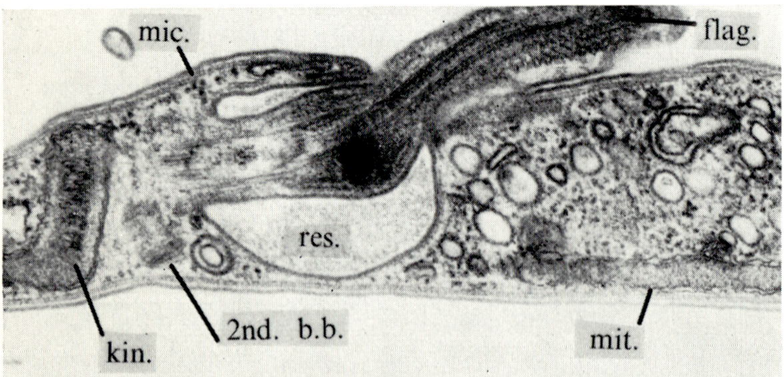

Fig. 3.5 *T. rhodesiense*. Longitudinal section of slender bloodstream form in the region of the base of the flagellum (*flag*.) showing the kinetoplast (*kin*.) and profiles of the mitochondrial canal (*mit*.) which lacks cristae. The second basal body (2nd b.b.) is shown in oblique section close to the reservoir (*res*.). (×34,000.)

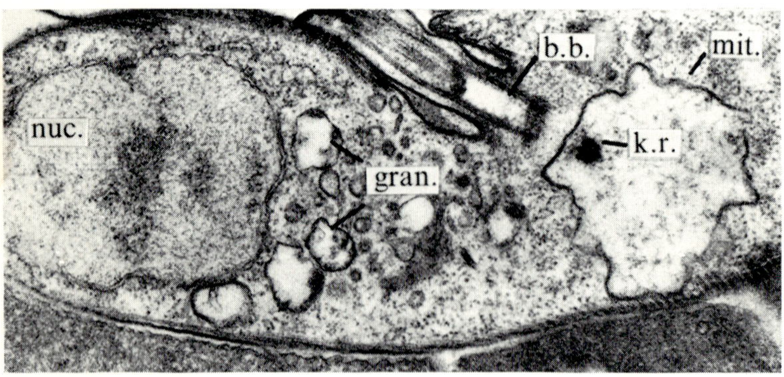

Fig. 3.6 *T. equinum*. Longitudinal section of part of posterior end to show the dense fibrous knot (k.r.) that replaces the kinetoplast in naturally akinetoplastic trypanosomes. The membranous mitochondrial envelope remains (*mit*.). Granules (*gran*.) lying close to the nucleus (*nuc*.) may represent the location of the L-α-glycerophosphate oxidase system. (×22,000.)

sections of trypanosomes (Vickerman, 1962) which show that the flagellum is bounded by a coated membrane similar in appearance to the pellicular membrane and that the two membranes are apposed, but not confluent, in the region of the undulating membrane (Fig. 3.1). A row of fibrous stud-like structures attaches the flagellum to the pellicle and so maintains contact while the flagellum is beating. In some sections the pellicle is seen to be thrown into a ridge along the line of attachment to the flagellum and it must be assumed tentatively that the undulating membrane that can be seen represents a deformation of the pellicle rather than one of the flagellum. The two internal rod-like structures of the flagellum have a characteristic sub-structure. One of them, the axial filament complex or axoneme, has a structure common to the flagella and cilia of almost all animal and plant cells, this consisting basically of nine tubule doublets arranged peripherally and two single microtubules centrally, as seen in cross section (Fig. 3.1). The other rod is known as the accessory filament complex or paraxial rod and has a lattice-like architecture.

The axoneme arises from the basal body which lies just below the floor of the flask-shaped reservoir or flagellar pocket (Fig. 3.2). The basal body is cylindrical and similar in its overall plan to the flagellum, but there are nine peripheral triplets and no central microtubules evident in transverse section. In the transition zone between the basal body and the axoneme the triplets become doublets but the two central microtubules arise from a double plate which traverses the flagellum slightly farther along the shaft (Figs. 3.2, 3.5). The paraxial rod is not represented in the first part of the flagellum which passes through the cavity of the reservoir and it appears only as the flagellum emerges to form the undulating membrane. How these various structures collaborate to produce contraction of the flagellum is not known. Trypanosomes are unusual in that waves of contraction proceed from tip to base instead of *vice versa* as in other flagella, yet no ultrastructural peculiarities absent from all functionally conventional flagella have been discerned in the trypanosome locomotory organoid. A second basal body, which lacks an appended flagellum, is often seen lying alongside the first, and this may represent a daughter basal body formed in anticipation of cell division.

During cyclical development of trypanosomes as seen with the light microscope the basal body is intimately associated with the kinetoplast. The nature of the latter was completely unknown until trypanosomes were studied by electron microscopy (*see* Steinert, 1960). The kinetoplast is unique as a cytoplasmic structure in containing readily stainable quantities of genetic material, deoxyribonucleic acid (DNA). DNA in such quantities is almost invariably found in the nucleus. Early electron micrographs of sectioned trypanosomes (*see*, for example, Clark and Wallace, 1960) showed a disc of longitudinally-orientated fibres in the kinetoplast region, the disc being enveloped by a capsule composed of two membranes, and the proximal end of the basal body lying close to (but not obviously attached to) the outer membrane (Fig. 3.2). A clue to the function of the kinetoplast came from the observation that the kinetoplast capsule was often seen to be continuous with canals having typical mitochondrial structure—that is with a double-membranous wall of which the inner membrane is drawn out into *cristae* (plate- or finger-like projections) (Fig. 3.3). It is now known from electron micrographs of serial sections (Mühlpfordt and Bayer, 1961) and from cytochemical staining (Vickerman, 1965) (Fig. 3.4) that the kinetoplast forms part of a single mitochondrion extending from one end of the trypanosome to the other (Fig. 3.7). In some trypanosomes (e.g. *T. vivax*) it is often difficult to distinguish a kinetoplast capsule region in the mitochondrion and it seems likely that the fibrous disc alone represents the kinetoplast as visualized by the light microscopist. This contention is borne out by the fact that the so-called akinetoplastic or dyskinetoplastic strains of trypanosomes retain the mitochrondrial envelope and lack the fibrous material (Mühlpfordt, 1964). At division the whole mitochondrion cleaves longitudinally, starting in the region of the nucleus, the cleft continuing forwards and backwards to split the expanded kinetoplast in two (Vickerman, 1966b).

Refined cytochemical and ultrastructural techniques have revealed the existence of small amounts of DNA in several self-perpetuating cytoplasmic structures, notably chloroplasts, mitochondria and the basal bodies of cilia (Vickerman, 1966a). The kinetoplast is a self-perpetuating structure for if lost it cannot be regenerated by the flagellate. The fibres of the kinetoplast are mensurally identical with those of the DNA in the mitochondria of higher organisms (Nass, Nass and Afzelius, 1965) and it seems more than likely that the kinetoplast represents the condensed DNA of the single massive trypanosome mitochondrion (Grassé and Pyne, 1965).

The form of the mitochondrion varies slightly from species to species but most strikingly from one stage in the life-cycle to another within the same species. The most dramatic changes are seen during the life-cycle of the polymorphic trypanosomes of the *brucei* group. Here in the slender forms the mitochondrion is represented by a simple canal passing forwards from the kinetoplast and a short post-kinetoplastic pouch (Mühlpfordt and Bayer, 1961; Vickerman, 1962) (Fig. 3.5). Internal *cristae* are almost absent at this stage, but they appear to be acquired as the flagellates transform through intermediate to stumpy forms (Fig. 3.7) and the width of the mitochondrial canal increases (Vickerman, 1965). In the trypomastigote forms of the tsetse fly midgut and proventriculus the kinetoplast moves to a more anterior position in the body and the mitochondrial system becomes transformed into a network of canals emanating from the kinetoplast in both directions and now having abundant *cristae* (Vickerman, 1962). The epimastigote (crithidial) forms of the salivary glands of the fly show a further forward advance of the kinetoplast to a prenuclear position (Fig. 3.8), and maintain this elaborate mitochondrial morphology (Vickerman, 1966). In the next stage the trypomastigote metacyclic forms show reduction of the mitochondrial network to a simple canal again, with reduced number of *cristae*, approaching the condition in the bloodstream forms.

This cycle of structural changes in the mitochondrion of *T. brucei*-like trypanosomes is of interest in interpreting the physiological and gross morphological changes which are known to occur in cyclical transformation. Mitochondria are concerned primarily with respiration, more specifically with the process of oxidative phosphorylation—the synthesis of adenosine triphosphate (ATP) as a result of oxidative reactions—to provide energy for the cell. In respiration, glucose is usually broken down by a series of reactions (glycolysis) to produce, largely, pyruvic acid: some ATP is synthesized (2 molecules for every glucose molecule) as a result of glycolysis and some reduction of pyridine nucleotide carriers takes place. The mitochondria contain the enzyme system (Krebs cycle) for the step-wise oxidation of pyruvic acid to carbon dioxide and water with the reduction of more pyridine nucleotides, and also the cytochrome chain of carriers which brings about oxidation of the reduced pyridine nucleotides in the presence of atmospheric oxygen. The energy from oxidation of the reduced nucleotides is used to synthesize several molecules of ATP (12 for each molecule of pyruvic acid, 36 for each original molecule of glucose).

Slender bloodstream trypanosomes appear to lack both the Krebs cycle of enzymes and the cytochrome chain components: pyruvic acid from glycolysis is excreted by these forms and reduced pyridine nucleotides oxidized by a non-mitochondrial pathway (the glycerophosphate oxidase system) with no concomitant ATP synthesis, so that all the flagellate's energy is derived from the small amount of ATP derived from glycolysis. To provide sufficient energy massive amounts of glucose from the host's blood must be taken in by the trypanosome and this wasteful utilization of respiratory substrate supported by an ample oxygen supply to satisfy the demands of the glycerophosphate oxidase system (Fulton & Spooner, 1959; Grant, Sargent & Ryley, 1961; Danforth, 1967).

On entering the fly the trypanosome finds itself in stagnant blood with diminishing glucose and oxygen supplies. It must cease its wasteful bloodstream metabolism and assume a more economical way of producing energy. This it does by synthesizing mitochondrial components (Krebs cycle enzymes, cytochromes) which enable it to oxidize pyruvic acid completely. This switch from a functionally inactive to a functionally active mitochondrion is registered by the structural changes described above—the appearance of *cristae* and proliferation of the entire mitochondrion into a reticulum. There is some evidence from both enzyme studies and ultrastructural observations that at least partial activation of the mitochondrion is initiated in the intermediate and stumpy bloodstream forms (Vickerman, 1965), so that these forms would be, by virtue of their metabolism, pre-adapted to life in the tsetse fly. Why the switch should begin here may become apparent when more is known of the stimulus eliciting the transformation of slender into stumpy forms. The mitochondrial regression that takes place in the salivary glands of the vector is presumably indicative of reduced mitochondrial activity, but as yet there are no detailed enzyme studies to support this part of the hypothesis.

Little is known of the metabolism of *T. congolense* and *T. vivax* but these monomorphic forms appear to resemble the stumpy forms of *T. brucei* in that they have a partially active mitochondrial tube with *cristae* (Fig. 3.3) in the bloodstream phase (Vickerman, 1965). Preliminary electron microscope studies show that their epimastigote forms in the tsetse proboscis have a much expanded mitochondrial network and so here too mitochondrial changes are a feature of cyclical development. It has been supposed (Vickerman, 1962) that the proliferation of the mitochondrial canal system within the confines of the trypanosome pellicle might be responsible for the shift in position of the kinetoplast when the trypanosome enters the fly. There is every indication from both

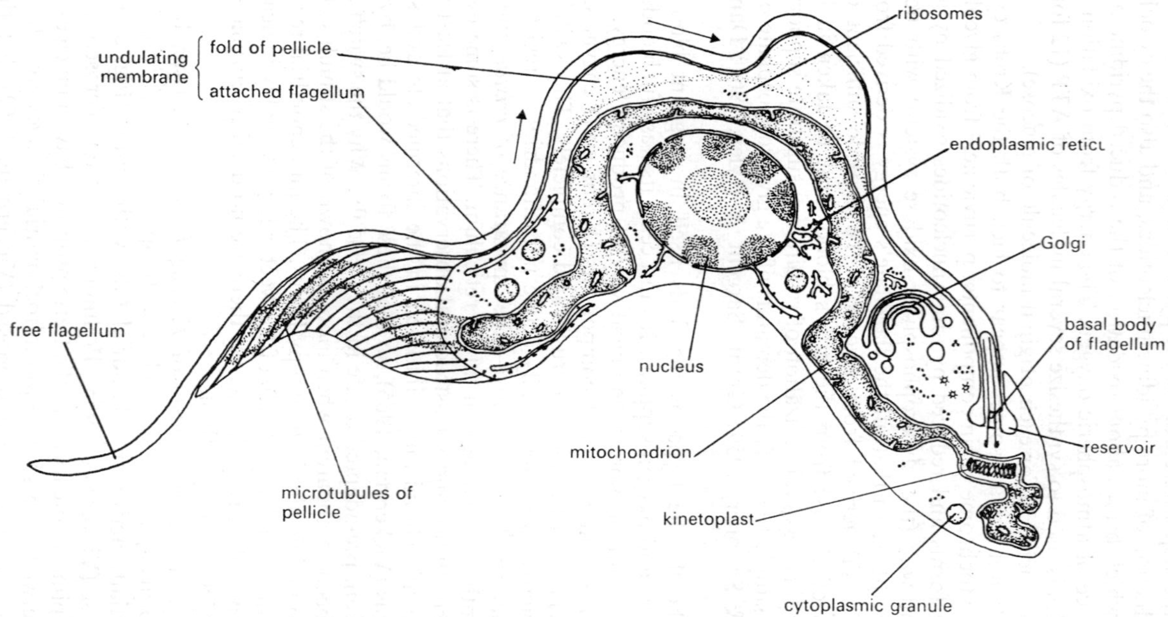

Fig. 3.7 Diagram of trypomastigote intermediate bloodstream form of *Trypanosoma rhodesiense* as seen at the level of the electron microscope. The arrows along the flagellum indicate the direction of travel of flagellar waves. Pellicular microtubules are shown only at the anterior end of the flagellate. Note the single mitochondrial canal.

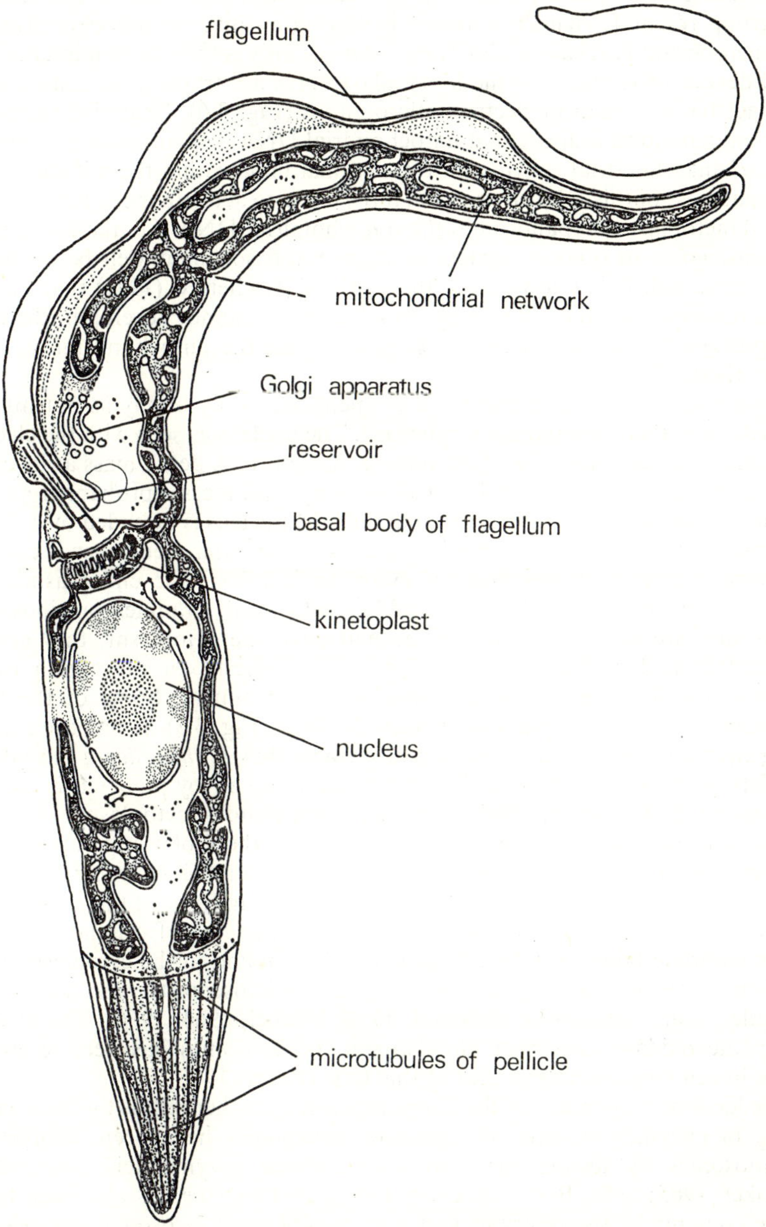

Fig. 3.8 Diagram of epimastigote stage of *Trypanosoma rhodesiense* as seen at the level of the electron microscope. Pellicular microtubules are shown only at the posterior end of the body. Note that the mitochondrion is now a well developed network of canals.

biochemical and ultrastructural studies that the trypanosomes of the *T. evansi* sub-group resemble slender *T. brucei* in having an inactive mitochondrion. In dyskinetoplastic *T. evansi* and in *T. equinum* not only is the simple mitochondrial canal devoid of *cristae*, but the kinetoplast fibres are transformed into a small compact body as seen in electron micrographs (Fig. 3.6). Extensive studies on yeast mitochondria indicate that mitochondrial DNA is involved in the arrangement of mitochondrial enzymes into functional units within the mitochondrion and intactness of this DNA is essential if the cell is to activate the mitochondrion. In dyskinetoplastic trypanosomes the mitochondrial DNA (i.e. the kinetoplast) has undergone an obvious structural change and so might well be no longer fully functional. It is known from the work of Reichenow (1941) that *T. gambiense* rendered dyskinetoplastic by drug treatment cannot develop in the tsetse fly—presumably because it can no longer activate the mitochondrion in order to live there.

Other trypanosome structures will be mentioned only briefly as not much is known about their functional morphology. The nucleus as seen with the electron microscope in sections shows little internal structure. A dense mass at its centre represents the karyosome and less distinct peripheral masses probably represent chromosomal material. As in all animal cells the nucleus is bounded by a double membranous envelope punctured by pores, and the outer membrane is continuous with a system of membranous cytoplasmic tubes—the endoplasmic reticulum. Many of these tubes are studded with small granules or ribosomes. Ribosomes are also found free in the matrix of the cytoplasm: they contain ribonucleic acid and are centres of protein synthesis. In the region of the reservoir membranous tubes and vesicles are prominent. Some of the latter may represent stages in pinocytosis (cell drinking, Fig. 3.3). It has been shown using electron dense protein (ferritin) as a tracer that *T. rhodesiense* can take up droplets of the surrounding medium from the reservoir by pinocytosis (Brown, Armstrong & Valentine, 1965). Another membranous cytoplasmic structure found in trypanosomes as in many other cells, is the Golgi apparatus—a pile of compressed sacks lying between the nucleus and the reservoir (Fig. 3.7), except in postero-nucleate *T. brucei* where it lies just in front of the nucleus. The Golgi apparatus of the cell is involved in the packaging of cellular secretions into membrane-bound vesicles. Several vesicles abound in the cytoplasm, some of them large enough to be seen by light microscopists who term them 'granules' (Bird, Molloy & Ormerod, 1966; Michel, 1964, 1966). The glycerophosphate oxidase system of bloodstream trypanosomes has been shown to reside in cell structures (Fig. 3.6) of this type (Ryley, 1966).

One identifiable product of the Golgi apparatus in other cells is the lysosome—a bag of enzymes involved in digestion. Lysosomes have been identified in trypanosomes by testing for their characteristic enzyme acid phosphatase (Brooker, 1965; Seed, Byram & Gam, 1967). This enzyme has also been found in the contents of the reservoir and it is possible that lysosomal enzymes are liberated into the reservoir to effect a certain amount of predigestion of material to be taken up by pinocytosis. Alternatively lysosomes may fuse with the pinocytotic vesicles and the enzymes effect digestion there.

Chapter 4

Techniques for the Detection of Trypanosome Infections

J. R. BAKER

DETECTION OF INFECTION IN MAMMALS

During the early stage of human trypanosomiasis, and throughout the infection of other mammals, diagnosis is dependent upon the demonstration of trypanosomes in the peripheral blood or lymph. The parasites may be sought by direct microscopy, using fresh or stained preparations. Often, however, particularly in human infections due to *T. gambiense* and infections of other mammals, parasitaemia may be so low that trypanosomes cannot be detected by this method even after attempting to concentrate the organisms present in the blood. It may then be necessary to use indirect methods of determining their presence—either by inoculating blood (or other fluids) into a suitable culture medium (cultivation *in vitro*) or into a susceptible mammal (cultivation *in vivo*). Failing this, evidence of the parasites' presence may be sought by serological and other tests.

In the more advanced stages of human infection with *T. rhodesiense* or *T. gambiense*, when the parasites have invaded the central nervous system, they may be looked for in the cerebrospinal fluid (CSF) by methods similar to those used in examining blood. Or, again, their presence may be inferred indirectly from their effect on the cell count and protein concentration. Although *T. brucei* is known to invade the CSF of at least some wild and domestic animals (McCulloch, 1967; Hornby, 1952), examination of this fluid is seldom if ever used as a diagnostic aid in animals other than man, partly no doubt due to the technical difficulties involved. These various techniques are described in more detail below and the practical application of them in the diagnosis of human trypanosomiasis is further considered in Chapter 35.

Blood Examination

Collection of Samples

Small amounts of blood, suitable for direct microscopic examination, are easily obtained from human beings by pricking a finger or ear-lobe: the skin should be sterilized with alcohol and allowed to dry before being pierced: the needle (unless disposable stylets are used) must be carefully cleaned and dried in the same way before use on the next patient. From other mammals, blood can often be obtained by similarly piercing a marginal ear-vein: from laboratory rodents and certain other small mammals, the tail-tip can be either pricked or cut off with scissors to obtain a few drops of blood. The preparation of smears for microscopical examination is described below (pp. 69–73).

Larger volumes of blood, such as would be required for inoculation into cultures or susceptible animals, or for certain serological tests, may be obtained by venipuncture performed under strict asepsis (in man, the median basilic vein at the bend of the elbow is often used). An anticoagulant is necessary unless serum alone is required: either sodium citrate (sterile 3% aqueous solution, used in the proportion of about 1 volume to 4 or 5 volumes of blood) or heparin, 1 unit of which is sufficient to prevent clotting of 5 ml. of blood (heparin is best prepared as a solution of 100 or 1,000 units per ml. of 0·9% saline; the syringe is then rinsed with this solution and enough remains in the nozzle and needle). If the blood is to be used for inoculation into a susceptible animal, the use of heparin is preferable to that of sodium citrate: blood collected for inoculation to Weinman's medium requires the addition of a special anticoagulant (p. 77). Blood collected with an anticoagulant is not suitable for the preparation of stained films.

Direct Examination

Fresh Preparations

A drop of blood is placed on a slide, covered with a coverslip and examined with a microscope for the presence of trypanosomes. It is advisable not to use an oil-immersion objective; a total magnification of about 400 diameters is adequate, as the actively motile organisms can be readily detected by the agitation they produce among the erythrocytes (care should be taken actually to see a trypanosome, however, since a rather similar agitation can be produced by exflagellating malarial microgametocytes or even, on a larger scale, microfilariae). The use of phase-contrast illumination is helpful, but is not essential: if direct illumination is used, the sub-stage diaphragm should be closed to a greater extent than normal. Fresh preparations should be examined as soon as possible after being made: if some delay is inevitable, drying should be prevented by sealing the coverslip to the slide with petroleum jelly, melted paraffin wax or nail varnish.

Stained Preparations

If the blood cannot be examined immediately, dried films must be prepared for subsequent staining and microscopic examination. Such films may be of two types—thin or thick. The former allow better preservation of the morphology of any trypanosomes (or other parasites) present, and hence are useful in morphological differentiation of species; the latter (*see* below, p. 72) are particularly useful in detecting infection when trypanosomes are too scanty to be discovered in a thin film.

PREPARATION OF THIN FILMS. To prepare a thin film, a drop of fresh blood (without anticoagulant) is collected on the narrow edge of a microscope slide: this edge is then placed on another slide lying on a flat surface, so that the blood drop lies in the acute angle between the two slides: the inclined slide is then pushed along the recumbent one so that the blood is pulled behind it and spread in a thin layer over the stationary slide (Fig. 4.1): the latter is then dried as quickly as possible by waving in air, or in front of a fan or air conditioner, or—in very humid conditions—by placing it in a desiccator: heat should not be used. The thickness of the film depends upon the amount of blood used and the angle between the two slides: the more nearly vertical the inclined slide ('spreader'), the thicker the film. Ideally, films should be prepared so that the erythrocytes are fairly close together but not overlapping. Thin films should be stained as soon as possible (within a day or two, especially in hot, humid climates): until this is done, they must be kept dry and protected from flies and other insects, which will rapidly eat the blood off an unprotected slide. If storage before staining is unavoidable, the slides should be wrapped in tissue paper and stored in a desiccator, preferably in a refrigerator (Shute & Maryon, 1966).

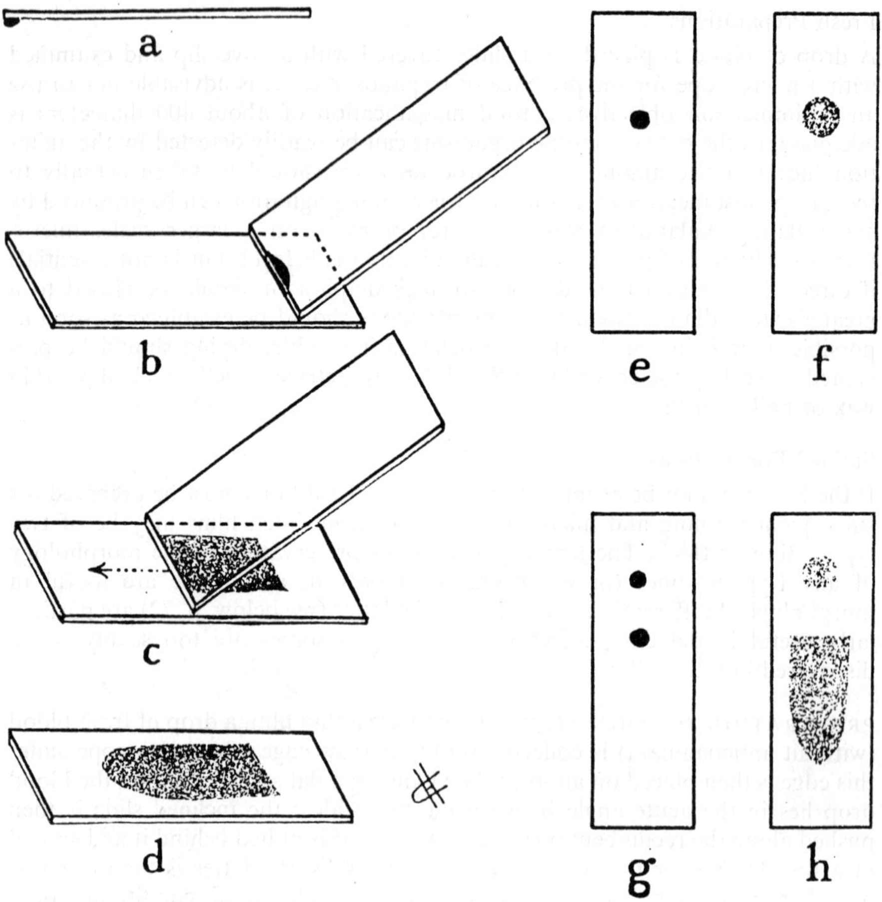

Fig. 4.1 Diagram illustrating the preparation of blood films. a–d. Thin films: a. drop of blood on end of spreading slide; b, c. spreading the blood; d. the finished film; e, f. Thick films: e. drop of blood on slide; f. the finished film; g, h. Thick and thin films on the same slide. (From Hoare, 1949)

STAINING. The best stain for general purposes is Giemsa's, though Leishman's and Wright's may also be used. Some brands of Giemsa's stain are less satisfactory than others.[1] Giemsa's stain can be purchased either in solution or in powder form. The former is more convenient to use but the latter is easier and lighter to transport and so its use may be indicated in certain circumstances. The powder can be dissolved as follows (Shute & Maryon, 1966).

> 3·8 g. of stain are added to a bottle or flask containing about 50 glass beads, together with 250 ml. of glycerol and 250 ml. of methanol (both liquids *must* be dry and pure: in particular, the methanol must be free from acetone). The bottle is closed, and shaken with a circular movement for 2–3 minutes every half-hour: it should be shaken at least six times. The stain should be stored in a tightly-closed bottle, protected from strong light.

The stock solution of stain is diluted for use with distilled water of pH 7·2–7·4: this can be prepared by adding lithium carbonate solution (0·5%) to distilled water containing a little bromothymol blue until the indicator becomes greenish-blue (nearer to green than blue), or even, if no other means is available, by boiling distilled water for ten minutes or more to expel the carbon dioxide. It is usually easiest, however, to prepare buffered distilled water as follows:

Na_2HPO_4	3·0 g.
KH_2PO_4	0·6 g.
Distilled water	1 litre

(7·5 g. of $Na_2HPO_4 . 12H_2O$ may be used if the anhydrous salt is not available)

This solution is stable but should be kept in the dark (or in a brown glass bottle) as algae grow readily in it. If distilled water is not available, filtered rain water is an acceptable substitute. Slides are preferably placed face downwards in the stain to avoid a deposit on the film: flat, square dishes to accommodate three slides with two ridges on the base to raise the slides slightly are convenient.[2] Otherwise, any form of staining dish may be used, or the slides may be laid face upwards on two pieces of glass rod resting across a sink: rinsing will, however, have to be done very carefully (though briefly) to remove most of the inevitable deposit. The method of staining is as follows:

1. Fix the thin film by covering it with (or immersing it in) methanol (which must be dry) for ½ minute or more (fixation is almost instantaneous).
2. Shake off the excess methanol and place the slide preferably face downwards into a solution of Giemsa's stain, 1 part and buffered distilled water, 10 parts.
3. Allow to stain for 50–60 minutes (or up to 90 minutes: it is difficult to overstain).
4. Remove the slide from the stain and rinse for 1 second (*not more*) in a gentle stream of tap water.

[1] 'Revector' brand (Hopkin and Williams, Chadwell Heath, Essex, England) is one of the better brands.

[2] Obtainable (made of polythene) from the Storekeeper, London School of Hygiene and Tropical Medicine, Keppel Street, London WC1, England.

5. Place the slide upright to dry (do *not* use heat to accelerate drying: an air current from a fan, etc., may be used if necessary).

It is usually unnecessary to cover thin films with a cover slip unless they are to be used repeatedly for demonstration purposes. The films may be examined directly with an oil-immersion objective (×100, or ×50 if available): if more rapid searching is required, a ×40 dry objective can be used, provided the unmounted film is covered with a thin layer of immersion oil, spread gently with the finger. After use, if the slide is to be kept, the oil must be removed with xylene (neutralized if necessary by the addition of calcium carbonate). If it is desired to use a cover-slip, mounting media with a canada balsam base should *not* be used, since they may become acid and decolourize the films. Strictly neutral media such as 'Euparal'[1] are satisfactory.

Stained films should be stored in the dark and in a reasonably dry atmosphere: in humid climates, storage in a desiccator may be advisable.

STAINED THICK BLOOD FILMS are useful for the detection of scanty parasites, though the latter's morphology may be less well displayed than in a thin film.

PREPARATION OF THICK FILMS. To make a thick film, 2–3 drops of blood are collected (p. 68) onto a clean slide and spread with a needle, or the corner of another slide, into an area about 1 cm. in diameter (Fig. 4.1). The resultant film should be of such a thickness that, when dry, small print (e.g. newsprint, or the figures on a wristwatch dial) can just be read through it. The preparation must be placed flat while it dries thoroughly, and protected from insects. Gentle heat during drying helps to prevent the film from floating off the slide during staining: 2–3 hours or more at 37°C (not higher) should be adequate, but Shute and Maryon (1966) recommend leaving thick films at 37°C overnight or heating over an electric lamp (at about 60–70°C) for 7 minutes.

When dry, the film is stained without fixation in Giemsa's stain. As the stain is in aqueous solution, lysis of the erythrocytes occurs and the contained haemoglobin escapes: thus it is possible to examine a much thicker layer of blood than would be possible with a fixed, thin film. If an alcoholic stain such as Leishman's is used (which is not recommended), the film must be first lysed in distilled water since the stain solution would itself fix the erythrocytes. Thick films should be stained as soon as possible after drying; if necessary they may be stored in the same way as thin films but should be lysed in distilled water before storage. If this cannot be done, lysis becomes progressively more difficult as the film ages. Such slides must be lysed before being stained, either in distilled water or—if that is inadequate—in a very weak solution of either lithium carbonate (a few drops of a saturated aqueous solution added to a staining dish full of water) or acetic acid (a few drops of commercial dilute acid per dish). The film should be washed in tap water after this treatment to remove the alkali (or acid) before being stained.

[1] Manufactured by GBI (Labs.) Ltd, Heaton Mills, Heaton Road, Denton, Lancashire, England.

STAINING. Giemsa's stain, diluted as described for thin films (p. 71), is used for about 30 minutes: it is helpful to agitate the dish gently from time to time during staining to disperse the liberated haemoglobin from the film (which has *not* been fixed). Washing of thick films after staining should be done briefly and *very gently*: they are less firmly fixed to the slide than are thin films. The morphology of trypanosomes is much better preserved if thick films are immersed in a 0·5% aqueous solution of methylene blue for 1 second and then rinsed gently and briefly with tap water before being placed in Giemsa's stain (MacLennan, 1957). If this is done, overstaining with Giemsa's stain is more likely to occur, so care should be taken to remove the films from the stain after not more than 30 minutes.

The remarks about examining, covering and storing thin films (p. 72) apply equally to thick films. For examination, select an area of the film which is as thick as is compatible with the retention of a sufficiently translucent, pale purple background; if the background appears dark blue or greenish, it is too thick. A thickness resulting in the appearance of about 10 leucocyte nuclei in each field of view using a ×100 objective is about right; this represents a concentration of about 10–15 times that of a thin film (Shute & Maryon, 1966). At least 200 fields of such a preparation should be examined with a ×100 oil-immersion objective before it is declared negative.

CONCENTRATING TRYPANOSOMES. Apart from the use of thick films, the trypanosomes present in a given volume of blood can be concentrated by repeated centrifugation: this technique ('triple centrifugation') may be useful in suspected early infections of human trypanosomiasis, especially those due to *T. gambiense*. Details of the technique differ slightly from different sources. The following procedure is recommended by Hoare (1949).

Collect 9 ml. of blood into 1 ml. of 6% sodium citrate in 0·9% saline and centrifuge it for about 7 minutes, starting at 900–1,000 r.p.m. and increasing gradually to 1,500 r.p.m. (on an ordinary bench centrifuge of radius 6 inches, this would result in accelerations of about 150–400 × G at the base of the tube): collect the supernatant plasma and the 'buffy layer' of leucocytes, and recentrifuge at 1,500 r.p.m. for 10 minutes. Collect the supernatant plasma and examine (fresh) a drop of the deposit: if trypanosomes are not seen in the latter, again centrifuge the plasma at 1,800–2,000 r.p.m. (650–700 × G) for 15–20 minutes and examine the final deposit, as before. Belding (1965) suggests that the second sediment be treated with distilled water or 2% aqueous acetic acid before the final centrifugation, to lyse any remaining erythrocytes: since the acetic acid (and possibly the water, depending upon the quantity used) would also kill trypanosomes, the final sediment would have to be stained and examined as a thick film. It is doubtful whether this suggestion would be worth adopting.

COUNTING TRYPANOSOMES. Provided the trypanosomes are sufficiently numerous, they are easily counted by diluting the infected blood 1:100 in a haematological pipette and placing the suspension in a haemocytometer: the volume examined (at a magnification of ×200–×400) can be varied according to the number of trypanosomes present so that a reasonably large number is counted. The number per mm.^{3} of blood can then be calculated by simple proportion. If the diluent used is physiological saline, the parasites will still be alive and the plane of focus of the objective will have to be changed when examining each square of the haemocytometer in order to see those flagellates which are swimming near the upper surface of the chamber: some difficulty may be experienced with organisms moving into or out of the square being examined. Some workers therefore use a fluid which lyses the erythrocytes and also kills and stains the parasites: for example, a mixture of 2 ml. each of formalin (40% formaldehyde), glacial acetic acid and Ziehl-Neelsen's carbol fuchsin, in 94 ml. of distilled water (Belding, 1965). Using such a fluid, blood in which trypanosomes are scanty need be diluted only 1:10 or 1:20 in a leucocyte-counting pipette. Numbers as low as about 100 parasites per mm.^{3} of blood can be counted in this way, if the entire 9 mm.^{2} area of a Neubauer haemocytometer is examined. Petana (1963) used Gram's iodine solution (iodine, 1 g.; potassium iodide, 2 g.; distilled water, 200 ml.) to kill and stain the trypanosomes. However, as this does not lyse the erythrocytes, the blood must be diluted to the same extent as when trypanosomes are counted alive.

Indirect Examination

Under this heading are included those methods of blood examination which do not depend on the visualization of the individual trypanosomes, but rather of their progeny or their effects. These methods are of value if the parasites are too scanty to be seen directly.

Culture of Trypanosomes

CULTIVATION *in vivo*. *T. brucei* and *T. rhodesiense* multiply readily in many mammals, including those commonly used in the laboratory such as mice, rats, rabbits, guinea-pigs, hamsters, and monkeys (both *Macaca rhesus* and *Cercopithecus* spp.). Thus inoculation of blood (or other material) into these animals is a useful diagnostic technique when parasitaemia is scanty. The rat and the mouse are most commonly used, being cheap, small, and easily handled. Both are equally, and highly, susceptible: one slight advantage of the rat is that it can tolerate the injection of larger volumes of blood.

The blood is inoculated intraperitoneally through a hypodermic needle (gauge 17 or 18): 3–5 ml. can easily be given to a rat, rather less (up to about 1 ml.) to a mouse. Fresh preparations of the blood of the rodents (obtained by pricking the tail tip with a needle or cutting a sliver off it with scissors) are then examined two or three times weekly, beginning perhaps 5–7 days after inoculation and continuing for 3–4 weeks (though mice are unlikely to be infected if parasitaemia has not developed within 10 days). Rats or mice infected with freshly-isolated strains of *T. brucei* or *T. rhodesiense* usually develop fairly long-lasting relapsing infections but always succumb eventually. With these two species the method is much more sensitive than the examination of thick blood films: in one study, only one half of the infections diagnosed by inoculation of blood from wild mammals into rats was detected by the examination of thick blood films (Baker, Sachs & Laufer, 1967).

T. gambiense develops much less readily in any mammal, so this method is of less value in its diagnosis. Young monkeys (*Cercopithecus* spp.) are among the more susceptible hosts. Recently Heisch *et al.* (1968) have shown that *T. gambiense* will develop readily if injected into the testis of a rabbit; this technique should certainly be tried as an aid in difficult diagnoses, if suitable animals are available.

Certain strains of *T. congolense* develop readily in rats and mice but others fail to do so. Godfrey (1961) has related infectivity for these animals with the mean length of the organisms—the longer strains being generally more infective. Unless cattle or sheep are available as recipients (expensive hosts for use on a large scale), cultivation *in vivo* cannot be relied upon to detect *T. congolense* although it should be used whenever possible.

T. simiae does not infect laboratory rats or mice: rabbits are sometimes susceptible, more regularly so after splenectomy (Desowitz & Watson, 1953a). *Cercopithecus* monkeys are often, but apparently not always, highly susceptible (Stephen, 1966a). *T. vivax*, *T. uniforme* and *T. suis* do not normally infect any small laboratory mammal. The only suitable diagnostic hosts for the two former species are sheep or goats. *T. vivax* has been induced to grow in rabbits (Unsworth & Nesbitt, 1952) and rats (Desowitz & Watson, 1952) by giving a supplementary injection of 5 ml. of serum from an uninfected sheep within twenty-four hours of the infective inoculum, but this technique is not sufficiently reliable for routine diagnostic use. As far as is known, *T. suis*, a very rare parasite, will develop only in Suidae (Stephen, 1966a).

CULTIVATION *in vitro*. Unlike the majority of trypanosomes of mammals and lower vertebrates, which can readily be grown *in vitro* in simple diphasic blood-agar media (Taylor & Baker, 1968), salivarian trypanosomes (Hoare, 1966) are very difficult to cultivate *in vitro*. For the isolation of *T. brucei*, *T. rhodesiense* or *T. gambiense* from blood, cerebrospinal fluid or lymph gland exudate, the medium described by Weinman (1960) is the most reliable: the preparation and use of this medium is described below (pp. 77–78).

A basically similar medium was earlier devised by Tobie *et al.* (1950) for the laboratory maintenance of these species, and has since (Tobie, 1958) been used also for *T. congolense*. Isolation of the latter (from laboratory rodents) has been achieved, with difficulty, if human rather than rabbit blood is used in the medium. The success of Weinman's medium is probably due, in part, to the use of an anticoagulant which is also anticomplementary (polyvinyl sulphuric acid or PVSA): the use of this or a similar substance in conjunction with Tobie's medium might well render the latter more suitable for the isolation of *T. brucei*, *T. rhodesiense* and *T. gambiense*. According to Weinman (1960), PVSA must be prepared in the laboratory by a rather lengthy synthesis. It is possible that the anticomplementary anticoagulant sodium polyanetholesulphonate known as 'Liquoid',[1] could be substituted for PVSA: 'Liquoid' was used by Brutsaert and Henrard (1938) with some success in the collection of blood for *in vitro* cultivation of *T. gambiense*.

Cultivation *in vitro*, therefore, is sufficiently reliable to be of routine use only with suspected infections due to *T. brucei*, *T. rhodesiense* and *T. gambiense*

[1] Marketed by Roche Products Limited, 15 Manchester Square, London W1, England.

(amongst the Salivaria), though further work may well show its applicability to *T. congolense* also. Since *T. brucei* and *T. rhodesiense* can readily be isolated by animal inoculation, the *in vitro* culture method is likely to be used mainly to detect *T. gambiense* and for this purpose Weinman's medium should prove to be very valuable. It must be stressed that this, like all *in vitro* culture methods for trypanosomes, must be performed under strictly aseptic conditions, using sterile media, apparatus and inocula; the parasites will not grow in the presence of bacterial contaminants. The organisms grow *in vitro* as the forms which develop naturally in the midgut of the tsetse fly, and are normally non-infective to mammals (including man). However, cultures of *T. rhodesiense* and *T. brucei* occasionally become infective, and the former species should therefore be handled with care. The development of infectivity has been investigated by Amrein *et al.* (1965).

No other species of salivarian trypanosome has been grown *in vitro* with the exception of *T. vivax* in cultures of tsetse-fly tissues (Trager, 1959): this is not a practical technique for diagnosis.

Cultivation Technique for Maintenance of *T. brucei*, *T. rhodesiense*, *T. gambiense* and *T. congolense*

(Tobie, von Brand & Mehlman, 1950)

Medium

Solid Phase

(a) Dissolve 1·5 g. Bacto-beef (Difco)[1]; 2·5 g. Bacto-peptone (Difco); 4·0 g. sodium chloride and 7·5 g. Bacto-agar (Difco) in 500 ml. distilled water (*see* Note 3). Adjust the pH to 7·2–7·4 with sodium hydroxide and autoclave (15 lb. for 20 minutes).

(b) Cool this mixture until it can be comfortably held in the hand (about 45°C); then add whole rabbit blood, which has been inactivated at 56°C for 30 minutes, in the proportion of 25 ml. of blood to 75 ml. of base. (Coagulation of the whole blood is prevented by using 0·5% sterile sodium citrate.)

(c) Dispense in amounts of 5 ml. or 25 ml. into test-tubes or flasks, respectively. The test-tubes are kept in a slanted position and the flasks upright until the base has solidified.

Liquid Phase

Sterile, modified Locke's solution of the following composition: NaCl, 8 g.; KCl, 0·2 g.; $CaCl_2$, 0·2 g.; KH_2PO_4, 0·3 g.; glucose, 2·5 g.; and distilled water, 1 litre. Add this to the solidified base in amounts of 2 ml. and 10–15 ml. respectively. The tubes and flasks are closed with cotton plugs which need not be capped since subcultures must be made before evaporation becomes serious.

[1] Difco Laboratories, Detroit 1, Michigan, USA. (British agents: Baird & Tatlock Ltd., Freshwater Road, Chadwell Heath, Essex).

Technique

After inoculation, cultures are incubated at 24°–25°C. Maximum population (about 21,000 per mm.³) is reached between 10 and 14 days after inoculation. Transfers to fresh medium are made every 1–2 weeks.

Notes

(1) Human blood can be used instead of rabbit blood but, except for the isolation of *T. congolense*, gives no better results.

(2) If used for isolation from an infected laboratory rodent, the first culture should be allowed to grow for 3 weeks before subinoculation.

(3) The solid components of the base (excluding the blood elements) are contained in Difco 'Nutrient Agar 1·5%' (Weinman, 1946): hence this product, 15·5 g. per 500 ml. water, can be substituted for the ingredients listed in paragraph (a) above.

Cultivation Technique for Diagnostic Isolation and Maintenance of *T. brucei*, *T. rhodesiense* and *T. gambiense*

(Weinman, 1960)

Medium

Preparation of Base

(a) Dissolve 31 g. of Difco 'Nutrient Agar 1·5%' (for composition see the medium described above) and 5 g. of plain agar in 1 litre of distilled water; dispense 5 ml. aliquots into screw-capped test-tubes and autoclave.

(b) Collect 400–500 ml. human blood into 75 ml. of 2·5% sodium citrate and separate the erythrocytes from the plasma by centrifugation: inactivate the plasma at 56°C for 30 minutes, wash the erythrocytes (by centrifuging) three times with at least three times their volume of isotonic saline, and then recombine the cells and plasma in equal parts by volume.

(c) When the autoclaved agar, (a) above, has cooled to 45°C, add the reconstituted blood (warmed to 45°C) in the proportion of 1 volume to 3 volumes of agar. Mix gently and allow to set in a sloping position.

(d) Incubate the tubes at 37°C for 24 hours; they may be stored in a refrigerator for up to 6 months. (Note: no overlay is added to this medium.)

Preparation of polyvinyl sulphuric acid (PVSA) (Chargaff *et al.*, 1936)

Suspend 1·04 g. dry polyvinyl alcohol in 24 g. dry pyridine and slowly add 6 g. chlorosulphonic acid to the *chilled* mixture. When the reaction abates, incubate the mixture at 21°C for 1½ hours. Decant the supernatant liquid and dissolve the rubbery reaction product in 20 ml. water (made alkaline with 2 *N* potassium hydroxide). Add 80 ml. ethanol to the solution, cool and collect the precipitate by centrifugation. Re-dissolve the precipitate in 75 ml. warm water, centrifuge the solution, filter through cotton wool and reprecipitate the product by adding 150 ml. alcohol. Repeat the precipitation process twice. Yield: 1·85 g. of the potassium salt of PVSA as a white, water-soluble powder. For use, dissolve 0·5 g. in 100 ml. physiological saline, adjust pH to 7·5 if necessary and sterilize by filtration.

Technique

(a) For diagnosis, blood is collected from the patient using polyvinyl sulphuric acid as anti-coagulant, 0·1 ml. of a 0·5% w/v solution in saline for every 1 ml. of blood. It is recommended to inoculate 2 ml. of blood and anti-coagulant to each of two tubes of medium: this must be done promptly since coagulation is inhibited for only about 15 minutes.

(b) Antibiotic (usually 0·5 mg. of dihydrostreptomycin sulphate or 2,000 units of penicillin, in 0·1 ml. of saline) is added to each millilitre of the inoculated blood.

(c) The blood is spread over the surface of the agar by tilting the tube a few times and the latter is then incubated at 25°C in the dark. Cultures should be first examined 5 days after inoculation: if not positive by 30 days they may be discarded. Examination should be made by washing the agar slope with liquid from the bottom of the tube, using a Pasteur pipette and finally withdrawing a drop of the fluid for microscopic examination: it is recommended that the agar should be gently rubbed with the tip of the pipette during the washing, since trypanosomes often grow as colonies on its surface.

Note

It is possible that 'Liquoid' (*see* p. 75) would be equally suitable as an anti-complementary anticoagulant: if so, the technique would be simplified since the preparation of PVSA could be omitted.

Determination of IgM Concentration

Recently it has been found that not only do the total serum proteins of man increase in concentration during trypanosomiasis due to *T. gambiense* but that the amount of one particular protein, IgM, γM or β_2-macroglobulin, increases rapidly and greatly (Mattern, 1964). This increase, while not entirely specific to trypanosomiasis, is highly suggestive of the infection. This work has been confirmed and extended for *T. rhodesiense* infection by Lumsden (1965 and personal communication) who found that increase in serum IgM was not typically associated with tuberculosis, leprosy, syphilis or kala-azar; it was, however, associated with trypanosomiasis and idiopathic splenomegaly, a condition apparently connected with chronic infection with *Plasmodium malariae*. Thus a raised serum IgM, while not pathognomonic for African human trypanosomiasis, is suggestive enough for persons having it to be subjected to a more thorough diagnostic examination: it may prove a particularly valuable indication in *T. gambiense* infection where parasitological diagnosis is less easy than it is with *T. rhodesiense*. Much less is known about the production of IgM in trypanosomiasis of animals other than man, though it is known to increase in monkeys (Mattern, Fromentin & Pilo-Moron, 1963; Collomb *et al.*, 1963), rabbits (Mattern, Duret & Pautrizel, 1963) and chimpanzees (Baker, 1968) experimentally infected with salivarian trypanosomes.

The amount of IgM in serum can be determined by an immuno-diffusion technique. The serum is placed in small wells cut in a layer of agar, which incorporates a specific antiserum to IgM. If the serum contains IgM, a precipitate forms in a ring around the well and the diameter of this ring is proportionate to the concentration of IgM in the test serum. By the use of standard solutions of known IgM concentration, the absolute amount of the protein in the test serum can thus be estimated by measuring the diameter of the ring of precipitate. Plastic trays ('Immuno-plates'), measuring 3 inches by 1 inch, containing a layer of agar (including antibody) with six wells cut in it, together with three different standard solutions of IgM, are obtainable commercially.[1] Full instructions for their use are supplied, and the method is simple and reliable. The manufacturers recommend leaving the plates for 16 hours at room temperature before reading. Lumsden (1965) recommended increasing this period to 65–72 hours. IgM concentrations in normal, healthy adults range up to about 3·5 mg. per ml., mean 1·36: in sleeping sickness patients, this level is raised rapidly (starting within 3–4 weeks of infection) to levels considerably (at least 8–16 times according to Mattern, 1964) above this. The IgM titre appears to fall to normal again fairly rapidly after treatment. A cheaper and easier variation of this technique has been devised by Cunningham *et al.* (1967). A drop of blood is collected on filter paper, dried and stored in a desiccator; such preparations last for up to two weeks and, if kept at − 20°C, for longer periods. Subsequently, a disc 3 mm. in diameter is punched from the dried blood and laid on the surface of a thin layer of 1% agar incorporating 0·01% anti-IgM serum, spread on a glass plate. A ring of precipitate is formed, the area of which is proportional to the concentration of IgM. The diameter of the ring is measured after 48 hours, by removing the discs and staining the agar for 5 minutes with amido black (1% in a mixture of glacial acetic acid, 2 vol.; methanol, 5 vol.; water, 5 vol.), washing and differentiating with the amido black solvent.

Complement-Fixation and Other Serological Tests

These tests are of value mainly in suspected cases of *T. gambiense* infection: with *T. rhodesiense*, diagnosis is usually more readily confirmed by discovery or isolation of the parasite. Their value (if any) in the diagnosis of trypanosomiasis of animals other than man is unknown.

COMPLEMENT-FIXATION TEST. According to Neujean and Evens (1958), a complement-fixation test using *T. equiperdum* as antigen is a reliable diagnostic aid in *T. gambiense* infection, being positive in about 95% of early cases: the percentage of positive results obtained drops a little as the infection develops and in patients relapsing after treatment is never higher than 80%. The test becomes positive 8–15 days after infection and remains so for 1–2 years after successful treatment. Falsely positive results, if they ever occur, are very rare. The test is performed in the usual way, details of which can be found in any standard work on bacteriology (e.g. Mackie & McCartney, 1953). The antigen is prepared as follows (Schoenaers *et al.*, 1953).

1. Rats are inoculated with 1 ml. of a 50% suspension of blood collected at the height of parasitaemia from another rat infected with *T. equiperdum* ('Watson' strain).

[1] Supplied by Hyland Laboratory Products Division, Baxter Laboratories Ltd., Caxton Way, Thetford, Norfolk, England; or Hyland Laboratories, Los Angeles, California, USA.

2. At peak parasitaemia, these rats are killed with ether and bled by cutting the neck: the blood of each rat is collected into 0·1 ml. of a 5% solution of 'Liquoid' (*see* p. 75).

3. The blood is filtered through glass wool and placed in thick-walled glass tubes, 27 × 90 mm., the lower end being closed with a rubber bung.

4. The tubes are centrifuged at 3,000 r.p.m. (presumably 1,500 × G) for 30 minutes. This results in the production of three layers in the tube—the lowest mainly erythrocytes, the middle one mainly trypanosomes and the upper one plasma.

5. The plasma is removed and the remainder frozen by plunging the tube into alcohol at − 40°C.

6. The bung is removed and the column of frozen blood allowed to slip out of the tube. With a scalpel, the upper white layer of trypanosomes is cut off and collected: about 0·5 g. 'purée de trypanosomes' is obtained from each rat.

7. This 'purée' is thawed and resuspended in a mixture of equal volumes of neutral glycerine and physiological saline, 2 ml. per 1 g. of 'purée'.

8. Immediately before use, this stock antigen is diluted 1:10 with physiological saline. The optimal amount to use in the test is determined by titration and lies between 0·05 and 0·1 ml.

Schoenaers *et al.* (1953) use as a source of complement a solution of alexine (source unspecified) diluted with an equal volume of Witte's solution (potassium sulphate, 10 g.; boric acid 4 g.; distilled water, 100 ml.): this is stored at 4°C. Test sera are inactivated at 56°C for half-an-hour, and used in the following amounts: 0·4, 0·2, 0·1 and 0·05 ml.

FORMOL-GEL TEST. Neujean and Evens (1958) found the formol-gel test (Napier's aldehyde test) a valuable indication in areas where leishmaniasis is absent: a positive reaction was given by about 85% of early cases of *T. gambiense* infection and about 70% of late cases, but only in some 25% of persons relapsing after treatment. Infection with leishmaniasis or leprosy also gives a positive result with this test. According to Hope-Gill (1938), the test when used to detect trypanosomiasis should be performed as follows. To 1 ml. of serum or plasma, contained in a narrow test tube, two drops of commercial formalin (40% formaldehyde solution) are added and the tube is shaken. If the mixture gels within 1 hour, the test is positive: very rarely, gelation may be more delayed, but if it has not occurred within 24 hours the patient is almost certainly not infected.

FLUORESCENT ANTIBODY TEST. The fluorescent antibody technique, though at present not adequately tested for the diagnosis of trypanosomiasis, shows every sign of being a valuable method in the future (Sadun *et al.*, 1963; Bailey *et al.*, 1967).

Lymph Examination

Collection of Samples

(i) From Chancre

Within the first few days after being bitten by an infected tsetse fly, a local swelling or chancre often develops: if this is pricked with a sterile needle or

Pasteur pipette (with aseptic precautions), the resulting serous exudate can be collected and examined for the presence of trypanosomes.

(ii) From a Gland

In suspected human trypanosomiasis, particularly that due to *T. gambiense*, lymph gland exudate should be examined for the presence of trypanosomes if they cannot be found in the blood. Evens *et al.* (1963) record that, in early infections due to *T. gambiense*, trypanosomes are seen in this exudate slightly less often than in thick blood films, although they may sometimes be seen in one fluid and not in the other: routine microscopic examination of both fluids fails to detect about 10% of even early *T. gambiense* infections.

Lymph is usually collected by puncture of posterior cervical lymph glands, which are often soft and swollen during the early infection: later, they become hard and fibrotic and gland puncture is unlikely to yield satisfactory material. After sterilizing the skin, the gland is grasped between the forefinger and thumb and gently massaged: a sterile, dry hypodermic needle, about 2·5–3 cm. long with a bore of 0·6–0·8 mm. (Hoare, 1949), is inserted into the gland and its tip is slowly moved around while the gland is squeezed. Some workers prefer to insert the needle before attaching it to a syringe, some insert the needle already attached to a syringe (Hoare, 1949; Belding, 1965) and some do not attach a syringe until after the needle is withdrawn (Craig, 1948; Manson-Bahr, 1966). Those who practise the first two methods use the syringe to aspirate a little of the gland's contents, all workers use the syringe to expel the juice collected in the needle. If difficulty is experienced in obtaining lymph, it may be helpful to inject a few drops of sterile physiological saline into the gland (through the same needle) before aspiration (Belding, 1965).

Direct Examination

Lymph may be examined either fresh or stained, as described above for blood (pp. 69–73). For stained preparations a thin film made with the spreading slide held at a wide angle gives a smear of suitable thickness. If the fluid obtained from a chancre is very clear, it may be stained as a thick film preferably fixed in methanol after drying.

Indirect Examination

Lymph may be inoculated into susceptible animals or cultures if enough can be obtained. If cultures are used, the aspirated material must be kept sterile and the cultures should be inoculated at once.

Examination of Cerebrospinal Fluid (CSF)

Collection and examination of the CSF is usually required in human trypanosomiasis as a means of determining the stage to which the disease has progressed or the manner in which it is responding to treatment. In very advanced infections, trypanosomes may not be demonstrable in the blood or lymph and diagnosis may depend upon the examination of CSF.

Collection of Samples

All authorities agree on the safety of lumbar puncture, the procedure by which CSF is almost always collected, though it should not be undertaken lightly and only under the highest attainable standards of asepsis. A full discussion of the risks and possible complications of the procedure is given by Craig (1948), and should be read by all who are about to do it for the first time.

Cisternal puncture is a possible alternative to lumbar puncture and although it may occasionally be necessary to resort to it in young children, it is emphatically not recommended as a routine. The technique, and the dangers, are described by Craig (1948) and will not be repeated here.

Lumbar puncture is performed with a special needle, about 8–10 cm. long with a bore of 1–1·5 mm., fitted with a stylet having a bevelled end matching that of the needle. The patient is usually laid upon his side, with knees drawn up to the chin; or he may be seated, bending forwards. The skin over the lower region of the spine is carefully sterilized. The puncture is usually made in the third lumbar interspace (between the third and fourth lumbar vertebrae), though the space below this (the fourth) can also be used and is advised in children (Craig, 1948). The third space can be located by drawing, with an iodine-soaked swab, a line across the back between the two iliac crests (Hoare, 1949). Having located the selected space with a sterile finger, the overlying tissues may be anaesthetized by infiltrating 2–2·5 ml. of 1% novocain into the deeper tissues and a few drops into the skin, but this is not essential. The sterile needle (with stylet) is then inserted in the midline and pushed steadily until a sudden cessation of resistance is felt: the tip should then be in the subarachnoid space. The stylet is withdrawn and CSF should drip out: if it does not, the stylet should be re-inserted to clear any blockage and, if necessary, the needle slightly withdrawn: if fluid does not appear aspiration should *not* be applied and the attempt should be abandoned. Usually, 5 ml. of fluid is allowed to drip into a centrifuge tube: the first few drops should be discarded since they may contain a little blood. The needle is then withdrawn, the puncture swabbed with iodine and a dressing applied. Craig (1948) recommends that the patient should lie down for at least three hours.

Direct Examination

(i) Fresh or Stained Preparations

A drop of CSF may be examined directly for the presence of trypanosomes or, if desired, it can be spread like a thick blood film and stained (*see* pp. 72–73), preferably after methanol fixation. The examination of fresh CSF for the presence of trypanosomes may be combined with the counting of the leucocytes present in the fluid (p. 84 below): often, however, the flagellates are too scanty to be seen without concentration.

(ii) Concentrating Trypanosomes

This is effected by centrifugation: Evens *et al.* (1963) recommend 3,000 r.p.m. (presumably representing about 1,500 × G) for 15 minutes at 4°C: using this procedure they were able to see trypanosomes in 42 out of 53 samples taken from patients with a CSF cell count of 20 per mm.^{3} or more, and in 45 out of 46 samples obtained from such persons relapsing after treatment. Hoare (1949) recommends centrifugation at only 1,800 r.p.m. (about 650 × G) for 5 minutes. The deposit is best examined fresh for the presence of motile trypanosomes: if desired, it can be made into a thin film and stained (p. 71). Stained preparations will reveal Mott's morular cells, if present.

Indirect Examination

(i) Cultivation *in vivo* and *in vitro*

If trypanosomes cannot be seen by direct examination, the CSF, either as withdrawn or as the deposit after centrifugation, can be inoculated into susceptible animals or (if all procedures have been done aseptically) into cultures (pp. 77–78).

(ii) Determination of IgM Concentration

This can be done as described above for blood serum (pp. 78–79).

(iii) Determination of Total Protein Concentration

There are several methods by which the protein concentration of biological fluids can be determined. The 'classical' method used with sleeping sickness patients is that of Sicard and Cantaloube. This method is simple to perform and does not require sophisticated apparatus; it has the disadvantage of being inaccurate, but, since the pathological changes produced in the CSF by trypanosome infection are considerable, this is of little practical importance. The merits and demerits of the Sicard-Cantaloube method have been discussed by Gall *et al.* (1955) who themselves evolved a standardized method of conducting the Sicard-Canteloube test which gives the highest attainable reproducibility and which is described below.

The test can be conducted using narrow (7 × 180 mm.) test tubes, graduated from 1 to 4 ml., with the first division being sub-divided into 0·2 ml. units. Alternatively (and preferably), special tubes (of these dimensions) can be used, marked at the 2, 3 and 4 ml. levels, below which they are graduated directly in milligrammes per 100 ml. of protein, in 5 mg. steps between 20 and 50 mg., and then (surprisingly!) at 56, 71 and 85 mg.

Four ml. of CSF are placed in each tube (less can be used, provided the final result is multiplied by the appropriate factor), and the tubes are placed in a sloping position in a water bath containing only about 1 inch depth of water (this ensures mixing by convection of the tubes' contents): the water is then brought to the boil and removed from the heat[1]: to each tube is added 0·6 ml. of 30% aqueous trichloroacetic acid, and after 5–10 minutes at room temperature, the tubes are replaced in the bath which is once more brought to the boil. The tubes are then removed and stood *vertically* for the deposit to settle. Each

[1] Gall *et al.* (1955) 'found that an excellent water-bath could be very simply made from two tins fitting loosely into one another. The larger tin, with its top and bottom removed and with holes bored for ventilation, fits over the spirit lamp and acts as a wind-shield and support for the smaller tin, which is suspended over the lamp on a pair of stiff wires passed through holes in the side of the larger tin.'

tube should be gently rotated six times between the palms of the hands as soon as the bulk of the precipitate has settled, and again 15–30 minutes later: they are then left (vertical) for at least 5 hours, or overnight, and the depth of deposit read off against the graduations. If tubes calibrated only in ml. are used, the following conversions are approximately correct:

Vol. of deposit (ml.)	Mg. % of protein
0·2	22
0·4	40
0·6	56
0·8	71
1·0	85

Gall *et al.* (1955) found that this method gave an approximately true result at 20 mg. %: below this level its results were high, and above it they were too low: accuracy is not greater than ± 5 mg. (95% confidence limits). It is usually accepted that, using the Sicard-Cantaloube procedure, values above 25 mg. % are suggestive of trypanosomal invasion of the CSF (Robertson, 1962). Gall *et al.* (1955) prefer a turbidometric method involving the addition of sulphosalicylic acid and the use of a photometer.

(iv) Cell Counts

These are very simply done by placing a few drops of undiluted, fresh, uncentrifuged CSF into an ordinary haemocytometer or, preferably, a special Fuchs-Rosenthal chamber (which is 0·2 mm. deep, instead of 0·1 mm. as is a haemocytometer). After allowing the cells to settle (which they do in 2–3 minutes), they are counted directly under the microscope (magnification ×200–×400): the whole ruled area should be examined unless the cell count is very high. If trypanosomes are seen, their presence should be recorded. The number of cells per mm.^{3} of CSF is then calculated by simple proportion. Care should be taken to distinguish and disregard any erythrocytes which may be present: these can be differentiated from leucocytes by their less granular appearance. If many erythrocytes are present, the CSF sample should be discarded. A leucocyte count of more than 5 per mm.^{3} is considered pathological by Robertson (1962).

DETECTION OF INFECTION IN TSETSE FLIES

Dissection

Before dissection, flies are killed with ether or chloroform: the wings and legs are then cut or pulled off. Dissected organs are placed in isotonic glucose solution (5%) or saline (0·9%): glucose is better as saline may interfere with subsequent staining (Hoare, 1949). Microscopic examination is usually made at a magnification of about ×400. The three organs which may be required for examination for salivarian trypanosomes are the proboscis, midgut (including proventriculus) and salivary glands: the hindgut will also be required if *T. grayi* is to be looked for.

(a) Proboscis

This dissection is best done *after* the salivary glands have been removed. The proboscis bulb is grasped with fine forceps, pulled off the head and mounted whole in a drop of glucose solution, beneath a coverslip, for microscopical examination. Trypanosomes can be seen (if present) through its chitinous wall, though, if desired, the labrum, labium and hypopharynx may be separated with needles.

(b) Gut and Salivary Glands

(i) Rapid Method

The head of the fly is grasped with fine forceps and pulled gently but steadily away from the thorax, in a straight line: the salivary glands are usually pulled out of the body still attached to the head, but if one or both should break they can be seized with the forceps and pulled out. The glands should be placed immediately in a drop of glucose solution on a slide for microscopic examination: it is convenient to do the dissection at one end of a slide and to place the glands in a drop of solution on the same slide and cover them with a coverslip. The proboscis can then be removed from the head as described above. Finally, the thorax is held with a needle or a pair of forceps and the last two or three segments are cut off the abdomen. The fly is then placed on its back on a slide with the tip of the abdomen touching a drop of glucose solution (or saline) and a second needle is placed horizontally across the abdomen and moved slowly backwards, squeezing out the viscera into the solution: a coverslip is placed on the viscera, which are crushed by gentle pressure before microscopic examination.

When examining salivary glands, the microscope must be focused on the lumen of each gland to avoid confusion with any flagellates which may have escaped from the ruptured intestine.

(ii) Alternative Method (simplified from that of Willett, 1955)

This method, though slower, results in cleaner preparations, is less likely to rupture the intestine and enables both salivary glands to be recovered consistently. This is the method of choice for detailed studies on the development of trypanosomes in the fly as distinct from the mere detection of infection but, if many flies are to be examined for the latter purpose, the rapid method (above) would be indicated.

1. Holding the fly in the fingers, pull off the legs and wings: with small scissors cut a very thin strip off both edges of the abdomen: pin the fly on its back on wax in a small dissecting dish and cover it with glucose solution (or saline).

2. Cut with scissors through the front end of the ventral wall of the abdomen (which is now uppermost), keeping the blade of the scissors lifted up as far as possible. Turn back the ventral abdominal wall, which has been cut on three sides, and gently pull back the abdominal contents.

3. Look for the salivary glands in the two front corners of the abdomen; they usually lie fairly deep, close to a trachea (*see* Fig. 4.2). Having found them

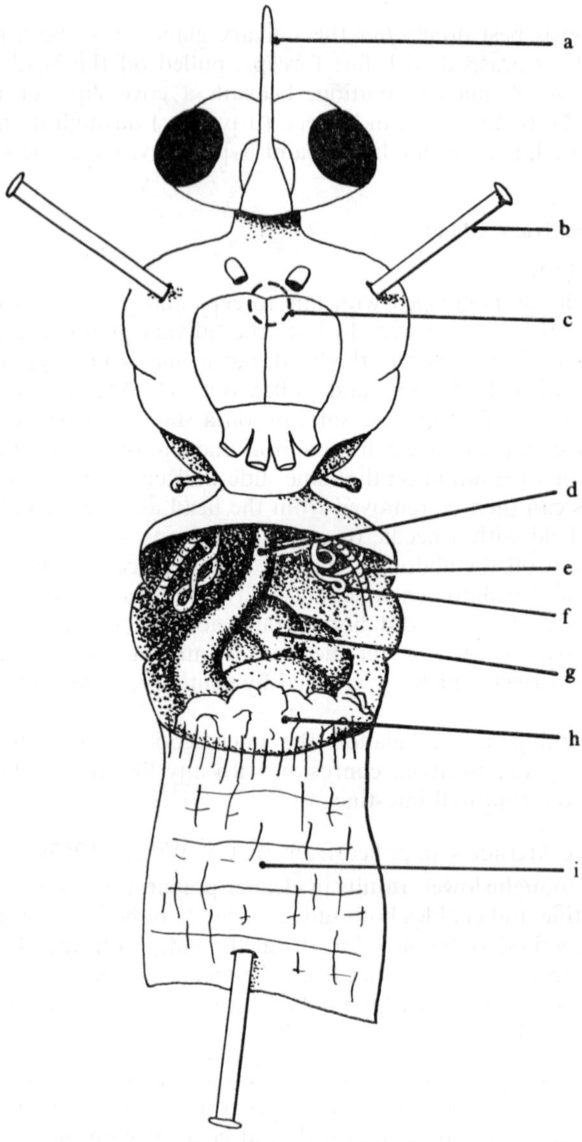

Fig. 4.2 Diagram illustrating general dissection of a tsetse fly: the fly is shown pinned supine to the wax in a dissecting dish. a. Proboscis; b. Pin; c. Position of proventriculus; d. Anterior portion of midgut; e. Trachea; f. Salivary gland; g. Coils of posterior portion of midgut (crop lies beneath); h. Reproductive organs and hindgut; i. Abdominal sternites, cut away and pinned back. (Diagram based on that of Willett, 1955)

grasp them firmly with fine forceps and pull them backwards gently, one at a time. Watch the glands under the dissecting microscope while they are being pulled out, to make sure they do not break or slip out of the forceps, and cover with a coverslip.

4. The midgut (and hindgut if required), proventriculus and proboscis can now be removed: the proventriculus is found by cutting away the floor of the thorax and carefully removing the nerve ganglion with forceps. The proventriculus lies dorsal to (i.e. beneath) this ganglion, and can be lifted out with forceps.

This dissection should be done under a dissecting microscope giving a magnification of about $\times 20$–$\times 30$.

Stained Preparations

Permanent preparations of flagellates obtained from any of the above dissections can be made by crushing the preparation by pressure on the coverslip, then removing the latter, spreading the fluid with a needle or another slide into a fairly thin smear, drying it in air and staining with Giemsa's stain after fixation in methanol (pp. 71–72).

Isolation of Infected Flies

(a) Feeding on Laboratory Rodents

Tsetse flies infected with *T. brucei*, *T. rhodesiense* or strains of *T. congolense* which are infective to laboratory rodents can be isolated by feeding them regularly, usually in groups of 10–20, on a suitable host (guinea-pigs are commonly used), keeping one rodent for each cage of flies. The rodent is examined regularly (two or three times per week) by means of fresh blood preparations (p. 69): if it becomes infected, it is clear that at least one fly in the cage is infective. The infective fly (or flies) can then be identified (unless it has previously died) by dissection or, if it is required alive, by feeding all the flies in the batch individually on rats and subsequently examining the latter for trypanosomes. Alternatively, the flies may be examined by Burtt's 'probing' technique (*see* below), which gives a result more quickly and is also cheaper, since it does not involve the use of several rats.

(b) 'Probing' Technique

By this method (a slight modification of that described by Burtt, 1946a) the use of large numbers of rats is avoided, infected flies can be identified more rapidly, and infections with trypanosomes which will not develop in rodents can also be detected. Each fly is kept individually in a 3 inch × 1 inch glass tube, the mouth of which is covered with mosquito or sandfly netting. Each tube is held in a retort stand, gauze end downwards, and a guinea-pig (or rabbit) is held close to the gauze-covered end of the tube. If the fly is hungry, it will protrude its proboscis through the netting in an attempt to feed; when this occurs, a glass microscope slide is interposed between the guinea-pig and the fly so that the tip of the proboscis touches the slide. As the fly probes, it salivates onto the slide, which is finally withdrawn, air dried, fixed with methanol and stained with Giemsa's stain (method for thin films, pp. 71–72). If present, metacyclic trypanosomes can be seen easily when the stained smear is examined with an oil-immersion objective: other developmental forms (epimastigote, and even long trypomastigote forms from the proventriculus) may also be extruded. If a circle of 1–2 cm. diameter is drawn on the slide with a grease pencil and the fly is allowed to probe only within this circle, the saliva will be more easily found after staining. If the slides are warmed to about 40°C, hungry flies will sometimes probe directly onto them, avoiding the need for a guinea-pig. It is *not* recommended to use the operator's hand or arm instead of a guinea-pig, in case the length of the proboscis is misjudged and the fly is infected with *T. rhodesiense* or *T. gambiense*.

Chapter 5

Techniques for the Manipulation and Maintenance of Trypanosome Strains in the Laboratory

P. J. WALKER

Research work on the biology of trypanosomes, including studies on virulence and response to inhibitory substances such as drugs or antibodies, necessitates the availability of suitable infections in laboratory animals. The methods employed for the maintenance to trypanosome strains vary in different laboratories and since they may influence the course of the infection in experimental animals it is important that the techniques used should be described in detail, at least until such time as standardized techniques have been developed and taken into regular use. The methods described below are those routinely used by the writer and are believed to be as simple and reliable as any others in common use.

SYRINGE PASSAGE

Until comparatively recently, the usual, and indeed the only practical, method of maintaining trypanosome strains in the laboratory has been serial passage in laboratory animals. This method involves the transference of material, usually blood but sometimes gland juice or other body fluid, from an infected to a clean host by means of a syringe. Syringe passage has certain inherent defects; biological variations such as changes in virulence or antigenicity are liable to occur. For example, *T. brucei* (NIMR 2) which is a virulent mouse-adapted strain, kills mice in three or four days if 10^6 parasites are inoculated but takes seven days to kill if only one parasite infects. It may be inferred that this strain is capable of a million-fold increase in about 3½ days, and so calculate that the generation (doubling) time is around four hours. Experienced technicians can influence the course of infection by varying the numbers of parasites inoculated (Walker, 1964). The amount of work involved may be reduced by transferring very few parasites so that passage need only take place once or twice a week but, after some weeks, the strain so treated becomes noticeably less virulent and it is probable that antigenic variation will have taken place. If passaged frequently, perhaps every other day, the virulence of the strain increases. In both circumstances considerable selection pressure has been exerted and the trypanosome strain responds by deviating from its original character. Methods for assessing strain characters are still very poor so that any technique which can be seen to create selection pressure should be avoided.

Experiments can usually be designed to take account of the hosts' response and antigenic variation. If, for example, healthy trypanosomes are required for subinoculation in known numbers of infective organisms into groups of mice, these may be obtained from young rats which have received massive inoculations of 10^7 or 10^8 parasites to yield a hundred-fold increase in only two days. These numbers are chosen because they will cause a fatal infection before the host can develop an immune response. Clearly, planning of experiments is required to provide enough infected rats to act as donors and they too should be infected for only two days. The course of infection of *brucei* group trypanosomes has been followed by direct counts and by infectivity titration (Cunningham *et al.*, 1963a). The results obtained by both methods of counting showed a rise in total number of parasites up to the third day but by the fifth day, although a maximum number of trypanosomes were circulating, less than one in ten thousand was infective. This loss of infectivity without parallel decrease in the total number of trypanosomes or loss of motility is a matter of concern, especially in syringe passage in the preparation of clones and in drug or antibody tests *in vitro*. In general, it is wise to passage from an early rising infection.

In experimental work with virulent infections it is sometimes desirable to inoculate relatively few healthy parasites. Blood from heavy two-day infections should be used and diluted appropriately to give only 10^3 or 10^4 parasites per inoculum. Slow-acting drugs such as homidium are best tested under such standardized conditions so that there is a sufficient time lag to allow careful observation at six- or eight-hour intervals before the infection overwhelms the host. The same principle applies in testing a vaccination procedure.

When syringe passage or experimental work involves less virulent strains such as those taken direct from patients or cattle, somewhat different procedures may be adopted. The parasites are usually few in number and already subjected to the action of antibody; in addition, the blood in which they are suspended probably contains antibody to the common antigens if not to the strain specific variable antigen. If time permits the best procedure is to dilute the blood with twice its volume of suitable medium (*see* below) to make about 10 ml. in all. Centrifugation in a small bench centrifuge at 1,500 r.p.m. (250 × G) for five minutes settles the red cells, leaving the white cells and trypanosomes mostly in suspension. The writer's practice is to stir the top of the cell layer gently to lift about one-eighth of an inch, a layer containing numerous trypanosomes, into the supernatant. This is pipetted off using a large bore (about 2 mm. at the narrow end) pipette into a fresh centrifuge tube. The suspended cells are centrifuged somewhat more vigorously at about 2,200 r.p.m. (550 × G) for five minutes and the supernatant is discarded. The cells are resuspended in a small volume of diluent and being more or less free from antibody are inoculated immediately. In the above procedure stress is laid on quick and gentle treatment of the parasites. The loss of a large percentage of parasites is of no consequence when dealing with virulent and heavy infections but extreme care must be taken when handling newly isolated and avirulent strains especially from groups other than the robust *T. brucei*.

As avirulent trypanosomes do not kill the host, such as the mouse, thick blood smears (tail) should be examined daily or every other day to observe the build-up of infection. As with virulent infections, it is important to subinoculate parasites taken from a rising infection. When the number of parasites is very low the first parasitaemia and one or more relapses may well be missed; with such strains the infection first detected may be a relapse and probably an antigenic variant.

One important practical consideration is the choice of diluent. This should be stable, autoclavable and capable of supporting infectivity over 12–24 hours. Low pH values are remarkably detrimental to trypanosomes (Lumsden *et al.*, 1965) and it is, therefore, advisable to incorporate a mild buffer and phenol red indicator in the diluent. It is also convenient to be able to use the diluent as an anticoagulant and, for this purpose, various workers have used citrate, heparin or ethylene diamine tetra-acetic acid (EDTA). For routine blood work using a wide range of trypanosome strains the writer favours EDTA, on the grounds that this substance is effective in preventing clotting of rat blood and is apparently non-toxic to trypanosomes, as judged by infectivity tests carried out after exposure for two hours at ten times the concentration necessary to prevent clotting. The reader's attention is however drawn to a comparison of anti-clotting agents used to dilute blood for feeding to tsetse flies through membranes (Southon & Cockings, 1963); EDTA was found to be more toxic to the flies than was heparin. In all comparative toxicity tests of this kind, the purity of the chemicals used should be considered as well as the stated results. Despite the extra expense the writer prefers to use only analytical reagent grade of chemicals for the preparation of media.

The medium used in the writer's laboratory consists of:

Sodium chloride	8 g.
Potassium dihydrogen orthophosphate, anhydrous	0·3 g.
EDTA	2·0 g.
Glucose	2·0 g.
Phenol red solution (phenol red 1 g., Sodium chloride 4 g. to 500 ml. with distilled water)	5 ml.
Glass-distilled water up to 1 litre.	

About 3 ml. of N sodium hydroxide solution are added dropwise until the indicator is at its mid-point (rose pink and pH 7·4) as seen in a $\frac{5}{8}$ inch diameter test tube. The bulk medium is conveniently dispensed into 50 Universal containers which are autoclaved at 10 lb. per square inch for 20 minutes. The medium may be stored at room temperature but should be discarded if the liquid becomes yellow. Small deviations from the above formulation (i.e. weighing errors of 5%) have not been shown to be significant so that it is unnecessary, and indeed inadvisable, to use very delicate balances.

For special purposes such as *in vitro* exposure to Antrycide (which precipitates with chloride ions) a Tyrode solution, based on nitrates, has been developed which has the following composition per litre:

Sodium nitrate	11·7 g.
Potassium nitrate	0·27 g.
Calcium nitrate ($4H_2O$)	0·43 g.
Glucose	2·0 g.

The solution is acid and should be neutralized cautiously with sodium hydroxide. After exposure in this medium for two hours, trypanosomes remain vigorously motile though infectivity is reduced.

PREPARATION OF CLONE STRAINS

Infections derived from single trypanosomes are of great significance when the homogeneity of a strain is in question and in experiments to measure the mutation rate in immunological or drug resistance studies. Two basic methods for preparing clones—dilution and micromanipulation—have been reported.

Dilution Method

If infected blood is diluted sufficiently and small quantities are inoculated into mice, it is found that only some of the mice develop infections. It has been presumed that these infections are derived from one trypanosome (Cantrell, 1958; Watkins, 1964; *see* also Walker, 1968) but while it is likely that many of them are clones, the dilution method must be regarded as unreliable.

Micromanipulation Method

This procedure involves the isolation of small drops of a highly diluted trypanosome suspension which are examined under a microscope to detect one which contains a single trypanosome. This drop is transferred to a mouse by intraperitoneal inoculation. The main practical difficulties are to prevent the drops from drying up and to ensure that the single parasite is not damaged during transference to an experimental animal. Many ingenious devices have been practised or recommended to overcome these difficulties including the use of high humidity boxes or even rooms, the use of plastic tape, or the placing of the drops on solid agar and removing a cube of agar with a selected drop on it for insertion into a mouse by surgical means. The writer considers these methods unnecessarily elaborate and recommends the procedure described in detail below.

Small centrifuge tubes are prepared by cutting and sealing Pasteur pipettes where the drawn part is 3 mm. in diameter and cutting the wide part (about 5 mm. i.d.) of the tube 5 cm. from the seal. The centrifuge tube is filled to within 5 mm. of the top with the medium described above (p. 91) but to which 10% v/v inactivated horse serum has been added. A mouse with an early rising infection is selected and the tip of its tail cut. After wiping away the first drop of expressed blood, a second small drop is allowed to form. The tip of the tail is inserted into the surface of the medium in the centrifuge tube. Without stirring, the tube is placed in a centrifuge and spun at 2,500 r.p.m. for one minute. A small quantity of the supernatant is withdrawn into a fine pipette which has been prepared from 2 mm. i.d. glass tubing by drawing down once. A microscope slide is flooded with liquid paraffin or silicone fluid (M.S. 550, Hopkin and Williams Ltd.) and placed under a dissecting binocular microscope. The fine tip of the filled pipette is inserted through the surface of the silicone fluid and touched on the slide; the briefest of contact is all that is necessary to cause a small drop of medium to be placed under the silicone. The drop assumes a flattened shape. Many such drops are spotted out and the slide is transferred to the stage of a microscope under a ×10 objective. The illumination is arranged so that a narrow cone of axial light illuminates the field. A micromanipulator[1] is set alongside the microscope and a pipette is mounted in the holder. This pipette is prepared from 2 mm. i.d. tubing but is double drawn to a very fine bore. The slide is searched for a drop with only one trypanosome in it. It is very easy to examine the whole of one drop if the diameter is less than the diameter of field of view. The tip of the pipette is moved over the drop and sharply lowered into it. The medium should rush in carrying the trypanosome with it. The pipette is removed from the holder and more medium mixed with 10% serum is sucked into it. The second drawn part of the tube is broken off and a rubber tube is fitted over the wide end. The fine point is used like a syringe needle to inoculate the contents of the pipette intraperitoneally by blowing through the rubber tube.

Despite the apparent complexity, the method in practice is simple and it should be possible to make inoculations every 3 to 5 minutes. The writer expects 80% success rate.

PRESERVATION OF TRYPANOSOMES IN THE FROZEN STATE

By 'freeze preservation' is meant the long term storage of frozen suspensions of parasites. It is to be distinguished from freeze-drying in which frozen suspensions are dried by high vacuum and may then be stored at room temperature. Freeze-drying, although extensively used for the preservation of bacteria and viruses, has not proved successful for protozoa (Merryman, 1966). The methods generally used for freeze preservation of trypanosomes are based on the work

[1] A convenient instrument is the Model D10P/S10 made by Research Instruments Ltd., which has a separate control for vertical (z) movement but a combined control for the two horizontal directions (x, y).

of Cunningham *et al.* (1963b) and have been reviewed recently by Walker (1966) and by Merryman and Weinman (1968).

Weinman and McAllister (1947) reported that trypanosomes and malaria parasites could be stored at the temperature of solid CO_2. Their method was simple: infected blood was frozen quickly and stored at a constant temperature of $-78°C$. Other workers quickly confirmed these results but the method did not prove to be as successful as it at first appeared. Although infection developed when thawed blood was inoculated into mice, it took a long time to establish itself. It became obvious that most parasites did not survive freezing and that infection resulted from the few that managed to survive.

When it was shown that the preservation of bull semen was improved by the addition of glycerol to the medium, it was natural that similar methods should be applied to trypanosomes. The work of Polge and Soltys (1957) provided a method which yielded good survival of trypanosomes in the frozen state; this method has been further developed and simplified.

The concern of current investigators is to achieve as near 100% survival as is possible so that selection for 'freezability' is avoided and to ensure long term (more than five years) survival.

Various aspects of freeze preservation are described below so that the prospective user may select the procedures best suited to his purpose.

Cold Storage Systems

The essential intense cold can be provided by liquid nitrogen, solid CO_2 or by an electrical refrigerator offering about $-100°C$. Experience has shown that liquid nitrogen is superior to the other systems in economy, reliability and lower storage temperature, providing supplies can be assured.

Union Carbide liquid nitrogen containers make suitable receptacles for a trypanosome 'bank'. Most have a maximum time between fillings of three weeks and can be considered safe for two weeks. It is sound practice to top up containers twice a week from a portable liquid nitrogen flask. A smaller type of liquid nitrogen flask is available for transport of strains. Airlines accept these flasks for transit, but they should be kept in the pressurized part of the aircraft and packed very carefully against mechanical damage.

Freezing Protective Agents

Glycerol and dimethyl sulphoxide are the two most commonly used freezing protective agents. Glycerol is more widely used and gives the most consistent results. It seems that glycerol (analytical reagent grade) is of a uniform high standard, whereas batches of dimethyl sulphoxide vary considerably but in a critical comparative experiment glycerol was found to be inferior to dimethyl sulphoxide (Walker & Ashwood-Smith, 1961). Strains vary in their ability to withstand freezing; trypanosomes of the *brucei* group are robust and freeze without a protective agent as also does *T. lewisi*. Although less experience has been obtained with *T. congolense*, *T. vivax* and *T. cruzi*, these appear to present greater difficulty and failure after long term storage is sometimes experienced. Opinions are much divided about the ability to preserve culture forms of trypanosomes and *Leishmania* over extended periods; it is difficult to assess the true situation as negative results are not usually published. The best advice is to freeze *T. brucei* and *T. lewisi* in glycerol because it has been shown to work but if facilities permit and the importance of the strain justifies it, parallel freezes should be made using both dimethyl sulphoxide and glycerol. The final concentrations which have been found suitable are 10% of glycerol and 7% of dimethyl sulphoxide.

The Choice of Container

Following the practice in semen preservation, ampoules holding up to 1 ml. were originally used but, while the quality of preservation was excellent, these ampoules required an unduly large volume of suspension and took up unnecessary space in the trypanosome bank. Glass lymph tubes or similar capillaries were introduced at the East African Trypanosomiasis Research Organization and have been successfully used since 1960; the volume of suspension required is only 25 μl. Capillary tubes have some disadvantages; owing to their small size the contents thaw out quickly (and sometimes explode) and care is needed to avoid overheating when sealing the tubes. An optimum procedure would appear to be to lay down, say, four ampoules and a sufficient number of capillaries to meet anticipated needs. The writer's practice is to lay down twenty-five capillaries which together with four ampoules fit one cane for the Union Carbide flask.

A Practical Method

To universal containers holding 20 ml. of the medium described previously, 4 ml. of glycerol or 2·8 ml. of dimethyl sulphoxide are added. The contents of the bottles are mixed well and cooled to 4°C. Blood is taken by cardiac puncture (small rodents) or by venipuncture (larger animals) and diluted with an equal volume of chilled medium containing protective agent. The suspension is cooled in ice water for about fifteen minutes and ampoules and capillaries are filled and sealed. Cooling should proceed at once at a slow rate of 2° per minute to − 40°C. This can be achieved by adding small pieces of solid CO_2 to the alcohol in which the ampoules are suspended, by placing the ampoules in a box thermally insulated from liquid nitrogen or solid CO_2, or by using a simple constant cooling rate device such as those described by Walker & Wilen (1967) or Goodwin & Thiel (1967).

When ampoules have reached − 30°C they may be transferred quickly to liquid nitrogen. It is more convenient to have a beaker of liquid nitrogen for this purpose than to attempt to fit the partly cooled ampoules into the bank.

One day after freezing, a capillary tube is withdrawn and placed in a beaker of liquid nitrogen pending preparations for the examination and inoculation of its contents. When all is ready the ends of the capillary are broken with forceps while the contents are still frozen and the contents are allowed to thaw out by holding the tube between the fingers; this procedure prevents explosion of the capillary upon thawing. Some of the suspension is examimined under a microscope for motility of the parasites. A small quantity is withdrawn from the capillary into a syringe containing normal diluent and inoculated into a mouse to test the viability of the strain.

This method of thawing is recommended for routine handling of capillaries. Ampoules are best thawed quickly by placing them in water at about 37°C; they appear not to explode so readily as do capillaries.

Nomenclature, Labelling and Indexing

Considerable confusion has arisen over the meaning of the word 'strain'. If, as is believed, the characters of a strain become altered when maintained by repeated syringe passage then the strain should not be known by its original name. The introduction of the freeze preservation technique has done away with the need for indefinite syringe passage and when a strain is preserved this is a unique event and should be known by one name or number. Lumsden and Hardy (1965a) proposed the word 'stabilate' to designate a single identifiable strain which is freeze preserved. The term has been well received and appears to be in general usage.

Opinions are somewhat divided on the method for identifying a strain; the word 'identifying' is used here in the cataloguing and not the systematic sense. The view held until recently was that the strain should be designated by its laboratory or place of origin, for example *T. rhodesiense* (Liverpool strain) or *T. congolense* (Buswale, 1). When relatively few strains were involved this was satisfactory but it is now considered that strains should be referable to an index held at most major trypanosomiasis research institutes. Thus *T. rhodesiense* (EATRO 118) identifies where a prospective worker should turn for supplies of frozen capillaries or for detailed information concerning the history of the strain. Lumsden *et al.* (1967) have taken the matter further in an attempt to introduce acceptable standardization in designation.

Chapter 6

Infection and Resistance

B. G. F. WEITZ

With a Section on Antigenic Variation by A. R. Gray

INTRODUCTORY

Immune reactions provide very convenient and sensitive methods for the study of the behaviour and the progress of parasites in the host. The complexity of the host's antibody response to parasitic infection is a reflection of the intricate nature of the antigens of the invading organisms. Antibodies may persist in the host in detectable amounts and for a sufficient length of time to provide a trail of evidence long after the parasite has been eliminated. The specificity of the antibody response is particularly important when antigen-antibody reactions are used for the diagnosis of the infection and for the study of immunity to infection.

The correct interpretation of immunological reactions depends on a precise knowledge of the mechanisms involved and of the behaviour and properties of the antigens which initiate these responses. For many years various immunological tests used for the diagnosis of trypanosome infections in man and in animals frequently gave confusing results because the underlying phenomena were incompletely understood. In recent years the many technical advances which have greatly increased the knowledge of immunology have been applied to various aspects of trypanosomiasis with varied success. Although the biology of trypanosomes can now be followed more accurately by using antibodies as markers of the parasites in the host, the progress of immunological studies on trypanosomes is still impeded by intrinsic difficulties, not the least of which is the difficulty of obtaining sufficient antigenic material for study.

Antigens are usually obtained from trypanosomes recovered from the blood of infected animals. Unfortunately, cultivated trypanosomes have so far been of little value in providing suitable antigenic material. For this reason much of the work on trypanosome immunology has been limited to the study of the species which proliferate rapidly in experimental animals. Thus, the trypanosomes of the *brucei* group have received most attention, although the adaptation of *T. vivax* to rodents (Desowitz & Watson, 1953) widened the scope of such laboratory investigations. New techniques designed to facilitate studies on species of trypanosomes which occur only in very small numbers in the blood of infected animals have made it possible to undertake limited investigations on species such as *T. congolense* and *T. vivax* as they occur in domestic animals. Work of this kind would be greatly facilitated if a method were available for the large scale cultivation of trypanosomes having the same antigenic nature as those occurring in the blood of infected animals or in the infective stages of the trypanosome in the tsetse fly.

IMMUNOLOGICAL METHODS

Serological tests applicable to the study of the immune reactions to trypanosomes fall broadly into two categories, namely, those which employ the antigenic components extracted from trypanosomes and those which require the living whole cell as a source of antigen. Antigenic extracts of trypanosomes have the main advantage of being easily standardized and fractionated into distinct chemical or physico-chemical components. Thus the nature and specificity of the antigen-antibody reaction can be relatively easily established. Living whole trypanosomes used for serological tests are difficult to standardize and their reaction with antibodies is limited to surface-active antigens. The relatively recent discovery that trypanosomes in whole blood can be preserved at low temperature (*see* p. 93) now allows repeatable samples of live antigens to be employed. Organisms producing only scanty parasitaemia are not suitable for antigenic extraction and therefore the use of whole living cells is essential. However, tests involving the whole cell are based on a complex reaction involving a wide variety of antigens.

Serological Tests applied to Trypanosomal Extracts

Complement Fixation Test

This classical test is very sensitive. When antigen and antibody react *in vitro* a substance called complement, usually added in the form of fresh guinea-pig serum, is used up or 'fixed' during the reaction. An indicator system essentially dependent on complement for its reaction, such as the haemolysis of sheep erythrocytes by anti-sheep cell serum, is used as a secondary test to determine the amount of complement which has not been used up by the specific antigen-antibody reaction. If no haemolysis occurs in comparison with suitable controls, the test is said to be positive because complement was fixed in the initial specific reaction and is no longer available for the haemolytic reaction in the indicator system. In practice several preliminary titrations are necessary to find the optimum amount of complement required and to ensure that the sera are not anti-complementary. All reagents except the source of complement (usually fresh guinea-pig serum) are heated to 56°C for half an hour to inactivate complement from any extraneous source. The complement fixation test was used extensively by early workers for the diagnosis of infections with *T. gambiense* in man. Various antigens were used but the most successful antigen was obtained from *T. equiperdum*.

Antigens obtained from trypanosomes in the deposits of centrifuged blood of rats infected with *T. equiperdum* were dried and sealed in ampoules *in vacuo* in which they maintained their activity for at least sixteen months (van Goidsenhoven & Schoenaers, 1944). To obtain better yields of trypanosomes from the animals, Evens *et al.* (1953) injected ephedrine to release the trypanosomes from the main organs before bleeding. Further improved extracts of the antigen were tested by Pautrizel *et al.* (1959) who obtained their best results with ultrasonically disintegrated trypanosomes stored at − 25°C.

Precipitation Reaction

When soluble antigens combine with homologous antibody, an insoluble antigen-antibody complex precipitates in the mixture. Precipitation occurs only under certain conditions of salt concentration and ionic strengths of the mixture and when the ratio of antibody to antigen is at its optimum. To obtain a visible precipitate a high concentration of antibody in the mixture is needed and therefore the reaction is most useful to detect small amounts of antigen. The test can be used for qualitative or quantitative estimations of either antibody or antigen by various techniques, some of which are best suited to the study of the antigen-antibody reactions of trypanosomes.

The precipitin ring test is a most sensitive technique to detect the smallest concentrations of antigens in solution. It has been used widely in the identification of the blood meals of tsetse flies (*see* p. 319). More usually gel diffusion precipitin techniques are used and although these may be relatively less sensitive than the ring test and take longer to react they have many other advantages in the qualitative analysis of antigens and antibodies. Single diffusion techniques allow the antigen and antibody to precipitate in tubes in the form of a ring at the site of the optimal ratio of antigen to antibody (Oudin, 1946). By using a blank portion of gel in the tube between the interface of antigen and antibody the double diffusion of both reagents in the gel occurs (Oakley & Fulthorpe, 1953; Preer, 1956). Most commonly the horizontal double diffusion, in petri dishes or on glass plates, is used for the analysis of antigens and antibodies (Ouchterlony, 1948; Elek, 1949).

Gels of various kinds are used, usually a 1% agar gel in buffered saline. Reagents are placed in pits or wells cut out of the gels and suitably positioned to allow the diffusing reagents to interact. Alternatively, troughs containing a common reagent are cut out in front of a row of small pits in which variable reagents are contained. Any patterns of pits or troughs may be used as required.

Precipitation lines appear through the points at which the antigen and antibody diffusing through the gel interact at their optimum ratio. The distance of the lines from the pits containing antibody varies with the concentration of the reagents, a feature which can be used for quantitative estimations.

Antigenic identities are evident when the precipitation lines between adjacent pits converge and fuse in front of a common pit containing antibody. Conversely, lines which cross each other and diverge from each other are produced by dissimilar antigens. It is thus possible to identify unknown antigen mixtures by allowing the precipitin lines to react with those from known antigens in adjacent pits. Conversely, the components in antibody mixtures can also be identified in this way. The number of lines reacting between antigen and antibody wells indicates a minimum number of antigens or antibodies in the reagents (Ouchterlony, 1964; Grabar, 1964). Crowle (1961) gives a comprehensive account of the subject and a complete guide to these techniques.

Gel diffusion methods are of great value for the analysis of soluble trypanosome antigens and for the estimation of the purity of such antigens or their respective antibodies. Unfortunately precipitins are not produced readily in the serum of some species of animals infected naturally or artificially with trypanosomes. However, the injection of soluble or homogenate trypanosome antigens into experimental animals such as rabbits, rats or guinea-pigs elicits good precipitating antibodies in the serum. Many applications of these techniques to trypanosome immunology have yielded valuable information on the nature of the antigens and these are discussed under that heading (*see*, for example, Weitz, 1960b; Gray, 1961; Brown, 1963; Gill, 1964; Miller, 1965). Tests for IgM protein in the serum and the cerebrospinal fluid of patients infected with trypanosomes are examples of the quantitative precipitin reaction (Mattern, 1962; Lumsden, 1965).

The further modification of the precipitin reaction in conjunction with the electrophoresis of the reagents (Grabar & Williams, 1955) provides a method of determining precisely the constituents of heterogeneous antigen mixtures or of characterizing the type of antibody which is active in the reaction. It was used for trypanosome immunological studies by Weitz (1960b), Mattern (1962), Williamson & Brown (1964) and the technique is in common use to determine the nature of antigenic mixtures or to assess the purity of antigenic components.

Passive Haemagglutination Reaction

Soluble antigens may be adsorbed on the surface of a variety of inert particles which are then agglutinated by suitable antisera. Because of the intrinsic difficulty of making standard suspensions of such particles (collodion, latex or resin particles) and of reading the tests, the technique has had only limited application. However, the use of normal erythrocytes as a vehicle for the soluble antigens has been more successful. Normal red blood cells of various species when treated with a dilute solution of tannic acid can be coated by a variety of protein antigens (Boyden, 1951) and are then agglutinated specifically by homologous antibody. The inhibition of the reaction with soluble antigens is a most sensitive and specific technique and was adopted for the identification of blood meals (*q.v.*) of tsetse flies by Weitz (1956). The stability of the test was greatly improved by treating the erythrocytes with bis-diazotized-benzidine (Gordon *et al.*, 1958) or with carbodiimide (Johnson *et al.*, 1966) before coating with antigen. Some antigens can be adsorbed onto red blood cells without previous treatment (Dodin & Fromentin, 1963).

The soluble trypanosomal antigens of *T. brucei* have been quantitatively assayed by the use of cells treated with tannic acid (Lee-Jones, 1961); although the test was difficult to standardize it required only very small quantities of antigen or antibody. Gill (1964) used the technique to assay the sera of animals infected with *T. evansi* and later used erythrocyte suspensions preserved in formalin instead of fresh cells (Gill, 1966). This test proved more sensitive for the diagnosis of surra in cattle and buffaloes than the complement fixation test. In human trypanosomiasis the supernatant from the liquid phase of cultures of *T. gambiense* in diphasic medium was adsorbed on normal red blood cells for use as a diagnostic test and was used with some success (Dodin & Fromentin, 1963).

Fluorescent Antibody Tests

This technique was introduced by Coons and his colleagues (Coons & Kaplan, 1950; Coons, 1956). The reaction can be used to determine the antigenicity of trypanosomes fixed on microscope slides but is difficult to apply on living material. Purified antisera conjugated with suitable fluorochromes (fluorescein or rhodamine compounds are most suitable) are applied to sections or fixed trypanosomes on glass slides. The antibodies specifically combine with antigens *in situ* and fluoresce when examined under the microscope with suitable UV light source and filters. Details of the techniques for the preparation of conjugated sera and for the testing procedures are given by Nairn (1964). There are two basic procedures applicable to the study of trypanosomes and their homologous antisera.

(i) THE DIRECT TECHNIQUE: Antisera specifically prepared against the trypanosomal antigen are conjugated with fluorescein. The fluorescent antibody is applied directly to fixed trypanosomes or frozen histological sections and after washing the preparation is examined under the UV microscope. Areas of specific fluorescence indicate where antibody has combined with antigen in the preparation.

(ii) THE INDIRECT (OR 'SANDWICH') TECHNIQUE: The specific unconjugated trypanosomal antisera are applied directly to the antigenic material. Their specific reaction with antigen is demonstrated by treating the film with fluorescent antisera against the γ-globulin of the species from which the specific antisera were derived. Thus if rabbit antisera are used, the combination with specific antigen is shown by adding anti-rabbit fluorescent antibody. Such fluorescent antisera must be carefully adsorbed to ensure they do not react with the contaminating serum proteins of the species from which the trypanosomes are derived. Anti-rabbit fluorescent antibody would be suitable for trypanosomes from any host other than rabbit. If the trypanosomes are derived from rabbits it is necessary to use specific antisera raised in a different species (e.g. rats or goats) and the fluorescent antibody against the γ-globulin of the species is prepared in rabbits. Proper control experiments are essential to ensure the specificity of the fluorescence.

The direct fluorescent antibody technique was used by Weitz (1963b) to demonstrate the specificity of antigens of *T. brucei* and *T. vivax*. By using specific antisera against *T. brucei* and *T. vivax* antigens conjugated with fluorescein and rhodamine respectively, individual organisms appeared green or red in mixed samples of the two organisms (Weitz, 1963c). These techniques have also been used for the detection of specific antibodies. The indirect fluorescent antibody test was used by Sadun and his colleagues (1963) to demonstrate antibodies in the sera of human patients with a history of trypanosomiasis. These antibodies cross-reacted with various species of trypanosomes irrespective of the species of the infecting organism but few non-infected sera gave positive reactions. Similarly, antibody was found in the cerebrospinal fluid of man and chimpanzees at different stages of infection with *T. gambiense* and *T. rhodesiense* (Lucasse, 1964). *T. brucei* obtained from infected rats could be used as antigen for the diagnosis of infections with *T. gambiense* or *T. rhodesiense* in rabbits (Williams *et al.*, 1963) by the fluorescent antibody technique. Similar reactions were obtained from samples of dried blood on absorbent paper and found to be a suitable field technique by Bailey *et al.* (1967).

The technique is of some value in diagnosis although it is likely to be less reliable in inexpert hands than other serological reactions and is probably less sensitive. A quantitative technique based on the measurement of the intensity of the fluorescence with soluble antigens adsorbed on to cellulose acetate membranes was developed by Toussaint and his colleagues (1965, 1965a) and was applied to trypanosomal antigens but this method needs rigid controls on account of the varied nature of the reagents used. It is also greatly influenced by the type of membrane used as a matrix to support the reagents (Weitz, 1967).

Serological Tests applied to Living Trypanosomes *in vitro*

Immune Adherence Tests

Rieckenberg (1917) found that when trypanosomes were incubated *in vitro* with rat blood platelets in the presence of antibody and complement, the blood platelets adhered to the trypanosomes. This was a manifestation of the immune adherence phenomenon which can be used to titrate antibody or complement in a variety of infections with bacteria (Nelson, 1953; Nelson & Nelson, 1959), protozoa (Duke & Wallace, 1930), soluble antigens (Turk, 1958) and viruses (Taverne, 1957).

Trypanosomal antibodies similarly cause the adhesion of erythrocytes of primates onto trypanosomes and were referred to as 'adhesins' by Duke and Wallace (1930). The reaction took place only in the presence of a complement-like substance (Wallace & Wormall, 1931). The sera of patients infected with *T. gambiense* caused adhesion of primate erythrocytes on the homologous trypanosome as well as on *T. rhodesiense*. After treatment of the patient the adhesins in the serum gradually disappeared. Cross reactions also occurred in the sera from animals infected with *T. congolense*. Although claims have been made that variant specific antibodies could be determined by this method (Leupold, 1928; Brown & Broom, 1938) it is difficult to assess the specificity of this reaction. It would seem profitable to evaluate this reaction for the analysis of the antigens of trypanosomes in the light of present day knowledge of the mechanisms of this phenomena (Turk, 1964). It is, perhaps, because of its complexity and undetermined specificity that this test has been largely superseded by more sensitive and specific serological tests.

Neutralization Test

The effect of antibodies on living trypanosomes *in vitro* can be assessed by inoculating into susceptible animals mixtures of trypanosomes and antibody after a period of incubation. Neutralizing antibodies either kill the trypanosomes or render them less infective. Lysis may occur in the presence of complement but workers who have used this test did not consciously add complement (Schilling & Neumann, 1932) and in this sense neutralizing antibody differs from lytic antibody. The technique is applicable only to trypanosomes which are infective to suitable laboratory animals and the infectivity of antibody-treated trypanosomes must be compared with untreated trypanosomes from the same source. It is not clear if the reduction of infectivity is due to the death of a proportion of the trypanosomes or if there is a general alteration of the infective nature of the trypanosomes under test. Soltys (1957), who developed a useful technique for the neutralization test, suggests that antibody-treated organisms although microscopically unchanged are perhaps more readily lysed or phagocytosed when inoculated into mice. He was able to show specific neutralizing antibodies for strains of *T. brucei*, *T. rhodesiense*, *T. gambiense* and *T. congolense*, and produced antisera containing such specific neutralizing antibody in rabbits vaccinated with formalin-killed organisms. The test has also been used to determine the presence of antibodies in infected cattle. This is a most useful test for the detection of antibody but is applicable only to trypanosomes which are infective to laboratory animals and therefore excludes *T. vivax*.

Cytolytic Test

Antibodies active against cellular antigens are able to lyse living cells containing the homologous antigens in the presence of complement. This 'trypanolysis test' was used first by Schilling (1902) and Lingard (1904) and later was found useful to characterize strains and variants of trypanosomes by a number of workers (Rosenthal, 1913; Russell, 1936; Lourie & O'Connor, 1937). A suspension of living trypanosomes is added to a mixture of antiserum dilutions and complement. After incubation at 37°C the action of the antibody on the organism is determined by microscopic examination of the mixtures.

Recently, Le Page (personal communication) revived and described an elegant technique for this test to identify the antigenic variants of *T. brucei* and *T. congolense* in mice infections. The main advantage of this technique is that the reaction can be observed with only very few trypanosomes, a most important factor in the study of species or strains which do not proliferate easily in laboratory or domestic animals. Thus it can be used to characterize the antigenic nature of trypanosomes derived in small numbers from human, animal or even insect infections. The presence of lytic antibodies in the sera of man or animals infected by different species of trypanosomes may be a reliable diagnostic method. Clarkson and Awan (1967) by means of this test were able to follow the antigenic variations in sheep infected with the rat-adapted strain of *T. vivax* (Desowitz & Watson, 1953). The revival of this test was long overdue and the technique should greatly facilitate antigenic studies on strains of trypanosomes which hitherto have received little attention.

Agglutination Test

Living trypanosomes are agglutinated by specific antibody *in vitro*. Care must be taken to ensure that the trypanosomes used in this test are fully active and motile, otherwise clumps simulating non-specific agglutination may occur. Washed trypanosomes fail to agglutinate because surface 'exo-antigen' has been removed. The density of the trypanosome suspension is also a critical factor in ensuring specific agglutination since well defined clumps do not form in scanty suspensions even after thorough mixing. This again limits the use of the agglutination test to species of trypanosomes which can be recovered in large numbers from infected animals. Soltys (1957a) found that the test was species specific when applied to each of two strains of *T. brucei*, *T. rhodesiense* and *T. congolense*. The sera of four patients infected with *T. rhodesiense* agglutinated his test strain of *T. rhodesiense* but not *T. brucei*. A standardized form of the test was described by Cunningham and Vickerman (1962) who used as the source of antigen frozen infected blood stored in capillary tubes. This has the great advantage that a suitable standard antigen ('stabilate') can be used to avoid the variations due to the many changes in the antigenic nature of the organism or to the physical condition of the trypanosomes in different circumstances. Such factors markedly influence the result of the test. The technique is also much simplified by this method and the suspension of trypanosomes can be applied directly from the capillary tube to the antibody mixtures. The final result is determined by examining the agglutination under the low power of the microscope after a suitable incubation period. The usefulness of this technique was clearly demonstrated in the antigenic analysis of the variants of *T. brucei* by Gray (1962, 1965) and for the study of antigenic relationships (Cunningham & Vickerman, 1962; Weitz, 1962). Unfortunately the technique is not applicable to many strains of trypanosomes which do not give a sufficiently high parasitaemia in infected animals to provide a suitable source of antigen.

Respiratory Test

The effect of antibody on the metabolism of trypanosomes can be measured by the effect on the oxygen uptake of trypanosomes *in vitro*. Desowitz (1956) evolved a most useful method of measuring antibody activity by this means. *T. vivax* was maintained under suitable conditions in a conventional Warburg respirometer for one hour at 36·5°C. Quantitative estimations of antibody concentration were made by adding various immune sera to the trypanosome suspensions and measuring the uptake of oxygen in comparison with normal sera. Estimated by this method antibody titres of the sera of Zebu, Muturu and N'Dama cattle which had been challenged with trypanosomes revealed a high immune response when these animals were born and bred in tsetse infested country (Desowitz, 1959). A decrease in oxygen uptake of *T. brucei* was also evident with specific immune sera (Thurston, 1958). Masseyeff and Gombert (1962) applied this technique to the sera of seventy-seven human subjects infected with *T. gambiense*. In all except three of these cases oxygen uptake was inhibited to some extent while in twenty-three uninfected controls there was no inhibition of oxygen uptake.

The test is a useful measure of antibody and a valuable research tool but has not been much used by other workers as a routine test because of the elaborate nature of the technique.

Immunity Tests

While serological tests indicate the response of a host to antigenic stimuli they give no certain evidence of the protection of the host against infection. The presence of humoral antibodies may coincide with a state of immunity but only extensive correlation studies are likely to show the relationship between antibody response and specific resistance to infection.

Immunity can be demonstrated in suitable hosts only by the results of deliberate infection with live virulent organisms. Varying degrees of immunity exist and these can be assessed by the severity of the challenge the host is able to resist. Artificial active immunity evoked by the administration of an antigenic stimulus indicates the presence of immunogenic ('protective') antigens in the inoculum and various laboratory procedures are employed to assess these reactions against trypanosome infections.

Methods of Immunization

The test host can be immunized in different ways before challenging with an infective dose of the test organism.

LIVE TRYPANOSOMES (live vaccine) administered to a susceptible host may be altered by decreasing the virulence of the organisms in some way or by administering specific drugs to modify the course of infection in the host. These procedures have the advantage that the organisms actively multiply in the host, at least for a period, and in such a fashion as to provide a continuing supply of immunogenic antigens to the antibody-forming apparatus.

KILLED TRYPANOSOMES injected parenterally into animals elicit an immune response the effectiveness of which depends on the presence of immunogenic antigens in the vaccine. Success in immunization also depends on the size of the dose given and on the frequency and the specificity of multiple doses of antigens. Killed vaccines, consisting of dead cellular material, contain all the available proteins to stimulate an immunity, and it is therefore necessary that the organisms should be killed by methods which do not damage the immunogenic antigens. To ensure that stimulation of the immune response is maintained adjuvants are commonly added to the inoculum and although these may act in different ways, they usually retard the absorption and the elimination of the antigens from the body, thereby providing a more prolonged contact with the immunogenic cells of the host. The most restricting factor is the difficulty of obtaining a sufficiently large number of organisms to provide the required antigenic stimulus. For this reason, such vaccines have not been tried extensively, particularly in large animals.

ANTIGENIC EXTRACTS OF TRYPANOSOMES derived from trypanosomes killed and homogenized in various ways obviously contain mixtures of antigens similar to those in killed vaccines. However, by chemical or physical extraction methods, defined components of the organisms can be isolated and used as immunizing agents. Such material can be stored without damage and is more suitable than killed whole organisms, as the study of the chemical nature of immunogenic antigens can be more easily standardized by chemical or physical methods. The metabolic product of the growth of trypanosomes can be used in a similar way. Adjuvants may be added to the extracts to enhance the immunogenic response. The same difficulties of obtaining the antigenic material from sufficient numbers of organisms have limited these studies to the trypanosomes which may be grown prolifically *in vivo* or *in vitro*.

Assay of Immunity

Various methods are available to measure the resistance of the host to a measured and defined infective dose of trypanosomes (the 'challenge'). They all depend on a significant alteration of the course of the infection in the immune host as compared with normal susceptible animals.

THE PREPATENT PERIOD. The time between the injection of the organisms into the host and the appearance of living parasites in the blood stream is a useful and objective measurement and is susceptible to experimental analysis. The length of this prepatent period depends on the character of the infective organism, the number of virulent organisms injected and the route and method of infection. The period can be determined with different challenges in a suitable number of susceptible animals and then compared with the prepatent period in immunized animals. Lumsden *et al.* (1963) used the prepatent period to determine the infectivity of various strains of trypanosomes. Although this may be a very reliable index it does not necessarily correlate with the further development of the infection. For example, in *T. vivax* infection of mice, a delayed prepatent period may be followed by a heavy parasitaemia and death and a short prepatent period may be followed by only a transient infection (Taylor, 1966). Thus it is not clear to what extent the prepatent period is a measure of immunity although it is likely to be an index of the early defence mechanisms of the host against infection.

PARASITAEMIA. The nature of the parasitaemia which follows artificial or natural inoculation of infective organisms is some measure of the host's susceptibility and of the virulence of the organism. In many natural trypanosome infections the parasitaemia is so low that it cannot be counted accurately, but may be assessed by the infectivity titre of the blood. Artificial infections in suitable animals with some species and strains of trypanosomes give rise to very high parasitaemia and a reduction or a delay of the height of parasitaemia may be used to assess the degree of resistance. The complete absence of parasitaemia is, of course, a clear indication of non-susceptibility.

CLINICAL EFFECTS OR DEATH. Some clinical symptoms of trypanosome infections may be a reliable guide to the progress of infection particularly in chronic disease. Deviations from the typical haematological picture or alterations in the constitution of the serum proteins are examples of objective and measurable factors for the assay of infection. In laboratory animal infections with trypanosomes which cause death of the animal, protection is indicated by the survival of the host or by a significant delay in reaching a fatal termination. This is probably the most effective measurement of immunity as it implies a resistance to a very severe infection.

Challenge Infection

The degree of immunity conferred on hosts by natural or artificial stimulation is assessed by the outcome of the infection following a challenge of the subject with a known infective dose of trypanosomes. The results in protected animals are compared with those in fully susceptible and strictly comparable hosts given an identical dose of trypanosomes. The infecting or 'challenge' dose can be varied to promote a predetermined effect for the assessment of the degree of immunity in the test groups. A severe challenge may overcome a weak immunity which would be capable of withstanding a relatively mild challenge dose. In challenge experiments it is therefore essential to measure accurately the load of the test infection.

Measurement of the challenge dose is too often based solely on the number of trypanosomes present in the inoculum; while this may be a valid and repeatable measurement for a given strain of trypanosome, it takes no account of the great variations in the virulence or viability of trypanosomes which may occur under different experimental conditions. It is essential that the challenge dose be measured by the effect it produces in a defined host and that a desired end point be determined by challenging individual hosts or groups of hosts with graded doses derived from a given suspension of trypanosomes. In effect, the grading of the doses is usually in terms of varying numbers of trypanosomes but the actual number of organisms in a dose giving a certain effect may vary considerably from one experiment to another because of differences in the quality of the suspension and of changes in the susceptibility of the test hosts however carefully they are chosen. Lumsden *et al.* (1963) have developed a technique to measure statistically the infective dose for mice based on the first appearance of trypanosomes in the peripheral circulation after infection with several dilutions of an infective suspension of trypanosomes. The end point (ID63) can be determined by standard statistical methods and is completely reliable and repeatable when a frozen batch of *T. brucei* suspension is used in a large number of experiments. This is a most accurate method of determining the infectivity of a trypanosome over periods for challenge of test animals and could be used equally for the measurement of different effects such as those described earlier (death, clinical symptoms, parasitaemia). Very small differences in the susceptibility of animals can be revealed by this accurate technique. Moreover, infective trypanosome suspensions which can be preserved and stored in the frozen state provide a standard challenge 'stabilate' dose giving reproducible results over long periods of time (Lumsden *et al.*, 1965).

The end point in such experiments should be determined before the infected animal produces antibody to the parasites received in the challenge dose. In practice the shorter the time of the observations the better, as irregular results may be obtained four days or longer after challenge because the immune response of the host to the test infection with trypanosomes becomes effective. This severely limits some experiments with species or strains of trypanosomes which have a prolonged prepatent period and which, for this reason, generally give irregular and unreliable results. Artificial challenge is most frequently effected by simple 'syringe passage' but there are occasions when challenge with metacyclic trypanosomes is desirable. Southon and Cunningham (1966) evolved techniques which enable a very accurate challenge to be made with the metacyclic infective forms of trypanosomes obtained from tsetse flies. These techniques are necessarily elaborate but they provide a practical method of infecting animals with a known infective dose of metacyclic trypanosomes, the characters of which are preserved by storage in the frozen state. When such material is used to infect experimental animals, the course of the resultant infection is both predictable and reproducible.

Artificial challenge by tsetse fly transmission is much less certain and extremely elaborate. Nevertheless, this method of challenge may be regarded as essential for the final testing of practical vaccination experiments in the laboratory. An estimation of the infectivity of tsetse flies fed on rats infected with *T. rhodesiense* indicates the variability of such challenge (Harley, Cunningham & van Hoeve, 1966). The assay of immunity in the field is far less precise because the severity of the challenge dose is unknown and extremely variable under natural conditions and can be estimated only empirically by including large numbers of suitable control animals in the test area. This problem has been a continual source of difficulty in the conduct of drug trials in the field. The difficulties are even greater in immunity experiments in the field because of the variable degree and nature of the immune state of the test animals. However the practical outcome of such field experiments is of great value in assessing the protection afforded to test animals on a realistic basis although the interpretation of results obtained can be considered valid only for the conditions pertaining at the time and are not necessarily applicable to other circumstances. Variable factors which influence these results include geographical and climatic differences, the species and density of *Glossina* in the areas, the presence of different hosts available to tsetse for feeding, the variations in the infectivity of the fly and of the antigenic nature of the trypanosomes transmitted cyclically. Typical experiments of this kind were carried out by Whiteside (1962), Chandler (1952) and Soltys (1955) to demonstrate resistance to natural challenge.

THE ANTIGENS OF TRYPANOSOMES

Nature of Antigens

The complexity of the antigenic structure of trypanosomes is evident from the various serological reactions which demonstrate different specificities. As the nomenclature of the characters of different trypanosomal antigens is confused, a few of the terms used in this text are defined below. The antigens of trypanosomes fall into two categories, (i) specific antigens and (ii) common antigens.

(i) *Specific antigens* are those which elicit antibodies reacting with the homologous antigens only and usually with the living strain of the trypanosomes from which the antigen was originally derived.

(ii) *Common antigens* elicit antibodies which react with antigens derived from trypanosomes of different strains or even different species from which the antigens are derived.

The characters of specific or common antigens are further described in accordance with their behaviour:

(a) Immunogenic antigens (often referred to as 'protective' antigens) are those which produce an immunity in the host. Thus, in theory, immunogenic antigens may be either specific or common antigens according to their behaviour but as far as is known only the specific antigens of trypanosomes are immunogenic.

(b) Other manifestations of the specific or common antigens are referred to by the nature of the trypanosomal antibody responses: e.g. agglutinogens produce agglutinins in the serum of the host and precipitinogens elicit precipitins, etc.

(c) Trypanosome antigens may be described also according to their source. Antigens which occur normally in solution in their environment (e.g. in the serum of an infected host) are referred to as *exoantigens*. The term soluble antigens is confusing in this respect as in fact most antigens are soluble whether they occur naturally in solution or not. The term *homogenate antigens* refers to solutions or suspensions of antigens obtained from the whole organism after the mechanical disintegration of the organism. Similarly, *flagellar*, *somatic*, *nuclear* or *surface antigens* refer to antigens derived from these particular structures or situations. Investigations on the nature of the antigens of trypanosomes are limited by the difficulty of obtaining sufficient quantities of trypanosomes for chemical determination. *In vitro* cultivated trypanosomes would, of course, solve the problem if methods of cultivation were devised which yielded trypanosomes with antigens of a kind similar to those present in infected animals. So far this has not been successful but new techniques of cultivation perhaps may yield better material in the future. For this reason more knowledge has been gathered about the *brucei* sub-group of trypanosomes than about other species which do not cause high parasitaemia in laboratory animals.

Source of Trypanosomal Antigens

Homogenate Antigens

There are two sources of trypanosomal antigens available from the blood of infected animals. The trypanosomes themselves can be separated from the blood collected by various means, washed and then mechanically disintegrated to give a solution of homogenate antigens. This method ensures that all available antigens are collected. Trypanosomes can be disintegrated in a number of ways such as mechanical shaking (Desowitz, 1959a), rapid freezing and thawing (Johnson *et al.*, 1963; Hughes, 1951; Weitz, 1960b) and sonic disintegration (Brown & Williamson, 1962); all have been successful methods.

Various methods to separate the trypanosomes from the blood are available. Simple differential centrifugation is practicable with many species of trypanosomes but the losses are heavy if a high degree of purity is required. To help the separation from the blood cells the red blood cells can be agglutinated by specific antibody against erythrocytes of the species or by the addition of non-specific erythrocyte agglutinating substances such as phyto-haemagglutinin (Johnson *et al.*, 1963) or normal horse serum, which commonly agglutinates the red blood cells of mice (Soltys, 1957, 1957a). The disadvantage of these methods is that the soluble substances added to the suspension cannot be eliminated easily from the solution and themselves elicit antibodies when the mixtures are injected into animals.

More sophisticated methods dependent on differential gradient solutions (Vaucel *et al.*, 1964; Ormerod, 1966) require complex apparatus not always available. Lanham (1968) developed a fractionation method through ion exchange columns. Heparinized infected blood passed through columns of TEAE cellulose or DEAE cellulose in a special buffer was completely freed of all blood cell elements and yielded infective and viable trypanosomes in a clean solution with very small losses. The method was applied with great success to *T. congolense*, a trypanosome difficult to separate from the blood cells by centrifugation, and also to *T. lewisi*, *T. vivax* and *T. brucei* laboratory strains obtained from rat and mouse infections. The method promises to be a most useful means of separating trypanosomes for antigenic studies as the organisms obtained are in a very pure state and fully viable.

Exoantigens

The cell-free serum of infected animals is another source of antigen (Weitz, 1960a and b). The soluble antigenic complex liberated from trypanosomes in the serum during the infection of animals was termed 'exoantigen'. Thillet and Chandler (1957) had shown that certain antigenic metabolic products of *T. lewisi* were found in the solutions in which the trypanosomes were maintained *in vitro*. The presence of exoantigen was very soon found in infections with many different species including *T. gambiense* and *T. vivax* (Gray, 1961), *T. congolense* (Dodin & Fromentin, 1963), *T. rhodesiense* (Seed & Weinman, 1963) and *T. evansi* (Gill, 1965) and it may be assumed that exoantigen formation is characteristic of some trypanosomes. To obtain the exoantigens, the parasitized blood is collected and allowed to clot and the serum is freed from trypanosomes by filtering through cellulose acetate membranes (e.g. Millipore filters). The infected serum containing the exoantigen can be used as the antigenic solution to characterize the nature of these antigens. Alternatively, both homogenate and exoantigen can be collected from the same infected blood. The blood is prevented from clotting by collecting into a suitable anticoagulant solution (1 part of 199 solution containing at least 10 units/ml. of heparin in 3 parts of infected blood). The cells are separated by differential centrifugation and the trypanosomes collected and repeatedly washed in 199 solution and finally centrifuged to produce homogenate antigens. All the washings of the trypanosomes are collected together, filtered, and finally concentrated by pressure dialysis. Such solutions contain all the exoantigens in the plasma.

The exoantigens being derived from living trypanosomes occur and are active on the surface of the cells. When the trypanosome cells are thoroughly washed to remove all surface exoantigens, and are then mechanically disintegrated, they release more antigens; some have the same properties as exoantigens, as would be expected since the organisms produce this antigen. It is, therefore, possible that the exoantigens which occur naturally in the serum of the infected host may be derived partially from cell autolysis. This, however, is not borne out by experimental evidence and indeed it is difficult to detect in solution in the serum any other antigens which are normally liberated only by breaking up the cells *in vitro*.

Biological Characters of Trypanosome Antigens

As would be expected on the basis of genetic relationships trypanosomes have a number of antigenic characters which are common to different strains or species. However, the common antigens appear to be limited to the homogenates as a source of material and are not usually present in the exoantigens. Common antigens are demonstrated by a number of *in vitro* reactions and by serological tests in which the whole antigenic make-up of the organisms is involved. They are not shown by serological reactions acting merely on the surface antigens of trypanosomes.

The cross reactivity of sera of infected humans or animals shown by the complement fixation test provides ample examples of the common antigens in different species of trypanosomes. Extracts made from *T. equiperdum* react with antibodies in the serum of patients infected with *T. gambiense* or *T. rhodesiense* (van Goidsenhoven & Schoenaers, 1944; Rodhain *et al.*, 1941; Evens *et al.*, 1953) and in cattle infected with *T. brucei* and *T. congolense*. However, common antigens of *T. gambiense* and *T. rhodesiense* and *T. vivax* were shown in the exoantigens of the organisms by precipitin tests and absorption tests (Gray, 1961) but perhaps this was due to contamination of the reagents used with homogenate antigen as in no other case were common antigens found in the exoantigens. Brown and Williamson (1962) showed common precipitinogens in homogenates of *T. rhodesiense* and *T. brucei* and Seed (1963) in those of related strains of *T. rhodesiense* and of the culture forms of the organism.

By precipitin and by fluorescent antibody tests common antigens in the homogenates of *T. brucei* and *T. vivax* were shown by Weitz (1962; 1963b). The agglutination test and the neutralization test, however, do not normally reveal common antigens of trypanosomes (*see* Soltys, 1957, 1957a; Gray, 1962) although Cunningham and Vickerman (1962) showed common agglutinogens in some strains of *T. brucei* and *T. rhodesiense* in rabbit infected sera but these were probably due to heterogeneous populations of variants. The Forsmann-like antigens of the *T. brucei* group of trypanosomes shown by Houba and Allison (1966) provide another example of common antigenic components. There is, therefore, ample evidence of the presence of common antigens in trypanosomes of different species or strains but these are limited to the homogenate antigens. However, the immunogenic properties of the homogenate antigens do not show any cross specificity. Seed (1963) and Miller (1965) were able to protect mice with homogenate antigens only against the homologous strain of trypanosome and Weitz (*unpublished*) was unable to immunize rats or mice against *T. vivax* with homogenate antigen from *T. brucei*. It is likely, therefore, that the immunogenic activity of homogenates is due to the exoantigen component which they normally contain.

The specific antigens, however, seem characteristic of exoantigens. These occur on the surface of the organisms as shown by the specific agglutination of live trypanosomes by antibody to the exoantigens (Weitz, 1960a and b) and also as is suggested by the concentration of exoantigen on the flagellum visible by fluorescent antibody technique (Weitz, 1963c). The presence of exoantigens in homogenates of trypanosomes is seen in gel diffusion tests to give lines of identity with sera infected with the same organisms containing the exoantigens only.

The specificity of these antigens is not confined to species but may extend even to antigenic variants and they are agglutinogenic, precipitinogenic and immunogenic. In animal infections the appearance of antibodies against exoantigens may be due mostly to the liberation of exoantigens in the serum. Miller (1965) has shown that the variant specific agglutinin of rabbits infected with *T. brucei* can be adsorbed specifically by the exoantigens of these variants. Clearly the exoantigen components are thus concerned with antigenic variation and may be the main variable constituent of the trypanosomal antigen. Immunogenically the exoantigen is specific and active protection is limited to the homologous strain or variants. Exoantigens thus produce an extremely limited immunity. As the common antigens of homogenate antigens appear to be non-immunogenic there is at present no suitable antigenic material for artificial active immunity experiments against a number of strains or variants of trypanosomes in the field.

Cultivated trypanosomes are also agglutinogenic and precipitinogenic (Seed, 1963) but do not immunize animals against related infective blood forms of trypanosomes, although some of the antigens of cultivated forms are common with those of the blood forms.

Trypanosome antigens can be properly characterized only when suitable purification of the antigens is possible. The present confusing state is mainly due to the difficulty of obtaining clearly defined antigenic components from infected animals.

From a practical point of view homogenates of trypanosomes, containing both specific and common antigens, are the most informative immunological material. However, the properties of the exoantigens suggest a specific function in the infection of the host. These antigens may be considered to protect the trypanosomes against the specific antibody defences of the host. The variation of the specificity of the exoantigens on the surface of trypanosomes defeats the antibody response of the host and allows the trypanosomes to proliferate under cover of different antigenic specificities. The possibility that the exoantigens also play some part in the pathogenicity of trypanosome infections should be considered. Although non-toxic and causing no apparent ill effects when injected into animals, it is possible that they may have affinities for certain tissues in the body and thus engender disease as a direct or indirect result of their contact with certain cells. Such considerations, although hypothetical at this stage of knowledge, deserve further experimental investigation.

Antigenic Variation (*contributed by* A. R. GRAY)

The instability of certain trypanosome antigens in infected animals limits the progress of research on immunity to trypanosomiasis. The real importance of antigenic variation lies mainly in the fact that the variable antigens include those which can stimulate the production of protective antibody, for example the exoantigen of *T. brucei* (Weitz, 1960a, b), the PR antigen of *T. rhodesiense* (Seed & Weinman, 1963) and the 4*S* and 1*S* antigens of *brucei* group trypanosomes (Brown & Williamson, 1962). Thus animals do not become immune when they are naturally infected, and no one has yet succeeded in inducing a high level of immunity artificially because the antibodies which animals produce are effective against only a few of the antigens which may develop in any strain.

Until recently, research on antigenic variation has often been difficult because of the lack of suitable methods for preserving the antigenic characteristics of trypanosomes during long-term experiments. The usual procedure adopted in the past was to subpassage the trypanosomes in rats or mice at two- to three-day intervals in the hope that the antigens would not change. The method had the disadvantage, however, that variants sometimes reverted to a 'parent' antigenic strain type when rodent subpassage was prolonged (*see* Lourie & O'Connor, 1937). The introduction of methods for preserving strains at low temperatures has removed this element of doubt from research on antigenic variation (*see* Walker, 1966). The antigenic characteristics of trypanosomes can now be preserved for years without any danger of non-experimental antigenic change.

The number of antigens which a strain of trypanosomes can produce has not yet been determined, but Ritz (1916) showed that a single trypanosome could give rise to at least twenty-two different antigenic types of trypanosomes. The ability of clone strains of trypanosomes to produce many antigens has subsequently been amply confirmed (*see* Lourie & O'Connor, 1937; Gray, 1965a). Strains of *brucei* group trypanosomes produce new antigens at intervals of two to four days in infected laboratory rodents, and in sheep and goats (Gray, 1965), but very little is known about the frequency of variant antigen production by trypanosomes in other domestic animals. There is no convincing evidence that any antigen of a strain is produced twice during an infection, and it seems that the total number of antigens produced in one host may be limited only by the length of time the animal lives. A strain of trypanosomes produces similar antigens in different hosts, but the antigens often develop in a different sequence. A number of antigens may develop at the same time and the antigenic character of a variant strain often results from a combination of the characteristics of several different antigens.

In relapsing infections, antigenic variation can be related to variations in the numbers of trypanosomes in the blood and to the formation of a series of variant-specific antibodies. Infection is followed by an increase in the parasitaemia which terminates in a crisis, coinciding with the appearance of antibodies in the serum of the animals and a reduction in the number of trypanosomes (Levaditi & McIntosh, 1910; Mutermilch & Salamon, 1928). Organisms of a new antigenic type soon appear and multiply until a further crisis occurs in association with the production of a second specific antibody; this process may be repeated at intervals of a few days until the animal dies. Crises and relapses, and variations in the numbers of organisms in the blood, become less obvious as infections progress, but antigenic variation continues until the animal dies.

The influence of antibody on antigenic variation has also been demonstrated in other ways. For example, Ehrlich *et al.* (1909) incubated trypanosomes with homologous antiserum *in vitro*, and showed that a new antigenic type of the strain developed when the incubated suspension was injected into an experimental animal, and Gray (1962) used specific antisera to suppress the development of selected antigens of a strain of *T. brucei* in rabbits. Inoki *et al.* (1956)

claim that they have induced variation in the agglutinogenic antigens of *T. gambiense* by exposing trypanosomes to immune serum *in vitro* but recent attempts to confirm their results have not been successful (Brown, 1963).

There is evidence that each trypanosome strain has an innate tendency to develop in one particular antigenic form which is relatively stable. This tendency is often noticeable when a strain multiplies in the absence of specific antibody. Thus, when a variant of a strain is maintained for a long time by repeated subpassage at intervals of a few days in laboratory animals, it may revert to one serotype, sometimes called the 'parent' antigenic type of strain (Mesnil & Brimont, 1909; Neumann, 1911). In addition, some authors have found that trypanosomes constituting the first relapse strains which develop after infected animals have been treated with drugs or serum, are of one antigenic type or a limited number of types (Ehrlich, 1911; Leupold, 1928; Raffel, 1934; Osaki, 1959; Inoki, 1960). It must be noted, however, that other authors have found little similarity among such trypanosomes (Neumann, 1911; Lourie & O'Connor, 1937).

Further evidence of the tendency of a strain to produce one particular antigen has been obtained in experiments on the effect of development in the tsetse fly on the antigens of variant strains. Trypanosomes of one strain transmitted by different tsetse flies have an antigen in common (Broom & Brown, 1940) which has been called the 'basic' antigen of the strain (Gray, 1965). When a tsetse fly ingests trypanosomes with the 'basic' strain antigen, the antigen persists for two or three weeks through all the morphological changes associated with cyclical development so that the fly transmits organisms with the 'basic' antigen when it becomes infective. When, however, a tsetse fly ingests trypanosomes with variant antigens there is a tendency for such antigens to be displaced during cyclical development. Thus cyclically transmitted substrains of a strain sometimes possess only the 'basic' strain antigen but they often possess a mixture of the 'basic' and variant antigens.

In addition to the 'parent' or 'basic' antigen, certain other antigens of each strain of trypanosomes tend to develop during the first few weeks of infection whenever a strain is introduced into a new host by syringe (Leupold, 1928; Osaki, 1959). These antigens have recently been called 'predominant' antigens to distinguish them from numerous other less prominent variant antigens which develop during the late stages of chronic infections (Gray, 1962). The 'basic' antigen associated with cyclically-transmitted substrains of a strain of *T. brucei* also behaved as a 'predominant' antigen when variants of the strain were transmitted to new hosts by syringe (Gray, 1965).

There is still considerable controversy as to whether antigenic variation results from random mutation and the selection of viable mutants, or whether the sequence of antigen synthesis is organized and the intracellular control system temporarily adapts in response to extracellular stimuli. Calculations of the mutation rates of *T. equiperdum* and *T. brucei* growing in rats and mice have shown that the mutation rates and populations of trypanosomes are great enough to account for the observed production of new antigenic variants (Cantrell, 1958; Watkins, 1964). In contrast, however, many features of antigenic variation seem to be more in keeping with a degree of organization rather than with a process of mutation. For example, variants of a strain tend to revert to a 'parent' or 'basic' antigenic type during blood-passage in experimental animals; strains persist in a 'basic' antigenic form, or tend to revert from variants to a 'basic' antigenic form during development in the tsetse fly; clones and variants of one strain produce the same antigens in different hosts and antigenic variation often occurs in a relatively fixed pattern. These facts seem to support an adaptive process as the basis for antigenic variation; an explanation in terms of mutation requires a much greater degree of 'back mutation' than seems possible.

Although previous studies have led to some understanding of antigenic variation, knowledge is by no means complete, and more work remains to be done on the fundamental nature of the phenomenon. Williamson and Brown (1964) have suggested that, as the variable antigens of trypanosomes are proteins, antigenic variation should be susceptible to analysis in terms of current knowledge of the intracellular control of protein synthesis. Their attempts, however, to explore this possibility were not successful, but their experiment has indicated lines on which work could develop in the future with profit.

A satisfactory theory of antigenic variation must account for the production of different variants during the course of a chronic infection, and for the occurrence of considerable differences between the variant specific antigens of different strains of the same species. It is possible that chemical and physical examination of the variant specific antigens will reveal the extent of change between different antigens, the number of sub-units in the molecule, and, most interesting of all, the production by the same strain of related, but not identical, proteins. It is the nature of graded chemical differences (as yet undetected) between variant specific proteins which will tell us most about the processes underlying the origin of new variants. Peptide fingerprint studies are being undertaken in conjunction with other methods in order to try to pinpoint the similarities and differences between purified protein antigens from a large number of clones of several strains of *T. brucei* (Le Page, personal communication).

Composition of Trypanosome Antigens

The accurate determination of the structure and composition of the antigens of African trypanosomes has been limited largely in the past by the serological techniques employed to assess their activities and by the lack of accurate physico-chemical techniques. The results of the early work of Kliger *et al.* (1940) and Ikejiani (1947) on *T. evansi*, *T. equiperdum* and *T. lewisi* largely suffer from such difficulties and their work remains inconclusive.

The extensive and complete analysis of the antigens of the *brucei* group of trypanosomes by Williamson and Brown is the main really valid contribution to this complex subject (Brown & Williamson, 1962, 1964; Williamson & Brown, 1964).

These authors studied the constitution of antigenic extracts of the homogenates of *T. brucei*, *T. rhodesiense* and drug relapse and antigenic variant strains derived from them obtained by lysis in water and disintegrated ultrasonically or mechanically. The material is thus most comprehensive and includes both specific and common antigens. Exoantigens would thus also be included and their character would be related mostly to the variant specific antigens described by these workers. However, their studies are limited to the antigenicity of trypanosomes in their capacity to form a precipitate in agar gel with antitrypanosome immune sera and it is just possible that immunogenic antigens which are not precipitinogens were excluded. Two components of unconjugated light-weight proteins were implicated as variant-specific precipitinogens. The major group (4*S*) consists of proteins with a molecular weight of about 4–8 $\times 10^4$ and a minor group (1*S*) of antigens of a molecular weight of 1–2 $\times 10^4$; this group was dialysable through cellophane membranes, fairly heat stable and only incompletely precipitated by trichloracetic acid. The chemical characters of both components indicate that they are predominantly protein; extensive search for lipid complexes or polysaccharides failed to reveal antigenically active components of this type.

The crude antigen protein was fractionated into eleven bands by starch gel electrophoresis. The active 4*S* protein was mainly in the cytoplasm or cell sap and only very limited activity was present in nuclear, microsomal and mitochondrial extracts. The 1*S* protein may be associated with nucleic acid although the antigenic activity was insensitive to the action of DNAase or RNAase. Two light-molecular-weight common antigens were associated with the nuclear fraction.

The results of Lanham (personal communication) are consistent with these findings. When homogenates of *T. vivax* were eluted on DEAE-Sephadex columns the first fraction obtained was characteristically protein in nature and free from nuclear compounds. This fraction reacted specifically with *T. vivax* antisera and not with antiserum against *T. brucei*. It was serologically distinct from later fractions, chiefly nucleic protein, and from a late protein component, all of which cross-reacted serologically. These late fractions are possibly the source of the common antigens of *T. vivax*. The first fractions were similar to the exoantigens which separated from infected rat serum on DEAE-Sephadex in the regions of globulins and albumin of normal sera. The immunogenic activity of exoantigens in infected rat sera was limited to the first fraction and to the supernatant obtained after precipitation with 65% saturation of ammonium sulphate.

Nature of Trypanosome Antibodies

There is no indication that the nature of the antibodies against the antigens of trypanosomes differs in any way from that of the antibodies to other infective agents. Moreover, the type of antibody produced probably varies considerably in different host species and at different times during infection or immunization depending on the experience of the host with previous antigenic stimulus. Thus no universal rule can be made applicable to all conditions.

The two main immunoglobulins concerned with antibodies are the IgG (otherwise known as γ-globulins or 7*S* globulins) and the larger molecular species IgM (macroglobulins extending from the faster moving γ-globulins and including the β-globulins and the slower α-globulins having a sedimentation rate of 19*S*). Antibodies of the same specificity and reactivity may be distributed in both types of immunoglobulins at the same time. The general decrease in the albumin/globulin ratio apparent in human trypanosomiasis is consistent with antibody formation but is a non-specific reaction also occurring in many infections, partly due to an increase of circulating antibody in the form of γ–globulin and partly to a reduction in the serum albumin content (Jenkins & Robertson, 1959; Evens *et al.*, 1963). Desowitz (1959; 1960) found similar changes in the serum proteins of cattle, gazelle, reedbuck and duiker and noted the presence of an extra γ–globulin component in the hyperimmune serum of N'Dama cattle. Increases in the serum β–globulins suggest that the antibody was present in the IgM immunoglobulins.

In man, the increases in IgM protein (*q.v.*) and the presence of this protein in the cerebrospinal fluid in infected patients also suggest an antibody response. However, no experimental evidence so far indicates that these macroglobulins may be limited to antibody; their presence may be due to a significant pathological alteration of the serum protein complex.

THE PRACTICAL SIGNIFICANCE OF IMMUNE RESPONSES

Serodiagnosis

The demonstration of the infective organism provides the only certain diagnosis of trypanosomiasis. The difficulties of isolating trypanosomes or observing them microscopically necessitate the use of other aids to diagnosis such as the demonstration of antibodies in the serum of the host. This method has the advantage that the persistence of antibodies in the blood during, and for some time after, infection makes it possible to obtain evidence of infection.

The various factors which markedly influence the presence of antibodies in the blood must be taken into account.

Presence and Persistence of Antibodies

Usually the appearance of humoral antibodies is delayed until about a week after infection and serodiagnosis is thus unsuitable for the very early stages of the disease. The rate of antibody formation varies with different hosts and different species of trypanosomes but is largely dependent on the intensity of the parasitaemia and other factors which affect the contact of the antigens with the reticulo-endothelial (lymphoid-macrophage) system. Similarly the persistence of the antibodies in the serum after recovery is variable and is probably influenced by the persistence of trypanosomal antigens in the tissues.

Antigenic Variation

The variation of the antigens of trypanosomes during infection promotes antibodies against each variant. Therefore, if specific antigens are used for the serological reaction, they can only demonstrate specific antibodies and these will be apparent only during distinct periods of the infection. To obtain a continuous and complete picture of all antibodies demands the use of a variety of antigens. This difficulty can be overcome by the demonstration of the antibodies to the common antigens, on the assumption that these will persist throughout the course of infection irrespective of antigenic variation.

Specificity of Serological Reactions

The diagnosis of trypanosomiasis can be made by demonstrating antibody which reacts with any trypanosomal antigen providing the reaction does not occur with antigens of different parasites. However, the species or strain of trypanosome causing the infection can only be ascertained by the demonstration of the specific antibodies.

The choice of diagnostic test is thus governed by a number of practical factors in addition to those governing the serological reactions described earlier. The demonstration of humoral antibodies provides strong, if not conclusive, evidence of trypanosomiasis but inability to do so does not prove freedom from infection since the antibodies may have fallen below a detectable level or the *in vitro* test may have failed because of the choice of an unsuitable antigen.

Serodiagnosis of Human Trypanosomiasis

The complement fixation test has been the most widely used test for the diagnosis of the human disease due to *T. gambiense*. Complement fixing activity may persist for two years after cure following drug treatment (Rodhain & van Goidsenhoven, 1944) but this persistence is obviously variable (van den Branden, 1941). The activity in the cerebrospinal fluid disappears soon after treatment (Rodhain *et al.*, 1941). Results vary with the complement fixation test but a reasonably good correlation with known infections of *T. gambiense* in man was obtained by most workers. Of 125 known infections 119 (95%) gave positive complement fixation tests and only 5 (4%) were negative (Schoenaers *et al.*, 1953). Occasionally a few false positive reactions occurred.

Results from the red cell adhesion test are less conclusive but as it appears that the basis of the test is dependent on the presence of complement ('adhesion') this is likely to prove of no greater value than the complement fixation test.

The detection of agglutinins in the serum of four patients infected with *T. rhodesiense* (Soltys, 1957a) suggests a possible diagnostic method, but in general the high sensitivity of the agglutination test makes this reaction unsuitable for widespread diagnostic purposes.

Fluorescent-antibody techniques may also be of some value; this antibody has been demonstrated in the sera of patients infected with human trypanosomes (Sadun *et al.*, 1963). The test is rather elaborate, easily subject to misinterpretation and is not very sensitive.

Perhaps the most promising serodiagnostic test for human trypanosomiasis is the detection of IgM (macroglobulin) which seems pathognomonic when raised levels occur in the serum and diagnostic when found in the cerebrospinal fluid.

In general it may be said that there is no foolproof serological test for the diagnosis of trypanosomiasis in man. As the usefulness of any test depends on good correlation with other diagnostic methods it would seem unlikely that any are of real practical value for general application except the presence of IgM. Nevertheless, if, by any test, antibodies to trypanosomes are detected in the serum of a patient, other methods should be applied to verify the diagnosis of trypanosomiasis.

Serodiagnosis of Animal Trypanosomiasis

There are very few records of serological tests extensively correlated with the infection of domestic animals. Most serological techniques have been tried on small numbers of sera from known infected animals but are too limited to be conclusive. The diagnosis of *T. equiperdum* in horses by the complement fixation test is probably the best documented technique in the field but it is still inconclusive. Desowitz (1960) showed respiratory inhibiting antibodies in hyperimmune cattle against *T. vivax*. The demonstration of precipitins in cattle and goats infected with *T. vivax* and *T. brucei* (Gray, 1961) and neutralizing antibodies in *T. congolense* infected cattle (Bolton, personal communication) might be of some value as a diagnostic tool particularly as the precipitating antigens are common to these species.

However, few studies on the usefulness in field diagnosis of various serological tests have been made and the general application of these techniques to field diagnosis cannot be regarded as reliable in our present knowledge. Cunningham and van Hoeve (1965) studied the serological reactions occurring in the sera of a herd of 114 cattle in Kenya of which 11 were known to be infected with *T. congolense* and 3 with *T. brucei.* Agglutinins to *T. brucei* were found in 28 cattle and precipitins in 17. These results were not always correlated with known infections and 4 animals known to be infected showed no antibodies. Precipitins occurred in 11 uninfected cattle and agglutinins in 20 such animals. Some animals infected with *T. congolense* had antibodies against *T. brucei.* These are the sort of results which can be expected when antigens of limited specificity are used for testing but they indicate the difficulty in interpretation when the infection status of a herd is unknown.

Serological reactions by themselves cannot yet be relied upon for the certain diagnosis of trypanosomiasis in man or animals. Much work is needed to establish the validity of tests for diagnostic purposes in relation to the time of development and persistence of the antibody, and also to the choice of suitable antigens. At present these tests must be regarded chiefly as experimental tools.

Immunity to Trypanosome Infections

There is no evidence showing unequivocally an acquired protection after recovery from the disease either in man or in animals which perhaps indicates the poor immunogenic response to the trypanosome antigen. Partial or incomplete protection is difficult to assess and cannot be measured satisfactorily in the field, so that, even if it exists, only total protective immunity is likely to be demonstrated. There are some indications that an immunity occurs for a relatively short time after recovery and its efficacy may be measured by the length of time such immunity may persist in the face of a suitable challenge.

Natural or Innate Immunity

Many species of animals are not susceptible to infection with various trypanosomes and man is susceptible only to some forms of the *T. brucei* group. The factors influencing the susceptibility of different species to infective organisms are varied. Intrinsic factors associated with the invasiveness (virulence) of the organism are probably the most important but the mode of entry of the organisms into the body, the constitutional factors of a potential host which affect the ability of trypanosomes to establish themselves, metabolize and proliferate in the body all play a part in the final outcome of the infection. In addition to such non-specific factors, a strong specific resistance to infection may occur in some animals and has often been referred to as an 'innate immunity' although there is little evidence showing that such a complex protective mechanism is in fact associated with, or due to, an active specific immunity in the strict sense. The insusceptibility of cotton rats to *T. vivax* infection has been attributed to a natural immunity because of the presence of humoral antibodies in the serum (Terry, 1957). The presence of such antibodies is obviously suggestive of a specific immunity but in no way proves it, because in many other instances humoral antibodies to trypanosomes are found in non-immune animals.

The laboratory rat is also insusceptible to *T. vivax* infection but a strain of this trypanosome, derived from infected sheep, was trained to live and proliferate in the rat by adding blood supplement from the original host (Desowitz & Watson, 1953). Gradually the strain became adapted to the rat in which it caused active parasitaemia and death; ultimately, it became infective to the rat without the blood supplement. This excellent example of a change in the strain which either overcame the host's resistance or became adapted to the host's metabolism indicates clearly that the change was in the strain and not in the host. As there is no indication of a change in the antigenicity of the adapted strain it is more likely that the organism evolved a metabolic activity suitable to its new host.

Whatever the nature of the change this adaptation exemplifies the principles involved and stresses the need for caution in distinguishing between insusceptibility and immunity.

The numerous examples of species of animals which are not susceptible to trypanosome infection are thus often misquoted as evidence of innate immunity; the terms 'resistant' or 'non-susceptible' are preferable.

The resistance of two native breeds of dwarf cattle in Western Africa, the N'Dama and the Muturu humpless cattle, appears to be, at least partly, due to an acquired specific immunity. These cattle when born and bred in tsetse areas tolerate trypanosomiasis far more readily than Zebu or Zebu cross cattle (Stewart, 1951; Chandler, 1952, 1958; Stephen, 1966) although they often become infected and sometimes may lose condition and die. This protection is probably the result of a more efficient immune response to trypanosome infection than to an innate immunity. N'Dama and Muturu cattle constantly produce a higher level of gamma globulins when born and bred in tsetse-fly country. However, animals born in the absence of trypanosome challenge show an immune response comparable to that of Zebu susceptible cattle (Desowitz, 1959). The practical aspects of breeding such naturally immune responsive animals are discussed elsewhere (*see* p. 759).

Premunity

The phenomenon of premunity described by Sergent *et al.* (1924) does not necessarily apply to trypanosome infections. In premune animals the persistence of the original infecting organisms affords protection against reinfection by organisms of the same antigenic nature. To demonstrate this process is impossible in the face of changing antigens in trypanosome infections. However, multiple infections are common and if the concept is accepted premunity could not protect infected hosts against any but the antigenic variants which they harbour. On general grounds, therefore, it seems that this concept cannot apply in practice to animal trypanosomiasis although it could perhaps have some effect on reinfection in man.

Acquired Immunity

NATURALLY ACQUIRED IMMUNITY. In the natural disease there is no evidence of an acquired immunity after cure and it is not uncommon for man to become reinfected some time after apparently successful therapy. However, it is possible that some of these cases were due to a relapse from the original infection. In domestic animals there is no evidence of a naturally acquired immunity with the exception of the N'Dama and Muturu cattle which may develop a clinical immunity in suitable environments.

EXPERIMENTAL ACQUIRED IMMUNITY. Laboratory animals or domestic animals have been frequently immunized with success against infection with trypanosomes. Live vaccine may be one of the most successful and practical methods of vaccination as it can be effected by a relatively small number of organisms and without damage to their antigenic nature. It is well known, for example, that rats or mice given a small non-infecting dose of the rat adapted strain of *T. vivax* survive any future challenge by doses which are fully infecting and rapidly lethal to rats not previously challenged in this manner. The danger of a relapse from the subinfecting dose, and the difficulty in assessing the right dose for different animals are perhaps risks too great to justify the use of this method in the field. Attenuated live vaccines were used by Schilling (1935) in calves and although partially successful the practical merits of this method were inconclusive in view of the limitations of these experiments. In any case animals immunized in this fashion are presumably resistant only to the homologous strain used for vaccination.

Although killed vaccines against *T. brucei* (Soltys, 1964) and against *T. congolense* (Johnson *et al.*, 1963) in laboratory animals gave reasonable protection against the homologous strain, the most precise immunizing agent is derived from extracts of trypanosomes because these can be standardized, chemically defined and stored more readily. The protective power of antigenic extracts from disintegrated trypanosomes has been amply confirmed in laboratory animals (Weitz, 1960a, b; Seed, 1963) but the immunity elicited is still only effective against the homologous species (Weitz, 1963b) or even against the homologous antigenic variant (Miller, 1965).

The main reason why so few experiments on artificial immunity of cattle have been done is the difficulty of obtaining sufficient antigenic material for vaccine trials. Apart from the early experiments by Schilling and his colleagues (1935) who immunized calves with killed trypanosomes with some success, the only known attempts to vaccinate cattle are those recently made by Neal (personal communication) who used *T. congolense* antigens with adjuvants but without great success.

Immunity Induced by Drug Therapy

Experimental laboratory animals cured by various trypanocidal drugs at the height of parasitaemia often remain immune to further challenge with virulent trypanosomes. Similarly, a temporary immunity occurs in young cattle after treatment which cured or mitigated infection (van Saceghem, 1938). Soltys (1955, 1958) found that cattle repeatedly treated with quinapyramine and maintained in areas infected with *T. congolense* acquired a resistance to reinfection for at least eighteen months. He attributed these findings to immunity induced by constant natural challenge under protection of the drug. Treated animals which were repeatedly challenged with virulent *T. congolense* by syringe inoculation were marginally more resistant than animals which only received the drug (Smith, 1958). Since the drug given alone in the absence of challenge has some lasting protective effect it is difficult to interpret to what extent the resistance which developed was in fact due to an acquired immunity in these experiments. The difficulty of standardizing experiments of this kind is probably the main reason for the somewhat contradictory nature of the results obtained in different experiments. Thus the effect of the drug depends on the intensity of the challenge. For example, the resistance of cattle lasted only two weeks in a heavily infected area but several months in an area where the incidence of tsetse fly was ten times less (Whiteside, 1962). Infected cattle treated prophylactically developed a brief immunity which was intensified after continued challenge in these areas. Whiteside also reports the possible transmission of such immunity to calves born from such immune dams.

Artificial Immunization in the Field

In our present state of knowledge the prospects for the effective immunization of livestock in the field by artificial means are not encouraging. It is not, as yet, feasible to produce vaccines prepared from antigenic extracts of trypanosomes or from the killed organisms themselves, even in sufficient quantities for small field trials. This practical difficulty will not be overcome until suitable techniques for the cultivation of trypanosomes have been developed.

The use of vaccines prepared from living avirulent or attenuated trypanosomes is perhaps a more promising approach but there are many practical difficulties in the preparation and use of living vaccines including standardization and distribution. Furthermore, available evidence indicates that, by their use, it is possible to achieve only partial protection and then against only a limited number of strains.

The development of effective immunity under field conditions is more likely to be achieved by exposing livestock to natural challenge while under the protection of chemoprophylactic agents. In the field trials to which this method has been subjected it appears that the protection conferred lasts little longer than that afforded by the drug itself. It remains to be shown whether continued treatment under constant natural challenge over long periods will increase the duration of protection. Calves born of dams protected in this way, if subsequently exposed to constant natural challenge, may perhaps develop a more durable immunity. The practical benefits to be derived from this measure would depend on local environmental conditions and the procedure adopted would have to be adjusted to suit local circumstances.

Any method of control which depends on the use of drugs carries the risk of producing drug-resistant strains in the locality concerned and of proliferating antigenic variants of the trypanosomes present in the area. The reaction of the trypanosomes to their environment may create additional problems. Gray (1965a) has shown that when tsetse flies become infected with antigenic variants, the trypanosomes, during cyclical development, revert to their original antigenic state ('basic' antigen) and that in a given locality, the trypanosomes transmitted by tsetse flies conform to a common type characteristic of that area. An effective immunity could then develop mainly against the basic antigens in restricted areas.

There are, however, at least two possible ways in which the immunity developed might prove to be ineffective. Firstly, new variant strains might emerge against which the immunity would not be effective; this would depend on the animal host's specific defence mechanism in the very early stages of infection as, if the metacyclic forms were immediately destroyed, variant forms could not develop. Secondly, mechanical (non-cyclical) transmission by biting flies other than tsetse is known to produce infection with trypanosomes of the variant and not the basic type. The number of variant strains is probably large and it is unlikely that immunity evoked by 'basic' antigen would protect against them. In such circumstances the incidence of trypanosomiasis in the herd would be greater where mechanical (non-cyclical) transmission was occurring (Weitz, 1964). These and other factors would require to be very carefully studied before adopting immunizing procedures to control trypanosomiasis in the field, particularly when dealing with closed communities such as herds of cattle.

It must also be remembered that the elimination of tsetse flies in a given locality might result in a lowering of the immune state of the animals present thereby rendering them highly susceptible to trypanosomiasis transmitted by mechanical vectors. The persistence of trypanosomiasis in certain parts of Africa from which tsetse flies have been virtually eliminated suggests that this may well be an important consideration. Similarly, the occurrence of trypanosomiasis in territories outside Africa, such as *T. evansi* infections in camels (*see* Hoare, 1957) or *T. vivax* in South America, exemplifies the persistence of trypanosome disease in localities remote from tsetse flies and the main reservoir of trypanosomes.

Chapter 7

Review of Chemotherapeutic and Chemoprophylactic Agents

J. WILLIAMSON

INTRODUCTION

General Considerations

The inception and early development of the specific chemotherapy[1] of infectious disease at the beginning of this century were largely concerned with the evolution of trypanocidal drugs. Of the many chemical agents which have subsequently been prepared and tested against experimental trypanosome infections, only a few of the active compounds have survived trial in natural infections of man or of domestic stock; even fewer have successfully withstood years of prolonged use in the field, during which the development of drug resistance is increasingly favoured and unsuspected forms of toxicity are sometimes revealed. The following account is intended to serve as introduction and background to the nature, development and function of therapeutic and prophylactic trypanocidal drugs. The clinical and field use of the relatively few drugs currently used for the prevention and cure of trypanosomiasis in man are described in Chapters 36 and 37 and of the animal trypanosomiases in Chapters 42 and 43.

Three major compendia document progress in the chemotherapy of disease overall: Fischl and Schlossberger's *Handbuch der Chemotherapie* (1932–4); Findlay's *Recent Advances in Chemotherapy* (1950–1) and Schnitzer and Hawking's *Experimental Chemotherapy* (1963–6). In each of these works, appropriate sections deal with the treatment of trypanosomiasis, but in addition there are a number of recent reviews dealing specifically with the chemotherapy of trypanosomiasis or special aspects of it, such as drug resistance and mode of drug action. The basis of the present condensed review is largely supplied by these texts and surveys, except where otherwise indicated, and especially by an earlier review (Williamson, 1962), together with those of Walls (1963) and Hawking (1963, 1966).[2]

[1] "What we want is a *Chemotherapia Specifica*, i.e., we are looking for chemical agents, which on the one hand will be taken up by and destroy certain parasites, and which on the other hand, in the amounts necessary for this destruction, will be tolerated by the organism without too much damage" (Ehrlich, 1907).

[2] For this reason, only references to work published since 1961, and such earlier references (given in small capitals) as are not easily accessible from these reviews, have been included in the bibliography.

Classification of Drugs

Several attempts have been made to classify trypanocides according to chemical structure and properties, or to various aspects of biological activity but no system is wholly satisfactory. The simplest practical division, into those drugs active against human and against animal trypanosomiasis respectively, will be followed here (Table 7.1), but the classes overlap, in terms of chemical structure (e.g. suramin and some diamidines are common to both), and of trypanosome group susceptibility (some drugs active in the *gambiense-rhodesiense* infections of man are generally effective also against the other members of the *brucei* group which infect animals).

TABLE 7.1

Activity of trypanocides*[1] *in current use

Chemical type	Human trypanosomiasis (*T. gambiense*/ *T. rhodesiense*)	Animal trypanosomiases	
		T. brucei/ *T. evansi*	*T. vivax*/ *T. congolense*
Acid naphthylamine	Suramin P	Suramin	
Aromatic arsenical	Tryparsamide Melarsen Mel B		
Diamidine	Pentamidine P [Berenil]	Berenil	Berenil
Nitrofuran	Nitrofurazone		
Quinaldine		Antrycide P	Antrycide P
Phenanthridinium			Ethidium Prothidium P Samorin P

[1] Common names are used in this introductory table. Recommended pharmacopoeial names, chemical names, and synonyms where applicable, are given in the appropriate sections of the text.

P indicates prophylactic activity.

Similar considerations apply to other attempted bases of classification, such as (a) Fischl and Schlossberger's simple division into 'metal-containing' (inorganic, aliphatic and aromatic compounds of arsenic and antimony) and 'metal-free' drugs (suramin, diamidines, nitrofurans, quinaldines and phenanthridiniums), (b) the ionic character of the drug at blood *p*H (Williamson & Rollo, 1959), and (c) the speed and mode of drug action (Hawking & Sen, 1960). System (b) has some relevance to cross-resistance behaviour and ability to pass from blood into cerebrospinal fluid, while (c) is useful in assessing the likelihood of a drug acting on respiratory or glycolytic processes, or on the more slowly reacting nucleic-acid-directed cell division systems (*see* p. 204).

Most of the overlapping in Table 7.1 can be avoided if the Salivarian parasites are split into only two natural groups: *T. gambiense/T. rhodesiense/T. brucei/T. evansi*, and *T. vivax/T. congolense*. Differential drug activity against these two parasite groups is defined more clearly, and accords more satisfactorily with known metabolic differences between them (*see* p. 200), but the system is of less practical convenience. No account is taken here or in the other systems, of the marked and important drug-refractoriness of *T. rhodesiense*, as compared with *T. gambiense*, in sleeping sickness patients.

CHEMOTHERAPY AND CHEMOPROPHYLAXIS OF TRYPANOSOMIASIS IN MAN

The Evolution of Trypanocidal Drugs

The effective drug control of human sleeping sickness in the last thirty years has rested essentially on three drugs: suramin (Fig. 7.17), tryparsamide (Fig. 7.18) and pentamidine (Fig. 7.27). The first two came into field use in the period 1920–5 followed by pentamidine in 1940–5. None was effective against late-stage *T. rhodesiense* or tryparsamide-resistant late-stage Gambian sleeping sickness; these infections came under control only with the later introduction of Friedheim's melaminyl arsenicals, especially Mel B (Fig. 7.24), in the period 1950–5.

The evolution of suramin and tryparsamide is of some historical interest in illuminating the early development of chemotherapy and its preoccupation with trypanosomes. These two drugs, established now for almost half a century, owe their origin to the convergence in the late nineteenth century, of a number of simultaneous technical innovations in optical microscopy, histology, haematology, sterile technique and the organic chemistry of new synthetic dyes available as cellular stains. Koch and Ehrlich invented some of these techniques and exploited the rest in an inspired way which, following Pasteur's earlier discoveries, revolutionized the recognition and isolation of microorganisms as causal agents of disease. At this time, medical and veterinary investigations which accompanied the opening-up of India and African colonial territories, were revealing the protozoal aetiology of an increasing number of tropical infections, especially the plasmodia of malaria and the trypanosomes of the animal diseases, surra, nagana and dourine. Simultaneously, the expanding German dye industry was making available a rapidly-widening spectrum of synthetic colours, following Perkin's synthesis of mauveine in 1856, and Griess's discovery of the diazo reaction in 1858.

Paul Ehrlich (1854–1915), an individual of exceptional genius, was thus uniquely placed, historically and geographically, as well as by training, inclination and experience, to seize the opportunity offered by the new dyes to establish principles of selective dye uptake by bacteria, protozoa, blood cells and animal tissues, and to extend these observations to a consideration of cell-fixed dyes as potential selective therapeutic agents in infected hosts. His use of Methylene Blue, first synthesized by Caro in 1876, is a pertinent example of this development. In 1881, in continuation of his student studies begun in 1877 on the use of aniline dyes as histological stains and in haematology, Ehrlich demonstrated the value of Methylene Blue as a stain for leucocyte granules in blood films, and with its aid, Koch discovered the tubercle bacillus in 1882. In 1886, Ehrlich showed that Methylene Blue was an intravital nerve stain, and as a result, was led to try the dye as an analgesic. The publication of this experiment in 1890 contained the prophetic statement of a principle now recognized as basic to modern rational 'metabolite-antagonist' chemotherapy, '. . . cellular therapy is a consequence of specific cell nutrition, as the cell can really be influenced only by those agents which, for what the expression is worth, are eaten by it'. Following Romanowski's introduction in 1890 of a Methylene Blue-Eosin stain for avian plasmodia, Ehrlich and Guttman showed that the recently discovered human malaria parasite took up Methylene Blue selectively at concentrations which did not affect white cells. As a result, they were stimulated to try the dye as a therapeutic agent for human malaria. Activity against tertian malaria was demonstrated in 1891, and in this report, the first example of selective chemotherapy evolved on logical grounds, Ehrlich drew attention to the need for a suitable experimental laboratory infection model if malaria chemotherapy was to progress. This vital requirement was not effectively developed for malaria chemotherapy until after the First World War when the use of *Plasmodium relictum* in canaries for drug-testing led to the first synthetic antimalarial, plasmoquine, introduced in 1926; appropriately enough, the chemical starting point for the evolution of this drug was the Methylene Blue molecule.

From 1893 onwards for a decade, Ehrlich was primarily occupied with establishing the quantitative basis of immunity, following von Behring's discovery of antitoxin in 1890. Serotherapy, though effective for some important bacterial diseases, did not appear promising for protozoal infections, and further development of the chemotherapy of both kinds of infection still had to await a convenient laboratory infection model. Two years after Bruce's report in 1896 that tsetse-borne trypanosomes caused nagana, this model was provided by Kanthack, Durham and Blandford, who showed that the causative organism, *T. brucei*, produced rapid, heavy and uniformly fatal infections in rats, mice and rabbits; trypanosomes also had the advantages over bacteria in being large enough to be seen easily in a wet blood preparation, to have much more intracellular organization, easily demonstrable by staining, and to be separable from infected blood by centrifugation. In 1902 in the Institut Pasteur in Paris, Laveran and Mesnil using the same strain of *T. brucei*, carried out the first successful experimental treatment of trypanosome infections in rats and mice. Of a large number of preparations tested, including Methylene and Toluidine Blue, only human serum and sodium arsenite were effective *in vivo*; with the latter, they made the first drug experiments on trypanosomes *in vitro*, and from the similarity of the involution forms rapidly produced by arsenic *in vivo* and *in vitro*, they drew the important conclusion that there was a direct action of the drug on the parasite. An effective start on systematic chemotherapy was now possible and from this time onwards, the new science in Ehrlich's Frankfurt laboratory and in the Institut Pasteur in Paris, progressed along two main lines, the testing against an increasing variety of trypanosomes of (i) synthetic dyes and related compounds, and (ii) organic arsenicals and antimonials. The first effective trypanocidal end-products of these two lines of development were respectively, suramin (1916–20) and tryparsamide (1919–25).

With his long experience of the chemistry of dyes and of their selective uptake and oxidoreduction by tissue cells, and using the fruitful concept of fixation by cell receptors which permeated his chemical approach to immunity, Ehrlich began by considering the new cotton-substantive dyes. These were derived from Congo Red (Fig. 7.1) introduced by Böttiger in 1884 and found to be the first synthetic agents capable of dyeing cotton directly. The parent structures, benzidine which was doubly diazotized and coupled to two molecules of a sulphonated naphthylamine, in this case naphthionic acid, were each capable of carrying a variety of substituent groups. A number of these dyes was available to Ehrlich, and for some years before his experimental chemotherapy work began, he had been particularly impressed with the long, non-toxic and vividly obvious retention of a Benzopurpurin dye closely related to Congo Red, in the skin and other tissues of mice which had been injected with it; such mice with their bright red ears were a showpiece for visitors and, microscopically, large cell areas showed the dye as granular deposits. Not surprisingly, Ehrlich's first

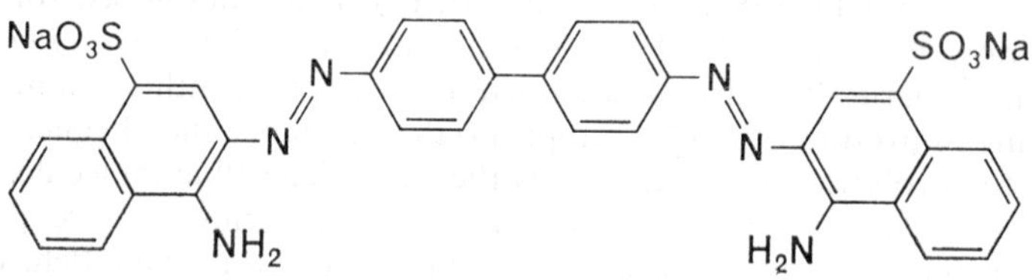

Fig. 7.1 *Congo Red*

choice of potential trypanocides included this group of benzidine azo dyes. With the collaboration of the Japanese bacteriologist Shiga, and of von Weinberg and Ullmann, two chemists in the nearby Cassella dyestuffs factory, he tested more than one hundred dyes in mice infected with *T. equinum*, the parasite of Mal de Caderas; at this time the test trypanosomes most easily available were those from animal diseases which were found to infect rats and mice more readily than those of the human infections. The first weak signs of trypanocidal activity were found in the dye Benzopurpurin (Fig. 7.2, a) (later known as Nagana, or Naga, Red). To promote speedier absorption, Ehrlich persuaded his chemist colleagues to introduce an extra water-solubilizing sulphonic acid (—SO_3H) substituent, in this case into the benzidine portion of the dye molecule. The resulting sodium salt, Trypan Red (Fig. 7.2, b), turned out to be both curative and prophylactic (Ehrlich & Shiga, 1904). This was the classic first cure of an experimentally produced disease by administration of a single dose of a synthetic organic substance of known chemical composition. These simple but carefully observed experiments enabled Ehrlich to emphasize a number of novel but essential features which were to set the pattern of all subsequent experimental chemotherapy: (i) the use of a suitable standard infection in small uniform laboratory animals; (ii) the application of 'intelligent empiricism' based on known chemical and biological properties of test compounds; (iii) the necessity of testing very large numbers of related compounds where, following indications of activity, however slight, molecular modifications could be made to select those which were desirable and to reject those which were not; (iv) the continual emphasis on 'Constitution, Distribution and Activity', and on 'parasitotropy' *versus* 'organotropy'; (v) the expression of activity as the relation of minimum curative dose to maximum tolerated dose; (vi) the recognition that, unlike sodium arsenite, the inactivity of Trypan Red *in vitro* and its slow activity *in vivo* might be due to the *in vivo* production of an active derivative; (vii) the demonstration of residual immunity after drug cure; (viii) the probable relation between tissue and plasma retention of the drug and its prophylactic activity; and (ix) the recognition that a drug may not be equally efficient against different trypanosome species. The last point was emphasized and extended by Laveran in the same year, using a sample of Trypan Red provided by Ehrlich, with which he demonstrated another basic chemotherapeutic principle, namely, the effectiveness of combined drug therapy. Trypan Red or sodium arsenite alone was only

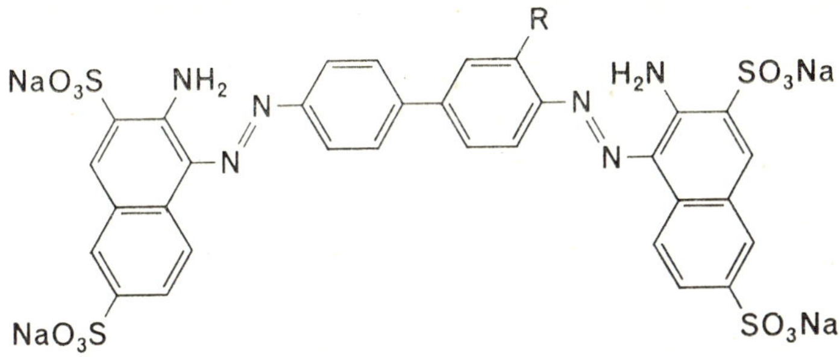

Fig. 7.2 (a) *Nagana Red* (R = H). (b) *Trypan Red* (R = SO_3Na)

weakly effective against infections with *T. evansi* in rats and mice but cures could be obtained with a combination of both drugs.

Within the next three years, apart from an increasing number of major trypanocidal drug discoveries, two fundamental phenomena of 'therapeutic biology' were established in Ehrlich's laboratory. In 1905 Franke, using Trypan Red, showed that relapse trypanosomes were 'serum-fast' i.e. serologically different from the organisms before treatment. Later, Franke, Roehl and Browning showed that trypanosomes could become resistant to drug treatment and that the resistance and cross-resistance of these strains was highly specific for different chemical groups of drugs; 'chemoreceptors' were postulated by Ehrlich for the three main groups separable in this way (arsenicals, benzidine-type dyes and triphenylmethane dyes). Practical implications were immediately drawn for therapy and these are still of paramount importance, namely, that continuous inadequate treatment with the same drug, or with different drugs of the same chemical type, is conducive to the emergence of resistant strains, so that *complete* sterilization of an infection should be sought, by *combined* or *alternating* treatment with drugs which attach to different chemoreceptors. Ehrlich's ingenious idea that the 'therapeutic sieve' of resistant strains might also be used by industrial chemical laboratories to assign provisional chemical structures to therapeutically active but uncharacterized compounds, does not seem to have been adopted extensively, but cross-resistance analysis has subsequently been of great theoretical and practical interest in studies of drug action (*see* pp. 211–217).

Progress in chemotherapy at this time was not restricted to Ehrlich's laboratory. In Bonn, Wendelstadt, in 1904 and later with Fellmer in 1906, discovered trypanocidal activity in the triphenylmethane dyes Malachite Green (Fig. 7.3, a) and Brilliant Green (Fig. 7.3, b). In Paris, Mesnil and Nicolle in a series of papers (1906–7) from the Institut Pasteur, systematically tested a very large series of dyes which, in the absence of synthetic chemical facilities in the Institut at that time, they collected mostly from the firm of Bayer in Germany but also from dye works all over Europe. They found two new trypanocidal dyes, later known as Trypan Blue and Afridol Violet, which were both related to, but more active than, Trypan Red. In Liverpool in 1905, Wolferstan Thomas made perhaps the most significant of all these new advances, by demonstrating the trypanocidal activity and low toxicity of an organic arsenical, Atoxyl (Fig. 7.7).

The rather toxic triphenylmethane dye series (Fig. 7.3) did not produce any

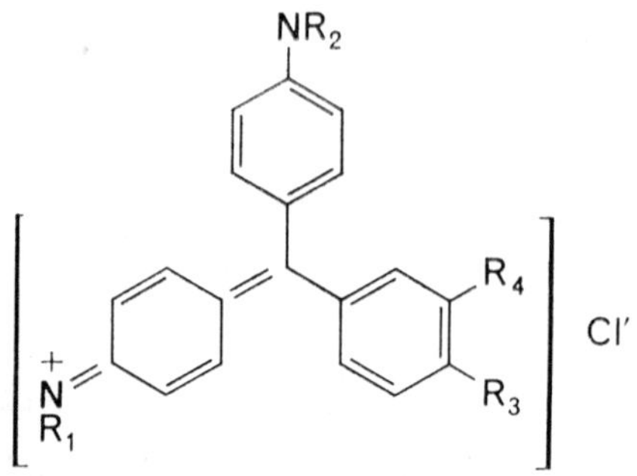

Fig. 7.3 (a) *Malachite Green* (R_1, R_2 = $(CH_3)_2$; R_3, R_4 = H). (b) *Brilliant Green* (R_1, R_2 = $(C_2H_5)_2$; R_3, R_4 = H). (c) *Parafuchsin, Pararosaniline* (R_1, R_2 = H_2; R_3 = NH_2; R_4 = H). (d) *Fuchsin, Rosaniline* (R_1, R_2 = H_2; R_3 = NH_2; R_4 = CH_3)

highly active trypanocides, but Ehrlich, with Shiga (1904) and later with Franke (1905), systematically examined the relation of structure to toxicity, in attempts to produce usable drugs. The simple Rosaniline with primary amino groups (Fig. 7.3, d) was known to be less toxic to the conjunctiva of the eye than derivatives in which there was alkyl substitution of the amino groups; the toxicity was also known to increase with increasing alkylation. Ehrlich and Franke showed a similar relation for the local necrotic toxicity at the site of subcutaneous injection in mice, and independently of Wendelstadt, Ehrlich and Shiga found that the less toxic acid-substituted (sulphonated, carboxylated) triphenylmethane dyes had no trypanocidal activity. Parafuchsin (Fig. 7.3, c) remained the only practicable drug in this series, although its weak activity was exploited only by enteral administration in animal food or by combined therapy with Trypan Red or Atoxyl. In 1909, Ehrlich and Benda, another Cassella chemist, produced a somewhat more active chlorinated derivative, Tryparosan, but neither Tryparosan nor Parafuchsin, although tested in sleeping sickness in man, was of clinical value, alone or in combination with the more active arsenicals.

The new trypanocidal azo dyes (A′, Cl and Ph) discovered by Nicolle and

Mesnil (1906–7) (*see* Tréfouel, 1962) and later known as Trypan Blue (Fig. 7.4, a), Afridol Blue (Fig. 7.4, b) and Afridol (Trypan) Violet (Fig. 7.5), respectively, were more active than Ehrlich's Trypan Red, especially against the animal trypanosomiases, but none came into field use as a trypanocide (although Trypan Blue, found to be active on piroplasms by Nuttall in 1909, was later used extensively for infections of this type in domestic stock). Figure 7.4 shows that Trypan Blue and Afridol Blue are based, like Trypan Red (Fig. 7.2, b), on a

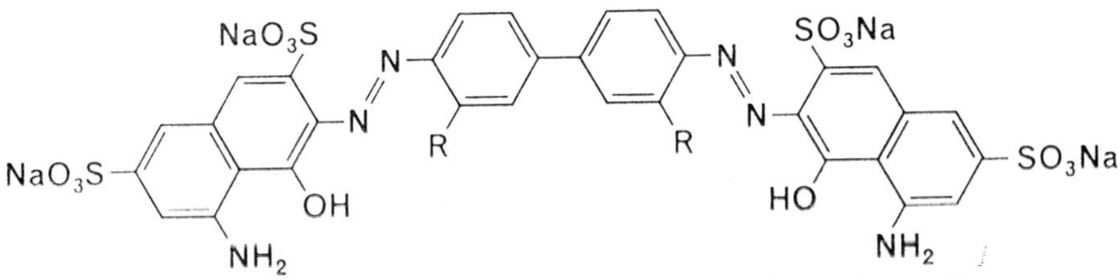

Fig. 7.4 (a) *Trypan Blue* (R = CH_3). (b) *Afridol Blue* (R = Cl)

central benzidine portion diazotized and coupled symmetrically to two naphthylamine sulphonates, which, unlike Trypan Red, are 'H-acid' (8-hydroxy-1-naphthylamine-3,6-disulphonic acid) moieties. H-acid (dye intermediate) moieties are also present in Afridol Violet (Fig. 7.5) so that all the known active drugs in this series were shown to carry sulphonic acid substituents in the 3,6 position of the naphthylamine residues. This apparent structural requirement for activity had been stressed earlier by Ehrlich and von Weinberg, who had prepared and tested about fifty different substitution products of Trypan Red without markedly improving the activity. The main point of interest is that Afridol Violet

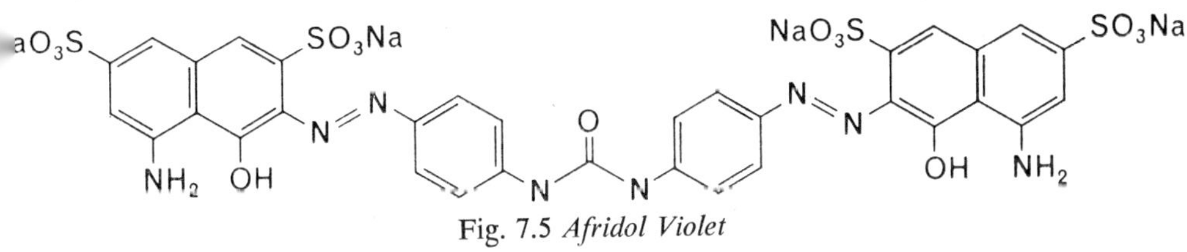

Fig. 7.5 *Afridol Violet*

differed from the other three benzidine drugs in being a symmetrical *urea* ($H_2N \cdot CO \cdot NH_2$) derivative, with diphenylurea in place of diphenyl as the central nucleus. In 1899 and 1902, new series of cotton-substantive dyes based on urea-linked sulphonated naphthalenes were patented, the earliest of which were colourless; Afridol Violet was one of the first symmetrical dyes produced in this series. Later in 1910–11, the introduction of *p*-aminobenzoyl moieties was found to favour production of colourless substances of this type which could be diazotized *in situ* on the cotton fibre. Highly coloured dyes have obvious disadvantages as therapeutic agents for man or domestic stock, and chemists of the Bayer firm under Heymann, who had collaborated originally with Nicolle and Mesnil, began to prepare from H-acid colourless *p*-aminobenzoyl-containing analogues of the trypanocidal azo dyes. One of the first active compounds (Fig.

7.6) was a colourless analogue of Trypan Red. In conjunction with the pharmacologist Roehl, Heymann and his colleagues, Dressel, Kothe and Ossenbeck, showed that trypanocidal activity, by analogy with cotton substantivity, could be increased by the introduction of further *p*-aminobenzoyl moieties, but only up to a point; if there were more than four, the trypanocidal activity was decreased (*see* p. 208). Over the period 1913–16, therapeutic activity was found to be

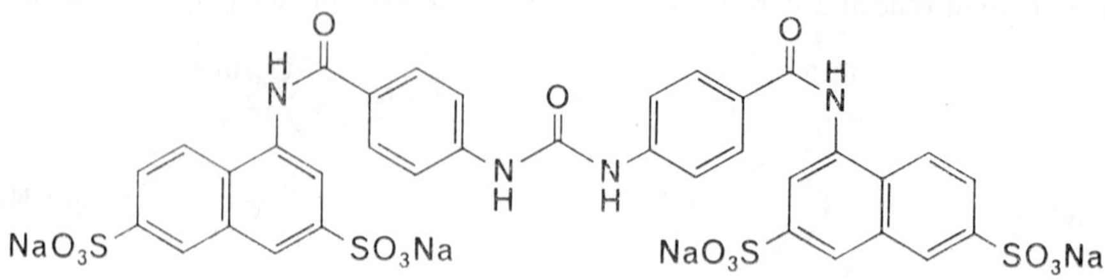

Fig. 7.6 *Suramin Precursor*

markedly favoured by two further major changes in the molecule: the introduction of 1-naphthylamine-4,6,8-trisulphonic acid, and of *m*- instead of *p*-aminobenzoyl moieties. The successful end-product of this work (Bayer 205, Germanin, suramin) (Fig. 7.17) was produced in 1916, but for wartime and post-war political reasons, the chemical constitution was kept secret until the French workers, Fourneau, Tréfouel and Vallée, elucidated the structure in 1924.

The introduction of the synthetic aromatic arsenical Atoxyl (Fig. 7.7) in 1905 was a pivotal point in the history of the therapeutic use of arsenic and the foundation of Ehrlich and Hata's work which led first to arsphenamine (Fig. 7.11) (Salvarsan) in 1910, and later to tryparsamide (Fig. 7.18). The extent of this chemotherapeutic revolution, which occurred in a space of fifteen years,

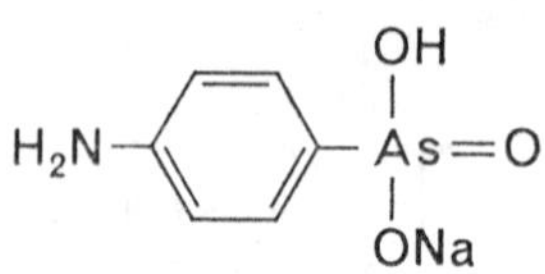

Fig. 7.7 *Atoxyl*

may be gauged from the persistence of the use of inorganic arsenic in medicine from the days of Hippocrates onwards for some 2,500 years. Both orpiment (arsenic trisulphide, first distinguished by Dioscorides in the first century A.D.), and Fowler's solution (of potassium arsenite, introduced for internal use in 1786), were used as adjuncts to the new benzidine dyes in the early stages of trypanocidal drug evolution. The revolution was less obvious in the treatment of African cattle trypanosomiasis. Tartar emetic (potassium antimony tartrate), first introduced into medicine by Paracelsus in the sixteenth century, was shown to be trypanocidal in 1908 by Plimmer and Thomson, but in this instance, although aromatic antimonial drugs were prepared in the following year, and later developed extensively for use in leishmaniasis, tartar emetic was still, forty years later, the only readily available treatment for the animal trypanosomiases in large areas of Africa.

Livingstone in his African missionary travels, although ignorant of the parasitic origin of nagana, had used Fowler's solution with some success in 1847–8 to treat a 'fly-struck' mare, and in 1893, Lingard in his Indian 'Report on Horse Surra', showed that the arsenite solution, together with cinchona alkaloids, had a therapeutic effect on the 'haematozoon' of surra. Bruce's report in 1896, which demonstrated tsetse-borne trypanosomes as the cause of nagana, also showed that the infection was susceptible to treatment by arsenious oxide or sodium arsenite. Arsenic treatment of this kind was naturally extended to the human infections as they became recognized, but the toxic reactions, acceptable in animals, were too severe for continued use in man.

Aliphatic compounds of arsenic, first prepared accidentally in 1760 by Cadet (in a study of 'sympathetic' (invisible) inks based on cobalt salts extracted from mineral cobalt arsenide), were later characterized by Bunsen in 1837, who showed that they were less toxic than inorganic arsenic. The compounds came into medical use in 1865 but as they were largely excreted by the lungs, they

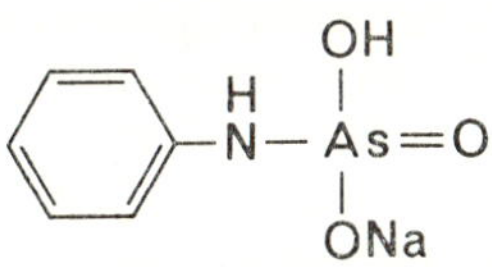

Fig. 7.8 *Atoxyl (original formula)*

soon fell into disuse because of the offensive garlic odour imparted to the breath. By a curious chance, Atoxyl, the first acceptable organic arsenical, originated as a by-product in the commercial production of the triphenylmethane dye, Parafuchsin. Arsenic acid (H_3AsO_4) was used in this process to oxidize a mixture of aniline and *p*-toluidine, and in the course of studying the conditions of the reaction, Béchamp in 1863 isolated a colourless compound which he regarded as an anilide of arsenic acid (Fig. 7.8). The sodium salt of this compound, under the name Atoxyl, was subsequently recommended at the turn of the century for anaemia and skin diseases. In 1902, Blumenthal found that it was forty times less toxic for rabbits than Fowler's solution, and in 1903, Mendel showed that Atoxyl was suitable for clinical administration, subcutaneously or intravenously.

In January of the same year Ehrlich and Shiga tested it in Frankfort, but Ehrlich, ironically enough, 'abandoned it because it did not exercise any destructive action on the parasites in the test tube'. In 1904, Wolferstan Thomas and Breinl began work in Liverpool on experimental trypanosomiasis, and in their memoir of 1905, *Report on Trypanosomes, Trypanosomiasis and Sleeping Sickness*, they demonstrated the superior trypanocidal action of Atoxyl *in vivo*; Thomas convincingly confirmed its lack of toxicity by giving himself high intravenous doses of the drug. As a result, Ehrlich, after visiting Thomas in Runcorn, again took up the study of organic arsenicals as trypanocides, and in his 'Chemotherapeutische Trypanosomen-Studien' lecture delivered in February 1907, stated that Atoxyl was not an arsanilide (Fig. 7.8), but that there was a diazotizable and therefore free amino group in the *para* position to the arsenic acid substituent which was directly attached to the aromatic nucleus (Fig. 7.7). Full details of this elucidation of the correct structure, established with the chemist Bertheim, were not published until later in the same year; in the meantime, Moore, Nierenstein and Todd in Liverpool, in the newly founded 'Biochemical Journal', independently gave chemical proof of the correct structure.

The new structure, unlike the old, showed that preparation of a wide variety of related arsenical compounds was now possible, principally by substitution of the free amino group, or by the use of aromatic amines other than aniline. Ehrlich showed that in this arsenical series, toxicities could be varied 1,500-fold by appropriate substitution. At this time, Atoxyl, after extensive use in man,

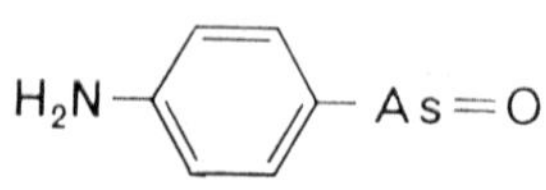

Fig. 7.9 *p-Aminophenylarsenoxide*

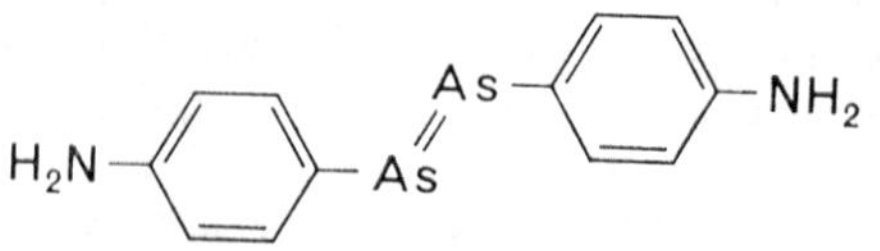

Fig. 7.10 *Diaminoarsenobenzene*

was being rapidly shown to have disturbing toxic effects, especially on the optic nerve, so that the synthesis of new and less toxic organic arsenicals was given increasing attention. By 1908, the likely assumption that the toxic and trypanocidal actions of pentavalent-arsenic-containing drugs like Atoxyl were due to their reduction *in vivo* to the corresponding trivalent arsenoxide form (Fig. 7.9), was reinforced experimentally. Ehrlich and Bertheim showed that chemical reduction of Atoxyl produced first *p*-aminophenylarsenoxide (Fig. 7.9) and then diaminoarsenobenzene (Fig. 7.10), both of which were several thousand times more toxic than Atoxyl; the phenylarsenoxide in particular was up to a million times more trypanocidal *in vitro*. Uhlenhuth in 1907 had shown that Atoxyl was active in spirochaetal infections, and as a result the anti-spirochaetal action of

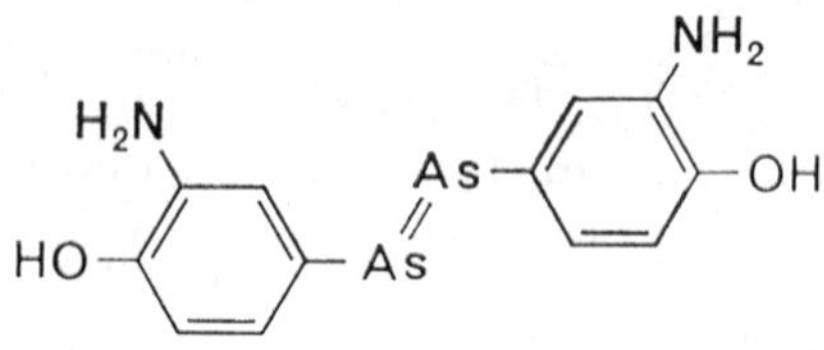

Fig. 7.11 *Salvarsan* (*Arsphenamine*)

organic arsenicals was tested by Ehrlich and Hata as intensively as the trypanocidal action; the culmination of this work was the major discovery in 1910 of the arsenobenzene compound Salvarsan (arsphenamine) (Fig. 7.11), active in syphilis. During this development, an early precursor of tryparsamide was prepared, *N*-phenylglycine-*p*-arsonic acid, which on reduction gave arsenophenylglycine (Fig. 7.12), a highly trypanocidal compound of low toxicity and of particular interest because of its activity against Atoxyl-resistant trypanosomes. In 1911, synthesis of aromatic arsenical and antimonial compounds was further facilitated by Bart's discovery that the metallic groups could be introduced into an aromatic nucleus by diazotization of primary amino groups.

Apart from these advances, subsequent work on aromatic arsenicals was largely directed to the improvement of Salvarsan. The 1914–18 war cut off the

German sources of supply of arsenical drugs to France, Britain and America, obliging these countries to take up research and production programmes of their own. The discovery of tryparsamide in 1919 was made as the result of war-time work by Jacobs and Heidelberger in the Rockefeller Institute, New York, who emphasized the necessity for working with readily accessible chemical types of similar general structure, allowing ready chemical modification by simple reactions to give water-soluble products. They chose the pentavalent aromatic arsenicals as best satisfying these requirements, rather than the trivalent compounds. Arsanilic acid (Atoxyl) (Fig. 7.7) '. . . the most accessible of the aromatic arsenical compounds, was naturally chosen as the fundamental substance'. In this instance the accessibility factor was complicated by war, as only the early work is stated to have been carried out with pre-war samples of arsanilic and other arylarsonic acids obtained from the German firms of Cassella and Farbwerke Hoechst.

From investigation of seven main structural groups, each containing large numbers of derivatives, Jacobs and Heidelberger, and their biological collaborators Pearce and Brown, found the most active to be the sodium salt of the

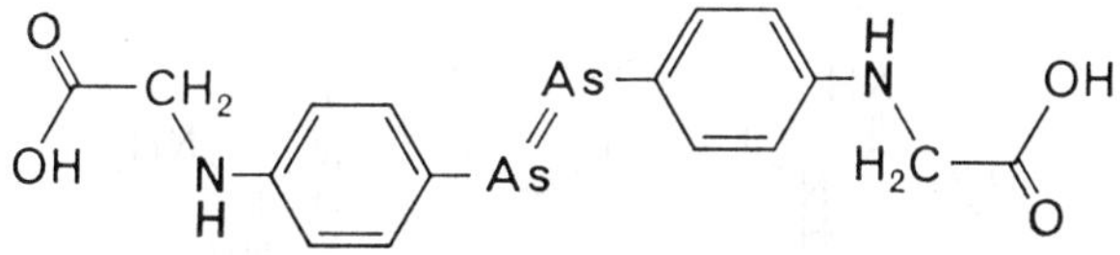

Fig. 7.12 *Arsenophenylglycine*

amide of *N*-phenylglycine-*p*-arsonic acid. This parent acid had been used to prepare arsenophenylglycine (Fig. 7.12), the active No. 418 in the long series of arsenicals (606) which led Ehrlich and Hata to Salvarsan. At that time also, the phenylglycine substituent had been chosen to replace the amino group of Atoxyl, because it was less easily hydrolysed *in vivo* than the acetamido (CH_3—CO—NH—) substituent, first introduced in early attempts to detoxicate Atoxyl. Sodium *p*-glycineamidophenylarsonate (later known as tryparsamide) (Fig. 7.18) is prepared by a simple condensation of Atoxyl and chloroacetamide; the product is easily purified, giving a crystalline and highly water-soluble neutral salt.

In 1920, trials of tryparsamide in human sleeping sickness were begun in the Belgian Congo, and by 1925, Pearce was able to report that the new drug was highly effective, especially in late-stage Gambian sleeping sickness for which it was the only satisfactory drug available. The successful conclusion of this work owed much to PEARCE AND BROWN's valuable reappraisal, in 1918, of the biologica lbasis of arsenical drug tests, especially their use of chroni cinfections in larger laboratory animals such as the rabbit.

The evolution of suramin and tryparsamide has been dealt with at some length in order to illustrate Ehrlich's prophetic dictum in 1907 that '. . . the discovery of any trypanocidal substance will always be the result of the interplay of chance and experiment . . .', and to show that most of the important principles and requirements on which all synthetic antimicrobial drug developments still rely, were laid down before the First World War, in a context primarily of experimental trypanosomiasis. The combination of 'intelligent empiricism', serendipity and reliance on industrial chemical facilities, characteristic of the development of suramin and tryparsamide, continued to be associated with the later discovery of other major trypanocidal drugs like pentamidine, although in this case, the basis of the first experiments appeared to be eminently logical.

The beneficial effect of glucose on trypanosome survival *in vitro* had been known since 1911, but the enormous extent to which pathogenic African trypanosomes metabolize glucose was not established until 1929 when Yorke, Adams and Murgatroyd in Liverpool elaborated a method for maintaining trypanosomes alive *in vitro* for extended periods at 37°C. Over the period 1925–35, trypanosome infection in various animals had been shown to be associated with host hypoglycaemia, although generally this appeared only in the agonal stage of the infection. The apparently probable connection between host hypoglycaemia and the high rate of parasite glycolysis, suggested to at least four different workers at different times, that induction of hypoglycaemia by insulin in infected animals might reduce or eliminate the trypanosome infection. In three cases,

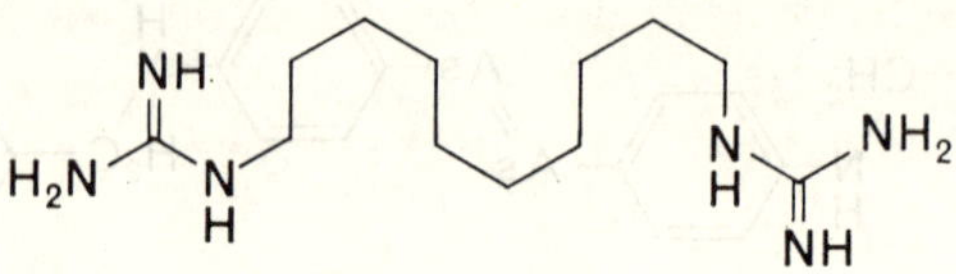

Fig. 7.13 *Synthalin*

insulin was shown to have some slight and variable therapeutic effect on the infective trypanosomes, but in 1935–6, von Jancsó and von Jancsó in Hungary, and Schern and Artagaveytia-Allende in Montevideo separately found that Synthalin, a synthetic substitute for insulin, had a marked therapeutic effect on experimental trypanosome infections. Although both groups of workers had used Synthalin to study the effects of deprivation of host glucose on trypanosomes, neither was able to exclude a direct action of Synthalin on the parasites. In 1937, the problem was resolved by Lourie and Yorke in Liverpool using Yorke's *in vitro* system. They showed that Synthalin had a powerful trypanocidal action *in vitro* of an order equivalent to that of the trivalent aromatic arsenicals. It was also active against drug-resistant strains, and under the same *in vitro* test conditions, was about 10,000 times more active than insulin.

This major discovery eliminated the indirect host-hypoglycaemia source of action, and focussed attention on the therapeutic potential of compounds related to Synthalin (Fig. 7.13) which is an aliphatic diguanidine (diguanidino-1,10-*n*-decane). A large number of related guanidines, *iso*-thioureas, amidines and amines were prepared by King in London and examined by Lourie and Yorke who found that the most active, which was superior to Synthalin, was a closely related aliphatic diamidine (diamidino-1,11-*n*-undecane) (Fig. 7.14).

Later collaboration with King and with Ewins of May and Baker Ltd., led to the selection of three aromatic diamidines with high therapeutic indices,

4,4′-diamidinostilbene (Stilbamidine) (Fig. 7.15), 4,4′-diamidino-diphenoxy-1,3-*n*-propane (propamidine) (Fig. 7.16) and 4,4′-diamidino-diphenoxy-1,5-*n*-pentane (pentamidine) (Fig. 7.27). From 1940 onwards these new drugs were tested against human sleeping sickness in West Africa and the Belgian Congo. Stilbamidine was found to be the most toxic, and did not come into extended use, but both propamidine and pentamidine were found effective, although only in the early stage of the disease. Their introduction at this juncture was timely, as they were active against 'arsenic-resistant' strains of *T. gambiense* which had become dangerously prevalent as a result of widespread arsenical medication

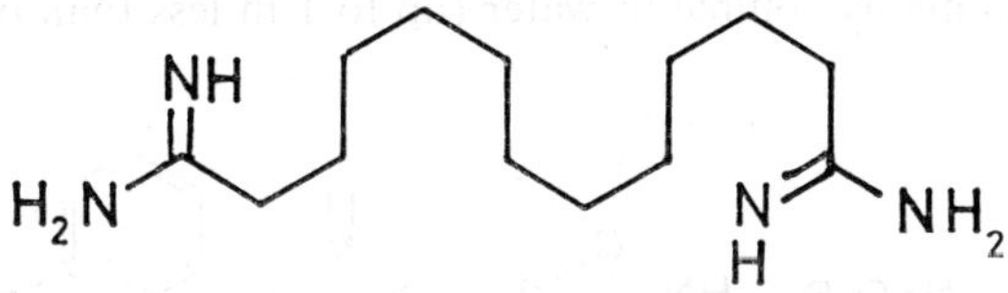

Fig. 7.14 *Undecane Diamidine*

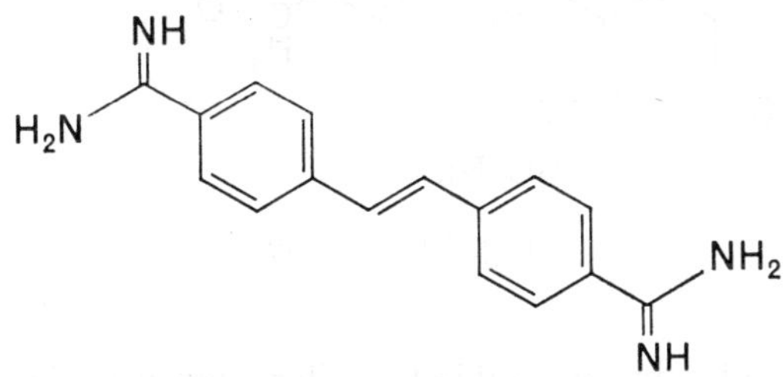

Fig. 7.15 *Stilbamidine*

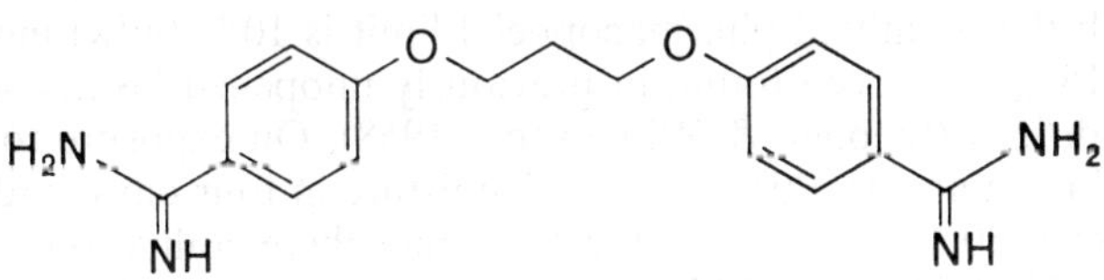

Fig. 7.16 *Propamidine*

over the previous fifteen years when *T. gambiense* epidemics were frequent. A major innovation in 1942 was the introduction by van Hoof of pentamidine as a prophylactic drug in the Belgian Congo, following earlier animal experiments in which this property was demonstrated; mass prophylaxis with pentamidine was subsequently practised on a vast scale and with great success, especially in the French and Belgian West and Central African territories. The value of the aromatic diamidines has not been restricted to sleeping sickness, as they were rapidly found to be highly active also in the treatment of kala-azar, and propamidine has continued in use as a valuable topical antiseptic.

Suramin

The principal member of the group of acid naphthylamine drugs is suramin *B.P.* (hexa-sodium 3,3′-ureylene-*bis* [8-(3-benzamido-*p*-toluido)-1,3,5-naphthalene sulphonate]) (synonyms: Germanin, Bayer 205, Antrypol, Moranyl,

Fourneau 309, Belganyl, Naphuride, Naganin, Naganol) (Fig. 7.17). Substances of related structure, such as Trypan Red, Trypan Blue, Afridol Violet and Pontamine Sky Blue 5 BX, have some trypanocidal activity, but suramin is the only representative which is clinically effective. Its therapeutic and prophylactic activity in human sleeping sickness in Africa has been established for almost fifty years, though its use is confined to early stages of the infection, usually in combination with tryparsamide.

Suramin *B.P.* ($C_{51}H_{34}N_6Na_6O_{23}S_6$; mol. wt. 1429) is an amorphous white, pink-white or faint cream coloured powder, odourless with an alkaline, slightly bitter taste. It is highly soluble in water (up to 1 in less than one part of water

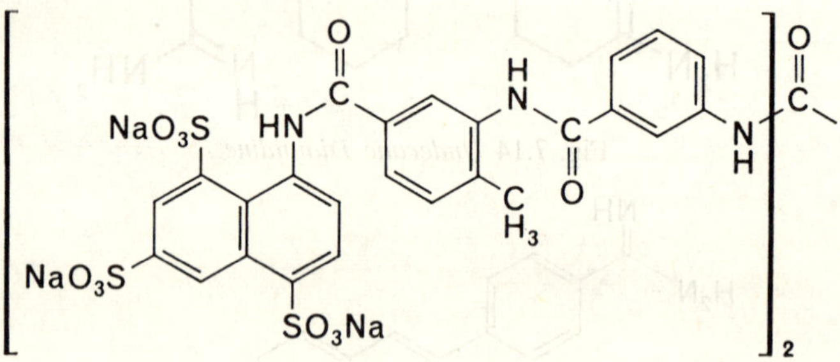

Fig. 7.17 *Suramin*

at 20°C) and the solutions are stable to boiling, but it is almost or wholly insoluble in alcohol, ether, chloroform or benzene. Suramin is highly hygroscopic, and although the permitted pharmacopoeial limit is 10% (w/w) moisture, contents of 14–15% have been found in previously unopened bottles stored under tropical conditions (Stephen & Williamson, 1958). On exposure to air, freshly dried suramin can absorb this amount of moisture in four days, and up to 20% in 5–6 weeks; at 30°C in a water-saturated atmosphere, anhydrous suramin will absorb 30–35% moisture in 24 hours and then deliquesce. Apparent decrease of toxicity of suramin on tropical storage, as reported by Nnochiri (1964), may well be caused by hydration of this kind.

Distribution and Toxicity

The chemical structure of suramin is highly specific in that removal of the two methyl groups, for example, virtually abolishes activity. Attempts to synthesize active analogues by replacing the naphthalene trisulphonate portion with heterocyclic nuclei have been unsuccessful (Adams, Ashley & Bader, 1956). Continued persistence in the blood for periods of up to three months is due to combination with plasma protein and is the basis of the prophylactic action of suramin (Dewey & Wormall, 1946; Wilson & Wormall, 1949). The structural requirements for persistence (Spinks, 1948) are much less specific than those for trypanocidal activity, and can probably be met by any symmetrical compound of high molecular weight with polysulphonated end-groups. The strongly anionic character of suramin, and its tendency to form colloidal aggregates in solution, are sufficient to account for its inability to enter red cells, to pass the 'blood-brain barrier' into the cerebrospinal fluid, or to be active after oral administration. These properties may also contribute to the nephritis which can occur as a delayed toxic reaction to the drug, as suramin is known to localize as granules in the epithelium of the kidney tubules of rodents (Jancsó & Jancsó-Gabor, 1952). Current evidence on the cellular localization of suramin in lysosomes (Smeesters & Jacques, 1968) would suggest that the kidney tubule granules are lysosomal depots of the drug.

Suramin is normally given intravenously in man because intramuscular or subcutaneous injection causes severe local irritation and necrosis. The possibility of reducing the toxicity of the acidic suramin by combination with a basic drug was first raised by Lourie's observation, during a sleeping sickness epidemic in Sierra Leone in 1939–41, that traces of suramin left in an imperfectly washed syringe gave rise to precipitation when the syringe was later filled with pentamidine solution. Subsequent investigation in Oxford by Guimaraes and Lourie (1951) showed that suramin could inhibit many of the pharmacological and toxic effects of pentamidine, primarily by the formation of an inactive and precipitable salt complex. The complex still retained its therapeutic activity and Guimaraes and Lourie considered that this work provided 'a basis of evidence . . . for a unique situation in therapeutics where two compounds tend to annul one another's pharmacological or toxic effects while acting in concert (if not synergistically) as chemotherapeutic agents'; the authors also indicated that the sparingly soluble salt complex was likely to be useful as a chemoprophylactic agent.

Further investigation in France (Beaudiment, Couvin & Leproux, 1954; Cosar, Ducrot, Gailliot & Baget, 1954) in conjunction with the firm of Rhône-Poulenc, showed that pentamidine-suramin mixtures ('lomidine-moranylate') were less toxic on intramuscular injection than either drug given separately, that there was a stoichiometric basis for salt formation (one molecule of suramin with six acid groups to three molecules of pentamidine, each with two basic groups), and that the product thus prepared showed not only a mutual reduction of toxicity but also a synergic access of prophylactic activity in experimental trypanosome infections. Later work revealed an unacceptable incidence (about 8%) of fairly severe local reactions after intramuscular injection in man, and further development was abandoned although simultaneous injection of intravenous suramin and intramuscular pentamidine was continued as a means of reducing any toxic side-effects of pentamidine (Neujean & Evens, 1958). Later exploitation of the principle of therapeutic and prophylactic suraminate formation for animal trypanosomiasis is dealt with below (pp. 172–174) but it may be noted that the principle has been extended into other fields: a prophylactic antimalarial chloroquine suraminate was patented by the Société des Usines Chimiques Rhône-Poulenc in 1961, and the later Parke Davis 'repository antimalarial' is a sparingly soluble salt of pamoic acid and the triazine metabolite of proguanil (Thompson, Olszewski, Elslager & Worth, 1963); the suraminate of Babesan is an active prophylactic for *Babesia* infections (Ryley, 1964).

Several reports (1950–4) of adrenal insufficiency in man (after suramin treatment had been introduced for pemphigus), together with the earlier results of suramin-treated rat experiments which showed adrenal damage, led Frisch and Gardner (1958) to re-examine the possibilities in rats more systematically. Careful histological examination failed to reveal any evidence of adrenal damage after suramin treatment.

One possible toxic effect of suramin in man appears to have been overlooked. Trypan Blue is actively teratogenic (GILLMAN, GILBERT, GILLMAN & SPENCE, 1948), and although this property appears to be sensitive to slight alterations in chemical structure (BEAUDOIN & PICKERING, 1960), closely related dyes are also active to a varying, if less extent. Suramin, as discussed earlier (pp. 133–134) is a chemical descendant of dyes like Trypan Blue, and trypanocidal cross-resistance occurs between the two drugs (pp. 211–215), so that the possibility of suramin being teratogenic cannot be dismissed, especially in view of the protean nature of its biological effects (pp. 208–210). In unpublished preliminary experiments which the writer has carried out in rats, using the technique of Beaudoin (1964), with Trypan Blue as control, results were negative although inconclusive, but WHITTEN (1956) has shown that suramin treatment can prevent or interrupt pregnancy in mice.

Tryparsamide

Although the use and synthesis of aromatic arsenicals and antimonials continue for a wide variety of purposes, their therapeutic use is largely for amoebic, leishmanial, trichmonad, coccidial and filarial infections, and for those non-syphilitic spirochaetal infections which do not respond to penicillin. Apart from

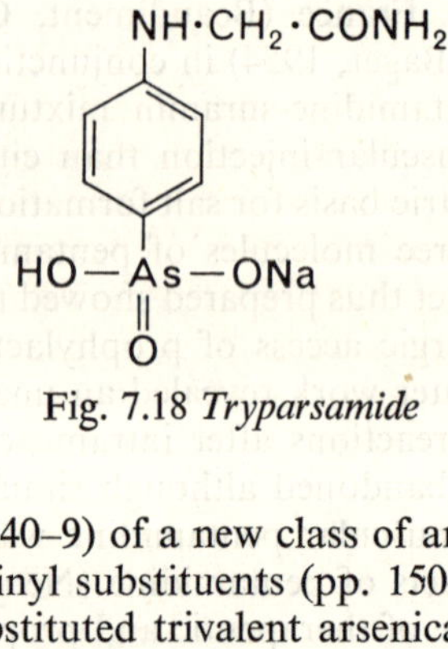

Fig. 7.18 *Tryparsamide*

the major introduction (1940–9) of a new class of aromatic arsenicals and antimonials with basic melaminyl substituents (pp. 150–156), and the discovery in 1945 of an active acid-substituted trivalent arsenical, Butarsen (Fig. 7.20), no organometallic drugs other than tryparsamide have been subjected to, or have survived, extensive clinical trial in human trypanosomiasis.

Within the chemical group of aromatic arsenical and antimonial drugs with substituents which are neutral or only feebly ionized at blood *p*H (pp. 211–215), the chief representative is tryparsamide *B.P.*, (sodium 4-glycineamidophenylarsonate hemihydrate; sodium 4-carbamoylmethylaminophenylarsonate hemihydrate) (synonyms: Glyphenarsine, Tryparsone, Tryponarsyl, Novatoxyl, Trypothane) (Fig. 7.18). Tryparsamide *B.P.* ($C_8H_{10}AsN_2NaO_4$, $\frac{1}{2}H_2O$; mol. wt. 305·1) is a white crystalline odourless powder which is slowly affected by light.

It is soluble in 1·5 parts water at 20°C, slightly soluble (1 in 3,500) in 95% alcohol and insoluble in chloroform and ether.

An equivalent compound, Orsanine (Fourneau 270) (sodium 2-hydroxy-4-acetamidophenylarsonate) introduced by Fourneau and his colleagues in 1923, has been used clinically by French workers since 1926, but with increasing replacement by tryparsamide (Schneider, 1963). Extensive use of tryparsamide, Orsanine (and even Atoxyl up to as late as 1945 in parts of French West Africa), ultimately produced arsenical-resistant strains of *T. gambiense* on a wide scale, but the situation was saved largely by the introduction of pentamidine which is active against these strains, at least in early infections (van Hoof, 1947). The ability of tryparsamide to pass into the cerebrospinal fluid is valuable only in late-stage Gambian sleeping sickness which is not already arsenical-resistant; in the case of the Rhodesian form, where the infection at all stages is radically more arsenical-resistant by nature, it is of little use (*see* pp. 690–691). The nature of this difference in sensitivity to arsenical treatment between the Gambian and Rhodesian forms of sleeping sickness is still unknown, but at least two possibilities may be suggested by the writer's (unpublished) observations on the differing drug sensitivity in mice of a recently isolated strain, and an old laboratory strain of *T. rhodesiense*. Both strains were equally susceptible at the minimal effective dose level to suramin, tryparsamide, pentamidine, Melarsen and homidium, i.e. to a dose sufficient to clear the peripheral blood of trypanosomes for at least twenty-four hours. With the sole exception of suramin, minimal curative doses which were effective for the old monomorphic strain were inactive on the fresh polymorphic strain; in the case of pentamidine and homidium, even maximum tolerated doses were not curative, and with tryparsamide and Melarsen, doses had to be increased by factors of 1·5–2× and 4×, respectively, to produce cure.

These results suggest that the polymorphic forms of *T. rhodesiense* are less drug-sensitive because they may be lodged in extravascular tissue sites inaccessible to the action of rapidly excreted drugs. Rhodesian infections in man are acute and Gambian infections are generally chronic so that immune defences are more likely to reinforce the action of short-acting drugs in the latter case, especially if both infections have tissue sites; the equal effectiveness of suramin on monomorphic and polymorphic *T. rhodesiense* is probably due to its persistence and to its interaction with the immune reaction (*see* pp. 219–220).

Distribution and Toxicity

Pentavalent aromatic arsenicals like tryparsamide are much less toxic and less rapid in action than the corresponding phenylarsenoxides; the latter can kill trypanosomes *in vivo* within half an hour of injection, while the former may take several hours to clear the infection. The latent period was assumed to result from tissue reduction of the arsonic acid group, and in a similar way the slow action of arsenobenzenes, which are less toxic than the corresponding arsenoxides, was assumed to be due to oxidation. Ehrlich and Bertheim in 1908 had provided a chemical analogy (Fig. 7.9 and 7.10) for the first process and in 1912 they also showed that arsphenamine (Fig. 7.11) could be oxidized in alkaline solution to *m*-amino-*p*-hydroxyphenylarsenoxide (Fig. 7.19). Ehrlich considered phenylarsenoxides as too toxic for clinical use and this compound was not developed further until Tatum and Cooper in 1934, introduced it as an effective agent ('Mapharsen', oxophenarsine) against syphilis.

Experimental support for the hypothesis of biological reduction of phenylarsonates in treatment of trypanosome infections was provided by Voegtlin and his colleagues (1920–5) (Findlay, 1950), by Yorke and his colleagues (1930–4) using their *in vitro* trypanocidal titre technique as a highly sensitive biological assay for serum drug levels, and finally, by Lourie, Murgatroyd and Yorke who showed in 1935 that red cells contained a very active heat-stable system for the conversion of phenylarsonates to the trypanocidal arsenoxide form. The evidence for reduction of phenylarsonates *in vivo* although highly circumstantial, was nevertheless indirect. The extent of reduction indicated by the sensitive trypanocidal assay was of the order of 0·1% or less, and thus not easily verifiable chemically. However, Crawford and Levvy (1947), using a precise chemical method

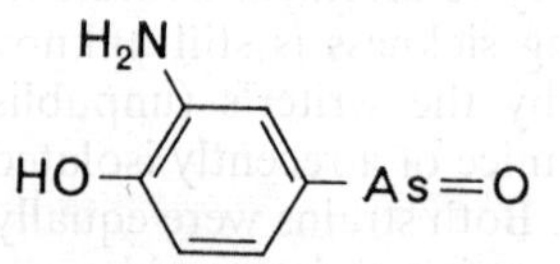

Fig. 7.19 *Mapharside*

which differentiated the valency states of arsenic, showed that in rabbits, over 90% of injected phenylarsonic acid was recovered in the urine after twenty-four hours (unchanged) together with up to 9% in the reduced phenylarsenoxide form; after seventy-two hours, approximately 50% of injected phenylarsenoxide was recovered in the oxidized phenylarsonic acid form. Pentavalent organic antimonials show similar rapid urinary excretion and low affinity for red cells, with some *in vivo* reduction; trivalent compounds bind to red cells and are retained for longer periods in the tissues, especially the liver (GOODWIN & PAGE, 1943; Otto, Maren & Brown, 1947).

In vivo formation of the trivalent phenylarsenoxide is generally accepted as necessary to explain the cytotoxic action of phenylarsonates and arsenobenzenes, but in considering the distribution and excretion of arsenicals, reductive and oxidative processes are only two of a variety of factors which make generalization difficult. Extensive studies by Hogan and Eagle (1944), Eagle, Hogan, Doak and Steinman (1944), Chance, Crawford and Levvy (1945), Doak and Eagle (1951) and Eagle and Doak (1951) established a few generalizations on distribution which appeared sound: (a) the toxicity of arsenic compounds, including inorganic salts, whether to the host or to the parasite, is quantitatively a function of the degree to which they are bound to tissue or to the parasite; in rabbits, LD_{50} doses of tryparsamide (700 mg./kg.), phenylarsonate (16 mg./kg.) and phenylarsenoxide (0·8 mg./kg.) all gave similar levels of tissue-bound arsenic, despite the 900-fold differences in dosage; (b) as a corollary to (a), the excretion rate of arsenicals is inversely proportional to their toxicity; (c) the red blood cell *in vitro* is a convenient model for tissue-binding of arsenic, most of which occurs in the liver and kidneys. The three major exceptions to rule (c) were the pentavalent phenylarsonates, the arsenobenzenes and some carboxyl-substituted phenylarsenoxides, all of which showed delayed toxicity attributable to metabolic conversion. Acid-substituted phenylarsenoxides were an apparent exception, in showing little binding to red cells *in vitro* and an initially rapid excretion followed by a sharp reduction in rate; a subsequent rise in tissue retention was reflected in delayed death at LD_{50} dose levels. The kind of conversion to a more toxic form which is suggested by these results is unknown. One member of this series γ-(*p*-arsenosophenyl) butyric acid (Butarsen) Eagle, 1945), (Fig. 7.20), had sufficient activity to warrant extensive trial in sleeping sickness in man. Despite its activity against arsenical-resistant strains, it is effective only in early cases and has not come into general field use.

The contribution of *in vivo* processes which promote oxidation of trivalent arsenicals may be more significant than is commonly realized. As Chance *et al.* (1945) indicated, the clearance of inorganic arsenite from the body is governed

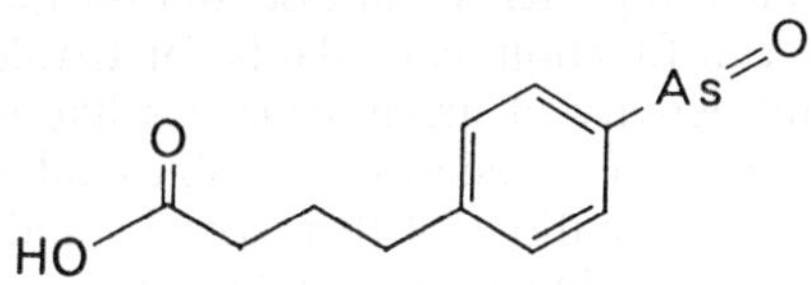

Fig. 7.20 *Butarsen*

by the rate of oxidation to the less toxic, less firmly bound arsonate and in their experiments, the more rapid excretion and lower toxicity of oxophenarsine, compared with unsubstituted phenylarsenoxide, was considered possibly to be due in part to readier conversion to the corresponding arsonate; the effect was unlikely to be caused entirely by nuclear substituents, because the unsubstituted phenylarsonate was excreted as rapidly as oxophenarsine. Although the ultimate cytotoxic effect of arsenicals is due to covalent binding of the arsenoxide grouping to essential thiol groups (*see* pp. 198–200), there is much evidence to suggest that this is preceded by an initial and reversible uptake stage, largely determined, in the case of aromatic arsenicals, by the nature of the substituents on the aromatic nucleus. This effect, combined with oxidative processes, could explain results such as those of Peters and Wright (1951), where the rapid inactivation of oxophenarsine given intravenously to rats, was assayed by chemical analysis of arsenic in blood, in parallel with estimations of trypanocidal activity; the latter decreased in four hours after drug injection and was lost in twenty-four hours, whereas the blood arsenic, after an initial fall, rose in twenty-four- and forty-eight-hour samples to higher levels than in eight- and twelve-hour samples; at eight hours the trypanocidal activity *in vitro* on an arsenic basis, was equivalent to only 1% of the level found chemically. Inactivation (probably oxidative) by rat blood *in vitro* occurred much more slowly, and extravascular tissues were therefore implicated as a major source of inactivation; slow oxidation to the less firmly bound and trypanocidally inactive arsonate, could account for the delayed rise in chemically determinable arsenic in the blood at a time when trypanocidal activity was reduced or absent.

COHEN, KING AND STRANGEWAYS (1932) indicated that attempts to determine arsonate-arsenoxide reduction potentials by titration with oxidizing or reducing agents were not feasible, nor was it practicable to estimate relative velocities of reduction of arsonates with a common reducing agent, as the reduction occurs in steps and the choice of suitable reducing agents is limited. They showed that it was possible to use the velocity of the reverse reaction, from arsenoxide to arsonate, as a comparative measure of the reduction velocity of different aromatic arsonates, and that cystine, containing a reducible disulphide bond, acted as an efficient oxidant in alkali. No straightforward correlation was found between reduction velocities of phenylarsonates and their toxicity; any expected correlation was considered likely to be masked by high excretion rate and the very small amount of reduction estimated to be necessary *in vivo* for production of a toxic concentration of the corresponding arsenoxide. Nevertheless, considerable interest attaches to the demonstration that the disulphide bonds of cystine, widely distributed in proteins and essential for their structural integrity and enzyme function, can function as oxidants for trivalent arsenic.

The distribution and activity of arsenobenzenes like arsphenamine are dependent among other factors, on oxidation. Aerobic oxidation of solutions gives rise to variable results in estimations of their toxicity and trypanocidal activity *in vivo* and especially *in vitro*, but when this factor is excluded or diminished, there is no doubt that arsenobenzenes are more slowly excreted than the corresponding arsonates. A slow rate of oxidation *in vivo*, coupled with the tendency of arsenobenzenes to form colloidal micelles by aggregation of arsenic linkages (Cohen, King & Strangeways, 1932), can explain the slow excretion which occurs, even with arsenobenzenes carrying hydrophilic carboxyl groups which promote rapid excretion in both phenylarsonates and arsenoxides.

Renewed interest in the distribution and metabolism of arsenicals has followed the first reports (1946–9) of the beneficial effects on livestock growth, of organic arsenic compounds, as well as antibiotics, when given as food additives. Frost (1967), in an interesting review of the varied and surprising biological applications of arsenicals, provides a useful guide to their nutritional use in animal production, and to subsequent related enquiries into the metabolism of arsenic. He is at pains to correct the historical 'blanket' condemnation of arsenic in any form as a carcinogenic tissue poison, and stresses that oxidative conversion of trivalent to the less toxic pentavalent arsenic is favoured by physiological *p*H. Recent experiments with ^{74}As-labelled and ^{74}As-, ^{14}C-double-labelled arsanilic acid (Atoxyl) fed to chickens (Overby & Frederickson, 1963, 1965), have shown that Atoxyl appears to be metabolically stable; it was more rapidly excreted than sodium arsonate, and unlike the latter, was not excreted by the lungs in any form. It was found unchanged in the excreta and no reduced arsenoxide forms were detected in the tissues, although in the later experiments, both sodium arsonate and Atoxyl gave rise to small amounts of unidentifiable metabolites in tissues. No reduced form was detectable in the livers of rats fed Atoxyl (Winkler, 1962), and in the same experiments, inorganic trivalent arsenic was largely oxidized and there was no detectable reduction of inorganic pentavalent arsenic. In cattle fed inorganic pentavalent arsenic for extended periods, urinary excretion of arsenic was rapid and the small amount of tissue-bound arsenic was in the unchanged pentavalent form (Peoples, 1964). 80–90% of Atoxyl and related phenylarsonates were excreted by hens in twenty-four hours after parenteral injection and nearly 100% in three days; there was no evidence of arsenic reduction or release of inorganic arsenic (Moody & Williams, 1962). Results were similar after feeding the drugs, but total excretion required nine to ten days. A further example of the metabolic stability of Atoxyl is considered by Frost (1967) to be its use by Landsteiner in 1936 as a serologically active hapten when coupled to protein to form an artificial antigen.

Reversible cellular uptake of pentavalent arsenicals is suggested by their detoxication by *p*-aminobenzoic acid (PABA) and related compounds (Sandground & Hamilton, 1943; Sandground, 1944), and by the more specific antagonism by PABA of the antibacterial and trypanocidal activities of Atoxyl, and by melamine of the trypanocidal activity of Melarsen (Peters, 1943; Williamson, 1959). Arsenic in atomic structure is a congener of phosphorus, and inorganic arsenate can substitute for phosphate in a variety of phosphorolytic and other reactions, even to the extent of incorporation into cock sperm DNA at a similar rate to phosphate, as demonstrated by neutron activation after Atoxyl feeding (Patrick, Voitle, Hyre & Martin, 1964).

Thus, despite the rapid excretion and hence relatively innocuous character of pentavalent aromatic arsenicals, they may not be entirely inert metabolically, and although the thiol-reactive arsenoxide group is not present, the arsonic acid group has an acid dissociation constant sufficiently low to be almost fully ionized as an anion at blood *p*H (as Moore *et al.* found with Atoxyl in 1907); in Melarsen, the cationic melamine substituent is also about 60% ionized at blood *p*H so that the drug molecule must exist mainly as a zwitterion *in vivo* (Williamson, 1959). Some form of ionic interaction with oppositely charged host or parasite receptors must occur, but the location and nature of these are unknown.

Drug Entry into Cerebrospinal Fluid

The ionic character of pentavalent aromatic arsenicals is of great interest in relation to their ability to pass from the bloodstream to the cerebrospinal fluid (CSF), *via* the 'blood-brain barrier'. The term 'blood-brain barrier' connotes at least two barriers, one between the blood and brain proper, consisting of brain capillary wall and a surrounding layer of glial cells, and the other, the choroid plexus epithelium between the blood and the CSF; the release of drugs or other substances from the CSF into blood is much easier than passage in reverse, and occurs mainly *via* the very permeable arachnoid villi (Schanker, 1962, 1966). Passage of drugs or other compounds into the CSF *via* a predominantly lipid phase is unlikely to involve active transport (Kurz, 1964), so that physical properties of the compounds assume great importance. Much conflicting evidence on the properties required has been rationalized by the demonstration (Brodie & Hogben, 1957; Brodie, 1967), that the ability depends on both the extent of drug ionization and the lipid solubility of the unionized drug molecules. In the case of tryparsamide and Melarsen, both of which can pass into the cerebrospinal fluid, the latter more effectively than the former (Rollo, Williamson & Lourie, 1949), it would seem that either ionic binding to elements of the 'barrier' is weak, or passage of the barrier occurs at an acid *p*H (e.g. in lysosomes), which would allow formation of unionized arsonic acid molecules; in the latter case however, increased dissociation of Melarsen as a cation would also occur. One inference is that ionic interaction gives rise to a more lipophilic product and the most probable receptor candidates are phospholipids. On this basis, inability of trypanocides like the aromatic diamidines or phenanthridinium compounds to pass the 'barrier' is difficult to understand, as these drugs can easily be converted *in vitro* into lipid-soluble forms by combination with common phospholipids (Williamson, 1965). Drug-lipid interaction models are however not always directly referable to cellular mechanisms (Cuthbert, 1967), and it may be that suramin, diamidines and phenanthridinium drugs having strongly acidic or basic substituents, and thus unable to exist in the undissociated form at any physiological *p*H, are bound more firmly at non-lipid than at lipid sites.

Other trypanocides which pass into the CSF have properties which conform to the Brodie requirements: nitrofurazone (Fig. 7.29) is poorly water-soluble, and melarsoprol (Fig. 7.24) with its highly reactive arsenoxide group masked by cyclic combination with a dithiol, is predominantly lipid-soluble. The apparently anomalous behaviour of the ionic trypanocides can however be reconciled with the Brodie theory if it is remembered that the dissociation constants (Williamson, 1959), imply that the percentage of the more permeable unionized molecules at *p*H 7·4 is 0·04% for Atoxyl and tryparsamide, and about 0·25% for Melarsen; although low, these amounts correspond to the estimate above that reduction of 0·1% of the dose to the arsenoxide form would be sufficient to account for the trypanocidal activity of phenylarsonates. Suramin, the diamidines and the phenanthridinium compounds are completely ionized at blood *p*H and would therefore be excluded from the CSF. The small amounts (approx. 0·2%) of lipid-soluble neutral pseudo-base formed at blood *p*H by the phenanthridinium drugs Ethidium and Dimidium (Watkins, 1952, 1961), although probably relevant to trypanocidal action in the blood, are unlikely to confer much activity on the CSF; Ethidium was found to be capable of entering the CSF of cats, but although active against *T. gambiense* in man, it did not warrant further trial (Hawking, 1963). Clinical trial of a related drug, Metamidium, in man (Onyango, De Raadt & Mbwabi, 1967) showed no effect on a Mel B-resistant *T. rhodesiense* infection of the CSF.

The penetration of tryparsamide and other arsenicals into the CSF in man was studied in considerable detail by Hawking, Hennelly and Quastel (1937), who used parallel estimations of total arsenic by chemical analysis, and of reduced trivalent arsenic, as measured by trypanocidal activity of the CSF *in vitro*. After intravenous injection of 3 g. tryparsamide, the total arsenic, measured chemically, was high (0·1–0·5 μg./ml.) after fourteen hours, falling to a minimum (0·05–0·1 μg./ml.) after forty hours with a later rise (to 0·2 μg./ml.) over the 60–80 hour period. By comparison, the trypanocidal activity of the CSF is low after fourteen hours, maximal after forty hours and falls to progressively lower levels over the period 60–80 hours; at these times, the corresponding amounts of active trivalent arsenic (as percentage total arsenic) were 3%, 18%, and 5%, respectively. The proportion of trypanocidally active arsenic was considered to be the resultant of three processes: (i) rate of drug penetration into the CSF, (ii) rate of reduction of the drug in the brain and diffusion of this form into the

CSF, and (iii) rate of inactivation of the reduced form. Similar results were obtained later with tryparsamide in sleeping sickness patients (Hawking, 1940). Reduction of the arsenical is assumed to occur in brain tissues, as CSF alone, unlike blood, is incapable of activating tryparsamide *in vitro*.

As oxidation of trivalent arsenicals by most tissues appears to be the more dominant if slower reaction, the pattern of CSF arsenic levels which Hawking *et al.* (1937) describe, could be elaborated as follows in the light of this and other recent work discussed above. Rate (i), which is dependent on the blood concentration of the unionized drug, is likely to be proportional to the dose administered, as appears in the results of Rollo *et al.* (1949) for tryparsamide and Melarsen in rabbits, and to be maximal (as shown by total arsenic levels) shortly after drug administration, i.e. before the rapidly excreted pentavalent form has disappeared from the blood, Adsorption and later reduction of the drug by brain tissue, and subsequent diffusion of the trivalent form in the CSF, could compete with rapid excretion of the unchanged drug *via* the arachnoid villi, so that the trypanocidal activity rises while the total arsenic level falls; the late rise in total arsenic, which occurs while the trypanocidal activity is falling steeply, may reflect a later re-oxidation of reduced drug subsequently liberated into the CSF. The low activity of therapeutic arsphenamine drugs in the CSF despite adequate penetration (Hawking *et al.*, 1937), suggests that excretion takes place before oxidation at tissue sites can release sufficient of the active arsenoxide form. Melarsen produces a higher level of CSF activity in rabbits than a comparable dose of tryparsamide, yet both are reducible to the same extent by red cells *in vitro* (Rollo *et al.*, 1949); in this case the difference is probably due to the higher proportion at blood *p*H of unionized molecules of Melarsen (approx. 0·25%), than of tryparsamide (0·04%).

Medication with tryparsamide and other pentavalent arsenicals has long been known to be responsible for ocular complications (Findlay, 1950), and even to have been implicated as an important source of blindness in the Belgian Congo (Debeir, 1953, 1954), where the incidence of ocular damage after treatment was of the order of 10–20%; this risk was to some extent diminished by mass pentamidine prophylaxis and the use of melarsoprol. The topic is dealt with in clinical detail in Chapter 36, but the present discussion of factors governing arsenical penetration into the CSF may be extended by noting the results of Hurst (1959) on central nerve changes in monkeys and rabbits after arsenical treatment. He found that tryparsamide, in addition to producing haemorrhagic and necrotic lesions at a number of sites in the central nervous system, characteristically produced further lesions in the cerebellar white matter and the optic tracts, the latter lesions involving considerable proliferation of glial cells. More specific effects are suggested by recent experiments with retinal cultures (Hansson, 1966) where thiol-blocking agents, including arsenicals, were shown to cause specific degeneration of rod cells. The apparent restriction of optic atrophy to pentavalent arsenicals could be taken as a reflection of the general inability of phenylarsenoxides to pass from the blood into the cerebrospinal fluid (Hawking *et al.*, 1937), but although Melarsen oxide (like oxophenarsine and Butarsen) does not penetrate the CSF of rabbits (Rollo *et al.*, 1949), it does so in monkeys (Hurst, 1959) and in man, and in the former it apparently does not give rise to ocular complications. Similarly, Melarsen is apparently less liable than tryparsamide to produce optic lesions (*see* Chapter 36), so that the melaminyl substituent appears to have some specific influence on cellular uptake of the melamine drugs in the central nervous system, as it seems to have on uptake by trypanosomes (*see* pp. 212–214). The more complex 'reactive encephalopathy' which occurs as a result of interaction between drug, diseased brain and trypanosome in late-stage sleeping sickness is discussed in detail by Robertson (1963, a, b); the reaction is apparently not restricted to arsenicals (De Raadt, 1967) but in the case of Mel B it may be reduced by pre-treatment with oral Berenil (Bailey, 1967, 1968).

Melarsen, Mel B (Melarsoprol) and Mel W

The novel class of phenyl-arsonates, -arsenoxides, -stibonates and -stibinoxides in which melamine (2,4,6-triamino-*s*-triazine) (Fig. 7.21) is coupled in the *p*-position to the metal-containing substituent, originated with Friedheim's publication in 1940 of the trypanocidal activity of Melarsen (disodium *p*-melaminylphenylarsonate) (Fig. 7.22).

FRIEDHEIM (1959) in an entertaining and illuminating essay on chemotherapeutic development, reveals that the discovery of the melaminyl drugs is another

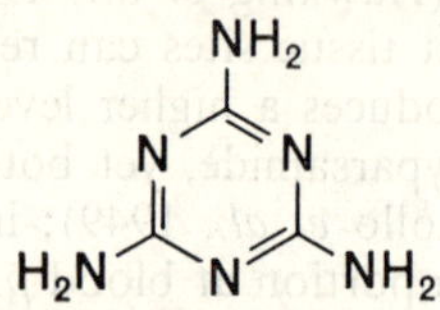

Fig. 7.21 *Melamine*

example of intelligent empiricism linked with industrial technology, in drug evolution: 'All arsenicals with significant trypanocidal activity contain nitrogen in one form or another . . . It therefore seemed reasonable to try compounds which cumulate various forms of nitrogen, and melamine chemistry, which was then coming to the fore in the manufacture of plastics, offered a convenient starting-point from *s*-triazine halides. In this way melarsen was developed, which contains one secondary amine, two amides and three nuclear nitrogens for one arsenic.'

Of the antimony analogues, the pentavalent compound corresponding to Melarsen (Friedheim & Berman, 1946; Friedheim, Vogel & Berman, 1947), can exist as a crystalline monomer, or as an amorphous polymer (MSb) which, unlike other polymeric stibanilates, shows increased trypanocidal activity and decreased toxicity, and in this form also has remarkable prophylactic activity (Mayer & Brousseau, 1946; Rollo *et al.*, 1949). The trivalent analogue (MSb3) corresponding to Melarsen oxide (the reduced form of Melarsen) does not polymerize and has no prophylactic activity; its trypanocidal activity is comparable to that of Melarsen oxide (Rollo *et al.*, 1949).

Following earlier experiments (Friedheim & Vogel, 1947), both Melarsen oxide and MSb3 were coupled with BAL (2,3-dimercaptopropanol) to give

Mel B (melarsoprol) and MSbB respectively (Friedheim, 1949, 1953; Le Rouzic, 1949).

Melarsen (Fig. 7.22) has been available as the disodium salt ($C_9H_9AsN_6Na_2O_3$; mol. wt. 370·16), (disodium *p*-melaminylphenylarsonate; disodium *p*-(2,4-diamino-*s*-triazinyl-6)-aminophenylarsonate) which is a white powder soluble in water, giving an alkaline solution; aqueous solutions are stable for up to three months at 45°C. The anhydrous salt hydrates to the tetrahydrate on exposure to air (Banks, Gruhzit, Tillitson & Controulis, 1944). According to these authors, a tetrahydrate is also formed in air by the sesquisodium salt ($C_{18}H_{18}As_2N_{12}Na_6O_6$), formed by crystallization of equimolar amounts of the mono- and disodium-salts; this salt is highly water-soluble and less alkaline than the disodium salt.

Although less attention seems to have been paid to Melarsen than to Mel B [van Hoof (1947) for example, recommended that it be abandoned because of its toxicity], the favourable immediate results obtained with it by McLetchie (1948) in Nigeria were confirmed by Duggan and Hutchinson (1951), and on the recommendation of the International Scientific Committee for Trypanosomiasis

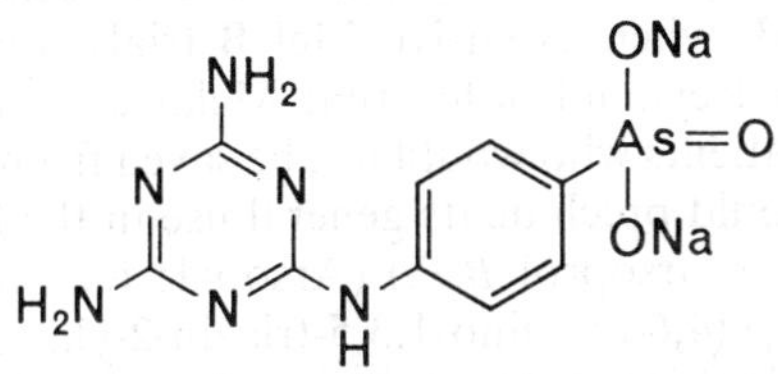

Fig. 7.22 *Melarsen*

Research, further Melarsen trials with adequately standardized products were undertaken (Hutchinson, 1956; Butler, Duggan & Hutchinson, 1957). Melarsen is much less toxic than Mel B, is water-soluble, easy to administer, and in Gambian sleeping sickness, a recommended course (eight injections of 15 mg./kg. at five-day intervals) is shorter than, and at least as effective as, an equivalent tryparsamide course (twelve injections of 3 g. at five-day intervals); it also has the advantage of being more active than tryparsamide in late-stage cases and of being active also against tryparsamide-resistant cases.

Activity against tryparsamide-resistant *T. gambiense* is of considerable importance. Van Hoof (1947) quoted almost 100% incidence of tryparsamide-resistant strains in certain areas of the Belgian Congo by 1947, and Friedheim (1949) stated that in 1946 in French West Africa, 80% of all second-stage cases of Gambian sleeping sickness were tryparsamide-resistant; the gravity of these figures was emphasized by the fact that of 50,000 new cases discovered in 1946, 60% were already in the second stage of the infection. The activity of Melarsen oxide against tryparsamide-resistant trypanosomes, demonstrated both in the field (van Hoof, 1947) and in the laboratory (Williamson & Lourie, 1948), and its ability to affect the cerebrospinal fluid infection in man, led to development, first of the less toxic BAL-compound Mel B, and subsequently of an apparently even less toxic and more water-soluble derivative, Mel W (Friedheim & De Jongh, 1959; De Jongh & Friedheim, 1959).

Melarsen oxide (Fig. 7.23) ($C_9H_9AsN_6$; mol. wt. 292·16) (*p*-melaminylphenylarsenoxide; *p*-(2,4-diamino-*s*-triazinyl-6)-aminophenylarsenoxide) is a white powder soluble in dilute alkali, and in propylene glycol. It was described by Friedheim (1944) and Banks *et al.* (1944), following an announcement of its activity against sleeping sickness in West Africa (Friedheim, 1941). Although it has been superseded by its BAL derivative, Mel B, early trials indicated its value

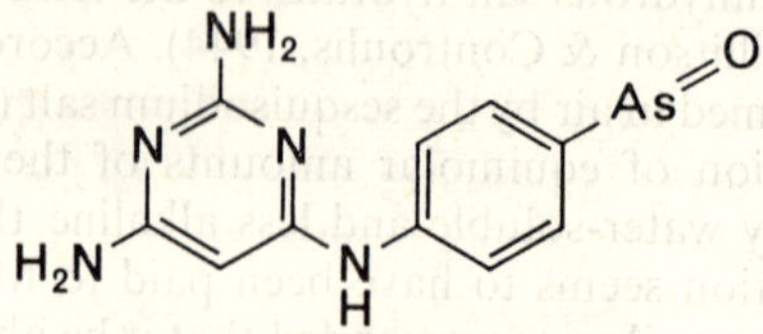

Fig. 7.23 *Melarsen oxide*

in late-stage Gambian sleeping sickness and its activity against tryparsamide-resistant infections, despite the drawback of considerable toxicity (Findlay, 1950). As late as 1953, when extensive Mel B trials were already under way, Jonchère, Gomer and Reynaud noted that Melarsen oxide could 'cure a considerable number of patients who would not be saved from death by other drugs', but that its toxicity would preclude its general use in the field.

Mel B (Fig. 7.24) (melarsoprol *B.P.*) (Arsobal; RP 3854) ($C_{12}H_{15}AsN_6OS_2$; mol. wt. 398·3) (2-*p*-(4,6-diamino-1,3,5-triazin-2-ylamino)phenyl-4-hydroxymethyl-1,3,2-dithiarsolan) is a pale cream powder insoluble in water, alcohol or

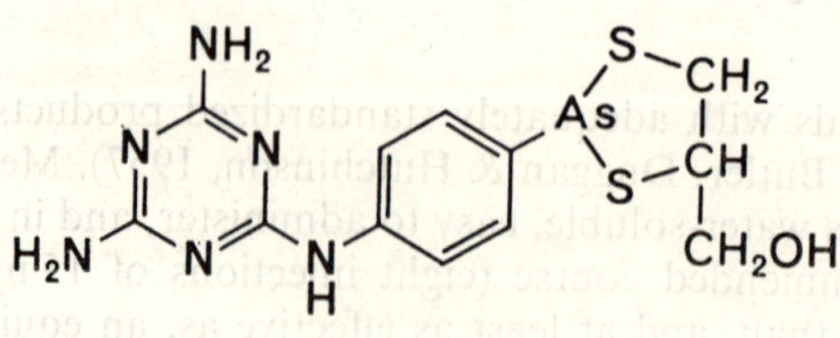

Fig. 7.24 *Mel B*

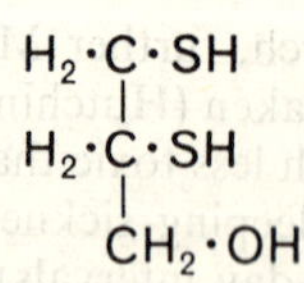

Fig. 7.25 *BAL*

ether, but soluble in propylene glycol (in which it is usually administered as a 3·6% solution); propylene glycol solutions are stable to autoclaving.

The discovery of British Anti-Lewisite (BAL) (dimercaprol; 2,3-dimercaptopropanol) (Fig. 7.25) by Peters, Stocken and Thompson (1945) and its ability to detoxicate trivalent arsenic by the formation of a highly stable ring compound, led to the combination of BAL with a number of phenylarsenoxides such as oxophenarsine, to produce the corresponding cyclic thiol derivative (in this case BAL-OXO; Peters & Stocken, 1947; Friedheim & Vogel, 1947). Several compounds of this type, including Mel B and MSbB, prepared by Friedheim, were tested against sleeping sickness in man in French West Africa by Le Rouzic (1949). As a result of these trials, Friedheim (1949) in his first account of the activity of Mel B, recommended a treatment course of daily intravenous injections of 3·6 mg./kg. for four days, followed by an interval of one week and a further course of four similar injections. A three-to-four day interval between injections was advised for very advanced cases, to avoid Herxheimer-type reactions due to sudden massive destruction of parasites in the central nervous system.

A related compound, Melarsen oxide dithiomalate (RP 3826), was much less effective than Mel B, and its inferior activity 'demonstrates clearly the advantage of cyclic over open chain arsenic dimercaptide structures' (Friedheim, 1951); thiomalate had in fact been used earlier by Ceccaldi, Trinquier, Pellissier and Arnoult (1949) to reverse the toxic effect of Melarsen oxide in man. The open chain dithioarsenite group (usually -As(S . CH_2CO . R)$_2$ where R = —OH, —O, -alkyl or —NH_2) has frequently been used with the aim of producing more soluble and less toxic derivatives of the free phenylarsenoxide (Cohen, King & Strangeways, 1931; Doak & Eagle, 1951); in general, the open chain derivatives

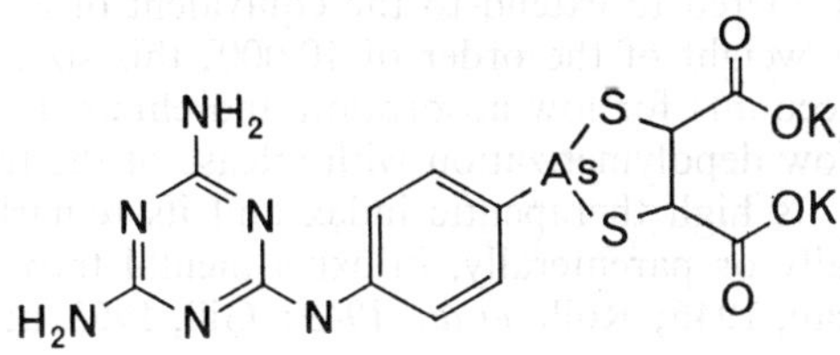

Fig. 7.26 *Mel W*

are less active, though less toxic, and usually more easily dissociable than the cyclic dithiol products of BAL condensation.

From 1950 onwards, Mel B came into wide use, to the virtual abandonment of its precursor, Melarsen oxide. Encouraging results, especially against tryparsamide-resistant late-stage *T. gambiense* infections, came from French, Belgian and Portuguese West and Central African territories, and dramatic effects were obtained by Apted (1953, 1957) for the first time among the formerly doomed late-stage drug-refractory cases of *T. rhodesiense* sleeping sickness in East Africa. Treatment was found to require hospitalization and care, and in the early period of its use, there was a considerable toll of toxic deaths and injuries for which BAL was later recommended as a helpful antidote. Essential factors for effective treatment are discussed in Chapter 36.

Mel W (Fig. 7.26) (Melarsonyl Potassium; Trimelarsan; 'Pentylthiarsphenylmelamine'; Melarsenoxide Dimercaptosuccinate; 9955 RP; Dipotassium 2-[*p*-(4,6-diamino-1,3,5-triazin-2-ylamino)phenyl]-1,3,2-dithiarsolan-4,5-dicarboxylate) ($C_{13}H_{11}AsK_2N_6O_4S_2$; mol. wt. 532·5) is a white powder soluble in water; aqueous solutions deteriorate and must be used immediately after preparation.

Mel W resulted from an ingenious attempt by Friedheim to produce a more water-soluble analogue of Mel B while retaining the latter's considerable activity. As described by De Jongh and Friedheim (1959) and Friedheim and De Jongh (1959), early trials in Gambian sleeping sickness cases gave encouraging results; the new drug had the considerable advantages of activity when administered by intramuscular instead of intravenous injection, activity against CNS infections and very short treatment time. NODENOT, RIDET, CHARTOL AND DESMOULINS (1960) and SCHNEIDER, LEVEUF AND TANGARA (1961) confirmed the activity of

Mel W in Gambian sleeping sickness but stressed the need for care in treating CNS cases. Subsequent experience in Gambian and Rhodesian sleeping sickness, has produced conflicting evidence of its activity and particularly of its toxicity as compared with Mel B.

Antimony Analogues of Melaminyl Arsenicals

The antimony analogue of Melarsen, called MSb (Friedheim & Berman, 1946; Friedheim, Vogel & Berman, 1947) is a polymer, of which the monomer resembles Melarsen 'in solubility, toxicity, immediate trypanocidal activity and rapid elimination' (Friedheim, 1959); its monomeric chemical structure can be considered identical to that shown in Fig. 7.22 if Sb is substituted for As. Polymerization through antimony-oxygen linkage, as occurs with other aromatic antimonials, is considered to extend to the equivalent of about 30 monomers, giving a molecular weight of the order of 10,000; this size, together with low water solubility, accounts for low absorption and elimination of MSb and for its low toxicity. Slow depolymerization with release of the trypanocidal monomer, accounts for its high therapeutic index and its remarkable prophylactic activity, either orally or parenterally, in experimental trypanosome infections (Mayer & Brousseau, 1946; Rollo *et al.*, 1949; Gill, 1962, a; Gill & Malhotra, 1963a).

The potential value of MSb in clinical prophylaxis in French Guinea was indicated by Le Rouzic (1949), but apart from an extended trial of its therapeutic activity against Gambian sleeping sickness in this area (Friedheim, 1953), no further clinical application has ensued. Production batch variation was considered to be an important cause of conflicting results in the experimental clinical trials of the melaminyl drug series (Lourie, 1952) and to be especially important in a polymerized antimonial like MSb. Effective biological standardization was urged (Lourie, 1952), and as a result, international biological reference preparations of both Mel B and MSb were set up in 1954 (WHO, 1960). A standardization procedure for MSb samples in terms of toxicity and therapeutic and prophylactic activity against *T. equiperdum* infection in mice was also described at this time (Edge, Hill & Stone, 1954), and indicated that batch variation was not perhaps so serious as had been previously thought. In view of the unique properties of this compound, which, of all trypanocides so far synthesized, would seem to correspond most closely, at least experimentally, to Ehrlich's ideal of a *therapia sterilisans magna*, it is surprising that its clinical development has not been pursued.

MSb3 and MSbB are, respectively, the antimony analogues of Melarsen oxide and Mel B. MSbB (Friedheim, 1953) was found to have comparable trypanocidal activity to Mel B, and given orally in man, in combination with the free acid form of MSb, cured 98 first-stage and 19 out of 26 second-stage cases; the advantages claimed were short treatment time and avoidance of risks of arsenical encephalitis. MSb3 has been used experimentally in the form of the dithioglycollate (Friedheim, 1947), but it is less stable and more toxic than the corresponding arsenoxide or the cyclic BAL derivative MSbB. TWSb (Stibocaptate), a dimercaptosuccinate compound of trivalent inorganic antimony, but much less toxic than the roughly analogous tartar emetic (FRIEDHEIM,

DA SILVA & MARTENS, 1954), had only a therapeutic effect on Mel B-resistant cases of *T. rhodesiense* sleeping sickness (Hawking, 1963; De Raadt & Kimber, 1966).

Toxicity and Pharmacology

In Friedheim's original 1944 study of a series of Melarsen analogues, the importance of two intact amino groups in the triazine ring is indicated by the sharp increase in toxicity (up to thirty-fold) which follows progressive substitution of one or both groups by alkyl substituents to form secondary and tertiary amino groups. This structural specificity is no doubt significant for such unique properties of the melamine drugs as their ability to act on trypanosomes resistant to other types of organometallic drug, and to show cross-resistance to non-metallic drugs such as the diamidines (Rollo and Williamson, 1951), but most of the central and peripheral nerve toxicity to which the melamine arsenicals can give rise, appears to be essentially similar to that caused by other arsenicals (Michielsen & Triest, 1954; Hurst, 1959). The typical symptoms of Mel B toxicity have been graphically described by Neujean and Evens (1958).

So far, no optic lesions have been reported, in contrast to tryparsamide which shows a characteristic pattern of nervous damage in experimental animals (Hurst, 1959). Kidney damage and resultant albuminuria are common symptoms of arsenical toxicity and have been reported for Mel B (Michielsen & Triest, 1954); in experimental animals, Melarsen oxide and its pyrimidyl analogue, compound 12,065 (Ainley & Davey, 1958), produced kidney lesions similar to those caused by organometallic diuretic compounds, and compound 12,065 was in fact found to be diuretic. In man, Mel B has also been found to produce myocardial damage and hypertension in a number of cases (Michielsen & Triest, 1954), and as a further instance of the care necessary in Mel B treatment, Janssens, Van Bogaert, Michiels and Van de Steen (1960) have shown that Mel B treatment is capable of aggravating encephalitis due to an intercurrent viral infection, especially in sleeping sickness cases where the patient's resistance is usually low.

Urinary excretion studies have shown that another contributory factor in Mel B toxicity is arsenic retention, which appears to occur particularly in long treatment courses (Monnet & Baylet, 1951). These authors have also shown that storage instability under tropical conditions is unlikely to contribute to Mel B toxicity, and demonstrated in mice the interesting point that, on the basis of equivalent arsenic content, Mel B was somewhat more toxic than the parent Melarsen oxide. This effect has been noted with other arsenoxide-BAL compounds and is discussed by Findlay (1950). The increased lipid solubility which the cyclic dithiol radical confers (Friedheim & Vogel, 1947) is probably responsible, and may account also for the ability of this type of drug to penetrate into the cerebrospinal fluid (*see* pp. 147–150).

Cross-resistance with diamidine drugs might suggest that the melamine ring opens *in vivo* by hydrolysis to a corresponding biguanide-type compound. This appears unlikely, as *p*-biguanidophenylarsonic acid (corresponding to an 'open ring' Melarsen), has been synthesized by Banks, Controulis and Holcomb

(1946) and found by McGeachin (1953) to have no trypanocidal activity; the toxicity appeared to be similar to that of Melarsen.

Hawking (1962a), using the trypanocidal titre bioassay method (Hawking, 1940; Hawking, Hennelly & Quastel, 1937), showed that although Mel B was 2–4 times as active as Mel W *in vitro*, both drugs, although given by different routes, produced a very similar degree of trypanocidal activity in the plasma of treated cases of Rhodesian sleeping sickness. With both compounds, the plasma concentrations fell rapidly within twenty-four hours of dosing to about 0·1–1 μg. drug/ml., but after three successive daily doses there was a moderate amount of accumulation which did not persist for more than 4–5 days. Only small amounts (approx. 1% of plasma level) of either drug were detectable in the CSF six hours after a three-dose course. Although these amounts must still be adequate to affect trypanosomes, they are very much lower than those recorded by Monnet and Baylet (1951) for total arsenic in CSF after Mel B treatment, or for trypanocidal activity of the drug after tryparsamide treatment (Hawking, 1940). Monnet and Baylet's maximum arsenic concentration in CSF (0·15 μg./ml.) corresponds to the plasma levels of Mel B estimated by Hawking (1962a) under comparable conditions and would suggest that Mel B passes freely into the CSF, but that inactivation in the CSF is rapid and extensive. As Hawking (1962a) indicates, there is still a strong case to be made for more intensive trial of the water-soluble pentavalent Melarsen in Rhodesian sleeping sickness; it appears to be at least as active as nitrofurazone (Fig. 7.29) after oral administration to rats (Bailey, 1967).

Although arsenicals have long been known to produce 'idiosyncratic' sensitization reactions, in view of the numerous and frequent toxic accidents which can attend the use of the melaminyl arsenicals, it would seem important that these drugs be subjected to investigations such as those of Frey, de Weck and Geleick (1966) on immunological sensitization to neoarsphenamine, especially as these authors describe cross reactivity to other aromatic arsenicals including Mel B.

Pentamidine

Pentamidine isethionate *B.P.* (Fig. 7.27) (M. & B. 800) 1, 5-di(4-amidinophenoxy)pentane di(2-hydroxyethanesulphonate) ($C_{19}H_{24}N_4O_2$, 2 $C_2H_6O_4S$; mol. wt. 592·7), is a white, or almost white, odourless, hygroscopic, crystalline

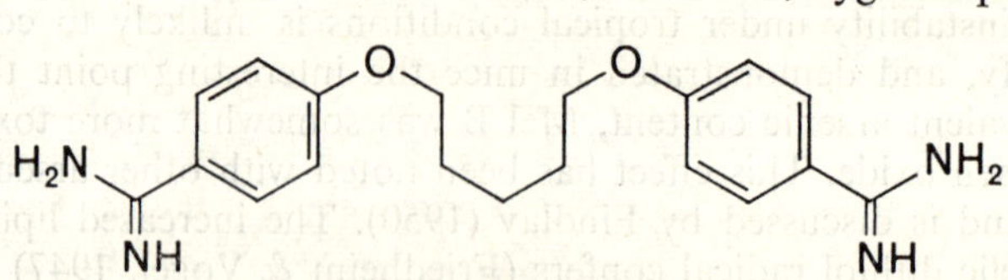

Fig. 7.27 *Pentamidine*

powder with a very bitter taste. It is soluble in water (1:10 at 20°C); a 1:20 aqueous solution has *p*H of 4·5–6·5. It is also soluble in glycerine, slightly soluble in alcohol, and insoluble in acetone, ether, chloroform, or liquid paraffin. Solutions deteriorate on storage.

The French equivalent, Lomidine (Specia, Paris) is the dimethanesulphonate salt (RP 212; pentamidine mesylate) (mol. wt. 532·7), where methanesulphonic acid (CH_3SO_3H) substitutes for 2-hydroxyethanesulphonic acid

$$\begin{pmatrix} CH_2OH \\ | \\ CH_2SO_3H \end{pmatrix}$$

in pentamidine isethionate. Lomidine is a white, or faintly pink, almost odourless, granular powder, a 1:20 aqueous solution of which has a *p*H of 4·5–6·5. It is slightly soluble in water, and almost insoluble in alcohol, acetone, ether, ethyl acetate, chloroform or benzene. For comparative therapeutic purposes, the drug weights of pentamidine isethionate and Lomidine which contain 1 mg. of pentamidine base are 1·74 and 1·56 mg. respectively. Occasionally the dihydrochloride may be used, of which 1·21 mg. contains 1 mg. of pentamidine base.

In the evolution of pentamidine (*see* pp. 138–139), the equally active Stilbamidine (Fig. 7.15) did not survive extensive field use, because of its instability in aqueous solution to light, *p*H and temperature, with formation of toxic products, mainly a dimer of *trans*-Stilbamidine ('photostilbamidine') (Fulton, 1948; Findlay, 1950). Unlike pentamidine it gave rise to a delayed neuropathy, mainly of the trigeminal nerve, but this disability has been turned to advantage in its use for the relief of tic douloureux (SMITH & MILLER, 1955). Its selective action on tumour cells, especially multiple myeloma, led to investigations on mode of action, and tissue distribution and retention, which have had useful application to the understanding of diamidine activity in trypanosomiasis. The less toxic 2-hydroxystilbamidine (Fulton & Yorke, 1942; Ashley & Harris, 1946) (Hydroxystilbamidine U.S.P.; Oxistilbamidine isethionate) is more stable to light and does not give rise to trigeminal neuropathy; like other aromatic diamidines it is fungistatic and has been used to treat blastomycosis in man.

Berenil (diminazene aceturate *B. vet. C.*) (Fig. 7.40) is the only new aromatic diamidine which has come into regular field use for trypanosomiasis since pentamidine was introduced. So far, Berenil has been used almost exclusively for animal trypanosomiasis (*see* pp. 185–188) but experiments with it in human sleeping sickness (Neujean & Evens, 1958; Hutchinson & Watson, 1962) suggest that it may also be of use in man, especially as activity after oral administration has been recently reported (Bailey, 1967, 1967a).

Mass Prophylaxis with Pentamidine

Mass prophylaxis is generally based on a single intramuscular injection of 2·9–3·3 mg. pentamidine base/kg. (Gall, 1954), given yearly or half-yearly; protection persists for at least six months.

The policy of mass pentamidine prophylaxis of Gambian sleeping sickness was vigorously and efficiently pursued by French, Belgian and Portuguese colonial health authorities especially, and in many areas with striking success, following its advocacy by van Hoof, Henrard and Peel in 1944. The use of pentamidine in this way was a major revolution in the control of Gambian sleeping sickness as will be evident from the full description given in Chapter 37.

Toxicity and Pharmacology

The toxic effects of pentamidine are considered to be mainly due to a combination of vasodepressor effect, a hypoglycaemic action and liberation of histamine (Gall, 1954). To reduce the incidence of these side effects, sleeping sickness cases are preferably treated in a prone position and rested in the shade for some hours after each injection; adrenalin is usually kept at hand and calcium (*see* below) has also been recommended (Gasq & Lapeyssonnie, 1949). Gross hypoglycaemic effects can be relieved by glucose, intravenously or orally (*see* Chapter 36 and 37). Transitory hyperuraemia, which has been suggested (Payet & Sankale, 1960) to be a more constant feature of pentamidine treatment of sleeping sickness than previously suspected, was apparently attributable only to the drug.

A number of isolated experimental studies with diamidines and diguanidines have some bearing on the clinical toxicity of pentamidine. The four best trypanocidal aromatic diamidines, including pentamidine, were intensively examined by Wien (1942) and Wien, Freeman and Scotcher (1942), who showed that all four drugs had a depressant action on the circulatory system, only partially reversible by atropine. The fall in blood pressure, mainly accounted for by peripheral vasodilatation, could be prevented by previous injection of calcium ion; serum calcium levels were otherwise rapidly lowered in treated animals. All four drugs had an ergotoxin-like action and reduced the effects of adrenalin; blood sugar was affected only at toxic dose levels, but lower doses, not affecting blood sugar, affected the kidneys, as shown by increased blood urea and non-protein-nitrogen values (*cf.* Payet & Sankale, 1960).

Stilbamidine shows curare-like action in nerve muscle preparations, and in low concentration, inhibits acetylcholinesterase (Bergman, Wilson & Nachmansohn, 1950); its known ability to release histamine may be related to its tendency to localize on mast cells where histamine production may occur (Fell, 1957). The hypoglycaemic activity of guanidines as a group has been recognized since the discovery of Synthalin (Fig. 7.13), which was used as a synthetic substitute for insulin; in experimental animals it produces specific hydropic degeneration of the α-cells of the pancreatic islets (Davis, 1952). These and other aspects of the diverse pharmacological activities of amidine and guanidine compounds are dealt with below (*see* pp. 195–220) and at length in reviews by SCHOENBACH AND GREENSPAN (1948) and Fastier (1962).

Experiments on the tissue retention of diamidines are of more immediate relevance to the prophylactic action of pentamidine in man. Snapper, Lieben, Greenspan and Schneid (1951) found that about one-third of injected Stilbamidine and 2-hydroxystilbamidine was recoverable from tissue deposits in the liver, kidney and adrenals, in man and experimental animals; the bulk of the deposit was in the liver in man and rabbits, and in the kidneys in mice. Liver and adrenal deposits in man were retained for extended periods; in one case, appreciable amounts were found twenty-three months after the last injection, and in another, marked traces were still present after three years and three months. Stilbamidine has been found in sheep liver up to three months after injection, and in rabbits, two months after injection; all organs were found to retain Stilbamidine including skin (Henry, Mansour, Watson & Zaki, 1952).

In these studies estimation methods based on the fluorescent properties of Stilbamidine were used, but Reid and Weaver (1951), using [^{14}C]-labelled Stilbamidine in mice, showed that although 70% was excreted within four days of intravenous injection, traces were detectable in many tissues six months later. Fulton and Mathew (1959) obtained similar results with [^{14}C]-Stilbamidine in rats, and showed that appreciable amounts (0·16%, 0·18% and 0·17% of injected drug in liver, kidneys and lungs, respectively) were detectable 230 days after intravenous injection; similar amounts in the kidneys, and traces in the lung and heart, were present up to 280 days after injection. LAUNOY, GUILLOT AND JONCHÈRE (1960), using [^{14}C]-pentamidine in rats, showed that after a small intramuscular dose (5 mg./kg.), drug was detectable in the liver for a month, and for seven months in the kidneys; none was detectable in the blood at any time, and only transitorily after a dose of 50 mg./kg.

Nitrofurazone

An entirely new structural type of trypanocide, based on the furan nucleus (Fig. 7.28) was developed from the discovery by Dodd and Stillman (1944) that some simple furan derivatives had bacteriostatic action.

5-Nitro-substituted derivatives were particularly active and the 5-nitro-2-furaldehyde semicarbazone (nitrofurazone) (Fig. 7.29) was later found to be

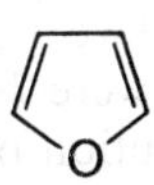

Fig. 7.28 *Furan*

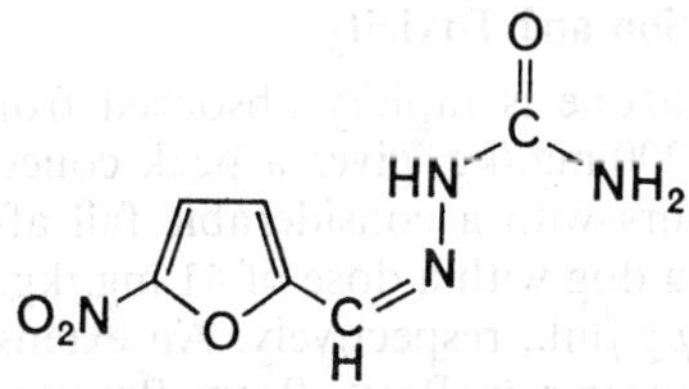

Fig. 7.29 *Nitrofurazone*

curative for experimental *T. equiperdum* infections in mice (Dodd, 1946; Giarman, 1951).

Nitrofurazone *B.P.C.* (Fig. 7.29) (Furacin, Furacilin, Nitrofural, Nitrofuran, Vabrocid, Vitrocin, Yatrocin, Chemofuran, Chixin, Furalone, Ibiofural, Otofural) ($C_6H_6N_4O_4$; mol. wt. 198·1) is a lemon-yellow odourless crystalline powder, with a bitter after-taste. It darkens on exposure to light and is only slightly soluble (1:4200) in water, giving a *p*H of 5 to 7·5. Solubility is 1:600 in alcohol, 1:300 in propylene glycol, and much lower in acetone and ethyl acetate; it is insoluble in chloroform and ether. The solubility can be increased to 1:100 for presentation by the use of Macrogol (polyethylene glycol) mixtures. All solutions should be stored in the dark.

Nitrofurazone appeared equally active by oral or parenteral administration (Giarman, 1951; Packchanian, 1955), and from its novel structure would be expected to act on trypanosomes resistant to the standard drugs. The continued incidence of late-stage sleeping sickness cases relapsing to suramin, tryparsamide, pentamidine and Mel B, prompted clinical trials of nitrofurazone on this type of otherwise hopeless case, especially as it had been shown to enter the

CSF of dogs after an oral dose (Evens, Niemeegers & Packchanian, 1957; *see* also Apted, 1960; Fierlafyn, 1960). Although results were encouraging in both Gambian and Rhodesian sleeping sickness cases, polyneuritis developed with raised blood pyruvate. Experimental work on isolated enzymes (Paul, Bryson & Harrington, 1956) had previously suggested that nitrofurazone interfered with pyruvate oxidation (*see* p. 210) and Robertson (1961) and Robertson and Knight (1964) have noted further examples of a beri-beri type of polyneuropathy and disordered pyruvate metabolism in Rhodesian sleeping sickness.

A related compound, Furaltadone (Altafur; Furmethonol) (a mixture of the L- and D-isomers of 5-morpholinomethyl-3-(5-nitrofurfurylideneamino)-2-oxo-oxazolidine) was tested by Adriaenssens (1960, 1962) on thirty-seven cases of Rhodesian sleeping sickness; thirty showed immediate clinical improvement, but later neurotoxic reactions were frequent and severe and caused three deaths. The L-isomer (NF-902) which appeared less toxic in animal tests, was later tested by Adriaenssens (1962a) in three Rhodesian sleeping sickness cases and by Robertson, Mbwabi and Bakari (1963) in seven similar late-stage cases, most of which were Mel B-resistant. Immediate results were favourable although variable, but most developed polyneuropathy and relapsed; Robertson *et al.* concluded that its action was uncertain in late-stage cases of *T. rhodesiense* infection, but that it could be reserved for cases relapsing after Mel B treatment.

Distribution and Toxicity

Nitrofurazone is rapidly absorbed from the intestine and in animals an oral dose of 200 mg./kg. gives a peak concentration in the blood of 6 μg./ml. after eight hours with a considerable fall after twenty-four hours. Two hours after treating a dog with a dose of 41 mg./kg., serum and CSF levels were 7·5 μg./ml. and 2·2 μg./ml., respectively. An extensive study of the distribution of various nitrofurans in rats (PAUL, PAUL, BENDER, KOPKE, HARRINGTON, ELLS & BUZARD, 1960) showed no evidence of tissue deposition or accumulation of nitrofurazone, probably because of rapid degradation of the drug by most tissues except blood. Nitrofurazone is bound by plasma protein to a slight extent (about 30% of the plasma drug level); forty-eight hours after treatment about 5% of the dose has been excreted unchanged in the urine.

Nitrofurans such as nitrofurazone have a specific cytotoxic effect on testicular tissue in animals (Nissim, 1957); nitrofurazone, because it causes degeneration of the seminiferous tubules, has in fact been used to treat disseminated seminoma of the testis in man (Wildermuth, 1955). This potential danger is overshadowed however, by observations which show that nitrofurazone and L-Furaltodone are capable of inducing an acute haemolytic anaemia in individuals with the heritable glucose-6-phosphate dehydrogenase deficiency trait (Gilles & Taylor, 1961; Robertson, 1961a; Robertson *et al.*, 1963). The incidence of this trait, which appears to affect erythrocyte integrity, is especially high (15–20%) in African negroes (Sonnet & Micheux, 1960), and in such deficient individuals, a number of important drugs such as 8-aminoquinoline antimalarials, aniline derivatives and *p*-aminosalicyclic acid, in addition to nitrofurazone, may precipitate haemolysis; this and other aspects of nitrofuran therapy of sleeping sickness are discussed further in Chapter 36.

The ability of nitrofurazone to penetrate the CSF after oral administration and its activity against trypanosomes resistant to other drug types (*see* pp. 211–214) are, despite the variety of unwanted side-effects, highly desirable properties which would suggest that other members of this expanding group (*cf.* Paul & Paul, 1966) might be more suitable for sleeping sickness therapy than either nitrofurazone or Furaltadone. Nitrofurantoin, for example, has survived lengthy clinical use for treatment of urinary Gram negative bacterial infections, without intolerable toxic side-reactions; inspection of its physical and chemical properties and its distribution, in the informative data tabulation of PAUL *et al.* (1960) shows that this compound and a related derivative, Furazolidone, would be suitable candidates for trial against late-stage drug-resistant Gambian or Rhodesian sleeping sickness.

CHEMOTHERAPY AND CHEMOPROPHYLAXIS OF THE ANIMAL TRYPANOSOMIASES

Drug Evolution

The development of chemotherapeutic and chemoprophylactic agents for use in livestock and other domestic animals is a more recent occurrence than in the case of human trypanosomiasis. At present, only a few active drugs are available for curative purposes and their value is often diminished by the rapidity with which drug resistance may develop. No completely satisfactory prophylactic agent has yet been introduced which can be relied upon to afford long term protection under field conditions.

Accurate estimates of livestock populations in Africa are difficult to establish and the tentative figures given below must be regarded as only crude approximations. The total cattle population of Africa is of the order of 114 millions but, as Buxton (1948) has indicated, the distribution of cattle and tsetse fly are 'to a considerable extent the converse of one another'. This observation is strikingly supported by the maps accompanying a report by Mittendorf and Wilson (1961) which show that tsetse distribution coincides with those areas in which, in 1957–9, the estimated meat consumption level was less than 8 kg. per person per year The population of sheep and goats is around 230 millions and is mainly concentrated in the more arid regions beyond the limits of tsetse distribution as are also the estimated 8½ millions of equines. The camel population of approximately 6½ millions is restricted to areas beyond the northern limit of tsetse distribution. About one half of the estimated pig population of four millions is exposed to the risk of trypanosomiasis. Apart from the tsetse-borne trypanosomiases of tropical Africa, camels and equines are liable to contract surra, a disease caused by *T. evansi*, and horses are often infected with *T. equiperdum* which causes a disease known as dourine. Of the tsetse-borne trypanosomes, *T. vivax* and *T. congolense* are mainly responsible for the disease in cattle and sheep among which losses in life and productivity can occur on a massive scale (Williamson, 1962). *T. brucei* is highly pathogenic for horses as well as contributing to the incidence of disease in cattle. *T. simiae* causes severe and often rapidly

TABLE 7.2

Summary of curative and prophylactic drugs used for the African trypanosomiases in domestic animals

Trypanocide	Type	Field use: Dose[1] (mg./kg.)	Field use: Animal	Field use: Infection	Toxic effects	Comments
Antrycide (quinapyramine) (Imperial Chemical (Pharmaceuticals) Ltd.) (quinoline-pyrimidine structure)						
(i) *dimethosulphate*	C	4·4 s.c.	Cattle	*T. congolense*, *T. vivax*	Curare-like. Aggravated by stress. Kidney damage	Possible induction of residual immunity
(quinapyramine sulphate *B. vet. C*)	C	3–5 s.c.	Equines	*T. evansi*, *T. equiperdum*	Equines more sensitive than bovines	
	C	3–5 s.c.	Camels	*T. evansi*		Active against suramin-fast infections
	?	3–5 s.c.	Pigs	*T. simiae*		Not curative in fly-induced infections
(ii) *chloride*[2]	P	50 s.c.	Pigs	*T. simiae*		3–6 months prophylaxis, depending on size of pig
(iii) (a) *pro-salt* (*dimethosulphate* : *chloride* 3 : 4 w/w)	P	11·7 s.c.	Cattle	*T. congolense*, *T. vivax*		Prophylaxis about two months, depending on challenge
(b) *pro-salt R.F.* (*dimethosulphate* : *chloride* 3 : 2 w/w (quinapyramine (prophylactic) *B. vet. C.*)	P	7·4 s.c.	Cattle	*T. congolense*, *T. vivax*		Similar prophylaxis to (iii) (a) but cheaper and less local reaction

Berenil (Farbwerke Hoechst AG) (diminazene aceturate *B. vet. C*) (aromatic amidine structure)	C	3·5 i.m.	Cattle	*T. congolense*, *T. vivax*		Rapidly excreted; resistance difficult to induce. Active against Ethidium (homidium)-resistant infections. Inactive against *T. simiae* Effects of higher doses in W. African cattle need investigation
Ethidium bromide (homidium bromide *B. vet. C.*) (Boots Pure Drug Co. Ltd.) (phenanthridine structure)	C	1·0 i.m.	Cattle	*T. congolense*, *T. vivax*	Local tissue damage if given subcutaneously	Chloride salt (Novidium) soluble in cold water; bromide salt soluble only in hot water. Possible alternating use with Berenil as 'sanative pair' to reduce incidence of drug resistance.
	C	1·0 i.m.	Horses	*T. vivax*	Liver damage only at high dosage	
Prothidium (pyrithidium bromide *B. vet. C.*) (Boots Pure Drug Co. Ltd.) (phenanthridine-pyrimidine structure)	P	2·0 i.m.	Cattle	*T. congolense*, *T. vivax*	Similar to Ethidium	Soluble only in hot water. Prophylaxis about four months or less depending on challenge
	C	0·2–0·4 i.m.	Cattle	*T. congolense*, *T. vivax*		

[1] s.c. = subcutaneously. i.m. = intramuscularly. i.v. = intravenously.
[2] Not available commercially.

C = curative.
P = prophylactic.

TABLE 7.2 (*continued*)

Summary of curative and prophylactic drugs used for the African trypanosomiases in domestic animals

Trypanocide	Type	Field use: Dose[1] (mg./kg.)	Field use: Animal	Field use: Infection	Toxic effects	Comments
'Samorin' (Isometamidium) (May & Baker Ltd.) (phenanthridine-aromatic amidine structure)	C, P	0·25–0·5 i.m.	Cattle	*T. congolense*, *T. vivax*	Similar to Ethidium	Less toxic than Ethidium. Soluble in cold water; heat-sensitive. Prophylaxis 2–4 months depending on challenge. Dose should be determined by challenge. Higher doses for drug-resistant infections, but doses above 1·0 mg./kg. less well tolerated.
Suramin (Sulphonated naphthylamine structure)	C	Approx. 10·0 i.v. (5 g./camel)	Equines Camels	*T. brucei* *T. evansi*		Suramin-resistant infections are susceptible to Antrycide. Hygroscopic drug.
Suramin-Antrycide complex[2]	C, P	40 s.c.[3]	Pigs	*T. simiae*	Negligible at this dose	3–6 months prophylaxis, depending on size of pig

[1] s.c. = subcutaneously. i.m. = intramuscularly. i.v. = intravenously.
[2] Not available commercially.
[3] Dose of basic drug in complex.
C = curative.
P = prophylactic.

fatal infections in pigs and it is not uncommon for piggeries to be decimated within a few days.

Because of the variety of domestic livestock which are susceptible to trypanosome infections and of the diversity of trypanosome species which are pathogenic for animals of economic importance, the problems of chemotherapy and chemoprophylaxis are even more complicated and formidable than in human trypanosomiasis.

The initial evaluation and ultimate application of an active 'cattle' trypanocide are complicated by these and other factors (*cf.* Whiteside, 1958), such as the apparent crude difference in the relative virulence of *T. vivax* and *T. congolense* in West and East Africa, *T. vivax* being more acutely lethal in West, and *T. congolense* the more virulent in East Africa. This difference appears to be reflected in drug susceptibility, as many new drugs seem to perform better against East rather than West African strains. Even tartar emetic was observed over many years in Northern Nigeria (Wilson, 1958), to be more active against *T. vivax* than *T. congolense* and extensive mass treatments with Ethidium and Novidium in the same area seem to have selected out the more resistant *T. congolense* as the predominant infection (Macgregor, 1966).

Comparisons of this type based on field practice or even on what appear to be adequately controlled field trials are difficult to establish, mainly because of the variations which can occur (a) in the tsetse fly (species, habitat, infective inoculum, infection rate, density, frequency of bite, etc.), (b) in the species and strain of trypanosome, (c) in the host animal (age, breed, sex, colour, weight, condition, nutritional status, intercurrent infection, management and herding) and (d) in the area (climate, season, vegetation and the interaction of these with (a) and (c) above). In attempts to control this variability, Smith and Rennison (1958) have defined trypanosome 'challenge' as 'the number of infective bites from a tsetse which a host receives in unit time', and have stressed the necessity for refining methods of assessing 'challenge' in the light of field experience and in particular of the work of Whiteside (1955), who showed that in cattle, for a given prophylactic drug, the greater the challenge the shorter the period of prophylaxis obtained. Whiteside also defined an index of trypanosome challenge for field use as the product of the number of non-teneral male and female tsetse per 10,000 yards (the Apparent Density), and their infection rate; in later work (Whiteside (1962a) recommended the use of a group of Berenil-treated cattle, in which fresh infections could be used as a simple index of natural incidence of infection (*see* also p. 187).

Attempts such as these to analyse, reduce and control the variables in the tsetse-trypanosome-animal complex are of the utmost importance for a satisfactory assessment of drug performance; many drug trials are models in this respect, and demonstrate the additional and more precise information that can be extracted from carefully controlled experimentation (e.g. Stephen, 1958; Smith, 1959; Smith & Brown, 1960). In Africa, where the resources for such experiments in cattle are so variable, a simple but highly desirable way of ensuring some measure of comparability among a number of therapeutic or prophylactic trials, carried out in different areas and under different conditions of challenge, is to incorporate at least *two* sets of control animals, one set untreated and introduced regularly into the experiment and the other treated with a well-tried drug such as Antrycide Prosalt or Berenil as a standard yardstick; both sets are exposed to the same challenge as the experimental animals.

The few active 'cattle' trypanocides which have become established in the field or have survived preliminary field trials are tartar emetic (Fig. 7.30) (the first active drug, used for over forty years but now displaced), Antrycide (Fig. 7.36), the phenanthridinium drugs, Ethidium (Fig. 7.37), Prothidium (Fig. 7.38) and Samorin (Isometamidium) (Fig. 7.39) and the diamidine, Berenil (Fig. 7.40); suramin (Fig. 7.17) has been used mainly for *T. evansi* infections and in the form of an Antrycide complex, has been recommended for treatment and prophylaxis of *T. simiae* in pigs and *T. evansi* in equines. Of these, only tartar emetic and Berenil have not readily given rise to drug resistance; this behaviour corresponds to laboratory experience where artificial production of trypanosome strains

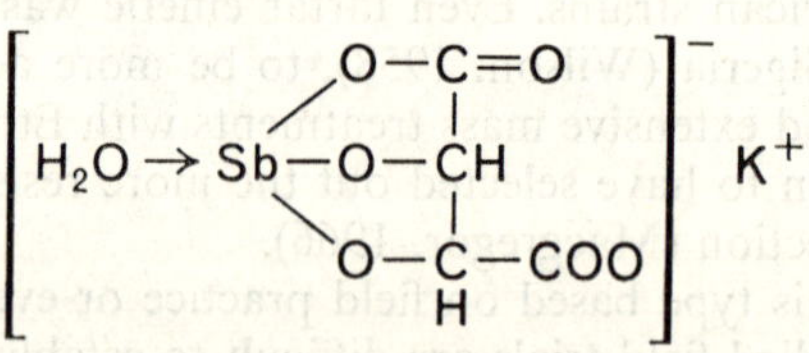

Fig. 7.30 *Tartar Emetic*

resistant to tartar emetic or to the aromatic diamidines is difficult or impossible (Yorke, Murgatroyd & Hawking, 1932; Fulton & Grant, 1955).

The trivalent antimony complex, tartar emetic (antimony potassium tartrate *B.P.*) (Fig. 7.30) and its more soluble and less irritant sodium analogue, were first shown to be active against nagana and surra infections of rats by Plimmer and Thomson in 1908. In the following year, Bevan, impressed by the curative activity of intravenous tartar emetic in sleeping sickness, demonstrated that it was also active in *T. congolense* infections of cattle in Southern Rhodesia; over the next eighteen years he treated 'many thousands of head' of cattle successfully (Bevan, 1928). Despite the introduction of Antimosan (Heyden 661) and its sodium salt, Stibophen, an analogous sulphonated pyrocatechol derivative of trivalent antimony which could be given intramuscularly but required repeated dosage (Uhlenhuth, Kuhn & Schmidt, 1924; Schwetz, 1933), tartar emetic continued to be widely used. Even up to 1950 in Northern Nigeria, where Dimidium (Fig. 7.33b), the first phenanthridinium drug, was never released for field use, tartar emetic was used on an increasing scale; 2,200 head were treated in 1930, 11,088 in 1938 and 34,200 in 1950. In the absence of other active drugs, tartar emetic held sway for forty years because, despite its toxicity (about 6% mortality), deaths in untreated animals might be as high as 50% (Wilson, 1958).

The modern phenanthridinium drugs owe their origin to Ehrlich's later work with dyestuffs based on the acridine nucleus. This work developed rapidly after the activity of the triphenylmethane dye, Trypanosan (*see* p. 132), was discovered to be due to an acridine compound present as an impurity. All available acridine dyes were tested, and in the process, activity was found especially in the dimethylated diamino dye, Acridinium Yellow, in which the ring N atom was quaternized; the trypanocidal activity of this compound led Ehrlich to persuade the chemist Benda to synthesize a homologous dye carrying only the amino groups. The new dye (2,8-diamino-10-methylacridinium chloride)[1] (Fig. 7.31), turned out to be much more active and was given the name Trypaflavine

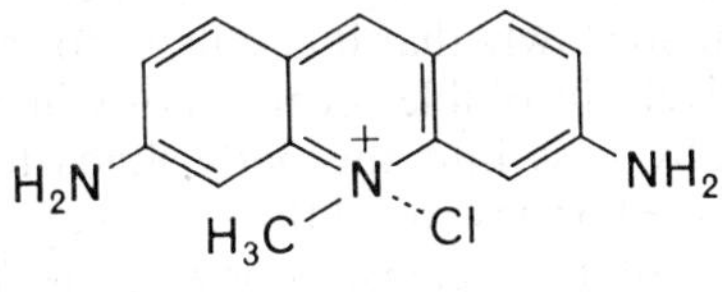

Fig. 7.31 *Trypaflavine* (*Acriflavine*)

(acriflavine). Although it did not come into field use for trypanosomiasis, Ehrlich's colleague, Browning, discovered that it was a highly active antibacterial agent (Browning & Gilmour, 1913), even in the presence of serum, and this antiseptic property was impressively exploited during the ensuing 1914–18 war (Browning, Gulbransen & Thornton, 1917). Later extensive attempts to associate antiseptic action with fragments of the acridine molecule, such as quinoline and pyridine (BROWNING, COHEN, GAUNT & GULBRANSEN, 1922), together with the discovery that the recently prepared group of quinolinium-type carbocyanine and isocyanine dyes, used as photographic sensitizers, were potent antiseptics (BROWNING, COHEN & GULBRANSEN, 1922), led to an examination of the simpler anil- and styrylquinolines. Some of these were first found to be powerful antiseptics, and later, in 1926, certain amino derivatives turned out to

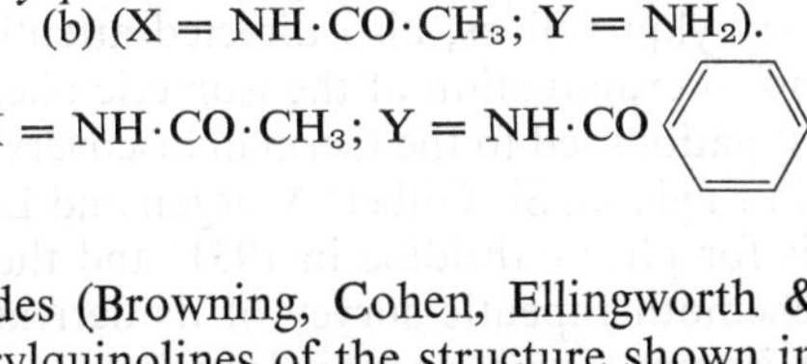

Fig. 7.32 *Aminostyrylquinolines.* (a) (X = NH_2, $N(CH_3)_2$; Y = $NH\cdot CO\cdot CH_3$).
(b) (X = $NH\cdot CO\cdot CH_3$; Y = NH_2).
(c) (X = $NH\cdot CO\cdot CH_3$; Y = NH·CO 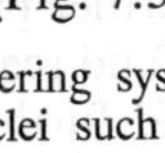 $\cdot NH_2$)

be active trypanocides (Browning, Cohen, Ellingworth & Gulbransen, 1926), especially aminostyrylquinolines of the structure shown in Fig. 7.32a and b.

Browning and his colleagues continued to exploit this series, but no derivative suitable for field use was evolved, although access of striking prophylactic activity was shown in compounds where *p*-aminobenzamido-type substituents were inserted in the quinoline ring, e.g. Styryl 245 (Fig. 7.32c). This and related

[1] Here and subsequently, the older Richter ring-numbering system is used which has advantages over the IUPAC system for heterocyclic nuclei such as phenanthridine and aeridine (Albert, 1966).

compounds formed a relatively insoluble tissue deposit after subcutaneous injection, and Styryl 245 conferred on mice '. . . longer protection than follows the administration of any other trypanocidal agent hitherto known' (Browning & Gulbransen, 1934). Many observations in this paper foreshadowed later experience with Antrycide and the phenanthridinium compounds. Requirements for prophylactic activity in a drug were detailed as '. . . (1) Its excretion or destruction may occur so slowly that it circulates for a long time in the body; (2) it may form a relatively insoluble local deposit in the tissues from which small amounts continually pass into the body fluids to act on the parasites; (3) although rapidly excreted or destroyed the drug may act as a stimulus leading to a persistent elevation of the defensive powers of the tissues . . .'. Early experiments with suramin, the only other prophylactic drug then known, had

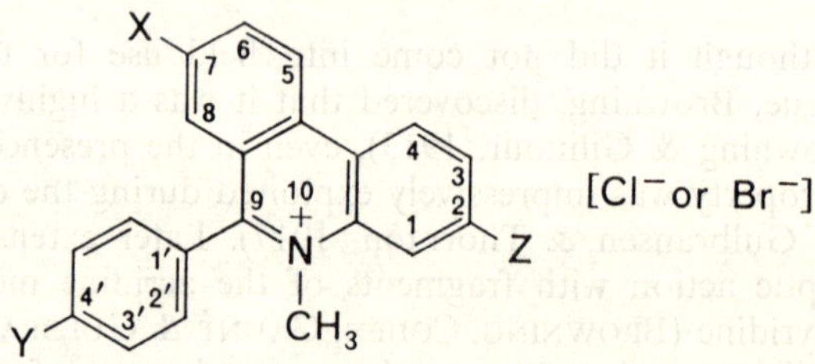

Fig. 7.33 (a) 897, *Phenidium* (X, Y = NH_2; Z = H). (b) 1553, *Dimidium* (X, Z = NH_2; Y = H)

shown no evidence for the third mode of action, nor was it found to be applicable to Browning's compounds. Like many of the later phenanthridinium drugs, the active styryloquinolines produced local dermonecrotic reactions at the site of injection and their effect on trypanosomes was similarly slow. The active prophylactic compounds were prepared as the methoacetate salts, as the chloride and iodide salts were too insoluble, suggesting that, as with Antrycide dimethylsulphate (*see* pp. 174–177), some precipitation by tissue fluid chloride may have been responsible for the insoluble deposit formation after injection.

The biological activity of aminoacridines like acriflavine, as well as stimulating Browning's work on styrylquinolines, also directed attention to possible antimalarial properties and to examination of the isomeric phenanthridine nucleus. The antimalarial investigations led to the German discovery of the acridine drug Atebrin in 1932, and in England, Sir Gilbert Morgan and L. P. Walls developed a convenient synthesis for phenanthridine in 1931, and thereafter collaborated with Browning in a chemotherapeutic survey of its derivatives. In addition to phenanthridine being isomeric with and analogous to acridine, Walls (1947) emphasized that other considerations were relevant; phenanthridine contained the quinoline ring system, present in quinine and Plasmochin (the first successful synthetic antimalarial), and the *iso*-quinoline system found in many biologically active alkaloids. A further practical advantage was that the synthesis was based on diphenyl, a cheap and readily available intermediate. Initial antibacterial and trypanocidal tests and further improvements in synthesis led to concentration on quaternized derivatives of phenylphenanthridines with two amino groups, as trypanocidal activity was found to be associated strongly with these structural features. In 1938, compound 897 (Phenidium chloride) (Fig. 7.33a) from this group was shown to have marked activity against *T. congolense* (Browning, Morgan, Robb & Walls, 1938), unlike the styrylquinolines which were active primarily on *brucei* trypanosomes. Later intensive field trials in African cattle up to 1944 confirmed this activity, but despite the advantages of a single injection and small dosage (about 0·3–0·5 g. per animal), the drug was not very

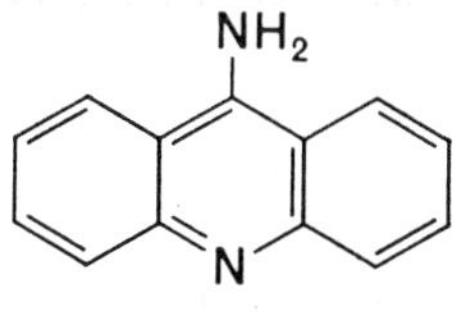

Fig. 7.34 5-*Aminoacridine*

water-soluble and the therapeutic index was low. Further work revealed a more active and water-soluble derivative with two amino groups in the phenanthridine portion of the molecule. This compound, 1553 (Dimidium bromide) (Fig. 7.33b) was later used extensively in cattle in East Africa until drug-resistance resulting from mass treatment became a problem, for example, in the Rhodesias by 1952; higher doses used to overcome resistance led only to mortality, delayed toxicity and photosensitization.

During the period of development of the phenanthridinium drugs in England, Jensch in Germany was struck by the tautomeric similarities of the 4-aminoquinoline nucleus with therapeutically active derivatives of 5-aminoacridine (Fig. 7.34) (such as the antiseptic Rivanol, which Jensch helped to develop in 1920, and the antimalarial, Atebrin (mepacrine)), which can be considered as a combination of two 4-aminoquinoline structures. As a result, a series of 4-aminoquinoline derivatives was found (Jensch, 1937) where two 4-aminoquinoline moieties were linked through amino substitution in the 6-position to a

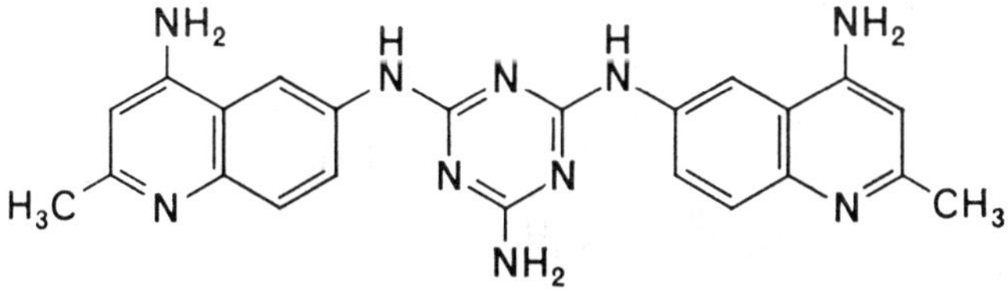

Fig. 7.35 *Surfen C*

central bridge, melamine in the case of Surfen C (Congasin) (Fig. 7.35), urea in the case of Surfen and a diallylmalonyl group in the case of Bayer 7602 (Ac). Surfen C (di(4-amino-2-methylquinol-6-yl) melamine) was the first metal-free drug to show marked activity against *T. congolense* infections in the field, Surfen was an active antiseptic, and Bayer 7602 had activity in the drug-refractory South American *T. cruzi* infection.

Unfortunately, African field trials revealed variable and unacceptable toxic reactions, although activity was generally shown to be of a higher order than that of tartar emetic or Antimosan. Nevertheless, Jensch's structural reasoning was later extended by Barrett, Curd and Hepworth (1953), who decided to eliminate the triazine bridge of Surfen C and to replace one of the quinaldine moieties by an aminopyrimidine system with similar tautomeric possibilities; the weak activity of the resulting compound was enhanced by quaternization, and after some difficulty a highly active *bis*-quaternary salt, originally considered an impurity, was isolated, characterized and later synthesized unambiguously (Ainley, Curd, Hepworth, Murray & Vasey, 1953). This salt was Antrycide

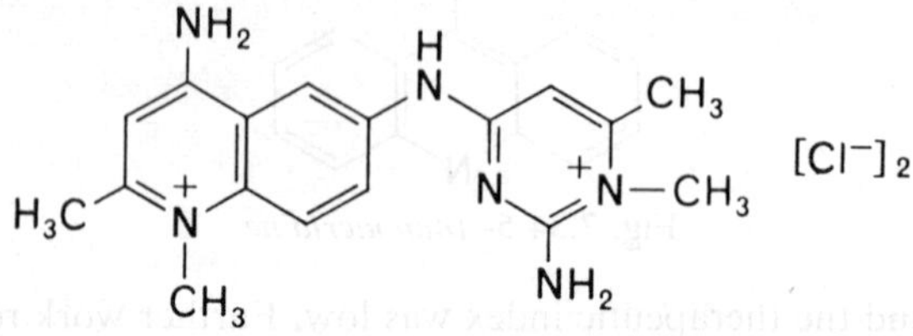

Fig. 7.36 *Antrycide Chloride*

chloride (Fig. 7.36) (Curd & Davey, 1949, 1950; Curd, 1950). Antrycide (quinapyramine, *B. vet. C.*) is used either in the form of the soluble dimethosulphate salt $(CH_3 . SO_4)_2$, or as a mixture of the dimethosulphate and the sparingly soluble chlorice to form 'Antrycide Prosalt' used as a prophylactic (*see* pp. 176–177). From its introduction into field use from about 1950 onwards, it was unique in being the first active prophylactic drug for cattle infections of *T. vivax* and *T. congolense.* Although its protective powers are not generally considered to extend beyond two months, and its use, like that of all other 'cattle' trypanocides except tartar emetic, has been dogged by acquirement of drug resistance, it is still a mainstay in field practice. Unlike its ancestor, Surfen C, Antrycide is

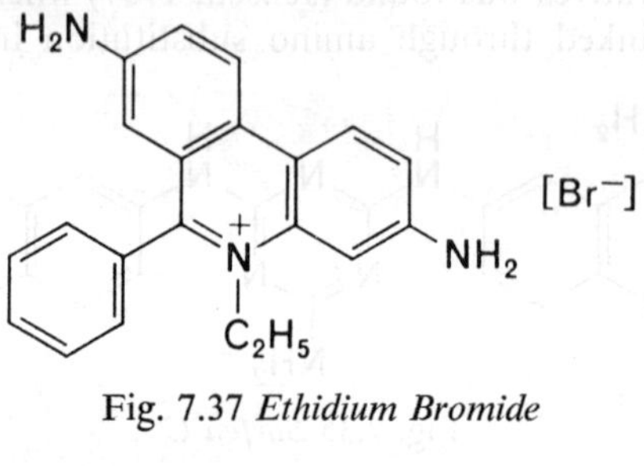

Fig. 7.37 *Ethidium Bromide*

active not only on the *congolense-vivax* group, but equally on the *evansi-equinum-equiperdum* group and to a lesser degree, on the *brucei* group trypanosomes.

The early years of its use in Africa coincided with the eclipse of Phenidium and Dimidium (Fig. 7.33), and the appearance of Ethidium (homidium) (Fig. 7.37) (Watkins & Woolfe, 1952), a much less toxic version of Dimidium. The impact of Antrycide and Ethidium on cattle treatment may be indicated by figures such as those of Larrat (1958) for the Upper Volta region of French West

Africa where the number of prophylactic Antrycide treatments rose from 6,206 in 1953 to 140,782 in 1957, and of Wilson (1958) for Northern Nigeria where the number of cattle treated with Antrycide and Ethidium rose from 45,000 in 1951–2 to 641,000 in 1957–8; subsequent decline to 25,000 in 1962–3 (MacGregor, 1965) was attributed to better discrimination and the overall reduction in infection by previous mass treatment, but in this area by 1963–4, treatments with Ethidium rose again to 320,000 (MacGregor, 1966); increasing and extensive incidence of Ethidium-resistant *T. congolense* infections (Jones-Davies & Folkers, 1966) appears to confirm the suggestion that this trypanosome is inherently less drug-sensitive than *T. vivax* (Williamson & Stephen, 1960) and has been selected out by mass drug treatment in areas where this has been applied. Such selection by Ethidium has also been demonstrated in East Africa (Mwambu, 1967) (*see* p. 179); an alternative explanation based on a differential immune response of the two species is discussed later (*see* pp. 217–220).

Rising treatment figures reflected the expansion of the cattle industry associated with increasing economic development, as in mainland Tanzania where, because of drug protection in the fly-belt fringes, the cattle population rose from about 6·5 million in 1946 to about 8 million in 1954 (Ford, 1965). Mass treatments have been inevitably followed by drug-resistance and Antrycide and the group of newer aminophenanthridinium drugs, Ethidium, Prothidium (Fig. 7.38) and Metamidium (Fig. 7.39), can all give rise to mutually cross-resistant strains in cattle (Whiteside, 1958). This cross-resistance (*see* pp. 211–217) was fostered by inclusion in the new drugs of moieties of other active drugs, e.g. Prothidium is essentially the early drug 897 (Phenidium) (Fig. 7.33, a) with the pyrimidyl moiety of Antrycide as a substituent, and Metamidium (or its active derivative, Samorin) is a form of Ethidium with a substituent consisting of the major portion of the *m*-amidino-substituent variant of Berenil (Fig. 7.40).

Berenil (diminazene aceturate) first introduced by Jensch in 1955, is proving in increasing measure to be the mainstay of control of drug-resistant cattle infections in both East and West Africa (Whiteside, 1962, a; *see* also Chapter 43). Because of drug-resistance, Antrycide and Ethidium were successively withdrawn from field use in Northern Nigeria in 1963 and 1965 respectively, and have been replaced by Berenil (MacLennan, 1968). It is active against strains resistant to other 'cattle' trypanocides, and its low toxicity provides a wide latitude in dosage variation; isolated reports of Berenil resistance have indicated resistance of a low order only, despite its widespread use over a long period, especially in East Africa. The drug is an aromatic diamidine like pentamidine, but does not seem to possess the latter's extensive prophylactic activity. It was devised as a result of Jensch's systematic dissection of the 4-aminoquinaldine Surfen C type of molecule and thus can be thought of as having its roots in both acriflavine and Synthalin.

The latest prophylactic drugs, Prothidium and Metamidium (1958–60) have not been as successful in the field as was originally hoped and the use of suramin complexes (1956) is now likely to be restricted to prophylaxis and treatment of *T. simiae* in pigs, and of *T. evansi* in equines. As in human sleeping sickness there is still an urgent need for new prophylactic drugs which will give longer protection, especially in areas of higher risk, without causing extensive cross-resistance, and for new curative drugs to increase the choice of those which do not cause resistance and which are active on resistant strains. Long-lasting prophylaxis is especially desirable, to promote land reclamation and agricultural settlement in conjunction with fly-eradication schemes, and to protect cattle during prolonged seasonal trekking through fly-belts in search of grazing. An alternative approach to prophylaxis is the possibility of drug-stimulated immunity (Soltys, 1955) but no clear-cut resolution of this complex problem is yet available (*see* pp. 217–220).

Suramin

Suramin (Fig. 7.17) has no pronounced activity on *T. vivax* or *T. congolense* infections of cattle, and only a therapeutic effect on *T. simiae* in pigs (Stephen, 1966a); its main use has been for *T. evansi* infections of camels, since its introduction for this purpose in 1925 until the later innovation of Antrycide (1946–50) (Knowles, 1925; Bennett, 1933; Evans, 1956; Larrat, 1958). Single intravenous doses of 5–10 g. suramin in aqueous solution were uniformly effective as a curative, but prophylactic activity was of short duration (1–4 months) and repeated use at small doses led to drug resistance. Fortunately, suramin-resistant *T. evansi* was susceptible to Antrycide treatment, although since its introduction, Antrycide-resistant strains have inevitably appeared (Rutter, 1967), for which Berenil appears to be unsuitable.

For equine trypanosomiasis (mainly *T. brucei* in tropical Africa, and *T. evansi* and *T. equiperdum* in North Africa) suramin has been used extensively for curative purposes, and has not been replaced by the newer cattle drugs which so far are either less effective or, like Antrycide, cause more severe toxic reactions in horses than in cattle; Mel B is apparently active and well tolerated in Indian ponies infected with *T. evansi* (Gill, 1964a). As Whiteside (1958) pointed out, the problem of equine trypanosomiasis in tropical Africa '. . . has declined in importance, for today horses and mules are rarely required to enter fly areas; their place has been taken by the motor vehicle'.

The principle of formation of a sparingly soluble suramin salt complex with pentamidine which has been described earlier (*see* pp. 139–142) has been extended to the 'cattle' trypanocides including Antrycide, Dimidium, Ethidium, Prothidium, Metamidium, Berenil, 'Cinnoline 528' and Tozocide (Williamson & Desowitz, 1956; Austin *et al.*, 1957; Wragg *et al.*, 1958). Maximal co-precipitation has a stoichiometric basis governed by the number of available ionized groups in the combining molecules (Williamson & Desowitz, 1956; Williamson, 1957); one molecule of suramin with six anionic groups combines maximally with six molecules of Dimidium or Ethidium, each with one cationic group, or with three molecules of Antrycide, Cinnoline 528, Berenil, Prothidium or Metamidium, each with two cationic groups.

Complex formation in this way considerably reduced the toxicity of the cationic drug component for rats by a factor varying from approximately 3× to 33× (Williamson, 1957). Similar reduction of toxicity, especially with Antrycide, was observed in the first prophylactic trial in cattle (Williamson & Desowitz, 1956; Desowitz, 1957).

The induction or enhancement of prophylactic activity in small animals by insoluble suramin complex formation, was considered to arise from 'depot' formation at the site of injection, and considerable prophylactic activity was in fact observed in African cattle exposed to regular and severe tsetse-borne *T. vivax* challenge. After a single dose, minimal periods of protection of 5½ months for Antrycide-suramin complex at 40 mg./kg.,[1] thirteen months for Ethidium-suramin complex at 10 mg./kg.[1] and nine months for Prothidium-suramin complex at 10 mg./kg.,[1] were obtained in small numbers of experimental cattle (Desowitz, 1957). High cost precluded further development of the Antrycide-suramin complex in cattle, but its marked prophylactic and therapeutic activity against the important *T. simiae* infection in pigs (Watson & Williamson, 1958; Stephen & Gray, 1960) continued to receive attention (Gray, 1961; Stephen & Gray, 1961; Stephen, 1962a) to the point where Stephen (1962a, 1963, 1966a) was able to recommend a schedule of treatment for pigs raised in tsetse areas. The schedule was based on extensive confirmation of the high therapeutic activity of Antrycide-suramin complex at a dose (40 mg./kg.) which will also protect adult pigs for at least six months (or growing pigs for at least three months) against severe fly challenge. Such drug treatment may also prove useful in view of reports that reservoir infections of *T. gambiense* may occur in pigs (Watson, 1963; Macario, 1963; Stephen, 1966a).

The Antrycide-suramin complex has also been shown to be highly active on *T. evansi* infections of rats (Gill, 1963) and to have marked prophylactic activity (Gill and Malhotra, 1963; Gill, 1964a). Subsequent trials on surra-infected ponies in India (*Vet. Bull.* (1966) 36, Abstr. 2437) showed that the Antrycide-suramin complex was well tolerated, curative at low dosage, and capable of inducing at least six to seven months protection (sufficient for the North Indian surra season which lasts three-and-a-half months); protection for thirteen months is now regularly obtainable (Gill, 1969, private communication).

The outstanding activity of the Ethidium-suramin complex shown in the preliminary field trial was subsequently bedevilled by the severe injection-site reaction which developed after subcutaneous injection (Stephen, 1958; Williamson & Stephen, 1961). Swelling, ulceration and sloughing, with consequent loss of drug depot, occurred in a high proportion of animals, and a variety of attempts to eliminate or decrease the reaction was unsuccessful. Trials in East Africa showed that lengthy protection could result in the few animals which did not lose their depot; in the remainder, the prophylaxis was, in general, equivalent to that of Prothidium.

Elsewhere, an intensive four-year trial of Ethidium-suramin complex, involving over 200 cattle in three former French territories (Republics of Chad and Cameroun, and the Central African Republic), was reported by SAUVEL, THOMÉ, MAGIMEL, BALIS AND FINELLE (1961). The unique prophylactic activity of this complex was confirmed in field conditions: six months' to a year's protection in forest gallery areas of high challenge and more than a year, even two years, in Western Sahara-type 'steppe' areas of moderate challenge. The injection-site reaction, despite ingenious and varied attempts to overcome it, was considered

[1] Quoted doses of suramin complexes refer to the amount of cationic drug present and not to the total amount of complex.

acceptable only under restricted conditions, and general use of the complex was therefore not recommended.

Both Prothidium and Metamidium, like all the active phenanthridinium and styrylquinolinium drugs, have dermonecrotic properties. To prevent or lessen this reaction, CAWDERY AND KNIGHT (1961) and Cawdery (1962) recommended incorporation of the drugs in a high viscosity oil base for injection with a modified grease gun, but extensive work was also directed, on the sparingly-soluble complex principle, to coupling the drugs with a wide variety of acidic substances other than suramin, in the hope of reducing local toxicity and extending prophylactic activity. BERG, BROWN AND LUCAS (1961) tried out over thirty pharmacologically suitable acids for combination with Metamidium; none was as effective as the suramin complex which had already been tested in Africa as M. & B. 4427 (Wragg, Washbourn, Brown & Hill, 1958; Gray & Stephen, 1962). The prophylactic activity of M. & B. 4427 at 10 mg./kg. varied from about three months in experimental West African trials (Stephen, 1960; Gray & Stephen, 1962) to about five months under natural conditions in East Africa (Smith & Brown, 1960) and Central Africa (Finelle, 1963). Attempts to control the injection-site reaction of M. & B. 4427 by altering its particle size (Smith & Brown, 1960), showed that the severity could be lessened by increasing the particle size to approximately 10 to 100 μ; a suspension of particles less than 3 μ was more toxic though more active prophylactically, in accordance with earlier work on the particle size of the Ethidium-suramin complex (Williamson, 1957; Stephen & Williamson, 1958).

Using Prothidium, Groves and Wilmshurst (1964) prepared insoluble complexes with a large number of acidic polysaccharides, ranging from heparin to seaweed products such as laminarin sulphate (which was sufficiently promising to warrant evaluation in East African cattle). The necrotic lesions normally following the standard injection of 2 mg./kg. of Prothidium into the dewlap were much reduced by combination with laminarin sulphate, but there was no extension of prophylaxis. The Prothidium-suramin complex, although much less toxic, generally and locally, than an equivalent amount of Prothidium alone, still produced unacceptable injection-site reactions, although extended protection was observed in animals which had not lost their drug depot (Stephen, 1962b).

Antrycide (Quinapyramine *B. vet. C.*)

Antrycide (quinapyramine *B. vet. C.*) is normally used either as the water-soluble dimethosulphate salt $(CH_3 . SO_4)_2$ (quinapyramine sulphate *B. vet. C.*) (4-amino-6-(2-amino-6-methylpyrimid-4-ylamino)-2-methylquinoline-1,1′ dimetho(methyl sulphate); $C_{19}H_{28}N_6O_8S_2$, mol. wt. 532·6) or as a mixture (Antrycide Pro-salt; quinapyramine (prophylactic) *B. vet. C.*) of the dimethylsulphate salt and the sparingly-soluble chloride (quinapyramine chloride *B. vet. C.*) (Fig. 7.36) (4-amino-6-(2-amino-6-methylpyrimid-4-ylamino)-2-methylquinoline-1,1′-dimethochloride dihydrate; $C_{17}H_{22}Cl_2N_6,2H_2O$, mol. wt. 417·3). The chloride is a white, cream or very pale yellow crystalline powder, odourless and with a bitter taste; the anhydrous salt is yellow. Water solubility is 1:850 at 20°C and about 1:50 at 100°C; solubility in organic solvents is almost nil. The sulphate resembles the chloride in appearance and is soluble 1:2 in water at 20°C; it is almost insoluble in organic solvents. Antrycide is the only member of the 4-aminoquinoline-type group to have come into general field use in Africa; the other members, Surfen C (Fig. 7.35), Cinnoline '528' (Lourie, Morley, Simpson & Walker, 1951) and Tozocide (Austin, Collier, Potter, Smith & Taylor, 1957) did not survive African field trial, but interest in the potentialities of the group has continued (Williamson, 1962; Barber & Berg, 1962).

The chloride form of Antrycide, like all the other halide salts prepared, is relatively insoluble in water, and after subcutaneous injection, is retained in the tissues as a 'depot' from which enough of the soluble form reaches the circulation to maintain a continuous, low but protective trypanocidal blood level. As Curd and Davey (1950) showed, surgical excision of this depot from treated rabbits abolishes the prophylactic effect. In field practice, after Prosalt treatment, the depot becomes encapsulated with fibrous and eventually calcified tissue; the blood supply is thus cut off, and prophylaxis is limited to about two months. Sufficient active drug is still present in the depot as demonstrated by experiments in cattle in which a fibrosed capsule has been excised, and its contents, after crushing and re-injection into another animal, have been shown to be capable of conferring protection for another extended period. Attempts to exploit this by crushing the encapsulated depot *in situ* have been unsuccessful (Whiteside, Fairclough & Bax, 1960).

Antrycide Dimethylsulphate

Following Davey's original field trials in the Sudan and East Africa (Davey, 1950), extensive field trials and increasing usage in all parts of Africa confirmed the efficacy of Antrycide dimethylsulphate as a curative drug, at the recommended field dose of 5 mg./kg.[1] (Davey, 1957). *T. evansi* infections in camels, even when suramin-resistant, have been successfully treated with Antrycide (Evans, 1956; Davey, 1957; Leach, 1961; Rutter, 1967). *T. evansi* and *T. equiperdum* infections in horses have also responded well (Davey, 1957), although equines in general appear more susceptible to Antrycide toxicity (Whiteside, 1958a) (*see* p. 172). In *T. simiae* infections of pigs, cures have been recorded at doses of 3–5 mg./kg. (Wilson, 1949) but these were blood-induced infections, possibly more susceptible to drug action; subsequent experience with tsetse-infected pigs (Unsworth, 1952; Watson & Williamson, 1958) showed that although high doses (up to 50 mg./kg.) of Antrycide chloride could be curative, the dimethylsulphate was not (*see* pp. 176–177).

One of the most promising applications of Antrycide dimethylsulphate treatment was the work of Smith (1958) and of Whiteside and his colleagues (Whiteside, 1958b; Whiteside, Fairclough & Bax, 1960) on the extensive residual immunity which was claimed by Soltys (1955) to develop in cattle after Antrycide Prosalt prophylaxis; residual immunity of this type (first noted by Ehrlich and Shiga, 1904), had in fact been observed in the field many years later with tartar emetic (Bevan, 1928). Whiteside *et al.* (1960) showed that with Antrycide Prosalt, this phenomenon might not be so much an acquired immunity as a residual

[1] Now 4·4 mg./kg. subcutaneously.

prophylaxis due to depots of the drug. To overcome this objection, they used curative regimes (Antrycide dimethylsulphate and Ethidium) and showed that even in an area of high trypanosome challenge, temporary immunity of five to twelve months duration followed a curative regime lasting seven months; a prophylactic effect of Antrycide dimethylsulphate treatment had also been noted in the Congo by Deom (1960). In some cases the immunity observed was apparent after as few as two Antrycide treatments and one Ethidium treatment. Antibodies were not demonstrable, and there was some evidence that the nature of the drug used affects the results, but an important point was that the infections which ultimately appeared were not resistant to the drugs previously used. Little further work on this important aspect of drug treatment has ensued, with the exception of a significant short report by Cunningham (1967), who controlled the two vital variables of drug retention and antigenic variation in a small number of infected and Berenil-treated cattle challenged at intervals with a homologous infection; 'drug-vaccinated' animals resisted challenge and showed neutralizing antibodies for periods up to eight months after treatment. This kind of approach requires much further expansion, in terms of analysis of curative drug protection against natural fly challenge; the reversion of large numbers of antigenic variants to a much smaller number of basic types after fly transmission suggests that immunological control combined with chemotherapy, may be more feasible than was once imagined (*see* Chapter 6). The complex interaction of drugs and the immune response is considered further below (pp. 217–220).

Antrycide Prosalt (Quinapyramine (Prophylactic) *B. vet. C.*)

On the basis of Davey's first field trial experience (Davey, 1950), it became clear that neither the dimethylsulphate nor the insoluble chloride alone would be useful for prophylaxis. The former was excreted too rapidly and the latter, although persistent, did not give blood levels high enough to cure an established infection quickly; these low blood levels appeared to be independent of dose size and were likely to encourage formation of resistant trypanosomes. A mixture of the dimethylsulphate (three parts) and the chloride (four parts) was therefore issued commercially by Imperial Chemical (Pharmaceuticals) Ltd., under the name Antrycide Prosalt; a standard dose of 11·7 mg./kg. contained 5 mg./kg. of the dimethylsulphate. Later, in 1958, a cheaper revised formulation (RF) was issued for trial, in which the chloride content had been reduced by one-half, the standard dose becoming 7·4 mg./kg. Preliminary results (Marshall, 1958; Whiteside *et al.*, 1960; Deom, 1960) indicated that the new form was at least equivalent to the old form; in Kenya, three-monthly treatment with either form was effective in areas of low fly challenge, two-monthly treatment was needed in areas of medium challenge but in high-challenge areas, this regime sometimes failed to give continued protection. In the Congo, Deom (1960) stressed that the new form seemed as active as the old and had the added advantages of less persistent local reactions and of lower cost.

Antrycide Prosalt is curative for, and has some prophylactic activity in, *T. simiae* infections of pigs (Wilson, 1949; Watson & Williamson, 1958), but better results are obtained either with high doses of Antrycide chloride alone

(50 mg./kg.) or with Antrycide-suramin complex at 40 mg./kg. (Watson & Williamson, 1958; Stephen & Gray, 1960) (*see* p. 174). Surra infections of cattle in Ceylon and the Philippines appear to be efficiently controlled by both Antrycide and its Prosalt, the latter providing up to twelve months' protection (Castillo, 1962; Lodha & Singh, 1963; Fernandez, Rico & Dumag, 1965). Prosalt has also been found effective for treatment and prophylaxis of dourine in Algeria (Favier, 1963).

Distribution and Toxicity

Antrycide dimethylsulphate, though freely water-soluble, is poorly absorbed from the alimentary canal, presumably as the result of formation of the sparingly-soluble chloride. After subcutaneous or intramuscular injection, absorption depends on the absolute amount injected; small quantities are rapidly absorbed and large quantities form a depot of the sparingly soluble chloride. Toxicity can be increased by reduction of the injected dose volume, as noted in mice by Lourie and Walker (1951). Using a sensitive method of fluorescence analysis Spinks (1950) showed that in mice, rabbits and in a calf, Antrycide was selectively localized in liver and kidney tissue and maintained there for some weeks after injection; within twenty-four hours of dimethylsulphate injection, plasma levels fell from a maximum of 4 μg./ml. to less than 0·01 μg./ml. The therapeutic blood concentration in cattle is believed to be not more than 0·03–0·3 μg./ml. and the suppressive concentration is probably below 0·001 μg./ml. (Hawking, 1963). High doses of Antrycide rapidly produce high levels of deposition in the kidney and later in the liver; severe kidney damage has been a characteristic feature of animals examined *post mortem* after Antrycide poisoning (Davey, 1957).

Antrycide chloride, because of its low solubility, is virtually non-toxic. The egg-like unabsorbed deposits which remain after repeated Prosalt treatment are unsightly and for that reason, injections are usually made into the extensive dewlap of African Zebu cattle to avoid damage to meat or hide; the deposits do not however produce any symptoms of general or chronic toxicity and are not diminished by hyaluronidase incorporation (Finelle, 1963).

Antrycide, as a *bis*-onium compound, has curare-like properties (Ormerod & Paton, 1950; Garner, 1950) both in small animals and in cattle and horses. Toxic symptoms such as excessive salivation, sweating, uncontrolled tremors and occasional temporary collapse, occur in a proportion of cattle treated with the recommended dimethylsulphate dose of 5 mg./kg. (Unsworth & Chandler, 1952; Davey, 1957), and these may be increased to the point of fatality if animals are treated while under stress from heat, fatigue, malnutrition, intercurrent infection or any of the numerous complicating factors which occur so commonly in African field conditions (Lawrence & Bryson, 1958).

Ethidium (Homidium Bromide *B. vet. C.*)

Ethidium bromide (homidium bromide *B. vet. C.*) (Fig. 7.37) (2,7-diamino-9-phenyl-10-ethylphenanthridinium bromide anhydrate) $C_{21}H_{20}BrN_3$, mol. wt. = 394·3; as monohydrate, mol. wt. = 412·3) is a dark purple, almost odourless, crystalline or amorphous powder with a persistent bitter taste. At 20° and

100°C the water-solubility is approximately 3·5% and 10% respectively; a 5–6% solution is stable for several days at 20°C. Solubility in chloroform is about 0·13%.

The production of Phenidium and Dimidium (Fig. 7.33, a, b) had demonstrated the association of high trypanocidal activity with phenylphenanthridinium salts containing two primary amino groups, preferably in the 2- and 7-positions; 3-amino-substituted compounds are less active. This was confirmed by later synthesis and biological tests of a comprehensive series of related derivatives (Brownlee, Goss, Goodwin, Woodbine & Walls, 1950; Walls & Whittaker, 1950a, 1950b), which also showed that trypanocidal activity was greatly reduced by modification of the primary amino groups, for example by acetylation or replacement with amidine groups; replacement with nitro groups did not reduce activity so markedly and 7-alkoxy derivatives were especially active against *T. congolense*. Trials of several of the most promising derivatives were carried out in West and Central Africa and the Sudan in 1952–3, but without success. The first improved substitute for Dimidium was Ethidium bromide, which differed from Dimidium only in possessing an ethyl instead of a methyl group on the quaternary nitrogen heteroatom (Watkins & Woolfe, 1952; Watkins, 1952; Woolfe, 1952). As Davey (1957) remarked: 'The difference in biological properties is therefore remarkable; it is equally remarkable that fourteen years went by before the attributes of the ethyl quaternization group were discovered.'

In experiments on mice (Watkins & Woolfe, 1952; Woolfe, 1952) with a homologous series of quaternary N-alkyl derivatives of Dimidium, the therapeutic activity varied enormously. The ethyl homologue was ten times and fifty times more active against *T. congolense* and *T. gambiense*, respectively, than the parent Dimidium, and the propyl homologue was thirty-five times more active against *T. brucei*, but this access of activity fell off sharply with higher homologues. The effect on toxicity was small by comparison and subsequent field trials in cattle confirmed that Ethidium was not only somewhat more active than Dimidium against *T. congolense* but also much less toxic; extensive use of Ethidium in the field has not produced the liver lesions and photosensitization which accompanied large-scale Dimidium treatment.

Similar enhancement of activity by changing the quaternary alkyl group was demonstrated experimentally in a number of other phenanthridinium derivatives, including Phenidium (Woolfe, 1956a, 1956b), but none of the compounds was sufficiently active to displace Ethidium. Ethidium bromide is readily soluble only in hot or boiling water, but this practical disadvantage was overcome by the use of the chloride (Novidium) (Wragg, 1955) which is soluble in cold water.

On the basis of trials in the Sudan, Kenya, Tanganyika and Nigeria against a variety of strains of *T. congolense* and *T. vivax* (Forde, Wilmshurst & Karib, 1953a, 1953b; Wilson & Fairclough, 1953; Wilde & Robson, 1953; Unsworth, 1954a, 1954b) a therapeutic dose of 1·0 mg./kg. was recommended. Intramuscular injection was advised by the manufacturers in order to reduce the local reaction which can occur at this dose given subcutaneously, because Ethidium, like most active quaternary ammonium-type trypanocides with the possible exception of Antrycide, has dermonecrotic properties; it is inactive after oral administration to rats (Bailey, 1967a).

Ethidium has been used primarily as a curative drug in cattle. A large-scale investigation of block-treatment (1 mg./kg.) of 11,200 head of cattle in 200 herds in Uganda (Mwambu, 1967) showed that these cattle, which were no longer responding to Antrycide curative treatment, improved in the two to three months after Ethidium treatment; the previous infection rate of up to 33% was much reduced or eliminated, feeding and milk yield were improved, and no clinical cases or deaths from trypanosomiasis occurred. A selective effect on *T. vivax* was noted, as this infection was predominant in the cattle before Ethidium treatment, but relapses were mainly to *T. congolense* (*see* pp. 170–171) Ethidium is not curative for *T. simiae* in pigs (Watson & Williamson, 1958) but at 1·0 mg./kg. in the horse it was well tolerated and curative for a fly-transmitted *T. vivax* infection (Stephen & Mackenzie, 1958). Extensive use in cattle rapidly led to the appearance of Ethidium-resistant strains (*see* pp. 170–172), especially of *T. congolense* in West and East Africa; this important aspect is discussed further below (*see* pp. 215–217). The toxicity and pharmacology of the active amino-phenanthridinium group of drugs are described below (*see* pp. 182–185).

Prothidium (Pyrithidium Bromide *B. vet. C.*)

Prothidium (pyrithidium bromide *B. vet. C.*) (Fig. 7.38) (2-amino-7-(2-amino-6-methylpyrimid - 4 - ylamino) - 9 - *p* - aminophenylphenanthridine - 10,1′ - dimethobromide) ($C_{26}H_{27}Br_2N_7$, mol. wt. 597·4) is a brick-red to reddish purple,

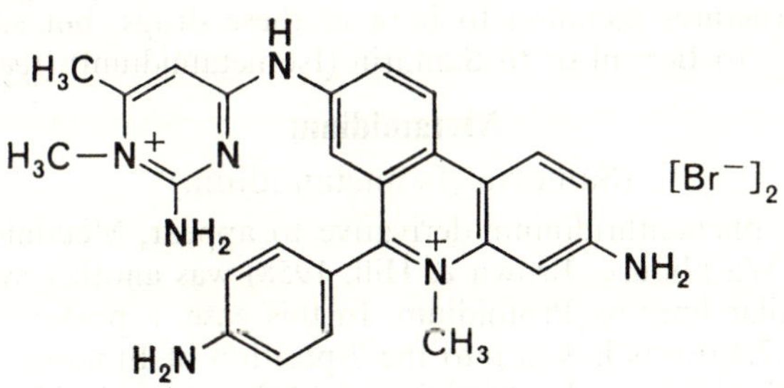

Fig. 7.38 *Prothidium*

odourless or almost odourless, hygroscopic powder, soluble 1/200 in water at 20°C. Prothidium solutions show a high degree of supersaturation, but a 2% solution prepared by dissolving in boiling water and cooling has a *p*H of 3 to 6, and is stable for about a week.

Having produced one successful new phenanthridinium derivative by the simple and original expedient of changing the alkyl quaternary group, Watkins and Woolfe (1956) then proceeded to effect an equally novel synthesis by substituting the pyrimidyl moiety of Antrycide (Fig. 7.36) into the 7-amino group of 2,7-diamino-9-*p*-aminophenyl-10-methylphenanthridinium chloride, a compound resembling Phenidium (Fig. 7.33, a), and one of four active compounds tested by Goodwin and Unsworth (1952). The resulting compound, Prothidium (Watkins, 1958) had remarkable curative and prophylactic activity.

Although most emphasis has been placed on its prophylactic activity, Prothidium is also an active curative drug; doses of 0·2–0·4 mg./kg. were curative for *T. congolense* (Whiteside *et al.*, 1960).

The general acceptance of Prothidium into field use was held up by the discovery in 1959 that glucose, used as excipient in the commercial production of tablets, was combining with, and partly inactivating, the drug component (Robson, 1961), but this interruption in use was only temporary. A useful summary of experience of Prothidium in field trials in different parts of Africa up to 1962 is given by Stephen (1962b) who ran a well-controlled trial in West Africa on both Prothidium and is suramin complex (*see* pp. 172–174). He confirmed previous experience that subcutaneous doses of Prothidium higher than 2·5 mg./kg. caused unacceptable injection site reactions and weight loss, and that even the 2·5 mg./kg. dose produced unsightly swellings. To avoid this, incorporation of Prothidium in high viscosity lanoline/olive oil mixtures was recommended by CAWDERY AND KNIGHT (1961), and Cawdery (1963) in an extensive study, has shown that subcutaneous dosage of up to 6 mg./kg. Prothidium into the dewlap may be acceptable in this vehicle.

Finelle and Lacotte (1965) found that Prothidium (2 mg./kg. intramuscularly) was a useful prophylactic for donkeys, giving eight to nine months' protection in an area of high *T. congolense* challenge where untreated animals became infected in 1½ to 4 months; in the same area, untreated cattle became infected in less than a month, but were protected by Prothidium for 4 to 6 months.

Prothidium-resistance has generally been found to develop rapidly, with cross-resistance to both Ethidium and Antrycide, as might be expected from possession of chemical structures common to both of these drugs, but such strains are usually sensitive to Berenil or to Samorin (Isometamidium) (*see* pp. 215–217).

Metamidium

(Samorin (Isometamidium))

The next active phenanthridinium derivative to appear, Metamidium (M. & B. 4404) (Wragg, Washbourn, Brown & Hill, 1958) was another synthetic hybrid devised on similar lines to Prothidium. In this case, a portion of the Berenil molecule (Fig. 7.40) was linked into the 7-position of Ethidium (Fig. 7.37) by coupling diazotized *p*-aminobenzamidine and Ethidium chloride in the presence of sodium acetate. Two isomeric *p*-amidinophenyldiazoamino derivatives were produced which had considerable trypanocidal activity, and further syntheses showed that the *m*-amidino-substituted product, also obtained as a mixture of two isomers, was the most promising of the series. This mixture was highly active, therapeutically and prophylactically, in experimental *T. congolense* infections and was named Metamidium.

The two isomers were provisionally considered as (a) 2-(*m*-amidinophenyldiazoamino-)-7-amino-10-ethyl-9-phenylphenanthridinium chloride hydrochloride and (b) 7-(*m*-amidinophenyldiazoamino)-2-amino-10-ethyl-9-phenylphenanthridinium chloride hydrochloride (Fig. 7.39).

The isomer (a) with the '*m*-Berenil' substituent in the 2-position is purple, relatively water-insoluble and less active than the much more soluble red isomer (b), the structure of which was later confirmed by Berg (1960; 1963) who announced that it had been isolated in pure form in sufficient quantities for field trial under the name of Isometamidium (M. & B. 4180A), now known as Samorin (Fig. 7.39) ($C_{28}H_{25}ClN_7 \cdot HCl$, mol. wt. = 531·5).

The original Metamidium preparation contained the purple and red isomers in the proportions of 55% and 45% respectively, and was much less toxic than Ethidium in mice and also more active against *T. congolense*. A dose of 1/9 of the LD50 of Metamidium protected mice from infection for up to sixteen weeks, but neither Ethidium nor Berenil at doses of 1/3 of the LD50 showed any appreciable prophylactic activity under comparable test conditions.

In African cattle (Fairclough, 1958), high subcutaneous doses (5 and 10 mg./kg.) produced toxic symptoms locally and in the liver, similar to those caused by Dimidium, but a dose of 1 mg./kg. appeared completely non-toxic. Intramuscular injections were better tolerated (Smith & Brown, 1960; Stephen,

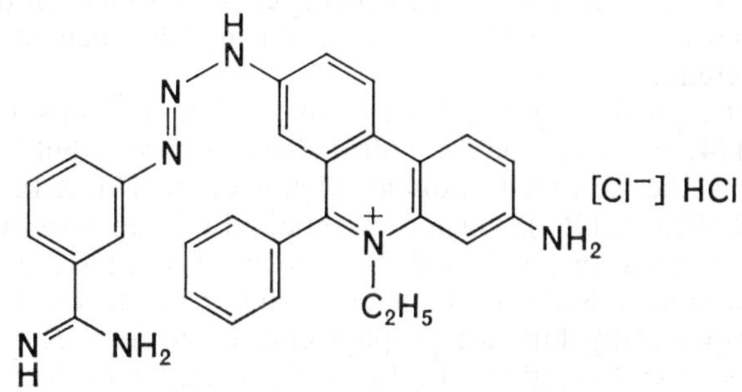

Fig. 7.39 *Samorin*

1960), but local reactions were observed even at 0·5 mg./kg. in some cases (Kirkby, 1960a).

Cures of *T. vivax* and *T. congolense* infections in both East and West Africa were achieved with doses down to 0·2 mg./kg. (Marshall, 1958), but the prophylaxis obtainable did not appear to be as great as was anticipated. In Kenya, in an area of low challenge, a dose of 3 mg./kg. gave protection similar to that given by Antrycide Prosalt (Whiteside *et al.*, 1960), and similar results were obtained at the same dose in Northern Nigeria (Kirkby, 1961b); in a West African trial with controlled infection, the same dose gave nineteen weeks protection (Gray & Stephen, 1962). In an area of high tsetse density, Metamidium at 4 mg./kg. gave significantly longer protection (average eighteen weeks) than Prosalt (average ten weeks) (Smith & Brown, 1960), and at a higher dose (5 mg./kg.), Stephen (1960) obtained protection against West African *T. vivax* infection for periods of over twenty-nine weeks. Like Ethidium, Metamidium was therapeutic but not curative for *T. simiae* in pigs (Stephen & Gray, 1961).

By 1961 the manufacturers were able to recommend use of the new Isometamidium (Samorin) as 0·5 mg./kg. (curative dose, normal strains), 1–2 mg./kg. (curative dose, drug-fast strains) and 2 mg./kg. as a prophylactic (all doses by deep intramuscular injection). Marked advantages of Metamidium had appeared to be its activity against strains resistant to Antrycide, Ethidium, Prothidium and Berenil, and the retention of Berenil-sensitivity by an experimentally-produced Metamidium-resistant strain which was cross-resistant to Antrycide, Ethidium and Prothidium (Whiteside, 1960).

Combination prophylaxis with small doses of Samorin, Prothidium and

Antrycide, taken in pairs, has been explored in cattle in East Africa (Robson, 1962); all three combinations (of doses about $\frac{1}{4}$ of the normal prophylactic) suggested potentiative synergism (*see* p. 215). Despite the danger of drug-resistance developing, further investigation of this kind of treatment would be desirable, perhaps the TWSb (Stibocaptate) (*see* pp. 154–155) or its sodium salt (Astiban), as a less toxic substitute for tartar emetic or Antimosan (*cf.* Williamson, 1960 (*see* also p. 218). Early hopes of the activity of Metamidium on Ethidium-resistant strains appear to have been over-optimistic, as Samorin at doses up to 0·8 mg./kg. has been shown to be only partially active in Northern Nigeria against *T. congolense* infections resistant to Novidium (Ethidium chloride), and to intensify rapidly the existing cross-resistance of these strains to Samorin (Jones-Davies & Folkers, 1967); fortunately such strains are fully sensitive to Berenil.

The difficulties of finding a suitable form of Metamidium-suramin complex (*see* pp. 172–174) have presumably applied also to Samorin, but trials have been carried out on the so-called 'double Metamidium' (M. & B. 4596), (Berg, Brown, Hill & Wragg, 1961), which is essentially Ethidium with two moieties of '*m*-Berenil' substituted in the 2- and 7-amino positions, instead of one in the 7-amino position as in Samorin. Experimentally, it was less active than Metamidium, therapeutically but not prophylactically, against *T. congolense* and apparently less toxic. In cattle trials, doses of 2·5 mg./kg. in the dewlap seem to have been well tolerated and prophylaxis of ten months against *T. congolense* in East Africa has been reported (Finelle, 1963, 1965); intramuscular doses of 2·5 mg./kg. and higher are less well tolerated, but have given prophylaxis up to five months in conditions of severe challenge. Subsequent experience has shown that it has no advantage over Samorin and no further development has taken place.

Toxicity and Pharmacology of Phenanthridinium Drugs

The use of Dimidium in African cattle caused a high incidence of delayed toxicity. About six weeks after treatment, symptoms resembling photosensitization frequently appeared, characterized by acute dermatitis, lachrymation, nasal discharge, emaciation and jaundice, and accompanied by damage to the liver parenchyma. The drug caused periportal fatty infiltration in the liver (Thorold & Plowright, 1952; Plowright, Burdin & Thorold, 1952; Burdin & Plowright, 1952a, 1952b; Plowright & Burdin, 1952) which appeared to be of central importance, but external factors such as climate, nutritional status, and incidence of photodynamic substances in the diet were also considered significant. In herbivora with liver damage, photosensitization can arise from the presence of phylloerythrin derived from chlorophyll, and this reaction may have been coupled with the Dimidium liver lesion. Burdin and Plowright (1952a, 1952b) suggested that the methyl-substituted quaternary nitrogen possibly interfered with transmethylation reactions in the liver; this theory was supported by the absence of liver toxicity in the ethyl-substituted analogue, Ethidium, but was contraverted, as Goodwin and Chandler (1952) pointed out, by the similar absence of liver lesions even after very high doses of the comparable methyl-substituted analogue, Phenidium (Burdin & Plowright, 1952b).

The compounds which have succeeded Dimidium (Ethidium, Prothidium and Metamidium), are also capable of producing liver damage, but unlike Dimidium, do so only at doses considerably higher than the therapeutic level (Ford, Wilmshurst & Karib, 1954; Wilson, 1954; Unsworth, 1954a; Robson, 1958; Fairclough, 1958), and delayed toxicity and photosensitization symptoms have not followed their use in the field. As with all 'cattle' trypanocides, toxic reactions are more severe in trekked or worked cattle in poor condition than in rested animals in good condition. Local tissue damage at the injection site can be severe with high doses of all active phenanthridinium drugs so far prepared, especially if given subcutaneously, and an investigation of the structural factors responsible for this histotoxic effect in the phenanthridinium and related series would be of considerable interest and importance.

Fluorescence in ultraviolet light is typical of active phenanthridinium drugs, and this property has been used to demonstrate the distribution of drug in the organs and tissues of anaesthetized experimental animals laparotomized, injected intravenously and then observed under ultraviolet light. Goodwin, Goss and Lock (1950) used this method in rats, rabbits and cats to show the rapid appearance in the bile, liver and kidney cortex of a phenanthridinium derivative active against *T. cruzi*. The predominance of biliary excretion was established by analysis, and similar techniques applied by Taylor (1960b) with Prothidium in rats, rabbits and cattle have shown that the bile is a major excretory route for this drug also. Both drugs were concentrated in the liver and kidneys and urinary excretion was negligible. The immediate distribution of Ethidium after intravenous injection in the rabbit appears to differ from that of Prothidium (Williamson & Stephen; *see* Nash, 1958), in that although the kidney cortex fluoresces with both drugs, the thyroid, lung and gall bladder rapidly become intensely fluorescent with the former drug only. In mice, 51 % of an intraperitoneal dose of Ethidium is excreted in the urine in twenty-four hours, with initially high accumulation in the liver and kidneys; some later accumulation occurs in skeletal and heart muscle (Kandaswamy & Henderson, 1963a).

The importance of tissue binding for the prophylactic activity of soluble trypanocides was first adumbrated by Ehrlich and Shiga's experiments with Trypan Red (*see* pp. 130–131) and later by Browning and Gulbransen in 1934 with their prophylactic styrylquinolines (*see* pp. 167–168). Deposits at the site of injection of relatively insoluble drugs are obviously of prime importance for prophylaxis, but with the discovery of Prothidium, the first soluble prophylactic active in the field, laboratory analysis (Taylor, 1960b) suggested that tissue binding of soluble trypanocides at the subcutaneous or intramuscular injection site might also be significant for prophylaxis; the prophylactic activity of Prothidium after subcutaneous injection did not appear to depend on retention by plasma protein, as with suramin, but to the formation of a local tissue deposit at the injection site, reinforced by strong binding of the drug in liver tissue. Examination of the late soluble prophylactic drugs, Metamidium and the related M. & B. 4596 (Bénazet, 1962), showed that these, like Prothidium and pentamidine, appeared in the blood of rats only in small amounts and for a short time after subcutaneous injection, but were detectable for up to eight months in liver tissue; organ-binding was concluded to be probably more important for prophylaxis than deposition at the injection site. The role of the tissue injection site was further explored by Hill and McFadzean (1963) using Samorin in mice and rats. A dose of Samorin which protected mice against infection for four or five weeks if given subcutaneously, gave only one week's protection after intravenous injection; drug fluorescence in the liver and kidneys disappeared after a week, but was detectable at the subcutaneous injection site for up to ten weeks. A protection period of sixteen weeks in rats, given by Samorin injected subcutaneously into the tail, could be reduced to one week if the tails were amputated twenty-four hours after treatment; drug fluorescence in intact tails persisted for at least thirty weeks. It was concluded that the tissue deposit of Samorin at the injection site was of prime significance for prophylaxis and that storage in the liver and kidney was of only secondary importance. In the same experiments, a methanesulphonate salt of M. & B. 4596 was found almost equally active prophylactically by the intravenous or subcutaneous routes; in this case, organ-binding was considered to be as effective as localization at the injection site, and the high tissue affinity was thought to be responsible for the relatively poor therapeutic activity shown after subcutaneous injection. Recent demonstration of anticancer activity in Ethidium (Kandaswamy & Henderson, 1962), Metamidium and Samorin has led to more intensive study of their tissue distribution (Philips, Sternberg, Cronin, Sodergren & Vidal, 1967) (*see* pp. 195–198); extensive and prolonged accumulation of Samorin occurred in the liver and kidneys of rats, dogs and monkeys.

The phenanthridinium trypanocides are in general poorly absorbed when given orally. The non-prophylactic curative drugs, Dimidium, Phenidium and Ethidium are excreted fairly rapidly, but as Ethidium has been shown to have a short-lived prophylactic effect in cattle, some tissue-binding no doubt occurs. Only low and transitory blood levels appear to be produced by the phenanthridinium drugs, whether prophylactic or curative (Hill & McFadzean, 1963; Hawking, 1963, 1966) but it is likely that the assay methods so far reported (chemical, radiochemical or biological) are insufficiently sensitive; new methods of isolating blood-free *T. congolense* suspensions (Williamson & Cover, 1966; Lanham, 1968) should facilitate more sensitive biological assay by infectivity titration.

The pharmacological activity of phenanthridinium drugs has not been extensively documented. Dimidium depressed both circulatory and respiratory rates, while Ethidium appears to have little effect on the cardiovascular system or on smooth muscle, although it can depress the respiratory centre to the point of fatality; high doses of Dimidium, Prothidium and Metamidium also appear to be capable of causing muscular incoordination in cattle (Hawking, 1963; Finelle & Yvore, 1963; Stephen, 1962b). Samorin causes reversible blockade of neuromuscular transmission and stimulation of cholinergic receptors (Philips *et al.*, 1967).

Chronic toxicity, manifest as progressive weight loss, can result from deep intramuscular injection of Prothidium or Ethidium preparations at doses which apparently cause only minor swellings. In the case of apparently well-tolerated doses of Ethidium-suramin complex, weight loss led to a number of deaths, but at post-mortem there were no obvious signs of organ damage to account for fatality other than the large sterile abscesses of fluid and drug at the injection site in the muscle (Stephen & Williamson, 1958). An intensive study of the local reactions of prophylactic phenanthridinium drugs (Cawdery, 1962) given by subcutaneous or intramuscular injection, illustrates in detail the tissue-irritant effects of Prothidium and Samorin which tend to be concealed by intramuscular injection; persistent fibrosed, necrotic, fluid-filled abscesses can cause extensive meat spoilage, as well as pain and restriction of movement in treated cattle, even at 1 mg./kg. doses of Samorin. Intramuscular injection of Prothidium and Samorin should be avoided for this reason, especially if repeated injections were contemplated, in favour of subcutaneous injection in the dewlap, where the reaction is externally visible and is normally resolved without symptoms of general toxicity. Local irritant action can be reduced by incorporation in a high viscosity oil-grease base, but the crucial requirement for retention of the drug depot seemed to be that no drug should be left in the track of the withdrawn needle, otherwise the drug reaction is sufficient to create a weak area where leaks and rupture subsequently develop; doses of Prothidium as high as 6 mg./kg. in a viscous base, gave acceptable reactions so long as the depot remained intact. This important detail is obviously applicable also to the irritant suramin complexes, the prophylactic activity of which is dependent on an intact drug depot. The problem is aggravated by the necessity to use large-bore needles with drug preparations of high viscosity but the development of a 'self-sealing' drug depot should not be technically insuperable.

Berenil (Diminazene Aceturate *B. vet. C.*)

The only new aromatic diamidine which has come into accepted field use since pentamidine is Berenil (Fig. 7.40) (diminazene aceturate *B. vet. C.*) (*p,p'*-diamidinodiazoaminobenzene diaceturate tetrahydrate; *N*-1,3-diamidinophenyltriazene diaceturate tetrahydrate; $C_{22}H_{29}N_9O_6 . 4H_2O$; mol. wt. = 587·6; mol. wt. base = 281·2). It is a yellow odourless powder, soluble 1/14 at

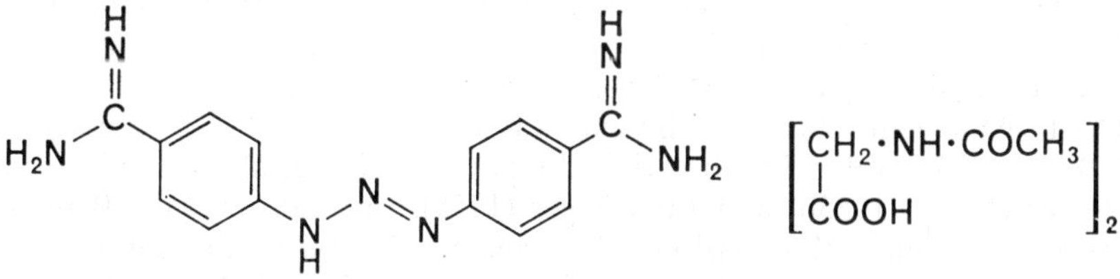

Fig. 7.40 *Berenil*

20°C in water, slightly soluble in alcohol and sparingly soluble in ether and in chloroform.

Though stable when dry, an aqueous solution in contact with air is stable only for two or three days; according to Fairclough (1963), antipyrine in amounts almost equivalent to that of the drug (Fairclough, 1963a), has been added by the manufacturers since 1959, as a stabilizer, and solutions are now stable for ten to fifteen days at room temperature. A more stable hydrazone form has been described (Jensch, Loewe & Bauer, 1958), in which the triazene 'bridge' is replaced by the isosteric hydrazone, —CH=N—NH—, but has apparently not so far replaced Berenil in the field. A sparingly soluble embonate salt has been described (Bauer, 1964) which was prophylactic but regularly gave rise to drug resistance: it is apparently effective as a prophylactic for *Babesia canis* in dogs (Bauer, 1966).

The chemical origins of Berenil are described in considerable detail by Jensch (1958) who shows how development proceeded by systematic dissection of the Surfen C 'bis-4-amino-chinaldin-Typ' molecule (Fig. 7.35) into chemically and therapeutically equivalent portions. The first '4-amino-chinaldin-Mischtyp' series consisted of a 4-aminoquinaldine nucleus linked with a guanidino-, amidino- or guanylformylhydrazone-substituted phenyl moiety. In the second 'guanyl-hydrazon-Typ' the phenyl ring was first omitted without loss of activity, and then the 4-aminoquinaldine nucleus itself was found to be replaceable by a guanidino- or amidinophenyl group without loss of activity, and in some cases with improved tissue tolerance. This led logically to the synthesis of symmetrical molecules of the 'bis-guanyl-phenyl-Typ', in view of the known parasiticidal activity of the aromatic diamidines. By varying the inter-ring 'bridge' grouping on the basis of experience in earlier series, maximal activity was found in Berenil, which consists of two amidinophenyl moieties joined by a triazene bridge.

The great interest of this work is the way in which biological activity was shown to be retained in chemically equivalent structures. As Jensch (1958) concludes: 'Der Pyridinanteil in 4-amino-chinaldin ähnelt demnach in seinen chemotherapeutischen, sowie in mancherlei chemischen und physikalischen Eigenschaften einer Amidino-, Guanidino-, oder Guanylformylhydrazonogruppe.'

Berenil, apart from its trypanocidal activity, is also highly effective against *Babesia* infections, an added advantage in veterinary usage in Africa; in the form of the dilactate salt it was, in fact, originally named 'Babesin'. High activity against *T. congolense* has been shown by Taylor, Terry and Godfrey (1956) to correlate with activity against *Babesia* in a series of 'cattle' trypanocides which included phenanthridinium derivatives and Antrycide. It is also an active bactericide, mainly against *Brucella* spp. and streptococci.

The trypanocidal activity of Berenil was reviewed in detail by Fussgänger and Bauer (1958), following the original reports of biological and clinical trials by Bauer (1955a, 1955b) and Fussgänger (1955). In small animals, Berenil is more active against *T. congolense* than against *T. brucei*; the curative subcutaneous dose for *T. congolense* in mice may vary from 1–2·5 mg./kg. up to 5 mg./kg. depending on the strain (Davey, 1957), but the maximum tolerated dose in mice is of the order of 100 mg./kg. In larger animals, the maximum tolerated intramuscular dose is correspondingly less, about 40 mg./kg. in the rabbit and at least 8–10 mg./kg. in sheep and cattle, although subcutaneous doses as high as 21 mg./kg. are reported as having been safely given to cattle in Kenya (Fairclough, 1963, 1963a).

On the basis of extensive treatment in Tanganyika, Portuguese East Africa, the Gold Coast, the Belgian Congo, the Union of South Africa and other areas, Fussgänger and Bauer (1958) claimed that a single intramuscular dose of 3·5 mg./kg. would cure *T. congolense* and *T. vivax* infections 'in allen Teilen Afrikas'. *T. brucei* infections were less susceptible (but see below) and required a dose of 5 mg./kg.; this dose in pigs was not curative for *T. simiae* infections. Subsequent and increasing usage has borne out the validity of these early results and the prediction that Berenil would be active 'in all parts of Africa'. In Kenya, for example, the average yearly consumption of Berenil doses rose from 2,000 in 1957 to 190,000 in 1961 (Fairclough, 1963), and in Northern Nigeria, Berenil has replaced both Antrycide and Ethidium (MacLennan, 1968).

There are three main reasons for the success of Berenil; it has a much higher therapeutic index in cattle than any other active curative or prophylactic drug, it is active against cattle infections resistant to other drugs (if the degree of resistance is not too high), and in over ten years of widespread use it has not given rise to any serious degree of drug resistance. If a prophylactic form of Berenil were available which retained these properties, it would fulfil most of the desiderata for the ideal cattle trypanocide. The rapidity with which Berenil is degraded metabolically, and excreted, usually within twenty-four hours of treatment (but see below), is probably responsible both for its lack of pronounced prophylactic activity (Fairclough, 1963, 1963a) and its apparent inability to give rise rapidly to serious levels of drug resistance. This last property, coupled with its activity against drug-resistant infections have formed the basis of Whiteside's invaluable 'sanative pair' system of control of trypanosomiasis in East African cattle (Whiteside, 1962a) (*see* pp. 215–217).

A further useful feature of Berenil's rapid excretion appeared to be that control animals, in a drug trial of cattle exposed to natural infection, could be treated whenever infected, to give an average time between treatments (the Berenil Index) which indicated the extent of trypanosome risk (Boyt, Lovemore, Pilson & Smith, 1962). Use of this principle to economize on the number of uninfected controls in a drug trial was advocated by Fairclough (1962) who found that in areas of heavy tsetse infestation, there was no apparent evidence of immunity developing as a result of repeated Berenil treatment. Later work has shown that a short but increasing period of apparent residual immunity can develop with repeated Berenil treatment (Whiteside, 1962) under natural conditions, although other, more slowly-excreted drugs, are more efficient in this respect. Biological assay of Berenil levels in cattle blood by the use of a sensitive *in vitro* method, measuring effects on the infectivity of *T. brucei*, has shown however that small amounts of Berenil are detectable for up to three weeks after an intramuscular injection of 7 mg./kg., and that repeated Berenil treatment of previously uninfected cattle can confer some weeks' protection on them when introduced into a tsetse fly area of high risk (Van Hoeve, Cunningham & Grainge, 1965) (*see* below and pp. 175–176).

Although Berenil is well tolerated in cattle, sheep, dogs and man, *T. evansi*-infected camels can apparently show severe toxic reactions to a 7 mg./kg. dose; the camel infections, presumed to be Antrycide-resistant, were not affected by the standard 3·5 mg./kg. dose (Leach, 1961), although satisfactory results in camels at this dose have been reported by Fussgänger and Bauer (1958). *T. evansi* infections in rats and Indian ponies are highly susceptible to Berenil, but a proportion of treated ponies showed pyelonephritis at *post mortem* examination

(Gill, 1964). *T. brucei* infections, originally thought to be less sensitive to Berenil than the *congolense/vivax* group, show equal sensitivity *in vitro* (Van Hoeve & Grainge, 1966), so that with activity also demonstrable against *T. gambiense* and *T. rhodesiense* infections in man (see p. 157), Berenil now qualifies, even more extensively than Antrycide, as a 'wide-spectrum' trypanocide, as first indicated by Fussgänger and Bauer (1958) who found curative activity even for *T. lewisi*. Detectable, but clinically insignificant, effects in *T. theileri* infections of cattle have also been reported (Wilson & Grainge, 1967). Its value in African cattle trypanosomiasis is enhanced by its high activity on *Babesia* infections, and like other active diamidines, by its marked antibacterial and antifungal properties.

Toxicity and Pharmacology

Berenil shows features of toxicity and pharmacological action which distinguish it from other active aromatic diamidines (Fussgänger & Bauer, 1958; Hawking, 1963) (*see* pp. 158–159). The latter affect respiratory control primarily, with hypotensive and hypoglycaemic effects, and by prolonged tissue retention, can cause chronic toxicity, whereas Berenil affects the central nervous system by causing tremor, nystagmus and ataxia, and at higher doses, convulsions, vomiting and death; at therapeutic dose levels, there appear to be transient effects on blood pressure (but only after intravenous injection), no effects on blood sugar and little or no evidence of chronic toxicity. Local reactions to subcutaneous or intramuscular injection are negligible even at six times the normal therapeutic dose in cattle (Fairclough, 1963, 1963a). Transient albuminuria after Berenil treatment of sleeping sickness cases (Fussgänger & Bauer, 1958), and evidence of nephritis in treated ponies (Gill, 1964a), probably reflect the rapid urinary excretion by which almost all of a parenterally-administered dose is eliminated in twenty-four hours.

Rapid urinary excretion is accompanied by a correspondingly transient maintenance of analytically determinable blood levels. Dogs treated intramuscularly with a 7 mg./kg. dose showed peak blood levels (by spectrophotometric assay) of 2 to 7 μg./ml. one to three hours later, falling to less than 1 μg./ml. in sixteen hours and to zero in twenty-four hours. 'Biologically-active' Berenil, as noted above, has been detected in cattle blood for up to three weeks, and in dogs, a 3·5 mg./kg. dose can protect against *B. canis* infection for a week (Fussgänger & Bauer, 1958). Maximum tolerated doses of Berenil were shown to protect mice from *T. congolense* for five weeks (Williamson, 1957), as confirmed more recently by Lumsden, Herbert and Hardy (1965b) using *T. brucei*, so that some degree of tissue retention of Berenil, as yet unlocalized, must occur.

New Drug Developments

So far, this review has been confined almost exclusively to established trypanocidal drugs, and their precursors, but it is desirable also to mention briefly a number of therapeutic compounds which, although unacceptable after field trial or insufficiently active to reach this stage, may indicate future trends; some of these have been or are likely to be, useful tools to dissect the complexities of drug-trypanosome interaction (*see* pp. 195–211).

In human trypanosomiasis there is still an urgent requirement for a cheap, simply administered and well-tolerated, preferably 'one-shot' drug which would be as effective a prophylactic as pentamidine, active therapeutically against all stages of the infection in both Gambian and Rhodesian sleeping sickness, incapable of inducing drug resistance and active also against strains with acquired resistance to other drugs. Possibly the two requirements of prolonged tissue retention (for prophylaxis) and ability to penetrate into the central nervous system are mutually exclusive, but with increasing knowledge of the structure and function of the so-called 'blood-brain barrier' (*see* pp. 147–150), this problem should not be insuperable. In *T. vivax*/*T. congolense* infections of animals, where CSF-penetration is not required of a drug, most of the primary requirements except prophylaxis—a single locally and generally well-tolerated intramuscular or subcutaneous injection, high therapeutic index, inability to give rise to drug resistance and activity against resistant strains—seem to be met by Berenil. As the emergence, whether rapid or slow, of drug-resistant strains appears to be inevitable, the necessity remains for a *selection* of equally active drugs, preferably of widely different chemical types, to be retained as 'stoppers' for drug-resistant strains. Similar requirements apply to prophylactic drugs, with the added necessity for prolonged tissue retention to be free from local cellular damage and chronic toxicity. None of the existing prophylactic 'cattle' drugs combines these properties, although Antrycide chloride or suraminate in *T. simiae* infections of pigs, or Antrycide suraminate in surra of Indian equines (*see* pp. 172–174) appear to be free of most drawbacks with the possible exception of expense and commercial availability.

Drug developments are indicated below under the heading of the relevant chemical (*see* Table 7.3) or antibiotic group.

Acid Naphthylamine

Suramin is the representative member of this group, which comprises the trypanocidal dyes Trypan Red, Trypan Blue and Pontamine Sky Blue 5BX. The structure of suramin is highly specific and attempts to replace the naphthalene trisulphonate portion with heterocyclic nuclei have been unsuccessful (Adams, Ashley & Bader, 1956).

Aromatic Arsenical/Antimonial

The therapeutic possibilities of this group of organometallic drugs (Hilmer, 1958; Hawking, 1963, 1966) are by no means exhausted. The aromatic arsonic acid group is comparable in ionization properties to the aromatic carboxyl group (*see* p. 147), but apart from pteroic acid analogues of this type tested for antitumour action (Angier, Gazzola, Semb, Gadekar & Williams, 1954) a similar approach on this basis or on phosphate-arsenate analogy, has yet to be made in trypanosomiasis chemotherapy; arsenical hybrids with other active molecules (tetracyclines, amidines) have not so far been successful, but apart from dangers of cross-resistance, this 'dual antagonist' combination synthesis (Bardos, Datta-Gupta & Hebborn, 1966) may justify further investigation. The acid-substituted arsenobenzene Spirotrypan (Hoechst, 10557) (FUSSGÄNGER, 1951; Hilmer, 1958) is active against both spirochaetes and trypanosomes, and like other acid-substituted arsenicals, also acts on trypanosomes resistant to 'neutral' aromatic arsenicals. Although active on *T. lewisi* and the blood forms of the 'arsenic-refractory' *T. cruzi*, it is inactive on *T. vivax* in cattle; *T. evansi* infections appear to be susceptible, especially in dogs (Fernando & Jayasinghe, 1965).

Detoxication of arsenicals and antimonials by combination with thiol-containing acids or BAL has continued, with most interest centred on Friedheim's melamine compounds (*see* pp. 150–156), but recent investigations by Ercoli (1967, 1968) suggest that dimethylcysteine combination is preferable. Therapeutic activity is unaffected while toxicity is reduced, unlike BAL, dimercaptosuccinate and cysteine, which all cause some reduction of activity; further reduction of toxicity results from chelate formation with excess dimethylcysteine, and derivatives of tartar emetic have been produced in this way, which are fully active yet non-irritant on intramuscular injection. This type of compound (*cf.* Williamson, 1960) could have a place in the treatment of drug-resistant cattle trypanosomiasis. Further investigation of *T. congolense* metabolism (*see* pp. 199–200) may indicate why this group is insusceptible to those organometallic drugs to which the *brucei*-group trypanosomes are so sensitive.

Diamidine, Aminoquinoline and Phenanthridine

These groups of drugs are intimately related chemically, in that they all deploy, in a variety of free, cyclic, or vinylogous forms, the —N—C=N— amidine type of linkage which occurs also in the melamine moiety of the melaminyl arsenicals. Extensive cross-resistance occurs among these groups of trypanocides (*see* pp. 211–217) which would appear to be associated with the amidine-type structural unit (*see* pp. 166–169).

A number of active variations on this heterocyclic theme have been produced, one of the most interesting of which was 2-amino-4,6-*bis*(*p*-amidinoanilino)-*s*-triazine (M. & B. 2242) (Ashley, Berg & McDonald, 1960) which, like Surfen C (Fig. 7.35) had melamine as an inter-ring linkage. This compound was prepared on the basis that the 4-aminoquinoline moieties of Surfen C could be regarded as vinylogues of 2-aminoquinoline, which is itself a cyclic amidine derivative; M. & B. 2242, with two amidinoanilino groups joined by an amino-triazine ring would thus be equivalent to Surfen C. M. & B. 2242 was in fact an active trypanocide, especially against *T. congolense*; it was less active than Antrycide or Dimidium but also much less toxic, but on field trial was found to be less active on drug-resistant strains than Berenil or Metamidium. Attempts to replace the quinoline nucleus of Antrycide with a variety of other bicyclic heterocycles (BERG & PARNELL, 1961) showed retention of activity only in the quinazoline, phthalazine and benzoxazole analogues (*see* p. 207). Several amidine-substituted aminoquinolinium and aminostyryl-quinolinium derivatives are trypanocidal and babesicidal (Berg, 1961, 1962); all these have formal resemblance to active drugs like Berenil and Samorin, and in some cases reflect their styrylquinoline precursors (Fig. 7.32). Related work (ASHLEY, BERG & LUCAS, 1960) uncovered the active babesicide, amicarbalide (*B. vet. C*), (N,N′-di(*m*-amidinophenyl) urea diisethionate); extra vinylogous —N—C=N— linkages which appear in this molecule may be associated with activity, as the corresponding *p*-amidino-substituted compound, which presumably would not allow such vinylogue formation, is inactive. The Ciba trypanocide (23889 Ba) (*p*-biguanidoacetophenone amidinohydrazone) (Hawking, 1962) has an extended series of amidine, vinylogous amidine and isosteric hydrazone linkages, and resembles the active trypanocidal diamidines in having little effect on infectivity and being inactive on a diamidine-resistant strain of *T. rhodesiense*; it has little effect on *T. congolense*.

Jensch, of Farbwerke Hoechst, the discoverer of Berenil, after almost a lifetime spent unravelling the complexities of structure-activity relationships in the 4-aminoquinoline series, died in 1956, unfortunately too soon to see the widespread adoption of his most successful synthesis. The influence of his work has been apparent on drug developments in other European and American

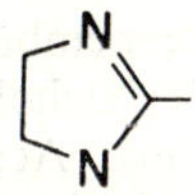

Fig. 7.41 *Imidazolyl*

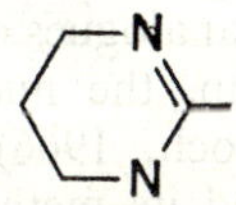

Fig. 7.42 *Tetrahydropyrimidyl*

chemotherapy laboratories, and it obviously continues both at Hoechst and elsewhere. Bauer (1963) described a *bis*-guanylhydrazone compound (2,3-hexanedione-*bis* [N-guanyl-N-(*p*-amidinophenyl)] hydrazone diaceturate) which was active against *T. evansi* in horses but rapidly produced drug resistance; a closely-related compound given to *T. evansi*-infected guinea pigs for 2½ years (Holz, 1965) also produced drug resistance and a loss of trypanosome virulence apparently associated with a change to short stumpy forms (*see* p. 218) 'Cyclic amidine' groups such as imidazolyl (Fig. 7.41) (first used as such by King, Lourie and Yorke (1937) in the search for Synthalin analogues) and

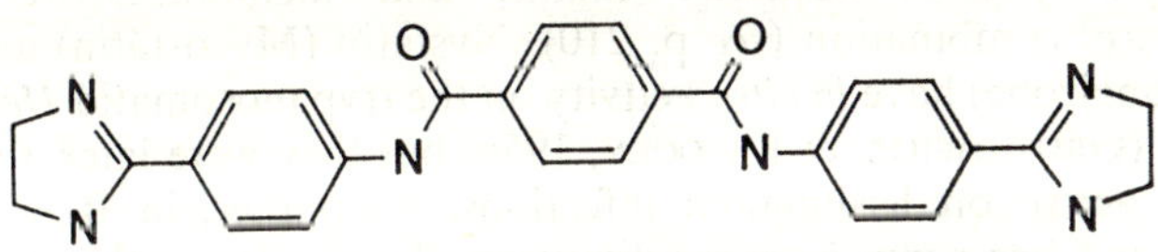

Fig. 7.43 *Terephthalanilide*

tetrahydropyrimidyl (Fig. 7.42), have been used to produce an interesting series of amidine/4-aminoquinoline type compounds some of which have high antibacterial, trypanocidal or specifically leishmanicidal properties (Loewe, 1964; Loewe & Urbanietz, 1965; Loewe, Urbanietz & Mieth, 1967).

Correspondences between the metabolism and chemotherapy of trypanosomes and cancer cells (*see* p. 203) have been further strengthened by the discovery that the terephthalanilide group of compounds (Fig. 7.43) (Bennett, 1965) which have antileukaemic activity (Hirt & Berchtold, 1961) also have appreciable trypanocidal activity (Schmidt, 1965).

The parent compound, derived from a central terephthalic acid (1,4-benzenedicarboxylic acid) structure, is essentially an aromatic diamidine, a group in which the possession of both trypanocidal and antitumour activity has been known since 1947 when Snapper used Stilbamidine to treat multiple myeloma.

Nucleoside and other Antibiotics

None of the commoner antibiotics such as penicillin, streptomycin or chloramphenicol is active against African trypanosomes. The general insusceptibility of protozoa, unlike bacteria, to antibiotic action may indicate a closer phylogenetic connection to the metazoa; certainly, almost all those antibiotics which have antiprotozoal activity are also toxic for the mammalian host. An increasing number of antibiotics, mainly from *Streptomyces* spp., has however been shown to possess both antitumour and trypanocidal activity. A number of these, including Puromycin and Nucleocidin which have been tested clinically in Africa, are close analogues of adenosine (Fig. 7.44) and are members of a closely interrelated group, the nucleoside antibiotics (Bloch & Nichol, 1965; Fox, Watanabe & Bloch, 1966). Of the remainder, Azaserine, Actinomycin D, Mitomycin C and its methyl congener, Porfiromycin, and Phleomycin (Jaffe, 1963, 1965, 1967a) are of varied and unrelated chemical structure; Pactamycin (Jaffe, *loc. cit.*) although of unknown structure, has chemical properties which suggest that it is not a nucleoside. Three other non-nucleoside antibiotics, also from *Streptomyces* spp., have trypanocidal activity; Amphomycin (Packchanian, 1956), Oxytetracycline (Terramycin) (Petana, 1964) and Paromomycin (Najarian, 1965). Terramycin is weakly active only on *T. congolense*, and another antibiotic ICI No. 13959 (Davey, 1961) derived from *Paecilomyces*, is also specifically, but much more highly active on *T. congolense*.

The polyene antifungal antibiotics (Kinsky, 1967) form another distinct group of structurally-related compounds, the more active members of which have antiprotozoal activity. The group is characterized by the possession of continuously-conjugated aliphatic chains, and membrane-lytic properties involving sterol combination (*see* p. 210). Nystatin (Mycostatin) and Amphotericin B (Fungizone) have *in vitro* activity on the trypanosomatid *Herpetomonas culicidarum* (GROSSOWICZ & RASOOLY, 1958) but they were later found to be particularly active on leishmanial infections. Amphotericin B is also active on *T. cruzi* and has some *in vivo* activity on *T. congolense*; this activity is increased with blockade of the reticulo-endothelial system (Actor, Wind & Pagano, 1962) where the drug is otherwise sequestered, and thus enabled to act on intracellular parasites of this tissue, such as *L. donovani*, *T. cruzi* and *Histoplasma*.

NUCLEOSIDE ANTIBIOTICS: These antitumour compounds are analogues of the purine nucleoside adenosine (Fig. 7.44) or of the pyrimidine nucleoside, cytidine, consisting of the purine or pyrimidine base and the sugar or ribose moiety linked to it by a glycosidic bond. Analogues are substituted either in the base or the sugar, or in both as in Puromycin (Fig. 7.45) the first of these antibiotics found to have trypanocidal activity; so far, only adenosine analogues have this property.

PUROMYCIN: This substance was originally labelled Achromycin by Lederle Laboratories Division, American Cyanamid Co. (Porter, Hewitt, Hesseltine,

Kupka, Lowery, Wallace, Bohonos & Williams, 1952). Subsequently the trade name was changed to Puromycin and then to Stylomycin, the label Achromycin having been assigned to a Lederle brand of tetracycline.

Originally isolated from *Streptomyces albo-niger* (Porter *et al.*, 1952), Puromycin (6 - dimethylamino - 9 - (3′ - *p* - methoxy - L - phenylalanylamino - 3′-deoxy-β-D-ribofuranosyl) purine) can also be degraded by loss of the

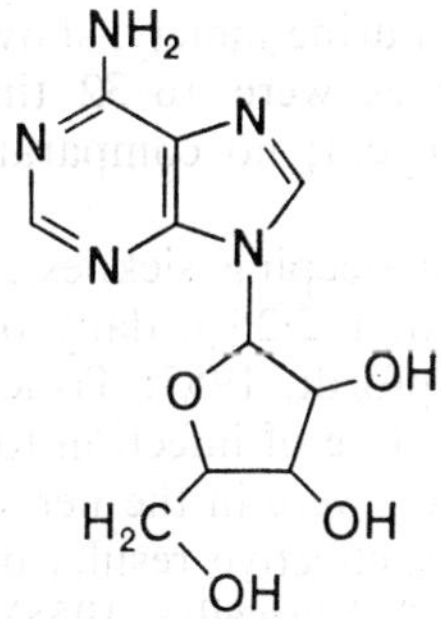

Fig. 7.44 *Adenosine*

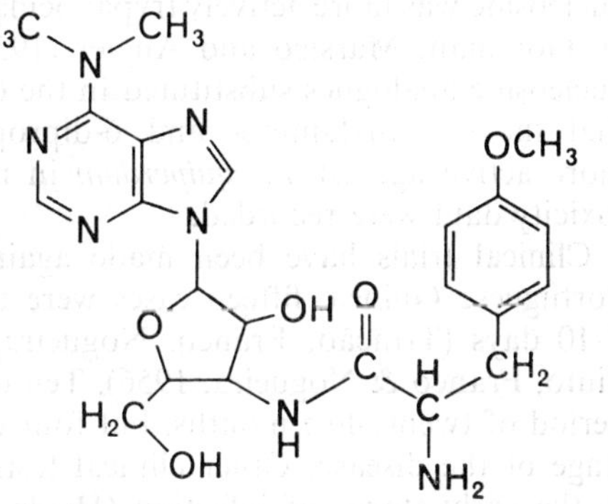

Fig. 7.45 *Puromycin*

phenylalanyl portion to a form known as Puromycin aminonucleoside (6-dimethylamino-9-(3′-amino-3′-deoxy-β-D-ribofuranosyl) purine (Fig. 7.46).

The striking resemblance of Puromycin to the terminal adenylic acid-amino acid 'tail' postulated for 'transfer' ribonucleic acid is commented on elsewhere (p. 202) but it may be noted that the trypanocidal action *in vivo* and *in vitro*

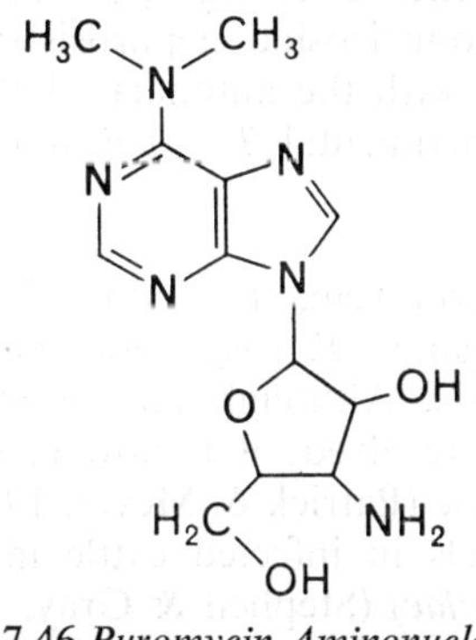

Fig. 7.46 *Puromycin Aminonucleoside*

can be selectively antagonized by adenine (Hewitt, Gumble, Wallace & Williams, 1954; Agosin & von Brand, 1954).

Porter *et al.* (1952) showed that Puromycin was curative for *T. equiperdum* in mice either orally or parenterally. *T. equinum*, *T. equiperdum* and *T. evansi* infections of mice are more susceptible to Puromycin than *T. gambiense* and *T. rhodesiense* infections (Tobie, 1954); *T. congolense* is particularly insusceptible. In a comparative study of fifty-two Puromycin analogues (Hewitt, Gumble, Wallace & Williams, 1955) none was found more active against *T. equiperdum* than Puromycin aminonucleoside. The trypanocidal activity in the series varied in a manner parallel to antitumour activity, and interference with nucleic acids or nucleoprotein synthesis was suggested to be a locus of drug action, in view of the reversal of this action by a number of purine derivatives (Hewitt *et al.*, 1954). Tobie and Highman (1956) concluded, in agreement with the earlier results of Hewitt *et al.* (1954) on *T. equiperdum* infections, that the aminonucleoside was more actively trypanocidal than Puromycin itself. Further studies by Goldman, Marsico and Angier (1956) on a variety of Puromycin aminonucleoside analogues substituted in the 6-position of the purine moiety, showed that the 6-diethylamino- and 6-dipropylamino-analogues were 16–32 times more active against *T. equiperdum* in mice than Puromycin; no comparative toxicity data were recorded.

Clinical trials have been made against *T. gambiense* sleeping sickness. In Portuguese Guinea, fifteen cases were treated orally with 1–2·25 g. daily over 7–10 days (Trincão, Franco, Nogueira, Pinto & Mühlpfordt, 1955; Trincão, Pinto, Franco & Nogueira, 1956). Ten of these remained free of infection for a period of twenty-five months, but four out of five relapses were in the nervous stage of the disease. Other clinical tests have also given effective results only in the early stages of infection (Heuls, Orio, Ceccaldi & Merveille, 1958) or have not been considered successful (Neujean & Evens, 1958). Puromycin thus appears unlikely to supplant existing drugs for the treatment of African sleeping sickness, but it is likely to be of considerable experimental value in studies on the mode of trypanocidal drug action (*see* pp. 202–204). Both Puromycin and its aminonucleoside are now established tools in experimental biochemical and physiological work, the former as a specific inhibitor of protein synthesis in mammalian cells and the latter as an agent for the artificial production of a nephritic condition ('aminonucleoside nephrosis'); in addition, the aminonucleoside, in combination with the antimalarial Primaquine, has a powerful suppressive action on experimental *T. cruzi* infections (Moraes, Farid & Fernandes, 1960).

NUCLEOCIDIN: Unlike Puromycin, this antibiotic isolated by Thomas *et al.* (1957), was more active against *T. congolense* than against *T. gambiense* in rats and mice (Tobie, 1957). Although known to resemble Puromycin, its structure was incompletely resolved; it is now considered to be 9-adenyl-4′-sulphamyloxypentofuranoside (Patrick & Meyer, 1968) and to contain fluorine (Morton *et al.*, 1969). Trials in infected cattle in West Africa (*T. vivax*/*T. congolense*) and pigs (*T. simiae*) (Stephen & Gray, 1960b, 1961) showed some therapeutic but non-curative activity at doses of 0·025–0·05 g./kg. The antibiotic is fairly toxic, which is not surprising in view of a recent description of it as the most active known inhibitor of protein synthesis *in vivo*.

CORDYCEPIN: The trypanocidal activity of the three adenine analogues above, and the apparent dependence of some pathogenic trypanosomes on an exogenous supply of adenine (Little & Oleson, 1951; Williamson & Rollo, 1952) suggested that other adenine analogues might be trypanocidal. A simple and unusually non-toxic analogue, Cordycepin (3′-deoxyadenosine) (Fig. 7.47)

(CUNNINGHAM, HUTCHINSON, MANSON & SPRING, 1951) has been found to be highly active on trypanosomes *in vitro* and to have high specific activity on *T. congolense* infections in mice (Williamson, 1966) with a possible therapeutic index of 36, compared with 15 and 25 for Antrycide and Ethidium tested under the same conditions. The upper limit of mammalian toxicity has not yet been determined (more than 900 mg./kg. in rats), but further development of this and the increasing number of related nucleoside antibiotics now becoming

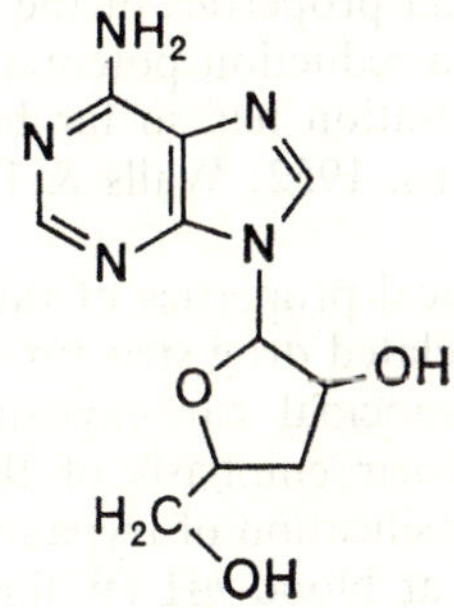

Fig. 7.47 *Cordycepin*

available, may be profitable for trypanosomiasis as well as tumour chemotherapy.

MODE OF DRUG ACTION

General

In none of the active drugs considered above is the mode of action precisely known. The cytotoxicity of the aromatic arsenicals is undoubtedly due to inactivation of metabolically active thiol groups by the trivalent arsenic substituent but, while this is an adequate explanation of lethality, it does not account for the high degree of structural specificity which governs both the degree of activity against the parasite cell, and the extent of inactivity against the cells of the mammalian host. Cross resistance and selective antagonism studies (Schnitzer & Grunberg, 1957; Bishop, 1959; Williamson & Rollo, 1959; Williamson, 1959a) and analyses of structure-activity relationships (King & Strangeways, 1942; Doak & Eagle, 1951) confirm the conclusions of Yorke *et al.* (1930, 1931a) that the observed specificity is controlled by the structure of the non-metallic portion of the drug molecule.

The postulate that drug action consists of at least two stages, a preliminary fixation, which may be reversible, and a subsequent lethal action (Clark, 1933; King & Strangeways, 1942), provides an acceptable basis for analysis of trypanocidal drug action and the related phenomena of cross-resistance behaviour. It is essentially the *chemorezeptor* hypothesis of Ehrlich, which, as Schnitzer and Grunberg (1957) remark 'has not been replaced by either a more lucid or more comprehensive working hypothesis' (*cf.* Waud, 1968). Tables 3–5 in Williamson (1962) (also reproduced in Hawking (1963) and Goodwin (1964)) represent an attempt to equate the chemoreceptors for trypanocidal drugs with sites of enzyme action, on the reasonable assumption that enzyme inactivation represents the final lethal action of the drug.

The preliminary fixation of a drug at the active site on an enzyme protein, and its passage thereto *via* membrane barriers such as those of the cell itself, and of its internal organelles, are determined by a multiplicity of factors. Many of these are susceptible to analysis (Albert, 1951b; Brodie & Hogben, 1957; Doorenbos, 1960), but elucidation of trypanocidal action in terms of structurally-determined physical properties of the drug, such as ionic dissociation, lipid solubility, oxidation-reduction potential, and intramolecular charge separation and electron distribution has so far been only partially successful (Brownlee *et al.*, 1950; Watkins, 1952; Walls & Beveridge, 1952; Williamson, 1959a, 1959b).

Systematic analysis of physical properties of this kind is most fruitful when applied to a series of closely-related drug structures, and the work of King and Strangeways (1942) on trypanocidal carboxyl-substituted phenylarsenoxides is a model in this respect. Their emphasis of the importance of ionization (*cf.* Albert, 1951b) led to a classification of trypanocides based on their neutral, cationic or anionic character at blood *p*H (Williamson & Rollo, 1959). This grouping shows a certain, though incomplete, correspondence with cross-resistance behaviour, with differential activity against human and animal trypanosomes, and with ability to pass from the blood into the cerebrospinal fluid; the last property is of considerable importance in the treatment of human trypanosomiasis. Membrane-permeative properties which are likely to affect equally the predominantly lipid barrier structures assumed to exist both in the trypanosome and in the central nervous system (*see* pp. 147–150), must obviously be delicately balanced to keep the toxic action directed selectively at the parasite; the neurotoxic effect on the human host of the few drugs active in late-stage sleeping sickness is sufficient evidence of this. Attempts to influence the passage of a number of trypanocides by the use of hyaluronidase and other substances have not been successful (Fromentin, 1957).

An alternative broad division of trypanocides into two groups has been proposed by Hawking and Sen (1960) on the basis of (a) the speed with which they kill trypanosomes *in vivo* and *in vitro*, (b) their ability to affect the infectivity of trypanosomes in the period before death, and (c) the extent to which they are absorbed by trypanosomes. Trivalent arsenicals, acriflavine and most diamidines are rapidly lethal, do not affect infectivity, and combine with trypanosomes in relatively large amounts, whereas suramin, Antrycide (Ormerod, 1951; Hawking and Thurston, 1955), and phenanthridinium compounds (Lock, 1950) including Prothidium (Taylor, 1960a), take much longer to kill trypanosomes, although they abolish infectivity at an early stage without much effect on motility, and are absorbed only in very small amounts. The localization of the second group on the trypanosome is mainly extranuclear, and interference with cytoplasmic protein synthesis *via* ribonucleoprotein appeared probable (but see below); the selective action of the cationic members of this group on the *congolense-vivax* trypanosomes suggests that other mechanisms may also be operative.

A recent major advance in the correlation of cell structure and function has been the characterization of the lysosomes as a distinct group of subcellular organelles, which consist of single-membrane-bound vesicles containing acid hydrolases (DE DUVE, PRESSMAN, GIANETTO, WATTIAUX & APPELMANS, 1955), and which are capable of rapid and selective uptake of a variety of drugs (Allison & Young, 1964; Allison, 1968). The first-stage 'receptor' for drug uptake postulated by Ehrlich (1908) and Clark (1933) would now seem to have a structural basis in the lysosome, which in various forms appears to provide the bulk of the essential digestive, transport and excretory mechanisms of all protozoan and metazoan cells. Living mammalian cells rapidly concentrate Trypan Blue, suramin, stilbamidine, Ethidium and Antrycide in the lysosomes (Allison, 1968). Lysosomal concentration of Samorin is also probable (Philips *et al.*, 1967), and interaction of trypanocidal drugs with the lysosomes of *T. rhodesiense* has been inferred from observations of drug effects on the fine structure (Macadam & Williamson, 1964; Williamson & Macadam, 1965; Macadam & Williamson, 1967, 1969). Antrycide and Ethidium are taken up by the large lysosomes of *T. theileri*, and suramin, which is taken up by liver lysosomes and inhibits some lysosomal enzymes (Smeesters & Jacques, 1968), appears to remain as electron-dense material in the lysosomes of *T. rhodesiense* during the terminal stages of attack by suramin *in vivo*; Trypan Blue shows a similar lysosomal deposition in the rat visceral yolk-sac (Lloyd, Beck, Griffiths & Parry, 1968).

All the representative trypanocidal drugs so far examined for their effects on the fine structure of *T. rhodesiense*, show a sequence of non-specific changes, of which the most marked is on cytoplasmic ribosomes which lose electron opacity, become reduced in number and ultimately disappear. Those drugs which show delayed action and seem to act primarily on cell division, rather than on respiration or glycolysis, stimulate proliferation of lysosomes, usually in the cytoplasmic area adjacent to the kinetoplast, where the pellicle forming the 'reservoir' pocket round the flagellar insertion is devoid of a subpellicular layer of fibrils, and may therefore be more permeable to drug passage; support for this inference is provided by observation of the selective passage of ferritin particles across this area in *T. rhodesiense* (Brown, Armstrong & Valentine, 1964). The slow-acting trypanocides such as Antrycide induce formation of 'chemotherapy granules' in trypanosomes (Ormerod, 1951, 1961; Ormerod and Shaw, 1963; Molloy and Ormerod, 1965) and formation of 'ribosomal aggregates' in *Crithidia* (*Strigomonas*) *oncopelti* (Newton, 1962), both of which are probably identical with drug-filled lysosomes, although Antrycide can aggregate isolated ribosomes *in vitro* (Newton, 1963). Ormerod (1962) later described the similar 'volutin granules' of *T. rhodesiense* as 'aggregated ribosomes surrounded by a lipoid membrane' (the typical appearance of a primary lysosome); a second type of granule (Molloy & Ormerod, 1965; Michel, 1964) does not appear to be lysosomal; Antrycide has also been reported to cause intense activation of the lysosomal 'marker' enzyme, acid phosphatase, in *T. evansi* (SEN, RAY & DUTTA, 1954).

So far, there is no experimental confirmation of the possibility that lysosomal interaction with trypanocidal drugs causes injury to the trypanosome, either by activation and release of lysosomal enzymes (such as acid ribonuclease), or by stabilization of lysosomal membranes and inhibition of mitosis, although stilbamidine, but not suramin, has been shown to have the latter effect (Weissmann, Davies & Krakauer, 1969). But lysosomal membrane composition may possibly play a part in the specificity of reversible initial drug uptake, the steric basis of which seems to be fundamental to the related phenomena of trypanocidal drug resistance and selective interference with drug action (*see* p. 211). The cationic nature of most of the slow-acting drugs, especially those acting on the animal trypanosomiases, suggests that membrane phospholipids are likely anionic receptors (Williamson & Macadam, 1965; Williamson, 1965), and several coloured or fluorescent drugs such as Antrycide, Ethidium and stilbamidine, are strongly bound *in vitro* by various common phospholipids. Thin-layer chromatographic micro-analysis of trypanosome lipids extracted from drug-treated cells suggests that more specific combinations can occur, and it seems likely that entry of these predominantly water-soluble drug cations into the lipid/lipoprotein phase of parasite cellular membranes is facilitated by this kind of interaction. Mammalian cell lysosomes are known to contain a cation-binding lipid constituent (Barrett & Dingle, 1967).

Analysis of the 'second stage' lethal loci of trypanocidal drug action in terms of enzyme inactivation (Williamson, 1962) suffered from a number of limitations, which have not subsequently been extensively repaired. The tabulated observations referred to enzyme activity from many different sources, only a few of which had been identified in trypanosomes. Of some eighty-eight references cited, only eight referred to known trypanosomal systems, and seven of these dealt with only four species of trypanosome in the *evansi-brucei* taxonomic group (*T. equiperdum*, *T. evansi*, *T. hippicum* and *T. rhodesiense*). Of these species only the last undergoes cyclical development in the tsetse, but the work referred to was done on a monomorphic, blood-passaged strain which differs in many ways, especially in drug sensitivity, from the natural fly-transmissible strain. Two important gaps were thus obvious at the outset; the *vivax-congolense* trypanosomes and trypanosomes capable of undergoing cyclical transmission.

The lack of work on the *vivax-congolense* group was mainly due to the technical difficulties of large-scale preparation of isolated erythrocyte-free suspensions, but two recent technical innovations have largely overcome this problem: the use of low-speed centrifugation of infected blood on linear sucrose density gradients (Williamson & Cover, 1966) and of filtration of infected blood on cation-exchange cellulose (Lanham, 1968). The necessity for improved ways of making blood-contaminant-free trypanosome suspensions for metabolic work has been emphasized by experiments showing that almost all the lactate dehydrogenase activity previously claimed for *T. rhodesiense* suspensions could be accounted for by blood platelet contamination (Dixon, 1966); defibrination followed by sucrose gradient centrifugation removed this source of error.

A second obvious feature revealed by the analysis was the concentration of effort on the effect of organometallic drugs on glycolytic enzymes. This is not surprising in view of the well-known high rate of aerobic glycolysis typical of African trypanosomes of the *evansi-brucei* group. Glycolytic enzymes are predominantly 'thiol' in character and thus susceptible to heavy metal inhibition, and aromatic arsenoxides are now conventional reagents for the detection of thiol enzymes (Johnstone, 1963). Lotspeich and Peters (1951), for example, indicated the possibility of distinguishing mono- and di-thiol reactive groupings by the use of appropriately substituted aromatic trivalent arsenicals.

Arsenicals

The susceptibility to arsenicals of key enzymes in phosphorylation (hexokinase and adenosine triphosphatase (ATPase)) seemed likely to be highly significant in the trypanocidal action of these drugs. Studies on the unique cytochrome-free terminal respiratory L-α-glycerophosphate oxidase system of bloodstream forms of *T. rhodesiense* (Grant & Sargent, 1960) showed that oxophenarsine was an inhibitor. Subsequent investigation of arsenical-sensitive trypanosomal enzymes revealed that the kinase group was especially sensitive to Melarsen oxide (Grant & Bowman, 1966; *see* Grant, 1966), and that phosphopyruvate kinase and glycerol kinase were most sensitive; the corresponding mammalian enzymes were some fifteen times less sensitive. ATPase did not appear to be significantly affected by Melarsen oxide.

Further intensive analyses of the mode of action of Melarsen oxide (Flynn & Bowman, 1968, 1969) showed that the terminal glycolytic enzyme of *brucei* trypanosomes, pyruvate kinase, was selectively inhibited *in vitro* by this drug and by the parent compound, phenylarsenoxide; the comparable host enzyme from rabbit muscle was less sensitive. Host and parasite enzymes were equally susceptible to non-selective thiol inhibitors, so that the specific parasiticidal action of active aromatic arsenicals could be due to differences in uptake by dithiol groupings participating in the formation of the enzyme-substrate complex at the active site of the enzyme; a similar differential sensitivity to trivalent antimonials by host and schistosome phosphofructokinase has also been observed *in vitro* by Mansour and Bueding (1954), and *in vivo* by Fisher, Bruce, Bourgeois, Bueding *et. al.* (1966). The pyruvate kinase of trypanosomes and the phosphofructokinase of schistosomes are strategic 'pacemaker' enzymes for these parasites, and even slight preferential inhibition of them may exert a profound influence on the overall metabolism of the parasites. The parasites depend primarily on glycolysis for energy production, like tumour cells, where the key 'pacemaking' glycolytic enzymes are considered to be hexokinase (glucokinase), phosphofructokinase and pyruvic kinase (Weber, 1968); trypanosomal hexokinase, as confirmed by Grant and Bowman (1966), although sensitive to thiol inhibitors, is not a rate-limiting factor in the glycolysis of *T. rhodesiense* or *T. gambiense* (Seed & Baquero, 1965).

Flynn and Bowman's work is also of interest in recognizing the desirability of studying polymorphic as well as monomorphic *brucei* trypanosomes (Bowman & Flynn, 1968). Using preparations of separated 'thin' and 'thick' forms, they showed that the 'thick' forms do not use pyruvate with concomitant uptake of oxygen, and that their oxygen uptake, with glucose as substrate, is insensitive to cyanide. The implication is that the 'mitochondrial' Krebs cycle and cytochrome systems which operate in the 'culture' or midgut forms of the tsetse, are not fully functional, as postulated by Vickerman (1965), on the basis of histochemical observations which suggested maintenance of 'mitochondrial' enzyme activity in the 'short stumpy' bloodstream forms of polymorphic *T. brucei.* Nevertheless, Flynn and Bowman found that conversion of glucose carbon to CO_2 and pyruvate was 5–10% and 40%, respectively, for a polymorphic *T. rhodesiense* compared with zero and 95% for the monomorphic strain.

Although incomplete glycolysis is typical of all African trypanosomes so far examined (Ryley, 1956), phosphorylative glycolysis of the Embden-Meyerhof-Parnas type has been established or implied only in the four *evansi-brucei* species mentioned earlier. This is a further difficulty in argument by analogy from drug action on non-trypanosomal systems, especially in the light of the suggestive experiments by Dickens (1934, 1939) where some correlation appeared to exist between the trypanocidal action of acridine, amidine and styrylquinoline compounds and their inhibiting activity on the Pasteur effect, which is known to involve phosphorylation. A similar correlation with inhibition of oxidative phosphorylation by Judah and Williams-Ashman (1951) suggested that this process might be a locus of action of the few compounds active against the arsenic-refractory *vivax-congolense* trypanosomes (Williamson, 1959). In the absence of relevant experimental evidence from this group of parasites and with the respiratory enzyme framework of all trypanosomes only partially established as yet (Fulton & Spooner, 1959; Grant, Sargent & Ryley, 1961), drug action in these terms can only be speculative, particularly as experimental demonstration of oxidative phosphorylation in *T. rhodesiense* has not yet been successful (Williamson, 1959; Grant & Sargent, 1960). The hypoglycaemic action of amidine-type drugs appears to involve respiratory phosphorylation (Falcone, Mao & Shrago, 1962; Schäfer, 1963) and is unlikely to be related to trypanocidal action.

Other difficulties in interpretation arise. Wide variation can occur in the reaction of the same enzyme from different sources, and a correlation between the biological activity of amidines and their inhibition of amine oxidase, originally shown by Blaschko and Duthie (1945, 1951), was subsequently invalidated for this reason (Blaschko & Himms, 1955). Again, although thiol inactivation may account for the ultimate lethal action of organometallic drugs in *evansi-brucei* infections, their specificity, degree of binding and drug resistance behaviour are largely, if not wholly, determined by the non-metallic portion of the drug molecule.

Aromatic arsenicals and antimonials, although active against the *evansi-brucei* group, are generally inactive against the *vivax-congolense* trypanosomes, although both groups of parasites show active aerobic glycolysis and hence might be expected to show a comparable sensitivity to the organometallic drugs, as they appear to do towards sodium arsenite (von Brand, Tobie & Mehlman, 1950; Desowitz, 1956). Here again, the non-metallic portion of the drug molecule would seem to control its lethal action, and it may be concluded that the so-called arsenic-refractory nature of the *vivax-congolense* group may in part be due to a different pattern of enzyme protein receptors in the region of the active thiol centres, rather than that thiol enzymes are reduced or absent.

Diamidines

Inhibition of glycolysis does not account completely for the mode of action of the large class of diamidine trypanocides, the specific lethality of which appeared from the earlier analyses to be exerted on protein and nucleic acid metabolism. The number of possible susceptible loci in the trypanosome has been reduced considerably by the intensive studies of Gutteridge (1966, 1967, 1969) on the action of pentamidine on the trypanosomatid flagellate *Crithidia fasciculata.* Biosynthetic processes, (DNA, RNA, protein and phospholipid synthesis), as in bacteria (Gale & Folkes, 1967), are more sensitive to growth-inhibitory concentrations of pentamidine than respiration, and in addition, the transport system for the basic amino acids, lysine and arginine, is pentamidine-sensitive. Higher concentrations of pentamidine affect respiration and cause loss of potassium and magnesium ions. Cation efflux is unlikely to be a primary lethal effect of pentamidine, as it does not occur at growth-inhibitory concentrations of pentamidine or of the related diamidines, 2-hydroxystilbamidine, propamidine and Berenil; it can also be produced by the unrelated cationic drugs, Antrycide and Prothidium. Some form of intracellular cation-exchange may occur, as the effect does not appear to result from membrane damage; pentamidine-treated organisms do not leak materials containing ribose, phosphorus or α-amino-nitrogen (Gutteridge, unpublished). In this connection, Wallis (1966) showed that pentamidine, propamidine and Stilbamidine, like Antrycide (Newton, 1966), could displace magnesium ion and polyamines from the ribosomes of *C. oncopelti in vitro*, although unlike Antrycide, extensive ribosomal aggregation did not occur either *in vitro* or *in vivo*; the possibility that the small amount of pentamidine bound to ribosomes could affect ribosomal protein synthesis was not excluded. The inhibitory effect of diamidines on a number of reactions involving amino acids may be due in part to the well-known facility of amidines to form insoluble salts with carboxylic acids, but more specific mechanisms must be operative as in the case of lysine/arginine transport in *C. fasciculata.* Amino acid incorporation in pathogenic trypanosomes is likely to be a vulnerable function, as transaminase activity is high in the few species examined, an intracellular free amino acid pool is maintained by a variety of species, and an energy-dependent amino acid assimilative mechanism is probably present (Williamson & Desowitz, 1961).

The loci of pentamidine lethality, although now considerably narrowed, are still far from precise specification. Among other of its manifold effects recently described are inhibition of thymidine phosphorylase activity in *C. fasciculata* (Gutteridge, unpublished), and a preferential fragmentation of kinetoplast rather than nuclear chromatin material in *T. rhodesiense* blood forms (Macadam & Williamson, 1969). The latter effect is also produced by Berenil and probably reflects the selective action of Berenil on kinetoplast DNA synthesis and on the buoyant density of trypanosome kinetoplast DNA in caesium chloride gradients (Newton & Le Page, 1967, 1968). Concentration of attention on kinetoplast DNA and its interaction with drugs can be expected to yield more results of interest and importance in view of the central function of the kinetoplast 'mitochondrion' in the trypanosome life cycle (Williamson, 1962; Vickerman, 1962, 1965; Mühlpfordt, 1964), and in relation to the long-established observation of the dyskinetoplasty induced by many trypanocidal dyes and drugs, especially acriflavine and pararosaniline, and more recently, Surfen C (Williamson & Rollo, 1959), Prothidium (RAY & MALHOTRA, 1960), Berenil (Killick-Kendrick, 1964) and Ethidium (Riou, 1967).

Nucleosides

Ormerod (1951) and Newton (1957, 1958, 1960) provided a valuable lead to the mode of action of Antrycide and Ethidium, and related drugs, by showing that they may act by interference with nucleic acid synthesis. Newton's demonstration that Antrycide and its pyrimidyl moiety inhibit purine incorporation into the nucleic acid of the trypanosomatid flagellate *Crithidia* (*Strigomonas*) *oncopelti*, focussed attention on what may be a significant but so far largely neglected biochemical consequence of parasitism in trypanosomes, the apparent inability of at least three important pathogens to synthesize the purine ring. *T. rhodesiense* requires preformed adenine (Williamson & Rollo, 1952), adenylic and ribonucleic acids have a stimulant effect on *T. cruzi* (Little & Olesen, 1951; Citri & Grossowicz, 1955) which is unable to synthesize its own adenine (Fernandez & Castellani, 1958), and *T. vivax* cannot synthesize nucleic acid from glycine (Newton, 1965). According to Guttman and Wallace (1964) '. . . Inability to synthesize purines *de novo* from glycine is emerging as a general property of the *Trypanosomatidae*, the block being somewhere between glycine and synthesis of the last imidazole precursor.'

The implications of this deficiency in terms of dependence on exogenous sources of vital adenine-containing cell constituents, other than nucleic acids, such as adenosine polyphosphates (ATP, ADP), and flavinadenine (FAD) and nicotinamide-adenine (NAD) dinucleotide coenzymes, suggest that this is a vulnerable area in the trypanosome which might be attacked preferentially to the host cell in accordance with the requirements of effective chemotherapy. The apparent success of the analysis of Puromycin aminonucleoside activity against *T. cruzi* in terms of adenine antagonism (Fernandes & Castellani, 1959), demonstrable also in *T. equiperdum* (Hewitt, Gumble, Wallace & Williams, 1954; Agosin & von Brand, 1954), was the first indication that therapeutic exploitation of a specifically trypanosomal metabolic deficiency might be feasible. The mechanism of action of Puromycin as a specific inhibitor of cellular protein synthesis, has been subsequently specified with some precision as the details of protein assembly on the ribosome have become established. 'Messenger' RNA (m-RNA), carrying genetic instruction from nuclear DNA, directs the order of assembly on the 'polysome' group of ribosomes, of incoming amino acids, each esterified to a specific soluble or 'transfer' RNA (t-RNA). Puromycin, as a close structural analogue of aminoacyladenosine, the terminus of 'charged' t-RNA, causes release of nascent peptides from the t-RNA bound to ribosomes, apparently by taking part in and terminating the peptide bond-forming reaction (*cf.* Bretscher & Marker, 1966).

Cell-free extracts of *C. oncopelti* (Chesters, 1966; Cross, 1966, 1968) and *C. fasciculata* (Kahan, Zahalsky & Hutner, 1968) have been used to construct ribosomal protein synthesis systems which appear to resemble the chloramphenicol-resistant 80*S* ribosomal models typical of mammalian cells, rather than the chloramphenicol-sensitive 70*S* ribosomal systems of bacterial cells, except that they are more sensitive to magnesium ion. The crithidial systems are sensitive to Puromycin, but inhibition of ribosomal protein synthesis seems unlikely to be the primary locus of trypanocidal action. The aminonucleoside of Puromycin is more actively trypanocidal than Puromycin (*see* p. 194) and also has greater antitumour activity (Olesen, Bennet, Halliday & Williams, 1955) although it has little effect on protein synthesis (Decker, Franz & Franz, 1964; Farnham & Dubin, 1967; Taylor & Stanners, 1968). The effects of Puromycin aminonucleoside on the Krebs cycle of the kidney cell, which have been adduced as a possible basis for the nephrosis induced by the drug (Yoshida, Yamashita & Metcoff, 1968), do not seem to be relevant to its trypanocidal action, and an increasing amount of evidence from its effects, and effects of analogues, on nucleic acid and nucleotide metabolism favours some form of competition with adenosine or a related metabolite.

Almost all of this evidence derives from analyses of the mode of action of antitumour adenosine nucleosides on tumour cells; its relevance to trypanocidal action is enhanced by (a) the similarity of metabolism of tumour cells and pathogenic trypanosomes (high rate of aerobic glycolysis resulting from an inefficient or non-functional mitochondrial system), (b) the antitumour activity of many established trypanocidal drugs, (c) the trypanocidal activity of several active antitumour adenine nucleosides related to Puromycin aminonucleoside, such as Cordycepin (Williamson, 1966), Nucleocidin (Tobie, 1957) and Tubercidin (7-deaza-adenosine) (Williamson, 1969) and (d) the reversal by adenine or adenosine of both trypanocidal and antitumour action (Hewitt *et al.*, 1954; Rich, Meyers, Weinbaum, Cory & Suhadolnick, 1965).

Puromycin aminonucleoside, Cordycepin and Tubercidin are readily phosphorylated in the cell to analogues of the nucleotides AMP, ADP and ATP (adenosine mono- di- and triphosphate) (Farnham & Dubin, 1967; Klenow, 1963; Acs, Reich & Mori, 1964), and Tubercidin has been shown to be incorporated, in place of adenosine, into bacterial NAD and hence to interfere with NAD-dependent glycolytic processes. The rapid inhibition of respiration and glycolysis of *T. rhodesiense* by low concentrations of Cordycepin (10^{-6}–10^{-7}M) (Williamson, 1966) suggests that interference with vital nucleotide coenzyme formation and function may well be significant for its trypanocidal action. A less rapid but equally damaging metabolic lesion may be the effects of incorporation of the active nucleosides into trypanosomal DNA and RNA as occurs in bacterial and tumour cells with both Cordycepin and Tubercidin (Fox, Watanabe & Bloch, 1966); inhibition of DNA and RNA function could be responsible for the aberrant multinuclear, multifissile forms of *T. rhodesiense* and *T. congolense* produced *in vivo* by Cordycepin treatment (Williamson, 1966). A lesion in the fine structure of *T. rhodesiense*, specifically produced by Puromycin, Puromycin aminonucleoside and Cordycepin, is the formation of large 'cytoplasmic clefts' which seem to be associated with the dissolution of endoplasmic membranes, promoted perhaps by the proliferation of lysosomes which appear in areas adjacent to the clefts (Macadam & Williamson, 1969); the metabolic basis of this unique lesion is as yet undetermined, but a superficial similarity to atheromatous plaque formation in blood vessel walls suggests interference with membrane lipid components.

The mode of action of Nucleocidin is less well-documented than the other antitumour nucleosides, but its inhibition of ribosomal protein synthesis differs from that of Puromycin (Florini *et al.*, 1966). In trypanosomes, its primary effect on fine structure is to produce a characteristic fragmentation of the nucleolus into the nucleoplasm with exaggerated peripheral clumping of nuclear chromatin (Macadam & Williamson, 1969). This lesion closely resembles those produced in various mammalian and tumour cells by drugs known specifically to interfere with nucleic acid synthesis, especially by inactivation of the DNA template primer of RNA polymerase, the enzyme which catalyses RNA formation (Simard & Bernhard, 1966; Lewin & Moscarello, 1968); this group of drugs includes the trypanocides acriflavine, Ethidium and Puromycin aminonucleoside. As the nucleolus is now considered to be the site of ribosomal RNA synthesis, the suggestive correlation of specific effects on structure and function indicated by these results is of great interest in view of a recent syncretic survey of the mode of action of drugs affecting nucleic acid metabolism (Waring, 1968). The recent demonstration (Siev, Weinberg & Penman, 1969) of selective inhibition of nucleolar ribosomal RNA synthesis by Cordycepin indicates that this site may be a primary locus of attack also for Nucleocidin and perhaps all active nucleoside drugs.

Ethidium

Biophysical observations on the interaction of acridines and DNA (Lerman, 1961; Brenner, Barnett & Crick, 1961) suggested that the intercalation of acridines between adjacent base-pairs in the DNA helix could be responsible, by consequent disturbance of base-pair sequence, for the known mutagenic effects of acridines; this effect could obviously have some relevance to their trypanocidal action. Lerman (1961) indicated that the mechanism could also accommodate large polycyclic compounds such as dibenzacridine, and stated that 'it is tempting to consider the well known requirements of planarity for the carcinogenic activity of polycyclic aromatic hydrocarbons . . . in terms of an intercalated complex with DNA'; an obvious extension of the mechanism in trypanocidal terms was to the planar phenanthridinium drugs (Williamson, 1962), also known to form complexes with DNA (Brownlee *et al.*, 1950; Seaman & Woodbine, 1955).

Following the demonstration by Elliott (1963) that Ethidium bromide inhibited a bacterial DNA-primed DNA polymerase at concentrations which Newton (1957) had shown to inhibit DNA synthesis in *C. oncopelti*, and that it formed a metachromatic complex with DNA, Waring (Fuller & Waring, 1964; Waring, 1964, 1965, a, 1966, a, 1968) proceeded to show that the effects of Ethidium on nucleic acid synthesis *in vivo* and *in vitro* were probably a direct consequence of the physical binding of the drug to DNA or RNA; strong primary binding occurs by intercalation between adjacent base-pairs of the double helical structure, while some secondary binding can occur by the tangential 'stacking' interaction known also to occur with acridine dyes. In addition, a survey of the sensitivity of a bacterial RNA polymerase system to a large variety of antibacterial and trypanocidal drugs (Waring, 1965) showed that the most active inhibitors, apart from Actinomycin D and proflavine (which were already known to be active), were Ethidium, Prothidium and suramin, all giving 100% inhibition at concentrations near 10^{-5}M; Antrycide and pentamidine, which gave substantial inhibition, precipitated the DNA primer at inhibitory concentrations in the range 10^{-2} to 10^{-3}M. The comparability of these concentrations with those known to affect the infectivity of *T. rhodesiense* and *T. congolense in vitro* (Williamson, 1969) suggests that this enzyme is an important locus for the secondary lethal action of the active metal-free trypanocides. Examination of the effects of some members of this group of drugs on the fine structure of *T. rhodesiense* lends support to the thesis, in the light of the nucleolar structure-function correlation established by Simard and Bernhard (1966). Acriflavine fragmented nucleolar chromatin more extensively than that of the nucleus or kinetoplast, although both of these were affected; Cordycepin and pentamidine also fragmented the nucleolus, although pentamidine, like acriflavine, caused in addition, severe damage to the kinetoplast chromatin core.

Despite this simplification, the mode of action of both Ethidium and Antrycide is still far from total elucidation. Since Newton's demonstration, in 1957, that Ethidium specifically inhibited crithidial DNA synthesis, the drug has been increasingly widely used as a metabolic tool, and has shown activity and use in a number of unexpected ways. Closely-related compounds had greater antiphage and antiviral than antibacterial activity (DICKINSON, CHANTRILL, INKLEY & THOMPSON, 1953) and Gram-negative bacteria were more susceptible than Gram-positive. Ethidium inhibits DNA synthesis preferentially in *E. coli*, as in *C. oncopelti*, but in the Gram-positive *B. cereus*, DNA and RNA synthesis are both inhibited (Tomchick & Mandel, 1964); there was no evidence for the intracellular 'compartmentation' suggested by Kandaswamy and Henderson (1962, 1963) for the action of Ethidium on tumour cells, where inhibition of incorporation of exogenous purines was observed in the absence of inhibition of nucleic acid biosynthesis *de novo* from endogenous substrates. Ethidium treatment eliminates the extrachromasomal elements responsible for transferable antibiotic resistance in enteric bacteria (Bouanchaud, Scavizzi & Chabbert, 1969). In yeasts, Ethidium inhibits nucleic acid synthesis preferentially (Kerridge, 1958) and irreversible photosensitized inhibition of animal viruses by Ethidium can occur (Vilagines & Atanasiu, 1967; Content & Cogniaux-Leclerc, 1968) mainly by binding to native DNA. Analysis of the mechanism of intercalation with DNA by Ethidium has had two useful practical results: the altered drug binding by the closed circular molecules characteristic of mitochondrial (and kinetoplast) DNA (*cf.* Newton, 1968) has allowed their selective isolation by centrifugal methods (Hudson & Vinograd, 1967; Bauer & Vinograd, 1968), and the enhanced fluorescence of DNA-Ethidium complexes has been used as a basis for an analytical assay method for nucleic acids (Van Dyke & Szustkiewicz, 1968).

So far, no specific nucleolar damage has been demonstrable in trypanosomes from Ethidium-treated animals, despite the demonstration of selective inhibition of bacterial DNA and RNA polymerases by Ethidium and of nucleolar changes which the drug induces in HeLa cells (Newton, 1964). The binding of Ethidium, like acriflavine, to DNA is not affected by base composition, except possibly at very low levels of binding (LePecq & Paoletti, 1967; Waring, 1966), so that preferential attack (as occurs with the diamidines) on kinetoplast DNA, known to have a base composition differing from that of nuclear DNA, might not be expected; the possible irrelevance of this prediction is stressed by the predilection of acriflavine for trypanosome kinetoplast DNA (Steinert & van Assel, 1967), the selective loss of kinetoplast DNA in Ethidium-treated *T. cruzi* (Riou, 1968) and the preferential inhibition by acriflavine and Ethidium of the mitochondrial, rather than the nuclear, DNA polymerase of rat liver cells (Meyer & Simpson, 1969). Other considerations, such as differential binding to the closed circular DNA of kinetoplast/mitochondrion structures, lack of the DNA-bound protein, histone, in the kinetoplast (Steinert, 1965) which might facilitate drug-binding in preference to the histone-containing nuclear DNA, and the ever-adduced but so far amorphous 'selective membrane permeability' mechanisms, cannot be excluded. Ribosomal aggregation (*cf.* Newton, 1964) does not seem to be of primary importance and Ethidium treatment does not induce cytoplasmic 'chemotherapy granules' as readily as other cationic trypanocides (Ormerod & Shaw, 1963).

The 'compartmented' action of Ethidium and other related drugs like Dimidium and Prothidium, on tumour cell DNA synthesis (Kandaswamy & Henderson, 1962, 1963; Henderson, 1963) was exploited effectively by showing that azaserine, a selective inhibitor of *de novo* purine biosynthesis, acted as a strongly potentiative synergist with Ethidium on ascites tumour growth (Kandaswamy & Henderson, 1962b), presumably effecting a concurrent blockade of purine nucleotide supply for nucleic acid synthesis; during the course of this work, the important observation was made that Ethidium was not metabolized by either normal or tumour tissue, so that the observed effects were due to the intact drug molecule (Kandaswamy & Henderson, 1963a). The differential inhibition of DNA synthesis observed in tumour cells is not found in *C. oncopelti*, and apparently not in trypanosomes, as a combination of azaserine with Ethidium produces no increased trypanocidal activity (Williamson, 1966a).

Kandaswamy and Henderson's demonstration of the antitumour activity of phenanthridinium derivatives has stimulated renewed interest in their distribution in animal tissues and cells, and in their mode of action against tumour cells. As emphasized in an earlier review (Williamson, 1962), much of this work is very relevant to trypanocidal action, in view of the metabolic similarities of tumour cells and pathogenic trypanosomes, and of the known susceptibility of tumours to trypanocidal agents such as styrylquinoliniums, diamidines and diguanidines and phthalanilides (*cf.* Philips *et al.*, 1967). Prior to a clinical trial of Samorin (p. 180) against leukaemia in man, Philips *et al.* (1967) reported an intensive study of the tissue and intracellular localization of the drug in rats, dogs and monkeys. Hydrolysis to Ethidium at the acid-labile triazeno group (*see* p. 185) occurred only in rats given the drug by intragastric intubation; parenteral dosage did not give rise to detectable amounts of Ethidium in any of the treated animals. Intracellular drug location by fluorescence, which mainly distinguished nuclear and cytoplasmic sites, differed considerably in various tissues; the variation in many cases could be ascribed to diffusion artefacts resulting in apparent nuclear localization. Subcellular fractionation of liver cells from drug-treated animals showed that the drug was predominantly localized in the lysosomal and mitochondrial fractions, corresponding to the fluorescent cytoplasmic 'granule' appearance of intact cells.

Antrycide

The mode of action of Antrycide has been studied intensively by Newton, using *C. oncopelti* and *C. fasciculata*, and the main results of his investigations have been embodied in a valuable review (Newton, 1966). Briefly, Antrycide differs considerably from Ethidium in not acting primarily on DNA synthesis or on the DNA-primed synthesis of RNA; it apparently reduces growth rate by aggregating and inactivating cytoplasmic ribosomes, from which essential magnesium ion and polyamines are displaced by the drug. This result with the crithidial system is consistent with observations of the action of Antrycide on pathogenic trypanosomes where, as with suramin, trypanocidal action is the resultant of at least two effects, damage and inhibited growth caused by the drug, and the consequent promotion of increased susceptibility to the host's immune defence system. Antrycide action on crithidia however, resembles that of Ethidium on tumour cells, in showing a 'compartmented' inhibition of RNA synthesis; it inhibits the synthesis of RNA from exogenous purines, but not the synthesis of DNA or RNA from purines synthesized *de novo*. Curiously enough, Antrycide has no effect on the adenine metabolism of tumour cells (Kandaswamy & Henderson, 1962). Structural dissection of Antrycide showed that selective inhibition of the incorporation of exogenous adenine, and of the aggregation of ribosomes in the crithidial system, were specific properties of the intact molecule. Antrycide, unlike Ethidium, is not a flat molecule and therefore intercalation into helical nucleic acid seems improbable; this assumption is supported by Waring's (1965) results which show that Antrycide inhibits RNA polymerase significantly only at concentrations which precipitate the DNA primer.

Experiments with *T. vivax* from African cattle (Newton, 1965) showed that although this trypanosome, like *T. rhodesiense*, cannot make its own adenine, the incorporation of exogenous adenine is not inhibited, but stimulated, by Antrycide; this effect, perhaps unexpected from the results on the crithidial system, has a suggestive parallel in the work of Waring (1965) where Antrycide and its hybrid Prothidium at low concentrations, showed a characteristic stimulation of AMP incorporation; this inexplicable effect, which also occurred with suramin, would seem to be of considerable interest and significance in trypanocidal action.

The complexity of the action of Antrycide, as revealed in these experiments, is further compounded by the observation (Newton, 1966) that a minor fraction of the crithidial total cell DNA synthesis from exogenous adenine was highly sensitive to Antrycide inhibition, suggesting that this fraction might be kinetoplast DNA. As with the demonstrations mentioned earlier, of selective inhibition of kinetoplast DNA synthesis by acriflavine and Berenil, this effect may be due to any or all of at least five possible factors (*cf.* Steinert & van Assel, 1967; Newton, 1968), none of which has yet been fully investigated. Interspecific differences in the drug reactivity of the kinetoplast can also occur; according to Mühlpfordt (1959) acriflavine causes direct expulsion of the kinetoplast in *T. lewisi* and *T. congolense* but disintegrates it in *brucei*-group trypanosomes; there is no effect on the kinetoplast of *T. cruzi*.

Suramin

The mode of action of suramin remains enigmatic even after more than a half-century of use, despite the intermittent attention of several groups of workers dating from ROEHL (1926) who, in reporting briefly the course of eleven years' work, delineated most of the important aspects of suramin action. He showed that suramin (a) *in vitro* affected trypanosome infectivity but not motility, (b) showed initially reversible binding to trypanosomes, (c) induced cytoplasmic granule formation, (d) combined with basic cellular proteins such as protamines and (e) depended on an intact host defence system for effective trypanocidal action. Subsequent work, reviewed by Findlay (1950), has added little to these observations, but some of the results are now of suggestive significance in the light of current knowledge of cell biology. Although suramin at concentrations up to 10^{-2}–10^{-3} M has little or no effect, even after several hours' exposure, on the motility, respiration or glycolysis of blood forms of African trypanosomes, the infectivity is slowly affected at concentrations as low as 10^{-5} M (Jancsó & Jancsó, 1934; Hawking, 1939; Dixon & Williamson, unpublished results). With this estimate as a basis, the significance of experiments on isolated enzyme systems can be assessed to some extent. The most sensitive enzymes examined appear to be hyaluronidase, inhibited at 10^{-5}–10^{-6} M (Beiler & Martin, 1948), fumarase, inhibited at *ca.* 10^{-7} M (Quastel, 1931b), urease at *p*H 5 (*ca.* 10^{-4} M), hexokinase (10^{-4}–10^{-5} M) (Town, Wills & Wormall, 1949b; Wills & Wormall, 1949) and RNA polymerase (10^{-5} M; stimulation at 10^{-6} M) (Waring, 1965).

Quastel's results are of particular interest in showing that the trypanocidal activity, fumarase inhibition and cotton substantivity of the series of symmetrical urea-linked *m*-aminobenzoyl structures composing the suramin molecule (*see* p. 134 and p. 140) increase *pari passu* as the number of these structures increases. The structural factor common to the drug-susceptible locus of trypanosomes, the active centre of fumarase and the configuration of cotton cellulose has still to be determined; investigations on the cotton substantivity of dyes (e.g. Bach, Pfeil, Philippar & Reich, 1963), which suggest that the mechanism involves incorporation of dye aggregates into the inner spaces of cellulose micelles, do not shed much light on the lethal locus of suramin in trypanosomes, and no fumarase is detectable in blood forms of *T. rhodesiense* (W. E. Gutteridge, personal communication). Four closely-related dyes of the suramin type, Trypan Blue, Azovan Blue, Pontamine Sky Blue 5BX and Pontamine Sky 6BX form two pairs, the first two having the same central dimethylbenzidine moiety and the last two, the same dimethoxybenzidine moiety, with one member of each pair being the *bis*-3,6-disulphonate and the other, the *bis*-2,4-disulphonate salt. In both pairs, only the *bis*-3,6-disulphonate is trypanocidal; it is also the member most strongly adsorbed on cellulose (Williamson & Rollo, 1959), possibly because of solubility differences between the two salt types which would affect their adsorbability on both protein and cellulose structures. The enhancement of cotton substantivity in azo dyes by the *s*-triazine nucleus

(Bradley, 1958) suggests a further link between trypanocidal action and affinity for cellulose.

Adsorbability to protein, especially plasma proteins, accounts for the long retention and consequent trypanoprophylactic activity of suramin, but this property may also be highly significant for drug transport into the cell. As Quastel (1931a) noted, dyes like Methyl Violet and Congo Red are more cytotoxic when protein-bound, suggesting the possibility '. . . that the presence of the protein has an effect on the permeability of the cell, making the entry of the dyestuff easier. . . .' This prescient observation has subsequently been validated by later work on pinocytosis, now known to be especially inducible by proteins and cationic dyes. JANCSÓ AND JANCSÓ-GABOR (1952) first showed that intracellular suramin could be localized histochemically in cytoplasmic granules which accumulated first in the epithelial cells of the proximal tubules of the kidney of treated rodents, and later in reticulo-endothelial cells; the drug was present in protein-bound form, and in the kidney, was assumed to arise from reabsorption of drug-carrying plasma protein. The granules observed would correspond to the phagosome-lysosome vesicles into which suramin now appears to be taken up both in mammalian cells and trypanosomes (*see* p. 197); suramin alone, as an anion, would be unlikely to stimulate endocytosis, so that its entry is presumably facilitated by carrier plasma protein. In rat liver cells, Smeesters and Jacques (1968) showed that suramin treatment markedly decreased the activities of the lysosomal enzymes β-glycerophosphatase, β-*N*-acetylamino-deoxyglucosidase (β-*N*-acetylglucosaminidase) and β-glucuronidase, but not of β-galactosidase, acid maltase or the protease cathepsin D. The greater activity *in vitro* of suramin on enzymes such as urease at *p*H 5 than at *p*H 7 (Town *et al.*, 1949) accords with its activity on the lysosomal acid hydrolases, and in general, the strong affinity of suramin for protein suggests that its enzyme-inhibitory effects are the result of binding to free cationic amino acid residues in the area of the active centre. An effect of this sort on the protein of the suramin-sensitive RNA polymerase (Waring, 1965) would seem more likely than an inactivation of the DNA primer, perhaps by competitive binding as a polyanionic inhibitor (Bernfeld, 1963), at the site of DNA attachment; a similar large anionic molecule, polyvinyl sulphate has recently been shown to compete with m-RNA for attachment to ribosomes (Shinozawa, Yahara & Imahori, 1968).

The structural requirements for protein-binding and consequent persistence in suramin-type molecules were examined by Spinks (1948) who showed that the property was not a sole prerequisite for trypanocidal activity and was apparently to be found in any symmetrical high-molecular-weight compound with polysulphonic acid end groups. No hydrolysis of suramin *in vivo* was detectable and in this respect it differs from its *bis*-azo analogues such as Trypan Blue, Evans Blue (Azovan Blue), Afridol Blue and Niagara Blue 2B which Lloyd *et al.* (1968) found to inhibit rat liver lysosomal enzyme acid phosphatase *in vitro*; further demonstration of the probable interaction of these dyes with lysosomal enzymes *in vivo* is complicated both by the chemical heterogeneity of the azo dyes and by their susceptibility to *in vivo* hydrolysis.

Among the many biological activities of suramin, such as its anticoagulant and anticomplementary properties, its 'protuberculous' effect may be of considerable relevance to trypanocidal action. REES AND D'ARCY HART (1956) showed that suramin treatment markedly enhanced mouse tuberculosis, and that this effect was probably associated with drug localization in macrophage cells. Certain surface-active polyoxyethylene ethers showed the same effect; neither these compounds nor suramin had any growth-inhibiting or enhancing effect on the tubercle bacillus *in vitro*. Some members of the polyoxyethylene series, such as the non-ionic detergent WR-1339, were antituberculous, anti-leishmanial and trypanocidal, and as all the agents, including suramin, tend to localize in lysosomes, varying interaction with macrophage lysosomal constituents has been postulated to account for the pro- and anti-tuberculous effects, now also demonstrable in infected macrophages *in vitro* (Hart, 1968). The activity *in vitro* of the polyene antifungal antibiotic Amphotericin B against *T. congolense* (Actor *et al.*, 1962) is demonstrable *in vivo* only after blockade of the reticulo-endothelial system; this drug, like suramin and the polyoxyethylene drugs, is sequestered in reticulo-endothelial cells, but in addition, is known to affect cell membranes specifically by interaction with the sterol components which are essential for membrane stability. Although unlikely to be of clinical value in trypanosomiasis, polyene antibiotics of this type may also prove useful tools to dissect the lysosome-drug-parasite complex.

Nitrofurazone

Nitrofurazone (p. 159) appears to operate by virtue of the readily reducible 5-nitro substituent. Much work, mainly on bacterial systems, indicates that the antibacterial activity at least, is related to this ability to act as an electron acceptor (Asnis & Gots, 1951; Brodie & Gots, 1952; Gots, Jordan & Brodie, 1952) which may interrupt NAD oxido-reduction (Asnis, 1957). The enzyme-inhibiting activity is fairly specific, as furacin, unlike the organic arsenicals, is not generally thiol-reactive (Green, Heath & Yall, 1951; Yall & Green, 1952). A similar interference mechanism possibly operates in its trypanocidal action, though this has not yet been demonstrated. A possibly cogent observation is that of von Brand, Tobie, Mehlman and Weinbach (1953) who found that an arsenic-resistant strain of *T. gambiense* showed a hypersensitivity to nitrofurans. This might imply that there had been an alteration in the oxidative metabolism of the resistant strain, and some evidence for an alteration of this kind (in dehydrogenase activity) has in fact been found in a Melarsen-fast strain of *T. rhodesiense* (Williamson, 1953). The decreased sensitivity to glyceraldehyde inhibition of the oxygen uptake of an arsenic-fast *T. gambiense* (von Brand *et al.*, 1953) might suggest that the active glycerophosphate-NADH oxidase system of Grant and Sargent (1960a, 1960b) could be a locus of enzymic alteration induced by drug-resistance. Oxidative alterations of this kind have already been suggested as a common factor in the otherwise inexplicable cross-resistance which develops between acriflavine and aromatic arsenicals (Williamson & Rollo, 1959).

Miscellaneous Observations

The reaction to drugs of culture and tsetse midgut forms of trypanosomes has not been studied extensively. Hawking (1963a) has repaired this omission in studies on *T. congolense*, *T. vivax* and *T. rhodesiense* using both *in vitro* cultures and mixtures of drug and cow blood fed to *G. palpalis*. In general, culture forms of *T. rhodesiense* and *T. congolense* were much less sensitive than the bloodstream forms to pentavalent and trivalent arsenicals, suramin, Berenil, Antrycide, Ethidium, Prothidium or Samorin. All the 'cattle' drugs were inactive at 0·1–1·0 mg./ml. on *in vitro* cultures and were lethal to *T. vivax* in the fly at concentrations of 0·1 mg./ml. (approximately 10^{-2}–10^{-3} M); Ethidium was toxic to the fly at 0·03 mg./ml. and below this concentration was not trypanocidal. Lehmann (1964) obtained similar results with suramin, tryparsamide, Melarsen and Mel W on cultures of *T. brucei* and *T. rhodesiense*, although the former appeared much more susceptible to tryparsamide and Melarsen than the latter.

The successful demonstration that the antimalarial activity of 2,4-diamino-pyrimidine compounds such as Daraprim (pyrimethamine) and Trimethoprim depends on specific inhibition of the malaria parasite enzyme, dihydrofolate reductase (Ferone, Burchall & Hitchings, 1969), has stimulated an intensive study of the distribution of this enzyme in the genus *Trypanosoma* (Gutteridge, Jaffe & McCormack, 1968) with a view to possible therapeutic exploitation. The sensitivity of the trypanosomal reductases to representative 2,4-diaminopyri-midine inhibitors was of a distinctly different pattern from that typical of the mammalian or bacterial enzyme, and within this pattern, the African trypano-somes differed from those of non-African origin. So far, none of the available inhibitors shows trypanocidal activity *in vivo*, but the search for new compounds to inhibit this enzyme, which is concerned in DNA synthesis, may well reveal active trypanocides.

The numerous and necessarily speculative points raised in the above dis-cussion of trypanocidal drug action are now mostly capable of experimental verification with currently available techniques and data from related fields of cell biochemistry. Given the necessary attention, this largely neglected but important field should yield results of considerable value, not only for an understanding both of trypanocidal drug action and of trypanosomal meta-bolism, but for cell biology in general.

DRUG RESISTANCE

Cross-resistance

The preceding sections give some indication of the complexity of drug action analysis in terms of drug constitution, and of enzyme inactivation, considered as the end stage of the parasiticidal reaction. Knowledge of the earlier stages of trypanocidal action, where reversible drug adsorption occurs in many cases, has largely been inferred from cross-resistance studies. This kind of analysis, initiated by Ehrlich over half a century ago, uses resistant strains as 'therapeutic sieves,' on Ehrlich's analogy, to sift out any common factors of activity not otherwise apparent among unrelated drug types (*see* p. 131).

An accumulation of the data of Ehrlich and his collaborators, Yorke *et al.* (1930, 1931a), Lourie and Yorke (1938), King and Strangeways (1942), Williamson and Rollo (1952), Fulton and Grant (1955), Schnitzer and Grunberg

(1957), Hawking (1958), Williamson and Rollo (1959) and Williamson (1966 and unpublished results) is presented in condensed form in Table 7.3.

Apart from the obvious absence of experimental data in some cases, Table 7.3 is incomplete in several other respects, and the more extended versions given by Schnitzer and Grunberg (1957) and Williamson and Rollo (1959) should be consulted for more specific detail on individual drugs. Nevertheless, Table 7.3 shows clearly that cross-resistance behaviour is not wholly explicable on an ionic basis. The possibilities of variation due to the use of strains of different origin (Goble, Ferrell and Stieglitz, 1959) have been reduced by the use of a single parent strain of *T. rhodesiense* in the study by Williamson and Rollo on which Table 7.3 is largely based. The latter workers showed that major inconsistencies in an ionic theory of drug resistance included (a) a marked difference in cross-resistance towards neutral aromatic arsenicals, aliphatic diamidines and quinapyramine between strains made resistant to the cationic metal-free drugs Surfen C and stilbamidine, (b) the restriction of cross-resistance to neutral aromatic arsenicals and Antrycide only, in a strain resistant to the cationic metal-free acriflavine, (c) the lack of complete cross-resistance among the members of the group of anionic trypanocides, and (d) the cross-resistance of the cationic stilbamidine-resistant strain to the anionic benzidine azo trypanocides. Similar inconsistencies in an ionic interpretation of resistance mechanisms have been noted by Wagner, Pedal and Schöneberger (1954).

Although amidine-type linkages form a common structural factor in the melaminyl arsenicals, the diamidines, the Surfens and Cinnoline 528, it is difficult to construct an appropriate receptor structure, common to these drugs, modification or loss of which would account for all the observed facts. An example is the ability of the Surfen C-fast strain to distinguish between aliphatic and aromatic diamidines, unlike the closely-related stilbamidine- and Melarsen-fast strains; in addition, strains resistant to one or other of the two types of diamidines differ in their sensitivity to neutral aromatic arsenicals, and it has been suggested (Williamson & Rollo, 1959) that this difference reflects the differing mode of action of aliphatic and aromatic diamidines observed on trypanosomes *in vitro* (Marshall, 1948). Some inconsistencies in the resistance behaviour of anionic and cationic drugs may be resolved by the assumption of ribonucleoprotein as a receptor site (Ormerod, 1951b) where the former drugs could be adsorbed by protein and the latter by nucleic acid; this site may represent a preliminary fixation receptor, rather than the locus of final lethal action (Ormerod, 1961).

Resistance to melaminyl arsenicals seems to be associated with changes in enzymic oxidative mechanisms (Williamson, 1953); Tobie and von Brand (1953) have also found that a tryparsamide-fast strain of *T. gambiense* showed some hypersensitivity to nitrofurazone which apparently acts by oxidation (*see* p. 210). The well known cross-resistance between aromatic arsenicals and acriflavine may have a basis in the known susceptibility to several oxidizing agents of the group of antibacterial 2-aminoacridines which includes acriflavine; bacteria become resistant to this group of acridines but not to other derivatives which are resistant to these oxidizing agents (Albert, 1951b). A relation between trypanocidal activity and oxidation-reduction potential can be demonstrated

Cross-resistance analysis of trypanocidal drugs

Drug group	Drug	Ionization at blood *p*H	Response of strain resistant to								
			Atoxyl	Acri-flavine	Mel-arsen	Stilba-midine	Surfen C	Quina-pyramine[1]	Butarsen	Suramin	Benzidine azo dyes
Neutral aromatic arsenicals, antimonials	Atoxyl	Feeble	+	+	+	+	−	−	+	−	+
Nitrofurans	Nitrofurazone		−			−				−	
2, 8-Diamino-acridines	Acriflavine	Cationic	+	+	+	+	+	+(1) −(2)	+	−	−
Melaminyl arsenicals, antimonials	Melarsen		−	−	+	+	+		−	−	−
(a) Aliphatic and (b) aromatic diguanidines, diamidines	(a) Synthalin		−	−	+	+	−		−	−	−
	(b) Stilbamidine		−	−	+	+	+	+(1) −(2)	−	−	−
6-Amino-quinoline-type	Surfen C		−	−	−	+	+		−	−	−
	Quinapyramine		−	+	−	−HS(2)	+	+	−	−	−
	Cinnoline 528		−	−	+	+			−	−	−
Aminophenanthridine-type	Dimidium		−	−	+	+	+	+(1) −(2)	−	−	−
Triphenylmethane dyes	Pararosaniline		−	−	+	+	+		+	−	−
Nucleosides	Puromycin		HS			+				HS	
	Puromycin aminonucleoside		HS			+				HS	
Carboxylated aromatic arsenicals	Butarsen	Anionic	−	−	−	−	−		+	−	−
Sulfonated naphthylamines	Suramin		−	−	−	−HS(2)	−	HS(1), (2)	−	+	−
	Benzidine azo dyes		−	−	−	+	−		−	+	+
Nucleosides	Nucleocidin		−			−				−	

+ = resistant. − = sensitive. HS = hypersensitive. [1] = *T. equiperdum*. (1) = Ormerod, 1952. (2) = Hawking, 1958.

by measuring the effect of a series of redox indicator dyes both on trypanosome motility and on the potentials of oxygen-free suspensions of isolated trypanosomes (Williamson, 1959b); although this property is likely to be important for a number of trypanocides, it is not obviously correlated with drug-resistance behaviour.

An analysis of the *p*H-dependent activity of the ionic trypanocides against normal and drug resistant trypanosomes *in vitro* suggested that this activity was less likely to be due to changes in the proportion of cell-permeable unionized drug molecules, as suggested for Butarsen by Doak and Eagle (1951), than to changes in the ionization of a cell receptor (Williamson, 1959b). The parallelism of the *p*H-activity curves with normal and resistant trypanosomes implied that the relative proportion of these ionic receptors was reduced in the resistant strain. A change of this sort could be caused by a shift in the isoelectric point of trypanosomal protein structures associated with drug uptake, and thus account for resistance to ionic trypanocides as envisaged by Schueler (1947). Electrophoresis of crude trypanosomal 'cytoplasmic' protein gave no evidence of such a shift (Williamson, 1961) although amino acid analysis of normal and stilbamidine-fast *T. rhodesiense* suggested that, in the latter strain, the ratio of 'anionic' to 'cationic' amino acids may be reduced (Williamson & Desowitz, 1961); the hypersensitivity of stilbamidine- and quinapyramine-resistant trypanosomes to the anionic suramin (Ormerod, 1952; Hawking, 1958) and of suramin-fast trypanosomes to the cationic nucleosides (Table 7.3) might be a consequence of this kind of change. Among the nucleoside group of drugs, ionic form appears to correlate with cross-resistance behaviour; the stilbamidine-fast strain, which is predominantly resistant to various cationic drugs (Table 7.3), is also resistant to the cationic Puromycin and its aminonucleoside, but susceptible to the anionic Nucleocidin. The activity of nitrofurazone against this strain may be due to the lipid solubility of the drug, as phenylarsenoxides with lipophilic substituents are known to be active against trypanosomes resistant to aromatic arsenicals with hydrophilic substituents (King & Strangeways, 1942).

The use of selective antagonists, capable of reversing trypanocidal action, has lent further support to the assumption that cellular structures associated with a reversible stereospecific drug adsorption phase are modified during resistance acquirement (Schnitzer & Grunberg, 1957; Williamson, 1959a). Thiols, such as cysteine and glutathione, antagonize neutral, cationic and anionic aromatic arsenicals equally, but do not antagonize the metal-free trypanocides. The neutral oxophenarsine is antagonized selectively by methyl *p*-hydroxybenzoate, but not by sodium *p*-aminobenzoate or melamine. The cationic melaminyl arsenicals are antagonized only by melamine, which also specifically reverses the action of the aliphatic and aromatic diguanidines and diamidines.

Thus each type of arsenical appears to have a different structurally-specific initial attachment site on the trypanosomes, as would appear from the cross-resistance behaviour within this group. The specific melamine antagonism of the melaminyl arsenicals and the diamidines also reflects the cross-resistance between these two important drug groups, suggesting the modification of a common receptor.

The results so far dealt with, have been derived from controlled laboratory experiments, and where applicable, have agreed in the main with clinical observations on human sleeping sickness. Early-stage *T. gambiense* infections with acquired resistance to tryparsamide, for example, have generally been found susceptible to treatment with suramin, diamidines, Butarsen, or melaminyl arsenicals. Cross-resistance between the diamidines and the melaminyl arsenicals has not so far become significant, in view of the difficulty of producing pentamidine-resistance either in the laboratory or in the field, and the, as yet, limited use of Mel B. The activity of Mel B against resistant trypanosomes was demonstrated by Friedheim (1953) in a unique case of human sleeping sickness which had become resistant over a number of years to repeated courses of tryparsamide, pentamidine, Butarsen, suramin and tartar emetic. Later, Friedheim, Geigy and Kauffman (1959) showed that Mel B was also active against the *T. rhodesiense* strain isolated from wild antelope by Heisch, McMahon and Manson-Bahr (1958); this historic strain was infective for man and its insensitivity to tryparsamide was natural, and not artificially acquired.

Cross-resistance behaviour, selective interference, hypersensitivity and synergism appear to be related phenomena in drug action, but compared to extensive studies in antitumour drug action (*cf.* BROCKMAN, 1961), little is known of the last two phenomena in trypanocidal drug action. The occurrence, in trypanosomes resistant to a particular drug, of hypersensitivity to a different drug, can easily be missed in the usual cross-resistance analysis experiment, and so far, the few known examples (Table 7.3) seem to involve suramin particularly. Stilbamidine-fast *T. rhodesiense* is hypersensitive to suramin and Antrycide, and Antrycide-fast *T. equiperdum* is hypersensitive to suramin (Ormerod, 1952; Hawking, 1958). Suramin-fast, and to a less extent, Atoxyl-fast *T. rhodesiense* strains are hypersensitive to Puromycin and its aminonucleoside but not to Nucleocidin. Both Puromycin and its aminonucleoside show potentiative synergic activity with suramin against the normal parent *T. rhodesiense* (Williamson, 1965), and a similar effect, but with additive synergism only, is shown by Puromycin aminonucleoside with neutral aromatic arsenicals (Williamson, 1966b); these categories of synergism are as described by GADDUM (1958). The interlinked hypersensitivity-synergism effects may be related to a change in balance of ionic receptors, as envisaged by Schueler (1947), either at the initial uptake (lysosomal?) stage or at subsequent susceptible enzyme (nucleic acid polymerase?) loci common to several types of drug.

The implied involvement of neutral aromatic arsenicals in this relationship is further supported by experiments which show that suramin and tryparsamide, used in combination for many years for the treatment of sleeping sickness, exhibit additive synergism (Williamson, 1966b), with a distinct bias towards potentiation. The possibilities of treatment with combinations of trypanocidal drugs, or of drugs with metabolic inhibitors (*see* p. 206), have not been extensively explored, and further investigation seems warranted.

The number of drugs active against the *congolense-vivax* trypanosomes has increased rapidly in recent years. In almost all cases, resistance to these drugs is difficult to produce in laboratory animals, and the subinoculation of resistant strains from cattle to small animals is either impossible or attended with changes in resistance; significant knowledge of their resistance behaviour has been obtained mainly from the work of Whiteside (1958a, 1958b, 1960, 1962) on large numbers of East African cattle maintained under controlled conditions. Systematic analysis of the cross-resistance behaviour of curative and prophylactic drugs led Whiteside (1958a, 1958b) to propose a third category, 'sanative' drugs, which are active against strains resistant to other drugs; the distinction is thus solely one of use. Table 7.4 has been constructed on the basis of the results quoted by Whiteside (1960, 1962) for some 1,400 cross-resistance tests done with curative and prophylactic drugs in cattle infected with resistant strains of East African *T. congolense* and *T. vivax*.

TABLE 7.4

Cross-resistance analysis of drugs used in cattle trypanosomiasis

Drug	Response of strain resistant to				
	Antrycide	Ethidium	Prothidium	Metamidium	Berenil
Antrycide	++	±	±	±	—
Ethidium	±	++	++	++	—
Prothidium	+	++	++	+	—
Metamidium	+	±	+	++	—
Berenil	±	±	—	—	++

+ = resistant to curative doses.
++ = resistant to higher doses.
± = partially resistant to curative doses.
— = sensitive to curative doses.

The extended sanative use of Prothidium or Metamidium at high dosage was not advised because their prophylactic properties were liable to induce further resistance development. Berenil and Ethidium were therefore recommended as a 'sanative pair'. Neither is significantly prophylactic, and there is no cross-resistance, either reciprocal or one-sided, between them. An alternative treatment scheme was suggested, whereby one of the pair was used until resistant strains appeared. At this point the second member was substituted for the first until the resistant strains had disappeared from both the cattle and the tsetse, and so on. Preliminary trials were reported to be encouraging (Whiteside, 1960), and practical costed treatment routines were later recommended (Whiteside, 1962a).

The cross-resistance pattern in Table 7.4 indicates the close-knit relationships of the three phenanthridinium derivatives, both among themselves and to Antrycide, as might be expected from structural considerations. Apparently, the inclusion of a portion of the *m*-isomer of Berenil into the Metamidium molecule has prevented the appearance of cross-resistance to Berenil itself in a Metamidium-resistant strain. The one-sided cross-resistance between Antrycide and Berenil which is evident in Table 7.4 is an interesting confirmation in cattle of the similar relation between Antrycide and stilbamidine demonstrated in Table 7.3 with experimental infections in rodents.

A similar cross-resistance analysis of *T. congolense* in mice (Hawking, 1963c) confirmed Whiteside's results in the main, with only minor differences where intermediate grades of resistance were concerned; mouse tests failed to show that Antrycide-fast strains were partly resistant to Berenil. Among other observations in this report, Berenil was found to be very active in mice against newly-isolated strains of *T. rhodesiense*, which are usually resistant to pentamidine (*see* pp. 143) and subsequent clinical tests (*see* pp. 157) have established this activity in human infections; a Mel B-resistant strain of *T. rhodesiense* showed cross-resistance to Berenil, in agreement with the known cross-resistance of a Melarsen-fast strain to other diamidines (Table 7.3). Experiments with '*meta*-Berenil,' Metamidium, and '*para*-Metamidium' showed that cross-resistance behaviour among these compounds was not affected by substitutional changes between the *meta* and *para* positions.

As with other diamidines, resistance to Berenil is difficult to produce by direct exposure in the laboratory or in the field, (Fussgänger & Bauer, 1960; Bauer, 1962; Whiteside, 1963; Hawking, 1963), but it can arise in trypanosomes made resistant to Antrycide. Fortunately for field control, the degree of such Berenil-resistance has not generally been high (Table 7.4) and there is a wide margin between curative and maximum tolerated doses for African cattle. In Northern Nigeria, where Ethidium had been in use for mass treatment since 1955, the prevalence of Ethidium-resistant strains led to its replacement by Berenil in 1965. Subsequently, low levels of Berenil-resistance have been found, mainly in strains of *T. vivax* (MacLennan & Jones-Davies, 1967; Jones-Davies, 1967, 1968).

Drug Resistance and the Immune Response

The effect of the defence mechanisms of the mammalian host on trypanocidal drug action is a large and complex field which has only recently begun to yield to systematic investigation, confined mainly to analysis of the immune response with modern techniques. The effect of the reticulo-endothelial (lymphoid macrophage) system on a number of trypanosome infections was intensively reviewed by Goble and Singer (1960), and there is no doubt that its phagocytic activity is a considerable accessory factor in drug action. Stimulation or depression of the system by anti-organ sera (Goble, Boyd & Singer, 1958) has a marked effect on *T. congolense* in mice, for example, and splenectomy and blockade decrease the effect of such drugs as suramin, Stilbamidine and Antrycide (Findlay, 1950; Sen, Dutta & Ray, 1955; Ormerod, 1961). The action of oxophenarsine is also influenced by phagocytic activity and an immune response, as Cantrell (1955) and Cantrell and Betts (1956) have demonstrated by the use of cortisone in *T. equiperdum* infections of the rat.

As in most other protozoal infections, the immune response in trypanosomiasis is typically weak because of rapid antigenic variation, but it may be of considerable significance for chemotherapy (*see* pp. 175–176).

Indications of the interplay of drug resistance acquirement and the immune response arise from a number of sources, but so far the evidence is fragmentary and suggestive (Schnitzer & Grunberg, 1957; Whiteside, 1962) rather than conclusive. Tobie and von Brand (1953) provided an example, so far unique in trypanosomes, of an association of acquired arsenical resistance and lowered pathogenicity which may have resulted from an altered immune response. Apparent reduction in virulence of trypanosomes which appear on relapse after prophylactic drug treatment, both in cattle (Stephen, 1962c) and in mice (Hill, 1962) may possibly be due to selection of less virulent and more drug-resistant variants. Similarly, strains of *T. congolense* which were resistant to both Ethidium and Berenil, maintained their resistance on fly-passage but appeared to show an unusually long development period in the fly (Gray & Roberts, 1968). Cantrell (1955) showed that *T. equiperdum*, during development of resistance to oxophenarsine passed through a transient intermediate stage in which agglutinating properties develop (Cantrell, 1955). Further work (Cantrell, 1958) on the antigenic analysis of an oxophenarsine-resistant trypanosome population showed that this consisted of a major antigenic type resistant to the arsenical and to tartar emetic, and at least two minor types, one of which was more resistant to tartar emetic than the major type. The characteristic multiplicity of antigenic types which had long been assumed for trypanosomes, was previously invoked by Cantrell and Betts (1956) in a study of the immune response of rats infected with *T. equiperdum* and treated with oxophenarsine; here also a major and one or more minor antigenic types were inferred. Cantrell (1957) also showed that oxophenarsine treatment could produce prolonged immunity so long as an antigenically homologous strain was used for reinfection tests.

Tartar-emetic-resistance cannot be induced directly; a population of trypanosomes already resistant to aromatic arsenicals must be used (Hawking, 1966a). Ercoli (1962) showed that trypanosomes exposed to nitrogen mustard *in vivo* (but not *in vitro*) became resistant to tartar emetic and aromatic arsonates; resistance to the latter was stable, whereas tartar-emetic-resistance was low and transient. Nitrogen mustard treatment induced relapse-variant antibody formation and although immunosuppressive effects were not excluded, the mutagen was considered to have affected trypanosomal genetic structures concerned primarily with aromatic arsonate sensitivity. The cytoplasmic inclusions resembling volutin granules which occur in certain trypanosomes and may be induced by a number of ionic drugs, appear to have some relation to the immune response (Ormerod, 1951a, 1951b, 1952, 1959, 1961a), but their precise function is not yet clear (*see* p. 197).

Some highly suggestive but limited experiments on drug-antibody interaction were made by Szabo (1950) and Soltys (1957, 1959). Szabo (*loc. cit.*) used mouse protection antibodies derived from the sera of rats immunized with the saline-soluble and insoluble portions of lyophilized trypanosomes which had previously been subjected to drug or antibody action. Treatment with inorganic arsenic, acriflavine and Synthalin modified and heightened the antigenic activity of the trypanosomes, and the saline-insoluble portion of the lyophilized parasites, which was non-antigenic in the normal strain, became antigenic (a) after pre-treatment with drug, (b) if obtained from trypanosomes passaged through a guinea pig or dog, or (c) if obtained from a drug-fast strain. The results thus imply that antigenic structures in the parasites are modified by drug or antibody action. Possibly antigenic structures and drug receptors may coincide; in many ways the complex stereospecificity of cross-resistance reactions resembles that of the antigen-antibody reaction. Antigenic structural modification, either as a selective adaptive response to drugs or to antibody, may thus be similar to the structural modification in initial drug fixation receptors postulated earlier as a basis for acquired drug-resistance. The work of Cantrell (1958) suggested a selective process among antigenic variants in the development of oxophenarsine-resistance, and acquired resistance to antibody action in trypanosomes ('Serumfestigkeit') has been familar since the days of Ehrlich.

Further investigations of antibody-resistance development in experimental *T. brucei* infections by Soltys (1957, 1959) revealed that resistance to suramin and Antrycide appeared simultaneously with the acquisition of antibody-resistance, in the absence of any contact with either drug. About fifty times more drug was required for *in vitro* pre-treatment to abolish the infectivity for mice of the antibody-fast strain. Much lower differences (about 3-fold) were found in the therapeutic responses of the two strains in mice, but prophylactic experiments in rabbits showed that protection against challenge by the antibody-fast strain was much less than that against the sensitive strain.

These results agreed with the known acceleration of experimental suramin- and Antrycide-resistance by splenectomy and reticulo-endothelial blockade. The difficulty of producing strains resistant to diamidines such as pentamidine or Berenil, either experimentally in rodents, or in man and domestic stock, suggests that the action of these drugs has less connection with the immune response (*see* also Bauer, 1964). Splenectomy appeared to have no influence on the effect of Berenil on *T. congolense* infections of the rat (Bauer, 1958) and in cattle, curative treatment with Berenil, unlike Antrycide and Ethidium, did not seem to produce much residual protective immunity (Whiteside *et al.*, 1960; Whiteside, 1962) but this view may require modification (Cunningham, 1967). On the other hand, *T. rhodesiense* pre-treated *in vitro* with stilbamidine can produce antibody in the rat (Fulton & Grant, 1956), but prolonged contact of trypanosomes with the drug markedly inhibits their ability to stimulate antibody formation.

The possibility of a relation between virulence, antigenic variation and drug-resistance suggested (Williamson, 1962) that, in human sleeping sickness, the naturally tryparsamide-fast *T. rhodesiense* may in fact be an 'antibody-fast' (or variant) form of *T. gambiense* developed by sojourn in an animal reservoir. In cattle trypanosomiasis, the possibility that drug-resistance contains a considerable component due to antibody-resistance, may renew interest in observations such as those of Morgenroth and Freund (1924) who claimed that small doses of suramin specifically inhibited the ability of *T. brucei* to become serum-resistant. Brown and Williamson (1962) found that suramin treatment of *T. rhodesiense*-infected rats appeared to affect the variant-specific 4*S* antigens of the trypanosome; chronic infections of *T. rhodesiense* in the rabbit became less sensitive to treatment with suramin, as Soltys had described, but not to other drugs such as Antrycide, Ethidium or oxophenarsine. Gray (1966) investigated more intensively this kind of interaction between antigenic variation and drug-resistance, using several variants of clones of *T. brucei*, and found clear differences in their susceptibility to suramin; no such differences were observable with Antrycide or Berenil tests, and examination of a tryparsamide-resistant strain gave no evidence that resistance-acquirement had involved major changes in the antigenic characteristics of the trypanosomes.

Brown and Williamson (1962) found that trypanosome antigenicity ('1*S*' and '4*S*' antigen groups) was associated with the bulk of the soluble cytoplasmic proteins and suggested a possible relation between variant antigens and soluble enzymes to explain the type of drug resistance-immunity interaction described above (*cf.* Turnbull, 1964). Njogu (1967) and Njogu and Humphries (1967, a) have shown that a variety of soluble dehydrogenases and diaphorases are associated with the variable antigens although the identity of antigenic and enzyme active sites remains to be established. Le Page (1967, 1968) examined the peptide structure of the 4*S* antigen proteins and found a remarkable total change of tryptic peptide composition from one antigenic variant to another. The absence of common peptides would imply extensive changes in the primary structure of the soluble antigen proteins; radical changes in enzyme protein activity might also be expected to ensue.

Origin of Drug Resistance

Investigation of the genetic basis of resistance to trypanocides has been limited mainly because of the technical difficulty of isolating resistant individuals and the absence of sexual reproduction. Argument as to the predominance of phenotypic adaptation or mutation-selection processes in resistance development in trypanosomes have thus been even more sterile than in the case of bacteria, and as Szybalski and Bryson (1955) surmised, it seemed likely 'that neither interpretation is tenable as an exclusive theory. Which one is correct depends on the sample. . . . Conceptually, the two theories are opposed, but operationally they may co-exist'. The theory of 'clonal variation with selection' proposed by Yudkin (1953) accounted satisfactorily for most observations on the development of acquired trypanocidal drug resistance, and the probability, which has been discussed above, that structurally specific receptors for the initial uptake of drugs are modified in resistant trypanosomes, may be taken to accord with the thesis of Sevag (1955) that resistance is a manifestation of altered states of enzyme proteins.

The development of an ingenious acriflavine photosensitivity technique (Walker, 1964) opened up a new approach to analysis of drug-resistant populations of trypanosomes. Hawking and Walker (1966) have shown that the development of resistance of *brucei* trypanosomes to the trivalent form of tryparsamide occurred rapidly and by selection of resistant individuals in a freshly-isolated strain, and by a series of steps in an old monomorphic strain, considered to be initially free of resistant individuals. Step-wise appearance of resistance was taken to reflect corresponding discontinuous changes in the genetic material of the trypanosome, and at least one of these spontaneous mutations was considered to be stable. According to Walker (1964), on the basis of analysis of clones prepared from resistant populations, the observations are fitted only by a hypothesis involving a system of diploid expression of the genotype and occasional genetic exchange.

Such genetic exchange has not yet been unequivocally demonstrated. Cross transfer of resistance does not occur between different and easily distinguishable resistant offshoots of the same trypanosome strain when they are mixed *in vitro* or *in vivo* (Amrein, 1957; Amrein & Fulton, 1959; Amrein, 1965, a; Hawking & Walker, 1966), and attempts to induce transformation of drug-sensitive trypanosomes to a drug-resistant form, by incubation with purified DNA from resistant trypanosomes, have produced suggestive but equivocal results (Fulton, 1960a, b). The release of transforming material by ruptured resistant trypanosomes could accelerate resistance development as Szybalski and Bryson (1955) have pointed out, but presumably in the early stages of resistance acquirement *in vivo*, transformation of resistant trypanosomes to drug-sensitivity would be equally, if not more, probable.

CONCLUSION

Tropical Africa is at the beginning of an era of major technological revolution, within which trypanosomiasis control, especially in domestic stock, will continue to demand more effective therapeutic and prophylactic drugs, and to maintain a pressing concern with drug resistance and the immune reaction. The rapid expansion of the pharmaceutical industry has produced the post-war 'drug explosion' (Modell, 1961) in which, of an estimated 140,000 medicaments in current use in 1955, some 75% had been introduced since 1945. Intensified research in related fields of chemotherapy, particularly of anti-cancer agents, where there is much common ground, both in the metabolism of malignant tissues and of pathogenic trypanosomes, and in the types of active drug, is already having considerable influence on the design of new trypanocides.

The extension of knowledge of cell biochemistry and ultrastructure by increased and improved instrumentation, such as the ultracentrifuge, the electron microscope and the use of radio-isotopes and refined chromatographic techniques, is already throwing new light on trypanosomal metabolism and its interaction with drugs. Studies of this kind in combination with the application to trypanosomes of recently developed immunological techniques, are likely to provide an increasingly secure basis for interpretation of drug action; the necessarily speculative nature of its interpretation in the light of current information will have been evident from the relevant section of this review.

So far as parasiticidal drug design is concerned, the era of intelligent empiricism is unlikely to be superseded until the balance of effort and expenditure on drug production is adjusted more favourably in the direction of research on the metabolism of pathogenic parasites and on the mechanisms whereby existing drugs exert their specific effects. In the meantime, in the words of Jensch (1937): 'Es lässt sich darüber streiten, ob man auf der Suche nach neuen Heilmetteln sich mehr von Einfällen oder von dem gesammelten Erfahrungsschatz leiten lassen soll. Eines aber lässt sich nicht bestreiten: dass in jedem Fall sich ein hohes Mass an Geduld hinzugesellen muss.'

Part II

THE INSECT VECTORS: THE GENUS *GLOSSINA*

Chapter 8

The Genus *Glossina*: Introduction

J. P. GLASGOW

MORPHOLOGY

All tsetse flies are very similar in appearance and they are all placed in the genus *Glossina* which comprises twenty-two living species. Four fossil species from the Florissant beds of Colorado have also been assigned to the genus (Buxton, 1955, p. 23). The shape of the adult fly is shown in Fig. 8.1. The smallest and largest species are respectively about 7·5 mm. and 14 mm. long, with puparial weights of 20 mg. and 80 mg. Colours are unremarkable, mottled brown-grey thorax, often with darker bands on the abdominal segments; these dull hues confer, to human eyes at least, effective protective coloration so that when the flies perch on trees and rocks of many different kinds it is not easy to see them. When at rest both wings lie horizontally over the abdomen in such a way that the apices of the two wings coincide, giving the fly a distinctive elongated appearance. In the middle of the wing is a closed cell of a distinctive shape (Figs. 8.1 and 8.3) which a powerful imagination can compare with a butcher's cleaver with the edge facing forwards. This is called the 'hatchet cell', and is a useful diagnostic character which may make it possible to identify badly mangled specimens as being certainly *Glossina*.

It is not proposed to describe the anatomy of *Glossina* in detail but to include only brief descriptions of those structures which have particular relevance to the subject matter of this work. Readers interested in the detailed anatomical structure of *Glossina* are referred to the publications cited below. According to Buxton (1955, p. 7), 'The anatomy of *Glossina* was dealt with in a masterly way by Newstead, Evans and Potts (1924), and under their influence in every subsequent book. Certain parts of the subject have since been elaborated (e.g. the mouth parts by Jobling, 1933; the digestive tract by Wigglesworth, 1929). The internal structure and histology were studied by Stuhlmann (1907). Early papers on internal and external anatomy are dealt with by Hegh (1929).'

In addition to the works cited above, important contributions to the subject have been made (1) by Patton (1934, 1936) whose 'detailed and exact studies' are regarded by Machado (1959) as 'constituting a fundamental contribution' to the knowledge of the morphology of the copulatory organs of *Glossina*; (2) by Machado (1954, 1959) who makes another invaluable contribution to the same subject (*see* also pp. 252–257); (3) by Hoffman (1954) on the intra-uterine development of *Glossina*; (4) by Hagan (1951) on the embryology of *Glossina*;

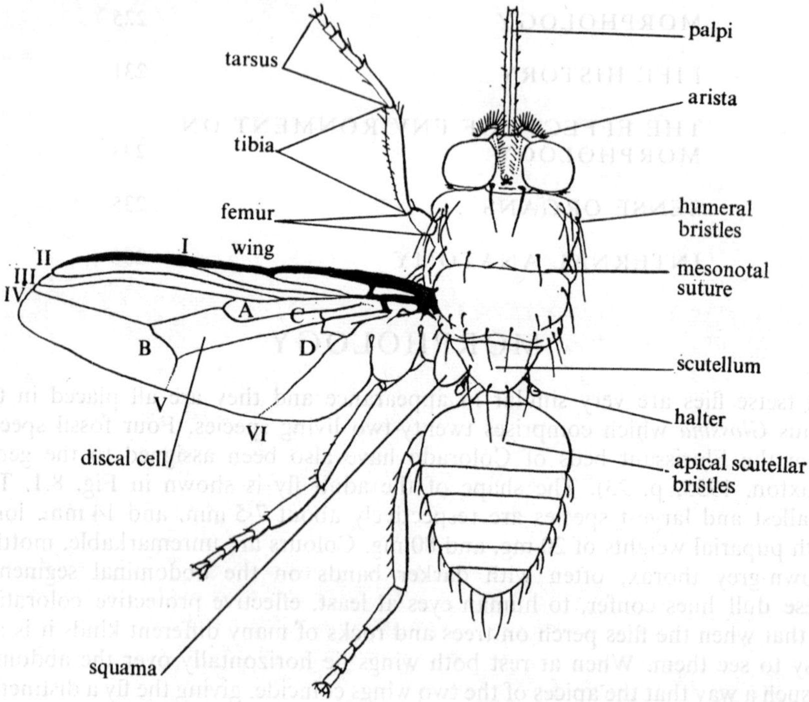

Fig. 8.1 Diagram showing external anatomy of a tsetse fly, with the palpi ensheathing the proboscis, longitudinal wing veins I–VI, and cross-veins of wings (indicated as follows: A, anterior cross-vein; B, posterior cross-vein; C and D, other cross-veins). (After Buxton, 1955)

(5) by Burtt and Jackson (1951) who have corrected previous views on the segmentation of the larva; (6) by Bursell (1955, 1958) who has further elucidated the structure of the polypneustic lobes of the larva and the intra-uterine and puparial development stages, establishing the existence of a fourth larval instar in addition to the three that have long been recognized (but *see* p. 343); and (7) by Saunders (1960b, 1961) who has revolutionized previous knowledge of the female reproductive system (*see* also pp. 327–344).

Table 8.1 lists the twenty-two currently recognized living species of *Glossina*, some of which are divided into sub-species. These are arranged in the three groups into which the genus is divided and to which some authors give the status of sub-genera or even genera (*see* further pp. 244–248).

In any sizeable sample of tsetse the males are on average smaller than the females, but the largest males are bigger than the smallest females. The males are readily distinguished by the presence of the hypopygium (Fig. 8.6) centrally at the tip of the abdomen. It is said that the male's eyes are larger, or alternatively that the space between the eyes is smaller, but this character is not distinctive enough for field use. In some species there is a secondary sexual character of

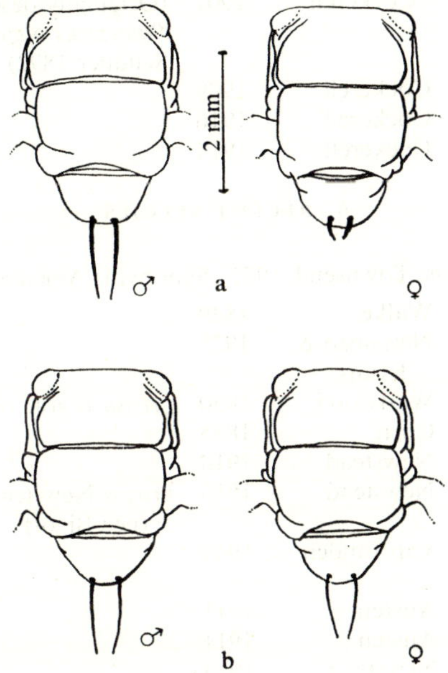

Fig. 8.2 Dorsal view of thorax of males and females of (a) *G. palpalis palpalis* and (b) *G. palpalis gambiensis*, showing relative lengths of apical scutellar bristles. (From Machado, 1954)

unknown significance; the bristles at the tip of the scutellum are shorter in the female (Fig. 8.2). This occurs rather haphazardly in the *fusca* and *morsitans* groups (Table 8.2), and throughout the *palpalis* group except for *G.p. gambiensis* (Fig. 8.2). According to Machado (1954) the tarsal claws are perceptibly longer in males, at least in the *palpalis* group.

The venation of the wings (Fig. 8.3) is constant throughout the genus. The cutting edge of the hatchet cell, roughly *k* to *d* in Fig 8.3, is sometimes measured with an eye-piece micrometer as an index of the size of the fly (Buxton, 1955, App. 2; Jackson, 1953a; Glasgow and Bursell, 1961; Glasgow, 1961c) but it is not a completely satisfactory index of size, a better one being a conventional measure of thoracic area (Bursell, 1960).[1] Supernumerary stub veins occur in

[1] This area is more precisely defined as that provided by the product of the distance between the points of insertion of each member of the outermost pair of humeral bristles (Fig. 8.1) and the distance between the mesonotal suture and the line joining the points of insertion of the two apical scutellar bristles (Bursell, *in litt.*, 1970).

TABLE 8.1[1]

The genus* Glossina*: species and subspecies* Glossina *Wiedemann, 1830

	Species and subspecies	Author	Date	Synonyms[2]	Length[3] (in mm.)
	a. EXTINCT SPECIES				
1	*oligocena* (Scudder)	Cockerell	1907	(Originally described *Paloestrus oligocena* Scudder 1892)	
2	*osborni*	Cockerell	1909		
3	*veterna*	Cockerell	1916		
4	*armatipes*	Cockerell	1918		
	b. RECENT SPECIES				
I	*Fusca* group (subgenus *Austenina* Townsend, 1921; Synonym: *Newsteadina* Townsend, 1921).				
1a	*fusca fusca*	Walker	1849		9½–13½
1b	*fusca congolensis*	Newstead & Evans	1921		—
2	*tabaniformis*	Westwood	1850	*grossa* Bigot, 1891	11–11¾
3	*longipennis*	Corti	1895		11½–13½
4	*brevipalpis*	Newstead	1910		10¼–13½
5a	*nigrofusca nigrofusca*	Newstead	1910	*grossa* Newstead, 1910 (nec Bigot)	12–14
5b	*nigrofusca hopkinsi*	Van Emden	1944		—
6	*fuscipleuris*	Austen	1911		10¾–11½
7	*medicorum*	Austen	1911		9–11
8	*severini*	Newstead	1913		10¾–12½
9	*schwetzi*	Newstead & Evans	1921	*schwetzi disjuncta* Potts, 1924	11–13½
10	*haningtoni*	Newstead & Evans	1922		10–13
11	*vanhoofi*	Henrard	1952		—
12	*nashi*	Potts	1955		10[4]
II	*Palpalis* group (subgenus *Nemorhina* Robineau-Desvoidy, 1830)				
13a	*palpalis palpalis*	Robineau-Desvoidy	1830	(*ventricosa* Bigot, 1885) (*bocagei* Franca, 1905) (*wellmani* Austen, 1905) (*maculata* Newstead, 1911) (*pallida* Simpson, 1918)	8–11
13b	*palpalis gambiensis*	Vanderplank	1949		—
14a	*fuscipes fuscipes*	Newstead	1910	(*ziemanni* Grunberg, 1912) (*angolensis* Vanderplank, 1949)	8–11

TABLE 8.1 (*continued*)

The genus* Glossina*: species and subspecies* Glossina *Wiedemann, 1830

	Species and subspecies	Author	Date	Synonyms[2]	Length[3] (in mm.)
14b	*fuscipes martinii*	Zumpt	1935		8–11
14c	*fuscipes quanzensis*	Pires	1948		—[5]
15	*caliginea*	Austen	1911		9–11
16a	*pallicera pallicera*	Bigot	1891		8½–10½
16b	*pallicera newsteadi*	Austen	1929		7½–10
17	*tachinoides*	Westwood	1850		6½–9
III	*Morsitans* group (subgenus *Glossina s. str.* Zumpt, 1935)				
18	*longipalpis*	Wiedemann	1830		9½–11
19a	*morsitans morsitans*	Westwood	1850	(*pallida* Shircore, 1913) (*paradoxa* Shircore, 1913)	8–11
19b	*morsitans submorsitans*	Newstead	1910	*ugandensis* Vanderplank, 1949	7¾–10[6]
19c	*morsitans orientalis*	Vanderplank	1949		—
19d	*morsitans ugandensis*	Vanderplank	1949		—
20	*pallidipes*	Austen	1903	*borgesi* Pires, 1960[7]	8½–11
21	*austeni*	Newstead	1912	*mossurizensis* Dias, 1956	7½–8½
22	*swynnertoni*	Austen	1923		8–9½

[1] This table largely follows that given by Glasgow (1963).

[2] The synonomy is taken from Haeselbarth *et al.* (1966).

[3] The measurements of length are from Zumpt (1936) and correspond mainly to those given by Newstead *et al.* (1924) taken to the nearest quarter of a millimetre, except for those as specified in the notes that follow; they can therefore be taken as 'the length of the fly in profile, exclusive of the proboscis'.

[4] From Potts (1955).

[5] Machado (1954) observes that *fuscipes quanzensis* is 'perhaps a little larger on the average' than the other two subspecies, and in order to give an approximate idea of their size he gives the following figures for the length of thorax: 3·8 (♂) and 4·2 (♀) as compared with means of 3·69 and 4·18 mm. for *fuscipes martinii*; the differences therefore must be very slight.

[6] Directly from Newstead *et al.* (1924).

[7] Considered by Machado (personal communication, 1968) to be probably a mere ecotype, perhaps even a local sub-race (or microgeographic race—*cf.* Mayr, Linsley and Usinger, 1953).

some individuals in some of the sites indicated in Fig. 8.3, a phenomenon studied by Glasgow (1960) and Welch (1960).

Some of the abnormalities have been found in every species which has been examined thoroughly, so that it seems likely that they occur thoughout the genus. The highest recorded incidence of any abnormality is 13 %, but usually they are much less common than this. In male *G. swynnertoni* the commonest abnormalities are *e* and *b*, in *G. morsitans morsitans d*, in *G.m. orientalis a.* Thus the pattern of occurrences is a sub-specific character, but not a character

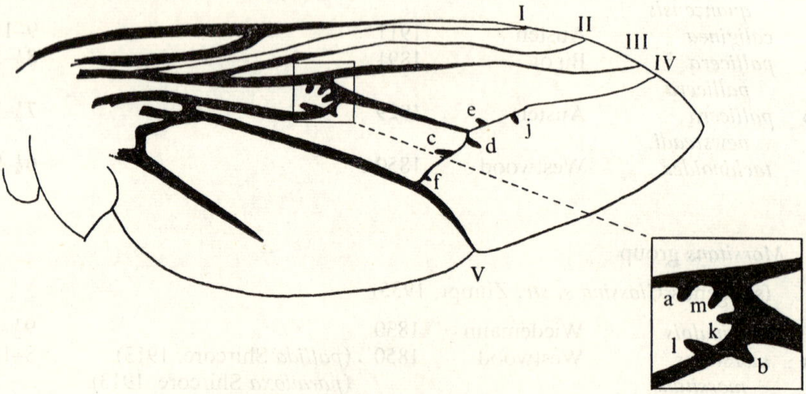

Fig. 8.3 Diagram of wing venation of *Glossina*. I–V, the main veins, conventionally numbered; *a–m*, the sites at which supernumerary stub veins have been seen in several species. Gaps sometimes occur in vein IV between positions *b* and *k*, and in the cross-vein between positions *f* and *d*. (From Glasgow, 1960)

usable for identifying individual flies. In *G. swynnertoni* the abnormalities are most common in the hot season and comparatively rare in the cool weather. If the puparial stages are incubated in the laboratory at 29°C there is a very high incidence of abnormalities in the emergent flies, far higher than any observed in nature, but if the puparial stages collected from the field (presumed to be on average half way through the puparial period) are incubated at 30°C the emergent flies do not differ from controls reared at 22°C. Evidently the abnormalities are affected by the temperature experienced during the puparial stages and the sensitive period is in the first half of puparial life. Since incubation at 29°C produced a level of abnormality never observed in nature, it seems fair to conclude that flies in the puparial stages do not experience this temperature under natural conditions.

It is possible that short exposures during the young puparial stage to a high temperature would induce abnormal venation (*cf.* Goldschmidt, 1938), but such experiments have not been tried.

TABLE 8.2

The development of a secondary sexual difference in the apical scutellar bristles as illustrated in Fig. 8.2 (from Glasgow, 1963 and Buxton, 1955)

	No regular or striking difference	Longer in males
Fusca group	*brevipalpis* *fusca* *fuscipleuris* *haningtoni* *schwetzi* *tabaniformis*	*longipennis* *nigrofusca* *medicorum*
Palpalis group	*palpalis gambiensis*	*palpalis palpalis* *caliginea* *pallicera* *tachinoides*
Morsitans group	*longipalpis* *pallidipes*	*austeni* *morsitans* *swynnertoni*

LIFE HISTORY

As in other Diptera, the female has a pair of spermathecae in which sperm acquired very early in life (often, probably, during a single mating) is stored and lasts the female's life-span. The two sexes emerge in equal numbers; it follows that if one mating per life is usual in females, males must on average mate only once. Young males are not usually potent, but laboratory evidence suggests that they are potent at the age of six days, and that they can mate every six days (Nash, Jordan & Boyle, 1966). A male that dies before it is six days old, then, is unlikely to mate, one that dies before it is twelve days old is unlikely to mate more than once, and so on. Table 8.3 assumes that the proportion of the male population which mates 0, 1, 2, 3 . . . times forms a Poisson distribution, and suggests that a mean male age at death of nine days would be sufficient for every female to mate once. Direct estimates of male longevity are about twice this figure: possibly male potency has been overestimated or possibly more than one mating per female is common, since Nash *et al.* (1966) have found evidence that after a single mating in the laboratory the supply of sperm may become exhausted in long-lived females. Females, of course, must live much longer: at 26°C, thirty days are necessary to produce two larvae, fifty days to produce four. Eggs are produced one at a time, and are retained in the uterus after fertilization. Recent work by Nash *et al.* (1967) suggests that fertilization does not always occur. It seems possible that poor nutrition of the female could inhibit the occurrence of fertilization. The egg hatches in the uterus. The resultant first-instar larva feeds by mouth on a secretion produced by 'milk glands' (Fig. 14.1). After a moult, the second-instar larva continues to feed on the same 'milk' (for further details *see* p. 337). After a second moult the larva is extruded; it is now in its third instar and weighs nearly as much as its mother. It behaves like most third-instar Cyclorrhapha: it burrows into the soil and assumes the shape of a barrel; its integument becomes rigid and darkens and is now known as the puparium.

TABLE 8.3

Hypothetical male mating regime, based on Poisson distribution for mean of 1, and one mating every six days (from Glasgow, 1963)

No. matings per male life	percentage	Mean age at death (days)	Product
0	36·8	3	110·4
1	36·8	9	331·2
2	18·4	15	276·0
3	6·1	21	128·1
4	1·5	27	40·5
5	0·3	33	9·9
	99·9		986·1

Mean age at death = 896·1/99·9 = 9 days

Within the puparium two moults take place: the first produces the pupa and the second the imago, a process often called eclosion of the adult (Bursell, 1958). There is a certain amount of confusion about the terminology of these immobile stages: thus *puparium* strictly means the third-instar integument after it has hardened and darkened, but often the term is used to include the puparial contents in whatever stage they may be.[1] The barrelling, hardening and darkening of the third instar integument should logically be called *pupariation*, but this term is not widely accepted and the process is often called *pupation*, although *pupation* should logically be reserved for the moulting of the fourth-instar larva to produce the pupa. *Pupa* has so often been used to mean 'puparium and its contents' that the cautious writer who wishes to signify 'pupa *sensu stricto*' often writes *true pupa. Pupal period* is tending to be replaced by 'puparial period' to indicate the lapse of time from pupariation to emergence of the imago. It varies from twenty days at 30°C to forty-seven days at 20°C.

Emergence from the puparium is effected by the extrusion of the ptilinum (Fig. 8.5) which breaks the puparium along three lines of weakness. Emergence

[1] Wherever appropriate the term 'puparial stages' is used in the text of this work to denote the puparium and its contents—Editor.

takes place between 1200 and 1800 hours, i.e. within a few hours of the daily maximum temperature. This rhythm is maintained under conditions of constant temperature, but displaced if the temperature rhythm is altered. On emergence the wings are crumpled, but they are expanded in about five minutes and the tsetse can fly in an hour or two. In some species the females are nubile immediately, even before the wings have expanded. Males, as noted above, commonly do not become potent until after the first meal. From emergence until they have had their first meal, which may be as much as forty-eight hours later, the tsetse are called *teneral.* This word is not used in exactly this sense with reference to other insects, but a special term is justified as the condition is unusual and not known in any other group of insects (*see* also p. 359). Teneral tsetse have a characteristic soft, empty feel, formerly attributed to delayed hardening of the integument. The abdomen by transmitted light appears fishy white, easily distinguished from the yellow of tsetse which have had a meal. Their flight is less noisy and determined than that of mature individuals (Jackson, 1933a). They are delicate, in that if they are caught wild, marked with spots of paint on the thorax, and released, they are seldom seen again, whereas numerous recaptures can be made of tsetse marked in the same way when mature.

Bursell (1961b) showed that the characteristic soft feel of teneral tsetse is occasioned by their flight muscles being only partly developed. One cannot usefully compare weights of whole tenerals with the weights of whole mature flies because the weight of mature flies depends largely on the time which has elapsed since the last meal. Thoracic weights, however, can be compared because the thorax contains only transmitting and not storage parts of the gut (Fig. 8.5). Bursell found that a mature thorax is nearly double the weight of a teneral thorax.

The increase in weight does not take place immediately after the first feed; two meals are required in males and three in females before full development is reached. The gain in weight is due to enlargement of the muscles which are functional shortly after emergence (Glasgow & Glasgow, 1962).

Many field workers have recorded the percentage of teneral individuals in their catches, *see* for example Fig. 15.3. These records have seldom led to any clear-cut conclusions; one reason for this may have been the simultaneous use of partly independent criteria. The soft, teneral feel is obvious as soon as one takes hold of the fly, but it may not disappear entirely until three feeds have been taken. Examination by transmitted light (i.e. holding the fly up to the sky) allows fed and unfed flies to be distinguished with certainty, and Bursell's (1961b) recommendation that the term 'teneral' should be reserved strictly for those which have never fed at all is being increasingly accepted by field workers (*see* also p. 344).

THE EFFECTS OF ENVIRONMENT ON MORPHOLOGY

We have already seen that the wing venation is affected by the temperature experienced during the puparial stages. Variations in size and colour are also under environmental control in at least some tsetse species.

Before discussing environmental control of size it is necessary to point out that the significance of size differences between various species is not perfectly understood. Each species has a characteristic size, and variation within each species is notably smaller than it is in other Diptera which have free-living larvae. This relative constancy of size is presumably a consequence of the method of reproduction, just described. Some physiological studies have revealed advantages in large size. Thus the puparial stages of *G. longipennis*, a large species, are able to develop successfully in dry air partly because their large size involves a more favourable ratio of weight to surface, but those of *G. swynnertoni*, a small species, can also develop in dry air by virtue of good waterproofing, and both these species are in fact found to occur in extremely arid, xerophytic environments. On the other hand, *G. brevipalpis*, a large species, and *G. austeni*, the smallest species of all, occur together in damp situations. We just do not know what the advantage of small size can be (assuming, that is, that the large size characteristic of the supposedly primitive *fusca* group is indeed a primitive character).

In Diptera with free living larvae (e.g. Tabanidae, Calliphoridae) well-fed larvae grow large and give rise to large adults, while poorly fed larvae do not get so big and give rise to smaller adults. The same is true of *Glossina*, although the range of variation is less. Laboratory-fed tsetse digest their meals much more slowly than their wild counterparts (Langley, 1967; *see* also p. 309) and are thus comparatively undernourished, and nearly all observers have found that they produce underweight larvae which give rise to undersize adults. In nature, the size of puparia is correlated with the nutritional state of their fathers (Glasgow & Bursell, 1961). The nutrition of the fathers is, of course, unlikely to affect the size of the offspring, but it is easier to measure than the nutrition of mothers and was taken as an index of maternal nutrition. Thus much of the annual variation in the size of tsetse, which is of the order of 5% by weight, is ascribed to variations in the nutrition of the maternal generation.

A very slight difference in size, but not in weight, has been found to be occasioned by the temperature at which puparia are incubated. Incubation at 25°C produces the largest adults: incubation at other temperatures produces slightly smaller adults with, however, the same weight (Bursell, 1960).

Differential mortality may affect the mean size of a tsetse population; sometimes the smallest members of the population are eliminated and sometimes both large and small are eliminated so that the mean size is not altered but the range of variation is reduced. The phenomenon is discussed in more detail by Glasgow (1963).

The humidity at which individuals of *G. pallidipes* are incubated during the puparial stages affects the colour of the dorsal surface of the abdomen of the resulting adults (Bursell, 1960a). Incubation in saturated air produces full pigmentation, incubation in dry air produces very pale individuals. Temperature has little effect below 28°C, but higher temperatures reduce pigmentation considerably. The same effect has been reported in *G. palpalis* (Roubaud, 1909), and Machado (1954) notes that examples of this species found in the equatorial forest and riverine gallery forests are darker than those found in less developed and less dense vegetation. Bursell (1960a) found that humidity had no effect on the coloration of *G. fuscipes*, *G. morsitans* and *G. longipennis* and only a very slight effect on that of *G. swynnertoni*, but the number of examples of *G. fuscipes* studied was small and in view of Machado's observation there is room for further investigation of this point. As pointed out by Glasgow (1963), there is no evidence as to whether these colour variations have any survival value. Bursell (1960a) made ingenious use of the colour-humidity relations of *G. pallidipes* to deduce seasonal changes in larviposition sites.

SENSE ORGANS

The antennae (Fig. 8.4) have two small basal segments and a third much longer one. Near the base of this third segment is inserted the *arista*, a long curved

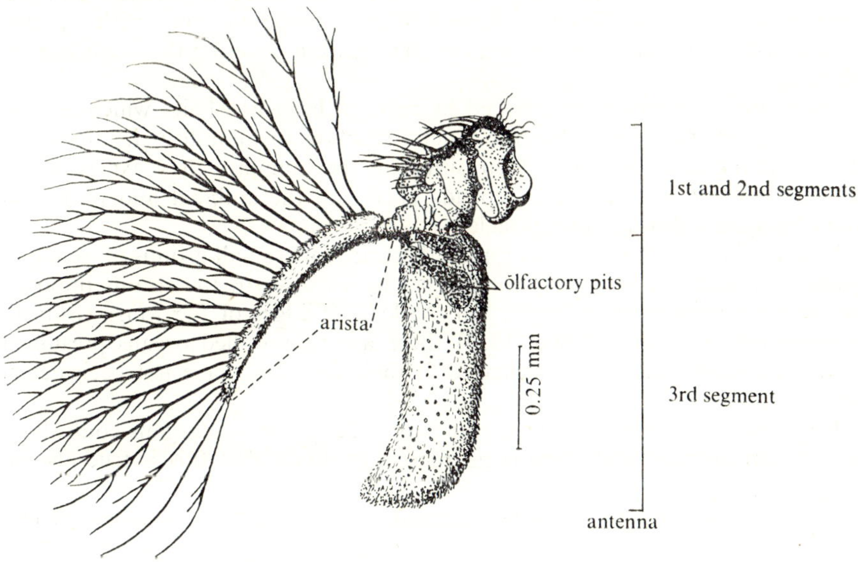

Fig. 8.4 Right antenna of *G. palpalis* viewed from side. (From Jobling, 1933)

structure with compound feathering along the anterior edge. This type of arista is peculiar to *Glossina*. In the third antennal segment rod-shaped and cone-shaped sensillae occur, some in pits and some on the surface. The antennae seem to be able to detect heat, odours and moisture, and the cone-shaped sensillae are believed to be the hygroreceptors (Johns, 1958a). According to Buxton (1955, p. 113) the antennae are erected in flight, which may expose some of the pits to the air stream. Vanderplank (1950) has suggested that the antennae may act also as airspeed indicators.

The maxillary *palps* combine to form a protective cover in which the piercing mouthparts are housed when not in use. This is their main function, although they may contain olfactory organs and doubtless carry tactile hairs like many other parts of the tsetse's body. The *labium* and the *labrum* are both well provided with what appear to be sensillae; it is likely that some detect relevant information about the skin of a potential host before probing and that others might come into use after probing.

The *compound eyes* are, as anyone who has tried to catch a wild tsetse knows, extremely efficient at detecting nearby movement. According to Bax (1937) *G. swynnertoni* responds to moving oxen at a distance of 150, but not 200 yards. The assumption that tsetse can respond to stationary objects at such distances must be treated with reserve, although it has to be borne in mind that when a tsetse is in flight the distinction between moving and stationary objects may disappear.

The three *ocelli* lie between the compound eyes. There seems to be no doubt that they are sensitive to light but their function is obscure. Bursell (1957) found that tsetse are much more active in dry air than in wet but that this effect disappeared in darkness. Covering the compound eyes with opaque paint had the same effect as turning out the light but covering the ocelli had no effect.

The *thoracic spiracles* are guarded by rows of branched hairs which are the hygroreceptors responsible for the kinetic reaction to humidity mentioned in the last paragraph. Owing to their situation the humidity they experience is not the ambient humidity but depends partly on the ambient and partly on water being lost through the spiracles.

Near the base of the wing membrane there are three small groups of 'remigial pores' (Newstead *et al.*, 1924) which may be sensitive to the strains imposed on the wing membrane by flight. On the leading edges of the wings (Bursell, 1957) and on the tarsi (Lewis, 1954) there are thin walled organs presumed from their appearance to be sensory but their functions have not been determined.

The *halteres* in other Diptera are known to be gyroscopic organs controlling equilibrium in flight and there is no reason to doubt that this is true also in *Glossina.*

No *organs of hearing* have been identified in tsetse and there is no completely convincing evidence that a sense of hearing exists. Vanderplank (1948), however, refers to 'mating notes' emitted by females which he believes to be a necessary condition of mating. Besides the organs of unidentified function mentioned above, there are, on various parts of the tsetse's body, many small tactile hairs, which are presumably sensitive to air movements and might be sensitive to sounds.

INTERNAL ANATOMY

Figure 8.5 shows the main features of the internal anatomy.

The *alimentary canal* is continued anteriorly as the lumen of the haustellum, or proboscis, which consists of three parts, the labrum, the hypopharynx, and the labium, shown unnaturally separated in Fig. 8.5. In section the labium is U-shaped, the labrum fitting across the top of the U to enclose a channel, the food canal; in this lies the slender, tubular hypopharynx, the function of which is to convey saliva down to the distal end of the haustellum and so into the pool

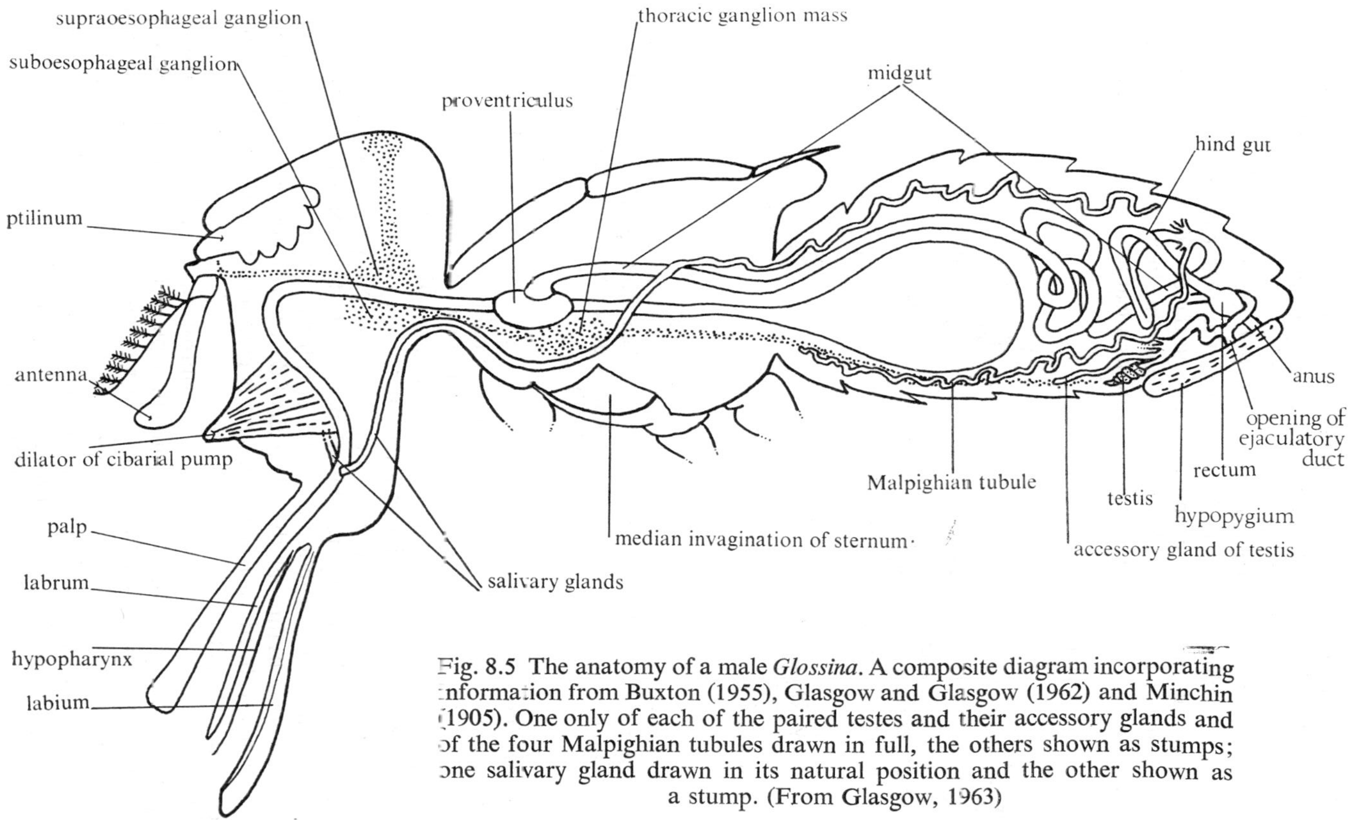

Fig. 8.5 The anatomy of a male *Glossina*. A composite diagram incorporating information from Buxton (1955), Glasgow and Glasgow (1962) and Minchin (1905). One only of each of the paired testes and their accessory glands and of the four Malpighian tubules drawn in full, the others shown as stumps; one salivary gland drawn in its natural position and the other shown as a stump. (From Glasgow, 1963)

of blood that provides the source of the fly's meal (*see* p. 306). The homologies of the mouth-parts are discussed by Buxton (1955), Jobling (1933) and Snodgrass (1944). A modification of the oesophagus forms the *cibarial* pump, consisting of a dilator muscle (Fig. 8.5) and a sphincter which can close the oesophagus. This sphincter can be seen in Fig. 8.8, which also shows how its innervation is closely associated with that of the dilator muscles.

Blood passes down the oesophagus through the proventriculus to the *crop*, a diverticulum of the foregut lying in the abdomen. In a hungry tsetse the crop is empty and the whole abdomen is as thin as a leaf and gives an impression of

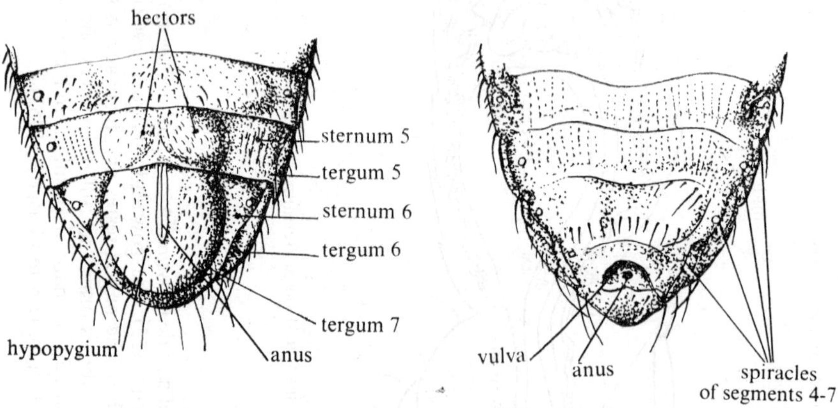

Fig. 8.6 Hind end of abdomen of male *Glossina*, viewed from beneath (left). Hind end of female *Glossina*, viewed from beneath (right), showing relative positions of vulva and anus, and spiracles of segments 4–7. (From Buxton, 1955)

utter emptiness when pressed with the fingers. Sometimes an otherwise empty crop contains a bubble of gas. A gassy condition of the abdomen can be produced artificially by tapping a tsetse rapidly and repeatedly between the eyes (Jackson, 1933a). Cottrell (1962) associated air-swallowing in *Calliphora* with the expansion of the insect after emergence, and Langley (1967a) regards the inflation of the tsetse crop as normally aiding expansion of the fly. When feeding begins all the ingested blood passes into the crop which swells enormously until the whole abdomen is almost spherical, the red colour of the blood being very obvious through the thin wall of the crop and the stretched abdominal wall; the convoluted part of the midgut is crammed with the hindgut into the back of the abdomen.

The muscular *proventriculus* (Fig. 8.7) controls the transfer of blood from the crop to the midgut, where digestion takes place (*see* Chapter 12). The proventriculus also produces the *peritrophic membrane*, a tube mainly of chitin, which invests the food in the midgut and extends from the proventriculus into the hindgut. The beginning of the membrane is shown in Fig. 8.8.

The *midgut* extends from the proventriculus to the junction of the Malpighian tubules (Fig. 8.5), and the hindgut from this point to the anus.

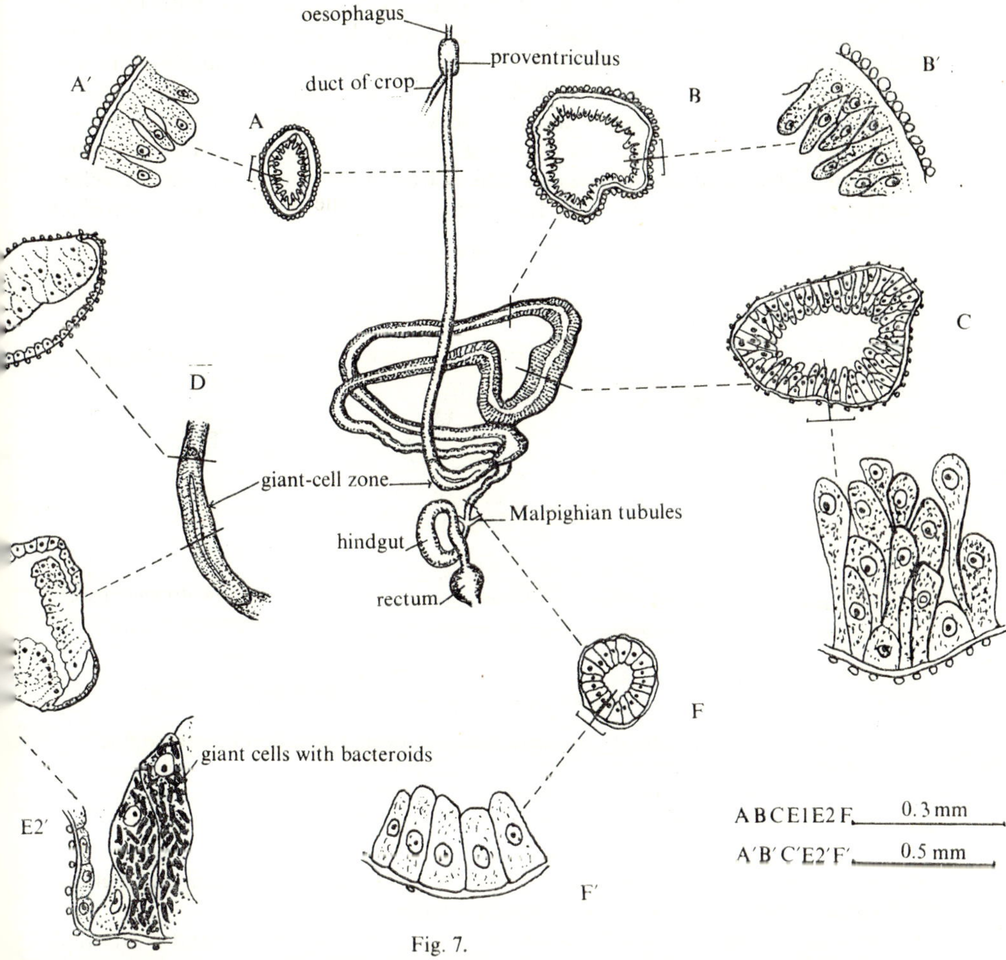

Fig. 7.

Fig. 8.7 Mid- and hindgut of fasting *Glossina*, showing normal relations of the coils and histological details of the midgut regions. A, A′, transverse section of anterior segment of midgut, just in front of junction with middle segment; B, B′, ditto of middle segment; C, C′, ditto of posterior segment; (D), details of giant-cell zone; El, transverse section through anterior end of giant cell zone; E2, transverse section through middle of giant cell zone and E2′ giant cells with bacteroids; F, F′, transverse section through terminal part of midgut. (From Buxton, 1955)

The *salivary glands* produce an anti-coagulant (Lester & Lloyd, 1928) which is discharged through the hypopharynx to mix with host blood as it is being ingested. If the salivary glands or the hypopharynx are infected with trypanosomes these may be discharged with the saliva. It seems that although the purpose of the saliva is to prevent coagulation of the blood sucked into the crop, not all of the saliva is sucked back—some remains in the host. Some trypanosomes may remain too and may survive and multiply in the host.

The *nervous system* (Fig. 8.9) has been studied by Langley (1965). In some details the arrangement in *Glossina* differs from that known in other Cyclorrhapha. Thus the recurrent nerve fuses with one of the nervi corporis cardiaci

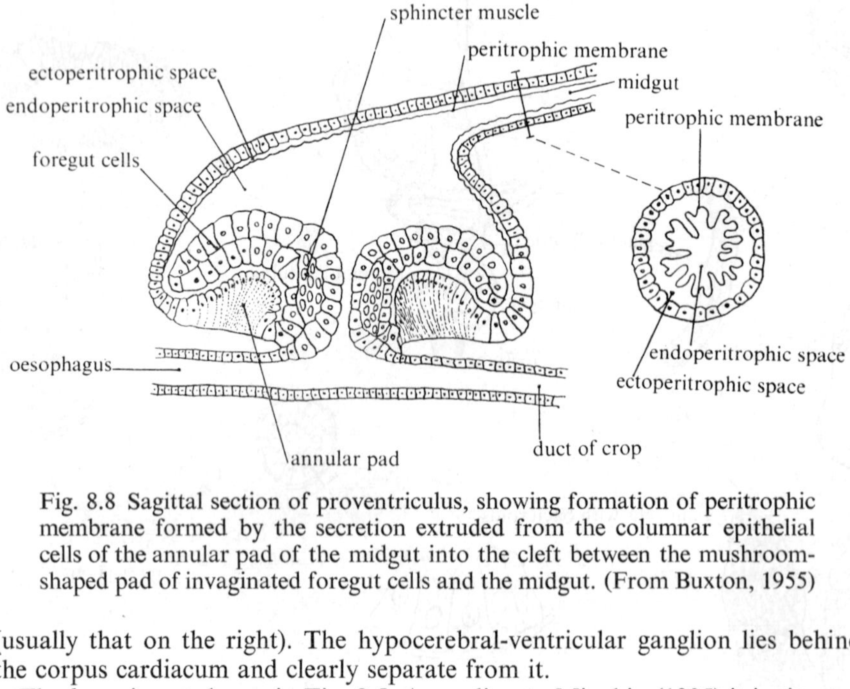

Fig. 8.8 Sagittal section of proventriculus, showing formation of peritrophic membrane formed by the secretion extruded from the columnar epithelial cells of the annular pad of the midgut into the cleft between the mushroom-shaped pad of invaginated foregut cells and the midgut. (From Buxton, 1955)

(usually that on the right). The hypocerebral-ventricular ganglion lies behind the corpus cardiacum and clearly separate from it.

The *heart* is not shown in Fig. 8.5. According to Minchin (1905) it is situated in abdominal segments one to five and is divided into five chambers. Each chamber has a pair of alary muscles and a pair of ostia, the muscles being small in front and large behind. Anteriorly the heart is prolonged as a tube of narrow calibre which enters the thorax and follows the midgut, proventriculus and oesophagus to the brain (Fig. 8.9). Imms' (1957) description of the hearts of *Musca* and *Calliphora* is very similar. Histologically, Minchin states that twenty-three pairs of giant cells, together with ten couples of smaller cells making up the five pairs of ostia, constitute the wall of the heart.

The *muscles* of the head are fully described by Jobling (1933). The main flight muscles, in the thorax, consist of six pairs of longitudinal muscles. Opposing these longitudinal muscles and situated farther from the median plane, are six pairs of dorso-ventral muscles (Glasgow & Glasgow, 1962).

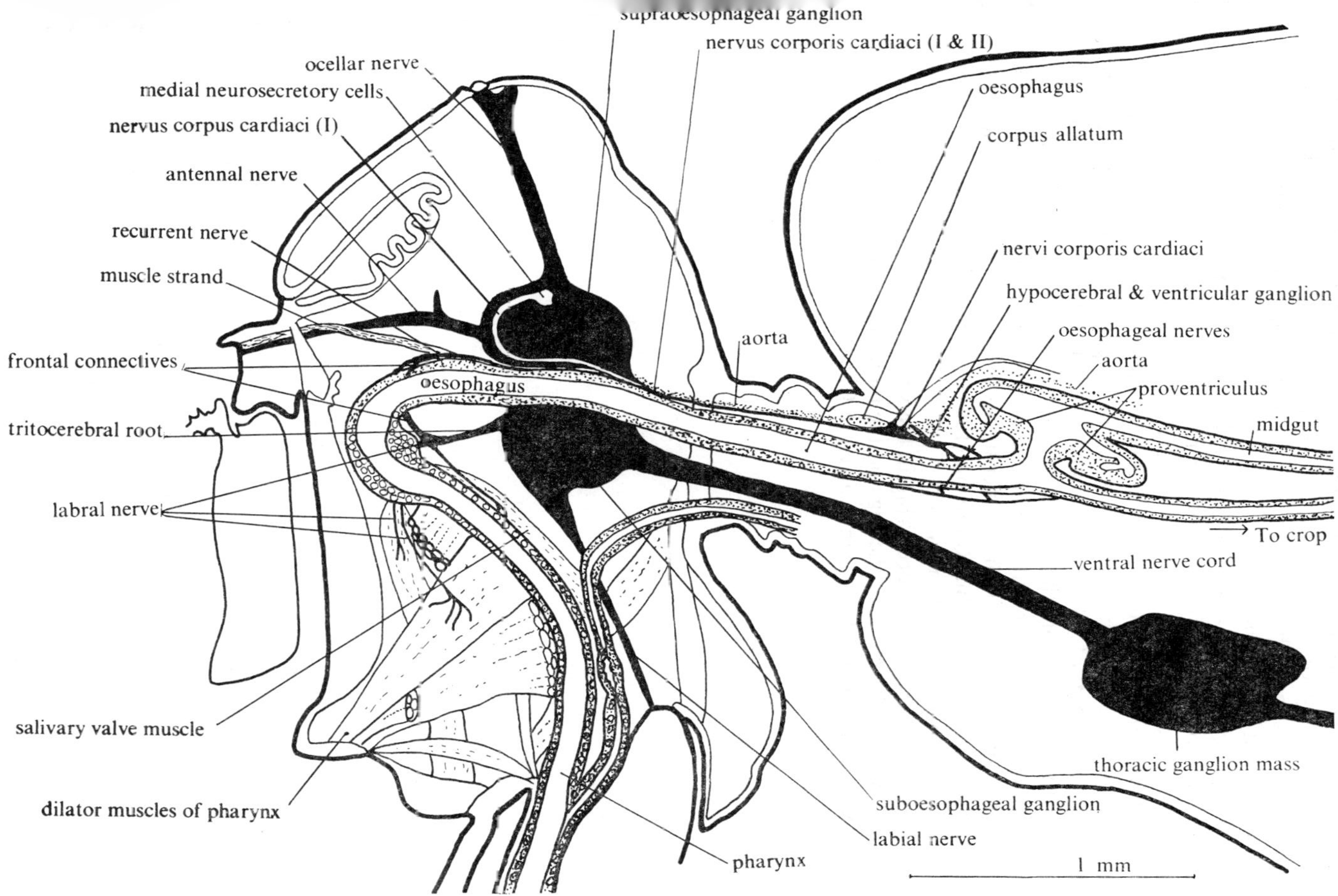

Fig. 8.9 Diagrammatic reconstruction of right half of head and prothorax of *G. morsitans* to illustrate the neuroendocrine system, the stomatogastric nervous system and associated parts of the central nervous system. (After Langley, 1965)

The *male reproductive organs* are shown in Fig. 8.5 and consist of a pair of testes and a pair of accessory glands. All these discharge into a single ejaculatory duct which passes round behind the rectum and then forwards to enter the penis, which is in front of the anus.

The *female reproductive organs* (described in detail in Chapter 14) occupy the same relative position as do those of the male, while the female is immature. During pregnancy the uterus bscomes very much enlarged to accommodate the enormous larva. When a meal is taken the crop becomes enromously distended and it follows that full meals are incompatible with late pregnancy. According to Nash *et al.*, (1967), if a female feeds the day before she is due to larviposit, the pressure from the crop may force the larva into such an awkward position that it cannot get out; under these conditions puparium formation may occur in the uterus and in their experiments this has always led to the death of both mother and puparium. Robinson (1964) has recorded what may be an example of this phenomenon in nature.

The *choriothete* is an organ occurring in the ventral side of the uterus, and is concerned with the hatching of the egg and the moulting of the first-instar larva. A detailed description of this organ is given in Chapter 14.

Chapter 9

Systematics and Identification of *Glossina*

W. H. POTTS

INTRODUCTORY

All tsetse flies belong to the genus *Glossina* Wiedemann, the species of which are found only in Africa, with the exceptions noted in Chapter 10 (Distribution). The genus is generally included in the Dipterous family Muscidae (e.g. Newstead, Evans & Potts, 1924; Imms, 1957), being placed either with the other blood-sucking species of the family in the sub-family Stomoxyinae or in a separate subfamily, the Glossininae. However, recently Haeselbarth, Segerman & Zumpt (1966) have followed Enderlein (1936) in separating *Glossina* from the genera of the true Muscidae in an independent family.

The principal characters of the genus *Glossina* are given in the work of Newstead *et al.* (op. cit.) as:

'Palpi spiny, completely ensheathing the proboscis; these organs are carried horizontally in front of the head when at rest. Antennae of three segments, the arista with a series of long bilaterally branched hairs arranged in regular order along the upper surface. Wings with the membrane slightly rilled; the fourth longitudinal vein curving suddenly upwards and uniting with the cross vein; in life, when at rest, they lie flat one over the other. Sexual dimorphism well marked. Length ranging from 6 to 14 mm.'

Although, as Buxton (1955, p. 10) remarked, 'Few would accept this statement [about sexual dimorphism], except insofar as this applies to the hypopygium', the passage as a whole stands today as a very good definition of the genus. The branched hairs of the antennal arista (Fig. 8.4) and the hatchet-shaped discal cell, formed between the fourth and fifth longitudinal wing veins by the upward curving of the fourth vein to unite with the anterior cross vein that joins the latter to the third vein (Fig. 8.1), are absolutely diagnostic for the genus. The identification of the fossil insects from Florissant, Colorado, as belonging to species of *Glossina* (Buxton, 1955, p. 23; Machado, 1959, p. 50) is based mainly on the last character and on the presence of a structure projecting from the head that closely resembles the palps and proboscis characteristic of the genus. A fossil specimen found earlier, now accepted as belonging to this genus, was described originally as a member of a new genus specially erected for it, *Paloestrus* Scudder, 1892, and so named because of the absence of the structure resembling the proboscis found later in the fossils which were undoubtedly of the same genus (Hegh, 1929, pp. 30–1).

It is not necessary to give a detailed account of the systematics of *Glossina* in this work. The interested reader can find all the details he requires in Newstead, Evans & Potts (1924) which still provides the basis for the systematics of the genus, and in Hegh (1929), which includes a reproduction of the original descriptions of the species published before 1900 and French translations of all the detailed descriptions to be found in Austen (1911) and the work by Newstead and his colleagues already cited. Later works that also give comprehensive accounts of the systematics of the genus are those by Zumpt (1936) and Gaschen (1945), the latter paying particular attention to the species occurring in French West Africa. More recent important contributions to the systematics of *Glossina* have been made by Machado (1954, 1959, 1964).

DIVISIONS OF THE GENUS *GLOSSINA*

Three well-marked groups of the genus were recognized by Newstead (1911), and the following definitions of them are taken from Newstead, Evans & Potts (1924, pp. 43–5); the species constituting each group are shown in Table 8.1.[1]

Group. I. The *fusca* group

'In the males of the species included in this group, the superior claspers are quite free, there being no membrane stretching between them (Fig. 9.1); the distal extremities of these appendages have either a single, large and bluntly-pointed, tooth-like extension, or they are bluntly bidentate; the harpes in all cases being markedly different in structure.'

'The external armature of the females (Fig. 9.2) consists of five plates—one pair dorsal, one pair lateral, and a single median sternal one; medio-dorsal plate absent. Internally the signum (p. 252) is generally well developed.'

This division includes the twelve largest species.

[1] In the following quoted passages, the Figure numbers within brackets refer to figures in this text, except where otherwise indicated.

Group. II. The *palpalis* group

'In the members of this group the superior claspers of the males (Fig. 9.1) are connected by a thin membrane which is deeply divided medially; in all cases the

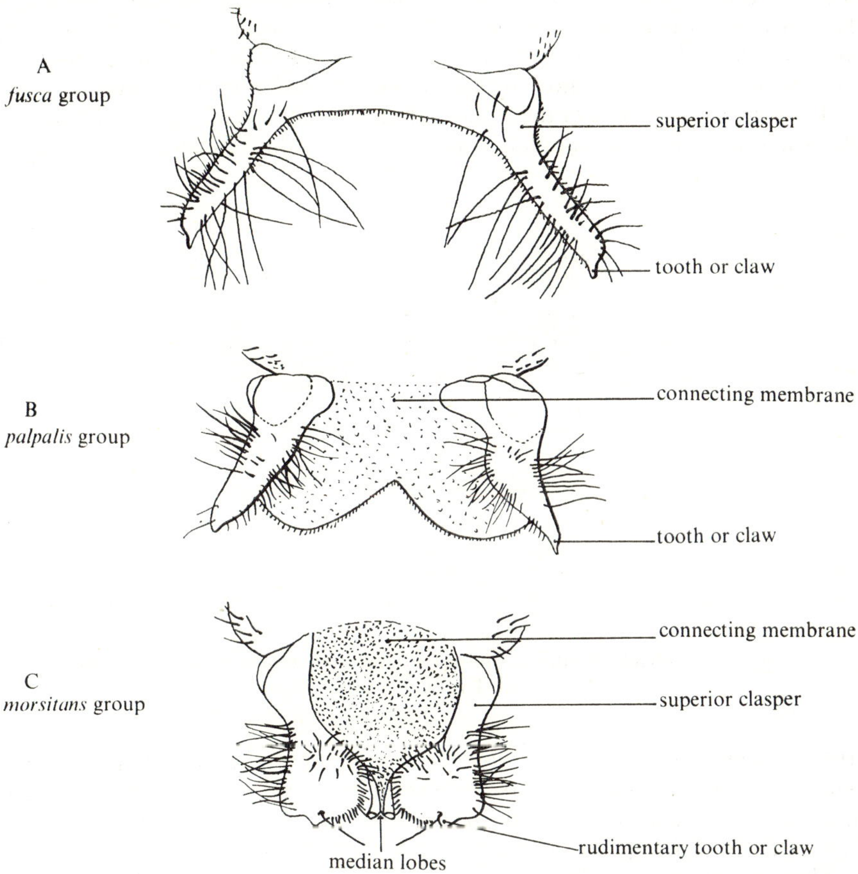

Fig. 9.1 Diagrammatic representation of typical forms of superior claspers of *Glossina* illustrating the three groups into which the genus is divided. (From Newstead, Evans & Potts, 1924)

distal extremities of the claspers are quite free and widely separated, but produced into a single more or less falciform or tooth-like process.'

'The external armature of the females (Fig. 9.6) consists of six plates. In addition to those present in Group I, there is a small medio-dorsal plate. A signum is never present.'

Group. III. The *morsitans* group

'In the members of this group, the superior claspers (Fig. 9.1) are completely united by a membrane and they are also fused medially at the distal extremity.

That they are a very remarkable form may be gathered by a glance at the illustration, their shape somewhat resembling the scapula of a mammal in miniature, and they are altogether much more complicated structures than those in either of the preceding groups. The blunt tooth-like extension on the distal margin of the superior claspers, which is most evident in *G. morsitans* and its race *submorsitans*, and also in *G. swynnertoni* is homologous with the terminal tooth of the superior claspers common to the species included in groups I and II.'

'The external armature of the females (Fig. 9.3) consists of a pair of fused anal plates and a median sternal plate (the function of which Nash and Kernaghan

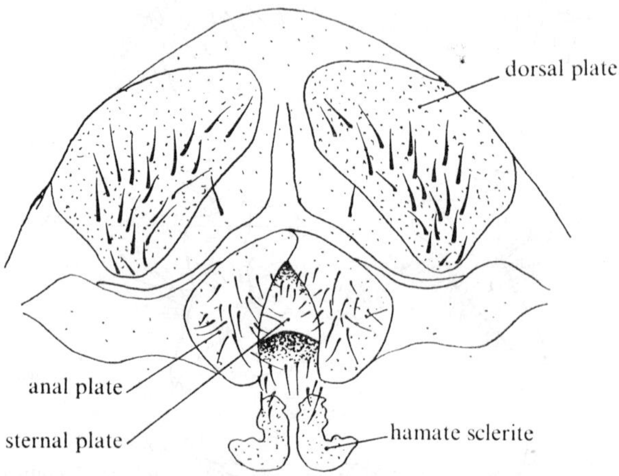

Fig. 9.2 External genital armature of *Glossina brevipalpis* (♀) (From Newstead, Evans & Potts, 1924)

(1965a) suggest is to keep the vulva clear of faecal matter). Dorsal plates are generally absent, but occur in a reduced form in G. *austeni* (and can be detected in a very reduced form in other species (Patton, 1936a, Figs. 20, 23; 1936b, Figs. 3, 5, 7)). There is no signum in any of the species.'

'Thus we see, in these three groups, forms which are so widely different as to lead one to assume, without taking the other external features into consideration, that they represent three distinct genera. Certain it is that these insects afford an interesting illustration of the fact that a high degree of differentiation in one set of morphological characters is not incompatible with the retention of others apparently of a more ancestral type.'

These groups are not only clearly differentiated by their morphological characters, as pointed out by Newstead, but are also characterized by marked differences in their requirements as to habitats. Thus, the species of the *fusca* group, with two exceptions, occur only in the great forests of West and Central Africa and in the gallery forests fringing the rivers of the grassed woodlands surrounding these forests; those of the *palpalis* group are generally confined to the forested edges of the lakes and rivers in close proximity to surface water;

finally, those of the *morsitans* group, with one exception, range widely through the grassed woodlands of Africa (*see* Chapter 10).

In the most recently published list of species of *Glossina* (Haeselbarth, Segerman & Zumpt, 1966, p. 40) these three groups are, as in Zumpt (1936),

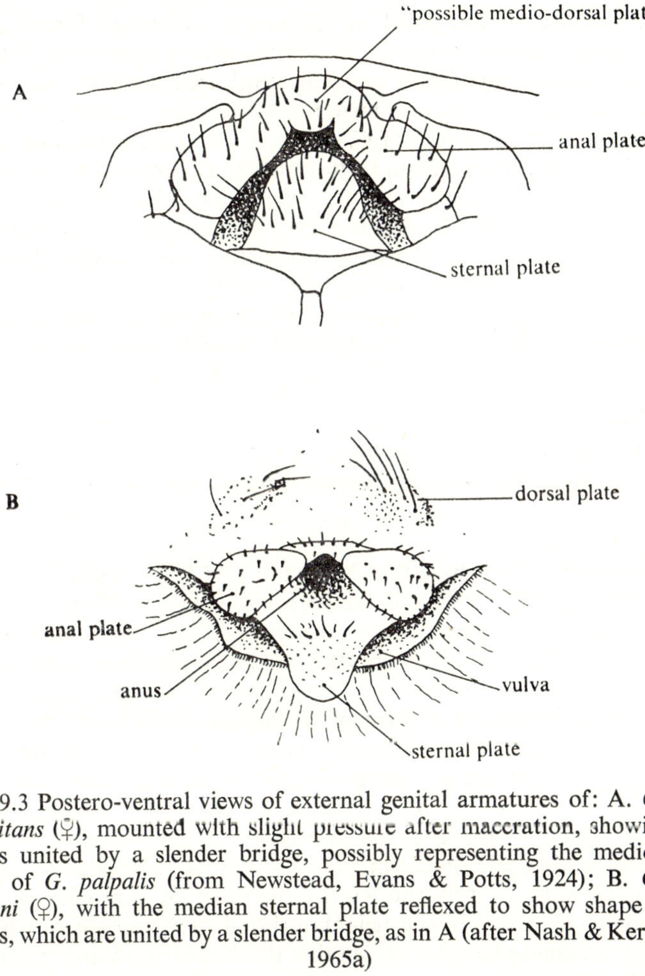

Fig. 9.3 Postero-ventral views of external genital armatures of: A. *Glossina morsitans* (♀), mounted with slight pressure after maceration, showing anal plates united by a slender bridge, possibly representing the medio-dorsal plate of *G. palpalis* (from Newstead, Evans & Potts, 1924); B. *Glossina austeni* (♀), with the median sternal plate reflexed to show shape of anal plates, which are united by a slender bridge, as in A (after Nash & Kernaghan, 1965a)

given the status of subgenera, under the names of *Austenina* Townsend, 1921 (for the *fusca* group), *Nemorhina* Robineau-Desvoidy, 1830 (for the *palpalis* group) and *Glossina sensu stricto* Wiedemann 1830 (for the *morsitans* group); it may be noted that van Emden (1944) wrote of the *fusca* group as 'a rather well-defined aggregate, to which subgeneric status may well be attributed'. Nevertheless, with Buxton (1955, pp. 16–17), we prefer to follow Newstead in regarding tsetse flies as forming a single genus, although as in Smart (1956) the subgeneric names are used in the key (pp. 259–272) and in the list of species in Table 8.1

(pp. 228–229). The list is substantially that given by Glasgow (1963, p. 4), except that the revision of the *palpalis* group by Machado (1954, 1959) is accepted completely.

I The *Fusca* Group

Machado (1959) discussed in detail the affinities of the species forming the *fusca* group, basing his discussion mainly on a study of the terminalia of the males, the genital armature of the females and the chitinized plate, the signum, at the distal end of the uterus. He recognized a western and central sub-group of closely related species consisting of *G. fusca, G. nashi, G. haningtoni, G. tabaniformis, G. schwetzi, G. vanhoofi* and *G. fuscipleuris*, as opposed to an eastern sub-group formed by *G. brevipalpis* and *G. longipennis*. The latter possess certain common characters which he considered relate them to the *palpalis* and *morsitans* groups, and which he therefore considered primitive. He described the characters of *G. nigrofusca* as intermediate between those of the two sub-groups, but those of *G. medicorum* as approaching those of the first sub-group rather more closely. He regarded *G. severini* as very much apart, though showing some primitive characters.

II The *Palpalis* Group

Following Machado (1954) *G. palpalis* (R.-D.) is split into two species, *G. fuscipes* Newst. being regarded as distinct from *G. palpalis sens. str.* (as it was originally by Newstead (1910)) and *G. newsteadi* Austen as a subspecies of *G. pallicera* Bigot.

It is appropriate to note here that Machado (1965) has shown very convincingly that it is not possible to sustain the suggestion made by Potts (1956) that the specimens of *G. palpalis* recorded by Austen (1903, p. 76) as collected by Sir John Kirk on the Zambesi River in 1864 might be ascribed to the subspecies now known as *G. fuscipes martinii*. These specimens have been shown by Machado to be examples of a form of *G. palpalis* transitional between *G. p. palpalis* and *G. p. gambiensis*, probably collected by Kirk during a visit to Freetown, Sierra Leone, on his voyage out to the Zambesi area. Neave (1909), discussing the distribution of *G. palpalis* in the Zambesi area, regarded these specimens as wrongly labelled; this conclusion is supported by Machado's demonstration that a male specimen from the Zambesi, labelled *G. longipalpis*, is indeed an example of this species (as recorded by Austen, 1903, p. 92), a species known to occur in the neighbourhood of Freetown but not in the Zambesi area. Machado has also shown that the record of a third specimen from the same collection (Austen, op. cit., p. 98), actually refers to a female of *G. medicorum*, again a species most unlikely to have existed in the Zambesi area but one which, although not recorded from Sierra Leone, is known to occur in the neighbouring territory of Liberia (*see* Chapter 10 for further information on the relationship and distribution of the species of this group).

III The *Morsitans* Group

In regard to the *morsitans* group, however, it seems better to follow broadly the system used by Glasgow, rather than to adopt the system proposed by

Haeselbarth, Segerman and Zumpt (1966, p. 40). Thus it is proposed to continue to regard *G. swynnertoni* Aust. and *G. morsitans* Westw. as distinct species rather than to consider the former a subspecies of the latter. Although it is true that Vanderplank (1948, p. 144) noted the occurrence of specimens he believed to be hybrids in some narrow areas of overlaps between the two species and that he (1947) concluded that *G. swynnertoni* and the various forms of *G. morsitans* inter-mate with varying degrees of readiness (see also discussion in Buxton, 1955, pp. 325–7), such matings are effectively sterile (Glasgow, 1963, p. 160). Few hybrids were observed to result from laboratory matings and the hybrids themselves were sterile. It would seem that the morphological and genetical relationships of the various species of the *morsitans* group and of the forms of *G. morsitans* need more thorough study before firm conclusions as to the taxonomy of the group (*cf.* Machado, 1954, p. 179) can be finally reached.

It also seems better to continue to recognize *G. pallidipes* Aust. and *G. longipalpis* Wied. as distinct species, rather than to follow Haeselbarth *et al.*, who, acting on a hypothesis put forward by Machado (1959, p. 59, f.n. 4), regarded the former as a sub-species of the latter. At the same time it should be noted that Vanderplank (1949a) was unable to agree that the position of the rudimentary claw or tooth of the superior claspers, whether subterminal (*G. pallidipes*, *see* Fig. 9.7, B) or terminal (*G. longipalpis*, *see* Fig. 9.7, A), is sufficiently constant to form a distinguishing character, as it was regarded by Newstead. This view has also been supported in a recent account by Pires and da Silva (1960) of the results of the examination of some thousands of examples of *G. pallidipes* from a number of localities in Mozambique extending from the northern most point of the range of this species in that territory to its southern limit there. These authors presented and described photographs of male terminalia in which they considered that the superior claspers appear to vary between those described as typical for *G. pallidipes* and for *G. longipalpis*, and even, in a few instances, to approach the form of those of *G. austeni*. They also noted the presence, in some examples, of median lobes that resemble apparently intermediate and aberrant forms described by Vanderplank (1949, 1949a).

Nevertheless, for the present it is considered preferable to continue the long established practice of recognizing the two species, *G. longipalpis* and *G. pallidipes*, distinguishing them by the contrast between the uniformly pale coloration of the last tarsal segment of the foreleg of *G. pallidipes* (whence its name) and the dark tip of this segment in *G. longipalpis*, in combination with the other above-mentioned characters. One may also mention the relatively narrow third segment of the antenna of *G. pallidipes* and the longer hairs of this segment, as compared with *G. longipalpis*, though again noting that Vanderplank (1949a) was unable to agree that the antennae of the two species presented constant differences. Machado also (in a personal communication, 1968; *see* also Machado, 1966), as a result of extensive studies of specimens from a large number of localities distributed widely through the range of the two species, concluded that the two mentioned characters are not sufficient for distinguishing between the two species for all the populations known at present; however, he considered that it is always possible to ascribe a given male specimen to one or other of the species, priority being given to the tarsal character and to a particular feature in the male terminalia (*see* also Machado, 1965, where a list of the principal characters distinguishing the species is given).

G. austeni, an aberrant member of the group (*see* also Chapter 10, p. 292), is easily identifiable, both by its external characters, and by the male terminalia and female genital plates. It is regarded as possessing primitive characters by Machado (1959, p. 51; *see* also p. 257 of this text). This view is certainly supported by the dark upper surfaces of the tarsal segments of the hind legs (reminiscent of the *palpalis* group and certain members of the *fusca* group), the tendency to a uniform coloration of the abdominal terga (as in the *fusca* group and most members of the *palpalis* group), the form of the superior claspers of the male (with their suggestion of that seen in the *palpalis* group) and the greater development of the genital plates of the female.

This leaves us with the forms of *G. morsitans* Westw. *sens. lat.*, and here it is proposed to follow the conclusions of Machado (personal communication, 1968). As a result of his comprehensive and widely based studies, *G. morsitans s. l.* may be regarded as constituted by four subspecies, *G.m. submorsitans* Newst., *G.m. orientalis* Vanderplank, the so-called *G.m. morsitans* Vanderplank[1] and *G.m. ugandensis* Vanderplank. These four subspecies occupy geographically distinct areas and can be defined by a combination of characters of the hypopygium (superior claspers and various parts of the phallic apparatus). The areas occupied by these four subspecies are, according to Machado, as follows: *G.m. submorsitans*—West Africa (north of the Congo forests), extending eastwards to the Bahr el Ghazal, Kordofan and the Faradje region; *G.m. orientalis*—Mozambique, Nyasaland, the lower eastern parts of Tanzania and the lower part of the Zambezi valley area, including the upper Luana valley; the so-called *G.m. morsitans*—the plateau of central Africa, including Angola, northern Botswana, part of Zambia (that approximately to the west of Broken Hill), the southern Congo, the high plateau of Tanzania and the southern fly belts of Uganda; *G.m. ugandensis*—the northern belts of Uganda (which are well separated from the southern belts) and portions of Abyssinia. As a result of examining Westwood's type of *G. morsitans* (in the Hope Department of Entomology, Oxford), Machado (personal communication, 1968) found that it corresponds to the subspecies *G.m. orientalis*, and this will involve nomenclatorial changes; nevertheless, until the full results of Machado's investigations are published, it will be better to adhere to the existing names as outlined above.

Although in the past it has been difficult to distinguish between *G.m. orientalis* and *G.m. morsitans*, the characters originally given by Vanderplank not having proved satisfactory in general practice, the two forms have long been considered to show certain differences in their ecology [Jackson in EATRO, 1954a (p. 25); 1955a (p. 22); Bursell, 1955a (p. 592)]. Further, two workers with considerable experience of both forms in the field (Drs Jackson and E. Burtt) considered them to show some differences in their appearance. Thus they maintained the eastern form to be paler in colour than the central one (Jackson in EATRO, 1954), particularly in regard to the ground colour of the wings, and to have somewhat shorter wings. In Table 9.1 are given some unpublished measurements made by

[1] *see* below

Dr Jackson, representing the wing lengths of samples of flies collected from eight localities in the eastern *morsitans* belt, ranging from Urungwe in Rhodesia through Zambia to Morogoro in Tanzania, and from six localities in the central belt, ranging from Mulungushi and Barotseland in southern Zambia through Bangweolu to Kahama in Tanzania. The means of the samples of the two forms

TABLE 9.1

Mean lengths of wings of samples of* G.m. morsitans *and* G.m. orientalis *as represented by measurements of the cutting edge of the hatchet-shaped discal cell (see Fig. 8.1)

Locality	mm.[1]	Flies
a *Western race, G. morsitans*		
Kahama District, Tanganyika	1·477–1·552	—
Bangweulu, N. Rhodesia	1·473	24
Mulwe road, Kawemba, N. Rhodesia	1·533	20
Malobazi railway, Barotseland, N. Rhodesia	1·483	20
West Lunga, N.W. Barotseland, N. Rhodesia	1·522	20
Mulungushi pocket, N. Rhodesia first collection	1·518	17
Mulungushi pocket, N. Rhodesia second collection	1·494	26
b *Eastern race, G. morsitans*		
Morogoro District, Tanganyika	1·365–1·412	—
S. of Mkushi, N. Rhodesia	1·407	16
Zambesi-Luangwa junction, N. Rhodesia	1·430	45
Luangwa R., left bank, N. Rhodesia	1·387	14
N. Lundazi, Luangwa scarp foothills, N. Rhodesia	1·417	26
N. Lundazi, Nyasaland border, N. Rhodesia	1·429	35
Locality 'E', S. of Mulungushi, N. Rhodesia	1·405	9
Between Msukwa and Rongatutu rivers, Urungwe, S. Rhodesia	1·430	30

[1] Length of cutting edge of discal cell.

do not overlap, varying from 1·365 to 1·430 mm. for the eastern form and from 1·473 to 1·552 mm. for the central form.

It is unfortunate that these figures are not now available in a form that would allow statistical analysis, and that the measurements of the wings are not related to any factor indicative of the body size of the flies (*cf.* Bursell, 1960). Machado (personal communication, 1968) has found that the variation in coloration and size throughout the range of *G. morsitans s. l.* presents a very complex picture, which he will discuss in detail in a forthcoming publication.

It is worth remarking here that Machado (1954, p. 179) is almost certainly correct in his suggestion that the specimens on which the race *congolensis* of *G.m. submorsitans* was based by Vanderplank (1949) in reality came from the north-east of the former Province Orientale of the Belgian Congo. The specimens were described as having been collected by B. D. Burtt 'in the neighbourhood of Stanleyville, Belgian Congo', and during the journey on which Burtt collected these specimens, he visited the elephant training establishment at Api in the Province Orientale; he would certainly have passed through areas in that region infested with *G.m. submorsitans* in doing so.

Haeselbarth *et al.* (1966) have drawn attention to a species of the *morsitans* group referred to by Pires and da Silva (1960) and described by Pires (1960) under the name of *G. borgesi.* They did not, however, include this species in their list, remarking that its status cannot be regarded as clear until it can be determined by examination of the type material, or of new material from the type locality, whether *G. borgesi* is to be regarded as a species or a subspecies or if it is valid at all. Machado has informed the writer (personal communication, 1968) that he has examined the Mozambique material including the type specimen and does not consider the species to be a valid one. It is therefore only included in Table 8.1 as a synonym of *G. pallidipes.*

IDENTIFICATION OF SPECIES OF *GLOSSINA*

Reference has frequently been made to the male terminalia and the female genital armature. These are the terms favoured by Machado (1954, p. 34 [f.n.], p. 48 [f.n.]) for features for which a variety of names have been used by various workers. Their appearance and situation is shown in Figs. 8.6, 9.2, 9.3, 9.4. Machado's nomenclature will also be adopted for the parts of the male terminalia and the female genital armature without further discussion of details, a description of which the interested reader will find in Machado (1954, pp. 33–50), together with two valuable tables showing the organization of the male terminalia and the various terms applied by different workers to the constituent parts, with special reference to the *palpalis* group. In a later paper, Machado (1959, pp. 33–9) discussed in detail the homologies of the parts of the male terminalia in the various species of the *fusca* group.

In the key for the identification of the species that follows, use will be made of these characters of the male terminalia and of the genital armature and signum of the female, for although it is possible to identify the species of the *morsitans* and *palpalis* groups largely by external characters such as coloration, shape of antennae, length of antennal hair fringe and so on, it is difficult to do so with any confidence for the *fusca* group or for some subspecies of the other groups. The signum is a chitinized structure found in this group on the inner side of the surface of the genital fossa, a thick symmetrical gelatinous area situated in the wall of the uterus towards its anterior end on the dorsal side (Fig. 9.4). The examination of the male terminalia and the female genital armature and signum entails the preparation of the terminal parts of the abdomen by maceration in potash, their mounting on a slide and examination microscopically, at least with a binocular dissecting microscope. The process has been described by Newstead *et al.* (1924, pp. 236–8; *see* also Chapter 19). It should be noted that unless this operation is carried out with care, erroneous conclusions may be reached. Although it may be useful that workers who have the opportunity to use such methods should do so, any specimens in doubt should be submitted to experts for examination. In making the preparations, it is most important that care should be taken to flatten the parts symmetrically, otherwise difficulties in interpretation are inevitable. A caution as to errors that may arise through the preparation and flattening of the material in mounting is sounded by Machado. Lambrecht (1954) showed in nineteen figures the varied appearance that was presented by the male terminalia of *G. morsitans* from a number of not very

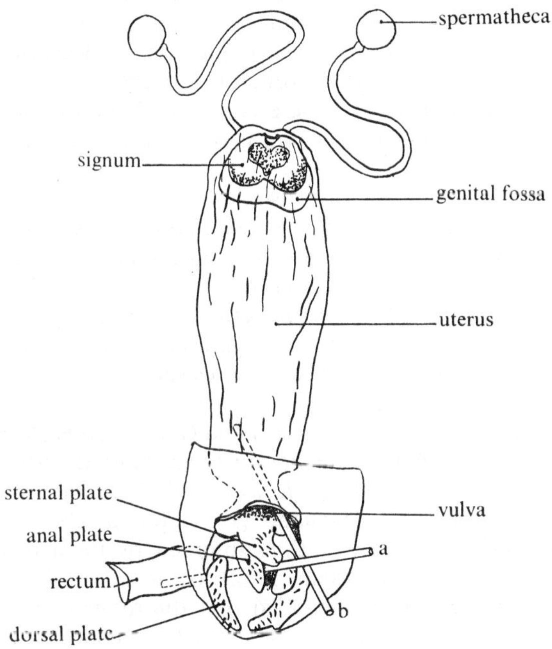

Fig. 9.4 Diagrammatic representation of external armature of *Glossina fusca* (♀), with extended uterus after maceration in caustic potash, ventral aspect, showing genital fossa and signum on the antero-dorsal wall of the uterus, with bristles (a and b) inserted into anus and vulva, respectively. (After Newstead, Evans & Potts, 1924)

widely separated places in the Ruanda-Urundi region, part of which might be accounted for in this way.

VARIATION IN *GLOSSINA*

Machado (1959, pp. 51–4) discussed geographic variation in the morphology of *Glossina*, and in course of this drew attention to the pairs of forms (*G. nigrofusca nigrofusca* and *G.n. hopkinsi*, and *G. pallicera pallicera* and *G.p. newsteadi*) in which the length of the fringe of hairs on the anterior edge of the third antennal segment is coupled with an accentuated curving and narrowing of the tip of that segment. To these couples can be added the pair *G. longipalpis* and *G. pallidipes* (see p. 249). He speculated as to whether these differences may have any functional significance. It is perhaps possible to hazard one for the last pair. It would seem that, although *G. longipalpis* and *G. pallidipes* are very similar in their habits and general choice of habitat and of host (*see* pp. 323–4), their distribution suggests that the latter species can exist in somewhat drier conditions than the former. The antenna, an organ believed to be concerned with the detection of atmospheric moisture (Glasgow, 1963, p. 17), is especially exposed during flight to currents of air. It may well be, therefore, that a thicker covering of hairs on the leading edge of the antenna, is an advantage in a species that is active in drier conditions. Whether such considerations might apply to the other pairs of forms is not known, but this could be a profitable subject for investigation. On the other hand, it might well be that these two characters are merely linked with some other constitutional character that is of advantage to one or other of the pair.

In his detailed discussion of the variation shown by the signa of the *fusca* group, Machado (1959, p. 55) made the useful point that a distinction must be drawn between geographical and individual variations. This is a distinction that is not always easy to make, and one that involves the study of a large number of specimens from a variety of localities covering as much as possible of the range of the species. Machado pointed out that, although variation in the signum has been referred to by various workers [in *G. fusca* (Newstead *et al.*, 1924, p. 94), *G. fuscipleuris* (*op. cit.*, p. 76; Evens, 1953, p. 9), *G. tabaniformis* (Patton, 1936, Fig. 18; Vaucel, 1943; Evens, 1953, p. 14) and *G. haningtoni* (Vaucel, 1943)], the only well worked-out instance of geographical variation described is that shown by the two subspecies of *G. fusca*, *G.f. fusca* and *G.f. congolensis*, and this was discussed in some detail by Machado (1959, pp. 52–3). Nash and Jordan (1959) described the range of variation observed by them in the signa of *G. medicorum*, *G. nashi* (*see* also Jordan, 1962), *G. tabaniformis*, *G. haningtoni*, *G. nigrofusca* and *G. fusca*. They concluded that the range of variation observed by them in a large number of specimens of *G. fusca* collected in Nigeria and a limited number from elsewhere was so great, individuals with genitalia intermediate between those of both the subspecies being common, that they could not recognize the validity of Newstead's subspecies. However, the work of Machado was followed up by Le Berre and Itard (1960) who gave a mensural basis to his conclusions, and later by Jordan (1965a) who, as a result of the study of the male genitalia as well as of the female signa, has confirmed the validity of Newstead's original recognition of *G.f. congolensis* as distinct from *G.f. fusca*. Jordan considered the two forms to be subspecies, the first a microphallic form, occurring in the eastern parts of the range of the species, and the second a macrophallic form, occurring in the western parts (*see* also Machado, 1959). Both subspecies are found in Ghana, where a search for intermediate forms would be worth while. He concluded that the Tago-Dahomey savanna gap is no longer a geographic barrier between these two forest dwelling forms, as Machado suggested it had been in the past, but that the separation between the two may be an ancient one and the penetration of *G.f. congolensis* into the forests west of the savanna gap a relatively recent phenomenon.

The macrophallism and microphallism of the two subspecies are reflected in the larger signum of *G.f. fusca* as compared with that of *G.f. congolensis* (*cf.* Machado, 1959, p. 53), and this supports the suggestion of Machado (*op. cit.*, p. 56) that the particular form of the signum of each species is related to the different forms of the male aedeagus. In this connection, he drew attention to the opaque concretions observed on the signa of certain of the *fusca* group (*cf.* Vaucel, 1943; Patton, 1936, Fig. 18, c,d; Nash & Jordan, 1959, Figs. 7, 9, 10 and 12), the nature and origin of which he discussed. He noted the resemblance of these internal concretions to the external mating scars ('ecchymoses nuptiales') observed in females of the *palpalis* group (Squire, 1951a; Machado, 1954, Fig. 9; Vattier, 1965) and to pigmented patches on the dorsal swelling of the uterine wall at the point of entry of the common oviduct (Machado, 1954, Fig. 11).

He suggested that all these phenomena may well be produced by the pressure of the hard processes of the male terminalia and pointed out how this accords with the account of the process of copulation given by Vanderplank (1948, p. 138 and Fig. 1), though he expressed some reservations about this account. In a later paper, Machado (1964) gave a detailed comparison of the position of these concretions on the signum of *G. fusca congolensis* with the disposition of the processes of the harpes of the male aedeagus, and demonstrated how the concretions correspond with the positions on the signum on which the aedeagal processes will press during copulation. In his 1959 paper, Machado noted the poor development or absence of the signum in certain species (*G. nigrofusca*, *G. longipennis*, *G. brevipalpis* and the species of the *palpalis* and *morsitans* groups), the males of which do not possess differentiated harpes or other pointed parts capable of exerting strong pressure on the internal genital tracts of the female, or in which such parts are feebly chitinized, as in the first-named species. He drew attention to the occasional presence of external scars on females of species of the *fusca* group, particularly of *G. longipennis* (see Machado, 1959, p. 42), the males of which have superior claspers with particularly well developed terminal claws) and of similar scars on males of the *palpalis* group, which suggest attempts of the males to copulate with one another, a phenomenon that the writer has observed to occur with *G. morsitans* and *G. swynnertoni* in nature. However, Machado now believes that these external scars are not mating scars but rather the results of attempts of predators to capture the tsetse (personal communication, 1968).

PHYLOGENY OF *GLOSSINA*

In a discussion of the phylogeny of *Glossina*, Machado (1959, pp. 49–51) reviewed the views of Newstead (1911, p. 9), Newstead *et al.* (1924, p. 43), Evens (1953) and Bursell (1958), who considered the *fusca* group to be the most primitive of the three groups. Machado suggested that Newstead's view was based principally on a consideration of the superior claspers of the male terminalia and that if he had taken as his basis other characters such as the structure of the aedeagus and the differentiation of the female armature, he would have come to another conclusion. It is perhaps unfortunate that Newstead wrote that his classification 'begins with the apparently primitive forms (the *fusca* group) and rises to the higher and more complex forms [the *palpalis* and *morsitans* groups]' (Newstead *et al.*, 1924, p. 43), for surely the course of evolution does not necessarily result in the production of more complicated structure, but may often proceed by a process of simplification. Thus, whereas the superior claspers of the three groups may be regarded as becoming progressively more complicated as one passes from the *fusca* group through the *palpalis* group to the *morsitans* group, the aedeagus certainly, as Machado suggested, cannot; this, however, does not necessarily prevent one from regarding the first group as the more primitive one. Indeed, whether one regards the superior claspers of *Glossina* as the anal cerci of other groups, as Patton (1934) appeared to do, or as flanges or lateral lobes of the ninth tergite, as Hardy (1944) suggested, it seems to the writer that the free condition and simple claw-like form of the claspers of the *fusca* group are much more likely to represent a primitive condition than that shown by the claspers of the *morsitans* group. Equally, one might regard the complicated aedeagus and its processes shown by the *fusca* group as having become simplified in the course of evolution to the somewhat less complicated conditions now shown in the other two groups.

One must, however, agree with Machado that one cannot accept the views advanced by Evens (1953) as to the closeness of the relationship of the fossil tsetse species found in the sedimentary shales of Florissant, Colorado, to the *fusca* group. On the age of the fossils there seems to be some doubt, but their assignment to the Oligocene period is perhaps the most well-founded (Machado, 1959, p. 50). One must also accept the conclusion of the latter that the palaeontological evidence allows one to say no more than that the genus *Glossina* is an ancient one, that it was already considerably diversified as long ago as, perhaps, the Oligocene, that its past distribution has included what is now part of the American continent and that there the genus existed under conditions probably considerably different from those in which it now lives in tropical and subtropical Africa.

Machado (1954, p. 178) remarks on the impossibility of knowing whether characters shared by two species or forms show a common inheritance or are merely the expression of similar potentialities, the phenomenon called paripotency by Haecker (*see* Mayr, 1942, p. 74; Huxley, 1942, p. 351). Machado expressed this conclusion after a consideration of the taxonomic status of the polytypic species *G. palpalis* and *G. fuscipes*. He noted that these species present an example of independent variation, in that a character that appears associated with certain other characters in one population, race or definitive species is associated with other different characters in another population, race or species. This results in a mosaic of characters that makes the determination of affinities of the taxa difficult, and he draws up an interesting table of the various degrees of differentiation manifested by the members of the *palpalis* group. Other instances of this are mentioned in the detailed consideration of the affinities of the species of the *fusca* group in Machado's 1959 paper (pp. 39–51). One must therefore agree with his conclusion that it is not possible to resolve with certainty which is the most primitive of the groups of *Glossina*. Nevertheless, the writer cannot avoid the suspicion that the balance of probability lies with the view that the *fusca* group represents the primitive condition of the genus *Glossina* in Africa, both in its morphology and in its way of life, and that the picture of the evolution of the genus in Africa suggested by Bursell (1958) may not be far off the mark. It is interesting, in view of the centres of tsetse evolution in the Congo suggested by Evens (1953), that certain members both of the *fusca* group (*G. longipennis* and *G. brevipalpis*) and of the *morsitans* group (*G. austeni*) possess what Machado regards as primitive characters (on the grounds that they are common to all the groups) and that these species are found at the extreme edges of the dispersal suggested by Evens. It might therefore well be that it is the passage of time involved in this dispersal that has allowed these species to adapt themselves to ways of life so different from those of the other members of their groups, rather than isolating barriers (on which Glasgow, 1963, p. 173, has cast a doubt).

THE GENETICS OF *GLOSSINA*

The study of the genetics of *Glossina* has received very little attention until recently. The only early information bearing on this subject was the reference by Vanderplank (1948) to an unpublished observation by Dr Slyzinski (of Edinburgh) to the effect that *G. morsitans morsitans* has two pairs of V-shaped autosomes and two sex chromosomes. The paucity of work on this subject has been due in part to the difficulty in establishing self-perpetuating colonies of *Glossina* in the laboratory and in part to the preoccupation of tsetse entomologists with objectives of a more patently practical nature. Recently, however, the successful establishment of self-supporting colonies of tsetse flies in the laboratory (*see* Chapter 20) and the increasing interest in the use of genetic methods of tsetse control (*see* Chapter 26) have made possible studies on the chromosomes of *Glossina* and stimulated interest in them. A preliminary picture of the chromosome structure in six species of the genus has now been obtained. These are *G. tachinoides*, *G. morsitans*, *G. palpalis*, *G. fuscipes*, *G. pallidipes* and *G. austeni*, on which the available information is summarized in Table 9.2.

It will be seen from Table 9.2 that whereas the chromosome numbers in species of the *palpalis* group are uniformly six, those of the *morsitans* group vary from six to fourteen. These observations have been discussed by Riordan (1968) and Itard (1969). The latter worker suggests that possibly the extra variable numbers of small chromosomes observed in the *morsitans* group may be supernumerary or B chromosomes. Such chromosomes, he remarks, have been observed to be present, at times, in some local populations but absent from others in different geographic zones; their presence or absence does not appear to affect the phenotype of the individuals concerned.

Chromosomes in mitosis have been found in the puparial stages by Riordan (1968), mostly during the first 18–24 hours, but even up to four days, after larviposition. Itard (1969) observes that the search for chromosomes is most often successful when the peri-oesophageal nervous tissue of twenty-four-hour old puparial stages (i.e. in the late third-instar larva) is examined and that meiosis is most readily detected in the testes of eight-day old puparial stages (i.e. in the early part of the pupal stage).

Methods used in the study of tsetse chromosomes are described by the two authors just cited and by Burchard and Baldry (1970) and Riordan (1970).

TABLE 9.2

***Summary of information on chromosomes in* Glossina**

Species	Somatic number	Nature	Mean length of pairs (μ)	Sources of tissue (all from larval or puparial stages)	Authority
G. tachinoides	6 (3 pairs)	Metaphase 1 (meiosis)	6·9, 5·5, 3·8[1]	Central nervous system, Malpighian tubes and testes	Itard (1966a)
G. morsitans[2] *orientalis*	10 (5 pairs)	Somatic tissues	{6·4 (2 pairs), 5·2, 1·9 (2 pairs)}	Central nervous system and Malpighian tubes	Itard (1966a)
		Metaphase 1 (meiosis)	12·4, 11·6, 8·4[3a] 3·2, 2·8[3b]	Testes	
G. morsitans morsitans	6 (3 pairs)	2 pairs V-shaped autosomes, and 2 sex chromosomes	?	?	Vanderplank (1948) [*see* also Itard (1969) through Curtis *in litt.*]
G. palpalis palpalis	6 (3 pairs)	Metaphase (mitosis)	5·1 (2 pairs) 3·6 (1 pair)	Central nervous system	Riordan (1968)
G. fuscipes fuscipes	6 (3 pairs)	Metaphase 1 (meiosis)	9·6, 8·1, 5·9	?	Itard (1969)
G. pallidipes	8 (4 pairs)	?	7·8 (2 pairs), 5·72,[4] 1·68	Central nervous system	Hulley (1968) and Itard (1969)
G. austeni	14 (7 pairs)	?	5·9–6·5 (2 pairs), 5·3,[5a] 2·7 (4 pairs)[5b]	Central nervous system and testes	Itard (1969)

[1] Two pairs metacentric, the third sub-acrocentric.
[2] Referred to by Itard as *G.m. morsitans*.
[3a] Two pairs metacentric and one sub-acrocentric.
[3b] Both pairs acrocentric.
[4] All three larger pairs metacentric, although in some preparations one seemed to be sub-acrocentric.
[5a] All three larger pairs metacentric.
[5b] All four smaller pairs acrocentric.

The three last named workers have also demonstrated the presence of polytene (banded) chromosomes in preparations of subcutaneous muscle obtained from newly deposited third-instar larvae of *G. palpalis* and in the midgut cells of larvae of this species deposited 36–48 hours previously. These latest observations foreshadow the possibility of preparing chromosome maps for the various species of *Glossina*, a development which would greatly facilitate taxonomic studies of local forms of *Glossina* and the evolution of genetic methods of tsetse control.

KEY FOR THE IDENTIFICATION OF *GLOSSINA*

The following key is based largely on those of Newstead *et al.* (1924), Buxton (1955) and Smart (1956). It has, however, been considerably modified from these. The modifications have been made in order to bring it into accord with the revision by Machado (1954) of the *palpalis* group and with the ideas of that author (1959), of Nash and Jordan (1959) and of Jordan (1965a) in regard to the *fusca* group. It has also been necessary to incorporate the two most recently described species of *Glossina*, *G. vanhoofi* (Henrard, 1952) and *G. nashi* (Potts, 1955; Jordan, 1962), not included in the earlier keys. At the same time, an attempt has been made to follow a more regular construction of the couplets. In these, with few exceptions, the use of the characters of the male and of the female genitalia is supplemented by the use of external characters such as coloration. It must, however, be emphasized that in cases of doubt the characters of the male and female genitalia will give the more certain identification. The terms used in the key for various structures are explained either by the figures or in the preceding text.

1. Pteropleuron (Fig. 9.12), bearing a few strong bristles of size equal to those on the sternopleuron, the bristles in both cases clearly distinguishable from the general vestiture of shorter setulose hairs of the pleural sclerites; hairs on edge of thoracic squamae (Fig. 9.12) curly and numerous, giving a woolly appearance; large species, 10·75–13·5 mm. long; males with the superior claspers free, not joined by a membrane, claw-shaped (Fig. 9.1, A); external genital armature of females consisting of five well-defined chitinous plates (Fig. 9.2). Subgenus *Austenina* or '*fusca* group' 15

Pteropleuron bearing only setulose hairs some of which may be larger than others but none of which equal in size the clearly differentiated bristles projecting from amongst the setulose hairs on the sternopleuron; hairs on edge of thoracic squamae fewer, not curly, giving a neat fringe-like appearance; smaller species usually under 11 mm. long; males with the superior claspers joined by a membrane (Fig. 9.1, B,C); external genital armature of female consisting of six well-defined chitinous plates (Fig. 9.6, D) or of less than five generally much reduced and indistinct chitinous plates (Fig. 9.3). Subgenera *Glossina* (*morsitans* group) and *Nemorhina* (*palpalis* group) 2

2. All segments of hind tarsi dark brown or blackish when viewed from above; abdomen generally dark brown with at most indistinct markings, but can have dark bands on pale yellowish background (*tachinoides*); superior

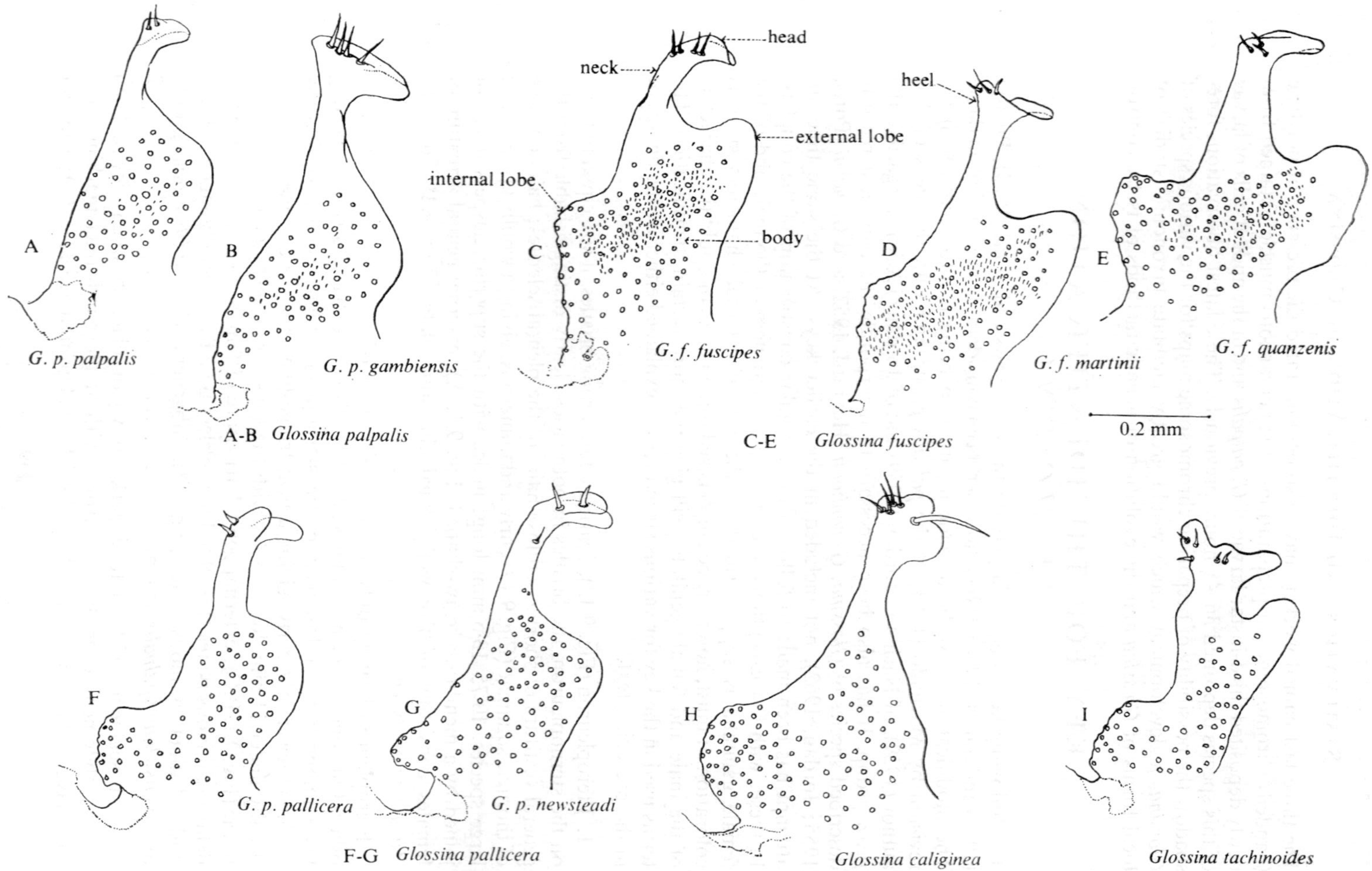

Fig. 9.5 Inferior claspers of males of *palpalis* group: A–B, *Glossina palpalis* subspp.; C–E, *Glossina fuscipes* subspp.; F–G, *Glossina*

claspers of male claw-shaped (Fig. 9.1, B); external genitalia of female consisting of six well-defined chitinous plates (Fig. 9.6, D). Subgenus *Nemorhina* (*palpalis* group) 3

Only apical two hind tarsal segments dark brown or blackish, basal three being paler brown except in some specimens of *austeni*, which may have all segments dark, as in *palpalis* group, but can then be distinguished by the reddish ochraceous dorsal surface of the abdomen, never with distinct darker bands; super claspers of male swollen distally (Fig. 9.1, C; 9.7); external genitalia of female consisting of much reduced and generally indistinct plates (Fig. 9.3, A), except for two small distinct dorsal plates in *austeni* (Fig. 9.3, B). Subgenus *Glossina s. str.* (*morsitans* group) 11

3. Fringe of hairs on anterior edge of third antennal segment a quarter of the antennal width or more; tip of head of inferior claspers of male bifurcated (Fig. 9.5, F,G); dorsal plates of external genitalia of female distinctly broader than tall (Fig. 9.6, G,H) (*pallicera s. l.*) 4

Antennal fringe a sixth of the antennal width or less; tip of head of inferior claspers of male not bifurcated (e.g. Fig. 9.5, A–E,H,I), at most notch giving a bilobed appearance; dorsal plates of external genitalia of female not markedly broader than tall (e.g. Fig. 9.6, A–F,I,J) 5

4. Third antennal segment unusually narrow and strongly curved at apex; antennal fringe nearly equal to antennal width; inferior claspers of male with internal lobe flat edged (Fig. 9.5, F). West Africa, Sierra Leone to Cameroon (Map 10.4) .. .. *pallicera pallicera* Bigot

Third antennal segment not unusually narrow or strongly curved at apex; antennal fringe a quarter to a third of the antennal width; inferior claspers of male with basal internal lobe pointed (Fig. 9.5, G). Gaboon, Ubangi-Shari, Belgian Congo, north-western Angola (Map 10.4) *pallicera newsteadi* (Austen)

5. Dorsal surface of abdominal segments light yellow in ground colour, with interrupted dark bands; inferior claspers of male with short necks (as broad as long) (Fig. 9.5, I); dorsal plates of external genitalia of female about twice as tall as broad, somewhat pale and without hairs on internal angles (Fig. 9.6, J). A small species, 6·5–9 mm. long; hinterland of West Africa to Sudan and Abyssinia; S. Arabia (?) (Map 10.4) .. .. .. *tachinoides* Westwood

Dorsal abdominal surface without any distinct banding; inferior claspers of male with long necks (plainly longer than broad) (Fig. 9.5, A–E,H); dorsal plates of external genitalia of female (Fig. 9.6, A–F, I) at most one and a half times as tall as broad 6

6. Dorsal surface of abdomen dark to sepia brown, hind margin of segments not narrowly paler than rest, a wide, more or less square median pale area on second tergite; superior claspers of male with free end very long, almost a third of the length of the clasper; inferior claspers as in Fig. 9.5, H; dorsal plates of external genitalia of female as broad as tall or nearly so, without hairs on internal angles, but medio-dorsal plate always broader than tall (Fig. 9.6, I). West Africa, from Ghana to Cameroon, Gaboon and Oubangui (Map 10.4) .. .. *caliginea* Austen

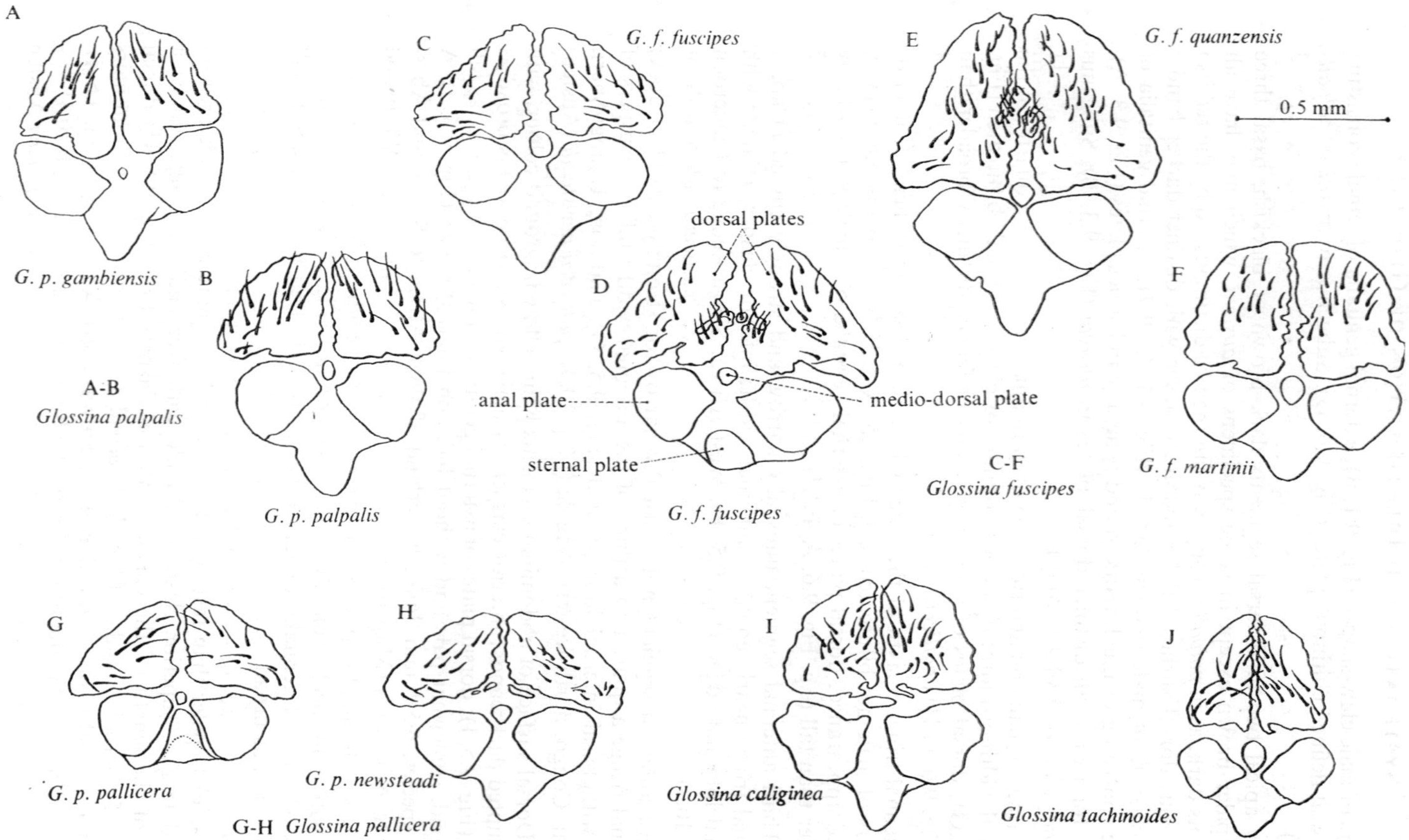

Fig. 9.6 Plates of genital armature of females of *palpalis* group: A–B, *Glossina palpalis* subspp.; C–F, *Glossina fuscipes* subspp.; G–H, *Glossina pallicera;* I,*Glossina caliginea;* J, *Glossina tachinoides*. (After Machado, 1954)

Hind margins of dorsal surfaces of abdominal segments narrowly paler, and the median pale area on the second segment narrow and elongated; superior claspers of male with free end short, distinctly less than a third of the length of the claspers (e.g. Fig. 9.1, B); inferior claspers not as in Fig. 9.5, H; dorsal plates of external genitalia of female often somewhat taller than broad, with or without hairs on internal angles, but medio-dorsal plate never broader than tall (Fig. 9.6, A–F) 7

7. Colour generally less dark; inferior claspers of male with external lobe not prominent and not projecting upwards, internal lobes absent (Fig. 9.5, A,B) dorsal plates of female close together, hairs more robust and absent from the internal angles and median space (Fig. 9.6, A,B) .. .. (*palpalis s. l.*) 8

Colour generally darker (except in *fuscipes martinii*); inferior claspers of male with external lobe prominent, projecting upwards, internal lobe prominent (Fig. 9.5, C E); dorsal plates of female well separated, hairs less robust and almost always present on internal angles and sometimes on median space (Fig. 9.6, C–F) .. ..(*fuscipes s. l.*) 9

8. Inferior clasper of male with terminal dilatation relatively small, its width less than length of neck, which emerges abruptly from the body (Fig. 9.5, A); dorsal plates of female about as tall as broad, internal angles projecting little, and anal plates not extending laterally as far as outer angle of dorsal plates (Fig. 9.6, B). West Africa, from Nigeria to S. Angola (Map 10.3) .. .. *palpalis palpalis* (Robineau-Desvoidy)

Inferior clasper of male with terminal dilatation relatively large, width more than length of neck, which emerges gradually from the body (Fig. 9.5, B); dorsal plates of female a little taller than broad, internal angles projecting markedly; anal plates extending laterally as far as or beyond outer angle of dorsal plates (Fig. 9.6, A). West Africa, from Senegal to Ivory Coast (with forms transitional to *palpalis palpalis* between Liberia and Ghana, at least) (Map 10.3) .. .. *palpalis gambiensis* Vanderplank

9. General colour pale; terminal dilatation of inferior clasper of male with marked heel (Fig. 9.5, D); anal plates of female extending laterally almost as widely or as widely as dorsal plates (Fig. 9.6, F). Congo, Tanzania, Zambia (from Upper Lualaba to Luapula rivers and Lake Tanganyika). (Map 10.3) .. .. *fuscipes martinii* Zumpt

General colour dark; terminal dilatation of inferior clasper of male without marked heel (Fig. 9.5, C,E); anal plates of female extending less widely than dorsal plates (Fig. 9.6, C–E) 10

10. Inferior clasper of male with straight thick neck (Fig. 9.5, E); dorsal plates of female appreciably taller than broad (Fig. 9.6, E). French Equatorial Africa, former Belgian Congo, Angola (Map. 10.3) .. *fuscipes quanzensis* Pires

Inferior clasper of male with curved thin neck (Fig. 9.5, C); dorsal plates of female about as tall as broad (Fig. 9.6, C,D). Central and eastern Africa generally (in the region of the great forest and the central African lakes) (Map 10.3) .. .. *fuscipes fuscipes* Newstead

11. Antennal fringe a fifth to a third of antennal width; superior claspers of male with outer lateral angle forming a blunt tooth (Fig. 9.7, A,B) .. 12

Antennal fringe length not more than a seventh of antennal width; superior claspers of male with outer lateral angle bluntly rounded or strongly produced and narrowly rounded, but not tooth-like (Fig. 9.7, C–E) 13

12. Front and middle tarsi uniformly yellow-brown; antennal fringe a third of antennal width, and length of third antennal segment about five times its width; tooth of superior claspers of male subterminal (Fig. 9.7, B). Central and eastern Africa, Somalia and Ethiopia to Zululand (Map 10.5) .. *pallidipes* Austen

Apical two segments of front and middle tarsi with sharply defined dark tips; antennal fringe length a fifth to a quarter of antennal width, and length of antennal segment about three and a half times its width; tooth of superior claspers of male terminal (Fig. 9.7, A). West Africa from Gambia to Cameroon (Map 10.5) .. .. *longipalpis* Wiedemann

13. Dorsal surface of abdomen reddish ochraceous with only indistinct transverse dark bands; all segments of hind tarsi dark, though last two sometimes slightly darker than the rest; outer lateral angles of superior claspers of male strongly produced and narrowly rounded (Fig. 9.7, E); external genital armature of female with strongly chitinized distinct dorsal plates and well-marked anal plates (Fig. 9.3, B). East African coastal regions, Somalia to Zululand (Map 10.6) .. .. *austeni* Newstead

Dorsal surface of abdomen light in colour and with distinct dark brown transverse bands medially interrupted; apical two segments of hind tarsi dark and sharply contrasted with the three pale proximal ones; outer lateral angles of superior claspers of male bluntly rounded and not strongly produced (Fig. 9.7, C,D); external genital armature of female without very distinct chitinized plates (e.g. Fig. 9.3, A) 14

14. Hind margins of transverse dark bands on abdomen rounded and tend to be somewhat indistinctly defined; median lobes of superior claspers of male with broad tips, turned outwards and generally ending level with or projecting slightly beyond the swollen distal portions of the claspers (Fig. 9.7, C). Western, central and eastern Africa (Map 10.6) .. .. *morsitans* Wiedemann[1]

Hind margins of transverse dark bands on abdomen angular and sharply defined; median lobes of superior claspers of male with small, pointed tips, not generally reaching level of distal edge of the claspers (Fig. 9.7, D). Kenya, Tanzania (Map 10.6) .. .. *swynnertoni* Austen

15. Palpi shorter than breadth of head or not exceeding this by more than one-ninth of their length 16

Palpi exceeding breadth of head by one-sixth to one-third of their length 20

16. Wings dusky; antennal fringe a quarter to a third of maximal antennal width; harpes of male terminalia with three pairs of long pointed lateral processes, each member of the third pair being bifid (Fig. 9.8, A); signum of female

[1] Four subspecies are recognizable (*see* p. 250) in different parts of its range, but, as the differences between them are slight, they can only be differentiated by detailed examination of the male terminalia.

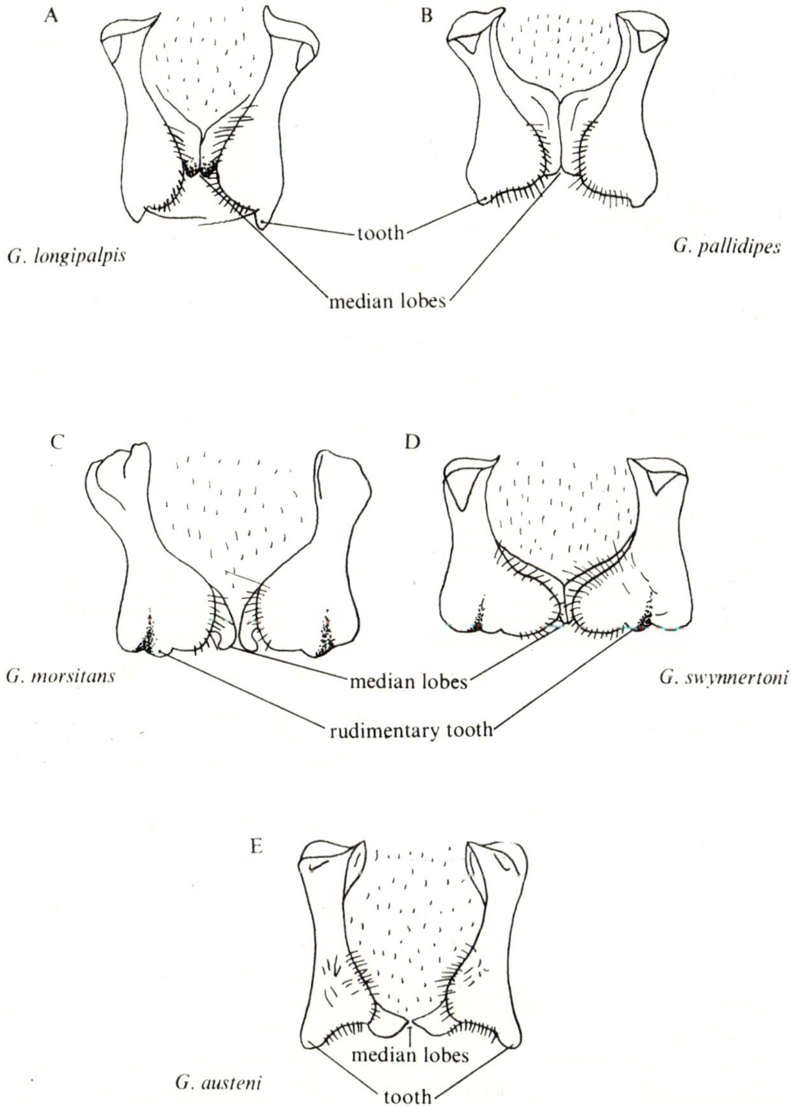

Fig. 9.7 Superior claspers of males of *morsitans* group: A, *Glossina longipalpis*; B, *Glossina pallidipes*; C, *Glossina morsitans*; D, *Glossina swynnertoni*; E, *Glossina austeni*. (After Newstead, Evans & Potts, 1924)

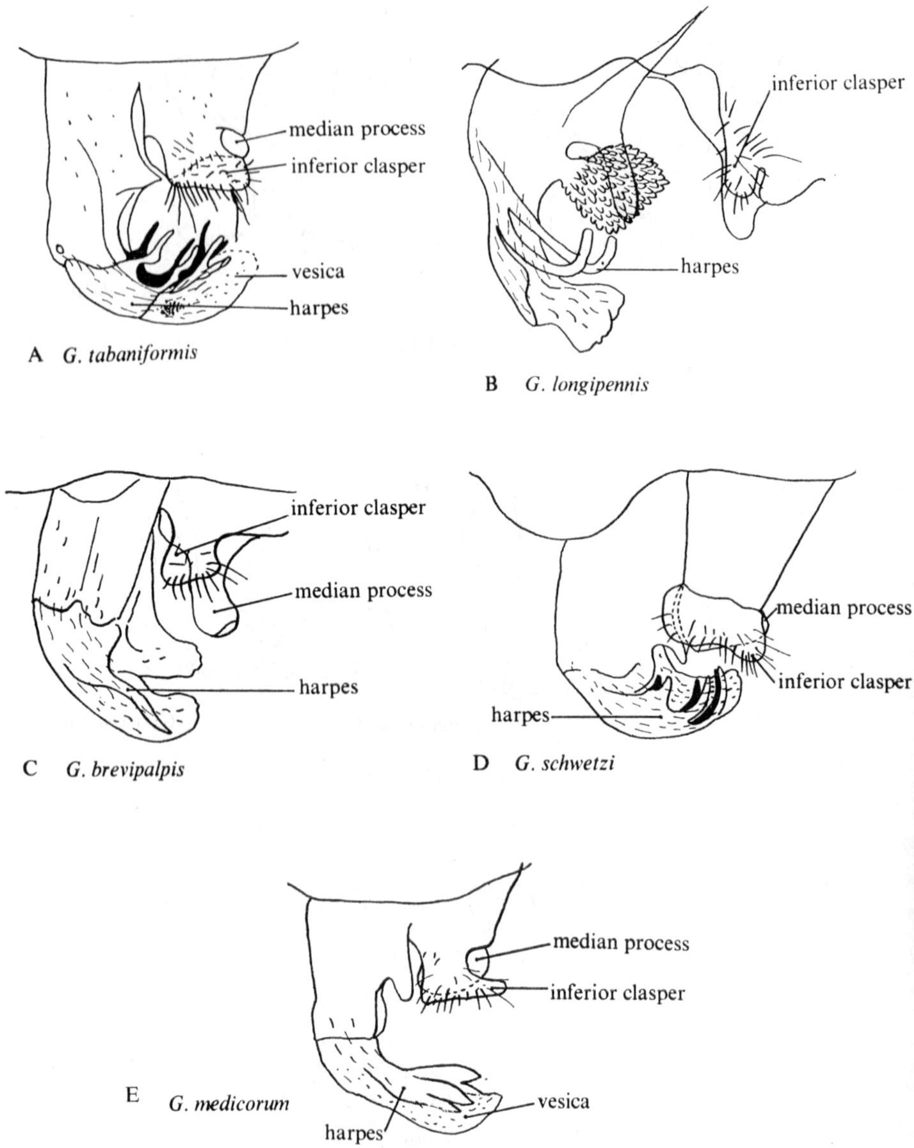

Fig. 9.8 Lateral views of male terminalia of species of *fusca* group: I: A, *Glossina tabaniformis*; B, *Glossina longipennis*; C, *Glossina brevipalpis*; D, *Glossina schwetzi*; E, *Glossina medicorum*. (After Newstead, Evans & Potts, 1924, with modifications based on Nash & Jordan, 1959, and Machado, 1959)

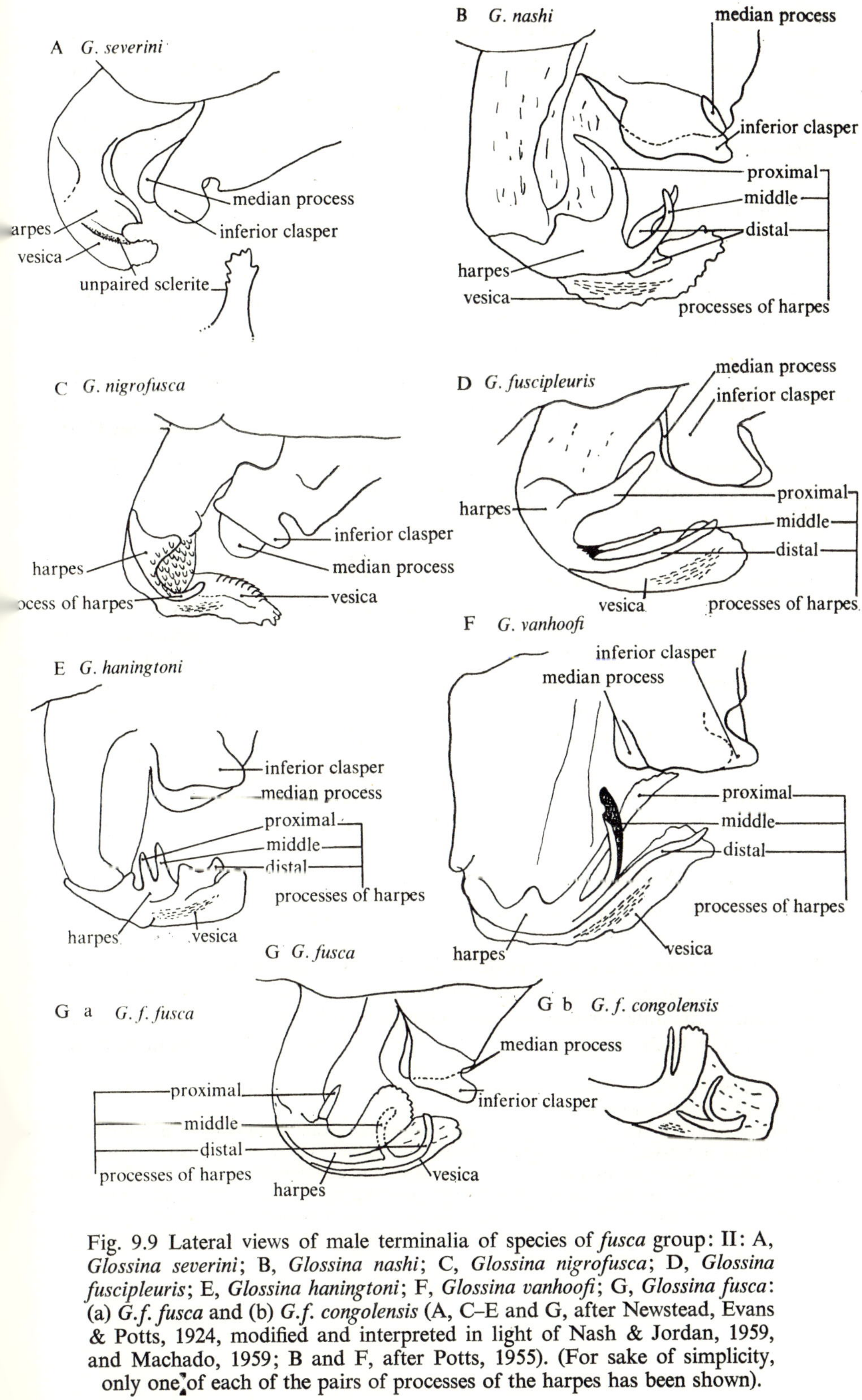

Fig. 9.9 Lateral views of male terminalia of species of *fusca* group: II: A, *Glossina severini*; B, *Glossina nashi*; C, *Glossina nigrofusca*; D, *Glossina fuscipleuris*; E, *Glossina haningtoni*; F, *Glossina vanhoofi*; G, *Glossina fusca*: (a) *G.f. fusca* and (b) *G.f. congolensis* (A, C–E and G, after Newstead, Evans & Potts, 1924, modified and interpreted in light of Nash & Jordan, 1959, and Machado, 1959; B and F, after Potts, 1955). (For sake of simplicity, only one of each of the pairs of processes of the harpes has been shown).

a thin somewhat lyriform unflexed plate, divided by a transverse constriction into two unequal parts, the distal one the larger and deeply bifurcated (Fig. 9.10, A).[1] West Africa, from Ivory Coast to former Belgian Congo and extending inland nearly to eastern boundary of latter (Map 10.1) *tabaniformis* Westwood

Wings pale; antennal fringe a fifth of maximal antennal width or less; harpes of male terminalia (Fig. 9.8, B–E) with or without paired lateral processes, but none with a bifid third pair; signa of females, when present, of varied form (Fig. 9.10, B–D) but never lyriform 17

17. A pale species, generally light yellowish brown, with a conspicuous dark brown spot in each of the four quarters of dorsum of thorax; harpes of male terminalia consisting of a pair of long undivided slender processes (Fig. 9.8, B); uterus of female with a reduced and often weakly chitinized signum (Fig. 9.10, B). Northern East Africa, including Sudan, Ethiopia and Somalia (Map 10.2) .. .. *longipennis* Corti

Dark brown or greyish brown species, without conspicuous dark spots as described above; harpes of male terminalia not as preceding (Fig. 9.8, C–E); signum of uterus absent or, if present, well developed (Fig. 9.10, C,D) .. 18

18. Anterior cross-vein of wing of both sexes with a thickened portion, strongly chitinized and darkened (Fig. 9.11, A); male terminalia with harpes poorly developed, lacking projecting paired lateral processes, and with a prominent median process projecting markedly from between the inferior claspers for more than twice their length (Fig. 9.8, C); uterus of female without signum and dorsal plates of external genital armature as in Fig. 9.2, the presence of the hamate sclerites being peculiar to this species. East and Central Africa (northern Kenya to Zululand, and south-eastern Congo) (Map 10.1) .. .. *brevipalpis* Newstead

Anterior cross-vein of wing with thickened portion not noticeably darkened in male (*cf.* Fig. 9.11, B); male terminalia with well developed harpes and with median process not prominent and not projecting markedly beyond inferior claspers (Fig. 9.8, D,E); uterus of female always with signum (Fig. 9.10, C,D) 19

19. Anterior cross-vein of wing with thickened portion noticeably darkened in female (as in Fig. 9.11, A) but not in male (Fig. 9.11, B); harpes of male terminalia with three pairs of processes (Fig. 9.8, D),[2] signum of uterus (Fig. 9.10, C) with a pair of dark, curved, chitinous thickenings and sometimes a posterior pair behind the anterior one. Western Congo and Angola, on the Congo River system (Map 10.2) .. .. *schwetzi* Newstead & Evans

[1] Considerable variation in the degree of chitinization of the signum is described by Vaucel (1943) and Nash & Jordan (1959).

[2] In certain more heavily chitinized forms and under certain conditions of mounting, the third pair of processes, which have been shown by Machado (1959) to be separated from the main body of the harpes, may appear to be joined with it, as originally described by Newstead and Evans (1921), and the median process may seem to project somewhat beyond the inferior claspers, as described by Potts (1924) when he named such a form as the variety *disjuncta*; these differences do not, as demonstrated by Machado, constitute characters that justify the maintenance of the variety as distinct.

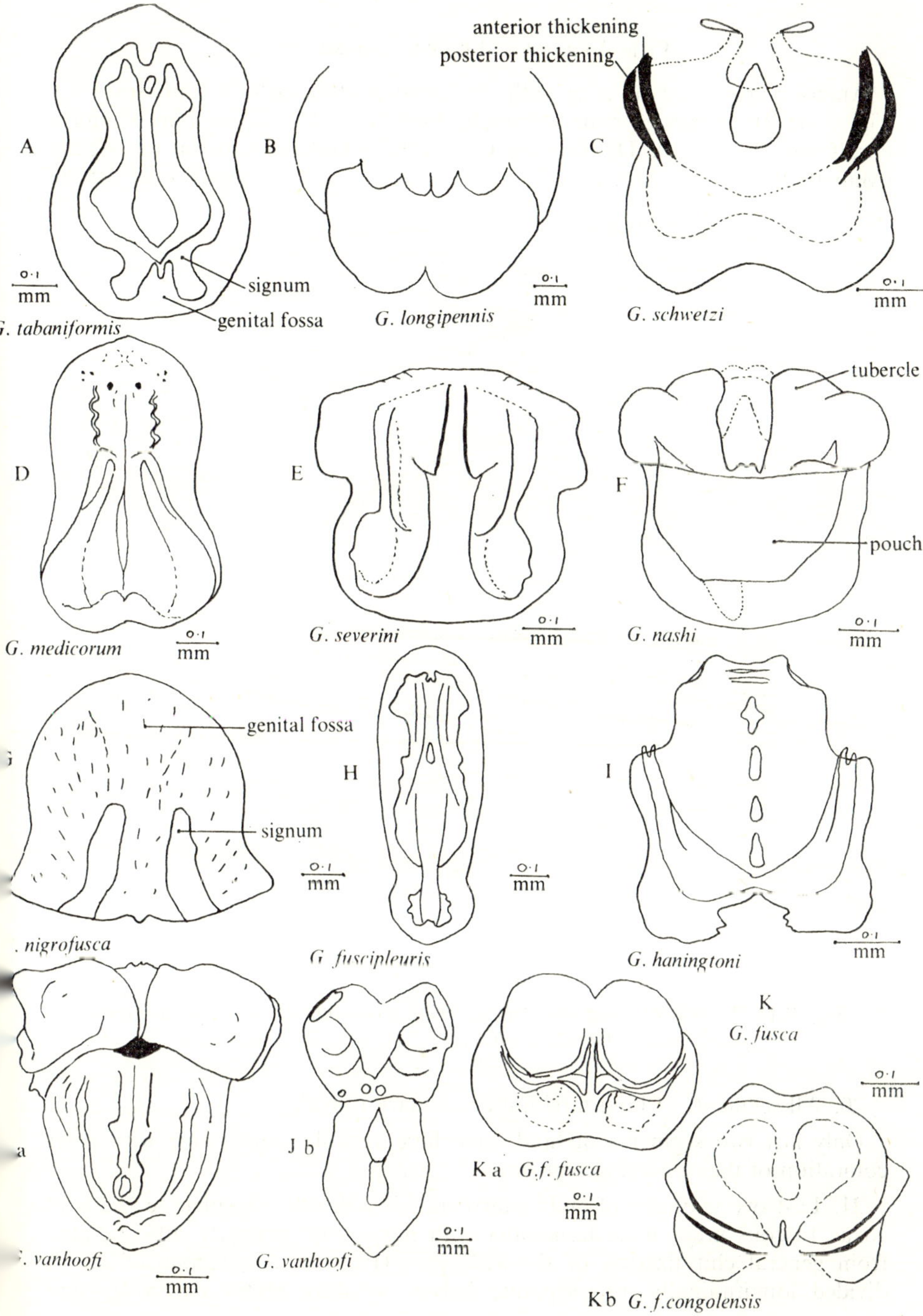

Fig. 9.10 Signa of females of species of the *fusca* group: A, *Glossina tabaniformis*; B, *Glossina longipennis*; C, *Glossina schwetzi*; D, *Glossina medicorum*; E, *Glossina severini*; F, *Glossina nashi*; G, *Glossina nigrofusca*; H, *Glossina fuscipleuris*; I, *Glossina haningtoni*; J, *Glossina vanhoofi*: (a) well chitinised specimen, (b) weakly chitinised specimen; K, *Glossina fusca*: (a) *G.f. fusca*, (b) *G.f. congolensis* (A, C–E, G–I and K, after Newstead, Evans & Potts, 1924; B, after Patton, 1934; F, after Jordan, 1962; J (a) after Henrard, 1952, (b) after Potts, 1955). (The genital fossa is not shown in B, C, E, F, I, J and K (b).)

Anterior cross-vein of wing with thickened portion pale in both sexes (*cf.* Fig. 9.11, B); harpes of male terminalia bifid (Fig. 9.8, E); signum of uterus cordiform (Fig. 9.10, D). Guinea Gulf Coast, Gabon, Liberia to Nigeria (Map 10.2) .. .. *medicorum* Austen

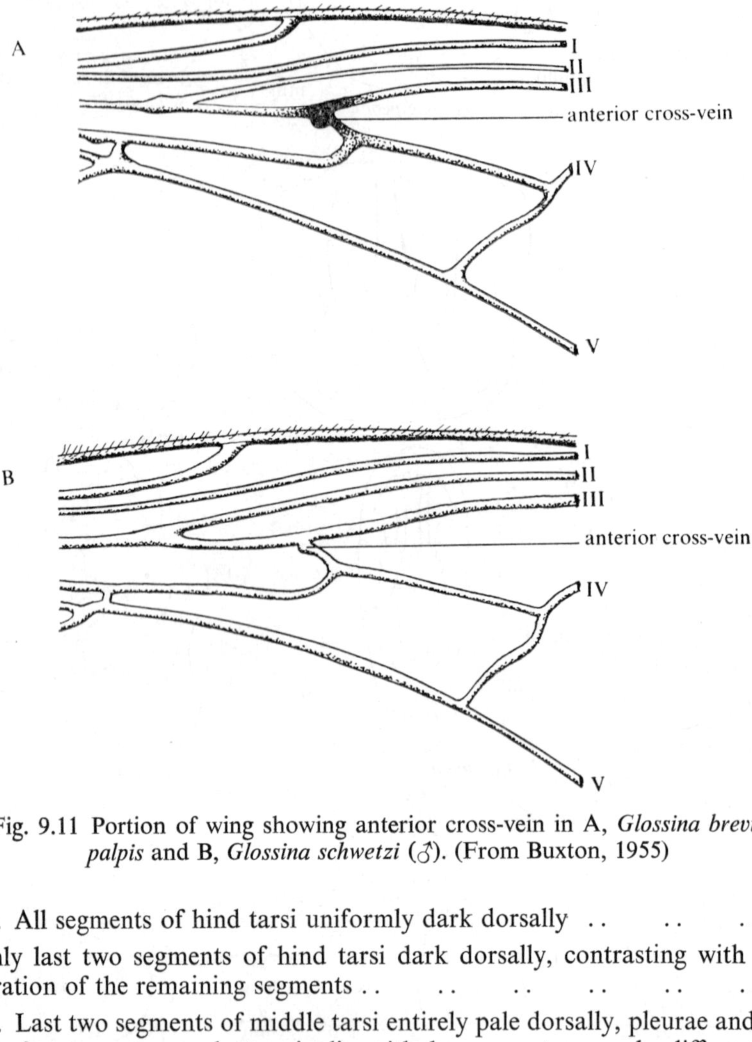

Fig. 9.11 Portion of wing showing anterior cross-vein in A, *Glossina brevipalpis* and B, *Glossina schwetzi* (♂). (From Buxton, 1955)

20. All segments of hind tarsi uniformly dark dorsally 21

Only last two segments of hind tarsi dark dorsally, contrasting with paler coloration of the remaining segments 22

21. Last two segments of middle tarsi entirely pale dorsally, pleurae and hind coxae fuscous grey; male terminalia with harpes not properly differentiated from general chitinization of the aedeagus[1] (Fig. 9.9, A); signum of uterus divided longitudinally into separate halves, of dark chitin outwardly and

[1] Machado (1959, pp. 37, 39 and Fig. 27, p. 48) regards the structure described as the harpes by Newstead *et al.* (1924) as an unpaired sclerite underneath the gonopore and considers the true harpes of this species to be undifferentiated and constituted by the structure labelled as the uxta by Newstead *et al.* (1924, Fig. 29, p. 81).

expanded distally (Fig. 9.10, E). Eastern part of former Belgian Congo (Map 10.2) .. .. *severini* Newstead

Last segment of middle tarsi entirely black and penultimate segment dark tipped, dorsally, contrasting markedly with paler coloration of rest of tarsal segments; pleurae and hind coxae pale to yellowish brown; male terminalia with well developed harpes having three paired processes of characteristic form

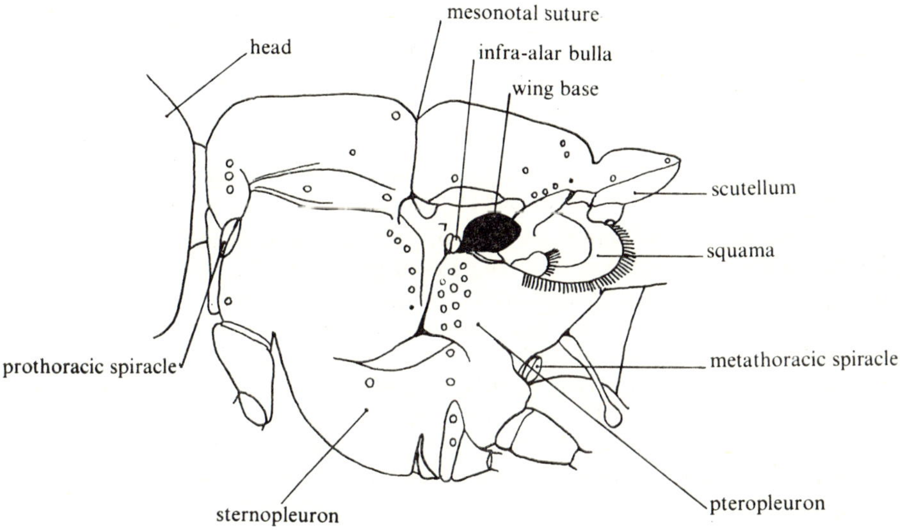

Fig. 9.12 Diagram of left side of thorax of *Glossina palpalis*. (After Buxton, 1955)

as in Fig. 9.9, B; signum of uterus with two anterior hollow bilobed tubercles tapering posteriorly into hollow stalks that lead into a sporran-shaped posterior pouch (Fig. 9.10, F). Southern Sardauna Province of Nigeria (former British South Cameroons), Central African Republic, Republic of the Congo, Gaboon and Angola (Belize, Kabinda) (Map 10.1) .. .. .. *nashi* Potts

22. Antennal fringe one half to three quarters of greatest antennal width; hind tibiae with broad dark suffusion in middle and much less distinct one at apex; harpes of male terminalia with one pair of processes only, as in Fig. 9.9, C; signum of uterus very slightly developed (Fig. 9.10, G), consisting of two lateral strips of pale yellow chitin studded to a greater or less degree with patches of brown chitin, the surrounding membrane of the genital fossae (p. 252 and Fig. 9.4) showing many intricate folds.[1] West Africa (Liberia, Ivory Coast, Ghana, Nigeria and along northern border of former Belgian Congo and adjacent portions of the territories to the north and west of this) (Map 10.1) .. .. *nigrofusca nigrofusca* Newstead

[1] The extent of chitinization of the signum shows considerable variation (*see* Nash & Jordan, 1959).

Antennal fringe less than one quarter of greatest antennal width; hind tibiae with or without dark suffusions; harpes of male terminalia with one pair of processes (as in Fig. 9.9, C) or three (Fig. 9.9, D–G); signum of uterus well chitinized (Fig. 9.10, H–K) (except in *nigrofusca hopkinsi*, *see* couplet 25) 23

23. Infra-alar bulla (Fig. 9.12) dark brown to fuscous, without any pale vertical streak in centre; harpes of male terminalia with three pairs of lanceolate processes, middle pair smallest, with dark base, rest of the process being very light, generally colourless (Fig. 9.9, D); signum of uterus elongate, about four times as long as wide, strongly flexed or bent double in middle of length, of characteristic shape, *see* Fig. 9.10, H. Central Africa (former Belgian Congo), southern Sudan, Uganda, western Kenya and (?) Botswana[1] (Map 10.2) .. .. *fuscipleuris* Austen

Infra-alar bulla testaceous, often with pale vertical streak in centre; male terminalia and signum of uterus not as preceding 24

24. Antennal fringe about one fifth of greatest width of antennal segment; harpes of male terminalia with three pairs of processes, the proximal two short and spine-like, the first slightly shorter than the other and the distal pair flattened and angular, as shown in Fig. 9.9, E; signum of uterus a somewhat rectangular flat plate with deep folds of dark chitin forming a horse-shoe shaped crescent, the arms directed anteriorly (Fig. 9.10, I).[2] West Africa, south-western corner of Nigeria to Republic of Congo, the Congo and Angola (Kabinda) (Map 10.1) .. .. *haningtoni* Newstead & Evans

Antennal fringe less than a sixth of greatest width of antennal segment; harpes of male terminalia with one process or, if with three, not as preceding; signum of uterus not as preceding 25

25. Hind tibiae with dark suffusion in middle, apical portion not infuscated, or only slightly so; harpes of male terminalia with only one pair of processes, as in Fig. 9.9, C; signum of uterus only slightly developed, as in Fig. 9.10, G. Extreme east of former Belgian Congo and extreme west of Uganda (Map 10.1) .. .. *nigrofusca hopkinsi* van Emden

Hind tibiae with or without dark suffusion and, if former, with a scarcely less distinct dark diffusion at apex of tibia; harpes of male terminalia with three pairs of processes (Fig. 9.9, F,G); signum of uterus well developed and highly chitinized (Fig. 9.10, J,K) 26

26. Male terminalia with pairs of processes of harpes unequal in size, middle (longest) broad and flattened, with serrated distal margins, distal pair sickle-shaped, proximal pair short, spine-like (Fig. 9.9, G); signum of uterus rounded, with deep or shallow emargination anteriorly, bounded posteriorly by a dark crescent-shaped sclerite (Fig. 9.10, K) 27

Male terminalia with all pairs of processes of harpes of about same size, slender and elongated and all, including middle pair, only slightly (if at all)

[1] Supported by the record of discovery of a puparial case (Dias, 1961a, 1962) in riverine forest on a tributary of the Lower Limpopo in Mozambique (*see* also Ford, 1970).

[2] Considerable variation in the extent of chitinization is described by Vaucel (1943) and Nash & Jordan (1959).

expanded distally, middle pair without serrated margins, proximal pair with serrated margins (Fig. 9.9, F); signum of uterus as in Fig. 9.10, J, not resembling the signum of any other species so far described.[1] Eastern edge of Equatorial Forest, in former Belgian Congo from its boundary with the Central African Republic to the Kivu area (Map 10.2) .. .. *vanhoofi* Henrard

27. A macrophallic form; proximal pair of processes of harpes reaching to about the middle of second pair, the members of which are broadly lanceolate distally and have relatively broad shafts, distal arm of sickle-shaped third paired processes as long as proximal one (Fig. 9.9, Ga); signum of uterus with halves of main portion sub-conical and separated by deep V-shaped depression anteriorly, chitinization generally complete, colour varying from deep ochraceous to black (Fig. 9.10, Ka). West Africa, Republic of Guinea to central southern Ghana (Map 10.2) .. .. *fusca fusca* Walker

A microphallic form; proximal pair of processes of harpes reach to tips of second pair, the members of which are truncated distally and have a relatively narrow shaft, distal arm of sickle-shaped third paired processes about half the length of proximal one or less (Fig. 9.9, Gb); signum of uterus with halves of main portion sub-rotund, separated anteriorly by only a shallow depression, chitinization generally incomplete, ochraceous petaloid area often surrounded by considerable colourless area (Fig. 9.10, Kb). West and central Africa, western south Ghana and Dahomey to western Uganda and former Belgian Congo, as far south as the south-eastern corner near the border of Angola (Map 10.2) .. .. *fusca congolensis* Newstead & Evans

[1] Described by author as 'formed of two parts: the upper part a hollow lobe, capping a truncated cone. The lobe is supported on an oblique axis, to left and right, by two chitinous bands. When extended, these bands form a V, of which the lower point is in contact with the sclerites formed at the centre of the truncated cone. These double parallel sclerites, forming a groove, are cut out in the shape of a spear head' (transl. from the original French, WHP). Two figures are given here (Fig. 9.10, J), (*a*) from Henrard (1952) and (*b*) from Potts (1955), the latter showing a very slightly chitinized specimen, probably from a recently emerged fly.

Chapter 10

The Geographical Distribution of *Glossina*

J. FORD

INTRODUCTORY

Six of the seven maps presented here bring up to date a series prepared in 1962 (Ford, 1963b). This was based upon Potts' (1953–4) maps and the additions and corrections to them which their preparation had stimulated glossinologists to produce in parts of Africa not previously well mapped. Cartographical revision has continued and mention should be made of a map, also prepared by Potts, to illustrate distribution of economically important groups of tsetse species as well as of the human trypanosomiases and mechanically transmitted trypanosomiasis of domestic livestock north of the *Glossina* belts (Regional Economic Atlas, 1965). Recent amendments used in the present series are due to the work of Finelle, Itard, Yvoré and Lacotte (1963) for the Central African Republic, of Gruvel (1966) and of Mouchet and Gariou (1966) for the Republics of Chad and Cameroon respectively. Touré (1967) has revised the tsetse map of Senegal and Baldry (1967) has added considerably to understanding of the southern limits of distribution of *Glossina tachinoides* in Nigeria and neighbouring countries. In Northern Nigeria the distributions of the belts of *G.m. submorsitans* have been revised according to the most recent map produced by the Veterinary Tsetse and Trypanosomiasis Unit (1965). Turner (*in litt.* 1967) has supplied amendments to the tsetse map of Tanzania.

The attempt made in the 1962 maps to show where recent extensions and retractions of the fly-belts had taken place has not been repeated. Thus Map 10.5 does not show the position of the former belt of *G. pallidipes* in Zululand in the South African Republic; it has undoubtedly been eliminated. The outlines have been drawn to fit the positions created by successful control operations, as far as they are known, but the changes so made when viewed on a continental scale are trivial in comparison with those that still emerge from entomological survey in country not recently explored by glossinologists. Baldry's new outline for *G. tachinoides* enlarges the area of distribution of that species to an extent that far outweighs any reduction due to its elimination elsewhere. It is almost certain that the distributions of many species are still far from fully known. This is true not only of the apparently rare *fusca* group flies like *G. nashi*, *G. vanhoofi* and *G. severini*, but also of some of the economically important species such as *G. pallidipes*, *G. longipalpis* and perhaps *G. austeni.*

The 1962 maps included the now fully accepted revision of the *palpalis* group by Machado (1954). They also indicated the location of those races created by Vanderplank's (1949) revision of *Glossina morsitans* Westwood which had not yet been seriously criticized by field workers. But it has become increasingly evident that much of Vanderplank's work is unacceptable. Nigerian workers, for example, have been unable to separate *G.m. submorsitans* collected in Nigeria from flies of the same subspecies from the neighbouring territories to the east, although according to Vanderplank these seemed to belong to the race *ugandensis.* The immense fly-belt that occupies most of the Central African Republic and much of the headwater country of the Bahr-el-Ghazal in the south-western portion of the Sudan Republic, must be attributed to *G.m. submorsitans.* On the other hand, Dr A. de Barros Machado (*in litt.* and verbally, 1968) informs us that certain of the northern Uganda *G. morsitans* show distinctive characteristics and that therefore the name *ugandensis* may yet be retained when his own revision of the species is completed. In the early years of the century two or perhaps three belts of *G. morsitans* existed in central and northern Uganda which subsequently coalesced after the removal of human populations from the Nile valley as a measure to control sleeping sickness.

On the authority of Ovazza (1956) the 1962 maps showed that *G. morsitans* in Ethiopia were *G. morsitans morsitans.* Balis and Bergeon (n.d.) now state that they are, in fact *G. morsitans submorsitans.* This attribution is accepted, since it is zoogeographically more probable.

Obscurities in Westwood's labelling of the type specimen of *Glossina morsitans* (Westwood, 1850) were discussed by Austen (1903). The label states that the insect was caught by Captain F. Vardon in the Lake Chad area of central Africa. Vardon did not visit Lake Chad and the type specimen must have been collected in the Limpopo valley in the Transvaal. There have been no *G. morsitans* near the Limpopo since about 1896 and abundant historical information exists to show that the Limpopo infestation was an extension of the eastern fly-belt and therefore it was to this geographical unit that Vanderplank should have allocated his type race. There was also another possibility of error. Newstead's creation of *G. morsitans submorsitans*, to which he at first gave full specific rank, was separated on the morphology of the genitalia; other characters admittedly overlap the patterns displayed by *G. morsitans* Westwood. In the paper in which he described that species Westwood also created *G. tachinoides*, the type specimen of which, although its label does not say so, might very well have come from Lake Chad. It was just possible that the Westwood type of *G. morsitans* might not have been an insect collected by Captain Vardon, but another collected in the same locality as the *tachinoides* type.

These points have now been settled. The genitalia of the Westwood type of *G. morsitans* were recently dissected by Mr D. N. Ackland of the Hope Department of Entomology, Oxford. It was at once clear that the specimen was not a *submorsitans* and that the Lake Chad label is wrong.

The more important point concerns the taxonomic affinities of the type. *Glossina morsitans* in eastern and south-central Africa extends southwards from near the equator in western Uganda to Mozambique and Rhodesia and, through Zambia, into the Katanga region of the Congo and thence into Angola. An outlier occupies the delta of the Okovango River in northern Botswana. The species forms several more or less discrete fly-belts, but the principal division is made by the line of highlands that stretches south-south-west roughly from Kilimanjaro to the northern end of Lake Nyasa and thence through Broken Hill to the Victoria Falls. In Vanderplank's (1949) revision, all *G. morsitans* west of this line were called *G. morsitans morsitans* and those east of it were called *G. morsitans orientalis*. No cognisance was taken by him of locality of Westwood's type (admittedly a subject of some confusion) and none of the historical studies (summarized by Ford, 1960a) which show clearly that the type locality, the Limpopo River valley, lay in the eastern or *orientalis* area. Vanderplank's *G. morsitans orientalis* should therefore have been designated by him as *G. morsitans morsitans* and the flies located west of the highlands divide should have received the new sub-specific name. Dr A. de Barros Machado (*in litt.* and verbally, 1968) who has been revising *Glossina morsitans* has concluded that although the characters given by Vanderplank for his '*orientalis*' subspecies are not valid, nevertheless there are constant and definable differences between the eastern and western *G. morsitans*. Dr de Barros Machado has now examined the genitalia of the Westwood type and has confirmed that it is, as historical and geographical evidence suggests, of the eastern or '*orientalis*' form. The problems of nomenclature raised by this conclusion cannot be dealt with here (*see* Chapter 9).

ZOOGEOGRAPHY OF THE THREE GROUPS OF *GLOSSINA*

Evens (1953) in an important paper excused his own speculations by remarking that one could not study the distribution of tsetse in the Congo, the country richest in species, without having the mind directed towards the problem of the historical evolution of the Muscidae. To the present writer Evens' excuse seems adequate. The exercise is no less fascinating because of the rapidity with which,

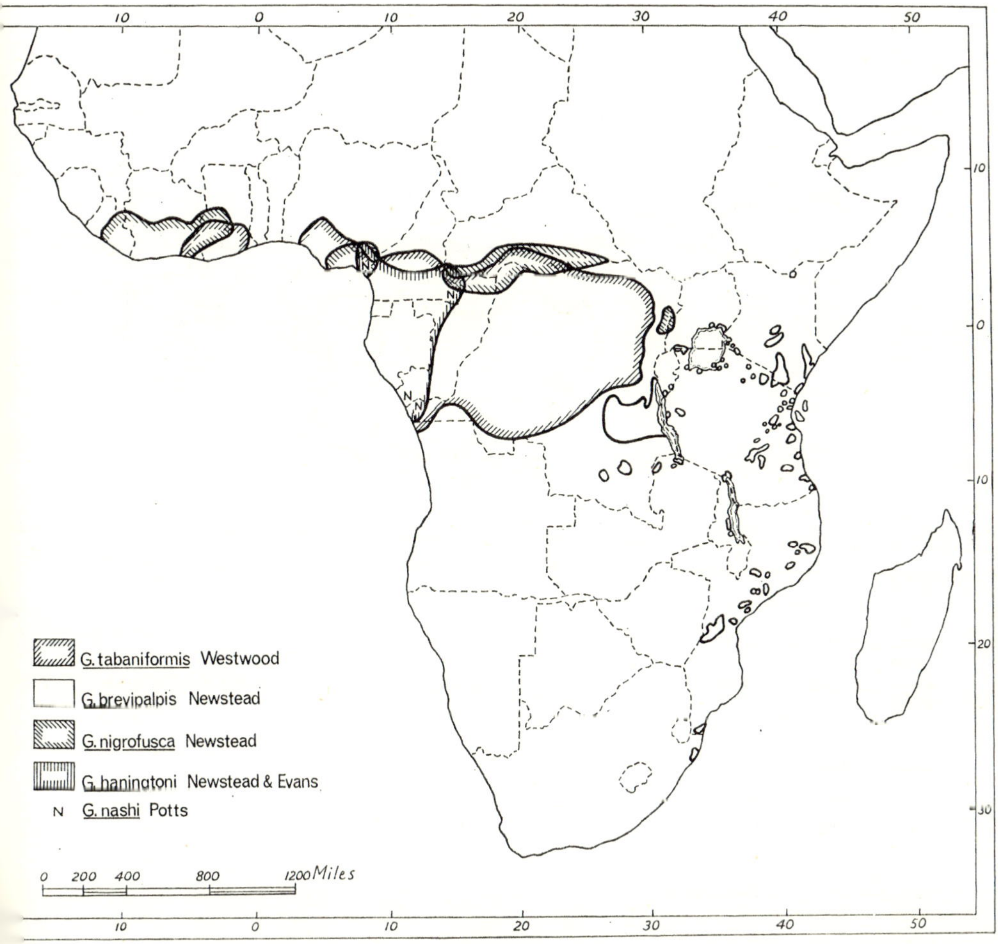

Map 10.1

Fusca Group. The rain forest species and *Glossina brevipalpis*

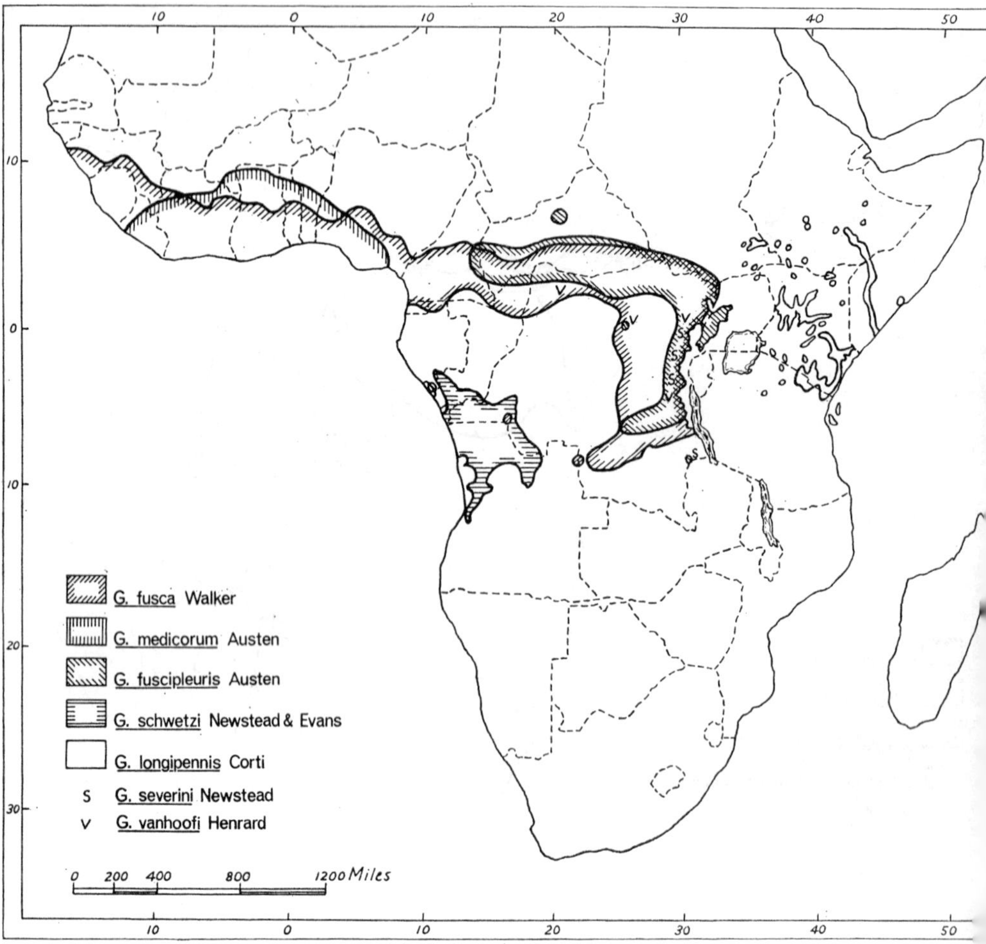

Map 10.2
Fusca Group. The forest edge species and *Glossina longipennis*

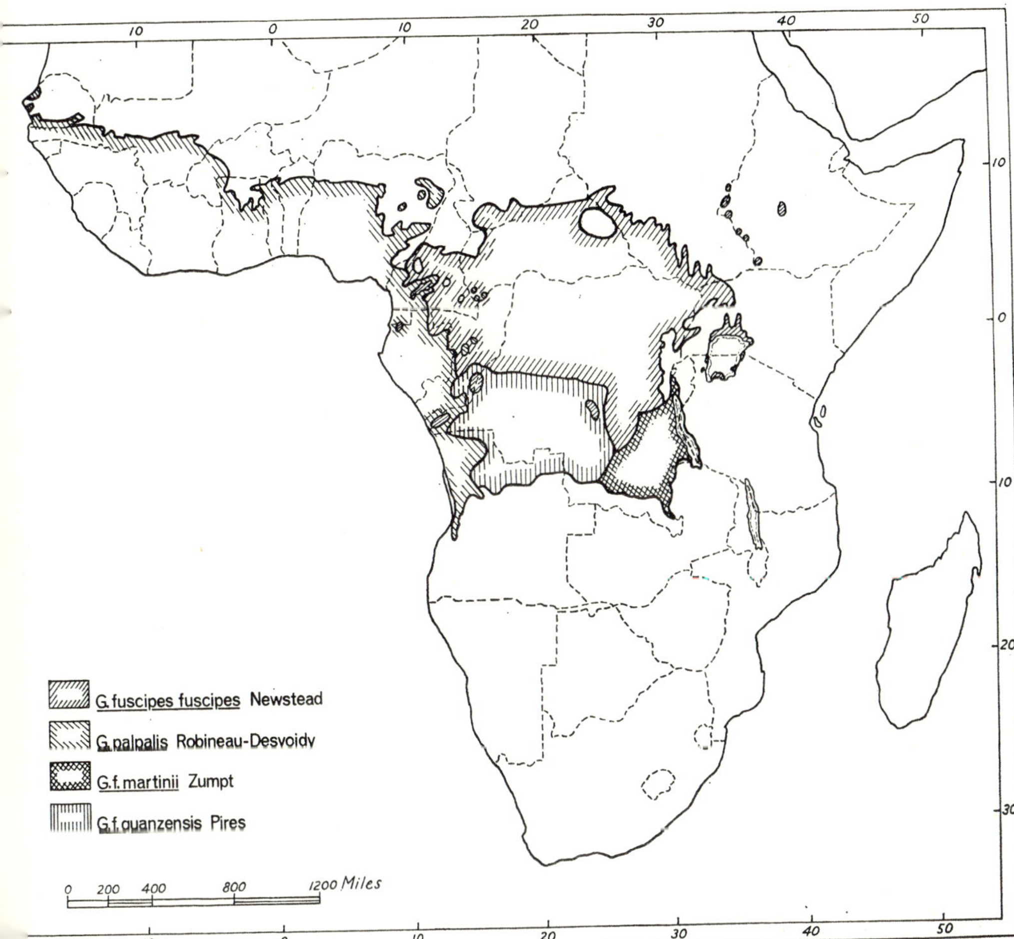

Map 10.3

Palpalis Group. *Glossina palpalis* and *Glossina fuscipes*

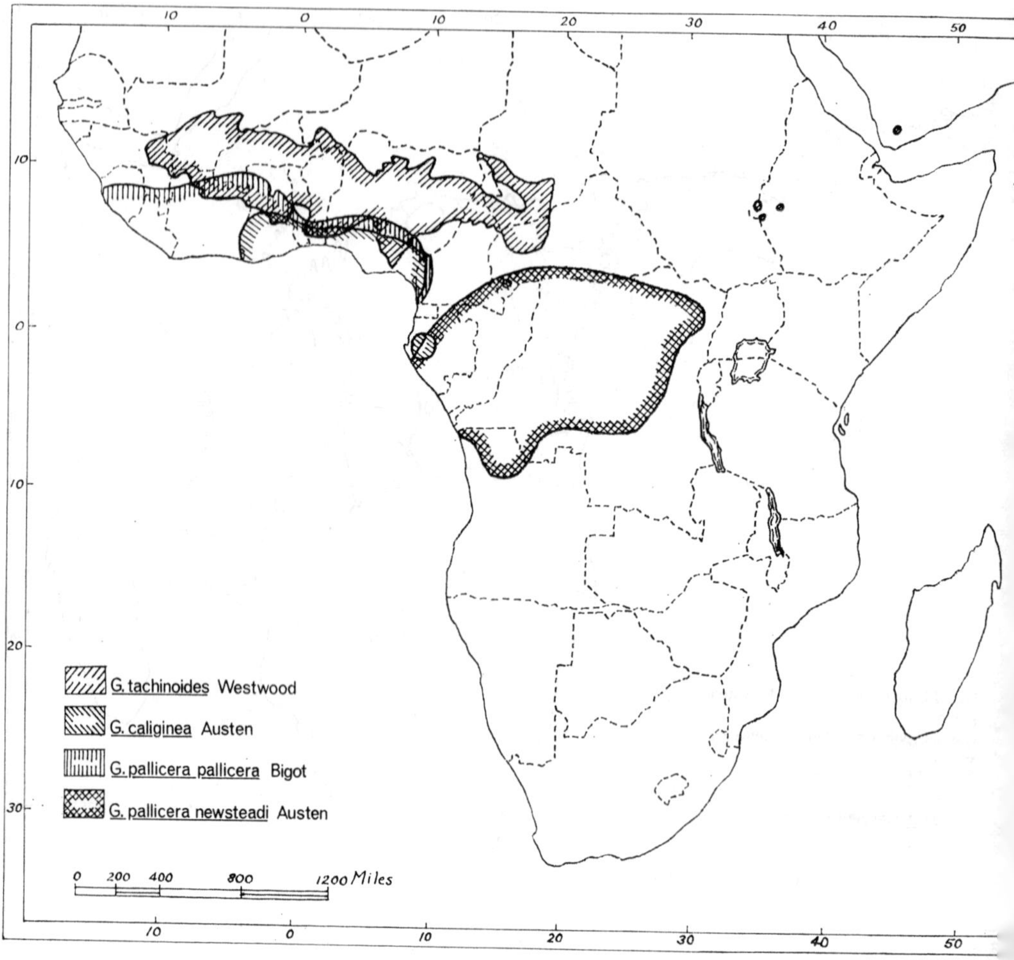

Map 10.4

Palpalis Group. *Glossina tachinoides*, *Glossina caliginea* and *Glossina pallicera*

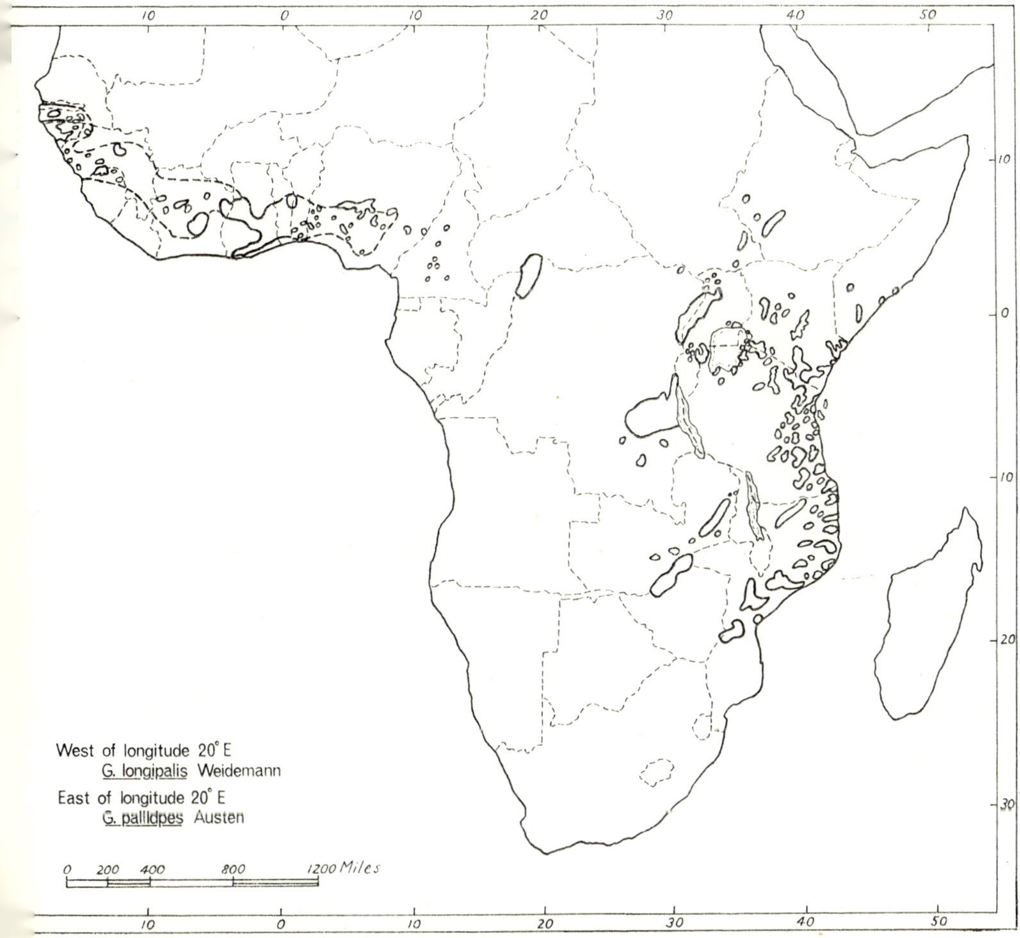

Map 10.5

Morsitans Group. *Glossina pallidipes* and *Glossina longipalpis*

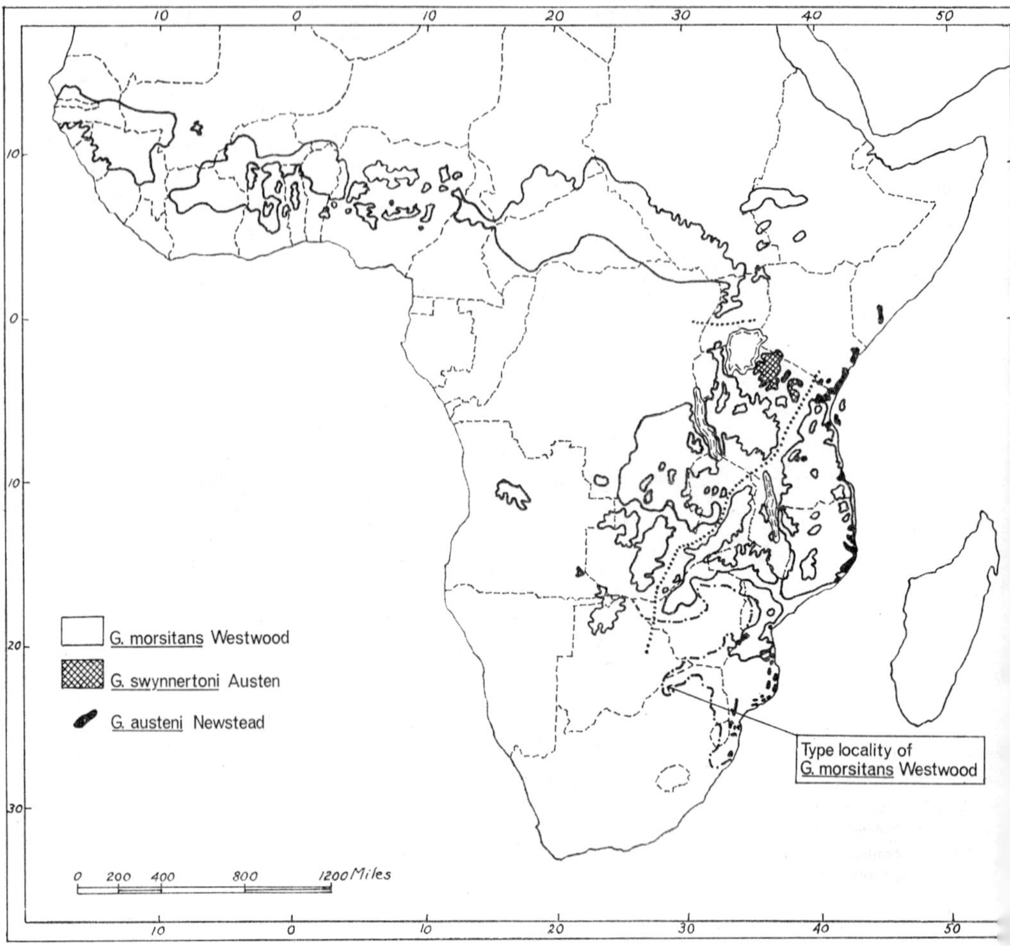

Map 10.6

Morsitans Group. *Glossina morsitans*, *G. swynnertoni* and *G. austeni*. The historical limit of tsetse in southern Africa is shown and also the type locality of *G. morsitans* Westwood. Dotted lines separate *G. morsitans orientalis* Vanderplank in eastern Tanzania, Mozambique and Rhodesia from *G. morsitans morsitans* as currently recognised and between the latter and *G. morsitans submorsitans* Newstead.

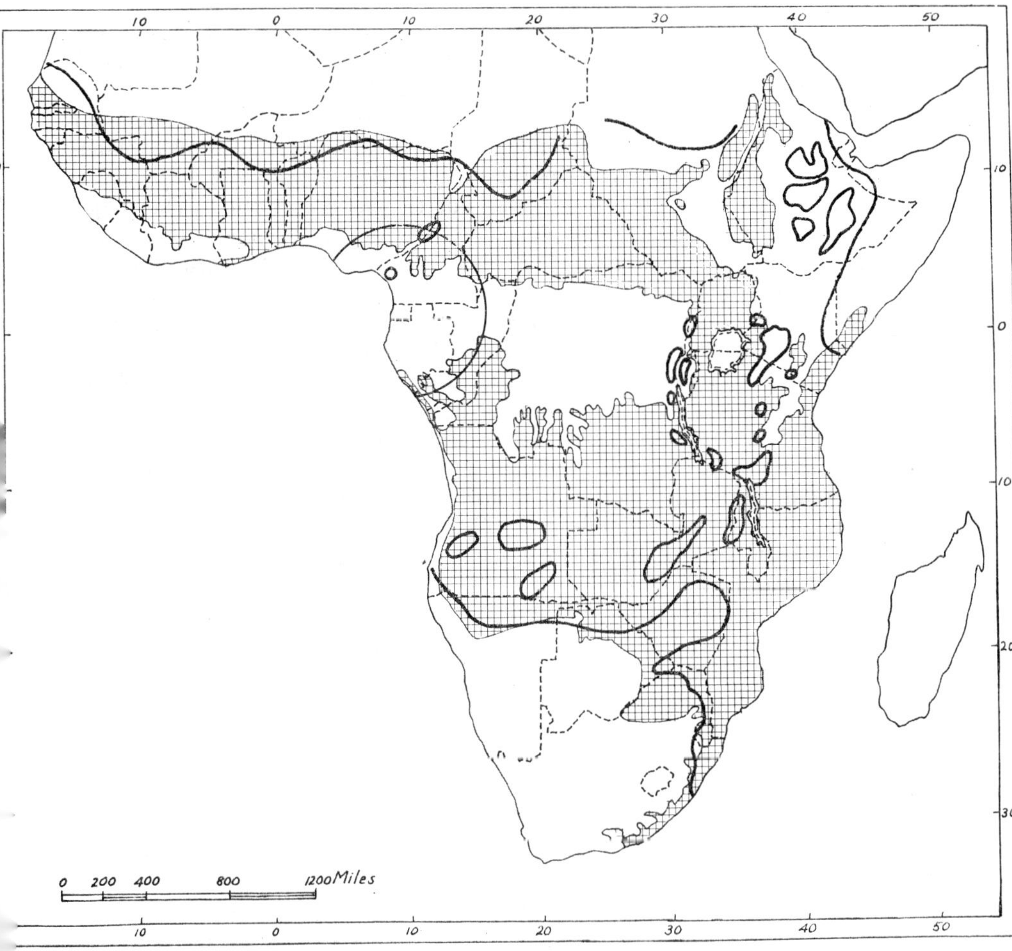

Map 10.7

The 'savanna' area of Africa (hatched) and climatic limits of *Glossina* based on Bursell (1960). The southern and internal isopleths indicate cold limits; the outer northern isopleth from the north Kenya coast to Senegal, the hot limit. The dispersal centre of *fusca* and *palpalis* groups after Evens (1953), indicated by incomplete circle, includes half the known species and subspecies of *Glossina*.

in recent years, knowledge about the African past, particularly the Quaternary, has developed. Much of the geographical isolation responsible for speciation in *Glossina* had its origin in the Quaternary; but Evens very rightly has drawn attention to the geography of the three groups into which the genus is divided and has pointed out that if one proposes to discuss that problem one's account must also explain the existence of the Florissant fossils in Colorado (Cockerell, 1918). This involves events much earlier than the Quaternary and Evens based his discussion on the ideas of Jeannel (1942; *see* also Jeannel, 1961). The latter studied the evolution of certain families of Coleoptera and founded his explanations upon the continental drift hypothesis.

This hypothesis is sufficiently familiar not to need description. The major lines of evolution of the Diptera developed during the Permian 200 million years ago. During this time the future continents were united (*Pangaea*) although inland seas broke up their surface and the movement of the earth's equator caused shifts in climates that were followed by movements in the flora and fauna associated with them. It is supposed that the Diptera appeared in *Laurasia*, the great northern land mass that later separated into Eurasia (*Angaria*) and North America (*Laurentia*). Evens has supposed that an *Ur-Glossina* that appeared in central *Angaria* spread westwards into *Laurentia* and so reached and, in due course, spread beyond the area in which the Florissant shales now lie. Another branch spread southward over what is now the Middle East into the southern portion of the continental land mass, *Gondwana*, and so became separated from the western branch by a sea associated with an east-west trough (the *Tethys* syncline).

If, indeed, the genus *Glossina* appeared during late Palaeozoic or early Mesozoic, then one must presume that its favoured hosts were reptiles. Baker (1963) has supposed that the adoption of the larger wild mammal fauna of Africa by trypanosomes as their natural vertebrate hosts is a comparatively recent development and that the adaptation to transmission by tsetse is a secondary phenomenon. But the stercorarian trypanosome, *T. grayi*, a non-pathogenic parasite of crocodiles, derives from a more ancient evolutionary event. Buxton (1955) deprecated Cockerell's suggestion that the disappearance of the Tertiary fauna of North America was due to trypanosome infection and Baker's hypothesis supports him; but may one not suppose that the relationship between *Glossina*, the crocodiles and *T. grayi* dates from before this epoch?

The Florissant fossils are Oligocene (Machado, 1959; *see* also Chapter 9) and thus about forty million years old. By this time tsetse must have been well established in Africa. It is wrong to think of the Colorado tsetse as primitive. There are four species (perhaps one is not a *Glossina*) and they show a bigger size variation than do modern tsetse. The wing lengths of 16 mm. for *G. oligocena* and 7 mm. for *G. osborni* compare with 13·5 mm. for *G. brevipalpis* and 8 mm. for *G. austeni*. Both the latter species are found in the same locality, although perhaps occupying different niches, over wide areas of East Africa. On the criterion of size, at any rate, the Florissant fossils were as much differentiated as are the modern African species.

Evens supposed that the Florissant species are fossil survivors of the western dispersal route that moved south with the equatorial tropics and entered

Gondwana perhaps in the neighbourhood of the modern Gulf of Guinea before the appearance of the Atlantic trough during the late Cretaceous. Such a view lends credence to a recent suggestion that *Glossina* may yet be found in the forests of the Amazon basin (Glasgow, 1967).

The two-pronged invasion of Gondwana led to the appearance of three dispersal centres. The *fusca* group established itself and spread out from a centre in the neighbourhood of the Gulf of Guinea. The same area served as a dispersal centre for the *palpalis* group that had derived from a branch of the eastern prong of the Gondwana invasion (Map 10.7). This had moved westwards around the southern shores of a Saharan sea. The third dispersal centre, from which the *morsitans* group was derived, arose in eastern Africa after isolation by the formation of the central Rift Valley. Another hypothesis for the origin of the *morsitans* group will be outlined below.

THE QUATERNARY AND TSETSE ZOOGEOGRAPHY

Potts (1937) invoked environmental changes during the Pleistocene to explain modern features of tsetse distribution. He supposed that the present widely interrupted range of *Glossina brevipalpis* (Map 10.1) was a relic of a much more universal distribution during the pluvial periods.

The advances in knowledge of geology, climatology and archaeology during the Quaternary have been so extensive in recent years and expert interpretations often so various that the glossinologist must hesitate to do more than indicate the sorts of changes that have occurred and to suggest how these may have produced modern distributions of tsetse flies.

Until recently, concentration of attention upon the successive pluvial periods that occurred, though not necessarily synchronously, throughout Africa has tended to suggest explanations in terms of alternating wetter and drier climates. This tendency was strengthened by the obvious importance of the atmospheric water content in the tsetse environment, e.g. the limitation of the dry season environment of *G. palpalis* in Northern Nigeria to a sharply defined microclimate controlled by the presence of residual pools in otherwise dry river beds as described by Nash and Page (1953). More recently Bursell (1960b) and Rajagopal and Bursell (1965) have discussed the effects of temperature on metabolic rate and the relationship of these interactions with the geographical limits of tsetse. This approach gains in interest from recent palynological studies of high mountain peats and of other organic remains in redistributed Kalahari sands. The fossil pollen profiles from the latter have been studied in Angola and results correlated with archaeological data from the Kalambo Falls at the southern end of Lake Tanganyika. During a dry interval in the Gamblian pluvial, dated by C–14 estimation at about 38,000 B.P., climate at that latitude was much the same as today and the country was covered by open *Brachystegia* woodland. By 14,500 B.P. the climate had become wetter and appreciably colder and there was a montane type of vegetation. The fall in temperature may have been equivalent to a rise in altitude of at least 500 m. (Van Zinderen Bakker & Clark, 1962). As this suggests a fall of between 3° and 4°C the present southern cold limit indicated on Map 10.7 might have shifted markedly to the north. Later, perhaps, during the Makalian wet phase (9,000 to 2,000 B.P.) with a warmer climate, tsetse may have reached somewhat to the south of its present limit.

In the Quaternary, the basic pattern of tsetse geography as suggested by Evens was modified by climatic cycles in which wetter pluvial periods alternated with drier inter-pluvials. There were also pronounced fluctuations in temperature. One cannot pretend to make any detailed reconstruction of former fly-belts; but there is sufficient evidence in contemporary or recent distribution records to show that the basic patterns of present tsetse distibution in Africa were laid down long before human society developed cultures and industries capable of making major changes in tsetse geography.

THE *FUSCA* GROUP

Geographically this group may be divided into three sub-groups. The first (Map 10.1) includes those species that may properly be described as rain forest species. They include *G. tabaniformis*, *G. haningtoni* and *G. nashi* and are confined to the Congo basin and the forests of Gabon, southern Cameroon and the Guinea coast as far west as Liberia. The continuity of this distribution is broken by the savanna gap between Lagos and Accra. *G. nigrofusca* in some areas is a true rain forest species (Jordan, 1961) but elsewhere is to be classified with the second sub-group (Map 10.2) comprising *G. fusca*, *G. medicorum*, *G. fuscipleuris* and *G. schwetzi* which tend to be associated with seral or relict forests and therefore are distributed peripherally around the fly-belts of the forest group. Some doubt attaches to *G. severini* and *G. vanhoofi*, but the location of records suggests that they also belong to this peripheral group. The third group contains the two species *G. longipennis* (Map 10.2) and *G. brevipalpis* (Map 10.1).

If one regards Evens' dispersal centre for the *fusca* group as a circle of radius of about 400 miles centred upon Rio Muni (*cf.* Map 10.7), all the species of Groups 1 and 2 are included except *G. severini* and *G. vanhoofi*. One may agree with Potts (1937) that *G. brevipalpis* is a survivor from a once very extensive East African rain forest. *G. fuscipleuris*, although mainly distributed around the northern and western edge of the Congo basin has some claim to inclusion in the same category. It survives in a small isolated fly-belt near the Mara River on the Kenya–Tanzania border and Buxton (1955) gives a record near Lake Nyasa just north of the Tanzania-Mozambique border. Santos Dias (1961a, 1962) found a puparial case (together with other cases of *G. brevipalpis* and *G. pallidipes*) in riverine forest on a tributary of the lower Limpopo in Mozambique. He believes that these must have been deposited prior to the extinction of *Glossina* in this area at the time of the rinderpest panzootic in 1896. Moreau's (1967) reconstruction of the Eastern African Pleistocene forest suggests that such a distribution is by no means an unlikely one and supports the view of Potts in regard to *G. brevipalpis*. *Glossina longipennis* is an anomalous case conveniently dealt with under another heading.

THE *PALPALIS* GROUP

The revision of the *palpalis* group by Machado (1954) reconstitutes Newstead's original *Glossina fuscipes* by bringing together three subspecies first erected for *G. palpalis*: these now become *G.f. fuscipes*, *G.f. martinii* and *G.f. quanzensis*. Essentially *G. fuscipes* occupies the Congo basin, but overflows it in the north and east to enter the basin of the upper Nile. *Glossina palpalis* is almost, but not completely, confined to the other rivers of West Africa (i.e. excepting the Congo) that drain into the Atlantic Ocean between Benguela and Cap Verde (Map 10.3).

Machado supposes that *G. palpalis* and *G. fuscipes* had a common ancestor, the distribution of which was divided by the elevation of the rim and subsidence of the centre of the Congo basin during the Miocene. The great inland lake which then formed persisted until it burst its bounds at Stanley Falls and the modern Congo began to flow into the Atlantic. In the meantime the ancestral *G. fuscipes* and *G. palpalis* had begun their respective evolutions inside and outside the Congo basin. Machado believes that *G. fuscipes fuscipes*, which occupies a far greater area than either of the other two *fuscipes* subspecies, is closest to the ancestral form. This hypothesis does not fully explain modern distribution. Islands of *G. palpalis* occur within the *G. fuscipes* area and of the latter in the *G. palpalis* area. Mouchet, Gariou and Rateau (1958) suggest that *G. fuscipes* is an invasive species pushing *G. palpalis* westwards off the main rivers into tributaries. Machado (1954) is also concerned to explain how *G. palpalis*, of which he recognizes two subspecies, can have moved westwards from one meridionally flowing river to the next along the Guinea coast. He therefore suggests, very tentatively, a past close association of the species with the coastal mangrove forests.

A large part of the Congo forests are rooted in Kalahari sands. There was an arid period 75–52 thousand years B.P. and perhaps another about 10,000 B.P. (Moreau, 1967). These dry epochs followed the emptying of the Miocene lake and reduced the peri-lacustrine forests, inhabited by the original *G. fuscipes*, to mere gallery forests. This process segregated the populations of *G. fuscipes* in the northern parts of the basin (the main Congo valley itself) from those of the Kasai and other great tributaries that take a meridional course across the Congo basin from the region of the present day Angola border. This isolation led to the development of *G.f. quanzensis*.

Lake Tanganyika, for long after its final formation in the middle Pliocene, was isolated from other hydrological systems and evolved its own unique endemic fauna. Later it overflowed intermittently into the Congo basin by the Lukuga River. This river was the route by which the shores of the lake and the rivers draining into it were invaded by *G. fuscipes*. Perhaps the Lukuga outlet was sealed off during the same dry period in the Quaternary which isolated *G.f. quanzensis*, and so also created the conditions in which *G.f. martinii* evolved independently. Later the Lukuga outlet reopened and the newly differentiated subspecies invaded the valleys of the Lualaba and Luapula. The continued separation of the three *fuscipes* subspecies has probably been assisted by the ecological differences between the ecosystems in which they now find themselves. *G.f. fuscipes* belongs to the great central rain forest of the Congo, although it has been capable of surviving in gallery forests in the north-east of the Congo, in Uganda and in small isolated relict belts in south-west Ethiopia. *G.f. quanzensis* is a gallery forest tsetse in derived savanna or forest mosaic and *G.f. martinii* is a gallery forest fly in *Brachystegia*-dominated woodland.

Machado (1954) drew attention to the paucity of intermediate forms along the interzones between the dispersal areas of the three *fuscipes* subspecies. Mouchet, Gariou and Rateau (1958) also noticed the absence of hybridization and of overlap, although they could not distinguish any environmental differences in the areas of occupation of the two species.

Possibly the solution is to be found in the work of Vanderplank (1948) who showed that, in his attempted crosses, 27% of female *G.f. fuscipes* died from injuries received when mated with *G. palpalis* males. When injury was prevented and mating was successful only a small proportion of inseminated females produced puparia. Few of these lived long enough to produce a second generation. If these effects occur in nature then overlapping and hybrid production would not be expected frequently (*see* Buxton, 1955, for further discussion).

The distributions of *Glossina pallicera* and *G. caliginea* shown in Map 10.4 do not call for special comment. However, in the same map, the distribution of *G. tachinoides* is of great interest. In terms of the physical and biotic characteristics of the habitats it occupies, it has a greater environmental range than any other tsetse. Latitudinally it has (or perhaps, more accurately, has had[1]) a wider distribution than any other species, stretching from Southern Arabia to the Niger headwaters in the Republic of Guinea. Machado (1954) believes that it evolved from the *G. fuscipes* ancestor when it became isolated in the basin of the Upper Niger or of Lake Chad. This lake reached a maximum (Mega-Chad) 22,000 years ago and remained the same size, with its shore line 400 miles north of its present limit, until 8,500 B.P. after which it began to shrink to its present dimensions. Further east the Nile sudd in the south of the Sudan Republic is a relic of another great lake. The existence of these vast Quaternary lakes could account for the spread of *G. tachinoides* and their survival in the rivers of western Ethiopia, but they do not explain the Arabian records, for the Bab-el-Mandeb was already open at the beginning of the Pleistocene. If the Indian Ocean flooded this strait in the Pliocene (Furon, 1962) the establishment of *G. tachinoides* in Arabia must have been very much earlier (one or two million years). Perhaps *G. tachinoides* should be thought of in terms of Evens' (1953) concept of the eastern invasion route into Gondwana, around the eastern shore of a Tertiary Saharan Sea.

One further point must be made regarding the geography of *G. tachinoides*. Nash (1948a) pointed out that it lives on rivers in the semi-arid Sahel bordering the Sahara that traverse country receiving as little as 380 mm. (15 inches) of annual rainfall. In the southern part of its range, in the Cross River basin of eastern Nigeria, it lives under a rainfall of 3,300 mm. (130 inches) per annum. Baldry (1965) demonstrated that, in its more northerly range, it is an indiscriminate feeder, but that it develops highly specialized feeding habits in its

[1] *G. tachinoides* was discovered in Arabia by Carter (1906) but its continued survival there to the present day requires confirmation.

southern, more humid, habitats. He has also shown that its distribution in the forest-edge areas of Nigeria is much more extensive than had formerly been supposed (Baldry, 1967).

FEEDING HABITS AND SPECIATION

Evens (1953) believed that the *morsitans* group evolved when isolated by the formation of the Rift Valleys that, from the Cretaceous into the Pleistocene, made a physiographical divide down the centre of the continent. But whatever its role in the past the central Rift has since been crossed, in both directions, by species of each group.

So far speciation has been considered as a response to orogenically derived isolation and to isolation produced by climatic change. No thought has been given to isolation due to adaptation to new hosts, yet this clearly has occurred, perhaps more than once. If we accept a late Palaeozoic or early Mesozoic origin for *Glossina* (and this seems necessary to account for the Florissant fossils) then we must also postulate an original dependence on large reptiles. During the Cretaceous the great land-dwelling reptiles flourished and then abruptly became extinct. By the Eocene, only snakes, lizards and some chelonians were living on land. The crocodiles and other chelonians remained aquatic or amphibious. There must have been a critical period at the beginning of the Tertiary when *Glossina* might either have remained committed to the crocodiles and large lizards in riverine or lacustrine environments or have branched out to attach themselves, as some of them did, to the now rapidly evolving mammals. Assuming that the habits of their ancestors were of the same nature as they are today one would look especially to the forest and the thicket pigs (*Hylochoerus* or *Potamochoerus*) and to large animals (like elephant, buffalo, rhinoceros or hippopotamus ancestors), in these habitats to provide the most easily available alternatives. Transfer of preference to such species would enable tsetse to move farther away from the aquatic reptile habitats, into the forests or to savanna forest interzones.

Weitz (1963), in his blood meal classification, grouped all Suidae together. It is here suggested that tsetse which had adopted a predominantly forest or thicket pig diet could, in appropriate situations, transfer their preference from *Hylochoerus* or *Potamochoerus* to *Phachochoerus* ancestors with little alteration in their feeding responses. Some support for this view may be found in the ideas, already mentioned, of Baker (1963). He believes that many Trypanosomatidae originated as gut parasites of annelids and thence became adapted to vertebrate hosts (fishes, amphibia, reptiles) *via* the leeches. In the latter they developed in the 'anterior station'. Insect trypanosomes originally developed in the 'posterior station' and used the stercorarian mechanism (as in *G. palpalis* and *T. grayi* or *Triatoma* and *T. cruzi*) to transfer to the vertebrate host. The pathogenic African trypanosomes were thus originally acquired by the mammal hosts from leeches and then found in *Glossina*, already carrying stercorarian trypanosomes, a new vector with a vacant anterior station.

This change in habitat of the trypanosomes can only have occurred in humid environments where encounters with leeches were frequent. The forest pigs seem to fit these requirements. Little is known about trypanosome infections in wild animals: but it seems that the wild Suidae, among the susceptible animals, are better adapted (Lumsden's 1962 term) than are most other species, save perhaps buffaloes, to trypanosome infection. When they are artificially infected, parasitaemia is transitory, while it is unusual to obtain positive blood smears from wild pigs (Ashcroft, Burtt & Fairbairn, 1959; Lumsden, 1962). On the other hand, the antelopes are much more productive of positive blood smears, while some, at any rate in captivity, are easily killed by trypanosome infection. It is tentatively suggested, therefore, that the acquisition of anterior station trypanosomes by *Glossina* was through the forest pigs and that from them tsetse turned their attentions to warthogs. The priority thus acquired by the Suidae has enabled them to achieve a greater degree of adjustment to trypanosome infection than is found in the antelopes. These essentially open country animals became 'secondary' hosts of tsetse of the *morsitans* group, after *Glossina* had invaded the savannas in the wake of the warthogs.

Weitz's (1963) five tables, after some rearrangement, are summarized below. All blood meals attributed to man or his domestic animals are excluded, for we are concerned with events that occurred before man developed habits that could have permitted him or his livestock to act as hosts (Ford, 1965) and only the fully identified records are used.

Lumsden (1962) summarized existing data on infections in wild animals and it is clear that among those which are preferred hosts, the pigs seldom display infections (10%). Among the bovids, bushbuck and situtunga (*Tragelaphus*) are outstanding both from their importance as tsetse hosts and as frequent carriers of trypanosomes in the peripheral circulation. It is notable that among those species which Weitz classified as Bovid feeders, but which in Table 10.1 are called Forest or Thicket Feeders (Group B), bovids other than bushbuck only supply 1·5% of all blood meals. Among the Savanna feeders only four bovids make a relatively large contribution to tsetse diet and of these only the giraffe (37%), kudu (45%) and eland (29%) show frequent infections. Nine remaining genera of bovids listed as supplying blood meals to the Savanna feeders together contribute only 4·0% of all blood meals. Of these some, like the waterbuck and reedbuck, frequently show trypanosome infections (52 and 43% respectively). Although their habits are such that they are not often bitten, they readily support infection. Other bovids, such as impala (11%), perhaps display few parasitaemias because they are not attractive as hosts and are seldom bitten. Feeding patterns and trypanosome infections together support the view that the bovids, in general, are less well adjusted to trypanosome infection than are the pigs, for there is a third group of bovids which, at least in captivity, may be unable to withstand infection (by *T. rhodesiense*) and die of trypanosomiasis. These include gazelle (Thomson's gazelle); duiker (*Cephalophus*) and dikdik (*Rhynchotragus*). To summarize the argument so far: tsetse were originally reptile feeders and, as such, became involved with the transmission of *T. grayi*, which persists between the *palpalis* group and the crocodiles. The anterior station trypanosomes entered the African Artiodactyla *via* leech attack on forest mammals, particularly Suidae (and, perhaps, the buffaloes). The prior acquisition of these trypanosomes has produced a greater degree of adjustment to infection (revealed by the relatively infrequent peripheral parasitaemias) in the pigs and buffaloes. The savanna-dwelling warthogs enabled *Glossina* to enter the savanna ecosystems, in which the *morsitans* group evolved as a separate entity and, during the process, the Bovidae and Giraffidae also became hosts to the trypanosome blood parasites to which they are, as yet, less well adjusted than the Suids.

Support for the view that Suidae were earlier hosts of tsetse other than Artiodactyla comes from the fossil record. It shows that non-ruminants of this order,

TABLE 10.1

Rearrangement and summary of blood meal analysis tables of Weitz (1963) excluding man and domestic animals

Lacustrine and riverine feeders			
palpalis group tsetse:		Reptile feeds	55·6%
		Bushbuck	22·3%
		Remainder	22·1%
Forest, thicket or forest-edge feeders			
Group A	*G. tabaniformis*	Bushpig & forest hog	74·4%
	G. fuscipleuris	Remainder	25·6%
	G. austeni		
Group B	*G. fusca, G. pallidipes*	Bushbuck	61·1%
	G. longipennis	Bushpig	11·9%
		Remainder	27·0%
Savanna feeders			
G.m. morsitans, G.m. submorsitans		Warthog	57·2%
G. swynnertoni		Buffalo	20·6%
		Giraffe & Kudu Remainder	22·2%
Specialized East African *fusca* group flies			
G. brevipalpis, G. longipennis		Elephant Rhinoceros Hippopotamus & Buffalo	70·9%
		Bushpig	17·6%
		Remainder	11·5%

of which living examples include pigs, peccaries and hippopotami, greatly predominated during the Eocene and Oligocene and that the ruminants, which now include the antelopes, giraffe and buffalo, only assumed their present importance during the Pliocene (Simpson, 1950).

From this phylogenetic viewpoint, Weitz's data display some anomalies. His group of species feeding mainly on bovids (which means, as we have seen, feeding mainly on bushbuck) includes *G. pallidipes* and *G. longipalpis*, the very closely related thicket or forest-edge species of the *morsitans* group, and *G. fusca*, type species of the *fusca* group, which is also a very widespread forest-edge or seral forest species. May one, perhaps, regard the first two of these as savanna species that have reverted to forest or seral forest habitats and *G. fusca* as a forest fly that has taken to the forest edge?

G. longipennis and *G. brevipalpis* are aberrant species to which attention has already been drawn. The most remarkable feature of their feeding habits is their reliance upon very large animals to provide their food. Elephants, rhinoceros and buffalo are fed on when sheltering in the thickets or secondary forest patches with which these flies are associated. *G. brevipalpis* is not invariably associated with hippopotamus-infested rivers, but when it is, the remarkable precision with which the male flies appear at sunset on the paths made by these animals as they leave the water, forcibly strikes anyone who has observed it (e.g. as described by Van den Bergh and Lambrecht, 1954). A key factor in the survival of the *fusca* group flies after the recession of the East African Pleistocene forests was the use made of relic forest islands or thickets as refuges by the very large mammals.

Finally, we have to consider *Glossina austeni*, a species which, like *G. brevipalpis*, recently extended its range within the East African coastal plain when abolition of slavery forced Arab farmers to abandon their plantations and turn to commerce. Weitz groups this tsetse with other mainly Suid feeders but in Table 10.1 it has been grouped with *G. tabaniformis* and *G. fuscipleuris* as a forest or thicket feeder on pigs. *G. austeni* provides a useful point at which to turn to another phylogenetic system, that of Bursell (1958) for he has found it necessary to postulate that this tsetse is one that, having adapted itself to an arid environment, later made a secondary return to evergreen, comparatively humid thicket habitats.

EVOLUTION AND GEOGRAPHY IN RESPONSE TO CLIMATE

Atmospheric Moisture

Bursell (1958) constructed a phylogenetic tree based upon his investigations into the water-proofing of tsetse puparia. He accepted the widely held view that the *fusca* group is the more primitive and that these large flies originally inhabited a humid environment as most of them do today. In these conditions they had no need to conserve moisture. *Glossina brevipalpis* and *G. fuscipleuris* cannot complete their puparial life at relative humidities less then 70%. On the other hand, *Glossina swynnertoni* and *G. morsitans*, dwellers in drier ecosystems, can complete their metamorphosis in atmospheres of 10% relative humidity. *G. morsitans submorsitans* requires a minimum relative humidity of 30%, while the thicket and riverine dwelling species, *G.f. fuscipes*, *G. tachinoides*, *G. pallidipes* and *G. austeni* require from 40 to 50% relative humidity. Water-proofing is related to size. A large puparium has a smaller surface to mass ratio. This is important in assessing the relative positions of *G. longipennis* and *G. austeni*. The former, a *fusca* group tsetse with a large puparium, has the most efficient water-proofing of all and can complete its development in dry air at

0% relative humidity. On the other hand, *G. austeni* has a small puparium which cannot survive at humidities below 45%, and lives in the same thicket that harbours *G. brevipalpis*, a tsetse requiring an atmosphere of at least 70% humidity. Bursell's supposition that *G. austeni* evolved under a drier climate and later reverted to a more humid habitat has been mentioned.

Machado (1959) finds it difficult to believe that adaptation to climate can be related in any way to the evolution of the morphological characters that are used by taxonomists to distinguish the three sub-generic groups. One may accept this view, but at the same time acknowledge that physiological adaptation is obviously of great significance in the geography of *Glossina* and, if one accepts that species evolution generally requires one kind or another of isolating mechanism, the physiological foundations of behaviour patterns may be of significance in creating them. If Maps 10.1 and 10.2 are compared, it will be seen that *G. brevipalpis*, which requires a humid atmosphere around its puparial stages, and *G. longipennis* which does not, both live in the same geographical region in the East African coastal plain between latitudes 1° and 5°S and also near Moyale on the border of Kenya and Ethiopia.

Temperature

It is wrong to consider behaviour, distribution, morphology and physiology in isolation from one another or from the environment. For purposes of discussion and investigation these analyses must be made, but the organism evolves in response to the evolution of the ecosystems of which it forms a component. It is therefore of some importance to define the limits of ecosystems in measurable terms. This was a vital question in southern African when *G. morsitans* was rapidly re-invading land that became free of tsetse after the 1896 rinderpest. Jack (1939) believed that the 20°C mean annual isotherm defined the limits to which *G. morsitans* could re-invade the valley of the Zambesi River. Bursell (1960b) demonstrated that the proportion of fat to other tissues (to residual dry weight) in teneral flies just emerged from puparia kept at 25°C, rose with increased residual dry weight. He also showed that the largest flies (and therefore those having the highest proportion of fat) were developed at an optimum temperature of about 24°C. He had previously also demonstrated (Bursell, 1959a) that when the fat content of the pharate insect was reduced to 4·4% of its total dry weight, eclosion could not take place.

At 16°C the pupal period is just over three months. At this temperature the smallest pupae will end their development with fat reserves below the critical level and of those tenerals that emerge, the smaller may have insufficient energy reserves to find the first blood meal (Bursell, 1960b). Similarly, above the optimal temperature, the critical level is reached at about 32°C, when the pupal period is just over eighteen days.

Later Rajagopal and Bursell (1965) modified these earlier conclusions and decided that consumption of nutrition reserves at higher and at lower temperatures were less rapid than had been supposed. But the principle established by the first paper, that the physiological basis of geographical limitation to dispersal of tsetse might be based upon over-exhaustion of nutrition reserves remains unassailed. In any event this factor is one that interacts with behaviour patterns that change in response to temperature variation. The work of Pilson and Leggate (1962a), Pilson and Pilson (1967) and of Edney and Barras (1962) has advanced the initial work of Jack (1939) and has demonstrated clearly how the behaviour of *Glossina pallidipes* and *G. morsitans* is adapted to the avoidance of critical temperatures by the adult flies (*see* also Ford, 1963; 1968a). Because of the existence of avoidance mechanisms, climate limitations suggested by laboratory studies will not fit exactly the geographical limits reconstructed from standard meteorological readings. On the scale of maps used here isopleths to indicate the limits of areas having winters of three months or more with mean temperatures at or below 16°C or with one or more months at or above 32°C, as postulated in Bursell's (1960b) paper, give a reasonably good fit when compared with the limits of contemporary or recently past infestation (Map 10.7).

THE *MORSITANS* GROUP: TSETSE AND VEGETATION

Map 10.7 shows the outline of deciduous woodland and savanna vegetations taken from Keay (1959). They form a band around the rain forests of the Congo basin and the Guinea coast. Outside them to the north and south, are the tsetse-free steppes and deserts. This band of vegetation is separated, in the map from which it is taken, into a number of zones that are most clearly shown between the northern edge of the rain forests and the southern edge of the Sahara. The forest savanna mosaics or derived savannas are artificial creations of human agricultural activity and if depopulated (as happened in Busoga on the northern shore of Lake Victoria after the 1900 *T. gambiense* epidemic) they revert quickly to forest. They surround the central rain forests and also replace most of the former East African coast forest. In West Africa the forest savanna mosaics give way to a zone of open woodland, the Southern Guinea Zone, still in a relatively moist climate. This stretches as far east as Lake Victoria, but south of the Lake it disappears except around an outlier of the Congo forest in north-west Angola. Elsewhere, south of the Equator, the forest gives way directly to 'miombo'. This vast deciduous woodland, dominated by Caesalpinaceae of medium height (twenty-five to fifty feet) is divided into two blocks. The southern block covers most of Africa between latitudes 5° and 20°S and is characterized by numerous species of *Brachystegia* and *Julbernardia*. The northern miombo, a band of woodland from 100 to 300 miles wide, is dominated by the closely related genus, *Isoberlinia*, and stretches from northern Uganda to the Republic of Guinea. It forms the Northern Guinea Zone of West African ecologists. Outside the miombo is a zone of generally lighter, more open woodland, wooded grassland or savanna, usually with smaller trees but with some communities of well-grown, variously dominated woodland. This is the Sudan Zone in West Africa. In southern Africa it includes a sub-division dominated by the unique 'mopane' (*Colophospermum mopane*). This fills the floor of the Zambesi, Limpopo and Luangwa valleys. At these latitudes much of the *Brachystegia* woodland lies above the altitude limit of tsetse, so that the distribution of *Glossina morsitans* tends to be especially associated with mopane. Further north, however, this tsetse has a similar relationship with *Brachystegia*,

Julbernardia and *Isoberlinia* woodlands, although it penetrates towards the central rain forests, even into the forest savanna mosaic. On the drier side, both north and south, it may be found in semi-arid savanna of the Sudan zone and in the mopane where annual rainfall may be as low as twenty inches annually. In these environments *G. morsitans*, in the hotter weather, may rely extensively on riverine thickets or forests for shelter.

The vegetational correlations that inspired so much of the earlier research on tsetse and led to the development of techniques of control by partial bush clearing, were principally worked out in studies of the *morsitans* group. It now seems likely that these correlations were not indicative of direct causal relationships but reflected the responses of tsetse to (a) host behaviour and (b) distribution of microclimates. However, taking Africa as a whole, there seems little doubt that the evolution of the *morsitans* group was a response to the development of savanna ecosystems, with their conspicuous and varied large mammal fauna. The behaviour of *Glossina morsitans* or its closely related *G. swynnertoni*, if described in relation to vegetation pattern, differs so much from one area to another, in diurnal activity, in resting behaviour, in larviposition and in response to movement (of men, animals or vehicles) that it has been impossible, so far, to find any common formula for control, either by bush clearing or by insecticides, that will fit all parts of its range. Only the preference for warthog, supplemented by a small group of other animals, is, with very few local exceptions, common from the Sudan Zone to the Zambesi River.

Similarly, the primary factor determining the distribution of *G. pallidipes* and *G. longipalpis* is not their dependence upon thickets but the attachment of bushbuck and a few other animals to this sort of habitat.

It is not implied that trees and shrubs do not play a vital role in the lives of tsetse flies. They provide perching places which are at once recuperative resting sites, shelter from adverse climates and from predators, as well as vantage points from which movement of potential host animals may be seen. The woodlands and savannas provide the habitats and food supplies of the host animals. The activities of some of the latter also contribute refuges from adverse climate (*see* Pilson and Pilson, 1967, on the use made of animal burrows as shelter for adult tsetse as well as for puparia).

The isopleths of Map 10.7 related to Bursell's study of pupal metabolism, but it is evident that similar lines could be constructed if some other physiological relationships were used. The mature *Glossina* can survive for short periods (one to three hours) at temperatures above 40°C. Screen temperatures well above this threshold are frequent in hot seasons near both the northern and southern limits of tsetse distribution. Exposure to these critical conditions is avoided by behaviour routines not encountered in the central portions of the fly-belts. Glasgow (1963) has summarized most of the laboratory work on climate thresholds and Ford (1968) has suggested that critical temperatures may be regarded as controlling the limits of tsetse population distribution by reducing the size of the effective habitat. *Glossina pallidipes* in the Zambesi valley escapes exposure to lethal temperature by retreating to refuges close to the ground in crevices of bark of big trees or by entering rot holes often high up on their trunks. The vegetation thus provides the material framework for carrying out these avoidance routines. Although the latter have been principally studied in relation to high critical temperatures it is possible that vegetation near the southern climate limit or at high altitudes nearer the equator also provides protection from cold (Goodier, 1960).

The isopleths of Map 10.7 were constructed from screen temperatures recorded at standard meteorological stations.[1] Some of their irregularities derive from the wide scatter of these stations in remote areas. They have been supplemented by lines drawn around high altitude areas where low temperatures, although not recorded, must impose a range limit. The distribution of apparently suitable vegetation does not everywhere coincide with boundaries to tsetse dispersal imposed by climate. This perhaps applies with greater force to distributions of tsetse hosts. Map 10.7 shows how cold areas associated with high altitude along the line of the eastern rift form the basis for the divide that separates the two belts of *Glossina morsitans* in East Africa.

The favourable conditions for intensive cultivation around many of these areas have obscured the natural pattern in recent times (i.e. the last 2,000 years). Before the advent of agricultural man, a continuous band of montane forest, especially along the heights associated with the eastern Rift, must have provided, on various occasions throughout the Pleistocene, an isolating mechanism between these two *morsitans* belts even more effective than the secondary grasslands or cultivation that now replace them.

The other, and more definite, division is that which separates *Glossina m. submorsitans* from the belts of *G.m. morsitans* and *G.m. orientalis* south of the equator. This division derives from the 'Lake Victoria Interval', a gap to be observed in many distributions of commoner trees (White, 1962) including some of the 'miombo' dominants and some, at any rate, of the larger mammals (e.g. rhinoceros, which does not cross the Kagera River from south to north). Lake Victoria was formed by a subsidence of the earth's surface during the Miocene. At the same time, between the area of the present lake and the western Rift an upthrust broke the drainages formerly running westwards and reversed the direction of flow in their upper reaches. They now ran into and filled the Victoria depression. The lake that formed was at one time much larger than it is now. During wetter epochs or simply as a result of orographical rain associated with the lake surface, a continuous forest link connected the montane forests of East Africa with those of the Rift mountains and so to the forests of the Congo basin. The savanna vegetation zone was therefore divided into northern and southern components and the savanna mammals, with their associated blood-sucking arthropods, were also divided into separate populations. The same process established continuity (perhaps on more than one occasion) between the forest dwelling species on both sides of the continent. This fluctuation provided the condition for establishment of the East African species of the *fusca* group as well as for the widespread, discontinuous distribution of the

[1] Observations by Jackson (1948), recently confirmed and extended by Harley (1968), suggest that temperatures recorded in this way have general relevance to the conditions in which tsetse are living although suggestions of avoidance behaviour might lead to the expectation that most of their time is spent in specially selected cooler ecoclimates, the lower temperatures in which would not be reflected by thermometer readings in standard screens.

forest-edge and thicket-haunting *G. pallidipes*. (The reader who wishes to speculate in greater detail about these events can conveniently start with Moreau's (1967) reconstruction of Pleistocene vegetation changes. But until tsetse systematics can be described in as much detail as can that of the African bird fauna, it seems unprofitable to try to elaborate further on the origins of the fly-belts.)

LIMITATIONS IMPOSED BY MAN

The geographical correlations between tsetse distribution and various aspects of human activity (as, indeed, of geology, soils, vegetation and climate) can now be very conveniently studied in the Regional Economic Atlas (1965).

The opportunity is taken to make a correction to Ford (1963b). In that paper it was stated that the Koalib fly-belt (now eliminated) in the Sudan Republic had been isolated as a result of a southward extension of the Sahara Desert. This overlooked Ruttledge's (1928) evidence of a former wider distribution to the east and to the south-west. The disappearance of *G.m. submorsitans* from the salient of savanna vegetation which stretches north-east into the centre of the Sudanese Republic (*see* Map 10.7), except from the Koalib Hills where it had become domesticated on man and his livestock, occurred in 1889–90. This was tentatively attributed to the effects of Arab hunting, but far more probably it followed the extermination of warthogs (not usually hunted by Muslims), kudu, buffalo and giraffe by rinderpest.

It is not proposed to examine recent changes in tsetse distribution. Discussions of the subject since Buxton (1955) are to be found in Ford (1958, 1960a, 1961, 1963b, 1964, 1965, 1970) and de Souza (1961). For changes due to the activities of tsetse control organizations reference may be made to numerous Department Annual Reports.

Chapter 11

The Search for Food

J. FORD

The commonly accepted explanation for the low percentage of females among tsetse flies attracted to man was put forward by Lloyd (1912) and Lamborn (1916). Females come to man only to feed; males, however, form following swarms in order to meet with females and therefore preponderate in the catch. When catching is restricted to feeding flies only, the sex ratio approaches more closely to unity. Nash (1930, 1933) and Jackson (1930, 1933a) added the concept of the feeding ground in which, it was stated, a higher than average percentage of females observed in certain vegetation communities was a consequence of the concentration in them of hungry flies. High apparent densities with a low female percentage indicated a well-fed population. The presence of numerous puparia in areas where this was observed showed that females, although unattracted by man, were present. This was the true habitat (Nash) or home (Jackson) of *G. morsitans* or *G. swynnertoni.* No real advance from this position was made in the next quarter of a century. In spite of its inability to explain all field observations, the 'feeding ground' theory with its corollary that the localized areas with high male apparent density (concentration sites) formed the 'home' of the fly, provided a basis on which several successful control schemes were founded. In them the concentration sites were destroyed by tree felling. Allied to this was the success of the fly-round (Potts, 1930) as an instrument for demonstrating the principles of the feeding ground theory throughout the *morsitans* belts. This was a sampling technique that could be used to measure temporal changes in population density as well as variation in its spatial distribution. In its former aspect it received strong support from Jackson's (1937) demonstration of a close correlation between seasonal change of apparent density measured by the fly-round and seasonal change of absolute population levels measured by his marked-fly-release technique. Soon the seemingly successful application of this research seemed to indicate a break-through in tsetse control (Bax, 1943–4; *see* also pp. 411–2, 548, 549).

Criticism of the fly-round technique leading, much later, to criticism of the 'feeding ground' theory perhaps had its origin in 1945. The present writer had been sent to Uganda to apply partial clearing techniques to the *G. morsitans* belt that for some years had been spreading through the *Acacia gerrardii* and *hockii* savanna of Ankole. After six months observation, using fly-rounds, he reported that no basis for this sort of clearing was discernible. So firmly established did the feeding ground theory seem that he concluded, not that it was inadequate to explain the Ankole situation, but that the fly-round was not a sufficiently precise instrument to demonstrate the distribution patterns that the theory demanded. Accordingly fly-rounds (which had been devised before the need for randomization in sampling had become familiar to all biologists) were now modified. Instead of paths designed deliberately to traverse all the major vegetation communities of the area, randomly placed transects divided into arbitrary fixed-length sectors were substituted. The new method was widely adopted and was successful in demonstrating distribution patterns in greater detail and also in giving added support to the feeding ground theory (e.g Jackson, 1955). One now sees that given the fly-round, in any form that used man as the bait, the feeding ground theory was almost bound to emerge as an explanation for the data it recorded. The Potts fly-round was so admirably suited to the task of survey in savanna vegetation and the feeding ground theory so well adapted to provide explanations for most aspects of tsetse behaviour observed by the fly-round, that together they formed the basis of many successful control operations and, indeed, in at least one country, still provide a foundation for extensive control schemes that seem perfectly satisfactory for the purposes for which they are designed.

The use of the term 'apparent density' implied that fly-round catches were resultants of actual population density and of response to catching parties. This idea led to the concept of availability (Jackson, 1954) as indicated by the ratio between apparent density, measured on a fly-round, and actual population density measured by the marking and release (or any other) method. At first it was thought that availability was a specific character. That of *G. morsitans* was 10% (i.e. one male per 10,000 yards of fly-round corresponds to a density of 10 per square mile), of *G. fuscipes fuscipes* [*palpalis fuscipes*] about 1% and of *G. pallidipes* 0·3%. This notion was no longer tenable after Harley (1958) showed that *G. morsitans* in south-west Uganda had an availability almost as low as that of *G. pallidipes* when measured in the Lambwe Valley in Kenya. Glasgow's (1963) interesting discussion of this subject defines availability as a quantity, 'such that the population is the product of the catch and the availability'. He concludes that the assumption that an availability estimated in one situation can be applied to another, should not be made lightly. In fact, a rigorous application of the idea of availability would make it difficult to attach any sort of population estimate to fly-round data. Thus in some areas, in the hot seasons, *G. morsitans* cannot be caught in mid-afternoon and whatever its availability during morning or evening catching periods, at 3 p.m. it may well be nil.

That fly-round data ought primarily to be regarded as measurements of response to a moving human bait rather than as population samples began to emerge from an examination of tsetse distribution patterns along fixed-length sector transects. It was shown (Ford, 1960) that the location of distribution peaks on these transects was, in part, controlled by the direction of movement of the observing team. The capture of a fly at a certain point did not indicate that it had been previously located there, but only that it had been taken at, or near, the point at which it had caught up with the catching party. In the open *Acacia* savanna of south-west Uganda the change in position of these peaks according to the direction of movement of the catchers, suggested that some of the flies had made approach flights of 2 to 400 yards. Elsewhere, good positive correlations between the sector catches and counts of trees in 2-metre wide transects along the transect paths, for example in parts of Karagwe in north-west Tanzania, in extensive stands of *Acacia hockii*, suggested that a flight response was only elicited when catchers approached quite close to previously resting flies.

In response to a suggestion by Buxton (1955) an account of transect fly-rounds, increasingly in use since about 1948, was eventually published (Ford, Glasgow, Johns and Welch, 1959). The collection of data for this paper prompted Glasgow (1961) to put on a formal statistical basis what had been known for a long time, namely the very large error that was attachable to estimates of mean apparent density. To this error the variability inherent in the population distribution evidently contributed far less than the time to time and place to place differences in response to the bait offered by the catching party.

In 1961 two papers were published that initiated new attempts to escape from the difficulties of fly-round interpretation. Leggate and Pilson (1961) realizing that fly-round catches were influenced by changes in environmental factors throughout the day determined, firstly, to use the catch made between first light and the cessation of all activity after sundown, as a single sample of the tsetse population. This eliminated effects of diurnal availability change. Secondly, their bait was a stationary ox, not a moving party of men; this eliminated variation due to behaviour differences associated with different areas. Thirdly, they captured and recorded only those flies that engorged themselves with blood from the bait ox; this eliminated variation due to different types of tsetse activity, the causes of which could not be fully understood. Feeding, however, was an obligatory process undertaken by all flies at more or less regular intervals. The 'feeding element' in the population might therefore be supposed to bear a fixed relationship to the actual population. Moreover, the stationary bait ox yielded female catches equalling or exceeding those of males. These authors have used their technique to study variation in trypanosome infection risk (Leggate & Pilson, *loc. cit.*), the seasonal and diurnal patterns of feeding activity and resting (Pilson & Leggate, 1962, 1962a), and, recently, the differences in distribution of a *G. morsitans* population between different vegetation communities (Pilson & Pilson, 1967; *see* also pp. 411, 549).

Bursell (1961a) made catches of *Glossina swynnertoni* in four different ways and then examined their mean nutritional states by fat extraction. By this means he was able to distinguish four activity phases in the male *G. swynnertoni* in which behaviour is related to successive stages in exhaustion of energy reserves, beginning with the undigested blood meal. These phases are in no way equivalent to the four hunger stages described long ago by Jackson (1933a) although they obviously comprehend them. One sequel to this work is that no longer can the use of hunger staging be justified as a tool for field research (and its disadvantages have long been apparent) but that the union of field study and laboratory analysis at length becomes obligatory.

So far Bursell's studies, especially his most recent collaboration with the Pilsons (Bursell, 1966a; Pilson & Pilson, 1967) have assessed mean nutritional states for population samples captured in different ways or in different environments. Thus a comparison is made between mean fat content of flies caught on a fly-round (moving human bait) and flies caught when about to probe the Pilsons' stationary bait ox. The latter are, by definition, in Bursell's activity Phase III or IV since they were all caught when about to feed. The former are treated as if they were all indulging in the following swarm behaviour characteristic of Bursell's Phase II. However, it is common experience that one may be bitten while at work on a fly-round and Jackson (1933a) long ago demonstrated that following flies that rested on a catching party (as opposed to following along the ground) could be divided into two behaviour groups: those settling 'head-up' having very little fat, as compared with 'head-down' flies in which it was plentiful. One may question the validity of comparing a sample of flies deliberately selected while in Phases III or IV (i.e. when feeding on the ox) with an unselected fly-round sample which, while it almost certainly comprises chiefly Phase II following swarm flies, may also include others from Phases III and IV.

The present writer, following up an unpublished observation of Bursell, has made a preliminary study of catches from three types of bait in which each fly is recorded separately according to its observed behaviour. Bursell had noted that the mean fat content of flies caught when about to probe a human being was very much less than that of flies caught when about to probe an ox; in fact the former flies were evidently within a few hours of death by starvation. This observation which suggests that man is an unwelcome host only used by this species under the compulsion of extreme necessity, has a double interest. It has an obvious epidemiological significance and, from the present view point, provides a link between studies of field behaviour and the blood meal analysis work on host preference by Weitz and his colleagues. It offers an explanation for the avoidance of animals like the impala which are rarely fed upon and perhaps only when starvation leads to suppression of discriminative sensory faculties.

The marked difference in the nutritional states of *G. morsitans* attacking man and ox was confirmed (in *G.m. submorsitans*) near Ilorin, Nigeria. Here the flies readily formed following swarms behind a moving party of men only, but hardly ever approached either to feed or to rest upon them. When the party was accompanied by a young bull, the following swarm was smaller and flies settled on the bull and fed. A marking experiment lent support to the view that flies that had exhausted a portion of their energy reserves in the following swarm behind the bull then alighted on it to feed. When the bull was absent they persisted longer in following, but eventually left the swarm without approaching the human bait. Experiments with single tubed flies provided evidence that as food reserves became progressively exhausted, so readiness to feed from man increased. These experiments also suggested that teneral flies show no preference for one species of host over another. Studies on the rate of pupal fat consumption (Bursell, 1960b; Rajagopal & Bursell, 1965) demonstrated that at all seasons rapid success in finding the first meal is of vital importance. Thus lack of discrimination in host choice by the teneral tsetse may have a survival value.

Ilorin lies on the northern edge of the forest-savanna mosaic zone. The field observations were repeated at Yankari in the Sub-Sudan zone which has a more arid climate. Here, the same species of *Glossina* readily attacked the moving party of men, provided no bait animal was present. If it was present, feeding flies were nearly all taken from it and very few from the accompanying men. The fat content of flies probing man was lower but, in contrast to Ilorin, not significantly so, than those about to feed from the bull. In both places flies that probed man were younger than flies that probed the bull. The differences between the feeding responses to man and bull in the two places, and at two seasons, are best summarized by comparing the rates at which probing flies were caught from the two hosts on different occasions (Table 11.1). Smaller, incidental catches of *G. tachinoides* indicated a similar effect (Ford, 1969).

TABLE 11.1

Season	Host	Ilorin: One fly probes every :	Ilorin: Ratios of probing intervals	Yankari: One fly probes every :	Yankari: Ratios of probing intervals
Wet June/July	Man	88·8 mins.	1 : 12·7	41·9 mins.	1 : 1·11
	Bull	7·0 mins.		35·0 mins.	
Dry February/March	Man	263·5 mins.	1 : 15·8	11·9 mins.	1 : 1·08
	Bull	16·7 mins.		11·0 mins.	

It would seem that work of this kind might usefully link the physiological and ethological approaches to field behaviour made by the Rhodesian workers with the host preference studies of Weitz and his colleagues, especially in the light of the observations of Baldry (1965) on feeding patterns exhibited by *Glossina tachinodes*. The conventional view of this species is that it is an opportunist feeder and will readily take whatever blood is available. But such a view is not tenable for those flies caught in the villages around Nsukka in eastern Nigeria, for here man (who is fed on frequently in the dryer north) is almost completely neglected in favour of his own domestic pigs.

One may speculate, vainly, on what might have been the course of tsetse-fly research had Nash and Jackson been able to develop their early comparisons of catches from human and domestic cattle baits. In particular Nash's (1933) deduction that man was distasteful to female *G. morsitans* foreshadowed the problem of host preference. However, although the unattractiveness of man was in some degree appreciated, workers tended to assume that there was no difference in kind between response to man and response to a favoured wild host. Harrison's (1940) striking observations on the neglect of zebra by *G. swynnertoni* (amply confirmed in Weitz's analyses) did not suggest changes in interpretation of fly-round data. In part difficulties were semantic. The frequent use of the word 'attack', for example, implied an understanding that the end point of all approaches to man was the blood meal. The use of the term 'feeding ground' was also unfortunate for it was clear, at any rate as regards females, that the flies that were taken in these relatively treeless areas were those that had failed, by some accident or other, to obtain a meal in the true woodland habitat. The point is discussed by Glasgow (1963). The deductions from fly-round data were not all wrong. In particular the conclusion that woodland areas with abundant, non-hungry males, among which females were rarely caught, was, in fact the true habitat where females were at least as abundant as males, seems to be well supported by the recent standing bait animal catches of Pilson and Pilson (1967).

The main inspiration behind earlier field study of *Glossina morsitans* and *swynnertoni* was the idea that the patterns of tsetse behaviour were governed by patterns of vegetation. This was expressed by Swynnerton's phrase 'the concurrence of requirements'. Research was directed towards discovering the uses to which the tsetse fly puts the various plant communities which together comprise its habitat. The notion derived partly from Swynnerton's early study of Zulu bush clearing methods, partly from the quasi-organismal concepts of the biotic community of American plant ecologists led by F. E. Clements. When failures with partial bush clearing began to occur, much effort was put into attempts at more precise description of vegetation community structure, in the hope that this would help to correct what was assumed to be faulty application of the basic idea that alteration of the aspect of the vegetation by tree felling would cause a disorganization of tsetse behaviour that would be fatal.

Newer research has not yet produced a successor to the feeding ground theory. In part this may be because the need for a comprehensive doctrine is not so acutely felt by control officers whose main weapon is now insecticides. More probably it is due to the great complexity of the events in the *Glossina* life that now have to be explained. The life of the individual tsetse will be described eventually in terms of energy consumption during the cycles of growth and reproduction, of food metabolism and of ageing. Although in the following pages these processes, all of which have been the subject of recent research, are examined separately, none is fully comprehensible without the others.

The mating behaviour of the male is clearly controlled by the rate of energy consumption in the following swarm and this in turn must affect the frequency of male feeding. That the size of feeds of females exerts a control over the larval weight in *G. fuscipes fuscipes* has long been known (Mellanby, 1937). Saunders (1962) has shown that the mean age of female *G. pallidipes* caught by a moving party of men (fly-round) is less than that of those caught on a bait ox and the latter, therefore, like young males, are less discerning in their responses to potential hosts. They are more ready to feed on man than are older flies. These observations recall those of Nash (1933) already mentioned and his suggestion that man was distasteful to female *G. morsitans*.

Saunders, in the same paper, pointed out the epidemiological significance of these studies. If man is fed on by flies younger than the mean age of the population as a whole then he must be subject to a lower frequency of bites from infected flies than a host acceptable to flies of all ages.

Glasgow (1963) has adequately disposed of 'the classical view that if there is enough food for 100 tsetse there is enough for 1,000'. In addition, the work of Weitz (*see* pp. 322–326) now shows that only a relatively small proportion of the whole wild game population can be regarded as normal food for *Glossina.* Studies of the kind briefly outlined in this section are gradually being related to the slowly growing knowledge of the differences exhibited by wild animals as hosts of trypanosomes. It is a return to the path set by the pioneers: Bruce, Roubaud, Rodhain, Kinghorn, Yorke, Johnson and others in regarding the tsetse primarily as the vector of trypanosomes.

Chapter 12

Feeding, Digestion and Excretion

E. BURSELL

Tsetse flies feed only on the blood of vertebrates and they show a variety of adaptations which can be specifically related to the blood-sucking mode of life. Anatomical aspects of such adaptations have been described in Chapter 8, where the structure of the alimentary canal and associated organs is described. In the present chapter consideration will be given to physiological processes associated with the intake of blood, the digestion of the blood meal, the absorption and subsequent metabolic manipulation of the digestive products, and the excretion of waste materials.

THE INTAKE OF FOOD

The act of feeding in tsetse flies is preceded by a disengagement of the haustellum from the palpi, and a swivelling of the mouth parts into a position normal to the plane of the substratum, a process which is often accompanied by the extrusion of droplets of salivary fluid. It appears that the most important factor in eliciting this feeding reaction is temperature (Dethier, 1954); flies can be induced to probe quite unsuitable surfaces, such as glass or paper, provided the temperature of the substratum is appreciably above ambient. Olfactory stimuli do not seem to play very much part, nor is there any evidence for the participation of tarsal chemoreceptors. The fact that flies can be induced to take up different blood fractions at considerable dilution, and even pure saline solutions (Lester & Lloyd, 1928; Langley, 1966a) and various other fluids including water (*see* also Buxton, 1955, pp. 68, 164), suggests that gustatory stimuli are not of major importance.

Penetration of the outer epidermal layers of the host is achieved by rasping movements of the cuticular teeth on the labella, and the flexible haustellum then explores the deeper epidermal layers, a process which is accompanied by intermittent ejection of saliva (Gordon, Crewe & Willett, 1956). When a blood capillary is ruptured by the labial tip, the extravasated blood is sucked into the food canal by action of the cibarial pump, and the fly starts to engorge (Gordon & Crewe, 1948; *see* also p. 236). This uptake of blood is also associated with periodic discharges of saliva. The mixture of blood and saliva is passed first into the anterior portion of the midgut, where concentration of the blood meal commences (*see* below). When this portion of the alimentary canal has been filled to capacity, the intake is diverted to the crop, which distends enormously to accommodate a blood meal that may weigh considerably more than the insect itself (Lester & Lloyd, 1928; *see* also Buxton, 1955, pp. 87–8). The speed with which engorgement is accomplished varies greatly, depending presumably on the rate of discharge at the source, and durations ranging from one to ten minutes have been recorded by Glasgow (1961a) for *Glossina swynnertoni* feeding on a calf.

The salivary secretion of tsetse flies has been shown to contain a strong anti-coagulant (Lester & Lloyd, 1928), which may facilitate the passage of blood through the fine tubes of the foregut, and prevent its clotting during storage in the crop. A number of amino acids and carbohydrates have also been demonstrated in the salivary secretion (Williamson, 1956), and histochemical tests have indicated the presence of protein and/or mucoprotein and of glyco-lipid (Fairbairn & Williamson, 1956), but the function of these materials is not known. According to Wigglesworth (1929) the saliva does not contain any digestive enzymes.

CONCENTRATION OF THE BLOOD MEAL

The intake of blood in quantities which greatly exceed the insect's own body weight presumably diminishes aerodynamic efficiency; the flight of newly fed flies tends to be sluggish. At this time the danger of predation would probably be high, and it is not surprising that a process of 'primary excretion' (Jack, 1939), which serves to eliminate excess water and thus to reduce the load, follows very quickly upon the act of feeding. It may even commence before the fly has fully engorged, and at a temperature of 27°C it is completed in less than two hours (Bursell, 1960c). The process appears to involve an absorption of water, and presumably of inorganic salts, from the anterior region of the mid-gut, and their elimination by the Malpighian tubules, along which a copious liquid flow can be observed in flies dissected soon after feeding. Once the excretory material remaining from the last blood meal has been flushed out of the hindgut, the primary excretion is voided from the anus as droplets of clear fluid.

The physiological mechanisms which form the basis of blood meal concentration have still to be elucidated, but a great deal of work has been done on quantitative aspects of primary excretion (Lester & Lloyd, 1928; Jack, 1939; Bursell, 1960c). The amount of fluid excreted is closely correlated with the size of the blood meal (*see* Fig. 12.1a) and for a given size of meal it varies according to the water content of the feeding fly, a subject that has been fully discussed

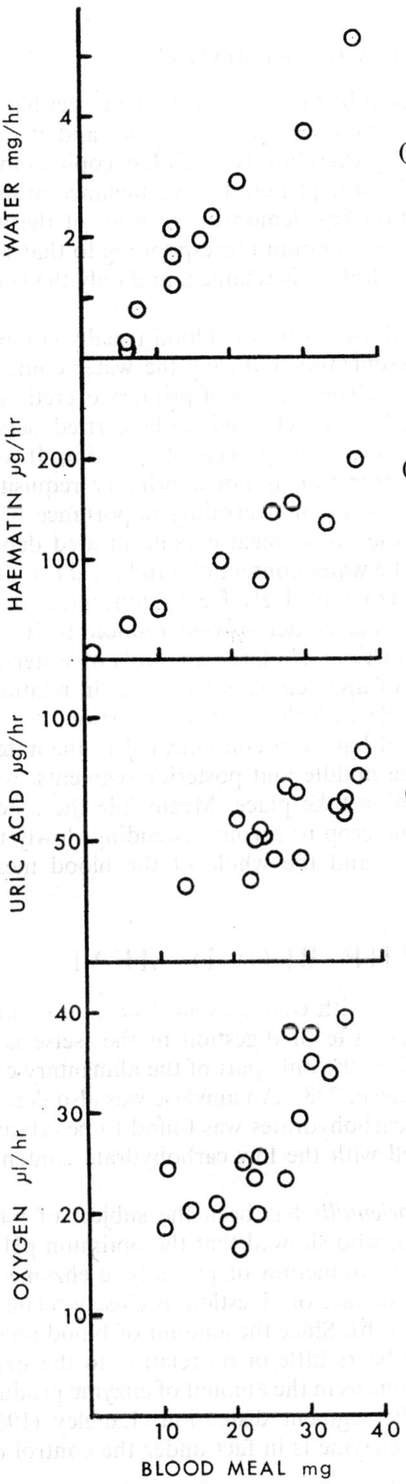

(a) The rate of primary excretion (from experimental data summarised in Bursell, 1960a)

(b) The rate of digestion, as reflected in the excretion of haematin (recalculated from Langley, 1966)

(c) The rate of excretion of uric acid (from Bursell, 1965a)

(d) The rate of respiration (from Rajagopal and Bursell, 1966)

Fig. 12.1 The relation between the size of the blood meal and the rate of different physiological processes associated with its digestion and assimilation.

by Buxton (1955, pp. 89–91, 103; *see* also Bursell, 1959a). If the insect has been exposed to low humidities during the preceding hunger cycle, and its water content in this way reduced, the primary excretion is much less copious than it is in flies whose water contents have been kept high by maintenance in humid air. Quantitative analysis of this relation has demonstrated that, of the water which is removed from the blood meal, an amount corresponding to that which is required to bring the tissues to full hydration is retained, and only the surplus is excreted.

The quantity of water which is withdrawn from the blood usually comprises about 45% of the water originally present, thus reducing the water content of the blood meal from 79% to about 50%. The process of primary excretion will therefore, in addition to lightening the load which needs to be carried, serve to concentrate the blood meal in preparation for the process of digestion. It would seem, however, that blood-meal concentration is not a primary requisite of digestion, and that water balance is a factor of overriding importance in this context, because the extent to which the blood meal is concentrated depends largely on the size of the blood meal. The water content of a full meal is reduced to about 50%, but partial meals are comparatively feebly concentrated, and with a meal size of one-fifth normal, water content is only reduced to 70%. In other words, the insect retains disproportionately large amounts of water after partial feeds, a phenomenon which is of appreciable significance in relation to water balance, but is difficult to reconcile with the needs of digestion.

When the first part of the blood meal has been concentrated in the anterior segment of the midgut, it passes to the middle and posterior segments, where the processes of digestion and absorption take place. Meanwhile the anterior segment is recharged gradually from the crop reservoir, distending slowly until the crop has been completely emptied, and the whole of the blood meal is accommodated in the midgut.

DIGESTION OF THE BLOOD MEAL

The early work of Wigglesworth (1929), with *G.m. submorsitans* and *G. tachinoides*, provided evidence that the main site of digestion in the tsetse is the middle segment of the midgut, since this is the only part of the alimentary canal that shows strong proteolytic activity (*see* p. 238). An amylase was also detected in this region, but the ability to digest carbohydrates was found to be relatively poorly developed, which correlates well with the low carbohydrate content of vertebrate blood.

The digestion of protein in *G. m. orientalis* has been the subject of recent investigations by Langley (1966, 1966a), who showed that the optimum pH for proteolytic activity is 7·5, and that the production of proteolytic enzymes by cells of the middle segment, and hence the rate of digestion, is closely related to the size of the blood meal (*see* Fig. 12.1, b). Since the amount of blood present in the middle segment at any one time bears little or no relation to the size of the blood meal, it would seem that differences in the amount of enzyme produced cannot be a direct response to middle segment distension. Langley (1966a, 1967a) suggests that the production of enzyme is in fact under the control of a neuroendocrine system, and that this control is mediated through the stomatogastric division of the nervous system (Langley, 1965; *see* also p. 240). The intake of blood could be signalled to this system by receptors monitoring crop distension, so causing the release of appropriate quantities of hormone which in turn exert an action on cells of the middle segment. The production of proteolytic enzyme was found to be stimulated to the same extent by whole blood and by dilutions of whole blood with saline, indicating that it is the volume of fluid ingested which controls the production of enzyme, rather than the quantity of protein in the meal. However, pure saline fails to elicit the production of enzyme, so it would appear that some blood factor is essential for the response of the middle segment cells. This factor has not yet been identified, but it has been shown to be associated with formed elements of the blood.

The secretion of proteolytic enzymes follows a regular pattern, with enzyme activity rising steeply during the first twelve hours after feeding, remaining high for the next twelve hours and then declining gradually to the level that characterizes the unfed fly. This pattern is accurately reflected in the rate at which haematin (a waste product of digestion, *see* below) appears in the excrement, a correspondence which suggests that the rate of digestion is closely controlled by the rate at which proteolytic enzymes are formed (Langley, 1967).

A marked difference in rate of digestion was demonstrated between flies captured in the field and flies maintained in the laboratory (Langley, 1967, 1967b). Field flies show extremely high initial rates, so that blood meal digestion proceeds rapidly to completion. Laboratory maintained flies show a later and much lower peak of digestion, and therefore take much longer to digest the whole blood meal, irrespective of the type of host (Langley, 1966). It would seem that laboratory maintenance causes some impairment of digestive function, and to this may perhaps be attributed the difficulties which are generally experienced in the laboratory maintenance of *G. morsitans*. Unfortunately, it has not yet been possible to identify the cause of this malfunction.

Before leaving the subject of digestion, mention must be made of the distinctive band of giant cells, packed with bacteroids, which form an oblique ring round the wall of the anterior segment of the midgut (Wigglesworth, 1929). No special investigation has as yet been made of the microorganisms contained in this region, but by analogy with the situation in other blood-sucking insects (Wigglesworth, 1965) it is reasonable to suppose that they serve in the synthesis of essential co-factors of metabolism, which would be deficient in the blood meal, and which the insect would not itself be capable of producing from blood meal constituents.

PRODUCTS OF DIGESTION

About 19% of the wet weight of vertebrate blood is protein, and the amino acids which arise from it will therefore constitute the main digestive products. By comparison, the concentration of carbohydrates (0·1%), of lipids (0·6%) and of other organic molecules (0·1%) is so small that these substances may be ignored for purposes of the present discussion.

The fate of amino acids, following their absorption from the last segment of the midgut, will depend in part on the age of the insect and on its sex. In immature flies taking their first or second blood meal, a considerable proportion of the digestive products are diverted to the synthesis of muscle proteins, which are required for the full development of thoracic flight musculature (Bursell, 1961b). Since the amino acid composition of the muscle proteins is not widely different from that of vertebrate blood proteins (Bursell, 1965a) the different amino acids will be utilized roughly in the proportion in which they appear as digestive products; the main exceptions are glutamic acid and arginine, which are relatively deficient in blood proteins, and histidine, which occurs in excess in blood proteins.

In mature males there will be little synthesis of proteins, but in the pregnant female large amounts of protein are required for the uterine secretion which serves the nourishment of larval stages. This secretion differs substantially from blood in the proportionate composition of amino acids, notably in respect of tyrosine, proline and glutamic acid, which are very much more abundant in nutritive secretion than in vertebrate blood, and histidine, which makes up a much greater proportion in blood than it does in nutritive secretion (Cmelik, Bursell & Slack, 1969). For the elaboration of this secretion extensive manipulation of digestive products must therefore take place, but quantitative aspects of this process have not been investigated.

Little is known of the fate of individual amino acids, except for arginine and histidine which will be discussed in the next section. Preliminary results suggest that a part of the proline and glutamate intake is oxidized directly to meet current energy requirements, while a part is diverted to the synthesis of triglycerides for storage in the fat body. A substantial fraction of the carbon of these amino acids becomes incorporated in uric acid, but the precise pathway by which this is brought about has not yet been elucidated (McCabe, personal communication).

THE EXCRETION OF WASTE PRODUCTS

The waste products of the tsetse fly are voided from the anus as a dark, semiliquid paste. They derive from two distinct sources:

(a) A portion represents undigested remains of the blood meal; these may be designated as faecal materials that have in a sense never entered the body of the insect.

(b) The major portion is excretory material *sensu stricto*, i.e. material which has been absorbed from the intestine following digestion, and has then been removed by the Malpighian system working in conjunction with the rectal glands, often following extensive metabolic transformation.

A list is given in Table 12.1 of the main components of the excrement of tsetse flies; together they comprise about 85% of its dry weight, the balance being made up of inorganic materials together with minor components such as urea, ammonia and amino acids other than arginine and histidine (Bursell, 1965a). Since the rate at which the waste products are produced is closely correlated with the quantity of blood ingested (*see* Fig. 12.1, c) values have been expressed in terms of the dry weight of the blood meal.

Uric acid is clearly the main nitrogenous waste product in the tsetse fly, as in most other terrestrial insects. The site and mode of its formation have not yet been established. It appears to enter the Malpighian tubules in soluble form and to be carried by bulk flow of tubule contents to the rectum. Here acidification occurs, the pH falling from about 7·2 to 6·0 (Berridge & Bursell, unpublished),

TABLE 12.1

The composition of the excrement of tsetse flies (from Bursell, 1965a)

	μg./mg. dry weight of blood
Uric acid	341·6
Arginine	33·1
Histidine	56·3
Haematin	28·2
Pigment	17·6
Total	476·8

with the result that most of the uric acid is precipitated. This precipitation is accompanied by a resorption of water, and probably of a variety of inorganic and organic solutes, until the rectal contents have been brought to a semi-liquid consistency, and as such they are voided.

Two amino acids, arginine and histidine, make up a substantial proportion of the dry weight of the excrement. These two substances differ from other amino acids in having a very high nitrogen content, close to that of uric acid itself. Their metabolic utilization would present a considerable problem for an insect like the tsetse, whose main excretory product is uric acid. Each of the four nitrogen atoms of arginine, for example, would have to be removed to make the molecule available for oxidative degradation. These nitrogens would then have to be incorporated into the uric acid molecule at the expense of substantial amounts of metabolic energy, so that the net gain in energy, if any, would be small. It is not surprising to find, therefore, that arginine and histidine are quantitatively eliminated, appearing in the excrement in the same amounts that they are ingested. Their elimination must be regarded as excretory, since they are routed *via* the Malpighian circuit.

The last two substances listed in Table 12.1 appear to be faecal materials as previously defined. Haematin, which is split off from the haemoglobin molecule during early stages of digestion (*see* also Buxton, 1955, p. 78), does not appear to be absorbed from the gut, since it cannot be detected in the haemolymph; the same applies to a yellow, fluorescent pigment, whose nature and origin remain obscure.

Before leaving the subject of excretory metabolism, mention should be made of the fact that the resorption of water from waste materials in the rectum appears to be regulated in close relation to the requirements of water balance (Bursell, 1960c). Flies which are maintained at high relative humidity excrete a waste material whose water content increases from about 60% to 85%; while for flies maintained in dry air, the percentage of water in the excrement drops from about 40% immediately after the completion of primary excretion to values as low as 25%. This ability to dehydrate the waste products has been shown to result in a very substantial saving of water, and is of great importance in relation to the general problem of water balance.

THE ENERGY BALANCE

The physiological processes discussed in this chapter have been summarized in diagrammatic form in Fig. 12.2. The situation which obtains during the first hour or so after feeding is shown in Fig. 12.2, a; the anterior segment of the midgut has been charged with blood, while the bulk of the blood meal is still accommodated in the crop. The main process which occurs at this stage is the cycling of inorganic salts and water from the anterior segment of the midgut into the haemolymph, from here to the Malpighian tubules and so to the hindgut, with resorption of certain solutes from the rectal papillae, and the excretion of a dilute urine (primary excretion). Although details of this process have not been worked out, there can be little doubt that it must involve the expenditure of energy for the performance of osmotic work, as indicated on the diagram.

Figure 12.2, b represents the situation during later stages of the hunger cycle, when the blood meal has been fully accommodated in the midgut, and the process of digestion has begun. At this stage substantial energy losses would be involved in the synthesis of triglycerides, and to a lesser extent of proteins, from amino acids, and in the detoxication of α-amino nitrogen by incorporation in uric acid. In addition, energy would be required for a variety of transport processes involved in the absorption of digestive products, and the recycling of water and inorganic salts through the Malpighian tube/rectal gland system.

Once digestion has been completed, and surplus digestive products stored as triglycerides in the fat body, the energy expenditure associated with feeding would fall away. Respiration would now be supported entirely by storage fats, and since these contain no nitrogen all of the energy trapped during oxidation would become available to meet the requirement for maintenance of the living state.

These, then, are the main processes associated with feeding in tsetse flies. The main purpose of feeding, in the tsetse fly as in other animals, is to obtain a

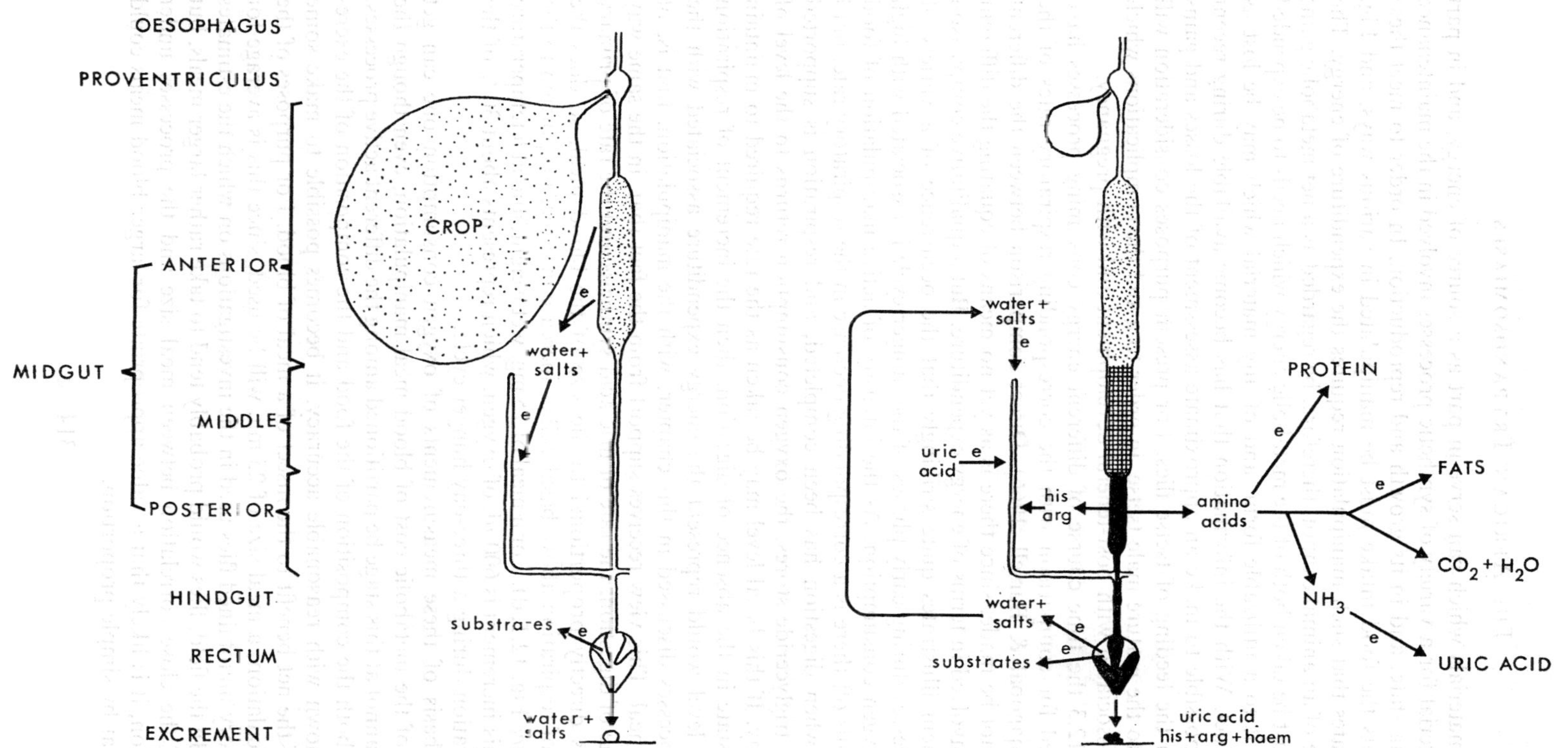

(a) The situation 1 hour after a blood meal

(b) The situation 24 hours after a blood meal

Fig. 12.2 A diagrammatic summary of physiological processes associated with feeding. Processes which are known, or thought, to require the expenditure of energy have been indicated (e). For further explanation *see* text.

supply of materials which can serve in part as a source of energy, and in part as raw material for a variety of synthetic processes involved in the maintenance of the living state, and in its growth and reproduction. In order to meet these requirements the food intake must be manipulated in various ways, and Fig. 12.2 illustrates that such manipulation requires the expenditure of energy. The food intake of an animal cannot, therefore, be regarded as a net metabolic gain; account must be taken both of the metabolic energy which needs to be expended to convert it to a utilizable form, and of any material which may be lost as waste product. With the information that has become available during recent years it is possible to make an approximate assessment of the losses and gains involved in the feeding of tsetse flies. For present purposes consideration will be limited to the mature male tsetse, in order to avoid the complications which would be associated with post-teneral development and with pregnancy.

In Fig. 12.3 the time course of different energy consuming processes have been plotted for comparison with the corresponding respiratory rates of the fed fly (Rajagopal & Bursell, 1966). Direct comparison between the different curves cannot be made, since there is as yet no means of equating the different processes involved in terms of energy expenditure. But a qualitative comparison between them illustrates quite strikingly that the occurrence of a variety of active processes during early phases of the hunger cycle is associated with high rates of oxygen consumption. As the intensity of active manipulation of food products falls off there is a corresponding decrease in the respiratory rate, until at a time when digestion has been completed, and respiration is supported entirely by triglyceride stores, the oxygen consumption returns to the level of the unfed fly. If this basal level may be taken as the rate required to maintain the living state in the absence of digestion, then the increment of respiration above this level would represent the energy expenditure associated with the sum of processes discussed in this chapter, with the manipulation, that is, of the blood meal. This view receives support from the fact that, in the same way that the rate of digestion, the rate of uric acid synthesis and the rate of primary excretion is directly proportional to the size of the blood meal, so does the increment of respiration above basal values increase in direct proportion to the meal size (*see* Fig. 12.1, d). For a meal of 25 mg. wet weight, and at a temperature of 25°C, this increment is 600 μl. of oxygen, which represents about 30% of the total respiration during a three-day hunger cycle.

On the basis of these measurements of oxygen consumption one can get some idea of the metabolic cost of blood meal manipulation, even though the total cost cannot at this stage be partitioned among the different active processes. And since both the composition of the food and the composition of the excrement is known with reasonable accuracy, it becomes possible to make some estimate of the net benefit to the insect of a meal of blood. For purposes of the present calculation, a meal size of 25 mg. will be used, since this is average for the laboratory-maintained flies used in the investigations on which the estimates are based. In the field, flies would probably tend to take rather larger meals, but in view of the close correlation between meal size and the processes under consideration, it is likely that a value appropriate for larger blood meals could be arrived at by simple proportion.

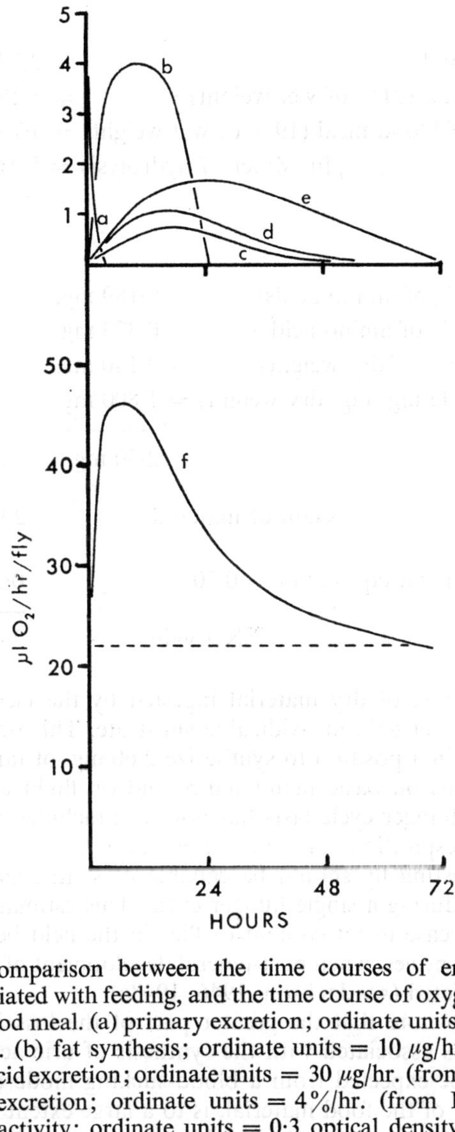

Fig. 12.3 A comparison between the time courses of energy-consuming processes associated with feeding, and the time course of oxygen consumption following a blood meal. (a) primary excretion; ordinate units = mg/hr. (from Bursell, 1960c). (b) fat synthesis; ordinate units = 10 μg/hr. (from Bursell, 1963). (c) uric acid excretion; ordinate units = 30 μg/hr. (from Bursell, 1960c). (d) haematin excretion; ordinate units = 4%/hr. (from Langley, 1966a). (e) proteinase activity; ordinate units = 0·3 optical density (from Langley, 1967). (f) oxygen consumption (from Rajagopal & Bursell, 1966) Interrupted line indicates teneral rate (23 μl/hr)

With a meal size of 25 mg. of fresh blood, the balance sheet would be as under:

Gain		
Wet weight of blood		= 25·0 mg.
Dry weight of blood (21% of wet weight)		= 5·25 mg.
Protein content of blood meal (19% of wet weight)		= 4·75 mg.
plus water of hydrolysis		= 5·41 mg. amino acids
Losses		
(i) Materials		
Arginine (3·5% of amino acids)	= 0·189 mg.	
Histidine (6·9% of amino acids)	= 0·373 mg.	
Haematin (2·7% of dry weight)	= 0·140 mg.	
Uric acid (0·342 mg./mg. dry weight)	= 1·800 mg.	
	2·50 mg.	2·50 mg.
Gain of material		2·91 mg.
(ii) Energy		
600 μl. oxygen; fat equivalent = 0·30		0·30 mg.
Net gain		2·61 mg.

Thus of the 5·25 mg. of dry material ingested by the tsetse fly, just under 50% constitutes the net gain in oxidizable substrate. This does not imply that the insect would be in a position to synthesize 2·60 mg. of fat, since the energy which the fly expends on basic maintenance and on flight activity during the three days that the hunger cycle lasts has not been included in the calculation. The maintenance respiration amounts to about 0·65 mg. of fat equivalent, suggesting that a resting fly should be capable of synthesizing 2·0 mg. of fat from a blood meal during a single hunger cycle. This estimate is in reasonable accord with the increase in fat content of flies in the field between the second and the third hunger cycles, when post-teneral development of thoracic musculature has been completed (*see* Jackson, 1946, 1948a).

It is interesting to note that the greater part of the loss involved in blood meal manipulation is associated with the synthesis of uric acid. It would seem that the benefit to be expected from a blood-sucking mode of life in terms of the easy digestibility of the food material, is to a large extent offset by the need to dispose of nitrogenous waste as uric acid.

Chapter 13

Hosts of *Glossina*

B. G. F. WEITZ

INTRODUCTORY

For many years it has been suspected that tsetse flies are selective in the choice of hosts from which their blood meals are obtained. Earlier studies on food preferences yielded inconclusive results because the methods available to determine food sources lacked precision and because observations were made in selected and usually restricted areas. In comparatively recent years extensive surveys have been made using more precise techniques and much valuable information has now been accumulated on the natural feeding habits of different species of tsetse in many parts of Africa.

METHODS EMPLOYED TO STUDY FEEDING HABITS OF TSETSE FLIES

Direct Observation in the Field

The direct observation of the act of feeding on wild animals is impracticable and unreliable and reports of this kind must be considered as mostly anecdotal. Some useful information was obtained from experiments on the feeding of captured or laboratory-bred flies on animals kept in captivity. Although the results obtained from this kind of study indicate some possible food sources they bear little or no resemblance to the feeding habits of *Glossina* under natural conditions. In addition, in view of the differences in the physiology of digestion of tsetse flies maintained in the laboratory compared with that of wild flies in their natural habitat, such experiments have certain important limitations. It is therefore very doubtful whether much valid information on feeding habits can be obtained by such means.

The use of live bait animals in the field to study the feeding habits also has similar disadvantages. Flies may be attracted variously to some bait animals depending on their state of hunger and many extraneous factors may influence the attraction of flies to different baits (*see* pp. 298 *et seq.*). Thus, although studies with bait animals may yield some useful information on the choice of tsetse hosts under special conditions, they do not reflect the selective feeding habits of the flies in their natural habitats. In any event the introduction of domestic animals or man as baits in tsetse-infested areas may itself significantly divert flies from their usual hosts. Buxton (1955) has reviewed the results of experiments up to 1952 and his full account, which virtually amounts to a plea for additional and more accurate information, should be consulted for the results obtained up to that date.

Identification of Blood Meals

The identification of stomach contents of flies caught in their natural environment provides the most objective method of determining the natural sources of food of tsetse flies. Blood obtained from the stomach of the recently fed fly can be identified by the examination of the cellular components or by the analysis of the plasma proteins.

Identification of Cells in the Blood Meal

In practice, examination of the erythrocytes in preparations made from the insect's stomach contents may provide a convenient means of identifying the source of the blood meal. Smears of the stomach contents may be prepared and stained for microscopical examination but in dried material there is usually some distortion of the cells. A more reliable procedure is to examine fresh preparations by phase contrast microscopy. In both cases it is important to ensure that the ingested blood is prepared for examination before there has been time for the insect's digestive processes to impair the morphological characters of the cells.

Avian and reptilian blood is readily identified by the presence of oval, nucleated erythrocytes. Blood from the Camelidae is easily distinguished from that of birds and reptiles by the absence of nucleated erythrocytes and from that of other mammals by the oval shape of the red blood cells.

When the ingested blood is sufficiently fresh it may be possible to distinguish the blood of different mammals by measuring the diameter of the erythrocytes under the microscope with the aid of a Vernier scale or with an eyepiece scale.

The measurements of the red blood cells of some hosts in Northern Nigeria were determined by Lloyd, Johnson *et al.* (1924) who classified the mammalian species into five groups according to the diameter of the erythrocytes. Jackson and Vanderplank (1941) found considerable variation in the size of the cells of individual species: warthog red blood cells varied between 5·9 and 6·7 microns in diameter and reedbuck cells between 4·8 and 5·9 microns. In general their results confirmed those obtained in Nigeria. Although these measurements may be of some value in excluding certain species, the reliable identification of the different species of mammals is not practicable in this way because many animals, having blood cells of similar measurements, are indistinguishable. However, under special circumstances, some early workers obtained useful data in this way.

Identification by Immunological Tests on Serum Proteins in Blood Meal

In 1904 Nuttall showed that the serum proteins of different species of animals were antigenically distinct and that these differences provided a practical means of identifying the sera of different animals as, for example, in medico-legal tests of blood stains. Later this principle was applied by several workers to study the blood meals of insects by the precipitin test.

(i) Precipitin Test

Antisera prepared by the injection of the serum proteins of different species into an animal of another species (generally a rabbit) react with the sera of these species to form an insoluble antigen-antibody complex which is visible as a precipitate. When the antisera are suitably prepared or absorbed they react specifically with the sera of homologous species and of closely related animals; for example, antisera prepared against human serum will usually react with other primate sera such as baboon or monkey.

The complex antigenic relationships of the sera of mammals have been detailed by Weitz (1952). All mammalian sera contain a number of antigens which are common to most species and although the various combinations of these 'mammalian antigens' are different in individual species, they overlap sufficiently to cause cross reactions on a wide scale. In practice antisera prepared in rabbits by multiple immunization with the serum proteins of one species of mammal contain antibodies which react with the sera of all other mammalian species but not with the sera of birds or reptiles. The specificity of such antisera can be improved by absorption with a mixture of sera from a relatively limited number of mammalian species (the sera of domestic animals form a suitable and convenient mixture) other than the homologous species. This procedure yields antisera which react only with the sera of animals closely related to the homologous species and can be used for the group identification of blood meals by the precipitin test (*see* Table 18.2, p. 422).

Theoretically, further absorption with the serum proteins of the closely related species should neutralize all the heterologous antibodies but, because of the resultant dilution of the antiserum, such absorptions yield antisera which fail to form a visible precipitate when allowed to react with the homologous serum proteins. The specific identification of the sera of closely related animals is therefore not practicable by the precipitin test.

These group specific antisera can be used, however, to identify single species when there are no closely related species within the group. For example, absorbed anti-rhinoceros or anti-hippopotamus sera react only with their respective homologous species because there are no species closely related to these animals. Similarly, such antisera can be used for specific identification when other species with which they react do not occur in the area of study. Thus anti-primate sera can be used to identify human feeds in areas where no primates other than man occur.

(ii) The Haemagglutination-Inhibition Test (H.I.T.)

The individual species of closely related mammalian sera can be identified by the passive haemagglutination-inhibition test (Weitz, 1956). For this test, which is based on the technique described by Boyden (1951), the antisera are diluted to such an extent that their absorption is greatly facilitated. The normal erythrocytes of rabbit are sensitized with serum proteins after treatment with tannic acid or bis-diazotized-benzidine (Gordon, Rose & Sehon, 1958) and are then used as the indicator system for antibody. These sensitized cells are agglutinated by high dilutions of antisera prepared against the serum proteins of the species used to coat the cells. The antisera may also agglutinate cells sensitized with a number of different species of mammalian sera but the reaction is inhibited specifically by low concentrations of antigens at appropriate pre-determined dilutions of antibody. Thus the blood meal extracts, used as absorbing antigens, can be identified by their ability specifically to inhibit the agglutination of sensitized cells by the homologous antisera. Full details of this test and examples of the serological identification of blood meals by its use are given in Chapter 18.

(iii) Other Methods of Identification

(a) PRECIPITATING AGAR GEL DIFFUSION TEST. A number of variations of the precipitin test have been used for the identification of insect blood meals. These are mostly techniques based on the agar gel diffusion method and the success of these techniques depends essentially on the quality of the antiserum employed. A modification of this method recently advocated by Cunningham, Kimber, Bailey and Harley (1967) incorporates the antiserum in agar gel on glass slides. The blood meal smears are applied directly to the gel and allowed to diffuse through the agar. The consequent reaction with the antiserum in the agar forms circular areas of precipitation around the smears. This technique is less sensitive than the precipitin test performed in vertical tubes (precipitin ring test, *see* pp. 416–7) as judged by comparative tests made by the writer (unpublished) about ten years ago in which equal portions of the blood smears of mosquito feeds received from the field were tested by both techniques using the same antiserum. In one series of sixty-four relatively poor smears which were all identified by the precipitin ring test, not one was identified by the gel tests and in another of twelve mosquito smears of good quality all were correctly identified by the standard ring test but only five were identified by the gel test. These results indicate the much lower sensitivity of the gel test. Further disadvantages are that the gel method is not easily automated for large scale tests and requires larger quantities of antiserum. The technique is, however, of great value when dealing with very small smears because it avoids the need to dilute the blood-meal as would be necessary for the ring test when it is extracted in saline solution.

(b) IMMUNE ELECTROPHORESIS AND MICROELECTROPHORESIS. Differences in the electrophoretic characters of constituent proteins of different sera can be demonstrated by immuno-electrophoresis in agar gels or on cellulose acetate paper strips. The differentiation of species can be established by such means in exceptional cases but insufficient information is available about the characteristic constituents of the sera of different mammals to enable this procedure to be used on a wider scale. This method is, however, a most valuable research tool for studies on the digestion of the blood in tsetse flies and other insects.

Assessment of Techniques Employed

Before putting any procedure to general use it is essential to define the sensitivity and the specificity of the techniques so that valid comparisons can be made between the results of tests carried out by different workers and with different reagents (*see* Weitz, 1960). In addition careful field control tests are necessary to ensure that such methods are effective with field material. Because of the differences in the digestion of tsetse flies in captivity and in the wild state (*see* Weitz & Buxton, 1953) it is not sufficient to prove the validity of techniques with tsetse flies which have been artificially fed or kept in the laboratory. Comprehensive field tests with marked flies (Weitz & Jackson, 1955), although extremely laborious, are necessary to establish the validity of the techniques selected for use in field studies.

The Collection of Blood Meals

The time after collection at which the feed can be identified may vary with the techniques of preservation. Ideally the whole undissected insect should be preserved immediately by freezing in dry ice or liquid nitrogen (Templis & Lofy, 1963). This method ensures immediate inhibition of any digestive enzymes present and optimal preservation of the proteins in the blood meal. The method is, however, seldom practical in the field where supplies of refrigerant may not be available and the samples, which must be preserved in vacuum flasks, are bulky and expensive to transport.

For this reason the more practical method of drying smears from the stomach contents on filter paper is usually employed. However, the rate of drying and the preservation of the smears vary considerably on filter papers of apparently identical quality so that some batches of smears are not easily eluted from the filter paper. The substitution of non-absorbent (plastic) sheets ('Velvetex' manufactured by Masons and Sons, Ltd., Colchester) as used by Cunningham (personal communication) may overcome such difficulties; the blood meal can be dissolved easily by adding a drop of diluent directly onto the paper itself and aspirating the solution with a pipette. However, there is the danger that the dried material may scale off the paper during transit.

Smears on filter paper or plastic sheets may be eluted by cutting out the portion containing the smear and dropping it into physiological saline solution contained in small test tubes. Although the serum proteins dissolve rapidly, the smears are usually kept in saline at 4°C overnight before use. A clear solution is usually obtained in this way, but should particles remain in suspension they can be deposited by centrifugation.

THE FEEDING HABITS OF TSETSE FLIES

As determined by the identification of blood meals, the feeding habits of *Glossina* are very characteristic for each species of fly. The results of many surveys of the feeding habits of tsetse flies in specified areas have been reported in detail elsewhere (Weitz & Jackson, 1955; Weitz & Glasgow, 1956; Weitz, Langridge, Napier Bax & Lee-Jones, 1960; Jordan, Lee-Jones & Weitz, 1961; Jordan, Lee-Jones & Weitz, 1962 and Weitz, 1963) but will be summarized here on a broad basis. At times, variations in the feeding patterns are evident from the results obtained in different areas, at different times of the year, under varying climatic conditions or in the presence of variable host populations. Although such variations must be taken into account it is possible to make certain generalizations about the feeding habits of different species of *Glossina* provided they are based on sufficiently large and representative samples. Samples should be collected on a random basis and should be obtained over a sufficiently long period to cover variations in climatic conditions and changes in the animal population of a given area. Likewise, it is necessary to obtain samples from a number of areas representative of the different climatic and host conditions occurring within the range of the species of *Glossina* concerned. It is important also to ensure that, for each species of *Glossina*, sampling should be representative of the age, sex and level of hunger of the fly population investigated. The results reported here are based on the identification of well over 25,000 blood meals from many parts of Africa and include only those collections which were judged sufficiently representative.

Broadly, different species of *Glossina* have specific feeding habits and available hosts are used discriminately as a source of food by tsetse flies. The feeding behaviour of some species of *Glossina* are largely similar and can therefore be grouped together (Weitz, 1963) according to the hosts most frequently used as a source of food (*see* Fig. 13.1).

Species of *Glossina* Feeding mainly on the Suidae

G. swynnertoni, *G. austeni*, *G. tabaniformis*, *G. fuscipleuris*

It is surprising to find the extent to which many species of *Glossina* select pigs as their main source of food, particularly as the numbers of wild pigs available represent only a small proportion of the accessible game population. About 65% of all feeds of *G. swynnertoni* in Kenya and Tanzania are derived from warthog (*Phacochoerus aethiopicus*) the remainder being obtained chiefly from large ruminants (22%) such as giraffe (*Giraffa camelopardalis* 8%) and buffalo (*Syncerus caffer* 8%) and from rhinoceros (*Diceros bicornis* 3%).

G. austeni uses bushpig (*Potamochoerus koiropotamus*) as its main source of food (about 60%), a finding consistent with the crepuscular habits of both fly and host. The fly is likely to be easily diverted to cattle for food if these animals enter their territory and duiker (*Sylvicapra grimmia* and other species) also contribute substantially (about 10%) to the diet of this fly.

G. fuscipleuris feeds mainly (65%) on the giant forest hog (*Hylochoerus meinertzhageni*) but, in certain areas, hippopotamus (*Hippopotamus amphibius*) provides nearly 20% of its diet.

In West Africa, the red river hog (*Potamochoerus porcus*) is the most important host (70%) of *G. tabaniformis*, a fly of the forest regions, and this fly also obtains nearly 25% of its feeds from the porcupine (*Atherurus africanus*).

These four species of fly typify the apparent predilection of some tsetse flies for suid blood, as was suggested by Jackson (1940). The various species of suids used are naturally those which inhabit the particular environment of the different species of fly but as they are certainly not the most available hosts in these areas, this habit can be regarded as a distinct food preference (Glasgow, Isherwood, Lee-Jones & Weitz, 1958).

Species Feeding Equally on the Suidae and Bovidae

G. morsitans morsitans, G.m. submorsitans, G.m. orientalis

Like the previous group, these flies feed freely on pigs but they do not show the same marked preference for suid blood and will as readily take the blood of large bovids. The suids (30–45% of all feeds) used are mostly warthog and the most common bovids (25–40% of all feeds) fed on are kudu (*Strepsiceros strepsiceros*), buffalo, bushbuck (*Tragelaphus scriptus*) and eland (*Taurotragus oryx*); the extent to which these species are used depends on the species of fly and the locality. The specificity of the feeding habits is again clearly shown by the distinct differences in the use made of hartebeest (*Alcelaphus buselaphus*) by these three sub-species. Neither *G.m. morsitans* nor *G.m. orientalis* appear to feed on this antelope in spite of its ready availability but, in contrast, *G.m. submorsitans* uses this animal relatively frequently (about 2% of all feeds). Other antelopes are occasionally used by this group of flies; reedbuck (*Redunca redunca*) and duiker form less than 1–3% of the feeds while other small antelopes are very rarely attacked.

Species Feeding Mainly on Bovidae

G. pallidipes, G. longipalpis, G. fusca

The East African species *G. pallidipes* and the West African species *G. longipalpis* have almost identical feeding habits, obtaining their food mainly from bushbuck which provides 80–90% of all feeds. This is a marked preference for this bovid as in many instances these flies overlap with *G. morsitans*. *G. fusca* also

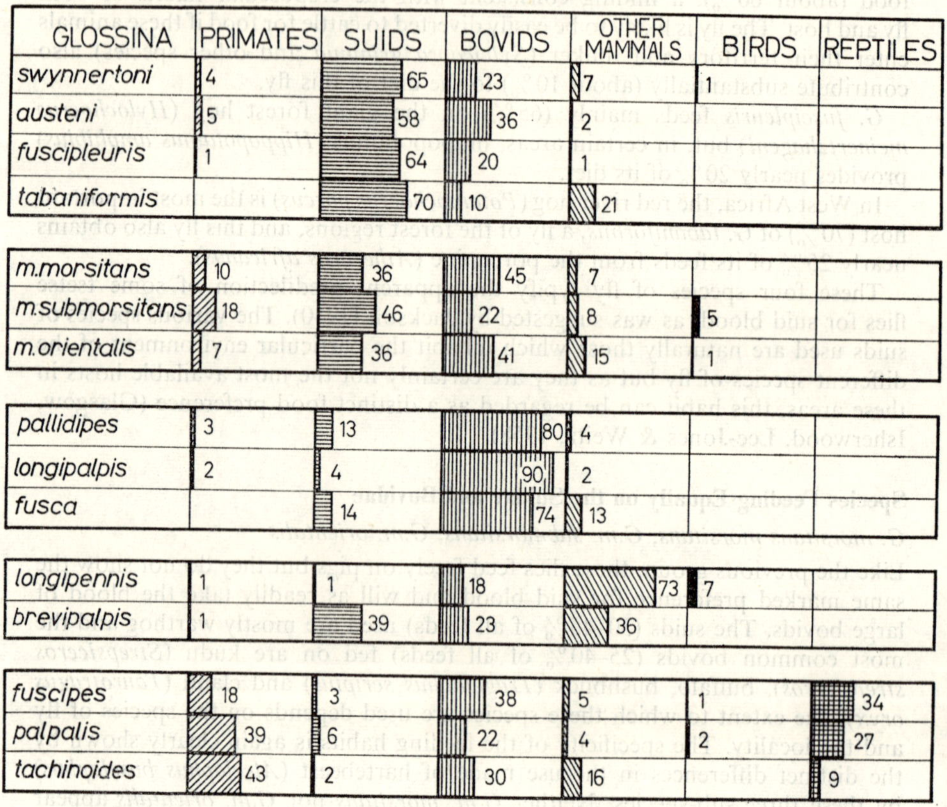

Fig. 13.1 Summary of the feeding habits of 15 species of *Glossina* obtained from the identification of approximately 25,000 feeds. The figures indicate the percentage of feeds of each species of *Glossina* derived from each category of host.

derives most (74%) of its food from bushbuck but the red river hog provides 13% and the aardvaark (*Orycteropus afer*) 12% of its blood meals.

Species Feeding Mainly on Mammals other than Pigs or Bovids

G. longipennis, G. brevipalpis

Although the feeding habits of *G. brevipalpis* are very similar to those of *G. tabaniformis*, the former is sometimes more dependent on hippopotamus for its staple diet (36%). Bushpig also form a large part (nearly 40%) of the diet of *G. brevipalpis* but this varies according to the availability of this host. Both buffalo and bushbuck are used frequently. Characteristically, *G. longipennis* depends almost entirely on rhinoceros (60%) for its food but elephant (*Loxodonta africana*) is an important host (12% of all feeds) when it invades the area; it appears to be the only species of *Glossina* which feeds to any significant extent (7%) on the ostrich (*Struthio camelus*) (*see* Weitz, Langridge, Bax & Lee-Jones, 1960).

Species Feeding on Man and Most Available Hosts

G. palpalis, G. fuscipes, G. tachinoides

Over the greater part of their range of distribution, species of the *palpalis* group are largely confined to the vicinity of water ('riverine tsetse'). Their sources of food are extremely variable and it is characteristic of these species that they can readily adapt themselves to whatever sources of blood are available. They are known to feed largely on aquatic reptiles (*Varanus*, *Crocodylus* spp.) and in undisturbed areas along the Nile these reptiles provide the main, if not the only, source of food for *G. fuscipes*. The latter species is the intermediate host of two protozoal parasites (*Hepatozoon pettiti* and *Trypanosoma grayi*) which occur exclusively in the Nile crocodile. The infection rate with *T. grayi* among wild *G. fuscipes* in the Upper Nile when correlated with that in experimentally infected flies provides strong evidence that the crocodile is the main source of food for *G. fuscipes* in this area (Hoare, 1962). Birds (probably aquatic species such as cormorants) form a significant part (1–2%) of the diet of this group.

Man is a variable source of food (8–40%) but is very frequently attacked when brought into close contact with the fly as, for example, at village water-holes or river crossings. Cattle also are frequently bitten in similar circumstances.

The liability of other animals to be attacked is dependent upon the extent to which they invade the flies' habitats. Thus pigs are not often used as a source of blood (3%) but antelopes such as bushbuck are commonly bitten (10–20%).

Baldry (1964) has made a special study of the feeding habits of *G. tachinoides* and has reported that, in close proximity to markets, this species will neglect all other sources of food to attack domestic pigs. A recent examination by Baldry of data relating to the hosts of this species in Nigeria has shown that six basic feeding patterns can be distinguished in different populations of *G. tachinoides*, one group feeding on most available hosts, four others mainly on Reptilia, Suidae, Bovidae and Primates, respectively, and a sixth almost exclusively on Bovidae. Such variation from the normally accepted feeding behaviour of a tsetse species may be of great importance in the epidemiology of trypanosomiasis and emphasizes the importance of detailed studies of local populations of tsetse.

CONCLUSIONS

Different species of tsetse flies have varying preferences for different hosts and all, apart from the *palpalis* group, seem to be highly selective. The most constant feature is a marked liking for the Suidae, out of all proportion to the available fauna.

It follows that different game species have very different roles in supporting different tsetse populations and that the control of tsetse flies by the removal of the most important sources of food does not necessarily entail the wholesale slaughter of all the fauna in the area.

The extent to which the tsetse fly may adopt new feeding habits in a changing host population is not clear, but overall, the constancy of the feeding patterns in different situations suggests that the fly might adapt itself to new hosts only relatively slowly. In Nagupande in Rhodesia, an area well populated with game of many species, *G. morsitans* was practically exterminated by the removal of the preferred hosts only (Cockbill, 1967). Elephant, buffalo, kudu, bushbuck and the Suidae were the only species destroyed or removed from the area while duiker, reedbuck, waterbuck and other small antelopes as well as zebra and very large herds of impala were allowed to remain. The success in starving out the fly by such means may well depend on the rapidity with which the normal hosts can be removed thereby denying the fly sufficient time to adapt itself to new hosts.

It is important to realize that certain species of game apparently play no part in supporting tsetse populations. Zebra, wildebeest and many of the small antelopes have never been recorded as hosts of any species of fly. Waterbuck, impala and hartebeest, although very numerous, are extremely rarely fed on by tsetse flies. The extent to which some animals are selectively used by tsetse flies is indicated by Glasgow and Wilson (1953) and by Lamprey, Glasgow, Lee-Jones and Weitz (1962) who calculated that warthogs lost between 13–27 g. of blood per day in providing food to *G. swynnertoni* and that in an area infested with *G. pallidipes* each animal (mostly bushbuck and bushpig) was bitten daily 291 times and provided 7·5 g. of blood. However inaccurate these calculations may be, they indicate the tremendous burden borne by some game species.

Chapter 14

Reproduction of *Glossina:* Breeding Sites

D. S. SAUNDERS R. J. PHELPS

Reproduction of *Glossina*

Introductory

The discovery by Bruce (1895) of the viviparous nature of reproduction in tsetse flies, together with the growing realization of the importance of tsetse flies as vectors of sleeping sickness, led to the publication of several reports on the anatomy of tsetse (Minchin, 1905; Stuhlman, 1907; Roubaud, 1909) which established the morphology of the female reproductive tract in such detail that only minor modifications have since been necessary.

The anatomy of the female genital system is adequately depicted in Fig. 14.1. It differs from the more typical oviparous Muscids in characters which are demanded by the viviparous habit: the ovaries contain a greatly reduced number of ovarioles, the common oviduct is enlarged to form a uterus in which the larva develops and the accessory glands are modified to produce the protein and lipid 'milk' from which the larva derives its nourishment. This form of reproduction is shared with the Pupipara and a few other Muscidae and is termed *adenotrophic viviparity* by Hagan (1951) because the egg contains sufficient yolk for embryonic development and the larva in the uterus is nourished by special maternal organs.

The consequences of viviparity are that only a small number of fully-developed larvae ($\sim$ 20) can be produced, a free-living larval stage is practically

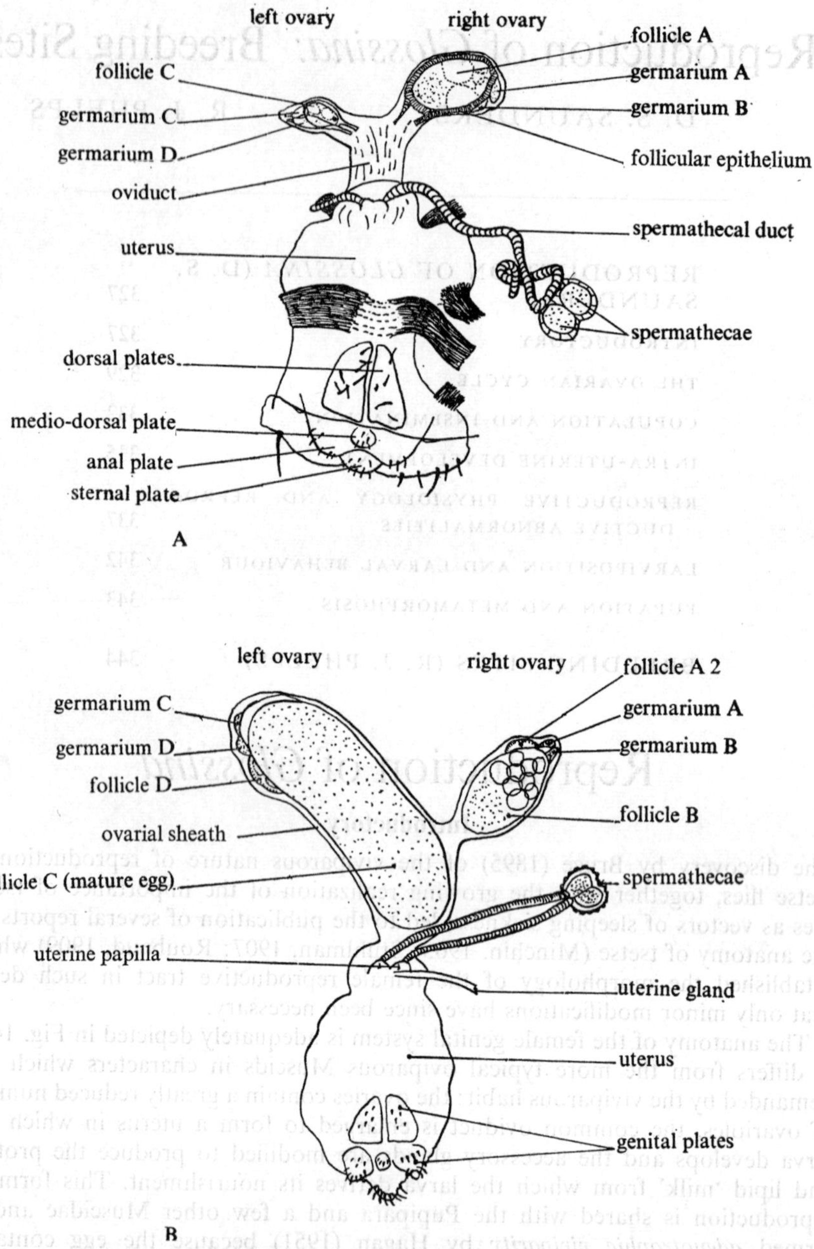

Fig. 14.1 The female genital system (*Glossina tachinoides*): A. Female 1-day old (uterine or milk gland removed); B. Female 20-days old just after first larviposition. Second egg (ovariole c) just descending into the uterus. Semi-diagrammatic. (From Itard, 1966)

eliminated and both adults and immature stages are dependent upon the same source of food (blood).

The Ovarian Cycle

The following account is based on normal fertilized females of *Glossina morsitans* maintained at 26°C, but, since only minor differences between species are known to occur, it may be taken as a general account.

Early investigators (Minchin, 1905; Stuhlman, 1907; Roubaud, 1909) came to the conclusion that only one ovariole was present in each ovary of *Glossina*; this often-quoted but erroneous view was perpetuated by subsequent authors (Mellanby, 1937; Hagan, 1951; Hoffman, 1954). However, it is now known that each ovary contains two polytrophic ovarioles (Saunders, 1960b, 1961; Itard, 1966) thus resembling very closely the condition seen in other adenotrophic Diptera (Pratt, 1899; Detinova, 1955; Saunders, 1964). In the newly-emerged female the four ovarioles are at different stages of development. Since only one egg is produced at a time the appearance of the ovaries in a teneral female reflects the sequence of the ovarian cycle (Figs. 14.2, 14.3).

The first follicle to develop is the larger one in the right ovary (A). Yolk deposition in this oocyte begins about seven days before the fly emerges from the pupa and continues in the unfed female (Saunders, 1961). Development is accelerated after the first bloodmeal and the first egg is fully developed by the 8th to 10th day. The mature egg then passes from the ovary into the uterus, embryonic and larval development follow (*see* below) and the first larva is produced on about the 18th to 20th day after emergence. Subsequent larvae are then produced at about 10-day intervals; the maximum number produced is uncertain but Azevedo and Pinhão (1964) have recorded twenty from a female of *G. morsitans*. Within hours of parturition the second egg in the sequence (from follicle C, left ovary) has reached maturity and is then ovulated. After the second parturition, the third egg (B) is ovulated from the right ovary; after the third parturition the fourth egg (D) is produced from the left ovary, and so on. The cycle is then repeated with ovariole A in the right ovary functioning for the second time. The sequence of ovulation can thus be described as, A, C, B, D, A_2, C_2, B_2, etc., and is illustrated in Figs. 14.2 and 14.3.

During ovarian development the follicular tube becomes greatly enlarged to accommodate the growing egg follicle so that, after ovulation, a large expanded sac is seen (Fig. 14.2, IV). Subsequently this sac contracts to a small dilatation at the end of the follicular tube which remains intact whilst the next egg follicle in the ovariole develops above it (Fig. 14.2, VA). This follicular relic marks the position of the first egg and is evidence that ovulation has occurred. Examination of the ovaries of wild-caught females for follicular relics, therefore, can be used to distinguish nulliparous from parous females. Furthermore, the number and position of such relics, together with the relative sizes of the four egg follicles and the contents of the uterus, may be used as an accurate method for the determination of physiological age (Saunders, 1962).

Serial follicular relics, as seen in Anopheline mosquitoes (Detinova, 1962), each denoting the position of a previous egg follicle, are not observed in the ovaries of tsetse flies. However, Vattier (1965), working with females of *G.*

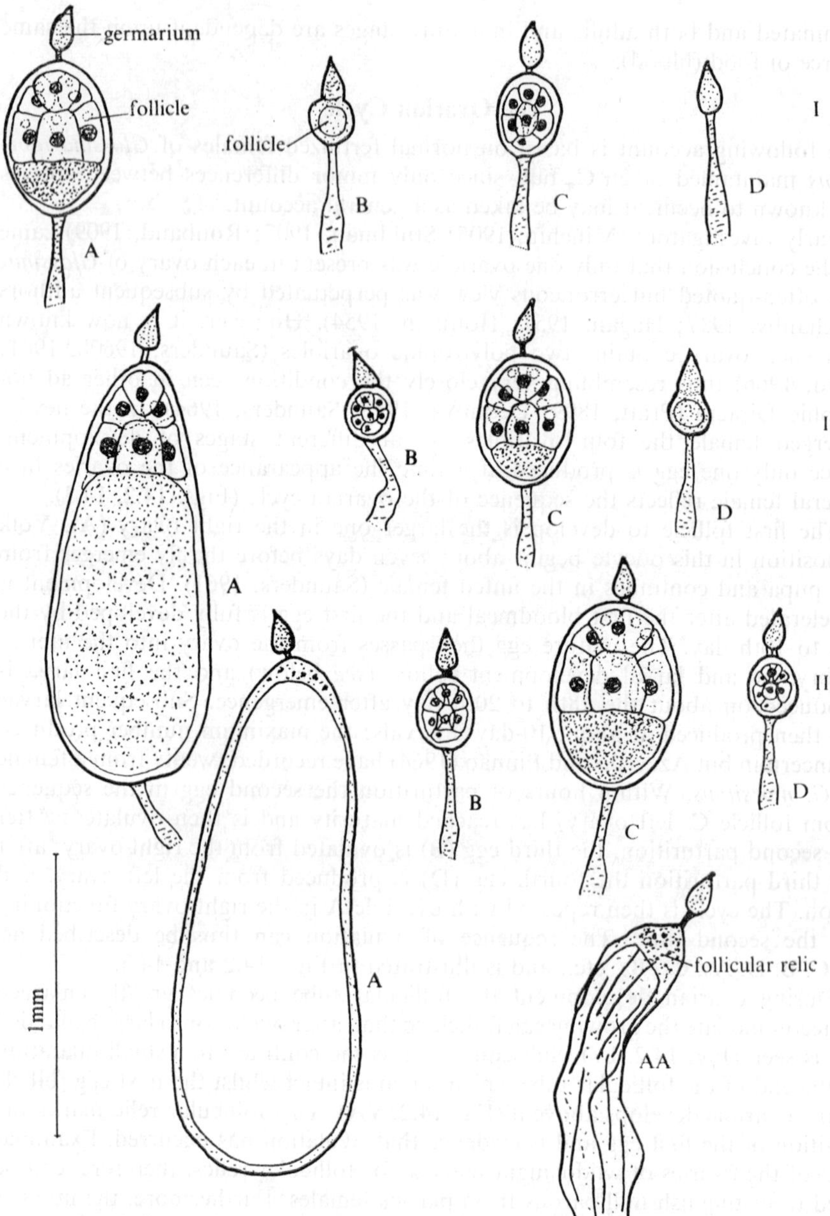

Fig. 14.2 (a)

The ovulation cycle in *Glossina morsitans*. The four ovarioles: A and B of the right ovary, C and D of the left: (a) I, in a newly emerged female, follicles of A and C descended from germarium, first signs of follicle in B; II, in a female 4 days old, first signs of follicle in D; III, in a female 7 days old, A with mature egg, follicle of D descended from germarium; AA—ovariole A immediately after ovulation, with follicular relic.

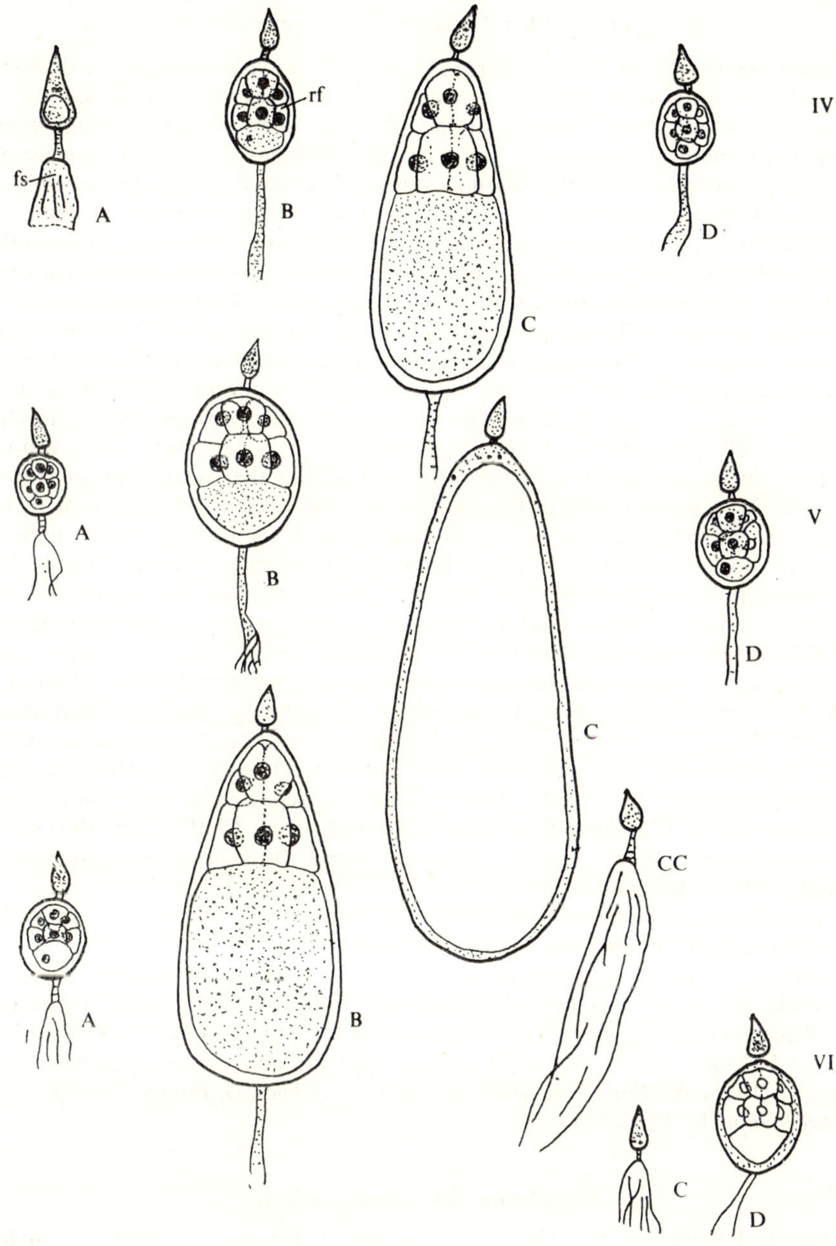

Fig. 14.2 (b)

IV, in a female 14 days old, largest follicle in C, A showing funicle stump from follicle 1 and first signs of follicle 2; V, in a female 20 days old, C with mature egg, A with fully developed follicle; CC—ovariole C 24 hours after ovulation, follicular relic passed out; VI, in a female 25 days old, largest follicle in B, funicle stumps on ovarioles A and C. (After Saunders, 1960b) *palpalis quanzensis*, and Challier (1964), with *G. palpalis gambiensis*, demonstrated the occasional existence of a small structure below, or at the side of, a newly-formed sac, recalling serial relics of mosquitoes. These structures were very rare in natural populations and Challier (1964) has shown that they are of abnormal occurrence. In the normal course of events the fully-developed egg breaks off the terminal part of the follicular tube during ovulation so that any follicular relic persisting from an earlier occasion is lost. Therefore, an ovariole in an old female shows only one relic even if it has produced more than one egg. Very occasionally, however, the mature egg is expelled through the *side* of the follicular tube so that the first or earlier relic is preserved. This is obviously too rare an event to be any assistance in the recognition of the older age groups.

The lack of any serial follicular relics constitutes a serious limitation of the ovarian method of age determination in its original form (Saunders, 1962). However, Challier (1965) extended and improved it by the simple observation that the ovarioles have a particular position within the ovary. For instance, ovariole A is internal to B in the right ovary, and ovariole C is internal to D in the left. Therefore, the sequence of ovulation involves not only an alternation of right and left ovaries, but also of internal and external ovarioles (Fig.14.4). By designating the four egg follicles, in order of size, by the numbers 1–4, nulliparous females were observed to show a configuration ('nombre repère') of 4213 when observed from the dorsal aspect. In this case the largest egg follicle (A) is in the internal position in the right ovary. After the first ovulation, follicle C (internal, left ovary) becomes the largest, and the 'nombre repère' becomes 3142; after two ovulations follicle B (external, right) is the largest, and the 'nombre repère' 2431; and after three ovulations D (external, left) the largest, and the 'nombre repère' 1324. The cycle is then repeated, females showing a configuration of 4213 after four ovulations, and so on. Challier was thus able to recognize eight age categories (0–7), to extend the method to include flies as old as 70–80 days and to obtain a more realistic age structure. However, categories 4–7 still contain a residue of older flies not differentiated by this method. For instance, all flies showing evidence of four ovulations and a 'nombre repère' of 4213 are either in classes 4, 8, 12, or 16, etc., and are designated 4 + 4n. Similarly, categories 5 to 7 are described as 5 + 4n to 7 + 4n. This method of age determination has been tested in a laboratory population of *G. tachinoides* by Itard (1966). It has also been used in wild populations of *G. palpalis* by Challier (1965) and Saunders (1967) and of *G. pallidipes*, *G. fuscipes* Newst. and *G. brevipalpis* by Harley (1966a).

Copulation and Insemination

Although females of *Glossina* may copulate twice (Nash, 1955) a single insemination is sufficient and is considered normal. In the field, females of *G. fuscipes* are inseminated as young tenerals before they emerge from the undergrowth whereas those of *G. pallidipes* are fertilized near the host whilst seeking their first bloodmeal (Saunders, 1962; Harley, 1966). This behaviour of *G. pallidipes* is probably typical of the *morsitans* group of species and probably explains the 'following swarm' of 'sexually-appetitive' males which

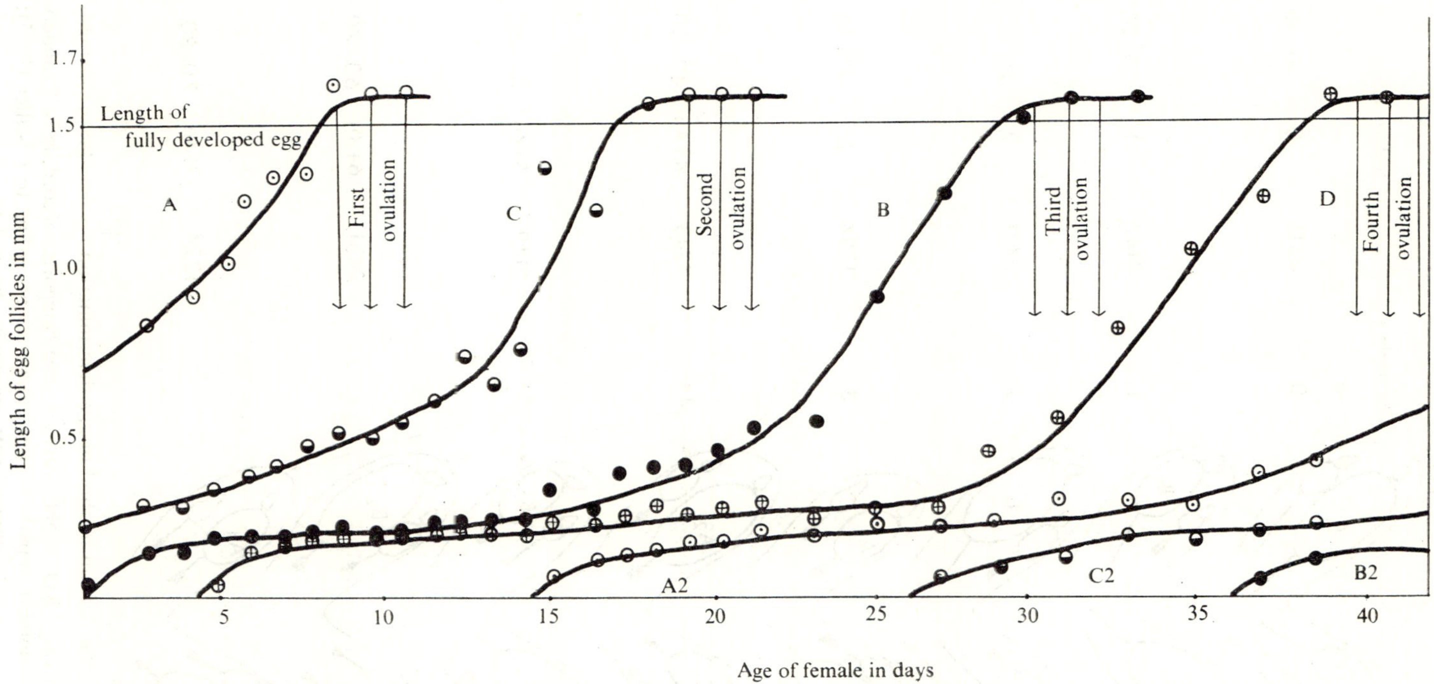

Fig. 14.3 The lengths of the egg follicles in *Glossina morsitans*, showing the sequence of egg development and ovulation at 26–27°C. A, B, C, D: first follicles in ovarioles A, B, C and D. A2, B2, C2: second follicles in ovarioles A, B and C. (From Saunders, 1960b)

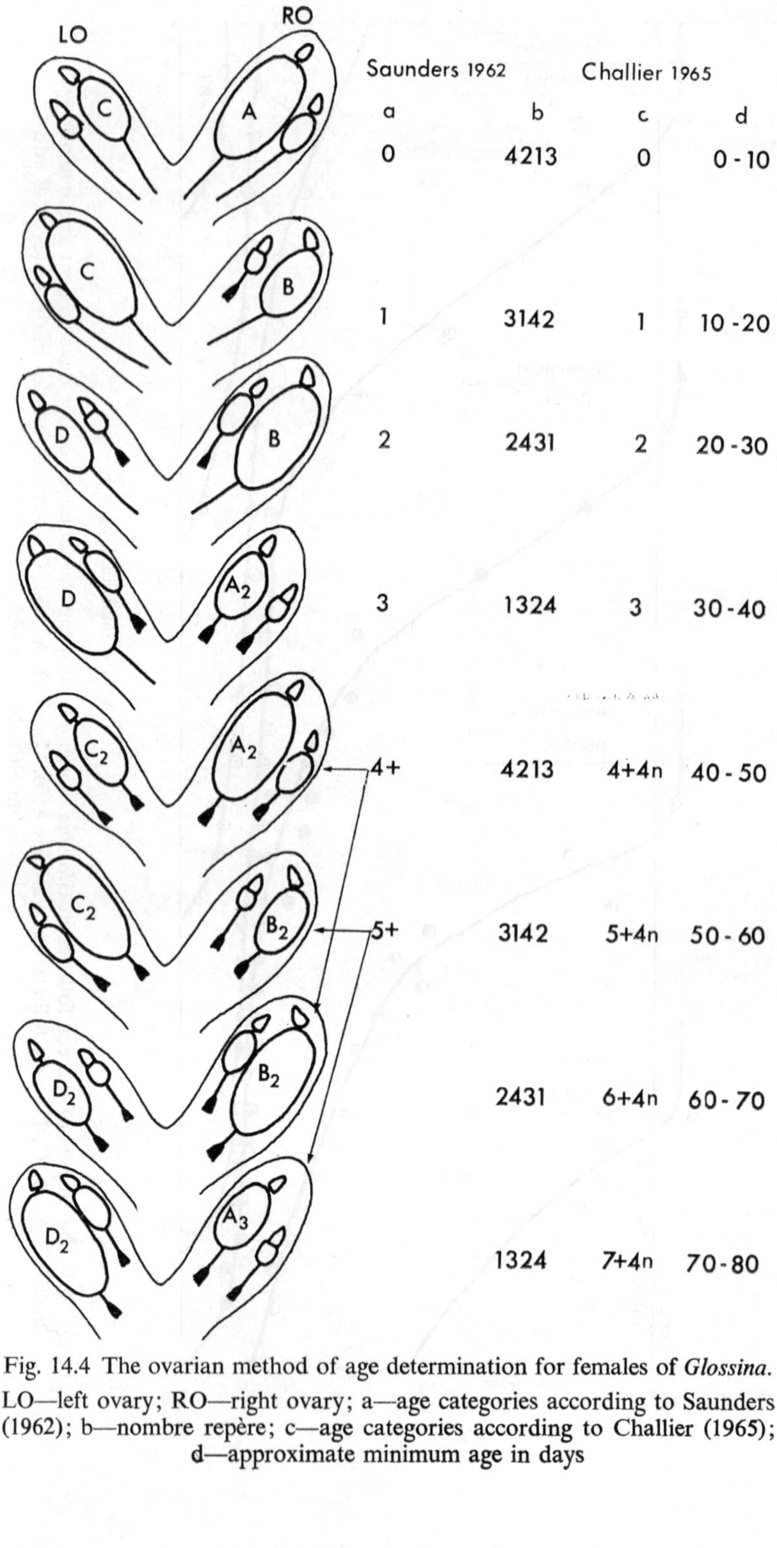

Fig. 14.4 The ovarian method of age determination for females of *Glossina*. LO—left ovary; RO—right ovary; a—age categories according to Saunders (1962); b—nombre repère; c—age categories according to Challier (1965); d—approximate minimum age in days

follow a host (Fiske, 1920; Swynnerton, 1936; Bursell, 1961a). Females of *G. palpalis* may show 'mating scars' after copulation (Squire, 1951a; Vattier, 1965).

In the laboratory it has been found that males are not fully potent until 4–7 days old and that more effective pairing is usually obtained with older (14 day-old) males and young (3–4 day-old) females. Working with *G. morsitans* Southon and Cockings (1963) showed that the male:female ratio as well as the age of the males was important. They found that a ratio of 2:1 with males aged 10–15 days gave fertilization rates of about 90%. Older non-virgin males are more potent than younger males, and pairing is very often more easily accomplished immediately after a blood meal has been taken by the female (Hoffmann, 1954).

Reproductive behaviour does not appear to be elaborate. When this is observed the male appears to seize the female, only to be brushed off if the female is unreceptive. Vanderplank (1948) refers to certain 'mating notes' which he claims are specific and essential if mating is to occur. These observations do not seem to have been re-examined.

Copulation usually lasts for 2 to 24 hours. Immediately after separation the sperm has filled the spermathecal ducts and partially filled the spermathecae (Hoffmann, 1954). Since only one insemination is necessary for the whole reproductive life of the female it follows that viability of the sperm is maintained in the spermathecae.

Intra-uterine Development

The ovulated egg of *Glossina* is about 1·5 mm. in length and is invested in a chorion with a characteristic reticulated pattern. It comes to lie in the uterus with the anterior or micropylar end near the point at which the ducts from the spermathecae enter the uterus. It is presumably at this time that fertilization occurs. The egg possesses sufficient yolk for the completion of embryonic development and this process, which seems to differ little from that in other Muscidae (Hagan, 1951; Hoffmann, 1954), is completed within 50–60 hours.

There are three larval instars. The first two and the greater part of the third occur in the uterus; the latter part of the third instar is spent in the ground. The mouth of the first-instar larva is provided with an 'egg tooth'[1] which serves to split the chorion at eclosion. The chorion is gripped and then removed by a special organ—the choriothete (Fig. 14.5)—lying in the uterine wall (Jackson, 1948b; Bursell & Jackson, 1957). The choriothete then re-attaches to the first larval cuticle and removes the exuvium when the larva moults to the second instar; it degenerates during the latter half of the gestation period, only to re-develop its full structure and function by the time the next egg descends from the ovary. The exuvium of the second-instar larva is not removed by the choriothete; it remains as a loose pellicle around the third-instar larva and is probably removed just prior to parturition, or during the act of birth, perhaps by the spines in the vagina. The empty chorion and larval exuvia are probably voided after the birth of the larva.

[1] Hoffmann (1954) was unable to find an 'egg tooth' in *G. palpalis*, although Itard (1966) observed one in *G. tachinoides*.

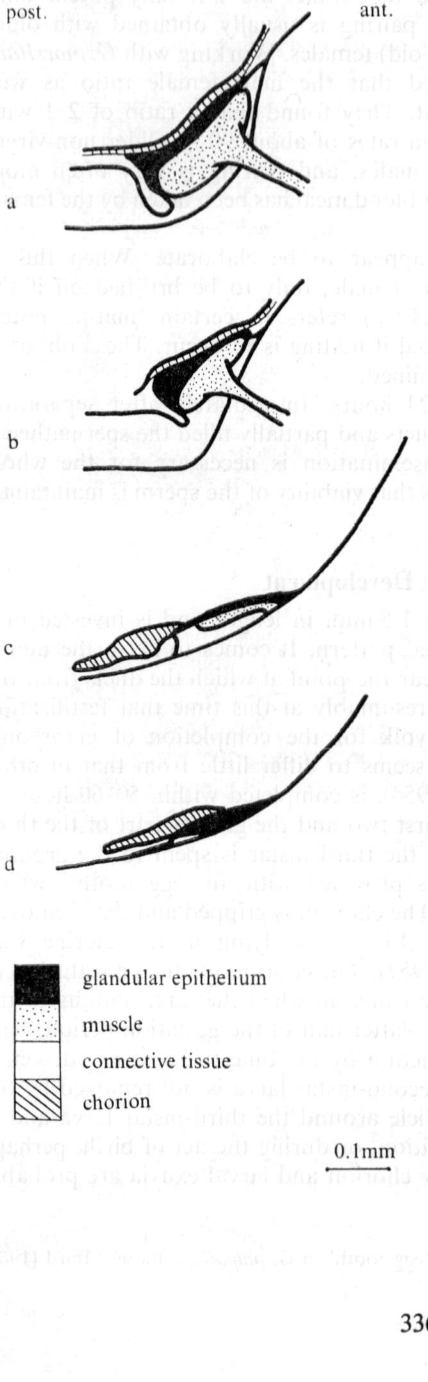

Fig. 14.5 Sagittal section of the anterior part of the uterus floor showing regressive changes of the choriothete during pregnancy. (a), (b), (c), (d)—2, 4, 6 and 9 days respectively after larviposition. The interlarval period at the time the sections were prepared was about 11 days. Horizontal shifts were determined with reference to the U-bend of spermathecal ducts above the dorsal wall of the uterus. (From Bursell & Jackson, 1957)

The larval instars have been described by a number of authors (Roubaud, 1909; Hagan, 1951; Hoffmann, 1954) and figured by Burtt and Jackson (1951). The first instar is of very short duration (Roubaud, 1909). The second shows the development of the respiratory lobes. Both first- and second-instar larvae have a cuticle clothed with short spines. The third-instar larva shows the full development of the polypneustic lobes and, anteriorly, an antenno-maxillary complex. The interpretation of the segmentation of the larva is discussed by Buxton (1955, pp. 372–3). The polypneustic lobes blacken about 1½ days before larviposition and in this condition may be seen through the body wall of the pregnant female.

The milk glands undergo a cycle of secretory activity during each gestation period so that, according to Hoffmann (1954), secretion of the 'milk' is confined to a sixty-hour period after the third day of development. Feeding commences in the first instar (Bursell & Jackson, 1957) and is practically completed in the second. Little food is taken by the third-instar larva and it is during this time that regression of the milk glands takes place. Roubaud (1909) was of the opinion that the larva attached itself by its mouth to a 'papilla' formed from the end of the milk gland ducts and assumed that the larva sucked from the papilla as from a 'teat.' However, Hoffmann (1954) and Bursell and Jackson (1957) pointed out that the 'papilla' is a transverse ridge on the dorsal wall of the uterus and that the mouth is too small to encompass this projection. For these reasons Bursell and Jackson (1957) make the much more reasonable suggestion that the 'milk' is poured freely into the uterus from which the larva sucks it up directly.

Although the pregnant uterus is well supplied with tracheae, respiration is accomplished in the larva, through the female genital opening, by means of the posterior spiracles. During the last third of intra-uterine life the larva develops a complex mechanism for the ventilation of the larval tracheal system through the polypneustic lobes. Bursell (1955) showed that the third-instar larva retains the second-instar exuvium as a thin pellicle until just before larviposition. This pellicle invests the polypneustic lobes and also lines the third-instar tracheal trunks, except for the posterior part where the second-instar spiracles open separately between the respiratory lobes (Fig. 14.7). Contraction of a respiratory muscle causes an intake of air through the supernumerary stigmata of the polypneustic lobes. This air is forced forwards between the second- and third-instar tracheae, backwards *within* the second-instar tracheae, and out *via* the second-instar spiracular openings. After larviposition, the second-instar pellicle is lost, so that respiration in the deposited larva is accomplished through the supernumerary stigmata of the respiratory lobes.

Reproductive Physiology and Reproductive Abnormalities

Of the many reproductive abnormalities described, abortion, egg retention in virgins and follicular degeneration seem to be the most frequent.

Examination of the literature reveals considerable disagreement on the subject of ovulation in virgin flies. For instance, some authors (Roubaud, 1909; Hoffmann, 1954) claimed that the first egg is never ovulated in virgins, others (Mellanby, 1937; Vanderplank, 1947; Saunders, 1960b) that the first egg may be retained for a time but that ovulation proceeds normally once that egg had

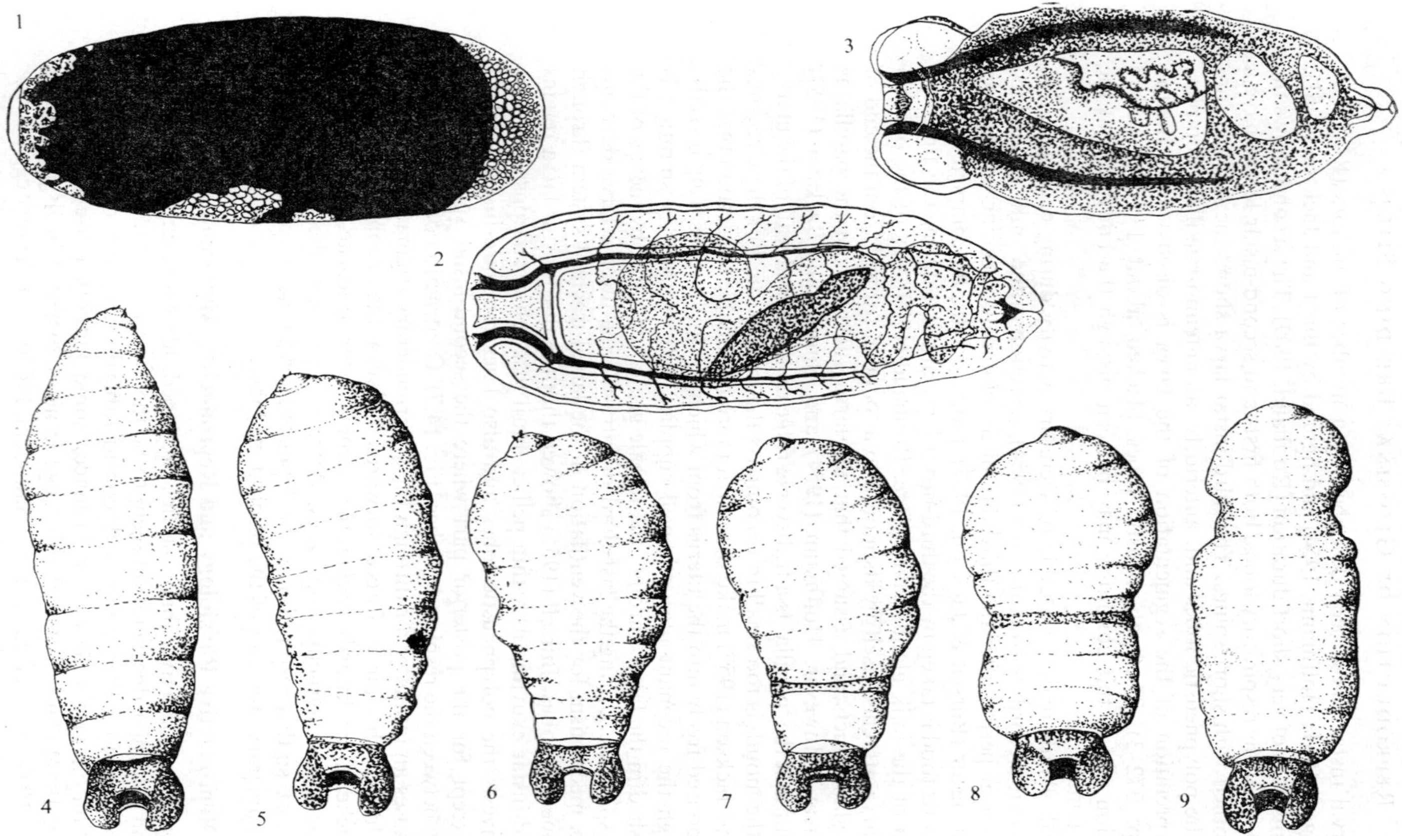

Fig. 14.6 (1) Egg viewed from dorsal aspect by transmitted light (×66). (2) First-instar larva from dorsal aspect (×66). Note tracheal trunks and branches, and egg-tooth in mouth. (3) Second-instar larva from dorsal aspect (×26). (4) Third-instar larva (×14), at 0 sec., completion of movement. (5) Third-instar larva (×14) at $\frac{1}{4}$ sec., retracting head. (6) Third-instar larva (×14), at $\frac{3}{8}$ sec., with respiratory lobes and hind end drawn forward, and lobes laid flat. (7) Third-instar larva (×14), at $\frac{1}{2}$ sec., with wave of contraction starting near hind end. (8) Third-instar larva (×14), at $\frac{3}{4}$ sec., with wave of contraction [illegible] (9) Third-instar larva (×14), at 1 sec., with wave of contraction nearly arrived at front end.

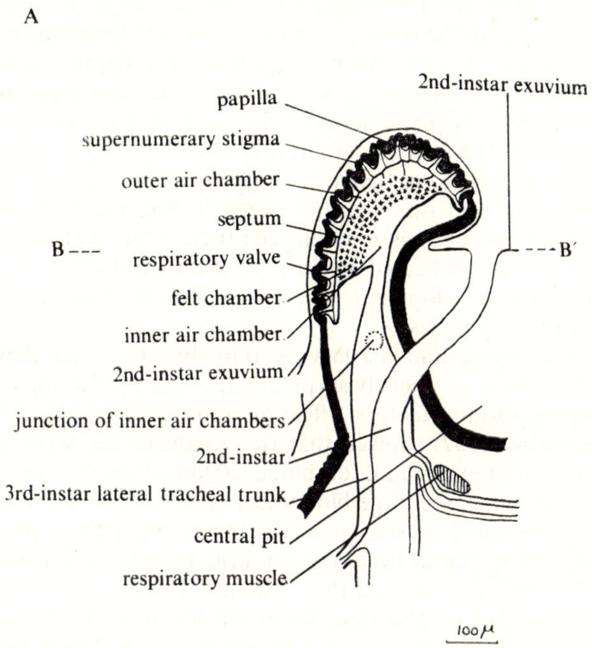

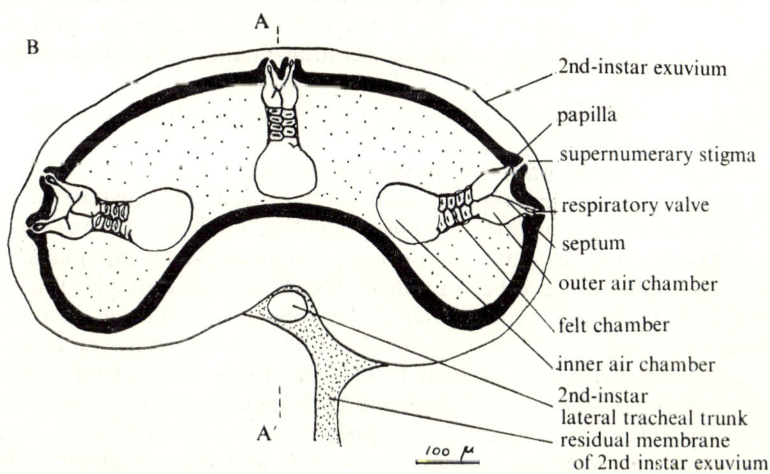

Fig. 14.7 Diagrams of sections of respiratory lobes of third-instar larva of *Glossina* before removal of second-instar exuvium. A. Longitudinal section; B—B^1, level of transverse section shown in B. B. Transverse section. A—A^1; level of longitudinal section shown in A. (From Bursell, 1955)

passed nto the uterus. Mellanby (1937) described females of *G. fuscipes* with severalifully developed eggs in the ovaries as well as several, in various stages of disintegration, in the uterus. On the other hand, Harley (1966a) found evidence of normal ovulation and abortion of infertile eggs in two specimens of *G. fuscipes* and one of *G. brevipalpis* in the field. Although retention of eggs in virgin females may be a problem in laboratory colonies, virgin females are very rare in natural populations, even at very low population densities (Teesdale, 1940). Provided that insemination occurs before the maturation of the first egg the reproductive cycle is not delayed; there is no evidence that, as in *Cimex*, egg *development* is affected by insemination (Mellanby, K., 1939; Davis, 1964); follicle A is developing at emergence and continues at the same rate in fertilized and virgin females.

Since both the adult female and the larva within the uterus are dependent upon the same source of food it is hardly surprising that the availability of blood is one of the most important factors affecting reproductive physiology in *Glossina*. Helen Mellanby (1937) showed that the weight of the larva at birth is closely correlated with the amount of blood obtained during pregnancy. Hoffmann (1954) found that three large bloodmeals were sufficient during each gestation period, the last being most beneficially taken about three days prior to parturition, i.e. before the larva becomes too large to prevent full extension of the crop. Mellanby (1937) also found that insufficient nutrition—interrupted or irregular bloodmeals—led to abortion, an event which is all too common in most laboratory colonies. Abortion may occur at any stage during the gestation period, from eggs to small third instar larvae which fail to pupate or which produce malformed and non-viable pupae. It is possible that abortion may be more frequent with females towards the end of reproductive life (Glasgow, 1963). Since fully-developed eggs lie in the ovaries until after parturition it is probable that abortion leads to an acceleration in the reproductive sequence (Saunders, 1960b).

In laboratory colonies very large larvae (50–70 mg.) which fail to be deposited, and which 'pupate' within the uterus, have been recorded (Hoffmann, 1954; Robinson, 1964; Nash, Jordan & Boyle, 1967b).

The various claims that reproduction is 'improved' by the type of blood taken (e.g. sheep blood superior to guinea-pig blood (Willett, 1953)) or pregnant hosts superior to non-pregnant hosts (Nash, Jordan & Boyle, 1966) have either not been confirmed or have been retracted (Nash, Jordan & Boyle, 1967a).

The ovarian cycle and the intra-uterine development of *Glossina* are temperature-dependent processes. The inter-larval period may vary between eight days at 30°C to about twenty-five days at 18°C (Jack, 1939). Under field conditions the inter-larval period of *G. pallidipes* and *G. brevipalpis* is about ten to eleven days (Harley, 1966a). In *G. fuscipes* complications in ovarian function seem to appear at constant temperatures of about 29°C and over (Mellanby, 1937), females being effectively sterilized and the ovaries contained 'no visible ova'. Similar abnormalities were observed by Potts (1958) in flies from irradiated pupae. Saunders (1960b) observed that females of *G. morsitans* maintained at 26°C sometimes developed ovaries of abnormal appearance; on dissection, follicles in various stages of degeneration (Fig. 14.8) were revealed which may

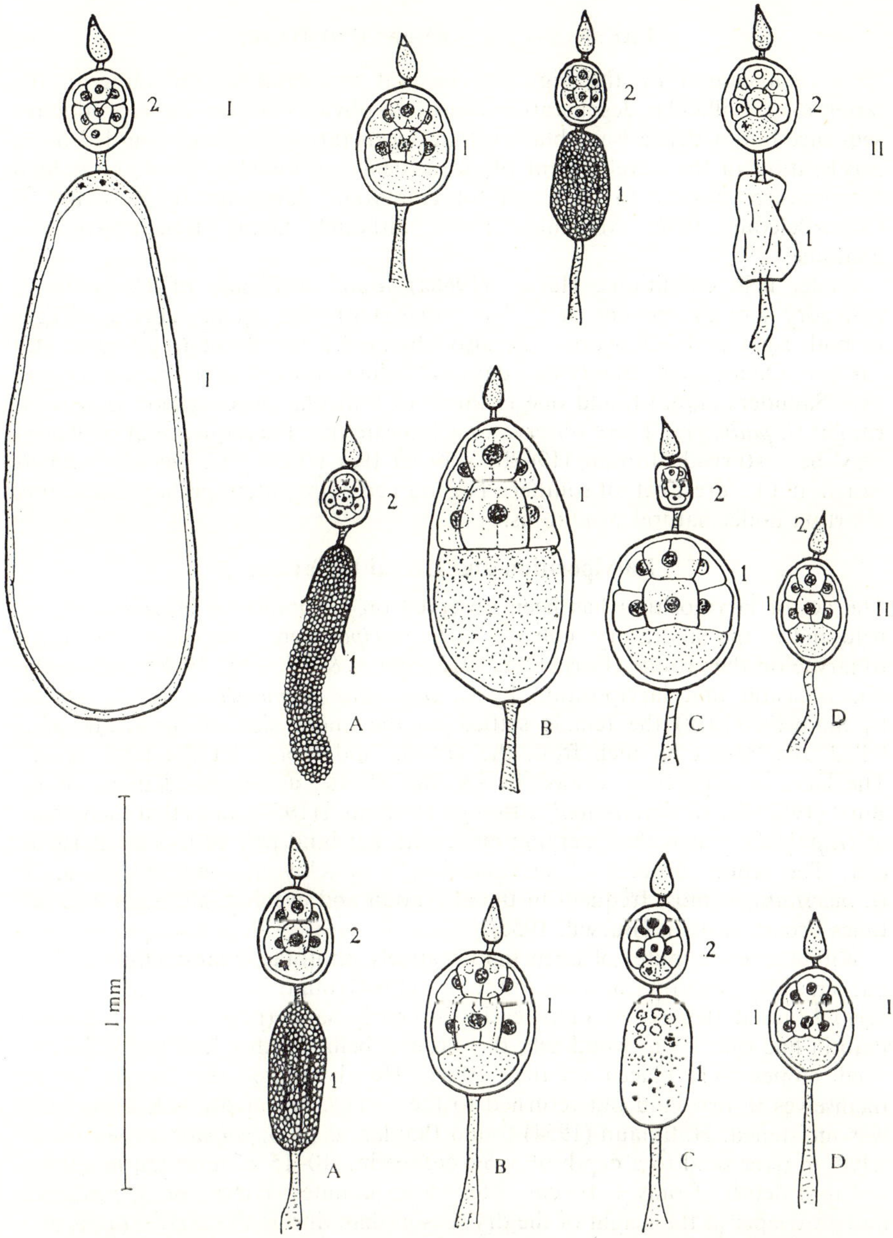

Fig. 14.8 Abnormalities in the ovarioles of *Glossina morsitans*. I, ovariole in virgin female, showing retention of mature egg (1) and development of second follicle (2); II, stages in degeneration of egg follicle; III, ovarioles of a fertilized female 15 days old, with first follicles in ovarioles A and C degenerated, showing accelerated development of the other follicles (degenerated follicle in A is broken); IV, ovarioles of a female 18 days old, showing follicular degeneration. (N.B. The pairs of ovarioles A, B are those of the right ovary and C, D those of the left ovary.) (From Saunders, 1960b)

have been caused by the high or constant temperatures obtaining in the laboratory. Follicular degeneration causes an obvious gap in the reproductive sequence but evidence was obtained that degeneration, like abortion, led to an acceleration in the development of subsequent egg follicles. Continuous high temperatures appear to be lethal for embryonic development (Roubaud & Colas-Belcour, 1936; Mellanby, 1937), although larval development can continue.

Under field conditions, Harley (1966a) found a female of *G. pallidipes* (category 4 or 5) and one of *G. brevipalpis* (Ob) with equally developed eggs in both right and left ovaries; he also observed a female of *G. fuscipes*, still category Oa although twenty-two days old, which showed no visible developing ova. Saunders (1962) found one example of follicular degeneration in a wild-caught *G. pallidipes*. These observations indicate that the sequence of ovulation may be disturbed. Jordan (1962b) showed that 60% of *G. palpalis palpalis* caught in the forest belt of southern Nigeria had empty uteri, perhaps indicating abortion under natural conditions.

Larviposition and Larval Behaviour

The act of larviposition has been observed on a number of occasions in the field and in the laboratory. Females of *G. fuscipes* were observed to give birth to larvae on the ground (Carpenter, 1912; Symes & Southby, 1938), and on the one occasion that larviposition by *G. morsitans submorsitans* was observed by Simpson (1918) the female settled on the under side of the trunk of a felled tree 'about an inch from the ground and thence let the larva drop'. The larva is apparently voided by its own efforts, as described in detail by Burtt (1952) for *G. swynnertoni*, although Hoffmann (1954) states that the female of *G. palpalis* grasps the emerging larva with her hind pair of legs to assist its exit. The whole process of larviposition is quickly accomplished and, in *G. morsitans*, is most frequent in the afternoon and evening, although it sometimes occurs at night (Bursell, 1958).

Within a few minutes of birth the negatively phototactic larva (Burtt, 1952; Parker, 1956a) burrows into the soil. Lewis (1934) found that larvae of *G. swynnertoni* buried themselves more easily in coarse sand (particle size 1–2 mm.) than in fine sand or in wood ash, this process being further facilitated if a few small stones were placed on the surface. He also noted that larvae buried themselves in dry sand but returned to the surface repeatedly unless the sand was moistened. Hoffmann (1954) found that larvae of *G. palpalis* buried themselves in river sand to a depth of 3–5·5 cm. within 10–15 minutes but in garden soil to a depth of only 1–1·5 cm. after 15–25 minutes. Larvae of *G. pallidipes* burrow deeper at the height of the dry season than during the early months and Bursell (1960a) showed that deeper burrowing was induced by high temperature, possibly accentuated by lower humidity. In a recent study of *G. morsitans orientalis*, Finlayson (1967) showed that larvae 'preferred' moist to dry air but showed no response to gravity. He also found that the length of time between birth and puparium-formation varied and was under nervous control. For instance, this interval was longer the earlier in the day that birth occurred, was greater in light than in dark, and least in those larvae which burrowed into sand in the dark. Suspension of larvae by a thread attached to the polypneustic lobes, however, resulted in a rapid puparium-formation. Finlayson (1967) attributes this to the mechanical stimulation received during the operation by handling, but Langley (1967a) considers that pupation begins early because tactile sensory inflow has ceased. Most authors agree that if a suitable material is not available, or if conditions are 'unfavourable', the larva is unable to burrow and puparium-formation may be delayed.

Pupation and Metamorphosis

Once the larva has buried itself in the ground the processes leading up to pupation begin. As in all other Cyclorrhapha the third-instar larva rounds up and the integument hardens and darkens (to a deep brown or black in *Glossina*) to form the puparium. This process is apparently completed in about 90–100 minutes in *G. palpalis* (Hoffmann, 1954). The insect then retracts itself from the inside of the puparium; this represents the larval-pupal apolysis (Jenkin & Hinton, 1966) and results in a cryptocephalic pupa, a stage which lasts from the second to the fourth day after puparium-formation (Bursell, 1958). At this time the insect still respires through the polypneustic lobes but the block between the mid- and hindgut is broken down so that the larval gut is emptied.

Five days or so after puparium-formation the head and thoracic appendages are everted to form the true or phanerocephalic pupa. The thin pellicle around the pupa at this stage is the inner endocuticle of the third larval integument and does not represent the cuticle of a transient fourth instar larva (Whitten, 1957; Hinton, 1968). Respiration is now accomplished by thoracic pupal spiracles (*see* Bursell, 1958) but air must enter the puparial space presumably through the polypneustic lobes rather than through the puparium itself. Neither the course of metamorphosis, nor the endocrine mechanisms controlling it, have been studied in detail. However, Langley (1967c) has shown that ligation of the larva behind the brain at any time after birth leads to an unexpected result, namely the hardening and darkening of the posterior part of the larva, whilst the anterior end remains larviform. This result is the opposite to that obtained in similar experiments with larvae of *Calliphora* or *Musca* ligatured before the 'critical period', and is explained on the grounds that sufficient ecdysone is present in the haemolymph at birth, but the central nervous system inhibits puparium-formation whilst the surface sense organs are stimulated. This result, therefore, agrees well with the observations on delayed puparium-formation by Finlayson (1967) described above. The alternative explanation that ecdysone is produced in the posterior part of the body is thought to be unlikely in view of the fact that the internal anatomy of the *Glossina* larva is similar to that of other Muscidae (Langley, 1967).

During the next twenty-one days of intra-puparial development the cuticle becomes pigmented; this is seen first in the compound eyes which change from yellow to reddish-brown, then in the bristles and finally in the general integument. These changes in pigmentation have been used as a basis for determining the age of tsetse pupae by dissection (Potts, 1933; Bursell, 1959). About two days before the fly emerges from the puparium, the pupal integument is loosened so that it appears dry and adheres to the inside of the puparium rather than to the adult cuticle. The entire period of pigmentation occurs after the pupal-adult apolysis (Hinton, 1968) and the insect at this stage is referred to most properly as the pharate adult.

The account given above makes it clear that the true pupal stage only occupies a short period of intra-puparial life; the first day is the quiescent phase of the third-instar larva and the last sixteen or so the development of the pharate adult. In consequence much confusion in terminology has arisen.[1]

Eclosion in *Glossina* is similar to that in other Cyclorrhapha, the young adult escaping from the puparium and then 'digging up' through the soil by means of the ptilinum. The newly-emerged fly is known as a 'teneral' and is still regarded as immature. The classical signs of a teneral fly are the soft feel of the thorax, the eversibility of the ptilinum and the white appearance of the abdomen when the fly is held up to the light (Glasgow, 1963). After the first bloodmeal the flight muscles begin to develop further and the thorax assumes a more rigid structure (Bursell, 1961b; Glasgow & Glasgow, 1962). This process continues over several bloodmeals but the teneral state is usually considered by tsetse workers to have ended with the first. It is therefore considered desirable to follow Bursell's suggestion and confine the term 'teneral' to flies that have not fed since emergence and to use the term 'immature' for flies that have fed but are still in the process of completing their post-teneral muscular development, thus freeing the terms 'young' and 'old' for use in regard to mature flies, according to the development of the reproductive organs, wing fray and other characteristics of age. If this muscular growth is regarded as a process which completes post-embryonic development, it can also be regarded as an adaptation to the viviparous method of reproduction (Bursell, 1961b). For instance, the development of the thoracic muscles may be a necessary prerequisite for the provision of sufficient power to carry the load of a fully-developed larva when the female is pregnant and, on the other hand, the lightened thorax of the teneral fly helps to keep the final weight of the larva down to a minimum since the final stages of growth are delayed until after eclosion.

Breeding Sites

The methods for collecting puparia outlined elsewhere (Chapter 17) require a knowledge of breeding sites and these are described below for the various groups of tsetse flies.

With the exception of *Glossina longipennis*, tsetse of the *fusca* group are tropical forest dwellers and so live in an environment which is relatively uniform in terms of climate. One would expect puparia to be widely scattered under such circumstances and this may account for the lack of breeding site records for most members of this group. Swynnerton (1936) recorded puparia of *Glossina brevipalpis* Newst. from humus beneath dense thickets, especially if there was low cover near the ground such as that given by lianes; Lamborn (1915a) found a similar pattern. In cases where *G. brevipalpis* is found outside its normal forest habitat, puparia are deposited in the same places as are those

[1] *See* footnote on p. 358.

of the prevailing species of tsetse fly. In deciduous woodland inhabited by *Glossina morsitans*, *G. brevipalpis* puparia were found together with those of *G. morsitans* under a fallen log (Lamborn, 1915a). Lewis (1939) found puparia of *Glossina fuscipleuris* in the same type of situation as those of *G. brevipalpis* in riverine forest or thickets, usually dense, not far from the forest. Puparia of *G. longipennis* which inhabits extremely dry country, have been found under logs and in the shade of a single tree, in open country, with larger numbers being found under logs in rather thicker vegetation (Lewis, 1942). No puparia were found in thick riverine bush which might have been expected to offer the most sheltered sites.

Tsetse of the *palpalis* group occur in a wider range of habitats than do those of the *fusca* group, but in general they may be considered as flies of the forests fringing large rivers and lakes. Several detailed studies have been made of puparial sites used by *Glossina palpalis* and its various forms and on those of *Glossina tachinoides*. A thorough investigation of the breeding sites of *G. palpalis* was made by Carpenter (1920) working on the shores of Lake Victoria and this together with a detailed study by Fiske (1920), provides a great deal of useful information. Dry sandy beaches shaded by dense vegetation provided the major breeding sites. Puparia were almost always found at ground level and it was observed that the larvae were deposited by females resting on the ground (Carpenter, 1912; *see* also p. 342). Fine vegetable matter under rock overhangs or the surface of well drained coarse sand provided a second category of breeding site. Such sites were sheltered by ferns beneath the forest canopy and Carpenter (1919) referred to them as 'loci' to distinguish them from the major 'sandy beach' type of breeding site.

In West Africa, workers on *G. palpalis* have emphasized the need for shade immediately above the puparial site and have found a high forest canopy alone to be inadequate (Nash, 1948a). The oil palm in West Africa has a growth form in which the old leaf bases hang down the trunk of the tree and reach the ground; the sheltered area formed round the trunk at ground level yields many puparia. Breeding in rot holes in trees, the holes being usually at ground level, has also been recorded.

The dry sandy beach site is, of course, available only in dry weather; in the wet weather puparia are scattered in 'loci' throughout the environment and are very difficult to find. Where *G. palpalis* occurs in true tropical forest it is difficult to find significant numbers of puparia at all seasons since, in the absence of climatic stress, the distribution of the fly is not restricted.

The only other member of the *palpalis* group on which an appreciable amount of work has been done is *G. tachinoides*. It was shown by Johnson and Lloyd (1923) that many puparia were deposited in sandy areas devoid of cover immediately above the puparia but shaded by a high canopy formed by large trees. Fallen trees and low shrubs yielded puparia in smaller numbers but Nash (1939) found these sites to be favoured in the rains when sand sites were largely unavailable. A small artificial puparial site consisting of dry sand under a low thatched roof was constructed by Johnson and Lloyd (1923) and yielded small numbers of puparia in the wet season, indicating that if dry sand were available it would still be used by *G. tachinoides* in wet weather.

The *morsitans* group of tsetse flies has been more fully investigated as regards sites for puparial deposition than either of the other groups mentioned above. Members of this group inhabit deciduous woodland and thicket and, in the dry season, puparia of some species can be collected in large numbers from what have come to be known as classical sites. In wet weather puparia are much more difficult to find and a number of workers have sought the wet season breeding sites without ever finding great numbers of puparia.

When dealing with the *morsitans* group it is particularly necessary to distinguish between a breeding *site* in the sense that it has been used above (the spot at which puparia are found) and the zones within which puparia are found in breeding sites which some workers term 'breeding areas'. Flies living in deciduous woodland tend to show seasonal fluctuation in population density in different parts of the woodland. In the wet season when the woodland is in full leaf they tend to be dispersed throughout the woodland thus approximating to the dispersal pattern of flies of the *fusca* group in forests. In dry weather, when the majority of trees are leafless, the flies tend to be rather more localized, although they are not as rigidly restricted to local patches of favourable environment as was at one time believed (Pilson & Pilson, 1967). The tendency to become localized results in large numbers of puparia being deposited in a relatively small area and it is this phenomenon that has lead some workers to define breeding areas on the basis of vegetation patterns. Actual breeding sites are likely to be present over the entire environment and it is the distribution of adult flies which determines the areas in which puparia are found.

The first discovery of puparia of *Glossina swynnertoni* was made by Swynnerton (1923) who recorded puparia under fallen logs, under rocks and under leaning trees. These breeding sites were generally in thickets, but overhead canopy was not essential and fallen logs in the open also yielded puparia. A study made by Lloyd (1935) gave similar results but he found puparia of *G. swynnertoni* more difficult to locate in terms of puparia per man hour than those of *Glossina morsitans*. It was not until Burtt (1952) investigated the breeding sites of *G. swynnertoni* that their wet season breeding sites were recorded. Puparia were found under fallen logs but the larvae had not entered the soil and puparia were found on top of flakes of bark and on top of leaves. Burtt also found that the sites in which puparia could be discovered were restricted to certain vegetation patterns, even in the wet season. The difficulty in locating the puparia in wet soil was shown to be very great but, after a short dry spell, many more were recovered.

Puparia of *Glossina pallidipes* have been found in a wide variety of environments within the considerable geographic range of this insect. In Zululand, puparia were found under leaf litter in thickets (Swynnerton, 1936; Du Toit, 1954). In East Africa, puparia of *G. pallidipes* were found in the same sort of breeding sites as *G. swynnertoni* in the dry season (Swynnerton, 1936), except that rot-holes in trees were apparently neglected by *G. pallidipes*. Swynnerton (1921) recorded puparia of *G. pallidipes* from the same 'fallen log' sites from which *G. morsitans* puparia were recovered in Mozambique. Recent work in Rhodesia (Phelps, *in preparation*) has shown that *G. pallidipes* uses the sand in river beds in the cool dry season and animal burrows in the hot dry season, in the same way as does *G. morsitans*. Wet season collection of *G. pallidipes* puparia have rarely been made but some have been found under fallen logs in thickets (Phelps, unpublished).

One of the earlier records of a breeding site of *G. morsitans* was that made by Jack (1912) who found a puparium at the base of a fig tree in Rhodesia. Jack and many subsequent workers have recorded puparia of *G. morsitans* under fallen logs, under decumbent trees, under overhanging rocks, and in rot-holes in trees (*see*, for example, Lloyd, 1914; Chorley, 1929a; Nash, 1933; Jackson, 1937; Harley, 1954; Jewell, 1958a; and Glasgow, 1961b). Some workers have recorded small numbers of puparia from animal burrows, generally holes dug by antbears (Lloyd, 1914; Chorley, 1929). Recent work in Rhodesia has shown that animal burrows provide major breeding sites in the hot dry season (Phelps, *in preparation*) and that the sandy beds of rivers are very favourable breeding sites in the cool dry season; the latter observation confirms that of Chorley (1929) and indicates a close resemblance to the sand breeding sites used by *G. tachinoides*. Sites under fallen logs, under overhanging rocks and under decumbent trees were regarded as obvious breeding places by Jackson (1952) who states that *G. morsitans* puparia can be found at all seasons in such sites and that similar sites are used by *Glossina austeni*. In wet weather the numbers of puparia found per searching hour falls off greatly in comparison to the yields in dry weather but Jackson's statement is certainly correct.

Very little is known of the breeding sites of *Glossina longipalpis*, a member of the *morsitans* group. Morris (1934) recorded puparia of this species from the bases of oil palms, the same site as is used by *G. palpalis*. Page (1959) found pupae of *G. longipalpis*, along with those of *G. palpalis*, *G. fusca* and *G. medicorum*, under logs, the pupae being readily found in the dry but not in the wet season; this is not in agreement with the statement of Morris (1934—on the authority of Pomeroy) that no breeding takes place in the dry season (*see* Buxton, 1955, p. 345).

Chapter 15

The *Glossina* Community

J. P. GLASGOW

RELATION TO ENVIRONMENT

The genus *Glossina* is confined to the African continent, including inshore islands such as Zanzibar and Fernando Po but excluding Madagascar and Pemba. There is a record of four extinct species from Colorado which have been variously ascribed to the Miocene or Oligocene periods (*see* p. 284) but so far as is known the genus is now extinct in the Americas. *G. tachinoides* was recorded from Southern Arabia by Carter (1906) but its presence there has not since been confirmed. The distribution of the species of the genus *Glossina* has been described elsewhere (*see* Chapter 10, Maps 10.1–10.7). Restriction of *Glossina* to Africa must be for palaeogeographical reasons (*see* also Chapter 10) for there can be little doubt that many species would find suitable conditions in other tropical regions. Within Africa, the distribution of some species clearly has a palaeogeographical basis—for example, the *palpalis* group is absent from land draining into the Indian Ocean and *G. austeni* is confined to that drainage—but the distribution of the whole genus has an edaphic basis. The northern limit is about 15°N, the southern limit about 29°S. The northern limit is the Sahara; the southern limit is the Kalahari in the west, but unlike the Sahara the Kalahari does not extend across the whole continent. On the non-desert east coast several species of tsetse extend (or did extend until recently) the range of the genus south until stopped by the end of sub-tropical conditions. In addition there are altitude limits; at the equator, areas more than 6,000 feet above sea level are free of tsetse but this limit decreases as the latitude increases. Before considering just what it is that stops the tsetse at the limits of its distribution it will be well to review what is known of the relations of the genus with its environment. This is such a large concept that one must break it down; the divisions used here are:

Physical (i.e. temperature, moisture, light; measured with instruments associated with physics).
Vegetational
Animal

Although these divisions are convenient for assembling the available information and for detecting gaps in our knowledge, they are interdependent. Thus the vegetation in any area is conditioned by temperature, moisture and light and by the herbivorous animals present; the tsetse whose environment is under consideration is itself part of the environment of these herbivores.

Physical Influences

Tsetse and Temperature

Tsetse seem to do best at temperatures near to 25°C. Departures from this favourable temperature have progressively deleterious effects, culminating in rapid death at 46°C and at sub-zero temperatures. Table 15.1 gives details of effects described by various authors on adults and puparia, observations of temperature effects on larvae being too few to be worth noticing. The third column of Table 15.1 gives the species used by each observer. There have been very few critical inter-specific comparisons, so that some of the apparent differences between species discernible in Table 15.1 may be unreal. At the same time it is not surprising that *G. morsitans orientalis*, investigated in Southern Rhodesia with its marked contrast between summer and winter, should tolerate wider temperature changes than *G. fuscipes fuscipes* investigated at Entebbe, a station with a notably equable climate on Lake Victoria and near the equator.

TABLE 15.1

(from Glasgow, 1963, with additions)

Centigrade	Stage	Species	Effect	Authority
46	Adult	*morsitans orientalis*	Killed by 5 minutes exposure	Jack, 1939
45	Adult	*morsitans morsitans*	Internal temperature 1·66° less than ambient	Edney and Barrass, 1962
44	Adult	*morsitans submorsitans*	Killed by 1 hour's exposure	Buxton and Lewis, 1934
44	Adult	*tachinoides*	Killed by 1 hour's exposure	Buxton and Lewis, 1934
43	Adult	*fuscipes fuscipes*	Killed by 1 hour's exposure	Mellanby, 1936
42				
41	Adult	*morsitans submorsitans*	All die if this maximum temperature attained	Nash, 1936
40	Adult	*morsitans morsitans*	Killed by 1 hour's exposure	Potts, 1933
40	Puparia	*morsitans morsitans*	Killed by 24 hours' exposure, but not by 8 hours	Potts, 1933
40	Adult	*morsitans orientalis*	Killed by 3 hours' exposure	Jack, 1939
40	Adult	*fuscipes fuscipes*	Killed by 3 hours' exposure, but not by 1 hour	Mellanby, 1936
39	Adult	*morsitans morsitans*	Thoracic spiracles open, cooling effect begins	Edney and Barrass, 1962
39	Adult	*morsitans submorsitans*	'Critical zone,' i.e. heavy mortality if this maximum temperature attained	Nash, 1936
38	Adult	*fuscipes martinii*, *morsitans morsitans* *brevipalpis*	Probing response elicited	Dethier, 1954
37				
36				
35	Puparia	*morsitans morsitans*	Cannot complete development if kept at this temperature	Potts, 1933
34				
33				
32	Adult	*morsitans orientalis*	Respiratory rate 5 times that at 16°	Rajagopal and Bursell, 1966
32	Puparia	*morsitans morsitans*	Approximate upper limit for successful completion of development	Bursell, 1960b, Rajagopal and Bursell, 1965
32	Adult	*pallidipes*	Becomes negatively phototactic at about this temperature	Vanderplank, 1948, Pilson and Leggate, 1962a
31				
30	Adult	*morsitans orientalis*	Becomes negatively phototactic at about this temperature	Jack and Williams, 1937 Pilson and Pilson, 1967
30	Puparia	*morsitans morsitans*	Mortality doubled (to 26%)	Potts, 1933
30	Puparia	*morsitans morsitans*	Adults from puparia incubated at this constant temperature infect more easily than those from puparia incubated at drying temperatures 2°–8° less	Burtt, 1946 and 1947
30	Puparia	*pallidipes*	Puparia incubated at this temperature produce pale adults	Bursell, 1960a
29	Adult	*fuscipes fuscipes*	Sterilized	Mellanby, 1937
29	Puparia	*palpalis*	Puparia incubated at this temperature produce pale adults	Roubaud, 1909
29	Puparia	*swynnertoni*	Puparia incubated at this temperature produce adults mostly with abnormal venation	Glasgow, 1960
28				

TABLE 15.1 (*continued*)

(from Glasgow, 1963, with additions)

Centigrade	Stage	Species	Effect	Authority
27	Puparia	*morsitans morsitans*	Puparia incubated at this and higher temperatures produce smaller but not lighter adults	Bursell, 1960
26		*morsitans*	Temperature chosen for laboratory colony	Azevedo and Pinhão, 1964
25·5		*austeni*	Temperature chosen for laboratory colony	Nash *et al.*, 1968
24, 23, 22 (bracketed)	Puparia	*morsitans morsitans*	Puparia incubated within this optimum range produce adults with maximum fat reserves at emergence	Bursell, 1960b
21	Adult	*fuscipes fuscipes*	Lowest limit of spontaneous flight, food-seeking and copulation	Mellanby, 1936
20				
19	Puparia	*morsitans morsitans*	Puparia incubated at this and lower temperatures produce smaller but not lighter adults	Bursell, 1960
18	Adult	*morsitans orientalis*	Normal, will copulate and breed, but feeds less often	Jack, 1939
17	Adult	*morsitans orientalis*	Can fly and feed	Jack, 1939
17	Adult	*morsitans morsitans*	Approximate lower limit for successful completion of development	Bursell, 1960b
16				
15	Adult	*morsitans orientalis*	Can crawl	Jack, 1939
14	Puparia	*pallidipes*	Approximate lower limit for successful completion of development	Bursell, 1960b, Rajagopal & Bursell, 1965
14	Adult	*fuscipes fuscipes*	Lower limit of flying when stimulated	Mellanby, 1936
14	Adult	*morsitans orientalis*	Able to crawl but somewhat ataxic	Jack, 1939
13				
12				
11	Adult	*morsitans orientalis*	Can move limbs but not crawl	Jack, 1939
10	Adult	*morsitans orientalis*	Almost immobilized	Jack, 1939
10	Adult	*fuscipes fuscipes*	Limit of crawling	Mellanby, 1936
8	Adult	*fuscipes fuscipes*	Immobilized, but recovers rapidly on warming	Mellanby, 1936
7				
6				
5				
4	Puparia	*morsitans morsitans*	Postulated real development threshold	Bursell, 1960b
3				
2				
1				
0				
−1				
−2				
−3				
−4	Adult	*morsitans orientalis*	Killed by 6 hours' exposure	Jack, 1939
−5	Adult	*morsitans orientalis*	Killed by 3 hours' exposure	Jack, 1939
−6				
−7				
−8	Puparia	*morsitans orientalis*	Some survived 3 hours' exposure	Jack, 1939
−9	Adult	*morsitans orientalis*	Killed by 45 minutes' exposure	Jack, 1939
−10	Puparia	*morsitans orientalis*	Killed by 3 hours' exposure	Jack, 1939

The reproduction of tsetse is affected by temperature in three ways—on it depend:

(a) the period from larviposition until the emergence of a new adult, loosely called the 'pupal period,' more properly the 'puparial period',
(b) the period from the emergence of a female until the first larviposition,
(c) the interval between successive larvipositions.

In Glasgow (1963, p. 40) the following formulae, based on those in the anonymous *Notes for field studies of tsetse flies in East Africa* (EATRO, 1955), are given for these three at a constant temperature t.

$$\text{Pupal period in days} = \frac{1}{0{\cdot}0323 + 0{\cdot}0028\,(t - 24)}$$

$$\text{First larva born on day} = \frac{1}{0{\cdot}0661 + 0{\cdot}0035\,(t - 24)}$$

$$\text{Inter-larval period} = \frac{1}{0{\cdot}0859 + 0{\cdot}0069\,(t - 24)}$$

From these formulae the curves of Fig. 15.1 have been drawn. The formulae have not been seriously challenged, although Saunders (1962) found a small specific difference between *G. fuscipes fuscipes* and *G. morsitans morsitans* in respect of the inter-larval period which is less in *G.f. fuscipes*.

According to these formulae, the time from deposition of a female larva until that individual can herself produce her second larva is eighty-three days at 20°C, thirty-nine days at 30°C. But the quality of the offspring as well as the speed of production is affected by temperature. Since larvae do not feed after birth, they must be born with an energy reserve sufficient to complete their development and to maintain the emergent adult until it finds its first meal. This energy reserve is in the form of fat and Bursell (1960b) found that puparia of *G.m. morsitans* incubated within the range 22°–24°C produced emergent adults with maximum fat reserves. Both higher and lower incubation temperatures produced emergent adults with progressively less reserve fat, until below 17°C and above 32°C emergence did not occur because the fat reserve was exhausted first. Using a different technique Rajagopal and Bursell (1965) repeated this work and concluded that the limits for successful completion of development are rather wider than those just stated. The general picture however is undisturbed.

Other entries in Table 15.1 record that incubation of puparia at temperatures different from the optimum has been shown to produce, in various species, smaller adults, paler adults, adults with abnormal venation, adults more liable to infection with trypanosomes. All this work has been done at constant temperatures—the effects of exposing the puparial stages for short periods to temperatures such as 40°C or 10°C, which are not lethal, but do not, if maintained throughout puparial life, permit successful completion of development, have not been explored. The work of Goldschmidt (1938) with *Drosophila* suggests that such experiments might be rewarding. None of these phenotypical variations has been shown to have adaptive significance, but of course this does not mean that they are useless to the tsetse. A demonstration that any of them increases the viability of their possessors would be so difficult that it is not surprising that no one has attempted it.

The temperatures recorded as lethal at the top of Table 15.1 were all determined before 1940 and perhaps require further examination, for Edney and

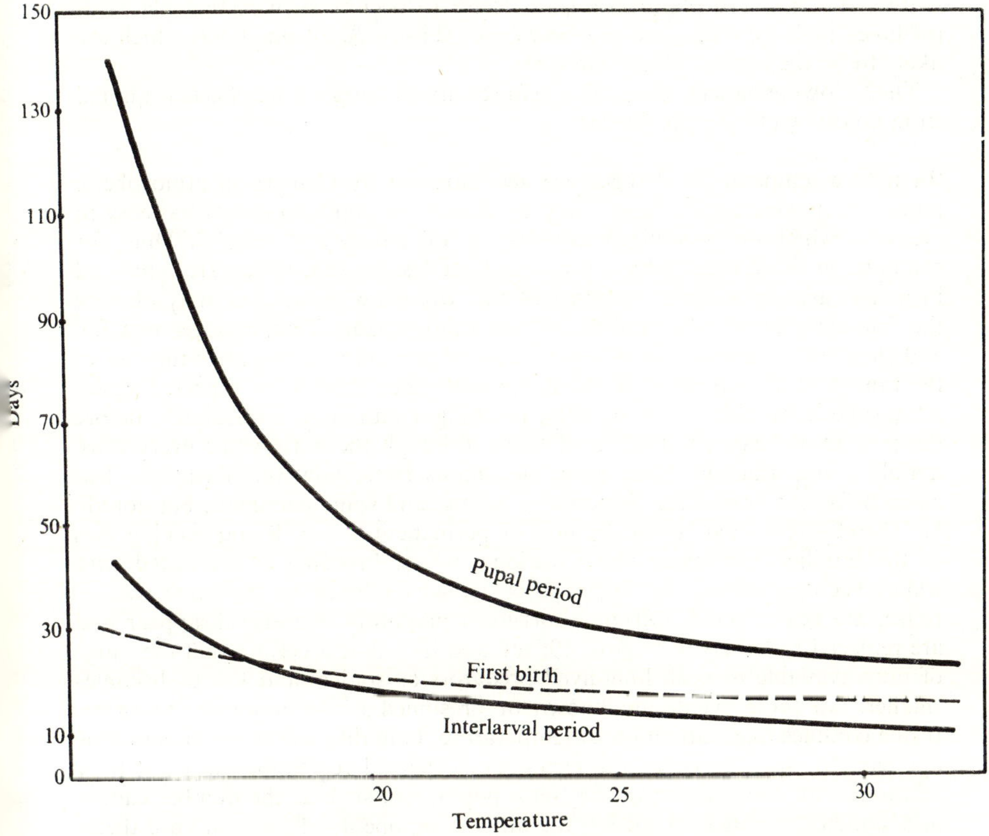

Fig. 15.1 The relation between temperature and the time from larviposition to emergence of the adult female (pupal period), the time of emergence till the first larviposition (broken line, first birth) and the interval between successive births (interlarval period). (From Glasgow, 1963, Fig. 9)

Barrass (1962) found that at temperatures above 41°C all four thoracic spiracles open and the internal temperature (measured by a fine thermocouple inserted into the thorax) became less than ambient, the difference being as much as 1·66°C at ambient 45°C. This effect is presumably brought about by evaporation of water, and must require an expendable reserve of water. Edney and Barrass doubted that this mechanism had an adaptive value, as they could not find field evidence of tsetse existing in ambient temperatures much above 40°C. However, it would be of interest to know if the internal temperature of tsetse rises in flight and how quickly the internal temperature rises as the result of insolation.

At temperatures below 30°C tsetse are positively phototactic, that is to say, if one has them in a cage they congregate on the side from which the light comes. At about 30°–32°C this taxis is reversed and tsetse move into dark places. In nature, this negative phototaxis leads tsetse to occupy such resting places as rot-holes in large trees, and ant-bear holes (Pilson & Pilson, 1967) which are likely to be the coolest places available.

The following passage describing field results on temperature effects is quoted from Glasgow (1963), pp. 68–73:

'In nature temperature changes are accompanied by changes in atmospheric humidity, in wind and in light. They are also bound up with effects less easy to measure, which one is obliged to think of collectively as "season". Thus, for example, in those areas with a prolonged rainless season, which are inhabited in many cases by various members of the *Morsitans* group, one may observe the following events after the end of the rainy season. Temperatures first fall and then rise, annual minima being recorded a month or two after the end of the rains and annual maxima about the time when the rain is expected again. Atmospheric humidity falls steadily, reaching a minimum immediately before the next rain. Leaves fall off most trees, although there are some evergreens, mainly along drainage lines. Some deciduous trees, however, flush into leaf again before any rain falls. Waterholes dry up, and some mammals, but not all, are thereby restricted to the vicinity of permanent water. Blood-sucking flies of the families Tabanidae and Culicidae, whose breeding is associated with water, become scarce, but Hippoboscidae, which breed in the same way as tsetse, are not affected. Certain short-lived predators of tsetse disappear and are replaced by others (Glasgow, 1961c), and it is almost certain that the range of prey available to such long-lived predators as spiders and lizards becomes smaller. All these events are known or presumed to be important to tsetse. If one confines one's attention to temperature, humidity and hours of sunshine one can, by making use of the technique of partial regression, sort out their relations with some aspect of the tsetse population such as the number caught in a standard manner. However, the other components of "season" are themselves bound up with temperature, humidity and hours of sunshine, but as they are difficult or impossible to evaluate on a numerical scale, they cannot be introduced into the partial regressions. Moreover, the experimental method is not usually applicable; for example, one cannot lower the temperature artificially over an experimental acre. It is, therefore, only exceptionally that one can have any confidence that phenomena observed in the field are caused by temperature and not by some other component of season (or day, as the case may be). We shall now notice some field observations which may plausibly be explained in terms of temperature.

'In Northern Nigeria it seems clear that the distribution of *Glossina* is limited by temperature. Nash (1942) studied the distribution of puparia of *G. morsitans submorsitans* in a "residual forest island". In December puparia having at the temperatures prevailing a life of about forty-five days in the ground, were found at the edge of the forest but not forty yards away in the centre of the island. In January small numbers were sometimes found in the centre of the island, and by April they had almost disappeared from the edge while large numbers were found in the centre. By this time the soil temperature at 1½ inches had risen to 28° in the centre, which would give twenty-three days life in the ground, and 29° at the edge. Meanwhile maximum temperatures (in a Stevenson screen four feet above the ground) rose to 41°. By sitting on the surface of the soil in the centre of the island, however, an adult fly could obtain considerable relief, since here the absolute maximum was 37°. Reference to Table 12 [Table 15.1] shows that 41° is lethal to some sub-species of *G. morsitans*, but not, according to Buxton and Lewis (1934) to the sub-species involved, *G. morsitans submorsitans*. Nash, however, states that "when batches of tsetse were caged in the hot weather, all the *G. tachinoides* would succumb if the day temperature reached 40·8°C, and all the *G. morsitans* if it reached 41·1°". This experiment would, one supposes, have exposed the flies to temperatures close to the recorded maxima for several hours, as opposed to the one hour of the experiments of Buxton and Lewis (1934).

'The mean temperature at 1½ inches depth in the soil at the edge of the forest, 29° in April, while below that which Bursell [1960b] regarded as limiting, is one which, it is apparent from his figures, is approaching the danger level. Although Nash was of course unaware of this relation, his very careful work supports this interpretation. He found that:

> puparia from larvae extruded in the centre of the forest island in March suffer no excessive mortality if buried in the forest edge, but puparia from larvae which have been extruded in the forest edge show a high mortality.

He also found that:

> from November to January the percentage of dead puparia in the forest edge which had died in pupal life ranged from 20% to 30%, but by March the range had risen to from 50% to 60%. No similar rise occurred in the middle of the forest. Admittedly the numbers are small, but much confirmatory evidence is available from other breeding grounds, which shows that at the time of evacuation the increased pupal mortality is invariably associated with a marked increase in the percentage of dead puparia which contain fully formed adults. This is particularly interesting because it is opposed to the general trend, which is for puparia to die early in pupal life in the dry season, but late in life in the rains.

'Nash was puzzled by these observations, but bearing in mind that the temperature experienced throughout the whole of pupal life is important, it seems reasonable to infer that the temperature at the edge of the forest was so high that a substantial proportion of the puparia exhausted their fat reserves before they were able to emerge. Such individuals would appear on dissection as almost completely formed adults. Puparia which began life in the centre of the forest would have passed through enough of their development in the cooler conditions there to be able to complete development at the edge without serious losses.

'Thus, by occupying the centre of the forest island these flies saved their own lives and those of their offspring. This was the "reason" for the move, in terms of survival. The actual stimulus which caused the individual flies to move into the centre was, however, the negative phototaxis operating at temperatures above 30°–32°C. Nash had recording thermometers at the edge of the forest and gives a table showing the number of daylight hours in which the temperature exceeded 32°C. In 1941, the "hot-hours" increased from 1 in the first week of February to 9·7 and 8·5 in the third and fourth weeks of March. By the end of March there were only about three hours a day during which the female would not be influenced by her negative reaction to light to larviposit in the darkest parts of the centre of the forest. As the cool hours occur in the early morning and larviposition occurs in the late afternoon, the negative light reaction seems to be a complete explanation of the disappearance of puparia from the forest edge.

'One concludes from this thorough study that adult tsetse moved into the centre of the forest because of the negative phototaxis operating at temperatures above 30°–32°, and that the results of this were two-fold: the maximum temperatures in the middle of the forest were safer for adults, and their offspring deposited there encountered mean soil temperatures which were safer for them. It is not possible to say whether one of these effects was more important than the other. Seasonal alteration of breeding sites has been reported by other investigators. In Shinyanga, during the wet season puparia of *G. swynnertoni* are in scattered situations on the surface of the soil where they are very difficult to find. In the dry season some, perhaps most, occur in large aggregations so that large collections can be made. "Foliage and shade are still abundant when dry season conditions set in, usually in May. Just over a week later pupae of *G. swynnertoni* abruptly appear again, not only under deciduous thicket but also in tree hollows" (Burtt, 1952). The sites used in the wet season would probably be dangerously hot in the dry season, but the way in which the change-over is mediated is not known. Harley (1954) describes a seasonal shift of breeding sites used by *G. morsitans*, which used warmer sites in the cool weather and cooler sites in the hot weather.[1] Again, the way in which this was brought about is not known.

'Another apparently clear temperature effect is mentioned by Nash (1937). He believed that *G. tachinoides* was most active at about 29°C. From October to February the mean maximum in the habitat of this species was 28°–31°, and during this season maximum catches were made in the middle of the day when temperatures were highest. In March-April-May maximum temperatures were about 36°. During this hot season the highest catches were made early in the morning and late in the afternoon, the fly being inert at midday. Smaller catches of *G. morsitans submorsitans* appeared to show the same cycle, but less clearly.

'When temperatures dangerously high were being considered, we could not determine whether adults or puparia were more affected. The same doubt arises

[1] Glasgow (1961b) records a similar shift, commenting on the dramatic suddenness with which the logs were abandoned in favour of rot-holes, and then in due course reoccupied.

with regard to low temperatures. *G. morsitans orientalis* can survive brief exposures to temperatures below freezing point, though I do not know of any temperature records showing that it encounters such temperatures in nature. Jack [1941a] published records from the Chipitani River Forest where the mean temperature in 1938 was 18·2°C. If puparia were exposed to this mean temperature the smaller ones were probably lost, although one must remember that the pupal period at 18°C is 65–68 days, so that a very brief cold season would be less harmful. The absolute minimum temperature recorded at Chipitani was 6°. A fall of 3° in temperatures would probably have destroyed the puparia without seriously affecting the adults. There is another possible effect of temperature, however, pointed out by Buxton (1955). Since even *G. morsitans* is inactive at temperatures below 17°, the time available for feeding is restricted to the number of hours of daylight in which this temperature is attained. At Chipitani the four coldest days (which occurred in early August) had a mean maximum of 19°C, so that the postulated reduction of 3° might have involved a few days of zero activity. In Southern Rhodesia (as in Northern Nigeria) the cold weather is dry. "A whole day with completely overcast sky is rare; the mean daily sunshine is about nine hours in winter, six hours in summer." (Kendrew, 1953, p. 128). It seems probable that it is the effect of cold on puparia rather than on adults which limits the distribution of *Glossina* in Southern Rhodesia. This may not be so in East Africa, where, in places, where tsetse approach their upper altitude limit, cloudy days are not uncommon in the cool season. For example, Jackson (1955) of a station at 4,500 feet altitude, wrote, "The mornings at Daga-Iloi were, however, often quite cold, especially in wet weather during the rains and on the generally very cloudy mornings that persisted during the next three or four months, and it was the practice not to start the fly-round until the temperature rose to 21°C or until 2 p.m., whichever was the earlier". On the other hand Bursell [1960b] mentions instances in East Africa where in mixed fly-belts the larger species tolerates the higher altitude, which suggests that it is the effect of low mean temperature on puparia which is critical.

'In general, it seems that with regard to temperature no stage in the life of *Glossina* is particularly susceptible. If temperatures are high, so that daily maxima approach the values lethal to adults, the means in the better insulated sites occupied by puparia are likely to be preventing the successful completion of development. If temperatures are so low that the period of diurnal activity is severely limited, again the mean temperature is likely to be imperilling the puparia.'

Tsetse and Moisture

From the moment it is born the immature tsetse does not feed and, as far as is known, it cannot absorb moisture from its environment. However, when given a choice, it will enter the moist air side of a chamber (Finlayson, 1967). The water reserve of the new-born larva must therefore suffice to complete pupal development and it must suffice the adult fly from the time of its emergence until its first blood meal which is generally taken one to three days after emergence.[1] These early stages of a tsetse's life are therefore more susceptible to dryness than the adult stage when water reserves are replenished automatically at every feed. Our knowledge of this subject comes from a series of papers by Bursell (1957, 1957a, 1958, 1959a, 1960a, b, c) which are summarized in the following pages. A fuller summary is given by Glasgow (1963).

Larval and Puparial Stages

At 25°C development takes 28–30 days from larviposition to eclosion of the adult. The larva which is deposited is in its third instar; it can lose water through its general integument and through the black polypneustic lobes at its back end. Very soon the integument of the larva becomes rigid and dark; no moult is involved so that the new puparium[2] so formed is still a third instar larva. A day later the larva shrinks slightly, leaving a narrow space separating it from the puparial shell. This shrinkage was regarded as an ecdysis, and the new surface inside the puparial shell as the fourth-instar integument. At this stage water vapour that passes through the new surface must afterwards diffuse through the puparial shell. Loss through the polypneustic lobes still goes on but, in addition, water is lost through anal excretion. This anal route is under control, less being lost from the puparial stages in dry air, more from those in moist air. The result is that when, after four days, pupation occurs, the water content is constant whether the animal has been in saturated air or in only 40% relative humidity (in the case of *G.m. morsitans*). Below 40% r.h. transpiration by other routes is so high that cessation of anal excretion cannot compensate for it and the water content of the pupae is below normal. When the pupa has appeared, still inside the puparial shell, it can lose water through the new pupal integument, through the pupal spiracle (which is controlled, very much as the losses from the larval anus are controlled) and water vapour from both these sources has to pass through the puparial shell to reach the environment. Finally, a day or so before eclosion the pupal apolysis takes place and the pharate adult is exposed (Chapter 14, p. 343 and Chapter 19, p. 438).

When the puparial stages of different species of *Glossina* are kept at controlled temperatures and humidities, a wide range of tolerance to dryness is found. Some are killed if the relative humidity is less than 80%, others withstand much lower humidities and a few will survive if kept over calcium chloride at zero relative humidity. Data exist for nine species, from which Bursell constructed a possible generic phylogeny (Fig. 15.2) assuming that the genus

[1] 'Although there is no precise information as to how long the teneral fly can survive without food, the writer (unpublished observations) found that when flies that had emerged from puparia collected locally were kept without food for seven days, a large proportion survived and were able to feed at the end of the period, whereas the few that survived for fourteen days were either unable to feed or died without digesting their first meal. The average periods that unfed teneral flies have been recorded as surviving without food have been reviewed by Jackson (1949) and these range from 2·3 to 12·5 days at various temperatures and humidities, but as these are for survival to death, they are difficult to relate to the actual ability of the newly emerged fly to survive and continue to live. This is a subject on which it would be valuable to have more precise information.'—W. H. POTTS

[2] As explained elsewhere (p. 232) the word 'puparium' in its strict sense refers to the dark rigid third instar integument. Here the meaning is extended to include its contents, using for clarity 'puparial shell' to denote the integument.

originated in damp rain forest conditions and that some species have become adapted to xerophytic conditions (*see* also pp. 292).

The systematist Machado (1959) does not accept this phylogeny, on morphological grounds (*see* also p. 255). Be that as it may, Fig. 15.2 is a convenient summary of the facts. The species named in the figure are there arranged in order of the tolerance of their puparia to dryness. If one considers instead the vegetational facies of their natural habitats, they fall into much the same order—*G. longipennis* occurring in low rainfall areas with a prolonged dry season and sparse xerophytic vegetation, whereas *G. fuscipleuris* is found in regions of high rainfall with vegetation akin to rain forest. The other species occur in intermediate types.

These observations explain why, for example, *G. fuscipleuris* cannot survive in conditions where *G. longipennis* flourishes, but not the reverse. There is no evidence of high humidities as such being harmful to any stage of *G. longipennis*; reasons for the absence of this and other dry-adapted species from moist habitats are not known but may have to be sought somewhere other than in the region of water relations.

The Teneral Fly

The young fly does not feed immediately after emergence. Depending on circumstances this stage lasts for 1–4 days. During this stage the fly is living on reserves of fat and water derived ultimately from its mother. If the development of the puparial stages has taken place under favourable conditions, the water content of the fly that emerges is 76–77% of the non-fatty wet weight. If this fly emerges into air at zero relative humidity it dies, and as it still has substantial reserves of unused fat it is reasonable to say that it has died of desiccation. On the other hand, the death of a fly that is kept from emergence in very damp air must be ascribed to exhaustion of fat; the critical fat content is 4·2% of the total dry weight in *G. pallidipes*, *G.m. morsitans* and *G. swynnertoni*.

Tsetse control the rate at which water is lost by closing the spiracles to a greater or lesser extent. In the resting fly, the stimulus is the actual ambient humidity; in flight, it is the physiological state of the insect. There are differences between species in this regard, and also some specific differences in duration of the teneral stage, that is, the time it takes to starve a teneral fly to death under standard conditions. These differences, however, could not be related either to the systematic groups or to the natural history of the various species.

The Adult Fly

Once a tsetse has taken its first meal it is no longer teneral and no longer dependent on reserves of fat and water derived from its mother. No water is taken as such, all water requirements being met from the blood meals, but as mammalian blood is 79% water there is in fact a surplus available. Indeed the first thing a tsetse does after feeding is to concentrate the meal, and reduce its weight, by excreting a clear fluid which contains little but water. Sometimes this process can be seen to begin at the back end while blood is still being ingested at the front end (Glasgow, 1963, *frontispiece*). In spite of this superfluity of water in the blood meal, Bursell (1960c) describes a number of interesting

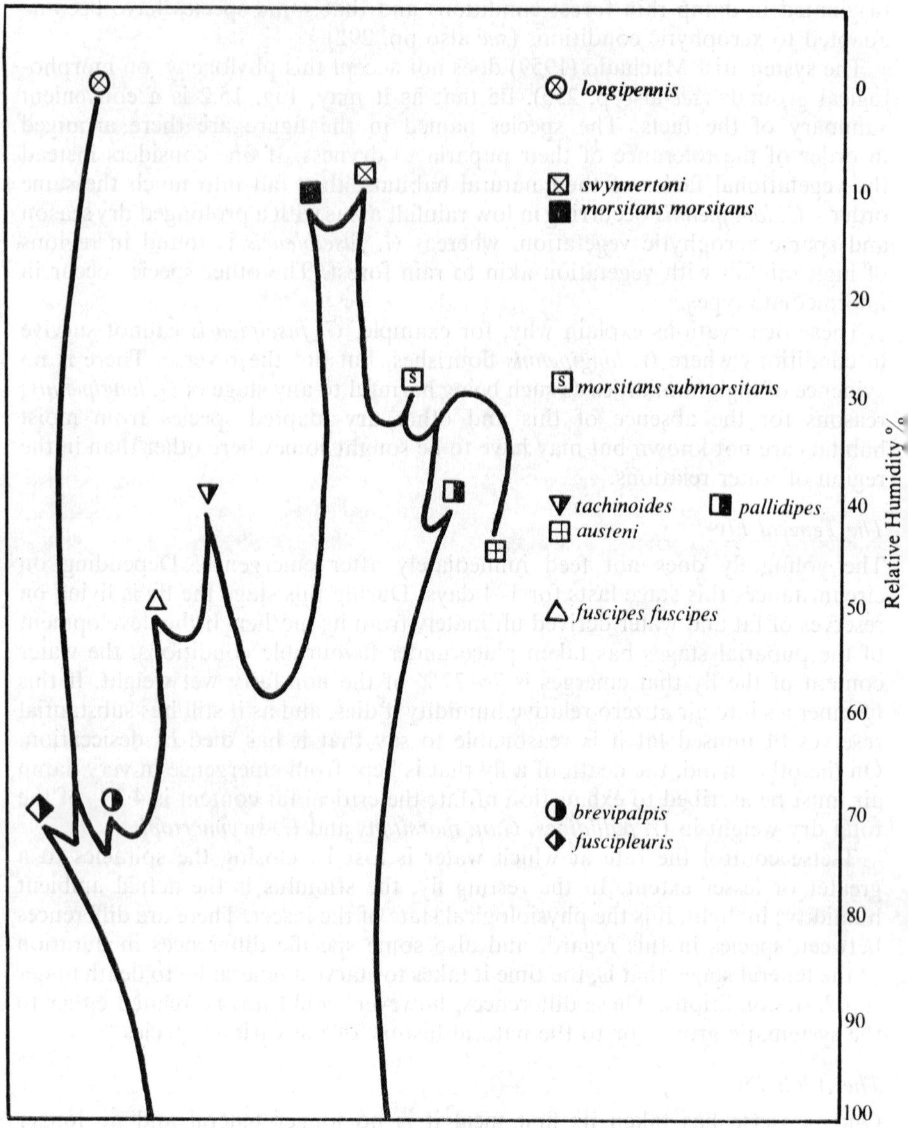

Fig. 15.2. A possible phylogeny of *Glossina*, based on pupal water balance. The genus is conceived as derived from a rain-forest ancestor dependent on high humidities, and the diagram indicates the relative effectiveness of all the adaptations to dry life developed by the puparia. The numerical scale denotes the minimum relative humidity (constant throughout development) tolerated by each species. Each species is denoted by a symbol which can be identified by reference to its name written at the same level on the right of the diagram. (After Glasgow, 1963, Fig. 16)

adaptations for water conservation. Thus the amount lost in the 'primary excretion' varied according to the degree of desiccation of the fly, and to the size of the meal taken. It was calculated that a fly which had been desiccated to the critical level (61% water) could become fully hydrated by taking a meal only 70% of a normal full one. This primary excretion was complete in about three hours. Production of faeces began the following day, and while the amount of solids produced was constant, the water content was greatly reduced in flies kept in dry air.

We have already seen that teneral tsetse, if not allowed to feed, may die of either fat exhaustion or desiccation according to the ambient humidity in which they are kept. Field experiments showed that under quite arid conditions it would be the fat reserves, not the water reserves, which gave out first. Adult tsetse are better off for water than tenerals, and so desiccation is unlikely to be an important cause of death. Of course tsetse starve to death if they do not find food, but it is probably the solid fraction which is critical, and dry conditions in themselves do not present an added hazard. Dry conditions may, of course, be associated with high temperatures and may actually cause a shortage of host animals, but that is another matter.

Field Results of Moisture Effects

In the history of tsetse research, much field work was done before the information summarized above was available. Investigators, naturally impressed by the spectacular changes associated with the seven rainless months characteristic of large portions of tropical Africa, sought for connections between numbers of tsetse and some measure of dryness. Two popular measures were the saturation deficit, which can be calculated from simultaneous readings of wet and dry bulb thermometers, and the rate of evaporation from the white porous sphere of a Livingstone atmometer. Nash (1937) combining observations of *G.m. morsitans* in East Africa with others on *G.m. submorsitans* in West Africa, concluded that optimum conditions were a mean monthly saturation deficit of 5–6 millibars and a mean evaporation of 20–25 millilitres per day as measured in a Livingstone atmometer (Scott, 1934). Deviations from this 'optimum zone' in either direction would be accompanied by a reduction in density. In a place where the minimum saturation deficit was about Nash's 'optimum zone', Jackson (1948) found a positive correlation between saturation deficit and death rate of *G.m. morsitans*. Jackson also measured weekly death rates and birth rates (by the technique of marking and recapture, *see* Chapter 17, p. 409) at two places eight miles apart in an extensive plain. He reasoned that if birth and death rates are really affected by saturation deficit or any other element of climate, then they should vary together in the two places. In fact he found very little agreement between the two places.

In another paper, Jackson (1953a) found that the mean size of three species of tsetse was negatively correlated with the mean saturation deficit of two months before. This was based on thirty-eight months' observations. Later, Glasgow and Bursell (1961) were able to continue the observations on one of the three species. The correlation was still there when the observations of 141 months were examined but it was weakened, not strengthened, by the additional data. They concluded that the correlation was fortuitous and meant no more than that nutrition (of which size is an indicator) was poor in the dry season when saturation deficits happen to be high. The dry season is important to the nutrition and to the size of the tsetse population, for it involves changes in the distribution of hosts, in the amount of shade, in the abundance of predators, in hours of sunshine and in temperature. It is perfectly conceivable that the tsetse was reacting to one or several of these, and still gave a correlation with saturation deficit, which is clearly one rough measure of season.

Tsetse and Light

Larvae of *G.m. orientalis* (other species are probably the same) avoid light and prefer damp air, the two reactions between them presumably leading the larva from the place where it is deposited to the place where it becomes a puparium. Puparium formation is delayed in light, from an average of forty-eight minutes to an average of 108 minutes (Finlayson, 1967). The puparium is black and presumably opaque and the puparial stages are normally passed underground, so that one would not expect any of them to be sensitive to light.

There is a lack of critical experiments on the effect of light on the tsetse imago. However, they are usually attracted to light, in the sense that they congregate on the light side of a cage in the laboratory or of the catching cage of a trap in the field. Some species can be caught in light traps at night and this is usually interpreted as evidence of nocturnal activity. As described above in the section on temperature, the positive response to light is reversed at high temperatures (i.e. above about 30°C) and in the field this reversal has the effect of taking flies into the coolest places available at a time when the ambient temperatures are getting dangerously high. In the case of females about to larviposit a similar reversal, at any temperature, seems likely, but has not been demonstrated.

Table 15.2 collects a number of references to nocturnal activity. It will be seen that the *fusca* group has earned more entries than either the *palpalis* or the *morsitans* groups; as the total volume of work on the *fusca* group is small, it may well be that night feeding is especially characteristic of this group. It can be seen that there is some disagreement about *G. pallidipes*. Harley's work is the most careful and quantitative; he caught thirteen *G. pallidipes* at night and 54,271 by day, but one would expect different results in hotter places. It is usually stated that *G. morsitans* is inactive at night, but Nash (1933) having found that catches made by the technique he was using fell to zero soon after sunset, recorded that 'many reliable observers have stated that they have been attacked while sitting up for game over water-holes on moonlight nights, or while walking along roads'. While it is true that night is not a fruitful time for collecting samples of tsetse, night feeding may well be of considerable importance to the flies.

Many workers (e.g. Nash, Kernaghan & Boyle, 1966) cover cages with a cloth when feeding tsetse. In nature, *G. swynnertoni*, at least, feeds more readily in shade than in direct sunlight (Glasgow, 1961a). It therefore seems that very bright light inhibits feeding. Foster (1957) found that captive *G. morsitans* would not feed without a minimum light intensity of 1–2 foot-candles, so that there is room for further investigation to clear up the anomaly between this observation and that of Nash (1933) noted in Table 15.2.

Bursell (1957) demonstrated that several species of *Glossina* are more active (i.e. move more often in a glass dish) in dry air than in wet. This orthokinesis disappears at low light intensities, and the disappearance is mediated by the compound eyes. For this and other reasons, field experiments involving blinded flies require caution in their interpretation. Thus Nash (1930) released 750 blinded *G. morsitans*, and a mile away recaptured seventy control but no blind

TABLE 15.2

Night activity of **Glossina**

Species	Observation	Authority
FUSCA GROUP		
brevipalpis	Caught all through the night on cattle	Harley, 1965
brevipalpis	Attracted to light, but not especially to ultra-violet light	Glasgow, 1956
fusca	Caught feeding off cattle at night	Jordan, 1962a
longipennis	Attracted to light	Lewis, 1950
tabaniformis	Caught feeding off cattle at night	Jordan, 1962a
MORSITANS GROUP		
austeni	Caught feeding off men at night	Moggridge, 1948
longipalpis	Sometimes comes to light	Morris, 1934
morsitans	Occasionally attacks man at night	Nash, 1933
pallidipes	Very few at night	Harley, 1965
pallidipes	Feeds on moonlight and on dark nights	Chorley and Hopkins, 1942; Moggridge, 1948
PALPALIS GROUP		
fuscipes fuscipes	None at night	Harley, 1965

flies. He concluded that this species hunts entirely by sight, a conclusion not justified by this experiment, for as we have seen their behaviour would have been altered, and their ability to avoid predators so seriously impaired that none may have survived for very long. Bursell (1957) found some specific differences in activity, *G.f. fuscipes* moving twice as often as the other species. This was interpreted as intolerance, by a forest fly, to high light intensity (not measured, but coming from a 300 watt lamp at a distance of 2 m.).

It may well be that light intensities, or patterns, are important differences between the habitats of various species of *Glossina* (Jack & Williams, 1937). Mellanby (1936) recalled the common observation that *G. palpalis* [*G.f. fuscipes*] is often seen perching in nature in flecks of sunshine at the boundary between shade and sun, and he succeeded in reproducing this phenomenon in a long cage, deeply shaded at one end and sunlit at the other. But the effects of temperature and light are not separated in this observation. Doubtless the internal temperature of tsetse sitting in the sun rises, and on a warm day it would not have to rise much to reach 30°C when the fly would presumably become negatively phototactic.

There is a need for critical studies of the responses of tsetse to light.

Vegetational Influences

Tsetse and Vegetation

The immature stages of most insects require food and conditions which may be different from those needed by the adults—the distribution of species is therefore conditioned by the needs of both adult and immature stages. In adopting adenotrophic viviparity tsetse have become free of the need to lay eggs on a larval food supply, but they are still restricted to some extent by the needs of their puparial stages. These must as a rule be in shade, because the temperature of unshaded soils may rise to lethal levels. This is seldom a restriction, as adult tsetse are woodland animals, spending most of their time perched on woody vegetation. In addition, puparial stages of some species perish if the ambient air humidity fall too low—while some can complete their development at a relative humidity of zero, others demand one of 80%. The air in the interstices of the soil is often moister than that above ground; nevertheless during prolonged dry seasons the air in the superficial layers of the soil becomes dry enough to destroy the puparial stages of many species (Bursell, 1960a). It seems likely that many species cannot occupy areas more arid than those they in fact inhabit because of the necessity of finding relatively damp breeding places. Such damper soils support vegetation which is relatively massive and non-deciduous, and the tsetse is then often said to be dependent on heavy evergreen vegetation. If the soils support vegetation which is relatively massive and non-deciduous, and the interpretation given above is correct, the tsetse is no more dependent on the vegetation than the vegetation is on the tsetse—both depend on the damp soil.

Other apparent correlations between tsetse and vegetation are less easy to explain. Consider for example two members of the *fusca* group, *G. brevipalpis* and *G. longipennis*, which occur side by side in eastern Kenya. *G. brevipalpis* is confined to evergreen vegetation associated with ground-water, while *G. longipennis* ranges far out into dry semi-desert. As we have seen, laboratory work has shown that puparia of *G. longipennis* can develop in quite dry air, whereas those of *G. brevipalpis* demand a high relative humidity. This one fact is enough to account for the restriction of *G. brevipalpis* to relatively damp habitats, but not the restriction of *G. longipennis* to dry habitats. In the diet of *G. longipennis* rhinoceros is prominent (*see* Chapter 13). Is this cause or effect? Nobody knows. It is thus with restrictions of other species of *Glossina* to xerophytic habitats.

In spite of these difficulties, there is a vast body of empirical data relating the occurrence of various tsetse species with various types of vegetation. The fact that there is little sound theoretical explanation of such relations in no way diminishes their value as aids to survey. The facts that more than one classification of vegetation types has been proposed (Buxton, 1955; Welch, 1960a) and that professional botanists tend to use words such as 'forest' with specialized meanings not obvious to non-botanists, are hindrances to communication between workers, but do not detract from the value of the experience of a skilled observer. With experience of a given region, one can predict with great accuracy, from purely botanical observation, which species of *Glossina* will be found in any place. By using aerial photographs, it is even possible to make valuable predictions about a place without visiting it (Ford, 1953). By considering the ecological succession a botanist may even be able to predict that an area currently free of tsetse may soon be suitable for a certain species.

How to Predict the Presence of Tsetse from Observation of the Vegetation

The circumstances described below refer to areas inside the geographical and altitude limits of *Glossina*.

Utterly treeless grassland cannot support tsetse. Grassland with a few scattered trees cannot do so either, but where grassland is interspersed by drainage lines with thicket or forest, tsetse disperse from the drainage lines for several miles in sufficient numbers to infect an appreciable proportion of cattle with trypanosomiasis. Such dispersal may be more noticeable in the presence of scattered trees; the species involved of course depends on the nature of the drainage line vegetation, but *G. pallidipes* and *G. longipalpis* are particularly associated with this situation.

Areas covered with grass and a few trees are called *wooded grassland.* As the quantity of trees increases until there is less than 50% of the ground covered with grass, we pass into *grassed woodland.* As grassed woodland commonly includes a number of small thickets (often associated with termite mounds) an alternative name for grassed woodland is *bushland and thicket.* In grassed woodland, and in all formations in which there is more woody vegetation and less grass, one expects to find one or more species of *Glossina.* This seems to the writer to be a fair summary of the facts but some other workers may not agree.

Grassed woodland is inhabited by one of the sub-species of *G. morsitans*, or in northern Tanzania and southwest Kenya by the closely related *G. swynnertoni.* The other members of the *morsitans* group, *G. austeni*,[1] *G. longipalpis* and *G. pallidipes* are associated with formations in which the crowns of the woody plants touch and grass is totally suppressed though the last two may be encountered outside this sort of formation. Such '*thicket*', as it is often called, is frequently associated with drainage lines, so that these species sometimes seem to have a linear rather than a two-dimensional distribution. But where low-closed-canopy woodland occurs in patches rather than lines these species are not confined to the edges. In northeast Tanzania and northern Kenya, in a very arid type of grassed woodland, occurs *G. longipennis*, an aberrant member of the *fusca* group. A belt of similar vegetation extends across Africa as one of the interzones between the dry Sahara and the wetter regions to the south, but *G. longipennis* does not occur much to the west of Lake Rudolph.

[1] *G. austeni* is confined to the Indian Ocean drainage.

Drainage line closed-canopy woodland is mostly evergreen. If low (less than, say, 30 feet high) it is inhabited, as noted above, by one of the *morsitans* group. If higher than this it may harbour one of the *fusca* group, *G. brevipalpis* in eastern Africa, *G. fuscipleuris* centrally, *G. medicorum* and *G. fusca* in the west. Belts of tall trees growing beside lakes or rivers have a certain resemblance to rain forest and such *ground-water forest* in places spreads away from the permanent water and is continuous with areas of rain forest. Under these conditions the members of the *fusca* group mentioned above may spread away from the waterside, or they may be replaced in the depths of the forest by other members of the *fusca* group, all of which seem to be creatures of the rain forest. Since there is much more rain forest on the west side of Africa, the majority of the *fusca* group are associated with the Atlantic drainage.

The *palpalis* group is not found at all in country draining into the Indian Ocean. Elsewhere, closed-canopy waterside vegetation whether high or low may contain one species of this group. Most of the species are fairly catholic, *G.f. fuscipes* for example ranging from low thicket in Kenya to noble forest in Entebbe. *G. tachinoides* is the most tolerant of dry conditions, and in northern Nigeria is found in thicket only 3 or 4 feet high. All members of the *palpalis* group tend to have a linear distribution, appearing reluctant to move far from water even though apparently suitable vegetation is widespread. This linear distribution, however, is not as rigid as was once supposed; attempts to eradicate *G.f. fuscipes* in Kenya by means of narrow waterside clearings have been clearly unsuccessful (Glasgow, 1954).

The above summary is intended to give a general idea of the way in which vegetation studies may help in tsetse survey. Space does not permit its expansion into a form which would provide useful field guidance to those faced with particular local problems.

Animal Influences

The most important other animal in the environment of tsetse is man himself. Besides being a source of food for tsetse, men kill tsetse by crushing them, modify their environment by various agricultural practices, deliberately destroy their environment by bush clearing or game destruction, and spread poison to kill them directly. These human activities are described in other chapters and will not be considered further. The remainder may be classified as:

Other animals of the same or nearly the same kind.
Other animals of different kinds.

1 Food
2 Rivals
3 Enemies

Other Animals of the Same or Nearly the Same Kind

Where tsetse are especially abundant the sexes have no difficulty in meeting. The insertion of a tsetse proboscis into a host may cause pain, and host animals are more likely to respond to many insertions than to few. In extreme conditions tsetse seek out favoured micro-climates in, for example, rot holes in trees (Pilson & Pilson, 1967). Although on one occasion thirty-two *G. morsitans* were caught from one rot hole, the Pilsons do not suggest that the hole was full. Although, then, one can imagine tsetse shouldering each other out of a micro-climate, there is no evidence of this in nature. Diseases of tsetse, especially if caused by specific parasites, must be supposed to be favoured by dense populations, but we have no information on this topic. We have anecdotes of a number of tsetse parasites, but quantitative information only about the parasitization of puparial stages by other insects. Such parasites would be expected to be favoured by dense tsetse populations, but scanty tsetse populations are so difficult to study, in this as in other respects, that there are in fact no comparative data.

The Reduced Chance of Mating in Sparse Populations

As in all Diptera, female tsetse have a spermatheca in which semen is stored and used as required. A simple dissection (p. 430) enables one to examine the spermathecae to see whether or not they are empty. In captivity, after a single mating, semen may become exhausted in long-lived females (Nash, Jordan & Boyle, 1966). In nature more than one mating may occur, but it seems most likely that they occur in quick succession while the female is young, since most writers have found that pairs captured while copulating consist of a teneral female and an older male. Squire (1951a) considered that elderly females may mate again and both Nash (1955) and Jordan (1958) obtained evidence of multiple mating in *G.p. palpalis* under laboratory conditions. More recently Curtis (1968) has established, by mating the same females of *G. austeni* with normal and sterile males, that multiple mating can occur, and found no evidence of changed 'receptivity' in the females between the first and second matings made, respectively, at age two and three days. Dame and Ford (1968) have also demonstrated by the same method that multiple mating is possible in *G.m. orientalis*. They also noted that, by exposing groups of males to successive groups of virgin females, the male complement of sperm could be depleted by heavy mating, and that fertility was never recovered.

It is reasonable to suppose that in dense tsetse populations the chances of the sexes meeting are better than they are in very sparse populations, and Teesdale (1940) and Glover *et al.* (1955) working in very sparsely populated areas, have dissected females to see whether an undue proportion were uninseminated. Teesdale investigated *G.f. fuscipes* in an area where the density had been so reduced that the average catch was only 1·12 flies per man per day. With a staff of forty men, however, this is over 1,000 flies a month, and in six months he dissected 1,737 females. Only 107, mostly tenerals, were uninseminated; 98% of non-tenerals were inseminated so that the mating machinery was working well.

Glover *et al.* (*loc. cit.*) worked with *G.m. morsitans*. First they excluded grass-fires, which measure was followed by a considerable reduction in their routine catches, and then they observed that most of the tsetse in their catches came from a particular kind of small valley. They therefore cut down the trees in these valleys, and this measure was followed by further falls in the catches and led ultimately to extinction of *G.m. morsitans*. During this final phase a number of uninseminated females was found, Table 15.3.

TABLE 15.3
Non-teneral uninseminated female* G. morsitans morsitans *caught near Abercorn, Zambia
(Glover* et al., *1955)

Year	Number dissected	Percentage uninseminated
1943	136	9
1944	152	20
1945	42	29

As to whether this rising proportion of uninseminated females was a cause or an effect of the decline in the population, there is no information. One cannot say whether real density, in terms of frequency of encounters between the sexes, was different in Teesdale's area from what it was in Glover's. Glover *et al.* (*loc. cit.*) mentioned the possibility that the valleys selected for bush clearing had been mating grounds of the tsetse, and the recent work of Pilson and Pilson (1967) makes this suggestion seem slightly more credible. Glover *et al.* (*loc. cit*) used a sampling technique (*see* p. 404) which produced mostly males in their sexually appetitive phase, and treated the places where such males were particularly abundant. The Pilsons used a sampling method which produces other elements of the tsetse population and found in at least some seasons that there are places which contain concentrations of males but not of other elements of the population. This discovery lends colour to the view (the writer's speculation, not the Pilsons') that 'mating grounds' may sometimes exist.

The Harassment of Host Animals by Dense Populations of Tsetse

The numbers of many wild animals are believed to be controlled, at least when they are numerous, by their food supply. Jackson (1933a) reasoned that the important thing for tsetse is the frequency of encounter with hosts. If host animals were scarce, hungry tsetse might die before finding a host and the tsetse population would become extinct. If hosts were more abundant, the average time taken to find a host would fall below the lethal level and the tsetse population would flourish. Since the amount of blood removed by a tsetse is small, there would be no question of hosts being sucked dry, and the important factor would be the time taken to find blood (presumably a function of the numbers of hosts) and not the volume of blood found.

This striking paradox has been found memorable by many writers, who have cited tsetse as an example of an animal whose numbers are, above a fairly low threshold, independent of its food supply.

To accept this paradox is to ignore a striking and well known piece of mammal behaviour. Here are some eye-witness accounts.

Giraffe: The long lashing tail is constantly in motion, hind hooves are scraping tsetse from their fore-legs, and above all the shudder of a giraffe, which must be seen to be believed, would dislodge the most tenacious insect. From these observations it was concluded that tsetse must follow for a considerable distance before they are finally satisfied (Harrison, 1940).

Warthog: Wild warthogs, watched on two occasions with a telescope at a distance of about twenty yards, and seen to have many tsetse attacking them, were taking continuous evasive action, using tail and all four legs to disturb flies from various parts of the body (Harley, 1959).

Lion: Rolled on their backs . . . trying to squash their tormentors (Adamson, 1961).

Cattle: The animal . . . nearly always attracted attention to biting flies by its attempts to drive them away (Harley, 1965).

The calf was hobbled and lying down; its reactions to tsetse bites included tail lashing, shuddering and rolling (Glasgow, 1961a).

None of these observations is quantitative, but it seems reasonable to conclude that whereas one hungry tsetse could alight on a host and feed quickly and easily, when a large number make the same attempt each one finds the process prolonged and dangerous.

The volume of blood lost by individual hosts is not easily determined. The present writer has been associated with two attempts on the problem (Glasgow & Wilson, 1953; Lamprey *et al.*, 1962). It is necessary to identify the host being used and to estimate its numbers; to estimate the numbers of tsetse feeding on these hosts, and to know how often they feed. Since there was some imprecision in the estimates of each of these parameters, the results must be treated with reserve, but as these results indicated that animals weighing about 100 kg. were losing 13–27 g. of blood daily, the old assumption that blood losses are always negligible requires re-examination. This is discussed at greater length by Glasgow (1963, pp. 134–5).

Other Animals of Nearly the Same Kind

Cross-matings have been made in the laboratory between various members of the *morsitans* group, and experiments indicate that the males cannot distinguish between females of their own and of a nearly related species, so that in mixed populations mating occurs at random (Vanderplank, 1944, 1947, 1948, 1949, 1949a, b; Jackson, 1945). The matings are in effect sterile, the hybrids produced being few and unable to breed. A female that mated only once, with a male of another species, would be in effect sterilized, and one may suppose that the effect prevents two nearly related species from occurring together. The three sub-species of *G. morsitans* do not overlap; *G. swynnertoni* and *G.m. morsitans* do overlap, but the overlaps are narrow, perhaps because of this hybridization effect.

Laboratory cross-matings have also been made within the *palpalis* group, where there is an additional mechanical barrier to cross-mating between

G. fuscipes martinii and *G.f. fuscipes* (Buxton, 1955, pp. 325–8; Machado, 1954, 1964). Male *martinii* have unusually large claspers, which piece the abdomen of, and kill, female *fuscipes*. According to Machado (1959) there is an overlap between these two forms on the Lualaba river, and we must suppose that this interaction between the two sub-species keeps the overlap narrow.

Other Animals of Different Kinds

Food of Tsetse

The only food taken by tsetse is the blood of vertebrates. Just which vertebrates are used is a difficult question which is examined elsewhere (Chapter 13). Here we shall merely note that feeding is seldom random. A list of the sources of blood actually ingested by wild tsetse in any place seldom corresponds with a list of wild vertebrates in that area. In most places there are a number of wild vertebrates whose blood is apparently seldom or never used, a very short list of hosts usually providing most of the food. It follows that the intensity of attack on favoured hosts is much greater than it would be if all the potential hosts in an area were attacked equally. There seem to be two possible explanations for this state of affairs:

(a) that there is a qualitative difference between the blood of different vertebrates such that tsetse flourish on some and not on others. It would follow that elimination of the favoured host, or of a very short list of host species, would eliminate the tsetse. In the laboratory, various mammals have been used for feeding cultures of tsetse, and differences demonstrated between rabbits, goats and calves, but it must be noted that an early suggestion that *G. austeni* reproduces better when fed on pregnant than on non-pregnant goats has been shown to be wrong (Nash *et al.*, 1966; Jordan *et al.*, 1966; Nash *et al.*, 1967a).

(b) that in any area certain trees will provide the best resting places for tsetse, and the most used host will be that one which sleeps under those trees. According to this view, elimination of a single host would have little effect, the tsetse readily feeding on an alternative host, especially if it came to occupy the preferred sleeping places.

It may well be that both these hypotheses must be invoked to explain all the observations.

Rivals of Tsetse

Other biting flies. Mosquitoes are very much smaller than tsetse, and they have a tendency to be nocturnal. No doubt there are occasions when their large numbers interfere with the feeding of tsetse, but I have seen no mention of this point in any account of a field study. Some members of the genus *Hippobosca* approach tsetse in size, and they can occur in large numbers. The writer has seen swarms of them round camels in Somalia and round cattle in Madagascar: in neither place were tsetse present, but they do occur in tsetse areas, and when numerous they must interfere with tsetse feeding.

Some members of the family *Tabanidae* are larger than tsetse, and in places with a marked contrast between dry and wet seasons they can occur in spectacular seasonal peaks (*see* for example Glasgow, 1946). According to Tinley

(1964) Tabanidae have a profound effect upon the diurnal activity of hippopotamus in north-eastern Zululand. The hippopotamus spends the daylight hours in water, and 'should a fly attempt to settle on the head parts, the animal submerges until the water is lapping against the base of the ears. The ears are then flickered in a circular movement, swirling the water up in fine droplets which prevent the flies from alighting'. Tsetse were not present in the area of Tinley's observations, but it seems clear that this reaction of the hippopotamus to Tabanidae would make it more difficult for tsetse to feed.

The following assessment of the interaction of Tabanidae with tsetse is quoted from Glasgow (1963).

'Fiske (1920) . . . describes an experiment in which the number of bites per hour (by wild *G. palpalis fuscipes*)[1] was counted on three cattle and on a monitor lizard (*Varanus* sp.). After a time biting flies of the genus *Tabanus* began to attack the cattle and caused them much annoyance. They would not permit the *Tabanus* to approach, and incidentally kept off the tsetse, so that the number of bites per hour fell to a fraction of its former value. The *Varanus*, however, was not attacked by the *Tabanus* and the number of bites by tsetse per hour recorded on it increased. I have myself noticed that on the approach of *Tabanus* sp. cattle become very restless and *G. swynnertoni* finds difficulty in feeding on them. Cattle are not important sources of food for either *G. palpalis fuscipes* or *G. swynnertoni* and one important point in Fiske's observation was that the *Varanus*, which *is* an important host of *G. palpalis fuscipes*,[1] was not attacked by *Tabanus*. Fiske made other observations on "several of the familar animals of Africa", of which only eland and zebra are named, in the Zoological Park at Washington. He noted that the animals varied in tolerance to biting flies, but none would tolerate flies which became too numerous and persistent. No figures are given but they would not be of much value since they would refer to exotic species of biting fly

'Lewis (1953), in a study of Tabanidae of the Sudan, concluded that these flies have a profound effect on the pastoral inhabitants, causing them to remove their stock from infested areas in the rains, and to undertake extensive migrations. The effect on *wild* animals is less clear. The views of Lewis are contained in the following quotation:

'Several observers have considered that Tabanids help to cause some of the migrations of game animals. . . . Balfour (1906) considered that Tabanids drove game north from Jebelein in the rains, and Tothill and others (1948, p. 147) mentioned wild game, as well as cattle, being driven north by biting flies. Tabanids are known to cause movements of wild animals in some other countries (Cameron, 1926; Darling, 1941, 1947; Edwards and others, 1939, p. 70). In Canada, caribou migrate in summer to places where there are few Tabanids. In Scotland Tabanids, more than anything else, drive the red deer to high grazing in July. The deer may receive thirty bites a minute from *Haematopota*, but it is the larger Tabanids which, partly by their buzzing, stampede the animals and may prevent grazing and milking. These flies are most active in sunlight

[1] Now designated *G.f. fuscipes.*

between 10 a.m. and 4 p.m. in hot still weather. Reindeer are among the animals affected in Europe.'

According to Cameron (1926), in Canada:

'the moose, deer and elk are so pestered by horse-flies during the summer months that they frequently betake themselves to the water of the numerous lakes to avoid annoyance.'

We note that the best established instances of migrations of wild animals being induced by biting flies are out of the tropics and that the migrations supposed to occur in tropical Africa do not involve tsetse areas. While it is a fact that migrations of some species of mammal do occur, their causes and significance are both complex and obscure, and it would not be easy to establish that blood-sucking flies were even a contributory cause in any particular case. Before claiming a migration as an example of other biting flies depriving tsetse of their food one would first require evidence that a migration of animals had resulted in hunger in tsetse. No unequivocal instance of this is known to the writer; the possible role of other biting flies may therefore be relegated to the status of an interesting possibility.

The alternative proposition is more plausible; that Tabanidae and other biting flies do not stampede host animals, but induce in them a state of irritation in which they defend themselves to such good effect that biting flies, including tsetse, have real difficulty in feeding. We have seen (pp. 368–9) that tsetse alone appear to induce such a state in their hosts, and it is easy to believe that when they are abundant the larger and clumsier Tabanidae would do so too. We may presume that this is one of the components of 'season', which has been shown to have a marked effect on the level of nutrition of *G. swynnertoni* and probably of other species as well (Glasgow & Bursell, 1961).

Predators and diseases of hosts. The artificial reduction of host numbers reduces tsetse populations, sometimes to the point of extermination (Potts & Jackson, 1952). Predators and diseases of hosts, which may reduce host numbers, are therefore adverse to the tsetse. The most spectacular and clear cut example of this is rinderpest. In 1890–6 a wave of this disease swept eastern Africa killing large numbers of cattle and of wild animals including wildebeest, kudu, sitatunga, buffalo, giraffe, eland, bushpig and warthog. After this (and as is now accepted, because of this) *G. morsitans* disappeared from the northern Transvaal and large areas in Southern Rhodesia and Tanganyika (Buxton, 1955; Ford, 1965). As rinderpest virus does not harm *Glossina* directly, it presumably acts by depriving the insect of food (Duke, 1919; Carmichael, 1933). Not all large mammals are destroyed by rinderpest; notable resistant species are elephant, rhinoceros and hippopotamus, but these were presumably too migratory, too few or too localized to support tsetse in the absence of other mammals.

The fact that this major change in numbers of wild mammals caused a major change in numbers and indeed in distribution of *Glossina* naturally makes one suppose that lesser changes in wild mammal numbers would cause lesser changes in numbers of tsetse. However, accurate studies of changes in wild mammal numbers are difficult and rare, and few have coincided with accurate studies of tsetse numbers. The situation studied by Fiske (1920) deserves mention. The Basesse people were evacuated from the Sesse Islands in Lake Victoria during the first decade of the century on account of an epidemic of Gambian sleeping sickness. Bush then grew up on the previously cultivated islands. Sitatunga antelopes, *Limnotragus spekii* invaded every island, but leopards, *Panthera pardus*, gained access only to some. On islands without leopards sitatunga and *G. fuscipes fuscipes* were very abundant, on those with leopards both were relatively rare.

It is reasonable to suppose that fluctuations in host numbers are often followed by corresponding fluctuations in numbers of tsetse, although it is only rarely that one is able to recognize cause and effect.

Enemies of Tsetse

Diseases of tsetse. There are no diseases of tsetse known to cause serious mortality. Foster (1963) collected from the literature twelve records of tsetse parasitized by Nematodes (7 *G. morsitans* and 5 *G. palpalis*). Foster found fifteen of 4,001 *G. palpalis* in Liberia infested with larval Mermithidae which he described and figured but did not identify. He thought that the tsetse probably became infected when resting on the ground. There is also a fungus disease (or diseases). Nash (1933) found a pathogenic Phycomycete infecting up to 20% of *G. morsitans* in one season in Tanganyika (*see* also p. 521). Van Hoof and Henrard (1934) lost whole boxes of *G. palpalis* from a fungus at Leopoldville. Lester (1934) recorded fungus infection rates of 33% in *G. morsitans* and 11% in *G. tachinoides* in Northern Nigeria in the wet season. Trypanosomiasis is, of course, from our point of view the most important infection of tsetse, since it is what this book is about. It is only doubtfully pathogenic and is considered in the next section.

Trypanosomiasis of tsetse. Certain species of the genus *Glossina* are liable to contract infection with trypanosomes. The infection is acquired when blood from an infected mammalian host is ingested. Under suitable conditions the parasite undergoes a cycle of development in the fly and, when this has been completed, the infection may be transmitted to a fresh vertebrate host when the tsetse feeds on it. The life cycle of the trypanosome in the invertebrate host and the groups of trypanosomes which are transmitted by species of tsetse have been described in detail in Chapter 1. So far as is known trypanosome infection is not in any way injurious to the fly and there has even been a suggestion (Baker, 1958) that, under comparable conditions, infected flies may live longer than uninfected flies. For further details of trypanosomiasis of tsetse flies the reader is referred to Glasgow (1963, pp. 101–5).

Predators of tsetse. An account of the predators and parasites of tsetse which have been investigated as possible methods of biological control of tsetse populations is given in Chapter 25. The subject of tsetse predators is also described in considerable detail by Glasgow (1963, pp. 109–17).

POPULATION DYNAMICS

Changes in Population Size

Regular catches of any species of tsetse in any one area are, of course, not constant. If one compares catches month by month, it may be that one detects a tendency for high catches to be associated with one season and low catches with another. Many investigators have reported long series of catches with such an annual rhythm; at least one has reported no sign of annual rhythm (Glasgow, 1954). An annual rhythm of catches has often been assumed to correspond with annual rhythmic population changes, but, as can be appreciated after study of the sampling methods described in Chapter 17, an alternative explanation of the observations could be that the population was constant, but annual rhythmic changes in the factors influencing the catching of tsetse produce annual rhythmic changes in catch. Some support for this extreme view is found in a study by Glasgow and Duffy (1961) of *G. pallidipes*: for eighteen months a population was sampled simultaneously by fly rounds and by traps, with such poor agreement that they did not feel justified in concluding that there had been real changes in the population. Jackson (1944), however, studied a population of *G.m. morsitans* by means of fly-rounds and simultaneous estimates of population by marking and recapture and found substantial agreement over fifty-eight months, concluding that 'catches of old males on fly rounds give at least a fairly good idea of concurrent changes in population'.

Jackson was not in this instance differentiating between population changes between and within years. Differences in catches between years can be ascribed to real changes in population more plausibly than can change within years; nevertheless the writer is inclined to agree that in many places there are regular changes in population with season, although these are less important than has often been supposed.

Fig. 15.3 shows monthly variations in apparent density of *G. swynnertoni* at Shinyanga, based on the unusually long run of twenty-two years continuous observation, 1935–56. The standard errors of the monthly catches are so large that not many of the months can be considered different. The November catch, however, is the lowest, and is clearly lower than that prevailing in the early part of the year. It is by no means certain that populations are lowest when catches are lowest. In another long investigation (1945–58) Glasgow and Bursell (1961) examined the size and fat content of the same flies. Fat content varied from month to month and was least in September; size likewise varied and was least in November. The puparial period and estimated mean age of the flies together totalled about two months, so that small flies in November suggested nutritional stress in September, when indeed low fat content had been observed. Nutritional stress may well be a cause of death, but it is likely to act immediately, not with a time lag. The coincidence of nutritional stress with high catches in September suggests that the stress conditions might have been making flies appear in the catches in relatively greater numbers than in other seasons, and makes it doubtful that the observed fall in catches from September to November corresponds with a change in the actual numbers of the population.

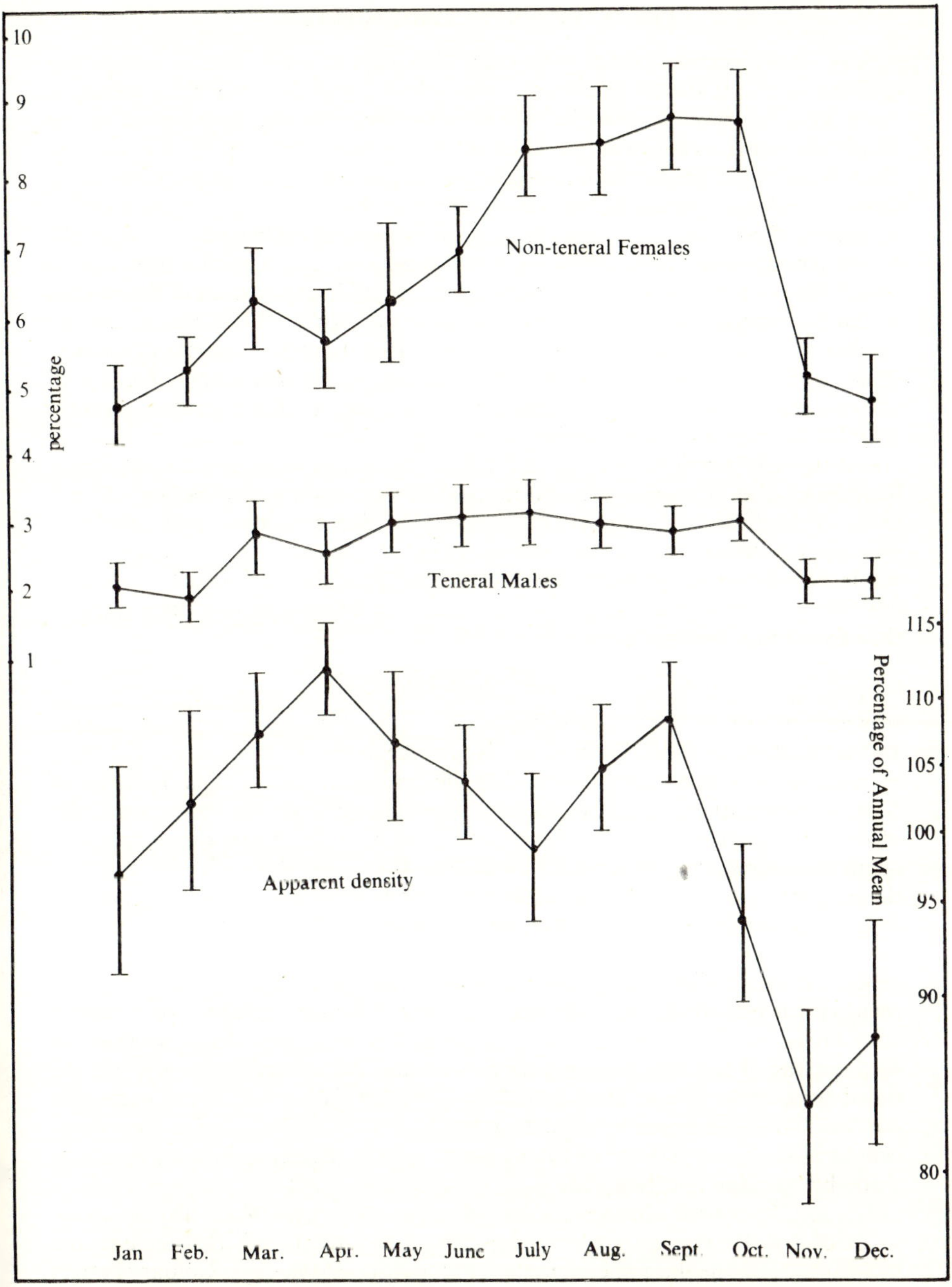

Fig. 15.3. *G. swynnertoni*, seasonal variations in apparent density, percentage of male flies that were teneral and percentage of non-teneral flies that were female. The extremities of each vertical line represent the mean value ± the standard error. The apparent density scale is logarithmic. (From Glasgow and Welch, 1962, Fig. 3)

Such considerations seem very much less cogent when one is comparing different years. If there are annual cycles which result in tsetse being easier to catch in some months than in others, such cycles would be expected to be much the same every year, so that it seems reasonable to ascribe marked changes in mean annual catch to changes in the size of the population being sampled, always provided that environmental conditions remain unchanged. If one interferes with the environment by, for example, destroying host animals, or the woody vegetation, then one would expect to alter the circumstances in which tsetse offer themselves to a catching party and interpretation of the catches would be accordingly complicated. Glasgow and Welch (1962) record annual catches of *G. swynnertoni* at Shinyanga from 1935 to 1957; this run of twenty-three years is believed to be the longest continuous observation of tsetse in any one place. The study area suffered a certain amount of interference, particularly in early years, from manipulation of grass fires, discriminative planting and clearing of portions of bush, and release of other species of *Glossina*. These happenings did not seem to make much difference to the catches, and do not seem to invalidate the main conclusion, that as the maximum catch, in 1954, was only eighteen times the minimum, in 1938, we were dealing with an unusually stable population of animals. This conclusion has been supported by Jordan (1965b) in a sixteen-year study of *G.p. palpalis*; here the maximum catch was less than four times the minimum.

Length of Life

It is not easy to determine the expectation of life, at birth, of any wild animal. Tsetse are no exception. Four methods have been used. Jackson (1948, 1953) by marking and recapture, showed that the death-rate was so high, in males of *G.m. morsitans* at least, that old age was seldom or never an important cause of death. Estimates of the death-rate indicated that the mean age of males at death was commonly between nineteen and twenty-six days. Confirmation of these figures was obtained by establishing the rate at which wings fray (Jackson, 1946). This was done by collecting large numbers of puparia of *morsitans* and *swynnertoni* and allowing them to emerge in each other's habitats. After emergence the exotic flies were collected at intervals—their age was known and a relation was established between age and the amount of damage to the trailing edge of the wing. There was much variation between individuals, so that the method was of little use for determining the age of any particular fly, but the mean age of a sample of thirty could be estimated with an error not exceeding one day. When Jackson applied this method to samples of *G.m. morsitans* caught in their own habitat he found estimated ages agreeing with his estimates made by marking and recapture.

Squire (1950) used changes in the colour of the wings of *G. palpalis* as an index of age. He recognized three age groups: smoky (blue), intermediate and tawny (old), but he did not equate the groups with ages in days. Colour changes occur in the wings of several tsetse species, and although the differences are small, it has seemed to the writer that the method should be capable of refinement. However, a shade matching expert was unable to see the difference between two extremes sent to him and the matter was not pursued.

Jackson's two methods of age determination were applicable only to males, females being caught in insufficient numbers either to estimate the death-rate or to calibrate the rate of wing fray. It was always clear that females must live longer than the three weeks or so which has repeatedly been estimated for males, since at 26°C a female will have produced only two larvae at thirty days and four at fifty days. However many may be the number of larvipositions necessary effectively to replace the mother and so ensure a stable population, this calculation in no way invalidates the estimates of male longevity, since the functions of the two sexes are quite different. If, as seems likely, only one copulation per life is normal in females, it follows (since equal numbers of the sexes emerge from puparia) that the mean number of copulations per male life is also one. This can be achieved in a life much shorter than three weeks.

Saunders (1962) has developed a method for determining the age of females by examining the ovaries. Details of the method are given elsewhere (Chapter 14). Working with *G. pallidipes* Saunders found striking differences in the age of different samples collected by different methods, those caught by hand as on a fly round being youngest, followed by those caught off a tethered ox, with trap-caught females the oldest. Of 287 females of *G. pallidipes* caught in traps, fifty-nine (21%) were in their fifth or a later ovulation cycle, and had presumably larviposited at least four times. The mean age of this sample was judged to be at least thirty-five days. This work, then, supports the general proposition that females must live considerably longer than the three weeks estimated for males. Since the sexes emerge from puparia in approximately equal numbers, it follows that, if females live longer, there must be more females than males in a wild population. Glasgow and Duffy (1961) found that of 42,000 *G. pallidipes* caught in traps, 78% were females; it is possible that the true female percentage in a wild population is not far from this figure.

Causes of Death

As we have seen, there is evidence that wild tsetse populations fluctuate in numbers, but not as much as other animals which have been studied in this respect. Although reproduction is slow, there is no doubt that tsetse populations could, if not checked, increase rapidly. In support of this statement, there are theoretical calculations (not completely satisfactory) by Buxton (1955) and Glasgow (1963) (*see* also p. 379); there is also a striking laboratory observation by Azevedo *et al.* (1964) of a fifty-fold increase in a laboratory colony in twelve months. Since such increases do not occur in nature, it seems that natural checks of some kind destroy tsetse in such a way as to keep populations very roughly constant. It is of interest to speculate as to what these important natural causes of death may be, but there is not much reliable information. The following facts seem to be important.

The limits of distribution of the genus are apparently set by temperature, lethal high temperatures on the edges of the Sahara and Kalahari, lethal low temperatures in Natal and the tropical highlands. Probably the distribution of individual species is likewise determined by climatic factors, the humidity experienced by puparia being critical in a number of species. It is easy to imagine that normal weather fluctuation saffect the edge of tsetse distribution, and cause populations to increase and decrease concomitantly, but there is little satisfactory evidence of this in nature.

Shortage of food can cause whole populations of tsetse to disappear, sometimes from large areas. Less serious shortages of food presumably cause populations to fall to a point short of extinction. When many tsetse attempt to feed on one host the host resists in various ways, so that there may well be a maximum number of tsetse which can live off a given number of hosts. This is perhaps the most plausible explanation of the relative constancy of tsetse populations. Shortage of food may act simply by starving unlucky members of the population, and also perhaps, in the case of females, by inducing abortions. Apparently ovulation occurs in alternate ovaries at intervals affected only by the temperature, but only properly nourished females can carry the resulting larva to full term. In the laboratory abortions are common: it is difficult to obtain a viable offspring from every ovulation. For example, the theoretical possible number of larvipositions by day 60 at 26°C is five; Nash *et al.*, in a long series of experiments give 2·0 viable offspring as the standard production after sixty days, and 4·3 as the result of one particular experiment. The balance had been aborted. Abortion has not been reported in nature. It is not surprising that direct observations of it have not been made, as natural larviposition of any kind has been seen only a very few times. Saunders' dissections, although they reveal the number of ovulations, do not reveal the number of full-term births. The laboratory evidence therefore makes it seem probable that abortions occur in nature, but no way of confirming this in the field has yet been devised.

Pupal parasites are sometimes an important cause of death, although quantitative work is not easy. Specific parasites such as some of the *Thyridanthrax* spp. may be supposed to become abundant when their host tsetse are abundant, and hence may control tsetse numbers, but this is pure speculation. Non-specific parasites such as *Syntomosphyrum* presumably fluctuate in numbers according to a complex of circumstances of which tsetse are only one, and consequently seem unlikely to control tsetse numbers. Several predators of tsetse puparia are on record (*see* Chapter 25); they have been invoked to explain the fall in tsetse numbers which sometimes follows the exclusion of grass fires (*see* also p. 566), but there seems little ground for supposing that they would destroy a greater proportion of tsetse puparia when tsetse were unusually numerous.

Web-building spiders are believed to eliminate tsetse from time to time on some small islands in Lake Victoria, but such elimination of tsetse by predators seems to be unusual. Another spider was shown to be an important cause of death of *G. swynnertoni* in Shinyanga (*see* p. 532), and there are many other animals which are known to prey on tsetse but whose predation has not been studied quantitatively.

It is clear that we are far from being able to assess the relative importance of different causes of death of even one species of *Glossina* in any one area, and there is therefore no point in attempting to generalize about the genus. It would be logical to attempt to augment any of the known causes of death with a view to eliminating tsetse. Conversely, diminution of any of the known causes of death must be expected to cause an increase in tsetse. Thus Game Parks must be expected to harbour tsetse as well as their hosts: one of the pleasures of visiting the Tsavo National Park in Kenya is to see *G. longipennis* and its favourite host *Diceros bicornis*. The use of non-specific insecticides involves the danger of destroying arthropod predators as well as tsetse: if the predators have powers of dispersal inferior to those of tsetse, there is a real risk of treated areas being invaded by tsetse which will find them temporarily more favourable than they were before.

If special importance is attached to identifying those causes of death which can be supposed to regulate tsetse numbers by killing a larger number in times of abundance, then food supplies and specific parasites seem, to the writer at least, to be the most likely candidates. This is in accordance with classical ecological theory, and seems reasonable and almost obvious. In the history of tsetse research, views which at one time seemed reasonable, and indeed obvious, have so often been disproved that one almost expects it to happen again.

The Innate Capacity for Increase in Numbers

A mathematical method for determining the intrinsic rate of natural increase of a population of animals was propounded by Birch (1948). The method was described by Andrewartha and Birch (1954) and its possible application to tsetse considered by Glasgow (1963). A quantity r_m is estimated, such that, beginning with a population of 1, the population alive after time t may be found from the value of $e^{r_m \cdot t}$.

For the estimation of r_m knowledge of two parameters is required; these are the female life table, that is, the probability at birth that a female will be alive at any given age and the fecundity rate at any given age. Since these quantities are affected by temperature and other conditions both must be determined for stated environments.

The mathematical treatment cannot well be presented in a condensed form and the interested reader is therefore referred to one of the authorities cited above. Glasgow (1963) noted that 'The innate capacity for increase has not been studied as such in tsetse but several workers have kept large colonies for experiments on transmission of trypanosomes and on insecticides. From their results and from physiological studies enough information is available to enable us to make at least a first approximation to the quantity r_m.' Information about the age-specific fecundity rate was unsatisfactory and two alternative values were adopted giving two alternative values of r_m. The first of these was undoubtedly the maximum possible and consequently yielded a maximum possible value of r_m. The second was based on experimental data and was considered to give a more likely value of r_m. Saunders (1967) has pointed out that as no laboratory cultures had, at that time, reproduced satisfactorily, the second assumed age-specific fecundity rate was probably too low as would be, therefore, the estimate of r_m based on it.

In the first two columns of Table 15.4 these two values of r_m are compared: it will be seen that if the higher value were correct, a tsetse population would double in fifty-three days and increase 117-fold in a year. With the lower value, 103 days are required for doubling and in a year the increase is barely twelve-fold.

TABLE 15.4

Comparison of the numbers of female tsetse alive after varying periods of time, calculated from two values of r_m ***(the intrinsic rate of natural increase, Glasgow, 1963) and two values of*** r ***(the actual rate of increase, Saunders, 1967)***

Days	r_m 0·0067113	r_m 0·013043	r 0·000177	r 0·006118
0	1	1	1	1
53	1·43	2·00	1·01	1·38
103	2·00	3·83	1·02	1·97
113	2·14	4·37	1·02	2·00
365	11·58	117·0	1·07	9·30

Saunders (1967) attempted to estimate r (the actual rate of increase) in a natural population of *G. palpalis palpalis* in Nigeria making use of his method of age determination by examination of the ovaries (p. 329) to estimate the life table. He obtained the values shown in the two right-hand columns of Table 15.4. In comparing these values with the theoretical maximum possible values given in the two left-hand columns, it is to be remembered that the two sets of values are not independent, as in the absence of new information about the age-specific fecundity rate Saunders was obliged to use the two extreme values given by Glasgow (1963).

As Saunders points out, the method is theoretically very attractive, since from a single observation one could, all being well, ascertain whether r is positive or negative: if it is negative the population is declining, a piece of information of particular interest when populations are being attacked. The term 'single observation' is used in a rather special sense, as Saunders dissected 117 females. However, a larger sample than this could be examined in a few weeks and if the results were reliable this would have clear advantages over the alternative methods of continually repeated sampling extending over many months.

Reliability is the difficulty. It is difficult to see how a reliable life table can be constructed until we know how to collect a sample of females which we can be sure is unbiased. Current work on laboratory maintenance of tsetse, in several laboratories, will probably soon produce greatly improved estimates of the age-specific fecundity rate but the problem of assigning fiducial limits to estimates of r is still unsolved. Until this can be done there will be reluctance to accept estimates of r, from however massive a single observation, as conclusive evidence that a particular population is declining or not declining.

Finally, it is perhaps worth quoting the reservoir analogy from Glasgow (1963). 'The reservoir gains water through a number of tributary streams and direct precipitation and loses water through the outlet pipe by leakage and by evaporation. If we could measure all these sources of gain and loss we could express the answer in the form of a single figure R, and if R were positive the level of water would rise, and if it were negative the level of water would fall. In a dry summer the level of water would fall but this would not be "explained" by saying that R was negative.' In other words, it is misleading to think of R, which is a measure of a large number of relevant factors, as being the cause of a decline. It is these factors, whose joint total effect is measured by R (or *r*) which are important, and are causal.

Chapter 16

Dispersal and Concentration of *Glossina*

E. BURSELL

INTRODUCTORY

To review the problem of tsetse dispersal it is necessary to go quite far back in history of tsetse research, since there has been little progress in this field during the past decade. Much of the early work was based on the recapture of marked flies and current stagnation may perhaps be attributed in part to a growing disenchantment among tsetse ecologists with this method of investigation. A great deal of time has invariably to be devoted to the careful organization of marking and recapture programmes, but the results obtained, in so far as they bear on the issue of dispersal, are often so few and of such questionable value that they seldom reach the stage of publication. The present review must therefore centre on the work of tsetse ecologists who wrote in more leisurely times, when brevity was not considered the essence of scientific communication, and to stay within the bounds of modern convention it has been necessary to adopt a selective approach. Attention will be concentrated on the work of Dr C. H. N. Jackson, which provides the finest example of the work of this period in point of sophistication, both of technique and of interpretation. A mass of information relevant to the problem of dispersal is furnished by other writers of the period but failure to incorporate such material will not significantly weaken the basis of such conclusions as may be drawn; it will, however, limit them to the savanna species of tsetse with which Jackson worked, but they are in any case the only ones for which a substantial body of information is available.

THE RATE OF DISPERSAL

The most direct evidence on the rate of dispersal of tsetse flies comes from the artificially isolated tsetse populations described by Jackson (1946, 1948a). Flies were released at a central release point as they emerged from their puparia, and the area surrounding the release point was uniformly sampled at daily intervals following release, to determine the average rate of dispersal. The mean distance of capture points from the release point, during successive weeks, is shown in Fig. 16.2b, and it will be seen that dispersal tends to occur at the rate of rather less than 200 yards per week, except for the first week during which substantially higher rates were recorded.

Similar values for dispersal rates were obtained by Jackson (1941a, 1944, 1948) during a long-term marking and recapture project carried out at Kakoma in central Tanganyika. Again there was a high initial rate of dispersal, with males travelling a distance of about 700 yards during the first week, but subsequently the rate dropped to an average of 200 yards per week.

A number of independent lines of evidence lends some support to the view that dispersal rates are of the order of 200 yards a week. The subject has been well reviewed by Glasgow (1963) and a brief summary will suffice for present purposes:

(a) the re-invasion of an area from which *Glossina morsitans submorsitans* had been eradicated by means of residual insecticide was found to take place at the rate of about one mile per month or 400 yards per week (Davies & Blasdale, 1960).

(b) The application of residual insecticide along parallel lines 200 yards apart took 1–2 weeks to produce a 95% reduction in the catch of *G. pallidipes*, suggesting dispersal rates of about 150 yards per week (Thomson *et al.*, 1961).

(c) An advance of *G. morsitans morsitans* into mature woodland was studied by Jackson (1933) who estimated the rate of advance to be 2–3 miles per year or about 100 yards per week, and similar rates have been reported for advances of *G. morsitans orientalis* in Rhodesia (Jack, 1914; Ford, 1961; Robertson & Kluge, 1968).

The concurrence of estimates based on such widely different methods of assessment inclines one to an acceptance of a weekly dispersal rate of about 200 yards as a well-founded fact of tsetse biology. It should not be overlooked, however, that each of these estimates is subject to its own particular type of error, and that the concurrence might, in fact, be spurious. The artificially isolated populations of Jackson, for instance, had, for purposes of identification, to be released in the habitat of another species of tsetse and it is possible that rates of dispersal would have been different in the species' own habitat; the necessity to mark flies in Jackson's other experiments may have had an effect on dispersal rate, though it had none on survival; the assessment of rates of advance into insecticide-treated areas was based on sampling techniques which are known to be unreliable when densities are low; and the rate at which a tsetse population invades a new habitat on a long term basis might be limited by factors other than dispersal. It would be an unlikely coincidence if these various sorts of error should all affect estimates of dispersal in the same way, to produce the same answer, but it would be just the sort of coincidence of which tsetse workers have learnt to beware. For purposes of the present discussion the estimate of 200 yards a week will be accepted, but not without reservation.

There is another kind of evidence which, while it provides no information about dispersal rate, yet confirms the image of the tsetse as an essentially local insect, with rates of dispersal which are low in relation to its powers of flight. This evidence is subject only to the error of biased sampling, from which no investigation of tsetse biology is free. It shows that samples of male *Glossina morsitans*, taken from areas no more than a few miles apart, can be distinguished on the basis of fat content and of size (Bursell, 1966a). Since the fat content of males reflects their success in host encounter during previous hunger cycles, and their size reflects the nutritional state of the females by whom they were deposited a month or more before capture, the results suggest that the exchange of individuals between parts of the population which inhabit closely adjacent regions of the general habitat is limited, as would be expected if dispersal rates are low.

THE ACTIVITY OF TSETSE FLIES

An estimate has been given above of the rate at which tsetse flies disperse through their habitat, and it would be instructive to compare this with estimates of the proportion of time that a tsetse spends in flight, and of the distance that it would be expected to cover in a given interval of time. Unfortunately there is very little information available on this point and what there is is of doubtful value.

Investigation of the behaviour of tsetse flies in the laboratory indicates that they tend to spend most of the time at rest. The frequency with which movements were recorded in a study of the effect of humidity on activity ranged from an average of once an hour in dry air to once in two hours in humid air for tenerals and hungry non-tenerals (Bursell, 1957), with the level of activity low at mid-day and higher during morning and afternoon periods. Automatic recording of the activity of tsetse flies in small cages showed considerable variability between individuals and a general increase in activity in the course of starvation with an average of less than 5% of the total time spent in activity (Bursell, 1959a). Recent experiments using flies tagged with radioactive material in large cages (Dean, Williamson & Phelps, 1969) confirm the impressions gained with small cages, that the frequency of movement is low. It is unfortunately not possible to estimate the extent to which, in all of these experiments, results may have been influenced by the abnormal conditions to which the flies were exposed. Earlier observations by Whiteside at Shinyanga, not published but mentioned by Potts (1950a), with several species of tsetse confined in small cages in the laboratory, support the observations described in the last two paragraphs.

Estimates of considerably greater relevance to the natural situation, but of correspondingly low accuracy, have been based on changes in the fat content of teneral flies and on the amino acid content of non-teneral flies captured in the field. The rate at which fat reserves diminish during successive days following emergence of *G. morsitans* from pupae exposed in the habitat of *G. swynnertoni* has been estimated by Bursell (1959a), and it has been calculated that a period of approximately fifteen minutes may be spent in flight during the course of a day. This would represent about 2% of daylight hours, in reasonable accord with results for caged flies, but in view of the errors involved to be taken as no more than a rough indication.

Unfortunately, a similar approach cannot be made to the activity of non-teneral flies because of the extremely variable fat content of flies that have had an opportunity to feed (e.g. Bursell, 1961). The only information which is available is that non-teneral males captured as they come in to feed at a bait animal have a very low content of proline, which suggests that they have been active for a period of not less than five minutes prior to capture, perhaps for much longer (Bursell & Slack, 1968).

In the, admittedly poor, light of these results it would seem that tsetse flies tend to be rather inactive, and that the daily duration of flight activity in hungry males exceeds five minutes and is possibly of the order of 10–15 minutes. During early parts of the hunger cycle the level of activity is likely to be substantially less and for purposes of the discussion which follows a value of ten minutes will be adopted as an estimate of the average daily flight period.

THE RELATION BETWEEN FLIGHT ACTIVITY AND DISPERSAL

The flight speed of tsetse flies has not been carefully investigated. It would undoubtedly vary considerably, depending on the type of activity in which the fly is engaged. As a matter of common observation it is known that flies following a catching party fly at about the speed of the party, which would be 2–3 miles per hour. On the other hand, it is usually necessary to drive at speeds in excess of fifteen miles per hour in order to prevent the entry of tsetse into motor vehicles. A flight speed of seven miles per hour would seem a reasonable compromise between these two extremes.

A tsetse fly travelling at seven miles per hour for a period of ten minutes would move a distance of some 2,000 yards; if it moved in a straight line its daily rate of dispersal would therefore be 2,000 yards as compared with estimated dispersal rates of about thirty yards per day. If this seventy-fold discrepancy is not to be attributed to errors in one or both of the estimates on which it is based, then it must be resolved on the basis of a consideration of the nature of dispersal. The pattern of movement of tsetse flies must be such, in other words, as to reconcile a very low rate of dispersal with a relatively high daily flight distance and there are a number of ways in which this could come about.

THE PATTERN OF DISPERSAL

One of the hypotheses which could be used to reconcile the discrepancy between flight duration and dispersal rate is firmly embedded in the tsetse literature and will be considered first. This is the so-called *feeding ground hypothesis* of tsetse behaviour as propounded and substantiated by Dr C. H. N. Jackson in a series of papers based on field investigations of *G. morsitans* and *G. swynnertoni* in central Tanganyika (Jackson, 1930, 1933a, 1937, 1941a, 1944, 1948).

The Feeding Ground Concept

The hypothesis envisages that the habitat of tsetse flies comprises distinct regions, in particular, areas of relatively open ground, which can be characterized as 'feeding grounds', and areas of homogeneous woodland which constitute the 'home' of the fly; and that there is a general movement of the tsetse population between these two regions, flies moving to one or the other depending on their state of hunger. Individuals could then be considered as moving in fairly well-defined 'ambits' restricted by different vegetation types and such a movement would clearly satisfy the requirement for long flight and low dispersal, in so far as flies might move far from their home to the feeding ground but they would tend to return to the place from which they came, and the rate of long-term dispersal would be low.

This interpretation of tsetse behaviour is supported by a wealth of observation and, in Jackson's later papers, by a critical analysis of marking and recapture records. It affords a satisfying explanation of much that would otherwise be puzzling; it has found fairly general acceptance among tsetse ecologists and it has stood well the test of time. During the last few years, however, results have accumulated which throw some doubt upon it as a general interpretation of tsetse behaviour. Since the question of its validity is crucial in relation to the problem of dispersal, it will be necessary to give some account of the objections which may be raised to the feeding ground hypothesis in the light of recent work, and to re-examine its theoretical basis and the evidence which supports it.

The work of Pilson and Pilson (1967 and in preparation) would appear to provide a particularly strong challenge to the feeding ground hypothesis. These authors investigated the biology of *G. morsitans* in an area south of Lake Kariba, using two different sampling techniques—the standard 'fly-round' sample (on which virtually all of Jackson's work was based), and the 'bait' sample, which comprised flies caught in the act of feeding from a stationary bait animal. In the region where they worked the tsetse population, as judged by sampling procedures, appeared to be strongly concentrated on riverine vegetation during the hot, dry season, and the situation would appear to be interpretable in the general terms of the feeding ground hypothesis. The shady riverine vegetation would constitute the home of the population, with adjacent and more open vegetation types serving as feeding grounds. Analysis of catches during the hot season, however, showed a spectacular difference between the two sampling methods. The fly-round catches were in accord with the traditional view of a strong concentration of flies in the riverine vegetation, but the bait catches suggested that, in fact, the population, and certainly the female population, was much more evenly dispersed through the different vegetation types. Even the barren *Colophospermum mopane* woodland, with not a blade of green, returned female catches off bait animals which were little if at all lower than those of the evergreen riverine vegetation.

These results raise the very serious question whether investigations of tsetse ecology have not been bedevilled throughout their history by a vicious sampling bias, almost reaching the dimensions of a practical joke. Virtually all of our activities have been based on the distribution of male flies as assessed by standard fly-round catches, and it now appears that these may have given a completely misleading picture of the distribution of the general population. One must hesitate to draw sweeping conclusions on the basis of a single investigation of *G. morsitans* in one particular part of its range, but the results are sufficiently startling to warrant urgent attention.

Beside this finding, of an even distribution of tsetse flies in their habitat, other objections which may be raised against the feeding ground concept may seem trivial, but they will be briefly listed since they support what seems now to be a convincing argument in favour of a re-assessment of the situation:

(a) In many areas where the apparent distribution of *G. morsitans* conforms to the feeding ground concept, the distances which separate different elements of the general habitat, between which the insects are supposed to move, are often substantial, and through woodlands which are often featureless. A movement in regular 'ambits' would, under such conditions, pose formidable demands on the tsetse fly's capacity for navigation.

(b) One of the most depressing features of investigations involving marking and recapture in local situations (e.g. Pilson & Pilson, 1967) is the relatively small proportion of marked flies which are ever recaptured. Percentage recaptures may drop to very low values compared with those which can be attained when the area involved is extensive (e.g. Jackson, 1937) or when flies are confined by natural barriers (Dr D. A. Dame, personal communication). If flies do move in ambits, and thus tend to return to the place where they were captured, one would not expect any substantial difference under these different sets of conditions.

(c) Recent work by Dean and his colleagues (Dean, Paget & Wilson, 1969) is also difficult to reconcile with the feeding ground concept. These authors reasoned that, if there were a tendency for flies to move in ambits and to return to the place from which they came, then there should be a possibility of building up a population of flies by providing a constant source of food in an appropriate region of the habitat. In the event it proved impossible to cause any detectable increase in fly densities by long-term, checker-board tethering of oxen, or by the herding of oxen in permanent paddocks.

It is not claimed that these considerations, taken singly or together, constitute anything like an unanswerable challenge to the feeding ground hypothesis. But in view of the difficulty of accommodating them within the framework of that hypothesis, it would seem worthwhile to re-examine its basis, and to consider whether the results on which it is founded would be capable of being interpreted in such a way as to embrace the later findings. For reasons of space it will not be possible to discuss every observation which may be adduced as evidence in favour of the feeding ground hypothesis, and consideration will be limited to what, in the writer's view, constitutes its main ground namely:

1. that a distinction can be drawn between parts of the habitat in which females and hungry flies predominate (the feeding ground), and other parts in

which males and less hungry flies predominate, in samples taken by standard catching parties (Jackson, 1937).

2. that flies marked in any particular place are often recaptured in another, and then re-captured near the place where they were originally marked (Jackson, 1937).

3. that the rate of emigration of marked flies from a marking area is high during the first week after marking, but falls thereafter to a low level (Jackson, 1941a); this is interpreted on the basis of 'ambits', which initially carry the flies out of the marking area but by which they later return.

In view of what has been said concerning the sampling bias which appears to be involved in fly-round catches, the first category of evidence cannot be considered to carry much conviction, especially since the weight of bias would be expected to vary in specific relation to nutritional state (Bursell, 1961). Results based on marking and recapture would, however, appear to be substantially free from such objection and what needs to be considered, therefore, is whether the second and third categories of evidence are capable of interpretation on a basis other than that of the feeding ground hypothesis. An attempt has been made to provide an answer to this question by consideration of a simple model of dispersal.

The Concept of Random Movement

The model to be considered is based on the assumption that the direction of movement of a tsetse fly in a two-dimensional system is random. On this assumption hypothetical displacements of a tsetse fly have been determined by dividing the circle into ten segments each of 36° (substantially the same result is obtained if 100 segments, each of 3·6° are used) and establishing the successive directions of movements by reference to a table of random numbers. An example of such a hypothetical track is shown in Fig. 16.1, a. From a number of such tracks it is possible to establish a relation between the number of displacements, each of one displacement unit (*see* Fig. 16.1), and the distance moved from the point of origin; in terms of the tsetse, this would be the relation between flight distance and dispersal.

Curve (i) of Fig. 16.2 (a) illustrates this relation for comparison with the rate of displacement which would have occurred had the movement been in a straight line from the origin or 'release point' (shown as curve (iii)), when the dispersal distance would equal the number of displacements. Two points of interest emerge from a consideration of these graphs:

(a) the rate of dispersal by random movement (i) is high to begin with, but falls gradually to what would appear to be a steady low value.

(b) the steady-state rate of dispersal is about 4% of the actual distance moved (as given by curve (iii)).

If curve (i) is compared with the actual dispersal of tsetse flies from a central release point, as established by Jackson (1946) in his main release (the only one which involved substantial numbers of recaptures during the first five weeks) a general similarity of pattern is obvious (*cf.* Fig. 16.2, a,b), which suggests that

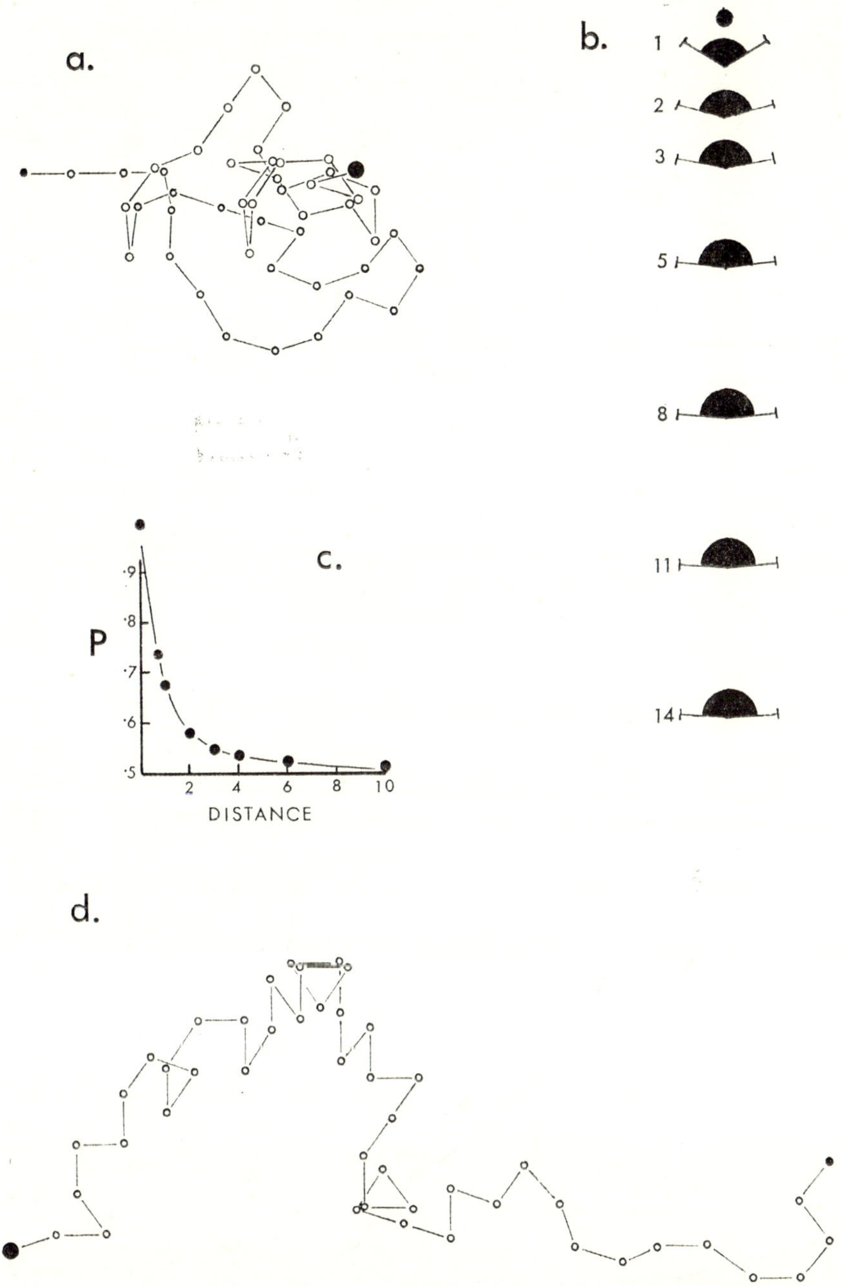

Fig. 16.1 (a) A hypothetical track showing displacement from the origin (•) by random movement. Successive open circles are separated by a distance of one 'displacement unit', which is the distance moved every time a movement is made. (b) Diagrammatic illustration of the progressive increase in the probability of movement towards a release point (●) as the distance from the release point increases. The filled-in angles give the probability of movement towards the origin; they are subtended by chords of one displacement unit's length drawn from points on the circumference of circles with radii of 1, 2, 3, etc., displacement units as indicated. (c) The probability (P) of moving away from the release point as a function of distance (in displacement units) from the release point. (d) A hypothetical track showing displacement from the origin during movement which is random except for a 10% bias towards the 'east'. For further explanation see text.

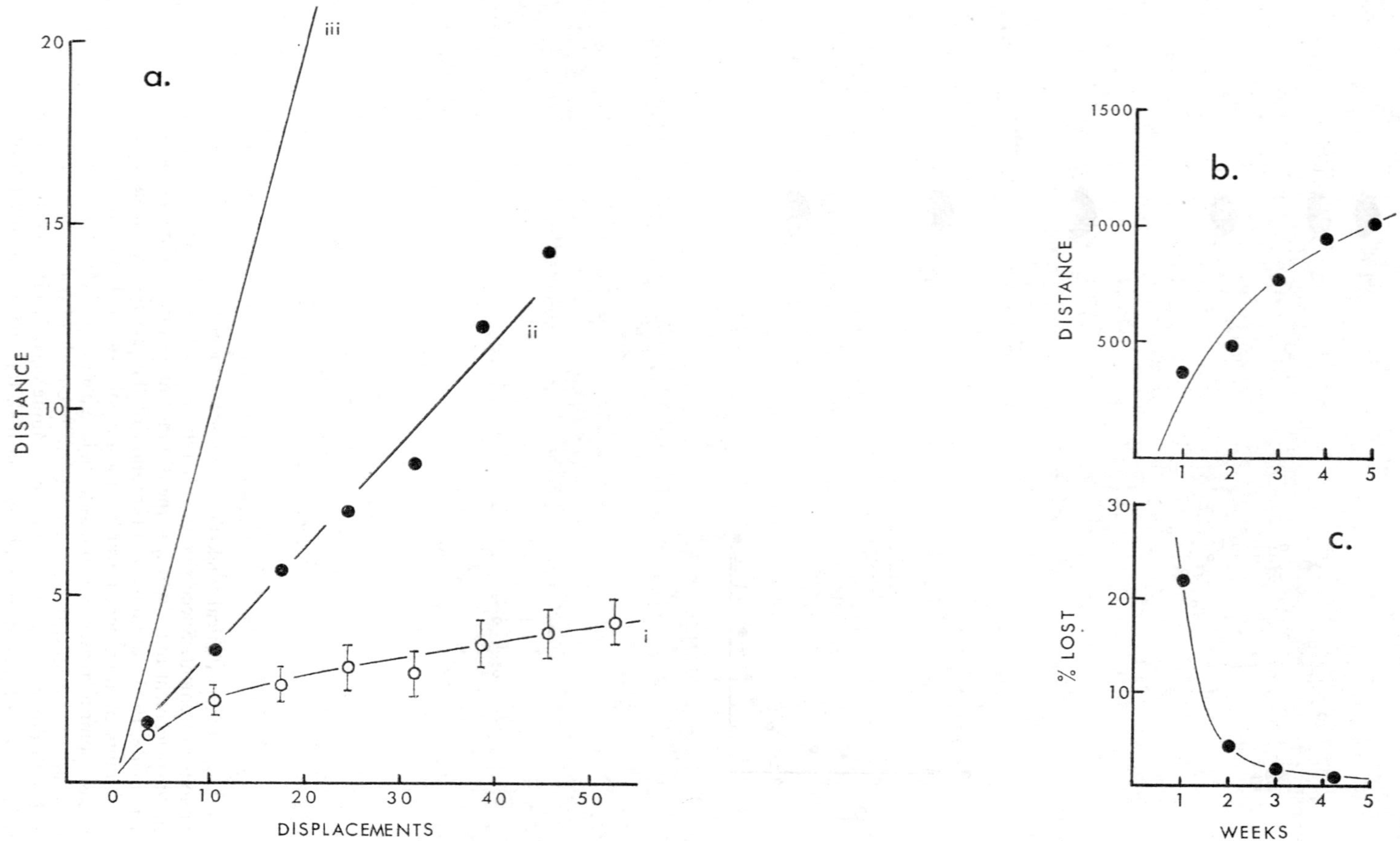

Fig. 16.2 (a) The relation between the number of displacements and the distance moved from the point of origin, both expressed in terms of the unit of displacement. Curve (i) random movement (95% fiducial limits are given by vertical lines through the means); (ii) movement with 10% bias; (iii) movement in a straight line. (b) The mean distance (in yards) moved by *G. morsitans*, released from puparia at a central release point in the habitat of *G. swynnertoni*, during successive weeks following release (data from Jackson, 1946). (c) The percentage of males of *G.* [illegible] (data from Jackson, (1940). For further explanation see text.

the model may not be entirely inappropriate. Furthermore, it would seem that the concept of random movement might be able to provide a basis of interpretation for one of the mainstays of the feeding ground hypothesis, namely the rapid initial emigration of tsetse flies from the marking area. However, both model and release experiments involve releases from a point, and the crucial question is whether the situation would be similar when flies are released in an area, as they were in Jackson's marking recapture experiment, rather than from a point.

It has already been pointed out by Glasgow (1963) that one reason for the rapid dispersal from a point during early phases is that initial movements of a fly can only be away from the point of release; it is only later that it can move either away from or towards the point of origin. It will be clear, however, from the illustration shown in Fig. 16.1, b, and the graph of Fig. 16.1, c which is derived from it, that the differential is not confined to the initial movement. The chances that a fly has of moving towards, or away from, the release point (given respectively by the angle which embraces the release point and the angle which excludes it in Fig. 16.1, b) do not become equal until the fly has moved sufficiently far from the release point to make its path along a circle centred on the release point effectively a straight line; and they remain grossly unequal so long as the fly remains within two displacement units of the release point (Fig. 16.1, c). In view of this it is clear that a general tendency towards rapid dispersal during early stages will characterize release from an area as well as release from a point, provided the area is not too large in relation to the unit of displacement.

In view of these considerations it becomes of interest to re-examine Jackson's data on the rate of emigration (Table 6 in Jackson, 1941a). The results are expressed as the percentage of male flies which are lost from the marking area during successive weeks, and since no seasonal differences could be detected, it has seemed legitimate to sum the results, and they have been plotted as such in Fig. 16.2, c. This shows that there is a progressive fall in the rate at which flies are lost from the experimental block, rather than the distinction which Jackson envisaged between a high rate during the first week followed by a steadily maintained low rate in later weeks. A progressive fall is, in fact, precisely what would be expected in view of the increasing chance that a fly has of moving towards the release area as it disperses away from it. It would seem, therefore, that the concept of a movement in 'ambits', by which flies leave and re-enter the marking area, might not be indispensable to an interpretation of the results. It may be mentioned, too, that the idea of an ambit associated with a hunger cycle which in the hot season averages no more than three days (Jackson, 1954b), as responsible for an exodus from the marking area that exceeds the five-day interval between marking and recapture, is not easy to accept.

The second main point in favour of the feeding ground hypothesis is the tendency for marked flies to return to the region of their first capture, and this has also been explored in terms of the model of random movement. Analysis of the twenty-two available tracks showed that ten 'flies' never re-visited an area within half a displacement unit's radius of the release point. Of the twelve that did, five returned after prolonged 'absences' (of more than ten displacement units) from the region. It would seem that it is not necessary to invoke a concept of 'ambit'-movement in order to explain the return of flies to a region near the point of original release after a visit to parts of the habitat which may be far removed from it.

Since the concept of random dispersal appears to be capable of furnishing a satisfactory basis for the observations which form the main evidence in favour of the feeding ground hypothesis, it remains to determine whether it is also in accord with those observations which cannot readily be interpreted on the feeding ground hypothesis, and most importantly, whether it can provide an equally convincing basis for a resolution of the discrepancy between flight distance and dispersal rate in tsetse flies.

If there is a random drift of individuals through the general habitat, as would be expected on the basis of random movement, then one would expect:

(a) a fairly even distribution of all elements of the population in the different vegetation types that comprise the habitat,
(b) that the rate of recapture in local situations would be low, and,
(c) that attempts to build up a fly population around a local concentration of bait animals would fail.

The hypothesis of random movement would thus seem capable of reconciling evidence which, on the basis of the feeding ground hypothesis, would be in conflict.

To examine the second question it is necessary to return to a consideration of the relation between flight distance and dispersal rate (Fig. 16.2, a), which showed that the rate of random dispersal is approximately 4% of the flight distance. With an estimated daily flight distance of 2,000 yards this would give a dispersal rate of some eighty yards per day, still somewhat high in relation to actual estimates of dispersal rates, but with the discrepancy reduced to manageable proportions. It is possible that the remaining discrepancy could be accounted for by taking into consideration factors that have not been incorporated into the theoretical model, but which would govern the actual movement of tsetse flies in their natural habitat. It is known, for instance, that the boles and branches of trees are often used as resting sites by tsetse flies (Pilson & Leggate, 1962a; Pilson & Pilson, 1967). It might not be legitimate to consider that an insect resting on the bole of a tree has an equal chance of taking off in any direction; in view of the obstacle which the tree would provide to flight in some directions, the insect might be more likely to take off in the general direction from which it has come than in any other. The introduction of such a to-and-fro bias would depress dispersal rates below the level which would be expected on the basis of a completely random flight direction.

It seemed of interest to investigate the consequences of introducing another kind of bias into the model, a bias such as might be associated with a tendency to orientate towards larger features of the environment, for instance an ecotone between vegetation types or a belt of riverine vegetation. To simulate such a tendency a 10% bias was incorporated, and an example of the sort of track which results is shown in Fig. 16.1, d. On the basis of an analysis of a number of such tracks the relation between flight distance and dispersal rate was calculated, and the results are plotted as curve (ii) in Fig. 16.2. It is clear that the introduction of even such a slight bias causes an enormous increase in the rate of dispersal, which now attains to about 30% of flight distance. This is of interest in two contexts. On the one hand it furnishes a theoretical basis for the very high dispersal rates which appear to characterize species of tsetse fly that inhabit 'linear' environments, such as *G. palpalis* (Nash & Page, 1953). On the other hand, it suggests that if the hypothesis of 'ambit' movement is to be sustained, it must be on the basis of an extremely accurate orientation to features of the environment. A general tendency to orientate in relation to massive features would produce a high rather than a low rate of dispersal. What would be required in order to confine dispersal within the limits of observed rates would be something much more akin to territorial behaviour, based on a 'knowledge' of minute details of the environment. In view of the featureless nature of many of the vegetation types inhabited by tsetse flies of the savanna species, such a concept could not easily be accepted on general grounds, nor could it be reconciled with the evidence of low recapturability in local situations.

CONCLUSIONS

A survey of the evidence on dispersal in tsetse flies has uncovered what appears to be a formidable discrepancy between the distance that a tsetse fly is thought to fly and the rate at which it is thought to disperse. Granted that it is a real one, and not based on erroneous estimates, this discrepancy is capable of being resolved on the feeding ground hypothesis, which postulates that there is a tendency for tsetse flies to return to the place from which they set out. This concept, however, is not easy to reconcile with recent findings, and it is for this reason that an attempt has been made to put forward an alternative basis for interpretation. The concept of random movement appears to be capable, in very general terms, of accounting for most of the results which have a bearing on the problem of dispersal. In putting it forward the writer would not like it to be thought that he, in fact, regards the flight of tsetse flies as being directionally random. Much work has been done to show that the flight of tsetse flies is influenced by visual stimuli (e.g. Barrass, 1960). But the writer would suggest the possibility that the direction of tsetse flight in the natural environment may be effectively random, in the sense that it is random in relation to the space/time co-ordinates which are appropriate to a consideration of dispersal; and that any directional tendencies are superimposed on such a general random drift. In view of the experimental work of Jack and Williams (1937) and of the field observations of Pilson and Leggate (1962a) one could imagine, for instance, that during the heat of the day tsetse flies might direct their flight towards dark and shady points of their immediate environment, with a return to lighter and more open regions during cool parts of the day, and that similar predilections might characterize different stages of the hunger cycle. But such local and temporary responses would constitute the fine detail of a longer term and spatially extensive drift, and it is this drift which is considered to be random in point of direction. In the writer's opinion this concept forms a better interim basis of interpretation than does the feeding ground theory. Unfortunately there seems to be little hope of putting these alternative hypotheses to any kind of crucial test, since it is doubtful whether it would be possible to design a marking and recapture experiment which could adequately distinguish between them. It may be that tsetse ecologists have long ago gone about as far as one can usefully go on the basis of marking and recapture programmes, and that significant progress in the study of dispersal, and perhaps of tsetse biology in general, must await the development of techniques which will enable individual flies to be tagged and followed continuously in their natural environment.

Chapter 17

Methods for the Collecting and Sampling of *Glossina*

J. P. GLASGOW, R. J. PHELPS

PUPARIAL STAGES

(R. J. PHELPS)

Methods of Collecting

The most usual way of locating puparia of *Glossina* is to search the soil in suitable sites by hand. This technique is tedious but workers become skilled in the recognition of sites likely to yield puparia and considerable quantities may be collected. The degree of success achieved by individuals varies widely and the subjective nature of the method makes it unsuitable for quantitative work.

In wet weather the yield of puparia in terms of man-hours of hand-searching drops to a small proportion of the yield under dry conditions. Two major causes for this are the more dispersed nature of the tsetse population in the rainy season (Nash, 1939), and the greater difficulty in detecting puparia when the soil is damp and adhesive (Burtt, 1952). It has often been suggested that unknown breeding sites are used by tsetse in wet weather but, while this cannot be ruled out completely, those puparia which have been found in wet weather have nearly all come from generally recognized breeding sites. It seems that the lack of climatic limitation on the movements of tsetse in wet weather enables them to use breeding sites which are less readily identified by collectors and so puparia are spread over many more breeding sites and are found only in small numbers, if at all, in each site. When tsetse are under climatic stress, the breeding sites selected conform more closely to the classical concept and are more easily recognized. Consequently, puparia are found in considerable numbers in some sites and as searchers tend to concentrate on such sites, many less fruitful sources of puparia are passed by and the numbers of puparia collected fall far short of the number actually deposited.

Some workers have attempted to improve yields of puparia by the use of sieves (Phelps, Simmonds & Parsons, 1966). This has not proved to be very effective as sieving of the soil is very time-consuming and more puparia can be found in the same period of time by hand searching. However, more ground will be covered by hand searching and undoubtedly many puparia will be missed (Jewell, 1958a) whereas conscientious sieving will recover all puparia in the selected plot. One situation in which sieves (No. 7 mesh) have been useful is in searching soil in animal burrows. Soil in these situations is often of very fine texture and sieving is rapid. Sieves also help in scooping soil out of burrows and, with the aid of a small sieve, searchers can reach into large burrows for distances up to 6 feet. Puparia are frequently collected from such places in the hot season in deciduous woodland (Phelps *et al.*, *loc. cit*).

Another technique which has been used is flotation in water (Abedi & Miller, 1963) but the method obviously depends on water being readily available. The method consists of pouring soil from breeding sites into a bucket of water and stirring. Puparia float to the surface and it is claimed that all present can be recovered. Subsequent emergence of flies from puparia collected in this manner is as good as that obtained from puparia collected by hand.

Potts (personal communication) has drawn attention to the possibility of using a combination of the flotation and sieving methods which would afford a useful device for searching the general woodland floor, especially during the wet season. A rather crude machine for this purpose was designed at the Tanganyika Research Station at Shinyanga some twenty-five years ago but a description of it was not published. By this means, one or two puparia of *G. pallidipes* were discovered during examination of a large area of surface soil in a thicket of *Euphorbia tirucalli* which had been planted as an experimental evergreen barrier against the passage of *G. swynnertoni*. Occasional adults of *G. pallidipes* had been known to occur in this thicket but it was not suspected that this species was breeding there.

The Breeding Site

The brief descriptions of the types of sites known to be used by various species of *Glossina* (*see* Chapter 14) indicate, as Buxton (1955) points out, that the requirements of all species are similar after allowance has been made for the difference in the habitats used by adults of different species. This contention is supported by the recovery from similar breeding sites of puparia of flies living in completely different regions, e.g. *G. palpalis* from sandy beaches in East Africa (Carpenter, 1920) and *G. morsitans* from sandy river beds in Rhodesia (Chorley, 1929). Further support comes from the fairly frequent reports of the occurrence of puparia of more than one species of tsetse in the same breeding site.

Experimental work on the selection of breeding sites by *G. palpalis* (Parker, 1956) has produced some interesting results. Preference was shown for dark vertical surfaces rather than dark horizontal surfaces, and dark soils were preferred to light ones. Leaf litter covering light soils made these more attractive than the same soil without the litter. Loose soil was preferred to compacted soil, a feature often commented on in the field, although in the laboratory larviposition and puparial formation takes place in glass tubes with no soil in them and Lloyd (1914) showed that in the field larviposition did take place on compacted soil. Damp soil was shown to be less attractive than dry soil and on waterlogged soil no puparial formation took place, which is confirmed by laboratory work by Burtt (1952). It is known from the work of Buxton and Lewis (1934) that puparia of *G. morsitans* and *G. tachinoides* do not survive two days in waterlogged soil. In the work done by Parker (1956) there was no evidence that the fly responded to any stimulus other than sight when selecting a site for larviposition. These results are important in that they show that the pregnant female selects sites for larviposition likely to be favourable for the development of the puparial stages and does not merely larviposit in resting sites which are attractive to the adult fly.

It was suggested by Buxton (1955) that puparial sites could be divided into two main classes, those above ground level which are mainly rot holes in trees and those in or on the ground. With the experimental evidence given by Parker (1956) and the relationship between response to light and temperature discussed by Jack and Williams (1937), it appears that a different form of breakdown might be made, namely that between breeding sites within cavities and those beneath objects. The former would present the darkest aspect to a fly and would be used in the hottest weather while the latter would present a less dark aspect which would be adequate in less extreme climatic conditions. Breeding sites under leaf litter, whether in thicket or on river sand, would fall into the 'beneath objects' category as would most fallen log, decumbent tree, and rock overhang sites. In the very hot season larger logs tend to be preferred (Harley, 1954), and these logs tend to provide a cavity-like situation. The same holds true for rock overhangs but the majority of fallen log and rock sites are small and do not resemble the cavity type of site. With such a breakdown of breeding sites, the seasonal shift from fallen logs to rot holes reported by Glasgow (1961b) for *G. morsitans* and the move of breeding sites of *G. morsitans* in West Africa into thicket in the hot season (Nash, 1939) would be due to the same response on the part of the fly. In the case of tsetse species living in equable conditions, there is no stimulus to seek the darkest breeding sites and leaf litter under low vegetation is adequate at all seasons. Similarly, for species living in deciduous woodland the wet season permits flies to use far less sheltered sites than are needed in the hot season. The cool dry season is intermediate, with flies being restricted rather more than in the wet season to more easily recognized breeding sites. The categories of sites used in the wet season tend to remain the same as those of the cool dry season and it is largely because examples of breeding sites less conspicuous to humans can provide adequate conditions that puparia become difficult to detect in wet weather. Some confirmation of this is found in reports of the use of breeding sites under fallen logs in wet seasons which have had poor rainfall (Jack, 1912; Burtt, 1952).

A sudden abandoning of the cavity type of breeding site in Tanzania by *G. swynnertoni* takes place in November (Burtt, 1952) and a similar shift is shown by *G. morsitans* in Rhodesia (Phelps, in preparation). Avoidance of breeding sites which are likely to become waterlogged is certainly of survival value to the fly but the conditions which trigger such moves are not clear. In the case of *G. tachinoides*, it appears that many puparia are destroyed by the first floods as sandy river beds are well used as breeding sites at that season (Nash, 1939) and there is no doubt as to the adverse effect of flooding on *G. morsitans* populations (Swynnerton, 1936). In Rhodesia, many deciduous trees flush before the first showers of rain, but this modification of the environment alone does not appear to make the flies stop using the cavity type of breeding sites. The first showers in the study area used by Burtt (1952) generally fell in October, as they did in Rhodesia, but these showers were very local and would not appear to have provided a stimulus for the general abandoning of the cavity type of breeding sites.

The soil in breeding sites varies from very fine silt to coarse sand and, provided it is loose, the texture of the soil does not appear to be a critical factor in determining breeding sites. When soils are waterlogged, larvae do not burrow but form puparia on the surface; the reason for this remains unknown. Burtt (1952) showed that lowering the temperature of dry soil from 24·5–26°C to 20°C resulted in a tendency for the larva to burrow less deeply—two out of eight pupated on the surface, an occurrence not observed at the higher temperature. This observation led Jackson (1955a) to suggest that failure of larvae to burrow during the cold season may be because they were insufficiently active when conditions were cool during rainy spells. Parker (1956), however, showed that evaporation of water from damp soils only lowered the temperature of the soil by about 1·5°C. Species of tsetse differ in their requirements as to the humidity of the soil necessary for survival of the immature stages in the breeding site (Bursell, 1958) and a gradient of humidity may occur in the hot dry season over the top 20 cm. of soil in tsetse habitats. Recent work by Finlayson (1967) has shown that larvae of *G. morsitans orientalis* prefer damp soil to dry soil and this may govern the depth to which the larva burrows before forming a puparium. The depth to which larvae of *G. pallidipes* burrow was shown to be related to temperature, and possibly to humidity (Bursell, 1960a). Generally, tsetse puparia are found in the top 4 cm. of soil in a breeding site. Any soil is suitable for tsetse breeding provided it is not waterlogged and is loose.

Several attempts have been made to collect large numbers of puparia by means of artificial puparial sites. The results of work by Carpenter (1923) on *G. palpalis* indicated that the best artificial sites yielded more puparia than the best natural sites and that, on average, artificial sites yielded more puparia than natural ones.

The artificial sites consisted of low sloping thatched roofs over suitable loose soil in places where flies were abundant. An extensive study of artificial breeding sites for *G. morsitans* was made by Nash (1933a) following work done by Lamborn (1916). Log sites were the best type of site to make and by adding a suitable screen of grass or bark round the log, these sites could be made more attractive than natural log sites at the same season. In the wet season the same log sites were used and they continued to yield puparia but they were improved by having drainage channels round them. It was noted that many good sites in the field, natural and artificial were never used, presumably because the area in which they occurred was not frequented by adult flies. Work in Rhodesia using artificial sites resembling natural cavity-type sites (Phelps *et al., loc. cit*) has shown that puparia can be obtained in such places but yields do not approach those of the best natural ones.

Quantitative Sampling of Puparia

It has been the experience of most investigators that the numbers of puparia which can be located in the field do not represent a population sufficient to maintain the numbers of adults known to exist and this has resulted in the frequently repeated claim that all types of breeding sites of tsetse flies have not yet been discovered. The first major study of this problem was made on *G. morsitans* by Jackson (1937) who concluded that 90% of larviposition took place in scattered, as opposed to classical, sites. These scattered sites in which very few puparia were found but which are relatively far more numerous than classical sites consisted of the bases of Borassus palms, tufts of grass and the bases of young plants or of standing trees, particularly if the trunk was irregular in form so as to give an overhang near the ground.

This investigation,[1] which involved searches of all the types of sites mentioned above within an area of some 8,000 square yards of woodland, was conducted over a considerable period of time. Only one intact and eighteen empty puparia were found so that it would appear that searches of this nature are not a profitable means of collecting large numbers of puparia. Jackson's work was followed by another investigation carried out in the same area by H. M. Lloyd during the rainy season (February–May) the results of which were not published. The woodland floor was marked out in 4-foot squares, the soil of 384 of which was examined to a depth of 2 inches. No intact puparia were found but seven empty puparia were collected from open unshaded sites, one from under a log and five from the vicinity of a fallen tree. This total of thirteen puparia in some 680 square yards of woodland floor would correspond to about 150 in an area of the size examined by Jackson and therefore suggests that a good deal of breeding takes place, at least during the latter part of the rainy season. These results further suggest that breeding occurs not only outside the traditional sites but also on the general floor of the woodland outside the scattered sites examined by Jackson. Indeed, Jackson (1949), as a result of these investigations, reported that he and Lloyd concluded that 'at all times the great majority of pupae were placed outside the classical sites', especially in the rainy season when 'many might be found in grass tussocks even with no overhead shade at all'.

[1] The writer is indebted to Mr W. H. Potts for the information given in this paragraph.

In following up this work, Jackson (reported by Potts, 1950), working in an area differing topographically and in other ways from that in which the earlier investigations were made was unable to repeat his earlier observations that puparia can be found at random in grass tufts or on the general woodland floor in the wet season. In this study, puparia were obtained from under overhanging rocks at all seasons. In a subsequent report, Jackson (1955a) gave figures showing that in the early dry season (June) in a third area differing in certain important respect from the other two, 10% of the predicted number of intact puparia of *G. morsitans* were found (the prediction being based on an estimated adult population) and a further 10% were accounted for in terms of puparia from which flies had emerged, leaving 80% unaccounted for. In the wet weather (March), 10% of the predicted number of intact puparia were found but no empty puparia were located, leaving 90% unaccounted for. The work done on *G. morsitans* by Harley (1954), in yet another area, showed a similar situation. Jewell (1958a), working in the same region as that of the 1955 studies, again obtained 10% recovery of puparia of *G. morsitans*, but it was pointed out that the confidence limits of the estimate of the adult population were wide and it was possible that a considerably larger proportion of the puparia had been found. In this study an attempt was made to assess the efficiency of the people searching for puparia. It was found that recovery of marked puparia was only 39% if the searchers were unaware that a test was being conducted and 88% if they had been informed beforehand. This low level of efficiency, together with the use of scattered sites in the wet weather, might well account for the failure to locate the predicted number of puparia.

In a study on *G. morsitans* in Rhodesia (Phelps, *et al.*, *loc. cit.*) careful monthly searches for puparia were made in a demarcated area which included a variety of vegetation types, and the yield from these searches was considerably more than would have been expected had the searchers covered an equal area on a less controlled basis. It appears that the problem is largely one of the degree of care taken in the search and with the large areas involved it is not surprising that puparia are located in relatively small numbers. Experimental and field results indicate that the sort of places suitable for tsetse breeding sites can be recognized but the distinctness, to humans, of the recognizable features grades from slight, under environmental conditions favourable to the tsetse, to fair under conditions where the flies are under climatic stress.

ADULTS

(J. P. GLASGOW)

One may wish to answer one of the following questions, for each of which a different sampling method is appropriate.

(1) Are tsetse present in a certain area?
(2) If tsetse are present, which species are they?
(3) Do they vary in number with time?
(4) Are they more abundant in, confined to, or dependent on, certain recognizable sub-areas within the larger area recognized in question (1)?

(5) What is the composition of the population in terms of sex-ratio and numbers falling into various age-classes and physiological states?

(6) Where do tsetse perch during their periods of inactivity?

These questions are arranged in order of increasing difficulty. The penultimate one, (5), though of basic importance for understanding both tsetse population dynamics and trypanosome transmission, has not often been asked, and has seldom been answered satisfactorily. Since different procedures are appropriate for answering the six questions, they are considered seriatim.

Methods for Determining the Presence of Tsetse

Some species of *Glossina* attack man very readily and there are some places where a brief visit is enough to provide a convincing demonstration of the presence of tsetse. But *G. morsitans*, and probably other species as well, can apparently survive at densities of 100 males—perhaps 300 flies of both sexes—per square mile. At this density one can catch on average only a couple of flies in a mile's walk, and since spatial distribution is far from uniform, a ten-mile walk without seeing a tsetse cannot be accepted as evidence of their absence. As other species of *Glossina* are even more reluctant than *G. morsitans* to show themselves to man, failure to catch them is even less satisfactory evidence that they are not there.

Convincing evidence of the absence of tsetse may indeed be difficult to obtain quickly. The presence of healthy herds of cattle means that the presence of tsetse is improbable but not impossible, since: (a) In areas with a prolonged dry season tsetse of the *palpalis* group often inhabit evergreen vegetation fringing permanent water. Cattle often co-exist in these areas, either because the *palpalis* group is an inefficient vector of the trypanosomes which are pathogenic for cattle, or because the herdsmen use tsetse-free watering places. (b) Many strains of cattle possess a certain tolerance to at least some trypanosomes (*see* Chapter 6). This is particularly marked in the N'Dama cattle of West Africa, but many 'native' breeds of cattle are more resistant to trypanosomes than are the exotic breeds which are introduced for the sake of increased productivity. (c) Drugs exist which, injected two or three times a year, protect cattle against the effects of infrequent inoculations of trypanosomes such as would be made by sparse populations of tsetse.

Thus, if cattle are seen to be living in an area, one may suspect that tsetse are absent, but to make sure, one would have to introduce susceptible animals (cattle are commonly used) and pasture them in the suspected area. If the way into the suspected area was not known to be free of tsetse it would be necessary to protect the test cattle, perhaps with a wire gauze cage, on their journey in. During the test it would be necessary to control the grazing of the animals, since if one of them did develop trypanosomiasis it would be important to know where it had been.

If a group of susceptible animals could be kept in an area for twelve months without developing an infection, that would be strong evidence of the absence of tsetse.

Glossina is an efficient transmitter of pathogenic trypanosomes, which are usually present in wild hosts, so that, if *Glossina* is present, susceptible cattle are unlikely to escape infection. An exception to this statement is that cattle may live sometimes in contact with tsetse of the *palpalis* group, and yet escape infection, perhaps because the wild hosts are reptiles not carrying mammalian pathogens (*see* Chapter 13).

If the test herd of susceptible animals does develop trypanosomiasis, this is an indication, short of proof, of the presence of tsetse. A special kind of animal trypanosomiasis (surra) occurs in North Africa, India and Central America in the absence of tsetse; it is transmitted non-cyclically by other blood-sucking insects. A competent protozoologist, however, does not confuse the causal organism of surra with the trypanosomes characteristically transmitted by tsetse, but it seems that even these trypanosomes are sometimes transmitted, especially from beast to beast within a herd, in a non-cyclical manner by blood-sucking insects other than tsetse (*see* Chapter 39). The only certain evidence of the presence of tsetse in an area, then, is the ability to catch tsetse there regularly.

Several species of the *morsitans* group, and *G. longipennis* in the *fusca* group, are attracted by moving vehicles, bicycles, cars or trains and carried on them into areas in which they would not otherwise occur. Regular catches of tsetse may therefore indicate a steady assisted immigration rather than a truly indigenous population. Sometimes 'de-flying posts' are set up to remove tsetse from passing traffic; a de-flying post may be simply a man with a net, or a chamber through which each vehicle is made to pass and submit to insecticidal spraying. The catches made at de-flying posts may be the only information available about some tsetse populations, but they are very unsatisfactory samples. As long as tsetse are being caught, even at the rate of one or two per year, one knows that tsetse exist somewhere in the vicinity, although their whereabouts may be uncertain. Long periods of zero catches from posts where tsetse were once caught encourage the belief that the tsetse have disappeared. But fluctuations in the size of the catch are difficult to interpret, since they depend not only on the tsetse population but also on the amount, composition and behaviour of the traffic and on the skill and diligence of the personnel of the de-flying posts.

Methods for Determining the Species of Tsetse Present

Since, as explained above, the only unequivocal evidence of the presence of tsetse is the capture of specimens, one might suppose that there was never any doubt about the identity of the species. But two or more species often occur together; so the fact that a certain technique produces catches of one species does not preclude the possibility of another technique producing another species.

The following survey techniques have been used:

(a) Reconnaissance
(b) Traps
(c) Searches for resting flies
(d) Searches for puparia

Each of these methods exploits different aspects of the tsetse's behaviour and therefore produces catches with different compositions.

Reconnaissance

Males of a number of species of *Glossina* are attracted to any moving object which approaches them. If then one walks through the habitat of one of these species at a suitable time of day it is easy to catch specimens with a small hand-net. Although where tsetse are numerous one may get an impression of intense attack, a little quantitative observation will show that only a small proportion actually attempt to feed. Examination of the tsetse caught will reveal that very few of them have fed recently—such flies have distended abdomens with visible red or black blood. The tsetse caught in this way, then, are males which are neither replete nor starving. They often alight on one's back so that reconnaissance parties should consist of at least two men. Sometimes the tsetse do not alight on the party, but on the ground or nearby vegetation. In this case the trick is to stop at frequent intervals and look about.

Sometimes it is useful to carry a 'screen'. This is a piece of cloth, usually sacking, but sometimes black cotton, rectangular, about 4 feet × 2 feet, attached along one of its long sides to a pole which is carried between two men on their shoulders. Its effect is presumably to increase the size of the target offered to the tsetse.

As to where to look, with experience one quickly gets ideas about the most likely places in which to search. Such ideas tend to be subjective and must be treated with reserve. It is always advisable to follow a grid to ensure that all parts of the study area are reconnoitred. The following species can usually be detected by this simple foot reconnaissance, with or without a screen:

The *palpalis* group as a whole (however, there is not much information about *G. caliginea* and *G. pallicera*).
In the *morsitans* group, *G. morsitans* and *G. swynnertoni.*
In the *fusca* group, *G. brevipalpis*, *G. fuscipleuris* and *G. longipennis*.

The time of day can be very important. Power (1964) caught *G. longipennis* in large numbers, but only at sunset. This sort of behaviour seems widespread in the *fusca* group. *G. tachinoides* can be caught in the middle of the day in the cool season, but only early and late in the day during the hot season (Nash, 1937).

In most cases larger catches will be obtained if one goes about in a motor vehicle, but this may not be so with *G. brevipalpis* and *G. longipennis*, which in some places are to be seen sitting on bare ground at sunset. The objection to motorized reconnaissance is that even four-wheel drive machines cannot go everywhere but, when used, 10 m.p.h. is a suitable speed. The airspeed of flying tsetse is thought to be about 15 m.p.h.; none will enter a vehicle travelling faster than this.

G. medicorum in particular has been studied by vehicle catches (Chapman, 1960). Jack (1939) also reports the results of catches of *G. morsitans* [*orientalis*] on lorries and Bursell (1961a) pays some attention to the composition of catches made by this method.

In Uganda a bicycle fitted with a sticky screen has been found useful for detecting *G. morsitans* where it is very scarce. The screen is of hessian or cloth, about 2 feet square, hung behind the back wheel. It is covered with banding grease or other suitable slow-drying sticky substance. The bicycle is ridden through suspected areas, after which tsetse may be found stuck to the screen.

If one takes a bait animal on foot reconnaissance the number of species caught increases. It is important to have an animal that will move when one wants it to move, and stand still while one is trying to catch flies. An ox is suitable and has been used more than any other animal.

The following species have been studied by means of foot reconnaissance with bait oxen:

In the *morsitans* group: *G. austeni*, *G. longipalpis*, *G. pallidipes*.
In the *fusca* group: *G. fusca*, *G. medicorum*, *G. nigrofusca*, *G. tabaniformis*, *G. brevipalpis*.

Traps

The main uses of traps have been in studies of detailed distribution and abundance, and in obtaining samples differing in sex-ratio and other points of composition from those obtained in other ways. For further information on the design and use of traps for tsetse the reader is referred to Chapter 22. They have been used in surveys for *G. pallidipes* and *G. palpalis*, and have the advantage that once in position they are at work throughout the hours of daylight, seven days a week. But minor changes of site have such a marked effect on the catch made by a trap that it would be very rash to assert that tsetse were absent from a certain area, merely because none had been caught in traps. It should be noted that traps have demonstrated the presence of tsetse when other methods failed (Thomson *et al.*, 1961).

Methods for Determining Variations in Numbers, Association with Sub-areas and Composition of Tsetse Populations

Do tsetse vary in number with time? Are they particularly associated with certain sub-areas? What is the composition of the population? These are three quite separate questions but as attempts have often been made to answer all three from the same set of field observations and as none of the field methods available is completely satisfactory for answering any of the three questions, it is convenient to discuss them together.

The following methods have been used:

(a) Moving catches (fly-rounds) with or without screens or bait animals.
(b) Standing catches.
(c) Traps.
(d) Searches for resting flies.

(a) Moving Catches

As mentioned above, if one moves about in the habitat of tsetse of several species, many males are attracted and can be caught. These males, which Bursell (1961a) terms 'sexually appetitive', are neither replete nor very hungry. It seems that their attraction to moving objects brings them into contact with teneral females which also are attracted to moving objects. Teneral females have not yet taken their first meal and are nubile.

If a route is marked by blazes on trees or by other suitable devices, and catches along it are repeated from time to time, it becomes a fly-round (Buxton, 1955, app. 5; Davies, 1967); the figures of the catches on fly-rounds have been regarded as samples of the tsetse population and changes in the figures have been regarded as indicating changes in the population.

Fly-rounds are usually carried out by parties of two or three men; their length tends to be what is regarded as a fair day's work. Depending on the length of the journey to the beginning of the round and other local factors, this length is often between three and six miles. It is unusual for all parts of a fly-round to be equally productive so that even if the primary purpose of a fly-round was to watch population changes in time, it is natural to examine the spatial distribution of the catches to answer the question: 'Are the tsetse particularly associated with certain sub-areas?'

In early days great attention was paid to the different vegetational communities of which the woodland was composed. For example, some areas might be recognized as dominated by trees of species A, others by trees of species B, others recognized by the presence of thickets, or of long grass, and so on. Care was taken to route a fly-round so as to pass through at least some examples of all the recognizable vegetation types in the area. The portion of the path passing through each different type of vegetation was called a section and demarcated with a number fixed to a convenient tree. Separate records were kept of the catches from each section. It was customary to arrange the fly-round on a roughly circular route with the end near the beginning so avoiding long unproductive journeys through the bush. This was how the term 'round' came into use.

Later it was realized that a more objective sample could be obtained by using a straight path, aligned on a compass bearing and divided into arbitrary short sections, from 25 to 200 yards long. Halts for catching tsetse, formerly at the discretion of the catchers, were now made only at the numbered posts demarcating the short sections. For further details of the method the reader is referred to Ford *et al.* (1959). Fly-rounds with such arbitrary short sections are called 'transect fly-rounds'.

One might suppose that the use of arbitrary short sections, with stops for catching made only at defined places, would produce less variable catches, but experiment shows that this is not necessarily so. In a study of the variability of fly-round catches of *G. swynnertoni* (Glasgow, 1961) three closely adjacent fly-rounds were worked simultaneously twenty-four times in twenty-eight days. Their total length was 21,200 yards and the total catch of non-teneral males varied from 315 to 720. On two of the rounds (Nos. 1 and 2) catching was at the discretion of the catchers, while on the third (No. 5) it was confined to numbered stopping places 100 yards apart. The variance between days was much the same on all three (compare the width of the bands indicating the fiducial limits in Fig. 17.1, a, b and c). It is worth noting that this day-to-day variation is very considerable. Fig. 17.1 shows, for each of the three fly-rounds, the mean catch over the twenty-four days, with fiducial limits. Fly-rounds are usually done once or twice a week. Data were therefore extracted for each day separately. Fig. 17.1 shows (a, b and c) that if the fly-rounds had been done once a week, the mean catches for four weeks (i.e. the mean catches on Mondays, Tuesdays . . .)

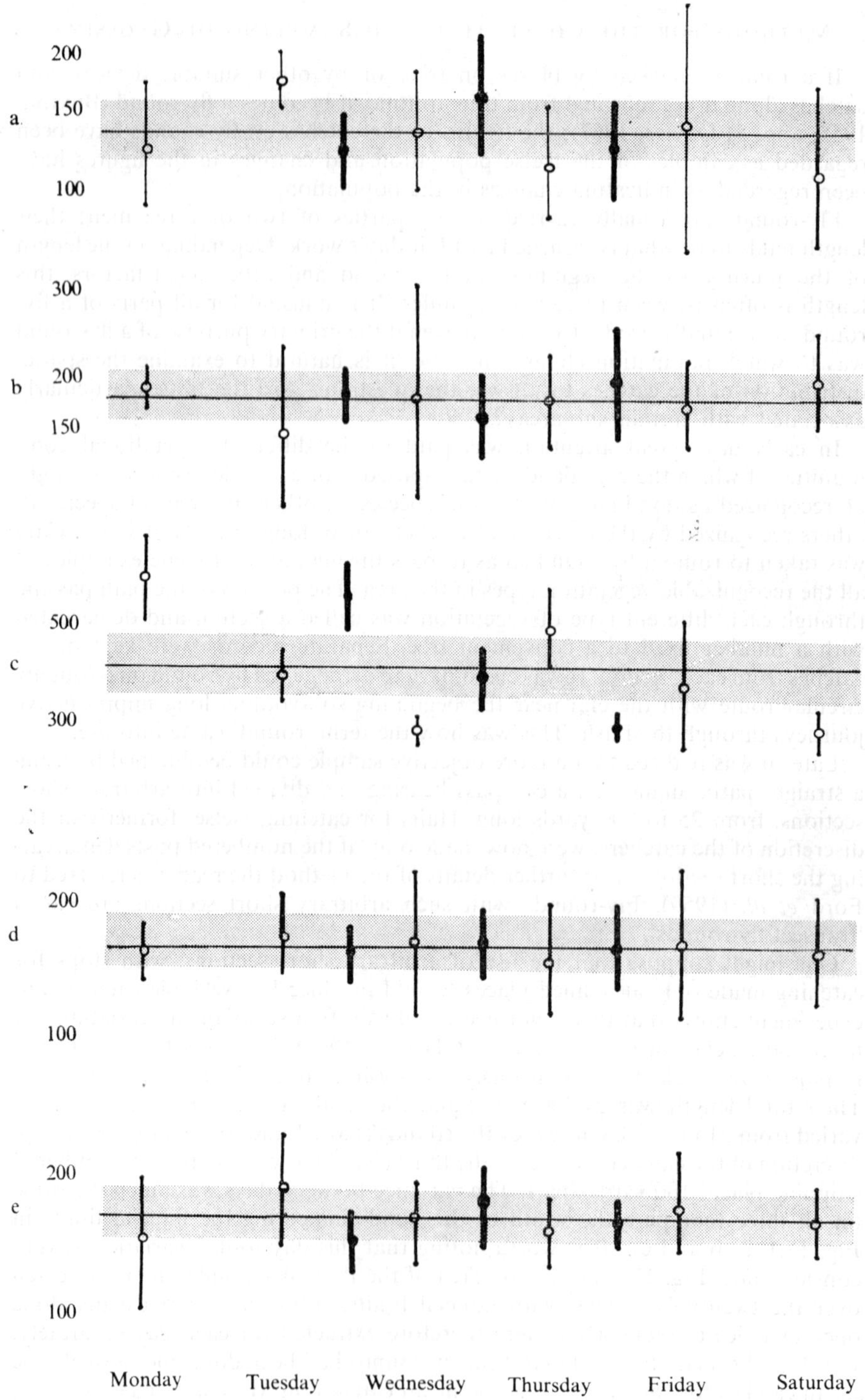

200
150
100
a.
300
200
150
b
500
300
c
200
100
d
200
100
e
Monday
Tuesday
Wednesday
Thursday
Friday
Saturday

Fig. 17.1

Fig. 17.1 The results of the fly-rounds expressed as Apparent Densities (catch of non-teneral males per 10,000 yards). The numbers are plotted on a logarithmic scale. The horizontal lines represent the means for the month, with their fiducial limits (± twice standard error) shown as shaded areas, and the vertical lines (thick and thin) represent the fiducial limits of the values (shown by circles ○ or dots ●) obtained by working only on certain days. (a) No. 1 fly-round: the six thin vertical lines give the result of each day's catch and the three thick lines of the Monday and Thursday catches combined, of the Tuesday and Friday catches combined, and of the Wednesday and Saturday catches combined. (b) No. 2 fly-round: symbols and thick and thin vertical lines as for (a). (c) No. 5 fly-round: symbols and vertical lines as for (a). (d) Nos. 1 and 2 fly-rounds combined and treated as one long fly-round: symbols and vertical lines as for (a). (e) The combined results from Nos. 1 and 2 fly-rounds carried out on successive days: circles and thin lines represent, in the Monday position, the results of fly-round 1 carried out on Mondays plus the results of fly-round 2 carried out on Tuesdays; in the Tuesday position, they represent the results of fly-round 1 carried out on Tuesdays plus the results of fly-round 2 carried out on Wednesdays; and similarly for the Wednesday, Thursday, Friday and Saturday positions. The dots and thick lines represent, in the position between Tuesday and Wednesday, the results of fly-round 1 carried out on Mondays and of fly-round 2 carried out on Tuesdays plus the results of fly-round 1 carried out on Thursdays and of fly-round 2 carried out on Fridays; in the position between Wednesday and Thursday, they represent the results of fly-round 1 carried out on Tuesdays and of fly-round 2 carried out on Wednesdays plus the results of fly-round 1 carried out on Fridays and of fly-round 2 carried out on Saturdays; in the position between Thursday and Friday, they represent the results of fly-round 1 carried out on Wednesdays and of fly-round 2 carried out on Thursdays plus the results of fly-round 1 carried out on Saturdays and of fly-round 2 carried out on Mondays. The bottom two rows of the figure represent the same amounts of work, the slight differences being due to the different arrangement of the data.

would be quite likely to lie outside the fiducial limits found by doing the fly-round six times a week. In the lower parts of the figure, labelled d and e, the data from two of the rounds have been combined to produce the equivalent of a round of 15,200 yards. If this long round were done twice a week, the variance would be so reduced that a mean of 100 in one month could be regarded as significantly different from a mean of 200 in another month. The last line of the figure shows the results of a procedure very likely to be adopted in practice when staff is limited, namely, working one half of a long round one day and the other the next (Fig. 17.1, e). Although comparison of the bottom two lines of the figure might suggest that this practice gives results slightly worse than the results of working both halves on the same day, analysis of the original data showed no significant difference in the variance produced by the two methods. It is therefore likely that no loss of precision would result from working two halves of a long fly-round on successive days.

By analysing catches in this sort of way it is possible to conclude that the *numbers caught* have been greater at one time than at another, or greater in one place, or in one set of circumstances, than in another. The inference, implicit or explicit, that changes in the numbers caught reflect changes in the absolute number in the population, or conversely, that no change in the catch means no change in the population, is on a much less certain foundation. It has already been mentioned that the majority of the tsetse caught on a fly-round are males which are neither replete nor hungry. It is in fact customary, when reporting fly-round catches as population indexes, to exclude all female flies and teneral males, and this has been done in the case of Fig. 17.1. The idea is that since these flies, which together often make up less than 10% of the total catch, presumably appear for reasons different from those causing the non-teneral males to appear, their inclusion would give a less accurate index of the total population. This idea has never been critically examined. Bursell (1961a) has examined the attraction of *G. swynnertoni* to a moving party of men. The flies take a very large meal every three or four days; between one feed and the next he recognized the following phases (which are not the same as the Hunger Stages of earlier writers, *cf.* Buxton, 1955, p. 707).

	Physiology	*Behaviour*
Phase 1.	Gorged.	Inactive.
Phase 2.	Digestion partly complete; fat reserve high.	Comes to moving party but not to feed. Most 'fly-round flies' belong to this phase.
Phase 3.	Little undigested material remains; fat reserve low.	Not attracted to moving parties of men. Most of the flies feeding off a tethered ox belong to this phase.
Phase 4.	Very empty, within a few hours of death from starvation.	Comes to moving party of men and attempts to feed. Many flies, especially in favourable conditions, never reach this phase, passing from Phase 3 back to Phase 1.

Thus only Phases 2 and 4 are caught on fly-rounds, and changes in the proportion of males in the various phases at any time could produce a change in the fly-round catch, although there had not been any change in the actual population. On the other hand, a reduction in the general level of nutrition, caused perhaps by an exodus of host vertebrates, would be expected to decrease the proportion in Phase 2 and to increase the proportion in Phase 4, and these two changes would tend to compensate for each other.

Female tsetse never enter Phase 2. Thus only those in Phase 4 are attracted to fly-round parties, and in well-fed communities this is a very small number. In taking the catch of males as an index of the whole population, one is assuming that the sex ratio remains constant, but this does not seem a very safe assumption. The sex ratio is about 1:1 on emergence from the pupae, but males have very much shorter lives, presumably because of the hazards they encounter during Phase 2, one of which is known to be predation by Asilidae (Robber flies). Changes in these hazards could have profound effects on the longevity of males, and hence on the sex ratio, without affecting females at all.

Another approach is to determine the absolute number of tsetse in an area and to compare this number with the fly-round catch. This gives rise to the concept of 'Availability', defined as the proportion of the population which is caught on the fly-round and to the calculation of conversion factors whereby the catch on a standard length of fly-round (10,000 yards is usual) is converted to populations of non-teneral males per square mile.

The absolute numbers given in Table 17.1 were determined by the method of marking, release and recapture. The theory of this is very simple. If one marks and releases, say, a hundred flies and, after giving them time to settle down, finds that 10% of a further catch is marked, evidently the total population is 1,000. The practice is much more complicated, because between marking and recapture flies are entering the population by birth and immigration and leaving by death and emigration. Also it is necessary to assume that marking does not alter the behaviour of the flies, and that the sample marked is a truly random one. Johns (1958) detected systematic errors which suggested that the sample marked was not random but contained at least some flies especially attracted to men and hence especially likely to be captured a second time. This effect would result in estimates of absolute population lower than the true value.

For details of the method the reader should consult Jackson (1948; also in Buxton, 1955, p. 726) and Jackson (1953). The only other method of determining absolute numbers is applicable only to small isolated populations, when it may be possible to catch all the tsetse (*see* under Hand Catching in Chapter 22). In one instance this has given results in agreement with the method of marking and recapture (Glasgow, 1953). Estimates of absolute population obtained by the recapture method have wide fiducial limits, and since mean fly-round catches also have wide fiducial limits the relation between the two is not as precise as a first reading of Table 17.1 might suggest. Attention is directed to entry No. 8, and the footnote.

The data from a transect fly-round can be transferred to a map and in this way the places where flies are caught, and where they are not caught, are readily displayed. The inference, that places where flies are caught are of exceptional importance to them, follows very easily. The practice of 'discriminative clearing' consists essentially of removing certain types of bush which fly-rounds have shown to be particularly productive of tsetse (the 'appetitive' males). Sometimes quite small discriminative clearings (some 5% of the total area) have been

TABLE 17.1

Determinations of 'availability' (from Glasgow, 1963)

The figures given are the populations of males per square mile calculated to correspond to a fly-round catch of one non-teneral male per 10,000 yards

Species	Place	Availability	Author
1 *morsitans morsitans*	Kakoma, Tanzania	7·5	Jackson, 1944
2 *morsitans morsitans*	Gedamara, Tanzania	11·2–7·4	Jackson, 1953
3 *swynnertoni*	Gedamara, Tanzania	15·1–7·2	Jackson, 1953
4 *morsitans*	Ankole, Uganda	526–50	Harley, 1958
5 *fuscipes fuscipes*	Port Victoria, Kenya	176	Glasgow, 1954
6 *fuscipes fuscipes*	Kuja River, Kenya	88	Glasgow, 1954
7 *fuscipes fuscipes*	Sari River, Kenya	150	Glasgow, 1954
8 *pallidipes*	Lambwe, Kenya	1,000–200	Johns, in Jackson, 1954

Entry No. 1 is the mean of 12 months' results, but variation between months was stated to be of minor importance. The variable results in entry No. 8 were related to abundance, the conversion factor 200 applying when tsetse were relatively scarce, and 1,000 when they were numerous.

followed by collapse and disappearance of a tsetse population (e.g. Glover *et al.*, 1955). But other discriminative clearings have not been successful, as will be seen below in the discussion of standing catches.

Most of the catch consists of males in physiological Phase 2 (*see* above). A very few newly engorged males are caught, apparently by accident, and very hungry males are taken as well; tenerals of both sexes are caught and a few very hungry females. Many workers have recorded the proportions of tenerals and of female non-tenerals in the catch, supposing that, since these classes clearly are ready to feed, high proportions of them would indicate that the population was short of food. Many workers also have divided the males into four 'hunger stages' (Buxton, 1955, p. 707) on the basis of external appearance and calculated a 'mean hunger stage' (*see also* Chapter 19). Others have recorded the position of each fly at the moment of capture, that is, whether it was perched on the moving party, or on the ground or on vegetation. Others have recorded whether the fly was 'head-up' or 'head-down' at the moment of capture but this, of course, cannot be applied to flies on the ground. Rather belatedly, Bursell and Glasgow (1960) attempted to assess the significance of some of these widely used criteria of hunger, working with *G. f. fuscipes.* As measures of the nutritonal status of the population they took size and fat content and the size of puparia contemporaneously produced. They found that the proportions of tenerals and of female non-tenerals could not be obviously related to nutritional status, but that the proportion of non-teneral males caught on the party was meaningful and sensitive. They did not examine the mean hunger stage since hunger staging is not considered satisfactory for *G. f. fuscipes.*

(b) Standing Catches

Most often a moving catch will return, at the end of a day's work, a larger number caught by this than by any other catching method, and therefore, if possible alterations in the size of the population with time are considered the chief object of the investigation, then moving catches will usually be preferred. But for answering other questions standing catches, especially with a tethered ox, have proved extremely informative. To establish the relation between activity and time of day one must get into position at a time of minimum activity, which usually means before dawn. If this precaution is neglected, the first catch will be swollen by tsetse attracted to the party on its way to the catching station, and the first catch is likely to be the biggest for the day. By recording separately, or confining one's attention to, those tsetse which actually feed, one gets an accurate sample of the tsetse potentially transmitting trypanosomiasis and some indication of the true sex ratio (Pilson & Pilson, 1967). The true sex ratio will not be the same as that observed by this method unless the interval between feeds is the same in the two sexes. By marking the flies as they engorge and waiting for them to return to feed again one can ascertain the interval between feeds (Glasgow, 1961a). By watching where flies go after feeding one can find their favourite resting sites at this time (Pilson & Leggate, 1962).

Pilson and Pilson (1967) studied *G. morsitans* by means of standing catches from a tethered ox and reached the following conclusions: 'The information derived from conventional fly rounds regarding the behaviour of *G. morsitans* has given rise to the idea that it concentrates in riverine vegetation and along vlei edges during the hot dry season but becomes more dispersed during the rainy season. The present results show that a wider range of vegetation types than had been supposed is frequented at all seasons. Feeding and resting flies were observed in leafless woodland under conditions of high temperature that have hitherto been regarded as intolerable to *G. morsitans*. It is concluded that the environmental conditions provided by semi-evergreen trees and double-storey vegetation are not essential to survival of the fly. If that is so, it may explain the failure to control *G. morsitans* in Ankole, Uganda, by clearing of upper-storey vegetation only (Harley & Pilson, 1961). Sampling of the feeding element of the population of *G. morsitans* by use of a stationary bait-ox has revealed that virtually no concentration of this species takes place in a specific vegetation type at any time of the year. The only exception is riverine fringe vegetation, which was particularly favoured by male flies in the hot dry season.'

In a complementary study, Bursell (1966a) found that the nutritional state was better in flies from leafless woodland than in those from riverine fringe vegetation. There seems to be no doubt that, in this instance at least, conventional fly-rounds (moving catches) had given rise to quite erroneous conclusions about the spatial distribution of the tsetse.[1]

Other species studied by means of catches from a tethered ox have been *G. pallidipes* (Smith & Rennison, 1961, 1961a, b; Harley, 1965), *G. brevipalpis* (Harley, 1965), *G. fusca and G. tabaniformis* (Jordan, 1962a).

(c) Traps

A very large variety of devices have been found to catch one or another species of *Glossina*; for details, the reader may consult Swynnerton (1936) and Buxton (1955). Swynnerton regarded traps as potential means of controlling tsetse but nowadays interest centres in their role as research tools. Morris and Morris (1949) believed them to be useful in the control of sleeping sickness by reducing local concentrations of tsetse (*see* also Morris, 1960b, 1961a, 1962), but they did not believe that traps could ever bring about eradication. Most writers agree that the siting of traps is of paramount importance. 'Identical traps can be placed in what appear to be equally good positions . . . perhaps only a dozen yards apart, yet one will make catches four or five times as high as the other' (Morris & Morris, 1949). This is a typical comment. It follows that testing variation in the design of traps is a tedious business, involving frequent interchanging of the traps between positions. In the absence of a satisfactory theory of the reasons for tsetse entering traps, most modern workers have adopted the Morris trap (described in the reference just cited) as one known to catch several species and to use it as a sampling method. The siting difficulty is best overcome by using a completely regular pattern; for example, a straight path is cut and traps are placed along it at exact intervals and left there for the duration of the experiment, whether individual traps are seen to be productive or non-productive. Comparisons of traps with other methods of catching *G. pallidipes* have been made by Smith and Rennison (1961, 1961a, b), Rennison and Smith (1961), Glasgow and Duffy (1961) and Harley (1967). Traps catch more females than males of this species. Smith and Rennison compared trap catches with fly-round catches and standing catches from a tethered ox, and found that the three were not correlated. Working from dawn to dusk, they found differences in the daily pattern of captures made by the three methods. Males in traps

[1] It is possible that in the area under investigation, the catching stations had been so sited as to provide samples only from 'feeding ground' areas in the riverside fringes and from the general woodland and that areas providing concentrations of appetitive males (on which partial clearings should be based) were missed. It is most important that these methods of study should be repeated in as many, and as varied, tsetse-infested regions as possible. In carrying out such studies consideration should be given to the discussion of the use of fly-rounds to detect concentrations (Ford *et al.*, 1959)—W. H. POTTS.

seemed to be less hungry than those taken off the oxen. Rennison and Smith found that, when the interval between emptying traps exceeded twenty-four hours, ants and perhaps other predators removed *G. pallidipes* without trace. They thought that this accounted at least in part for site variations, but Glasgow and Duffy (1961) found site variations in traps cleared daily. Table 17.2 gives an interesting comparison made by these workers.

TABLE 17.2

(from Glasgow and Duffy, 1961)

Comparison of catches of* G. pallidipes *made by two traps and a standing party of 3 men on the east edge of thicket habitat of the tsetse, each catching 11 hours daily

Period	Traps		Men	
	Males	Females	Males	Females
10–14.7.56	50	137	47	1
17–21.7.56	42	119	30	1
Total	92	256	77	2

They found evidence that traps in the open did not attract flies from distances as much as 100 yards, and accordingly used them to measure dispersal into open grassland, which is difficult to study by other methods. They concluded that 'traps are valuable because they catch a high proportion of females, thus affording information not given by fly-rounds, and operate continuously at a higher over all catching rate than that of men, thus facilitating the study of sparse populations. Nevertheless, site effects and day to day variability are both large with traps, so that reproducible results are difficult to obtain'.

To sum up: for detecting population changes in time, trap catches should not be ignored. The fact that trap catches are not correlated with catches made by other methods may mean that one of the methods being examined is faulty, but we do not know which one. If traps are used for investigating whether certain areas are particularly associated with tsetse, a positive result might mean an area containing a large number of productive sites rather than absolutely large number of tsetse. For studying the composition of the tsetse population traps are invaluable in giving large samples of females, but while there is reasonable certainty that, in Table 17.2 for example, the trap catches are a less biased sample than the man catches, the possibility cannot be rejected that the trap catches are biased to some extent.

(d) Searches for Resting Flies

All the methods considered so far have involved catching, by one means or another, tsetse which are active, whether spontaneously or in response to some stimulus presented by the investigator. Hence the term 'density-activity' has been used to describe such catches in order to emphasize that the size of the catch is a function of the absolute number of tsetse present and equally a function of the activity which brings them to the catcher.

A radically different approach is to do all the work oneself, to go out and look for tsetse in their non-active stages, just as one might walk on the sea shore and collect a sample of limpets.

This is not easy. The dull colours and muted patterns of all species of tsetse turn out to be very effective protective coloration—one may search for resting tsetse for days and, until one's eye is trained, never see one. While searching, one is a moving object in a tsetse habitat, and therefore attracts male flies, some of which perch on trees and get counted as resting flies. The maximum numbers to be expected are not large. The highest estimate by marking and recapture of a tsetse population which has been made was fifteen males—say forty-five flies—to 100 square yards, in an area of thicket with 144 woody stems per 100 square yards (Glasgow, 1963, p. 143). It must be emphasized that this was an unusually high population; densities of one hundredth of this figure are more usual.

Because of these factors the size of the catch of resting tsetse is unusually dependent on the skill and assiduity of the collector and all in all one would not attempt to use such catches to detect variations in the numbers of tsetse in a population. For determining whether the tsetse are particularly dependent on certain sub-areas one might use catches of resting flies to supplement other observations, but results have to be treated with caution. For example, there are thickets which one can penetrate only on one's hands and knees. Such vegetation, especially if it contains thorny elements, is difficult to search thoroughly, yet it may contain important and popular resting sites.

As a sampling method, searches for resting flies are of most use for studying the composition of a population. It is the only way of getting appreciable numbers of recently fed tsetse, and almost all the information in Chapter 13 has been obtained by analysis of the gut contents of tsetse collected in this way.

To obtain an unbiased sample of female tsetse is a difficult problem. Even in those species in which males are attracted to a moving party, females are usually not attracted in the same numbers and those that are attracted are all ready to feed. Besides the cycle of feeding and digestion, repeated every four days or so, females are throughout their lives subject to the cycle of pregnancy and larviposition which is repeated approximately every ten days. It would not be surprising if the pregnancy cycle also affected behaviour and Saunders (1962) has evidence that this is so. He collected samples of a population of *G. pallidipes* by three methods and found a different pregnancy ratio from each method: hand-caught, 51%; bait-caught, 62% pregnant; trap-caught, 79% pregnant. One might reasonably hope that females caught resting would provide an unbiased sample, but hope is not certainty. Quite small differences in, for example, the height of perch selected by the fly might make a large difference to the ease with which certain females at certain stages of their reproductive cycle were found.

Resting catches, of course, are the only sampling method likely to answer the last question in our list—where are the inactive flies? Pilson and Leggate

(1962a) and Pilson and Pilson (1967) have introduced a useful device to overcome the intrinsic difficulty of finding tsetse. Their observations are made in conjunction with standing catches with a tethered ox. The flies are allowed to engorge, then caught, given individual marks and immediately released. The marks make the flies much easier to see, a telescope being used at times for examining high level sites. Once found, a fly can be identified from its mark without being caught, so that the time elapsed since feeding is known. One may suppose that the knowledge that a certain number of marked tsetse are almost certainly in the near vicinity of the ox is an encouragement to the searchers. These workers also found tsetse lying up in the heat of the day in holes too small for the catchers to enter. The entrances to these holes were closed with fine nets; in the evening the tsetse came out and could be counted.

In attempts to discover the resting places used at night, tsetse have been marked with fluorescent paint and then sought with ultra-violet light (Jewell, 1956, 1958; *see also* Chapter 19). This method has been superseded by the use of paint which reflects visible light (Rennison *et al.*, 1958; Pilson & Pilson, 1967) or by small pieces of reflecting tape stuck to the thorax. The flies were marked and released in the daytime, and beam torches were then used in night searches.

Several workers have identified resting sites, and then applied insecticide to them (e.g. Chadwick, 1964; Chadwick *et al.*, 1964; Finelle, 1967; Finelle *et al.*, 1963; Yvore *et al.*, 1963). Should such an operation result in local extermination of the tsetse, that is evidence that one has treated sites used by all of the tsetse some of the time. There may still be other important sites used by the flies at another time, for example, at night or in the heat of the day. The problem of where all of the tsetse are all of the time is indeed difficult to resolve.

Chapter 18

Methods for Identifying the Blood Meals of *Glossina*

B. G. F. WEITZ

SEROLOGICAL TESTS FOR IDENTIFICATION OF BLOOD MEALS

Precipitin Test

Preparation of Antigens for Immunization

Equal volumes of undiluted serum and 10% potash alum solution are mixed and allowed to precipitate. The *p*H is adjusted to 6·5 with NaOH solution and the suspension is finely ground up in Griffiths tubes (or mechanically). The antigens are prepared fresh before inoculation.

Immunization of Rabbits

5 ml. of the above suspension are inoculated intramuscularly in each leg. The doses are repeated weekly on three occasions and seven days after the last injection the rabbits are test-bled. If the titres are satisfactory 25 ml. of blood are withdrawn by cardiac puncture. The animals are allowed to rest for a week or ten days after bleeding before being re-inoculated with a single dose of the same antigen. The rabbits can then be bled 7–10 days afterwards. The procedure can be repeated many times depending on the health of the rabbit

and the titres of the serum; some animals can maintain this regime for more than a year. The blood collected is allowed to clot and the serum from several bleedings or animals is pooled and stored at −15°C until required for testing for potency.

Tests for Sensitivity and Specificity

The highest dilution of the homologous serum which gives a positive ring test (*vide infra*) with undiluted antiserum is the titre of the serum. Animals with homologous titres of less than 1/50,000 are discarded.

The absorptions of the antisera are made as described by Weitz (1952, 1956) until the antisera fail to react with 1/10 dilution of heterologous sera. A suitable antiserum should react at a dilution of 1/50,000 to 1/126,000 of the homologous sera (or those of closely related animals) and should show no trace of reaction with a dilution of 1/10 of any heterologous sera after absorption.

Preservation of Sera

In order to produce crystal clear solutions for the precipitin test, the lipoproteins are extracted by freezing at −25°C in equal volumes of ether and the ether layer is removed from the serum after centrifugation. The process is repeated two or three times until all the fats are removed by the ether. Finally, the serum is filtered through a sterile membrane, ampouled under aseptic conditions in suitable volumes (0·5 to 5·0 ml.), freeze dried and sealed in dry nitrogen. Dried ampoules are opened and reconstituted with the equivalent volumes of distilled water immediately before use.

Method of Testing

The principle of the precipitin ring test is to superimpose a layer of antigen above a column of undiluted antiserum without allowing mixing of the reagents, in a narrow tube, thus forming an 'interface' between the antigen and the antiserum where the reaction occurs. The precipitate formed as a result of the combination of antigen and antibody appears as a whitish ring at the interface.

Many different devices may be used to layer the antigen over the antiserum. For identification tests on a large scale, an apparatus was devised by Weitz (1957) which allows twelve tests to be carried out simultaneously. By such means it is possible to manipulate several hundred tests an hour.

A common method used for small-scale work is to introduce a drop of the antigen in the bottom of a narrow conical (Dryer's) tube and to underlay the heavier serum by allowing it to flow along the sides of the tube, thus preventing mixing and forming an interface with the antigen in the conical part of the tube. Alternatively the reagents may be introduced into capillary tubes by suction or by capillarity but the narrower the interface the less visible the precipitate. The diameter of the interface should be about 2–3 mm. for optimum results consistent with the use of minimum volumes of the reagents.

Whichever method is used, the reaction is allowed to take place at room temperature for 1–2 hours and the interface is then examined for the presence of a 'positive white ring' in a suitable viewing box or across incidental light against a dark background.

Positive and negative controls consisting of suitable dilutions of known sera, or preferably identified or known blood meals, should always be included in the tests and the potency and specificity of antisera should be checked at regular intervals.

Haemagglutination-Inhibition Tests (HIT)

Antisera

These are prepared by the same method as for precipitating sera but are not absorbed. Usually the most useful sera for the HIT are obtained in the early stages of immunization (second or third course of immunization) because the specific inhibition is less sensitive in the later stages.

Tests for Specific Inhibitory Activity

The highest dilution of the homologous serum which *specifically* inhibits the agglutination by the antisera of sensitized cells is referred to as the titre of inhibition. Satisfactory antisera have an inhibition titre of at least 1/1,000–1/5,000 (*see* below) and these are then dispensed into ampoules and dried from the frozen state as the precipitin antisera but the lipoproteins are not extracted.

Sensitization of Red Blood Cells

Normal healthy rabbits are bled from the ear vein into an equal volume of Alsever's solution and the blood suspension is stored at + 4°C for not longer than twenty-four hours before use. Four times the volume of the suspension finally required is centrifuged at 1,500 r.p.m. for 5 minutes and the supernatant is discarded. This procedure is repeated two or three times in equivalent volumes of diluted saline solution. The final washing is discarded and the packed red blood cells are resuspended in an equal volume of chilled physiological saline solution.

A predetermined concentration (usually about 1/200) of the antigen (normal serum of the species under test) is diluted in saline and 30 parts are added to 1 part of the suspension of red blood cells. Five parts of a freshly thawed solution of *bis*-diazotized benzidine (prepared as described by Gordon *et al.* 1958) diluted 1/5 in phosphate buffer is added to the mixture which is left at room temperature for about 15 minutes and the mixture is gently shaken occasionally. The cells are separated by centrifugation at 1,200 r.p.m. for 5 minutes and are washed twice in 1% normal rabbit serum (NRS) in phosphate buffer. They are finally resuspended in NRS to the original volume of antigen and stored at 4°C until required but not longer than 6 hours.

Inhibition Test

The antiserum is diluted in NRS in saline to the optimum concentrations which are determined by a preliminary test (*see* Table 18.1). For example, an antiserum agglutinating the red blood cells sensitized with the homologous serum at a titre of approximately 1/50,000 can be used satisfactorily at dilutions of 1/500, 1/1,000 and 1/2,000.

Control system: it is essential to control the test with as many different antigens of the closely related species as practicable. For example, when testing for a particular species of bovid, at least all the other bovids which could act as hosts must be included in the control systems in addition to the homologous serum. (In the example in Table 18.1 only two species are included as no other Suidae occurred in the area from which the blood meals to be identified were obtained.)

Volumes of 0·05 ml. of each control serum in dilutions ranging between 1/10 and 1/128,000 are added to equal volumes of each concentration of the anti-serum. The unknown blood meal solutions are similarly added to each concentration of antiserum in equal volumes of 0·05 ml. After a period of incubation at room temperature for 1 hour, 0·05 ml. of the sensitized red blood cell suspension is added, mixing well, to each tube containing the control antigen dilutions and the unknown blood meals. The tubes are allowed to stand at room temperature for at least 1 hour to allow the red blood cells to settle on the bottom of the tubes.

Results

Non-agglutinated cells settle on the curved bottom of the tube in a small heap, giving the appearance of a dense spot or tight ring in the centre of the bottom of the tube viewed from beneath by means of a mirror. Fully agglutinated cells cover the whole bottom of the tube and are evenly distributed, appearing as a diffuse pink surface with no dense edges. Intermediate agglutination is indicated by the appearance of a dense edge surrounding the agglutinated cells. In the examples in Table 18.1, the results are recorded as – indicating no agglutination of the red blood cells (complete inhibition) and + to +++ depending on the degree of agglutination.

Interpretation of the Results

The identifications can be made only if all the controls are consistent. Table 18.1 shows the results obtained by the Haemagglutination-Inhibition Test on ten suid feeds with the anti-warthog system and the converse anti-bushpig system. As the concentration of the antisera is decreased the test becomes more sensitive and weak feeds are only identified in the most dilute antiserum concentration (e.g. feed No. 2 and No. 7). Too concentrated feeds will inhibit agglutination even at the low dilution of antiserum but may also show some inhibition in the high dilutions of the opposite system (e.g. feed No. 5 and No. 9). Very weak feeds may not inhibit either system and must remain 'unidentified suid feed' (e.g. feed No. 10).

Apart from indicating the concentration of the feed, the use of three dilutions of antiserum in the test ensures that each feed is tested three times for each system.

When larger groups of closely related animals are suspected hosts, it is necessary to carry out tests with antisera for each species. Thus bovid feeds which may be derived from as many as ten different bovid species will be tested thirty times (three dilutions of antiserum for each species) and the results obtained must be consistent throughout before a valid identification can be made.

TABLE 18.1

Identification of blood meals of tsetse flies by the inhibition of haemagglutination test. (Warthog identification)

Antiserum: Dilution	Inhibiting Antigen	Dilutions									
		1/10	1/100	1/1,000	1/2,000	1/4,000	1/8,000	1/16,000	1/32,000	1/64,000	Nil
anti warthog 1/500	Warthog serum	±	—	—	—	±	+++	+++	+++	+++	+++
anti warthog 1/500	Bushpig serum	+++	+++	+++	+++	+++	+++	+++	+++	+++	+++
anti warthog 1/1,000	Warthog serum	—	—	—	—	—	±	+++	+++	+++	+++
anti warthog 1/1,000	Bushpig serum	++	+++	+++	+++	+++	+++	+++	+++	+++	+++
anti warthog 1/2,000	Warthog serum	—	—	—	—	—	—	+	+++	+++	+++
anti warthog 1/2,000	Bushpig serum	—	++	+++	+++	+++	+++	+++	+++	+++	+++
	Unknown Blood meals no.	1	2	3	4	5	6	7	8	9	10
anti warthog 1/500		+++	+++	±	+++	—	++	+++	+	—	+++
1/1,000		+++	+++	—	+++	—	+	+++	—	—	+++
1/2,000		+++	+++	—	+++	—	—	—	—	—	+++
Identification		B	B	W	B	W	B	W	W	W	US

Cells sensitized with warthog serum were added to all tubes.

B = Bushpig W = Warthog US = Unidentified Suid.

TABLE 18.1 (*continued*)

Identification of blood meals of tsetse flies by the inhibition of haemagglutination test. (Bushpig identification)

Antiserum: Dilution	Inhibiting Antigen	Dilutions									
		1/10	1/100	1/1,000	1/2,000	1/4,000	1/8,000	1/16,000	1/32,000	1/64,000	Nil
anti bushpig 1/500	Bushpig serum	—	—	—	±	++	+++	+++	+++	+++	+++
anti bushpig 1/500	Warthog serum	±	+++	+++	+++	+++	+++	+++	+++	+++	+++
anti bushpig 1/1,000	Bushpig serum	—	—	—	—	—	++	+++	+++	+++	+++
anti bushpig 1/1,000	Warthog serum	—	+++	+++	+++	+++	+++	+++	+++	+++	+++
anti bushpig 1/2,000	Bushpig serum	—	—	—	—	—	+	+++	+++	+++	+++
anti bushpig 1/2,000	Warthog serum	—	+	++	+++	+++	+++	+++	+++	+++	+++
	Unknown Blood meals no.	1	2	3	4	5	6	7	8	9	10
anti bushpig 1/500		±	+++	+++	+	+++	—	+++	+++	+++	+++
1/1,000		—	++	+++	—	++	—	+++	+++	++	+++
1/2,000		—	±	+++	—	±	—	+++	+++	±	+++
Identification		B	B	W	B	W	B	W	W	W	US

Erythrocytes sensitized with bushpig serum were added to all tubes.

B = Bushpig W = Warthog US = Unidentified Suid.

TABLE 18.2

Procedure for the identification of tsetse fly blood meals

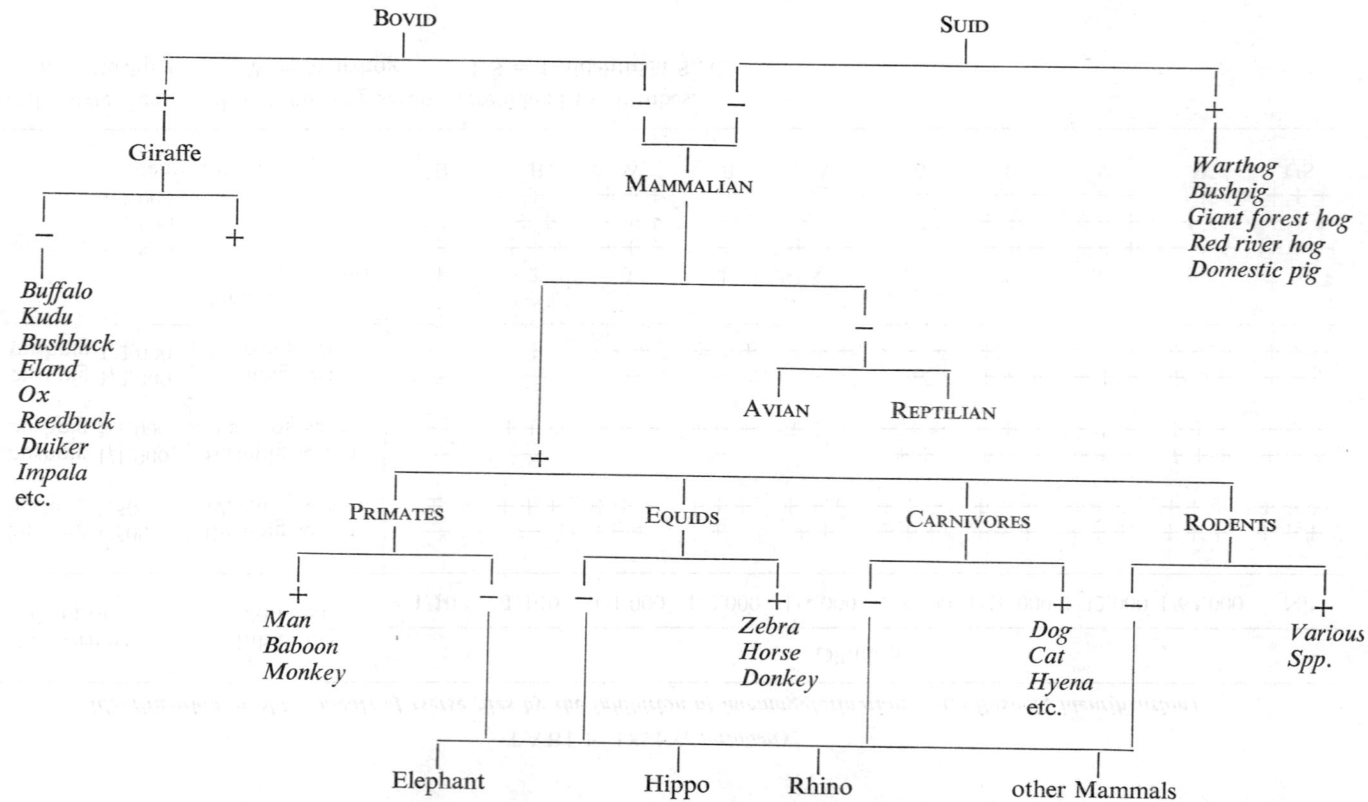

Antisera used to identify groups by the precipitin test are shown in capitals.
Antisera used to identify species by the precipitin test are shown in roman type.
Antisera used to identify species by the Haemagglutination-Inhibition test are *italicized*.

General Testing Procedure

To avoid wastage of the blood-meal solution, it is usual to test all blood smears for the most common hosts first (*see* Table 18.2) i.e. suids and bovids, by the precipitin test. All suid positive feeds are then tested by the HIT to identify the species of suid, e.g. warthog, bushpig or domestic pig as the case may be. Similarly all bovid feeds are tested for the individual species by HIT. The feeds which were negative with anti-suid and anti-bovid sera by precipitin test are then tested with anti-mammalian serum. Positive feeds can then be further tested by precipitin test for other groups of hosts, e.g. carnivores, primates, etc., and subsequently the species identified by the relevant HIT system. Feeds which did not react with anti-mammalian serum are tested with anti-avian and anti-reptilian sera. It has not usually been practicable to identify individual species of birds or reptiles but those feeds giving positive reactions could be further tested by the HIT for this purpose when required. Feeds which fail to react with any antiserum by the precipitin test must be regarded as unsuitable for identification unless there is good reason to suspect that other groups are involved (e.g. amphibian blood).

An example of the procedure commonly followed is shown in Table 18.2, but the schedule is altered according to the hosts available in the area studied and the results expected. If the material available for testing is insufficient, it may not be possible to identify the host, but at least many host species can be eliminated or the group reactions should give an indication of a limited number of hosts from which the feed was derived (e.g. suids). As these tests may have to be done over a long period, it is essential to ensure proper storage of the blood-meal extract at −20°C throughout the testing procedure.

Chapter 19

Miscellaneous Techniques Used in the Study of *Glossina*

W. H. POTTS

DISSECTION OF MALE TERMINALIA AND FEMALE GENITAL ARMATURE

The traditional methods for dissecting, preparing and mounting these parts have been described by Newstead, Evans and Potts (1924, pp. 236–38). The directions given for the removal of the male terminalia from dried, pinned specimens allow this to be done without destroying their usefulness for comparison with other specimens. After removal, the terminalia are boiled for 15 minutes in 10% caustic potash to dissolve the body fats and soft tissues which are then squeezed out, leaving the chitinous structures clearly visible. The chitinous structures are flattened dorso-ventrally for the *palpalis* and *morsitans* groups but laterally for the *fusca* group. After clearance with xylol, the preparations are mounted in Canada balsam on a glass slide, under a coverslip, with the ventral aspect uppermost. Nash and Jordan (1959) prefer dorso-ventral flattening and mounting for the *fusca* group also; male terminalia of the West African species of this group, mounted in this way, are illustrated in their paper and the results are compared with those obtained from laterally compressed specimens mounted according to Newstead's method. Machado (1954, pp. 18–20; 1959, pp. 56–7) points out that dorso-ventral flattening and crushing may result in grave distortion of some features of the terminalia; this makes the method unsuitable for critical taxonomic studies, although he concedes its usefulness for speedy mass identification of specimens from species in which the characters of the terminalia are well known. For critical work, Machado recommends a solution of chloral hydrate and acetic acid in water as a softening agent and states that potash should not be used for this purpose. He also advises that the terminalia should not only be mounted flattened *without crushing* but should also be examined unflattened; in addition, certain parts of the terminalia should be dissected out, examined from various angles and then mounted, again without crushing. Mounts of the various parts should also be made which permit them to be viewed from several different aspects. It is necessary, in Machado's opinion, to examine numerous specimens collected from the same locality.

For examination of the female genital armature, Newstead, Evans and Potts (*loc. cit.*) recommend the removal of the two distal segments of the abdomen in the case of the *palpalis* and *morsitans* groups, in which only the external genital plates are required; the segments are macerated in potash to remove the soft tissues and are then mounted dorso-ventrally, venter uppermost, as for the male terminalia. For the *fusca* group, it is necessary to remove the last four segments of the abdomen or, if the presence of a larva is apparent, the entire abdomen should be removed so that the whole of the uterus, with the signum at its anterior end, may be obtained. The genital fossa with the signum can then be isolated and mounted along with the external genital plates, again to give dorso-ventral views. Machado (1954) notes that although the dorsal plates of the females are not subject to grave distortion by flattening and crushing, as are the male terminalia, the anal plates can be so distorted.

TECHNIQUES FOR MARKING ADULT *GLOSSINA*

Scott (1931) was the first to review the methods used for marking tsetse flies. He records that the earliest worker to use marked flies was Bagshawe (1908) who, followed by Carpenter (1912), amputated a leg in the middle of the femur or tibia so that a simple but limited marking system was evolved by severance of different legs in different places on different dates. It was argued that, in nature, breaks in the legs of tsetse would occur only at an articulation between segments. By the use of this simple system, some conclusions were drawn as to the length of life of *G. palpalis* [*G. fuscipes*]; a male was recaptured on the 250th day after marking and a female on the 182nd day. As indications of possible longevity in *Glossina* these conclusions must be accepted with reserve because, in nature, legs might be broken at points other than articulations as, for example, by the bites of predatory ants. At the same time, it must be remembered that these estimations of longevity in wild flies have been closely approximated among flies kept in the laboratory.[1]

Apart from its doubtful reliability, the amputation method of marking is incapable of yielding the complicated information needed when something more than simple observations on length of life is sought. More complete information is essential when investigating the rate of dispersal of tsetse flies and, more particularly, when attempting to determine the absolute number of flies by marking, releasing and recapturing them (*see* pp. 408–410); it then becomes important to be able to distinguish, from a distance, a fly that has already been marked. These requirements led to the introduction of a method of marking by applying[2] small spots of paint to the thorax of the tsetse, and since then various systems of marking by this means have been devised and used.

In the marking system devised by Jackson (1933a), spots of two colours, changed every collecting day, were placed in any of five positions on the dorsum of the thorax, namely, the centres of the four quarters of the scutum and the centre of the scutellum. The two colours indicated the day on which the fly had been captured and released and the disposition of the spots showed the place of capture, the hunger conditions of the fly at the time and any other particulars desired. As two, three or four spots could be applied, it was possible to use a considerable number of two-colour combinations. It was found practicable to use thirteen different colours (dark blue, light blue, dark green, light green, red, pink, orange, white, yellow ochre, brown, purple and grey), all of which could be obtained by mixing, in various combinations, four basic paints (deep ultramarine, vermilion, chrome-yellow-mid and flake white, in the artist's series of oil paints); other colours and the student's series of paints were found to be unsatisfactory. This method permitted different assortments of colours to be used on seventy-eight separate days. On recapture, the pairs of colours of the day of recapture were placed peripherally on a clock system, one colour representing the hour and the other the minute (5-minute intervals being used). The fly thus received, on recapture and re-release, a unique individual mark. For example, a fly marked originally with two light spots on the left and one red spot on the right of the thorax might be taken as originally marked as

[1] Jack (1939) recorded 185 days as the maximum life of the male of *G. morsitans* at 18°C and 233 days as that of the female.

[2] A suitably robust dry grass stem was originally employed to apply the paints but later a thin spindle of wood tapered to a fine point was preferred. When a two-colour system is used, it is convenient to taper both ends of the spindle and to use one end for each colour.

hungry in locality A; the same fly, recaptured on a white-yellow day, would then be re-marked white and yellow, possibly by placing the white spot in the right fore corner of the thorax and the yellow spot mid-way up the left-hand side; this would be recorded as 1·45. If a second fly with the same original marking were recaptured on the same day, it would receive differentially positioned peripheral marks in white and yellow with, for instance, the marks at 3·35 or 4·40 or other appropriate situations.

Jackson (1953) introduced another system of marking by which it was possible to give individual marks to more than 25,000 flies. In this system, only the first nine colours listed above were used as it had been found that, with ageing, the remaining four were difficult to distinguish from some of the other colours. Again, the day of capture and release was indicated by pairs of colours but only two spots were used in the original marking, these being placed round the periphery of the dorsum of the thorax in two of ten selected positions. Two of these were situated medially, one immediately behind the head and the other on the scutellum, indicating the figures 0 and 5, respectively. Proceeding clockwise from 0, two further sites were selected on the right-hand side in front of the transverse mesonotal suture in the middle of the thorax (Fig. 8.1) to denote 1 and 2 respectively; the corresponding sites on the left-hand side indicated 8 and 9, and the remaining four positions, similarly disposed behind the transverse suture, denoted 3, 4, 6 and 7. In addition, four other sites were selected in the centre of the thorax, two immediately in front of the transverse suture and two immediately behind it. The left-hand position of the first pair was assigned 0, the right-hand position 1 and, proceeding clockwise, the pair immediately behind the suture, 2 and 3, respectively. The first of the colours of the day, placed in one of the last three central positions, indicated the hundreds (up to 300); in the peripheral position it denoted the tens (10–90). The second colour of the day, placed peripherally, indicated the digits. By this means, 360 flies could be differentially marked with one pair of colours (multiples of 11 could not be indicated as two spots could not be placed in the same position). By varying the order of the pairs of colours used to denote the day of capture and release (e.g. yellow-white, white-yellow, etc.), seventy-two colour combinations were available and thus, with the 360 positional markings mentioned above, it was possible to assign individual marks to over 25,000 flies.[1]

Buxton (1955, Appendix 6, pp. 721–3), in a critical discussion on the use of paints for marking tsetse, was not completely satisfied that this procedure was entirely harmless to the flies. He pointed out that the handling involved in applying paints might be harmful, that some paints or their solvents might be

[1] A good account of this system is given in a pamphlet (EATRO, 1955). This useful publication also describes several other techniques of value to field workers including detailed instructions for conducting reconnaissances, setting out fly-rounds, carrying out other methods of sampling tsetse populations (*see* also Chapter 17), diagnosing hunger stages (*see* also Chapter 17), recording vegetation types and identifying the East African species of *Glossina* by external characters only. A similar publication (Davies, 1967), written in simple language for the use of junior staff and having particular application to West African conditions, contains much general information about tsetse flies as well as an account of the bionomics of *Glossina* and of the measures used for their control.

toxic and that certain marks might make flies conspicuous to their enemies and so result in a higher mortality in the field as compared with unmarked or less conspicuously marked flies. Vanderplank (1947b) claimed that certain paints (particularly green ones) containing arsenic and chromium were injurious to the flies and Jackson had earlier noted that whereas the cheaper 'student's' paints were deleterious, the more expensive 'artist's' colours were not (*cf.* EATRO, 1955). Scott (1931) was satisfied that the paints used in his work were not injurious to the flies, as was Jackson (1941) for his paints from observations on the survival time of marked and unmarked flies kept in the laboratory. However, in critical experiments, Jackson (*loc. cit.*) showed that, although handling had little effect on the survival of released flies, the application of paint slightly shortened the survival time. Later, Jackson (1948) found that the paints appeared to have a slightly deleterious effect on freshly emerged flies but not on older flies. At the same time, he demonstrated that in the rainy season there was no difference in the frequency with which flies were recovered as between those conspicuously or inconspicuously marked with paint but that, in the dry season, the former were less frequently recovered than the latter. In a later series of investigations, Jackson (in EATRO, 1952, p. 16) liberated two groups of *G. swynnertoni* in an area from which this species was absent; in one group the flies were neither handled nor marked and in the other they were both handled and marked, but no difference was found in the survival period of the two groups. It would seem, therefore, that a further critical exploration of the subject would be useful (*see* also Chapter 17).

A more recent development has been the use of fluorescent paints for the study of the nocturnal resting places of tsetse flies (*see* also Chapter 17) and of ulta-violet light for their detection (Jewell, 1956, 1958; McDonald, 1960, 1961). Fluorescent powder has been used to mark *Musca autumnalis* De Greer by shaking the flies in a jar or paper bag containing the powder (Turner & Gerhardt, 1965). Flies marked in this way could be detected at night in ultra-violet light and, in daylight, they could be detected for days at a distance of at least 50 feet. In another method, used in East Africa, a reflecting paint containing microscopic glass beads was applied which allowed the detection of flies at night by reflecting the light of an ordinary electric torch (Rennison *et al.*, 1958; Southon, 1959). A modification of this method was used in Zambia by Robinson (1965); the flies were marked by affixing a patch (about 2 mm. square) of a white, reflecting material, Scotchlite, which made them visible at night, in the light of an electric torch, from a distance of 20–30 feet.

An ingenious method of marking tsetse flies or other blood-sucking insects, without the need to handle them, has been devised by Knight and Southon (1963). Flies were allowed to feed on an ox which had received an intravenous injection of 4 g. trypan blue in aqueous solution. *G. morsitans*, in batches of six, were fed on the ox and their blood meals were examined for the presence of the dye at intervals after feeding. In the batch that fed on the ox on the day on which it was injected, the dye was detected in all of the six flies examined two days after their meal and in four of the six flies examined eight days after their meal. In groups that fed on the ox on the twenty-fourth day after injection, the dye was detected in all of the six flies examined two days after their meal, in three of six flies examined three days after feeding and in one of six flies examined four days after feeding on the ox.

Another method, evolved for marking (without handling) flies that emerge from puparia buried in the ground, has been used in the study of tsetse flies. This method depends on the flies picking up a marker as they emerge from the buried puparia. MacLeod and Donnelly (1957) arranged that emerging blow-flies passed through a layer of vermiculite mixed with a fluorescent powder. For work with tsetse flies, Dame, Dean and Ford (1965) modified this method slightly, using as a marker a powdered blue dye that adhered to the everted ptilinum (*see* pp. 232, 344, and Fig. 8.5) as the flies made their way to the surface; the powder was retained when the ptilinum was withdrawn. Flies so marked were readily detected when their heads were squashed on a filter paper wetted with acetone.

Much use has been made of radioisotopes for marking insects in the study of their dispersal and range of flight but the method does not allow individual insects to be distinguished. The usual mode of administration of isotopes for this purpose has been in food or drinking water (e.g. for *Lucilia*, MacLeod & Donnelly, 1957; Donnelly, 1958: for house-flies and blow-flies, Wharton *et al.*, 1962) or, for mosquitoes and other insects with aquatic stages, in the water in which these stages are reared. In such instances, the isotopes generally used are those giving 'soft' radiations (beta rays) such as radioactive phosphorus (^{32}P); these have only feeble penetrating powers and a small range of detection. Marked insects are detected by scanning, with a Geiger counter, samples captured after the release and dispersal of the marked insects. The 'harder', more penetrating radiations (gamma rays) have been used to follow the movements of soil insects (Jenkins, 1962), the marker being incorporated in paints or, where the nature of the isotope lends itself to this mode of use, as metal labels. Even these more penetrating radiations cannot be detected at a range of more than a few feet. None of these radioactive methods has so far been applied to studies on *Glossina* but they may find a place in the investigation of adult resting places, especially the last mentioned.[1]

Southwood (1966, pp. 57–74) has given an exhaustive account of the marking of insects in connection with ecological studies, and Muirhead Thomson (1968) has reviewed this subject with particular reference to the investigation of insect vectors of disease.

Although it does not involve the actual marking of tsetse flies themselves, a brief reference may be made here to the latest development in a related field which has relevance to studies on *Glossina*. In Rhodesia, miniature radio transmitters, attached to warthogs, have been used in an attempt to relate the patterns of behaviour of these hosts of *Glossina* to those of the flies themselves (Anon., 1968). This is a line of research that the work of Weitz and his co-investigators has shown to be an essential prerequisite for intelligent and economic attack on tsetse flies through interference with their sources of food.

[1] But Dean, Williamson and Phelps (1969) attached radioactive Tantalum wire (^{182}Ta) to the thorax of individuals, of *G. morsitans* which they liberated in large cages in natural woodland; the flies were located by radiation monitors at a range of 5 to 12 feet.

DISSECTION OF FEMALE *GLOSSINA* TO OBTAIN THE OVARIES AND SPERMATHECAE AND TO DETERMINE INSEMINATION

In the notes for field studies published by EATRO (1955), two methods (methods A and B below) are described for dissecting female tsetse flies for the examination of the spermathecae to determine whether or not insemination has taken place; either of these methods serves also for the examination of the ovaries and uterine contents. In both methods the wings are removed and, in the writer's view, it is advantageous to remove the legs also.

METHOD A. Two cuts are made with a scissor-forceps so as to shave off an extremely narrow margin on each side of the abdomen, the cuts extending from the broadest part of the abdomen to about three-quarters of the way to its tip; the abdomen is then severed at the top of these cuts and placed back downwards in a drop of saline solution on a glass slide so that the ventral wall can be folded backwards to expose the abdominal contents. The spermathecae, uterus and ovaries can then be separated from the gut and freed from fat bodies and tracheae.

METHOD B. The extreme tip of the abdomen is removed by scissor-forceps, care being taken not to damage the uterus by removing too much. The abdomen is then cut off a little above its broadest point and placed on a slide with the venter uppermost. With a dissecting needle held in one hand, slight pressure is applied so as to cause the tissues to protrude slightly through the opening at the tip of the abdomen; the uterus, which can then be seen, is pulled out with a dissecting needle held in the other hand, bringing with it the ovaries and spermathecae. This method has the advantage that little subsequent dissection is needed since the organs come out with only a small amount of attached tracheae and fat-body.

Saunders (1962) advocates a small cut on each side of the sixth abdominal segment from which the tip of the abdomen is dragged away bringing with it the reproductive system and a short length of gut.

The writer favours a slight modification of the Saunders' method in which the incisions, directed inwardly and slightly anteriorly, are made at about the junction of the sixth and seventh abdominal segments; in addition, narrow margins of the abdominal segments are shaved off, as in Method A, to facilitate the withdrawal of the organs.

Similar methods can, of course, be used to obtain the reproductive organs of male specimens.

Examination of the spermathecae for insemination should be made microscopically, a low power being used with transmitted light. If the female has been effectively paired a mass of sperm will be observed, whereas if pairing has been ineffective the spermathecae will appear clear and transparent (Mellanby, 1936; Buxton, 1955, Pl. 33). No difficulty is experienced in detecting full insemination but uncertainty may arise if there is only partial insemination. Nash (1955) has paid a great deal of attention to this subject and, in the course of an investigation of fertilization in females of *G. palpalis* kept in captivity, he has examined different degrees of insemination in detail. He noted that females might be only partially impregnated and did not regard a female as fully impregnated (or inseminated) unless both spermathecae were dark and completely opaque. Thus, one spermatheca might be full and the other empty, or one might be half full and the other quarter full. Nash devised a rating for the degree of impregnation which he termed the mean spermathecal value; a fully impregnated female would rate as 2 (1 + 1) whereas in the other instances specified above the rating would be 1 (1 + 0) and 0·75 (0·5 + 0·25), respectively. Investigating the age at which females were most readily impregnated, Nash found that, when females were given the opportunity to mate during the first ten days after emergence, the proportion inseminated ranged from 60% (of those mated on the ninth day) to 84·4% (of those mated on the third day); significantly more females were inseminated during the first five days after emergence than during the second five days. Nevertheless, the mean spermathecal values were all either 1·8 or 1·9, indicating that all of the females impregnated during the first ten days after emergence would be nearly fully impregnated. Nash's observations were largely confirmed by Jordan (1958). Dame and Ford (1959), investigating multiple mating in *G. morsitans orientalis* (*see* Chapter 26, p. 539), tested the ability of males to continue effective insemination. They recorded that the sperm content of spermathecae varied from 10–15% to 100% of capacity, as shown by ordinary microscopic examination; they also used phase microscopy to detect smaller amounts of sperm which they recorded as sub-normal insemination.

METHODS USED FOR THE STUDY OF THE METABOLISM OF *GLOSSINA*

Methods used in the study of the metabolism of *Glossina* in the laboratory and in the field have been discussed by Buxton (1955, Appendix 2) with the object of achieving some degree of standardization[1] of the techniques employed. The headings under which these methods are discussed by Buxton are (1) hunger stages, (2) estimation of the proportion of dry matter, (3) estimation of water and fat, (4) estimation of size. In the following account, the salient points made by Buxton under these various headings are recapitulated and later developments are included.

Hunger Staging

Buxton considered it valuable to record the degree of repletion of wild flies and advocated the use of the four hunger stages described by Jackson (1933a; 1937) as a convenient conventional classification. These four stages are applicable only to non-teneral males; teneral males (Chapter 8, p. 233; Chapter 14,

[1] In support of Buxton's campaign for the standardization of techniques, the attention of investigators of the activity of tsetse flies in the field is drawn to the concept of catch time described by Lumsden (1952). In this, 1,800 hours is taken as constantly co-incident with sunset.

p. 344) and females (in which the development of the larva obscures the manifestation of the hunger cycle) are excluded. The four hunger stages, as crystallized in the notes for field studies of tsetse flies published by EATRO (1955), are described below.

Stage 1. Gorged: abdomen distended with red or blue-black blood clearly visible from outside; entirely opaque when viewed against the light; dissection showing recognizable red blood (corpuscles sufficiently intact to be measured).

Stage 2. Replete: abdomen slightly convex but no red or black colour visible, entirely to two-thirds opaque when viewed against the light (measurement from front end of hypopygium (*see* Fig. 8.6) to front end of abdomen); no wrinkling of underside of abdomen; recognizable blood corpuscles on dissection.

Stage 3. Intermediate: abdomen not swollen, may be slightly concave; a quarter to two-thirds opaque, viewed against the light; no trace of recognizable blood corpuscles on dissection; underside may show wrinkling.

Stage 4. Hungry: abdomen concave or flattened, underside often wrinkled, a third or quarter opaque to entirely clear, and yellow (not white as in the teneral fly) when viewed against the light.

Flies may be encountered that are difficult to classify, usually because they have taken only partial feeds. Flies that cannot definitely be classified as Stages 1, 2 or 4 should be assigned to Stage 3 (intermediate).

An estimation of the mean hunger stage (MHS) of a sample of flies can be made in the following manner. Flies in Stage 1 are disregarded (on the grounds that they have recently been in Stage 4). The number of flies in Stage 2 is multiplied by two, the number in Stage 3 is multiplied by three and the number in Stage 4 is multiplied by four. The sum of these numbers is divided by the sum of the numbers of flies assigned to each of these stages. This gives, for the MHS, a figure of between 2 and 4; a figure below 3 indicates some degree of hunger in the sample and a figure above 3 indicates some degree of repletion.

The value of the information obtained from an investigation of these hunger stages varies with the species of *Glossina.* The stages are readily distinguishable in *G. morsitans* and *G. swynnertoni* but, as most of the flies of the *fusca* group are taken in Stage 4, little information about hunger in this group is obtained by this method; similarly, in some situations, this technique is not very useful with *G. pallidipes.* Owing to the dark colour of the integument of *G. palpalis*, the hunger stages in this species are not easy to distinguish.

An alternative but somewhat cruder measure of hunger is based on the behaviour of flies encountered by the collecting party (EATRO, 1955). Hungrier flies tend to settle on the catchers head-up, whereas less hungry flies tend to settle head-down or in some position other than head-up, or even to sit on the ground nearby. The number of flies recorded in each position gives some indication of the degree of hunger of the sample of flies collected and this information can be used instead of, or to supplement, the method by which the flies are assigned to four hunger stages. Advantages of the behaviour method are that it is simpler to use and that it obviates the constant checking of the criteria in current use to ensure that these are not gradually changed. With *G. morsitans* and *G. swynnertoni*, a proportion of 80% or more non-teneral males caught on the ground indicates a sample of not very hungry flies (MHS of 3 or less) whereas a proportion of 50 to 80% indicates a more hungry sample (MHS of 3–3·5) and a proportion of less than 50% indicates a very hungry population (MHS of 3·5 or over). An even simpler and better procedure is to record the percentage of flies that settle head-up, as most of the flies doing so are anxious to feed; high percentages of flies that settle head-up indicate hungry communities and lower percentages less hungry communities. With *G. palpalis*, the proportion of non-teneral males captured on the catching party, irrespective of whether they settle head-up or head-down, may be taken as an indication of hunger; a high proportion indicates a hungry population and is generally associated with a high percentage of females and teneral flies.

In recent years, hunger-staging methods have been critically examined and compared with the more sophisticated methods of assessing the state of nutrition of flies (*see* also pp. 305–316). Bursell (1961a) has compared samples of *G. swynnertoni* obtained by different methods of catching and, from the results obtained, he concluded that four phases were discernible in the behaviour of males during the hunger cycle: (1) a phase of inactivity following the blood meal (also postulated by Jackson, 1933b), (2) a phase of activity characterized by attraction to moving objects and believed to be directed to the achievement of mating, (3) another phase of activity, directed to the satisfaction of hunger, manifested by attraction to potential hosts, and (4) a final phase of activity, again directed to the satisfaction of hunger, characterized by flies in a state of inanition in which they are again attracted to any moving objects. Standard catches, on the collecting party, consist mainly of flies in the third phase but with flies in the fourth well represented. The standard methods of sampling do not, according to this view, provide a representative sample of the fly population (*see* also pp. 388, 408–9, and Bursell, 1966a).

Estimation of Proportions of Dry Matter, Water and Fat

The methods used for these estimations consist essentially of ascertaining the wet weight and the dry weight of the flies and of extracting the fat by means of a suitable solvent. The weights (wet, dry and fatless) are usually obtained by means of a torsion balance (which can, if desired, be used in the field). Dry weight is ascertained after the flies have been dried in an oven until a constant weight is obtained. Fat is estimated by extraction with ether or chloroform. This is effected by repeated immersion of the dried flies in the solvent and weighing until a constant weight is again obtained. Jack (1939) showed that this method of estimating fat content gave results that approximated closely to those obtained by the use of the more sophisticated Soxhlet apparatus.

Buxton (1955, Appendix 2) has criticized these methods; nevertheless, valuable information is still being obtained by their use. Bursell (1959a) studied the water balance of flies at rest and of freshly emerged flies in the field (*G. morsitans* and *G. swynnertoni* in the habitat of the latter) and concluded that there was no relation between resistance to desiccation and habitat; he suggested that the water balance of the adult tsetse has been no obstacle to the invasion of semi-arid and arid habitats. From a study of newly emerged flies in the field he came to the tentative conclusion that flies tend to make use of microclimates in which the relative humidity is high. Parallel studies on the puparial stages have been described and discussed elsewhere (*see* pp. 358–9 and Fig. 15.2).

From further studies on the water loss of *G. morsitans*, Bursell (1960c) concluded that, although the mechanism for the conservation of water reserves under conditions of desiccation is present, the fly does not always make the fullest use of it unless its water reserves are threatened. Bursell and Glasgow (1960), investigating the relation between fat content and size, found a correlation between size and the saturation deficit of the atmosphere two months previously; they did not consider this to be a simple causal relation. The work of Bursell (1961) indicated that hunger may be a more important factor in determining the survival of the fly than desiccation. This led to more sophisticated studies on the metabolism of the fly, involving the use of chromatography to investigate the amino acids involved in its protein metabolism (Bursell, 1963, 1965, 1965a, 1966; Bursell & Slack, 1968); these studies are still in progress and are yielding valuable results (*see* also Chapter 12).

Measurement of Size

The size of tsetse flies, as distinct from their weight, is sometimes a matter of considerable importance. Jackson (1946) based his method of measuring fly size on the length of the cutting edge of the discal (hatchet) cell of the wing, that is, the distance between 'a' and 'd' in Fig. 8.3. Bursell (1960) has discussed methods for determining the size of flies critically and comprehensively. He found Jackson's method inconvenient in that it necessitated the removal and mounting of wings and, more importantly, that it was unreliable in that the discal cell measurement is poorly correlated with the residual dry weight of unfed flies. After testing a number of different methods, Bursell concluded that the most reliable results were obtained by measuring a defined area on the dorsal surface of the thorax; the area was calculated by multiplying the distance between the points of insertion of each member of the largest pair of lateral pronotal spines (humeral bristles, Fig. 8.1) by the distance between the base of the scutellar bristles (Fig. 8.1) and the mesonotal suture. These measurements were made, by means of a micrometer eyepiece and a low power objective, on the fly mounted on a vertical pin and correctly aligned in relation to the optical system. Bursell (1959a), however, found that this method was unsuitable for work on transpiration, as its use gave widely divergent rates of water loss from samples of resting unfed flies (*G. morsitans*) that had developed at different times of the year, although the composition (water content and fat content) was practically identical. For work on transpiration, therefore, correction for size should be made on the basis of residual dry weight, which gave a rate of water loss independent of size.

DETERMINATION OF THE AGE OF *GLOSSINA* IN ADULT AND PUPARIAL STAGES

Methods for Determining the Age of Adult Flies

The Wing-fray Method

Information as to the length of life of adult tsetse flies under natural conditions has been obtained from many investigations in which the flies have been marked, released and recaptured. Buxton (1955, pp. 459–63) has discussed the results of these investigations at length and has compared them with data obtained for flies maintained in captivity or kept in cages in a natural environment. By the recapture of unmarked teneral individuals of *G. morsitans* or *G. swynnertoni* released in localities in which the species did not occur, Jackson (1945a, 1946, 1948a, 1950) obtained information about the calendar age of the flies, this age being known to within ± 1 day, and the flies being liberated within 3d ays of emergence. Jackson related these ages to the degree of wear or fraying observed on the hind margin of the wing. According to the degree of damage or wear, he assigned flies to one or other of the six categories described in the terms given below, which are based on his (1946) description:

(1) wings perfect, hind margin intact and without any triangular notches;
(2) hind margin showing very slight or doubtfully genuine damage such as might be caused in the net during capture;
(3) definite evidence of wear, too extensive to be accidental, but with the notches confined to the proximal portion of the hind margin, between the fifth wing vein and the base of the wing;
(4) some wear or fraying on both sides of the fifth vein but with long sections still undamaged;
(5) hind margin presenting a saw-edged appearance and no longer showing long undamaged sections;
(6) hind margin showing heavy damage, rounded as well as triangular notches being present or large portions of the wing missing, giving a 'tattered' appearance to the wing.

In the notes for field studies published by EATRO (1955), the following directions are given for estimating the mean age of a sample of tsetse flies by this method.

One wing from each of thirty flies from the sample is examined microscopically under low power. It is convenient to place about ten wings between two glass slides for this purpose. Each wing is examined and assigned to one or other of Jackson's six categories. The mean age of the sample can then be estimated by multiplying the number of wings in each category by the factor assigned to that category in accordance with the following system. For categories 1, 2 and 3, the factors are 1, 2 and 3, respectively; for categories 4 and 5 they are 4·4 and 5·5, and the factor for category 6 is 6·9. The sum of the products (category × factor) is divided by the number of wings examined to give a mean value for the sample and from this the mean age of the sample can be obtained by reference to the table provided which is reproduced in Table 19.1 below.

TABLE 19.1

***Showing age in days under* (b) *and corresponding mean wing-fray value (MWFV) under* (a)**

(a) MWFV	(b) Age	(a) MWFV	(b) Age	(a) MWFV	(b) Age	(a) MWFV	(b) Age
1·6	11	2·8	21	3·9	31	5·1	41
1·8	12	2·9	22	4·0	32	5·2	42
1·9	13	3·0	23	4·2	33	5·3	43
2·0	14	3·1	24	4·3	34	5·4	44
2·1	15	3·3	25	4·4	35	5·5	45
2·2	16	3·4	26	4·5	36	5·6	46
2·3	17	3·5	27	4·6	37	5·8	47
2·4	18	3·6	28	4·7	38	5·9	48
2·6	19	3·7	29	4·8	39	6·0	49
2·7	20	3·8	30	5·0	40	—	—

Table 19.1 should only be used with male flies, as the wings of the females fray much more slowly. Jackson (1950) found no difference between the rate of fraying in the cooler wet season and that observed in his earlier work carried out in the hotter dry season. It appears therefore that the rate is not affected by temperature.

In his investigations on *G. palpalis* in Sierra Leone, Squire (1950, 1951, 1954) used the wing-fray method combined with wing colour to designate three age-groups: (1) a young age-group with smoky wings, (2) an intermediate age-group with tawny wings, and (3) an old age-group with wings both tawny and frayed. These age-groups were used in connection with studies on seasonal emergence from the puparium and on the natural infection rate of the fly with *T. vivax*; flies in the youngest age-group showed virtually no evidence of infection.

The Ovarian Dissection Method

The ovarian cycle in *Glossina* and its value in determining the physiological age of tsetse flies have been described in Chapter 14. By observing the contents of the uterus and the relative sizes of the follicles in each of the two ovaries and in each of the two ovules that constitute each ovary, it is possible to recognize eight age categories based on the ovarian cycles. This is illustrated in Figure 14.4 which records observations made on *G. morsitans orientalis* kept at 26°C. Saunders (1962) has shown how age can be determined with even greater precision by sub-dividing the eight categories according to the actual size of the follicles and other details. Thus, he sub-divides category (0), which in this instance lasts eight days, into two groups: (0a) in which follicle A measures less than 0·6 mm. in length (age 1–4 days) and (0b) in which follicle A measures more than 0·6 mm. in length (age 4–8 days). Category 1 is subdivided into three groups: (1a) in which ovariole A has an open sac and the uterus contains an egg (age 8–12 days), (1b) in which ovariole A has a follicular relic and the uterus contains a small larva (age 12–16 days) and (1c) in which ovariole A has follicle A_2 fully descended and a follicular relic and the uterus contains a third-instar larva (age 16–20 days). Similarly, category 2 is subdivided into three groups representing ages of 20–24 days, 24–27 days and 27–30 days. The same procedure can be followed for categories 3, 4 and 5. The fifth ovarian cycle (category 4) is the last recognizable with certainty, as serial follicular relics (such as are found regularly in mosquitoes) occur too irregularly to be relied upon. In this cycle, therefore, an indeterminate number of flies will be included from later cycles (e.g. 4 + 4n in Fig. 14.4) and the same holds true for the next three cycles shown in Fig. 14.4. Category 4 will therefore contain an indeterminate number of flies older than 30–40 days; similarly, later categories will contain indeterminate numbers of flies older than is shown in the figure.

Despite this complicating factor, it is believed that there would be so few of these older flies in a field sample that the correctness of the assessment of the average age of the sample by this method would not be appreciably affected. This contention is supported by the results of dissections of laboratory-reared females of known age (Itard, 1966) and of recaptured flies in release and recapture experiments in which freshly emerged flies were used (Saunders, 1962; Harley, 1966a) as well as by the ovarian age categories obtained by the dissection of wild flies the age of which had also be assessed by Jackson's wing-fray technique (Saunders, 1962; Harley, 1967a). Nevertheless, Harley, as a result of his work with *G. fuscipes* at Lugala near the northern end of Lake Victoria, considered that the extension of the ovarian dissection method to include even females flies of 70–80 days was insufficient to give a reliable assessment of the age-composition of the female population in that locality. He contrasts his findings with the results reported by Challier (1965), working with a population of *G. palpalis* in West Africa, and concludes that with a population so short-lived as that in the Chad area of West Africa (presumably short-lived because of the unfavourable climate) results of greater value may be obtained.

The assessments of the ages of individual females by means of ovarian dissection and by the wing-fray method have confirmed Jackson's belief that wing fray occurs at a slower rate in female than in male flies, doubtless because of the relative inactivity of the female in the field (*see* also Saunders, 1962). It must also be remembered that, as Harley (1966) has pointed out, a rise in temperature will result in an increase of the ovulation rate so that a fly assigned to a particular physiological age category as determined by ovarian dissection will be younger in calendar age in the hotter dry season than a fly assigned to the same physiological age category in the cooler wet season.

Saunders (1962) investigated the age of samples of *G. pallidipes*, *G. fuscipes* and *G. brevipalpis* collected by the standard fly-round technique (by a party of men only), by catching on a tethered ox and by catching in traps. He showed clearly that different sections of the fly population were sampled by these different techniques, as indeed was suggested by the earlier work of Jack (1939,

1941, 1941a) and as has been discussed in Chapter 17 (Adults). Harley (1966, 1966a, 1967, 1967a) has used this technique to examine the relation between the physiological age of tsetse flies and their infection rate. Later, Harley (1968) used the same method to follow up an earlier tentative suggestion by Jackson (1946, 1948a) that flies in the field were living at a temperature fairly close to the mean temperature as recorded in a Stevenson screen, but whereas Jackson's observations were made on *G. swynnertoni* and *G. morsitans*, Harley worked with *G. pallidipes* and *G. brevipalpis*. Having established the ovulation rates of the flies kept at known temperatures in the laboratory, Harley determined the physiological age of females recaptured at various intervals after their release in the field as newly emerged flies, and found that these indicated ovulation rates reasonably close to those that would have been expected at the screen temperatures recorded during the period. Saunders (1962), using a similar approach, compared the length of the ovarian cycle observed in a wild population of *G. fuscipes* on an island in Lake Victoria with the cycle previously found in *G. morsitans* maintained at 26°C in the laboratory. He concluded that the *fuscipes* population was living at a temperature somewhat lower than 26°C.

In a study of *G. palpalis* in the Niger Province of Nigeria, during the wet season of 1966, Saunders (1967) determined the age composition of the female population. By working out the probable number of flies in each ovulation cycle and by assuming a logarithmic adult death rate, he calculated a survival curve for the population which indicated a female adult life of 234 days. Further, by making a number of assumptions about the population and by using two extreme figures for the age-specific fertility, he made two estimates which, he considered, represented the limits for the population at the time of the investigation and from these he concluded that the population was slowly increasing. Saunders also suggested that this method would have general application in estimating the rate of change of a *Glossina* population in the field.

The instances cited above illustrate the various ways in which observations on the ovarian stages can be used to determine the age of female tsetse flies. This new technique has been used, and can with further advantage be applied, not only to increase our knowledge of tsetse population dynamics but also to assess the progress of control measures directed against the vectors of trypanosomiasis.

Methods for Determining the Age of the Puparial Stages

Fiske (1920, p. 412), working with the puparial stages of *G. palpalis* [*G. fuscipes*] collected in the field, assigned them to one of two categories: (a) an early stage 'showing no colour except on the eyes', and (b) a late stage 'showing the grey colour of the adult'. Potts (1933), working with *G. morsitans*, carried the classification of the puparial stages further and defined four categories each of which would, he considered, occupy roughly a quarter of the whole period of their development: (a) from formation of the puparium until three regions could be distinguished corresponding to the head, thorax and abdomen, the contents of the puparium remaining very watery and blue-white in colour throughout the period; (b) thence until the appendages and the form of the imago were discernible but no pigment was apparent, the puparial contents were no longer watery and their colour was creamy white; (c) from the time pigment first appeared as a pale orange tint in the eyes until the body hairs also became pigmented, though its general colour remained creamy white; (d) thence to the completion of the development of the imago in the puparium.

Bursell (1959), also working with *G. morsitans*, described an even more refined classification of the stages of puparial development. This recognizes three main categories the third of which includes six subdivisions, as under:

	Duration[1]	Mean Age[1]
I (quiescent stage of third instar larva): contents intimately associated with puparium at all points	1	0·5
II cryptocephalic pupa: contents bounded by a fine membrane [pupal skin] associated with puparium only at hind end of gut	3	2·5
III [phanerocephalic pupa (1) and pharate adult (2–4)] imaginal buds evaginated and all adult appendages recognizable:		
(1) No pigmentation	7	7·5
(2) Only the eyes pigmented:		
(a) eyes yellow	2	12
(b) eyes reddish brown	6	16
(3) Eyes pigmented and bristles black ..	3	20·5
(4) General integument pigmented (visible first on dorsum of thorax)		
(a) pupal skin moist and entire ..	3	23·5
(b) pupal skin dry and adhering to puparium [i.e. after pupal apolysis and preparatory to larval-pupal ecdysis]	2	26

The early categories I–III (1) are very fragile and in order to observe them great care must be exercised; it is recommended that the front half of the puparium be embedded in a block of paraffin wax. The later stages can readily be exposed by squeezing the puparium between the fingers until it breaks, when the pupa or pharate adult will be exposed.

Categories (a), (b), (c) and (d) of Potts correspond with categories I and II, III(1), III(2) and III(3) and (4) of Bursell, respectively. For a developmental period of about twenty-eight days (i.e. at 25°C) the categories of these two systems would correspond reasonably well except that Potts' first category would last for four instead of the seven days which he postulated and his last three categories would each last a day longer to compensate.

[1] Duration and mean age (at 25·5°C) given in days, the latter being formed by adding the full duration of the previous stages to half the duration of the latest stage.

METHODS FOR THE MEASUREMENT OF THE TEMPERATURE AND RATE OF DEVELOPMENT OF *GLOSSINA*

Measurement of the Temperature of *Glossina*

Edney and Barrass (1962, 1962a) described an apparatus for measuring the temperature of tsetse flies, the essential part of which consists of a thermocouple made from 47 SWG (0·051 mm.) constantan wire against 45 SWG (0·071 mm.) nickel-chromium-iron wire. The latter was selected because it was sufficiently rigid to allow easy insertion in the fly. They found that flies were not harmed by insertion of the thermocouple or by the Lepage 'Bondfast' glue used to affix it to the body of the fly; those flies not killed by the temperature to which they were exposed were able to fly and to feed after release from the apparatus.

Vanderplank, working in Shinyanga, devised an ingenious method for obtaining a very finely pointed thermocouple (unpublished but described in a thesis presented to the University of Bristol in 1947). The 'hot point' was obtained by reducing the end of a piece of 10 SWG constantan wire (the only gauge available to him at the time) to a fine tapering point by repeated dipping in nitric acid, the process being completed under a lens. The constantan wire was covered with graphite to within one millimetre of the tapering point, fine copper wire was twisted round it and the point was copper-plated under binocular magnification.

It was shown, by both of these methods, that tsetse flies are capable of depressing their internal temperatures appreciably under certain conditions. Edney and Barras (*loc. cit.*) demonstrated temperature depression amounting to 1·66°C at 45°C in dry air but observed none in moist air. They considered that the lowering of temperature even by this small amount might have some survival value during the hottest time of the day, but did not regard the adaptive value of the mechanism as proved.

Formulae for Calculating the Rate of Development of *Glossina*

As the rate of development of *Glossina* depends on temperature and not on humidity, the formulae given below for calculating this rate at different temperatures may be useful. These, based on the work of Jackson, are given in a corrected form in Glasgow (1963, p. 40).

If the temperature (t) is measured in degrees centigrade, the number of days required by a freshly emerged female to produce her first larva is about:

$$\frac{1}{0{\cdot}0661 + 0{\cdot}0035\,(t - 24)},$$

the number of days between successive larvae is about

$$\frac{1}{0{\cdot}0859 + 0{\cdot}0069\,(t - 24)},$$

and the number of days taken by a female to undergo development in the puparium is about

$$\frac{1}{0{\cdot}0323 + 0{\cdot}0028\,(t - 24)}.$$

The puparial period of the male is about 6% longer than that of the female.

Chapter 20

Methods for Rearing and Maintaining *Glossina* in the Laboratory

T. A. M. NASH AND A. M. JORDAN

INTRODUCTORY

An abundant supply of tsetse flies is an essential requirement for many aspects of research on trypanosomiasis and for studies on the insect itself; but, until recently, attempts to establish productive colonies of flies in the laboratory to meet these demands have, at best, met with only partial success. The technique for rearing tsetse flies described in detail below has been evolved after much experimentation and is believed to be the most successful so far devised. A brief account is first given of earlier work on this subject most of which, whether successful or otherwise, has contributed in some measure to the eventual emergence of a satisfactory method for tsetse colonization.

In almost all cases, attempts to colonize tsetse flies have relied on the use of living animals as sources of food. The approaches made fall under two main heads. Most investigators have attempted to establish a colony from a single importation of wild material (the closed colony) while others have maintained a large population of tsetse flies, by frequent importations from the field, with which they have experimented in the hope of developing techniques capable of producing a self-supporting colony.

WORK ON CLOSED COLONIES OF TSETSE FLIES

The first promising work on the colonization of tsetse flies was undertaken in Paris by Roubaud (1917). Of the flies which emerged from a batch of *G. morsitans* pupae collected in Senegal only one female was productive but from this single fly a colony was established which was maintained for three years and which reached a maximum population of thirty-two flies. The flies were kept in cages in an incubator maintained at 25°–27°C and 50–55% relative humidity and were fed on the shaved under surface of guinea-pigs or rabbits. The ultimate collapse of this colony was associated with a great increase in the proportion of male flies and evidence of degeneration of the females.

Mellanby (1936), working in Uganda, observed that to achieve maximum fertilization during mating it was necessary to ensure a preponderance of males over females. Mellanby and Mellanby (1937), working in England, succeeded in breeding four generations of *G. palpalis* and at the termination of the experiment the fly population was slowly increasing. They believed it to be essential to coax flies to feed individually. Attempts to enable flies to feed at will by confining them in the same cage as the host were unsuccessful, as were endeavours to apply cages containing a number of flies to the host.

Rodhain and van Hoof (1944) maintained a colony of *G. palpalis* in Antwerp for some six generations until the work was interrupted by the war. The colony was kept in a climatized room in glass tubes (12 × 5 cm.) each containing one male and three female flies. The flies were fed on guinea-pigs or rabbits.

A major advance in colonization was made by Geigy (1948) in his laboratory at Basle. He kept eight female and six male *G. palpalis* in each Roubaud cage and devised ingenious racks which enabled eight cages to be applied to the flanks of four guinea-pigs; 45 minutes was allowed for feeding on each day of the week except Sunday. A further labour-saving refinement was the use of 3 mm. mesh netting which enabled the larvae from four to six cages, kept in enamel bowls, to escape and pupate on the floor of the bowls from which the pupae were readily collected. In October, 1945, Geigy flew from Brazzaville with fed adult *G. palpalis* in cages packed in an ice box (8°–10°C). These flies together with their progeny and adults which emerged from pupae imported at the same time provided about 375 flies to initiate the colony. Flies were maintained at 26°C and 80% relative humidity. Within sixteen months the fly population had increased to 1,400 but, because of inadequate temperature control, the population then fell to some 250 flies. Air conditioning was later installed and losses were sustained and recoveries made from time to time. The colony was maintained for five and a half years but latterly showed signs of deterioration (personal communication). Geigy believed that colonies are best started by the importation of adults, as four attempts to start colonies with pupae failed.

Willett (1953) working at Shinyanga, Tanzania, studied the performance of flies kept under varying conditions and made a notable advance by recording the mean length of life of adult flies, the mean number of pupae deposited per female fly and the mean pupal weight. The technique employed was to keep flies (10 per Roubaud cage) over water in an open-sided, grass-roofed hut. All flies were offered a blood meal daily for at least 30 minutes. The best results were achieved with a colony of *G. swynnertoni* fed on sheep, the first generation of which consisted of thirty wild-caught female flies of unknown age. In subsequent generations each female was paired immediately after her first feed with a male aged not less than nine days. Thereafter the sexes were segregated. Pupae were kept singly in tubes in the laboratory at 90% relative humidity which greatly reduced weight loss during the pupal stage. By the start of the fourth generation the female population had increased to fifty-two. Subsequently (EATRO, 1953) the colony flourished up to the eighth generation but deteriorated seriously during the two subsequent generations, probably because of the adverse effects of an exceptionally prolonged and hot dry season. Similar experiments using *G. morsitans* were less successful, the colonies dying out at the fourth or fifth generation. Attempts to colonize *G. pallidipes* failed because the flies could not be induced to mate.

Willett (1953) also initiated a colony with eighteen female *G. austeni* but it died out at the fifth generation owing to adverse climatic conditions. In its earlier stages, however, this experiment yielded the valuable information that, under laboratory conditions, *G. austeni* has a long mean life and a high rate of pupal production; the average yield from seventeen females was 6·8 pupae whereas the highest yield from *G. swynnertoni* was only 4·5 pupae.

At Arusha, Tanzania, Foster (1957) started four colonies of *G. morsitans* from wild pupae. These were kept singly in tubes under varying conditions of temperature, humidity and frequency of feeding. Data for three of these colonies are given for the first generation only; the fourth colony virtually died out in the third generation. Foster also initiated a colony of *G. austeni* which, despite unsuitable maintenance conditions, yielded better results than did *G. morsitans*.

McDonald (1961a) established a colony of *G.m. submorsitans* at Kaduna, Nigeria, under partially controlled climatic conditions. The flies were kept in large wooden boxes, with front and back panels of gauze, providing a cubic capacity of 6,900 c.c. per fifty female flies. Flies kept in these boxes produced more and heavier pupae than those kept singly in 3 × 1 inch tubes, but the latter survived for much longer periods; better results were obtained from daily than from alternate-day feeding on sheep. In the first generation the mean pupal yield was only one per female, whereas by the fourth generation the mean pupal yield per female had risen to nearly seven and the mean pupal weight had increased from 27·6 to 33·2 mg. Thereafter, a high death rate among newly-emerged flies tended to nullify the high reproductivity. In this very promising attempt to establish a self-supporting colony, the yield and quality of pupae must be regarded as outstandingly good, but it was not a closed colony in the strict sense in that male flies from the main stock were often used for mating. Fifteen months after the colony was started and when it was entering its sixth generation McDonald left Nigeria and the colony subsequently died out.

In Lisbon, since late 1959, Azevedo and Pinhao (1964, 1968) have most painstakingly built up a closed colony of *G. morsitans*. A summary of this valuable work is given below but some difficulty has been experienced in its preparation owing to apparent discrepancies in their publications, possibly because of inaccuracies in translation.

In the Lisbon colony each fly is kept singly in a Roubaud cage and is fed on guinea-pig using the Geigy feeding rack. Originally the cages were applied for 45–60 minutes but this was later reduced to 20–30 minutes; blood meals are offered daily (Sundays excepted) and any flies which do not feed for one or two days are allowed a longer time. For mating, one male and one female are kept together for two to three days. Initially each pupa was kept singly in a glass tube but later practice has been to place damp sand inside the tube. The stock is kept in a small room maintained at 26°C and 70% relative humidity and illuminated (550 lux) for 12 hours daily.

The initial (standard) colony originated from twenty-one male and twenty-two female flies which emerged from pupae imported from Mozambique in 1959. During the first four years the total population fluctuated between ten and seventy-five flies but, starting in 1963, the population increased to about 1,000 flies in little over one year. This striking rise was attributed, at the time, to keeping pupae in damp sand but later experiments showed that there was no difference in the emergence rate between pupae maintained with or without damp sand. It has been suggested that the sudden increase in population may be due to genetic selection, the first four years representing a phase of 'adaptation' followed by a phase of 'growth and stabilization'.

By January 1967, the colony had reached the thirty-sixth generation. The mean female longevity for the first twenty generations (covering the 'adaptation' phase and the first year of the 'growth' phase) was 64·4 days (personal communication), whereas about ninety to one hundred days is now considered normal. For the first twenty generations an average of 5·3 larvae per fertile female was recorded.

It seems worth while to mention two misfortunes which befell the Lisbon colony. In 1964, through plant failure, the temperature rose to 30°–32°C for 2 hours resulting in a loss of 20% of the flies. In 1966, a second misadventure resulted from the application of dieldrin to the walls of the guinea-pig room. Despite removal of the animals before spraying and thorough washing of the walls and floor of the room before their return, 623 flies out of a total stock of 2,216 flies were lost in two days. The vitality of the colony was adversely affected for six months as indicated by a fall in the emergence rate, refusal of young flies to feed and early deaths. The number of flies in the colony fell to 200 but a year later had increased to 1,200.

A colony of Nigerian *G.m. submorsitans* was started in Lisbon in 1965 and a colony of Rhodesian *G. morsitans* was initiated in 1966.

Itard and Maillot (1966) described the technique which they used to establish colonies of *G. morsitans* and *G. tachinoides* in Paris. Up to twenty flies are kept in each Roubaud cage at 24°–25°C. Pregnant female flies and male flies over ten days old are kept in the fly-feeding room at 65–70% relative humidity with 3 or 4 hours of light daily, while young flies and pupae are kept in a small room at 80–85% relative humidity with 12 hours light daily; pupae are kept in tubes with dry sand. The sexes are not mated before the females are three and the males seven days old; after three or four days the sexes are separated and transferred to the drier room. In their hands the fly-feeding apparatus devised by Jacquemin (1956) has proved superior to that designed by Geigy (1948). Flies are offered food daily for 30 to 45 minutes except young flies which are allowed only 20 minutes.

The *G. morsitans* colony was started from 135 flies which had emerged from pupae collected in Tanzania and after thirteen months (eighth generation) the population had nearly doubled itself. Emergence rates for the first four generations ranged from 90·4 to 93·4%; the fourth generation produced 4·1 pupae per female.

The *G. tachinoides* colony was initiated from flies emerging from pupae sent from Tchad and had been maintained, with difficulty, up to the eleventh generation. Survival and reproduction improved at the eleventh generation (Itard, 1968a) when feeding on guinea-pigs and chickens was replaced by feeding on rabbits' ears as described by Nash, Jordan and Boyle (1966a).[1]

The need for extreme care of the fly colony environment was again emphasized by the heavy fly mortality which followed the repainting of a fly-room despite subsequent airing for four days.

Dame and Ford (1966) described a method for feeding *G. morsitans* on guinea-pigs, and Dame (1968) has made reference to two self-sustaining colonies of the same species, one of which had then been established for two years.

WORK ON REPLENISHED COLONIES OF TSETSE FLIES

To meet an annual demand for some 8,000–13,000 *G. palpalis* by workers at the West African Institute for Trypanosomiasis Research, attempts were made to establish a colony at Kaduna, Nigeria, in 1950; about half of this demand was met from laboratory-reared females. A major difficulty was to achieve adequate environmental conditions in the presence of an ambient temperature range of from 10°C to 39°C.

Initially, the method described by Geigy (1948) was used but this was abandoned when it was found that female longevity, reproductivity and pupal weight increased when the flies were fed on goats. Flies were kept in Bruce boxes (Prates, 1928) which were applied manually to the flank of a recumbent goat. Further experiments showed that female flies are most readily fertilized on the third day of life, that older male flies (nine to thirty-three days) are much more virile than younger flies and that for mass mating a preponderance of males to females (two to one) are all-important factors in increasing the fertilization rate.

[1] Itard has recently reported that, using rabbits' ears, he is now breeding *G. tachinoides*, *morsitans* and *austeni* in large numbers—Editor.

The rate was increased to 88% by adding five seven-day old males to each box of twenty newly 'fertilized' females (Nash, 1955). Jordan (1958) found that mating was maximal with female flies aged two to three days. It was also found that reproductivity decreased with age and that under the maintenance conditions employed it was uneconomic to keep females over one hundred days old. Pupae were kept in open-ended glass containers (made from jam jars), the ends of which were covered with spun rayon. Pupae were placed on a layer of dry sand (1·5 cm. in depth) and the jars kept 7 cm. above trays of wet sand thus ensuring that the pupae were maintained in a very humid atmosphere without becoming wet. The emergence rate from 33,000 fly-room pupae, bred in one year, was 94%. The yield of pupae per female per month showed a marked increase when these procedures were adopted in place of Geigy's method. Full details of this work are recorded by Nash, Page, Jordan and Petana (1960).

Evens and Niemegeers (1954) describe work carried out in Leopoldville in which large numbers of both laboratory-bred and wild caught *G. palpalis* were used. Large numbers of flies were kept in modified wooden Bruce boxes but, in the absence of equipment for climatic control, it is not surprising that survival and fecundity were disappointing. Mean female survival in the laboratory was twenty-two days for wild flies and 21·4 days for laboratory-bred flies.

TECHNIQUE FOR THE LARGE-SCALE REARING OF TSETSE FLIES AT LANGFORD, BRISTOL

The technique for rearing tsetse-flies in the laboratory, described in detail below, has been evolved by the writers and their colleagues over the past five years in a laboratory specially designed and equipped for this purpose (Nash, Jordan & Boyle, 1968). The primary objective is to meet demands from research workers in the United Kingdom and elsewhere for large numbers of uninfected flies for experimental work. Since so many of the earlier attempts, based on the importation of one or two batches of pupae or adult flies, had met with only partial success, it seemed wise to enage in large-scale experimentation, using regular massive importations of wild pupae, until a satisfactory technique had been devised. Using specially designed containers (Kernaghan & Nash, 1964), 49,000 *G. austeni* were imported from Zanzibar between June 1963 and April 1966, since when no further batches have been received. A population explosion took place in December 1965, but imports had to be continued for a further four months to complete a series of experiments based on females emerging from Zanzibar pupae. Since then the problem has been to keep down the number of flies in a rapidly expanding colony to manageable proportions. There is no reason to postulate that success has been due to the production of a a laboratory adapted strain; the introduction of improved techniques, based on experimentation, coupled with precautions against contamination by insecticides or other noxious agents, are sufficient to account for the success achieved. The decision to use *G. austeni* was based on its slightly shorter interlarval period, the encouraging results obtained from preliminary trials by both Willett (1953) and Foster (1957), and the likelihood that a species which lives in nature under equable climatic conditions would more readily adjust itself to constant temperature and humidity in the laboratory.

The self-contained Langford colony is now yielding pupae on a far larger scale than has been previously recorded as will be evident from the fact that during 1967 demands for over 13,000 pupae were met, and to reduce the numbers, over 22,000 flies, more than half of them females, were destroyed. The corresponding figures for 1968 were 34,000 and 40,000, respectively.

Fertilization

As indicated by the dissection after death of 740 females, the current insemination rate is 98·6%. Virgin females are offered food on kids. Those that have definitely fed are mated on the third day of life, but those that have not—about one tenth—are placed in a 'reserve cage' and are offered food twice daily; a worthless one fifth die in this cage but the rest are mated after feeding.[1] The fed female is placed in a 7·5 × 2·5 cm. tube for 24 hours with a male which is over fifteen days old and has not mated for five days; to obviate sperm exhaustion a male is usually used twice and never more than four times. Of 9,240 females only 1·7% died during mating, but when mass mating was undertaken in a large cage with an excess of males, only 89% of females became inseminated, and 8·5% died during mating (Nash, Kernaghan & Boyle, 1966).

Adult Maintenance

The type of cage used is a considerably modified version of that used by Roubaud (1917) and Geigy (1948). It consists of a shallow, rectangular frame constructed with ⅛ inch (3 mm.) diameter stainless steel wire, and is made in three sizes:

Size 25, to house twenty-five females at 4 cubic inches (65·5 c.c.) per fly.
Dimensions—10 × 5 × 2 inches (25·4 × 12·7 × 5·1 cm.).
Used for flies fed on goats (Nash, Jordan & Boyle, 1966b).

Size 10, to house ten females at 4 cubic inches per fly.
Dimensions—6 × 3·4 × 2 inches (15 × 8·5 × 5 cm.).
Used for flies fed on rabbit ears (Nash, Jordan & Boyle, 1966a).

Size 1, to house one female at 4·5 cubic inches (74 c.c.).
Dimension—2 × 1·5 × 1·5 inches (5 × 3·8 × 3·8 cm.).
For studies of the individual and the infected fly (Nash, Jordan & Boyle, 1967).

In cage sizes 25 and 10, one end is closed with a piece of hardboard sewn to the four corners with monofilament nylon; a one inch diameter cork-hole is drilled in the hardboard to facilitate removal of dead flies. All cages are covered with black Terylene netting—black because it is easy to see through and Terylene (Tergal) because it is not brittle and is non-absorbent. The type of cage and space per fly are factors of major importance; use of the right type

[1] The 'reserve cage' technique can be discontinued once an expanding colony has been achieved.

of cage may increase pupal production by 70% and mean pupal weight by 1·7 mg. (Nash, Jordan & Boyle, 1966b). Cages (sizes 25 and 10) are kept in 2-inch deep enamel trays with the closed end just resting on the tray-edge so as to permit faeces and larvae to fall through the netting of one of the narrow faces onto sand. When the contents of two cages holding flies of similar age have dropped to half, the combined contents are placed in a clean cage, the old cages are stripped, the frames boiled and then re-covered.

The climate is maintained at about 25°C and 70–80% relative humidity. For 12 hours of the day, the fly-racks receive light intensities which range, according to situation, from 0·5 to 2·5 foot candles (5·4–26·9 lux).

Flies are never touched by hand. New emergences are released in a box 31 × 31 × 31 cm., with glass top, netted sides and a sleeve, and are caught in tubes for transfer to cages.

Bitter experience has shown the need, when working in Europe, to guard against contamination with sub-lethal dosages of insecticide which reduce survival and fecundity without producing any of the classical symptoms of toxicity (Nash, Kernaghan & Boyle, 1966). All newly purchased animals, materials and articles which will come in contact with tsetse are washed in hot water and soft soap (*Sapo mollis*, BP) which is the only agent used for washing tubes and the floors of the controlled climate rooms. No chemicals are allowed in the fly rooms.

All flies are offered food for 15 minutes daily, Sundays excepted; seven-day feeding has been shown to improve survival and reproduction, but is impracticable with a small staff (Jordan, Nash & Boyle, 1966).

Most of the stock is fed on goats. The beasts are mounted on trolleys in the heated animal house and wheeled into the large controlled climate room, where four cages, each initially holding twenty-five flies, are fastened to the flanks of each adult goat (Nash & Kernaghan, 1964). In cold weather, cages should not be applied until the animals have warmed up. Each goat is used twice a week on a 3, 4, 3, 4-day rest cycle to allow tissue damage to be repaired; about 500 flies are applied on any one day; new goats are conditioned by progressively increasing the number of flies applied to 200 at the end of the first month (Nash, Kernaghan & Wright, 1965). The flanks are close-clipped at fortnightly intervals, and the beasts washed every two months with soft soap and hot water to guard against a build-up of insecticidal contamination and to remove tsetse faeces, scurf, etc.

A small proportion of the female stock is fed on the ears of lop-eared rabbits. The rabbit is placed in a specially designed box, with platforms for the ears; a size 10 cage is strapped to each ear (Nash, Jordan & Boyle, 1966a). A rabbit is used twice a week, when up to 160 females a day are applied.

To determine the suitability of the hosts employed for feeding flies, two-day old, unfed males are used as test organisms (Nash, Jordan & Boyle, 1968). Two (size 25) cages, each with ten males, are strapped onto the flanks of a goat which has been in the hot room for at least one hour; on removal, after 15 minutes, the flies are carefully examined by two observers. If there is a discrepancy in the number considered to have fed, a figure is agreed after re-examination (small feeds are not readily recognizable). Five counts are made over a period of several months. The proportion fed is established from a hundred males examined, and is referred to as the 'host suitability index'. Each goat is tested at about four-monthly intervals. The results indicate that newly purchased goats are uniformly attractive to the flies, but that later some may become unsuitable. A low host-suitability index has been found in a few cases and is associated with skin thickening or a hide-bound condition which may be due to the application of too many flies or to a susceptibility to tsetse saliva. Other individuals have continued to be satisfactory hosts after five years of regular use. Of forty goats tested, thirteen fell in the '90% and over' index range, eighteen in the 80–90%, and five in the 70–79% range; the figures for the remaining four beasts were 61, 47, 46 and 18%. (It was the chance inclusion of these four very unsuitable goats in the control herd which gave rise to the erroneous conclusion that female tsetse perform better when fed on pregnant goats, *see* Nash, Jordan & Boyle, 1966b).

Convincing evidence has recently been obtained which refutes earlier claims as to the value of host pregnancy (Nash, Jordan & Boyle, 1967a). Using two teams of goats having almost identical suitability indices, the performance of female flies fed on four male goats was found to be very similar to that of flies fed on four non-pregnant female goats. Using the same eight goats, the experiment was repeated after the four females had been fertilized; there was still no significant difference in fly performance. In all, 1,800 flies were used in these two experiments.

It is believed that periodic tests on hosts are essential for both experimental and practical rearing purposes. The present mean host suitability index for the Langford stock of goats is 91%.

Pupal Maintenance

For mass-production purposes the pupae are collected from the sand-filled trays at three-week intervals; the sand is poured through loosely stretched netting sewn onto a flat ring of wood placed over a bowl; the pupae are collected from the netting with a brush and teaspoon and are never touched by hand. In earlier work the pupae were buried in sand in pots having bottoms and tops of open-mesh Terylene voile; the pots were placed on grids just above wet sand (Nash, Kernaghan & Boyle, 1966). Using this method, in 1967 the overall emergence rate from 19,250 pupae was 97·6% but as 10·9% of the emergences failed to develop their wings, the effective emergence rate was only 86·9%. It has recently been discovered that 'crippling' is due to disturbance of the newly-emerged flies by those with expanded wings. By placing pupae on sand on the floor of a large emergence cage, kept in semi-darkness, only 2·9% of emergences from 9,900 pupae were crippled. By providing an illumination of seven lux on the soil surface for twelve hours daily, the rate has been further reduced to 0·7%, giving an effective emergence rate from 11,444 pupae of 98·0%. The emergence cage is 12 × 12 × 15 inches with netted top and sides. Up to 2,500 pupae are spread on dry sand, suspended over wet sand, on the floor of the cage. The pupal maintenance temperature is about 23·5°C (Nash, Jordan & Boyle, 1968).

To meet demands for pupae of known age some of the depositions are kept in dated pots, but before emergence they should be transferred to large cages.

Efficacy of the Technique Described

The key to the successful rearing of *Glossina* lies in nutrition and in factors which facilitate nutrition. A simple method of gauging female nutrition is to weigh large numbers of pupae individually. In 1964, it was found that the mean weight on pupation of pupae deposited by females which had emerged from wild pupae and had been fed on adult goats, was 4 mg., or 17% lower than the estimated mean weight for such pupae deposited in Zanzibar (Nash & Kernaghan, 1965); by 1967, using goat-fed females from the self-maintaining colony, the deficit had been reduced from 4·1 to 0·9 mg. This remarkable improvement was due to a number of factors including the adoption of the modified Roubaud cage with its open, shallow construction which facilitates location of the host, and to the resting or culling of unsuitable goats (Nash, Jordan & Boyle, 1966b, 1968).

The mean weight of nearly 3,000 pupae from females kept in Roubaud-type cages and fed on rabbits' ears was 23·6 mg. which is exactly the estimated mean weight of pupae deposited in Zanzibar (Nash, Kernaghan & Boyle, 1966).

Currently, the average yield of pupae per initial number of goat-fed females is 9–10; since 2·5 pupae must be retained to maintain the colony, the distributable surplus is 6·5–7·5 pupae. Comparable figures from rabbit-fed females are 11·4 giving a surplus of nearly nine pupae per female (Jordan, Nash & Boyle, 1967).

Under present conditions the mean age of goat-fed fertilized females at death is about 120 days. The figure for rabbit-fed females was 139 days (Jordan, Nash & Boyle, 1967).

Pupal production at Langford is running at about 109,000 per annum, despite the monthly reduction in stock due to distribution of pupae to other workers and the monthly destruction of adults required to keep numbers to manageable proportions. The use of goats as hosts, enabling up to 400 flies to be fed per beast per hour, is certainly a good large-scale method; 93% of the Langford pupal stock derives from goat-fed females. The use of rabbits as hosts, enabling up to eighty flies to be fed per beast per hour, is undoubtedly an excellent laboratory technique. If a large enough colony of lop-eared rabbits could be maintained, the method should be applicable for large-scale rearing.

Available evidence suggests that *G. austeni* can be infected in the laboratory with *T. rhodesiense* (Mshelbwala, 1967), with *T. brucei* and *T. gambiense* (R. A. Ward, personal communication) and with *T. vivax* and *T. congolense* (M. J. Clarkson, personal communication).

The technique described above should be basically applicable to other species of tsetse. Starting with ninety-four female *G. morsitans*, from pupae sent from Rhodesia, the female population has increased more than seven-fold in fifteen months, despite maintenance under the humid conditions employed for *G. austeni*.[1]

[1] The authors have subsequently reported that, in 1969, 145,600 pupae were produced of which 80,500 were given away, almost half of them *G. morsitans*—Editor.

CONCLUSIONS ON THE REARING OF TSETSE FLIES FED ON ANIMAL HOSTS IN THE LABORATORY

Stringent precautions must be taken against possible contamination of fly stock with insecticides or other noxious agents, bearing in mind that sub-lethal dosages are very difficult to detect but may be disastrous to the colony.

Using the Roubaud cage, and modifications of this cage, *G. palpalis*, *G. morsitans* and *G. austeni* have been bred in the laboratory with considerable success.

An adult maintenance temperature of about 25°C appears to be optimal, with a relative humidity varying from 60–80% according to the species' natural environment. For pupal maintenance a similar or slightly lower temperature is advisable, and for at least some species of tsetse the pupae should be kept dry but in a very high humidity. Emergence should take place in a large cage. The provision of a diurnal light rhythm is believed to be advantageous.

After taking their first blood meal the females should be mated with older males. Mating isolated pairs of flies gives better results than mass mating in large cages.

Female nutrition is a factor of major importance which can be most readily gauged by the individual weighing of pupae. Tsetse should be offered food daily for 15 minutes or longer. Recent work shows that it can be important to test the hosts used for individual variation in suitability.

ATTEMPTS TO REAR TSETSE FLIES USING OTHER METHODS

Insectaries in the Natural Habitat

In 1929, an insectary measuring 15 × 12 × 7 feet high (4·6 × 3·6 × 2·1 m.) was built in *G. morsitans* woodland in Tanganyika Territory (now Tanzania) and was covered with wire netting lined with cotton gauze. Shade was provided by overhead and lateral screens. The interior was furnished with log and rock breeding sites; a sheep was introduced to provide food. The insectary was stocked with newly-emerged flies from wild pupae. The investigation was of short duration, but it was noted that although the flies mated readily none became gravid, nor was a single pupa found (Nash, 1930). In the light of modern knowledge it seems that failure to breed was associated with inadequate feeding.

Harley (EATRO, 1966), working at Lugala, Uganda, has had some success in obtaining pupae for experimental purposes. A small thicket on the edge of forest was enclosed in a 20 × 20 × 10 feet high (6 × 6 × 3 m.) insectary of plastic gauze into which large numbers of tsetse were periodically introduced. Initially, mortality was very high. Predatory arthropods, in particular ants, had to be removed and hyperactivity had to be reduced by screening with hessian; sheep were found to be unattractive and were replaced by part-grown cattle restrained in a crush. In one month pupal production by an unknown number of wild females was 404 pupae of *G. pallidipes*, 619 of *G. palpalis* [*G. fuscipes*] and 1,255 of *G. brevipalpis*.

Attempts are being made in Rhodesia to breed *G. morsitans* in eight feet high (2·4 m.), quarter acre (1,000 square m.) wire-mesh insectaries, which enclose the lower vegetational canopy; oxen are usually provided as hosts. It is understood from G. J. Dean that survival is only two to three weeks, and that predation by ants of inactive tsetse flies is a serious problem, as is the seasonally high ambient temperature.

Substitution of Membrane Feeding for the Animal Host

The only prolonged investigation into the possibility of rearing tsetse by feeding them through membranes was made by Cockings. Because of difficulties experienced in getting *G. pallidipes* to mate in captivity, wild females of *unknown* age had to be used. Nearly 3,000 female *G. pallidipes* were fed through membranes on defibrinated ox blood; after fifty days 2,529 females had produced 3,608 pupae over 30 mg. in weight and 312 flies were still alive (EATRO, 1961). In later work, using *G. morsitans* which had emerged from wild pupae, it was found that the mean life of all flies fed on defibrinated blood was 58% of the mean life of flies fed directly on cows (EATRO, 1963a), results which were in accord with earlier findings (EATRO, 1963).

Chapter 21

Introduction to Control Methods

J. FORD

Various methods have been devised for the reduction or eradication of tsetse populations but only those which are currently in use or under investigation will be considered here.

Until about 1950, virtually only two methods of tsetse control had been used with any degree of success, namely, the destruction of the larger wild mammals on which some species of tsetse are largely dependent for their food, and modification of the bush cover of the land, usually by felling trees, so as to deprive tsetse of habitats suitable for their survival. In Rhodesia, since 1930, some 10,000 square miles of country have been freed from tsetse by shooting the large wild mammals in the Zambesi basin. The same method was widely used in Uganda between 1950 and 1960. For a long time it seemed that the simple word 'starvation' provided an adequate explanation for the undoubted success of game destruction in Rhodesia but it now seems that this is an over-simplification. It is, in any case, now a virtual certainty that the destruction of many of the species shot was unnecessary and that the same result could have been achieved with less slaughter. Since 1955, the use of bush clearing and insecticides and, quite recently, the confinement of shooting to hosts favoured by tsetse has greatly reduced the number of wild animals killed each year. Elsewhere, numerous very much smaller areas have been 'reclaimed' by modification of the bush cover, sometimes by its complete removal (total, sheer or ruthless clearing) and sometimes by removing only part of it (partial or selective clearing). These techniques were developed empirically and much of the effort of research glossinologists has been devoted to explaining their successes or failures. It is still impossible to state with certainty why a tsetse population disappears when the trees growing in its habitats are cut down but, during the last decade, some progress has been made in the elucidation of this problem.

In comparatively recent years, the most significant advance in the control of tsetse populations has been the use, on an increasing scale, of insecticides. Pyrethrum sprays have long been used in deflying chambers but it was not until the introduction of powerful residual insecticides, of which DDT was the first, that their full potential for tsetse destruction became apparent. During the past twenty years much research has been done on insecticide preparations and formulations, on methods of application and on the means of assessing their effects after use in the field. Their introduction was responsible for the revival and expansion of research on the resting habits of *Glossina*, hitherto much neglected. This has greatly enlarged understanding of tsetse behaviour as well as leading to economies and increased efficiency in use of insecticides.

Another possible means of controlling tsetse populations which is currently being investigated and which has been successfully used against other insect pests, is the release of male flies which have been sterilized by gamma-radiation or chemically; a suitable technique has not yet been developed to the stage of practical application in the field. The method was anticipated many years ago by Vanderplank who showed that the closely related *Glossina morsitans* and *G. swynnertoni* would mate and produce sterile offspring. An attempt to eliminate a small belt of *G. swynnertoni* by releasing in it large numbers of *G. morsitans* failed because the introduced species took up a different niche in the habitat and so did not mix with the indigenous population. Chemosterilized males should not do this when introduced into their own natural habitat.

Much of the difficulty in effecting control of tsetse populations is logistic. Whatever method, or methods, are used for this purpose, certain commitments are inescapable. The areas to be controlled are usually remote from centres of human population and economic development so that arrangements must be made for the introduction and maintenance of the staff and labour forces necessary to carry out the work. This entails the construction of roads, the provision of water supplies, the erection of houses and the organization of services for the supply of food and fuel. This heavy burden may sometimes be reduced if control is to be effected by the aerial application of insecticides but, for this purpose, light aircraft of limited range must be used and this, in turn, necessitates the construction of landing strips and of the roads needed to bring in insecticides, fuel, and ground staff to assist in the operation and assess its effects.

On rare occasions tsetse control may be a relatively simple matter. A successful attack against *G. fuscipes* was accomplished by an entomologist and his assistant operating from a small boat with a crew of one. The boat was floated down a narrow stream and as each tree overhanging the bank was passed insecticide was applied by pressing the trigger of a pressurized spray gun. This simple task was repeated on six occasions at fortnightly intervals and, for some months until the stream was re-invaded, the population of *G. fuscipes* was eliminated. Usually, however, the work is difficult, exhausting, lonely and protracted and achievement is not easy to assess. It may be as hard to prove that tsetse elimination has been achieved as to bring about reduction of the tsetse population to a level at which flies are virtually undetectable by ordinary survey methods; this is especially the case with tsetse of the *morsitans* group where it is necessary to operate over areas usually to be measured in hundreds of square miles.

In the past, much ingenuity has gone into devising techniques for the control of tsetse and for measuring their effectiveness. The need not only to experiment but to achieve control at the same time has made these tasks even more difficult; to add to these difficulties the relative virtues of experimental reclamation measures were hotly debated. Today, the practical control officer uses a whole range of techniques simultaneously to achieve his objective; this principle of attacking the tsetse at every possible point was first admirably demonstrated over fifty years ago when *G. palpalis* was eliminated from the Island of Principe (Da Costa *et al.*, 1915). When Principe was re-invaded by the same species of tsetse in 1956, the operation was successfully repeated (Azevedo *et al.*, 1962).

It is convenient to classify methods of tsetse control as 'direct' or 'indirect'. The destruction of individuals by violence (catching and squashing), trapping or poisoning by insecticides falls into the former category as also attempts to exterminate or reduce a population by augmenting its burden of parasites. Indirect methods often involve the use of destructive techniques not against the tsetse themselves but against their food supply or their habitats so that physiological and behavioural routines cannot be properly carried out; the slaughter of host animals and various types of bush clearing come into this category. The release of sterilized males to compete with wild males can also be classed as an indirect method of attack.

It is probable that all indirect methods of tsetse control act by reducing the net reproduction rate, irrespective of how this is achieved. It may be brought about by shortening the life span of the female tsetse so that insufficient larvae are produced to maintain later generations, or by preventing fertile mating, or by exposure of tsetse at any stage to increased predation or to lethal conditions of climate.

The various methods available for the control of populations of *Glossina* are described in detail in the chapters which follow.

Chapter 22

Control by Hand-catching and Traps

J. P. GLASGOW, W. H. POTTS

HAND-CATCHING OF TSETSE FLIES

Hand-catching is the most ancient method of insect control, and must be supposed to have been in use since the earliest Primate developed an opposable thumb. It has two important advantages (shared to a large extent by trapping) over all other methods of destruction—it is absolutely specific, i.e. nothing but the insect under attack is killed, and one can obtain an exact record of the number of insects destroyed. In the case of tsetse, hand-catching has been found effective against some species, but more expensive than chemicals, and it has therefore fallen into disuse. Nevertheless hand-catching experiments throw clear and important light on insecticidal attack in general.

Hand-catching was first tried in about 1913 against *G. palpalis* in the Portuguese island Principe, and against *G. palpalis* [*G. fuscipes*] by the Germans on an island, Riamugasire, on Lake Victoria. There is an account of the Principe operation in Austen and Hegh (1922); the Riamugasire work is described by Koch (1914). The Principe operation was a success and the island was free of *G. palpalis* for many years afterwards. The Riamugasire operation was not a success, no doubt because the island was not sufficiently isolated. Further failures to reduce populations of *G.f. fuscipes* to zero by hand-catching have been reported by Symes and Vane (1937), Symes and Southby (1938) and Glasgow and Duffy (1951). In each case the reason for the failure was non-isolation of the treated areas. Glasgow (1953) analysed the failure of the last experiment. It was done in a block of narrow riverine forest a mile and a half long, which was isolated by an upstream clearing 2 miles wide and a downstream clearing which was wider. Before the hand-catching began, intensive marking was done in the block until nearly half of the total population of 4,000 *G.f. fuscipes* was marked. As no marked flies could be found outside the block it was concluded that the clearings were effectively isolating the block. Hand-catching was begun, but in spite of an unprecedentedly large catching force exceeding fifty men, catches stabilized after ten months at 0·1 flies per man-day. By various means it was shown that about half a dozen flies a day were crossing the clearings. It is not known why the preliminary marking experiments failed to reveal this immigration. These flies would in any case have had a negligible effect on the population dynamics of the original population, but they were enough to prevent hand-catching proceeding to a successful conclusion and to re-populate the block of forest when hand-catching ceased.

Glasgow and Duffy (1947) describe an experiment in hand-catching *G.f. fuscipes* which ended in extermination. The experimental area was a strip of riverine thicket and forest 15 yards wide and 3,800 yards long, measured along the stream. The twenty-four catchers employed caught 400 tsetse in six months, the vast majority in the first three months. The block was isolated by a 3-mile clearing from other bush containing *G.f. fuscipes*. It was thought that the mere isolation of such a small area might adversely affect the tsetse and accordingly a 'control block' was isolated by similar clearings. *G.f. fuscipes* persisted in the control block for two years: it was considered that they would persist for ever if nothing further was done, and as the tsetse were believed responsible for a number of cases of *gambiense* sleeping sickness they were removed by another hand-catching operation. It is regrettable that a further experiment was not undertaken: eight parties of men in 3,800 yards of narrow bush must have had an effect on the hosts of *G.f. fuscipes*, but the effect of introducing this concentration of men, without nets, was not explored. Perhaps if the tsetse had not been caught their hosts would have been driven away and they would have died of starvation.

However that may be, the catchers did get rid of the tsetse, and although it is possible that half the number of men would have done nearly as well, even at the concentration of men employed the measure was cheaper than clearing of the bush would have been. It is probable that the first few weeks' operations removed all the tsetse old enough to be capable of transmitting sleeping sickness, so that as a disease control measure hand-catching is swift. It cannot be claimed as a permanent measure: it is naïve to suppose any more that clearings of 3 or even of 30 miles can be maintained as absolute barriers for ever. The truth of this assertion is well exemplified by the island Principe; this was rendered tsetse-free in 1914 and remained so for forty years. In 1956 it was found to have been repopulated by *G. palpalis* which were extremely numerous. The immigrant tsetse were believed to have been transported from the neighbouring island of Fernando Po, over 200 kilometres of sea.

Clearly one could not undertake a hand-catching operation except in an area isolated either naturally or artificially. Glasgow and Duffy (1947) also studied the reinfestation of a number of areas in which *G.f. fuscipes* had been made rare by hand-catching some ten years before. The reinfestation had been slow in that the population levels were still quite low, although there is no information as to whether low populations can be neglected as vectors of sleeping sickness. One could not in any case rely on this happening again—information from elsewhere indicates that tsetse populations can on occasion reach high levels in a short time.

Almost all hand-catching operations have been directed against members of the *palpalis* group, in conditions where the tsetse were living in narrow strips of lakeside or riverine bush. In these conditions it is easy to confine the attention of the catchers to concentrations of the tsetse which normally coincide with the water's edge. Operations against savanna tsetse would be much more difficult: the only attempt known to the writer was against *G. swynnertoni* in Shinyanga (Swynnerton, 1936). Although the operation was followed by disappearance of the tsetse, other measures were in operation at the same time and the experiment is difficult to evaluate.

Those hand-catching operations which have failed have used rather small numbers of catchers; for example, Koch on Riamugasire used four catchers on an island with a circumference of 4,000 yards, whereas Glasgow and Duffy used fifty catchers on 4,000 yards of river, and although the latter number may have been excessively high, it is clear that hand-catching would always require a large labour force especially if large areas were to be attacked. It seems unlikely that hand-catching could ever be preferred to insecticides if suitable insecticides were available, but if for any reason insecticides could not be used, hand-catching would be left as a possible measure to achieve swift control of trypanosomiasis transmission in isolated areas.

Even isolated areas will be reinfested. In estimating the cost of a proposed hand-catching operation, then, one is estimating the cost of an operation which will have only temporary benefits. The environment is not changed by the operation and remains suitable for tsetse. If there is a possible alternative, such as converting the tsetse bush into pasture, which would make the environment unsuitable for tsetse so that they could not return, this circumstance must receive attention before the method of attack is settled.

These considerations apply also to other insecticidal operations.

TRAPS AND ATTRACTANTS

Traps

Screens covered with bird-lime have been used for catching tsetse flies from the very early days of tsetse investigation (Maldonado, 1910; Da Costa *et al.*, 1915; Shircore, 1916; Swynnerton, 1923). Traps in the sense of devices into which tsetse flies can be attracted consist of an attractant part and a cage, usually designed on the principle of the lobster-pot, into which the flies are enticed but from which they cannot escape. The first of these were the famous traps invented by Harris (1930) by means of which very large numbers of *G. pallidipes* were caught in Zululand. The design of the Harris trap was suggested by his field observations on the response of tsetse flies to visual stimuli, particularly light and shade and objects of compact bulk and conspicuous outline showing total contrast with the surroundings. Such objects, Harris noted, were more attractive when extended in the horizontal rather than the vertical plane, that is, when they suggested a quadruped rather than a biped. Swynnerton (1933), stimulated by Harris's success, described a number of different traps which were tested against *Glossina* in Tanganyika Territory but neither these nor models of the Harris type were as successful in Tanganyika as were the original Harris traps in Zululand. Chorley (1933) also described some very simply constructed traps which he used against *G. palpalis* [*G. fuscipes*] in Uganda. Buxton (1955, pp. 500–22) discusses the design and operation of a number of the traps that have been invented and used from time to time. As he aptly writes, '. . . our present knowledge of the insect's [*Glossina*] behaviour fails to explain why it should pass downwards and enter the under surface of a hollow box (such as the Harris or Lewillon traps), and then travel upwards through a dark space towards a lighted cage from which it cannot escape'. No attempts to control *Glossina* by means of traps have so far succeeded though Harris's original work in Zululand seemed to come very close to eliminating *G. pallidipes* and, indeed, he and others at one time thought that this had been achieved. However, the time came when the fly population in the area where the traps were operating began to increase and continued to do so; it then became obvious that the traps had failed. Du Toit (1954) attributed the initial success of the traps to their use at a time when, following a game destruction campaign, the fly's food supply was drastically reduced; this was followed by a three-year period of drought which might be supposed to be favourable to the operation of the traps and at the same time unfavourable to the fly. Du Toit also noted that the increase in the fly population followed a period of increased rainfall over several years.

More recently, Morris and Morris (1949) introduced a fairly simple type of trap which they called 'the animal trap' because it was designed to suggest an animal. They used traps of this type against *G. palpalis* and *G. tachinoides* in West Africa but came to the conclusion that these traps could not compare in efficiency with selective clearing, although they might be useful as a subsidiary means of control. Later, Morris (1960b, 1961) regarded traps as a more efficient means of sampling tsetse populations and of surveying their distribution than the conventional fly-round. He observed marked local reductions in fly incidence in areas where traps were in operation and he advocated their use, combined with settlement, for reclaiming country from *G. pallidipes*. Morris (1961a) again concluded that traps were more efficient than hand collections for survey purposes when working with *G. palpalis* in Liberia, and the same worker (1962) claimed that trapping could provide a valuable means of controlling human trypanosomiasis in broken forest country. He based this claim on the proposition that traps could reduce fly populations to a level at which sleeping sickness is not transmitted. These investigations, however, had to be terminated before the validity of this claim could be demonstrated. Foster (1964), who also worked subsequently in forest country in Liberia, came to the conclusion that, owing to uncertainty of operation, 'animal traps' were unsuitable for quantitative assessments of populations of *G. palpalis* in forest and that, for this purpose, they were less reliable than hand catching. Foster also noted that M. G. Morris (1950) and Morris (1961a) recorded an escape rate from the traps of about 30%. The writer's experience of traps with other species of *Glossina* in East Africa, led him to the conclusion that they were too uncertain in operation to be likely to provide a reliable means of control, and that the difficulties of siting them so as to give consistent and comparable catches are too great to provide a really effective method of investigating the number of tsetse flies present. Nevertheless, traps may yield valuable information as to the constitution of fly populations by providing samples of portions of the population which differ from those obtainable by other methods of sampling (Smith & Rennison, 1961, 1961a;

Glasgow & Duffy, 1961). It would, therefore, appear that, generally speaking, the use of traps is an unsatisfactory method of controlling tsetse flies and that opinion is divided on their value as a means of investigation (*cf.* p. 413).

Attractants

When considering attractants for *Glossina*, especially in connection with control measures, it is natural to think first of all of attracting flies from a distance. It is, however, worth bearing in mind that attraction from a short distance may also be concerned, even though it is sometimes difficult to distinguish long- from short-range attraction to stimuli to such specific actions as feeding or larviposition, or from simple arrestants. Even long-range attractants may, of course, be concerned with specific behaviour patterns such as have just been mentioned rather than with behaviour of a more general nature. It is, therefore, possible that the study of short-range attractants, or even of stimulants and arrestants, may contribute significantly to the elucidation of the long-range attractants that is so vital to modern developments in tsetse control.

Buxton (1955) in his chapter on 'Sense organs: Discovery of Hosts' (*Ibid.*, pp. 110–35) has examined this subject very fully and has discussed exhaustively the work of numerous investigators. He concludes that the senses of both sight and smell are important in guiding the flies to their hosts from a distance, but continues . . . 'We do not know how the fly brings these two senses into use; whether it flies at random in suitable areas or sits at a favourable spot;' nor, he points out, can we tell which sense is the more important. The situation remains very much the same today. In a consideration of behaviour on and after alighting, he concludes 'The evidence leads one to think that the stimulus of scent affects *Glossina* in two ways; it may be effective from a distance and this leads to taxic behaviour of the insect in flight; it is also influential at close quarters and this leads to movements of orientation on the host, and to such activity as piercing and sucking'.

It would appear to the writer that scent must essentially be a short range stimulant, although it is undoubtedly capable of operating at a distance by carriage down the wind. Bax (1937), for example, found that *G. swynnertoni* reacted to the unseen passage of a party of men and cattle to windward at a distance of 180 feet, but not at twice that distance; this contrasted with their reaction in a glass-sided cage to the visible passage to leeward of cattle and men past a gap in a grass screen up to 450 feet, but not at 600 feet even in a bright light. It is also conceivable that a scented trail, such as might be left by a game animal or herd of game animals, could lead tsetse from a distance to a source of food, while the smell is still acting as a short-range attractant. Langridge (1961) has demonstrated the possibility of this by showing that catches of *G. pallidipes* were five times as great on paths through vegetation that had been sprayed with an emulsion containing benzene extracts of pig hair and skin scrapings or smeared with a sheep-wool grease (lanolin). More recently, Persoons (1967), at Lugala in Uganda, applied extracts in petroleum spirit from hot-water washings of pigs to the hessian screens of traps twice weekly, and found that this increased the catches of the traps 2·7 times for *G. pallidipes* and 2·4 times for *G. fuscipes*; the catches, however, fell to nearly the level of the traps with untreated screens a week after treatment ceased. Incidentally, it has been general experience that traps freshly covered with new hessian tend to catch more flies when first taken into use than after they have been in use for some time; this has been attributed to the strong smell of the new hessian, at first readily perceptible to the human nose but becoming almost imperceptible fairly soon after the traps have been exposed to the weather.

These experiences suggest that useful guidance to the evolution of attractants suitable for field trial might be obtained by observing the effects of exposing tsetse flies to the emanations of a variety of potentially attractive compounds; the attractant quality might be revealed by observing the activity of the flies, or their biting responses, or even the activity of the olfactory nerve on the lines of the sophisticated approach used by Burtt and Catton (1956) in investigating visual responses of the locust. This type of approach is at present under investigation by C. T. Lewis at the Silwood Park Field Station of the Imperial College of Science and Technology, London. Some earlier work of a preliminary nature on the responses of tsetse flies to odorous substances has been described by Hughes (1957); this suggested that a compound having low vapour pressure, low dielectric constant, and possibly high dipole moment, is likely to be a good olfactory stimulant.

Dethier (1954) made an interesting study of the biting responses of *G. palpalis*, *G. morsitans* and *G. brevipalpis*, from which he concluded that heat is the prime stimulus to feeding and the antenna the principal site of the thermoreceptors concerned. This would explain the numerous instances that tsetse flies have been observed to probe the trunks of trees heated in the mid-day sun, or the warmed tyres of motor vehicles. Dethier found that neither odour nor chemicals in contact with the tarsi of tsetse provided effective stimuli, in spite of the fact that Lewis (1954) has described the presence of numbers of specialized hollow setae on the ventral surface of tarsi of *G. palpalis*, of the same type as those shown to function as chemoreceptors in the blow-fly, *Phormia* (Protophormia) *terranovae* R.-D., and the house-fly, *Musca domestica* L. Buxton (1955), also, remarks that although tarsal organs of taste are known on many Muscid and other Diptera, there is no indication of the existence of such organs on the tarsi of *Glossina*, but notes that one must suppose that the rich and varied supply of sensillae on the haustellum functions in this way during the acts of piercing and sucking. He also notes that there is nothing to suggest that a sense of hearing is used by *Glossina*, although he remarks that the elaborate arista of the tsetse fly might perform such a function, as in many insects the hairs on the antennae or even the whole of the flagellum are supposed to be particularly responsive to vibratory movements of the air and to respond to a wide range of tones. Glover (1965), in a discussion of the senses of *Glossina*, recalls that Vanderplank (1948) refers to 'mating notes' which he presumed to be produced by the wing beat and which he believed to be of primary importance in mating. Glover also records that Langridge (in an unpublished departmental report of 1964) describes the making of tape recordings of the sounds made by female tsetse flies, and says that these seemed to attract the male flies, but Glover doubts whether these can be of any importance as attractants except at very close range.

A good deal has been published as to the colour on which most tsetse flies will settle. This is very relevant to any study of attractants and of considerable importance in considering the subject of sampling. The most critical and careful investigation of this nature is that described by Barrass (1960), carried out in the Zambesi valley in Rhodesia; most of the flies concerned were *G. morsitans* but small numbers of *G. pallidipes* were also present. A comparison was made of the numbers of flies settling on black, dark grey, light grey and white screens, the reflecting powers of which were measured. The investigation was therefore one rather of preferences for dark over light surfaces than for colours; it would be worth while carrying out a similar careful investigation of colour preferences. In his account Barrass gives a useful brief review of earlier work and also of similar work on other biting Diptera. The results he obtained are a little puzzling. Thus he found that, although flies preferred to settle on the darker of two screens, they settled on the sunny side of a screen rather than on the shaded side. This, one would think, might well lead to dangerous exposure to insolation. The flies thus caught, however, may be regarded as 'active' flies, for he remarks that all were not hungry flies and therefore cannot be regarded as flies seeking food. They thus behave differently from 'resting' flies, which are found during daylight hours on the shaded side of a tree (Nash & Davey 1950; *see* also Nash, 1952) or the underside of a branch (Isherwood 1957). Another interesting finding was that the breaking up of a black surface with white stripes, even narrow ones, reduced its attractiveness; this may possibly explain the very few feeds that have been recorded from zebra.

Another recent investigation of the senses used in host-finding by tsetse flies is that on *G. medicorum* in Ghana, described by Chapman (1960). In this, field and laboratory studies were combined. He found the flies to be stimulated by a moving screen, the stimulation becoming less and less when the screen was stopped and re-started for short periods and fell off less rapidly when it was kept in continuous motion. The bearing of this on the possibility of the fly losing contact with its host appearing and disappearing through thick vegetation is discussed. *G. medicorum*, a fly of the forests, unlike *G. morsitans*, a savanna woodland fly, did not respond to objects more than 25 feet away; his figures for *G. submorsitans* in northern Ghana, also showed a shorter visual range than did those of Bax (quoted earlier), as he failed to get a response beyond 150 feet. The smell of a guinea pig or a goat failed to elicit any response, but the vapour of dilute acetic acid produced a strong reaction. As did Bax with *G. morsitans*, Chapman observed a very strong response to the smell of cattle which were not visible to the flies; he also observed a tendency to fly up-wind in a wind-tunnel, even with flies that had been blinded by covering their eyes with black cellulose paint. Chapman concluded that this species must find its host mainly by scent. In the writer's opinion, this is likely also to be true of *G. pallidipes* and probably of any species living in thick vegetation.

An understanding of the basic principles of what constitutes an attractant for tsetse flies, probably a very complex matter, is one of the most important of the unsolved problems in tsetse work. It is surprising that more attention has not been paid to it. Not only would its solution make a very important contribution to investigation, for much of the sampling done depends on the attraction of the flies to the sampling party or mechanism, but it is also vital for the efficient and economic application of insecticides on a selective basis. The way would also be cleared for the wider use of the newly discovered chemosterilants; at present, their lack of specificity of action precludes their safe usage except on a very limited scale and under particular conditions. This knowledge would be of no less value in discovering the presence of a sparse population of fly, a vital necessity in assessing the success or failure of tsetse control schemes; at present, the only really reliable means of demonstrating the absence of *Glossina* is to maintain test herds of uninfected cattle in the area and to observe their freedom from typanosome infections throughout a year (*see* p. 401, and Wooff, 1965).

Chapter 23

Control by Insecticides: General Considerations

G. F. BURNETT

DEVELOPMENT OF THE USE OF INSECTICIDES FOR TSETSE CONTROL

The use of insecticides in various branches of medical and veterinary entomology was practised for many years before they were used against *Glossina*. This was because tsetse cannot be attacked with the chemicals which were available before the introduction of DDT (dichlorodiphenyl trichloroethane). Mosquitoes have a vulnerable larval stage that can be asphyxiated with oil or poisoned with metallic salts whereas the larvae of *Glossina* are shortlived and widely dispersed and the pupae safe below ground. The adults, especially the females, pay the briefest possible visits to their food source where they feed through the skin of the host and then disperse once more into the woodland. They are thus invulnerable to stomach poisons and to the washes and lotions used for sedentary ectoparasites, and indeed to the pyrethrum space sprays that have been used with some success against mosquitoes. In fact the only use for insecticides against tsetse before 1946 was of pyrethrum sprays in de-flying chambers. When DDT and BHC (benzene hexachloride) became available for experimental use in 1945 their possible uses were explored with great urgency and, by 1949, at least preliminary trials had been made of all the methods that were later used with considerable success, and some others that have not so far been developed for economic use.

Much of this early work was not adequately published, no doubt because a high proportion was inconclusive. Accurate laboratory work to precede and support field trials was very difficult because tsetse were not easy to maintain in the laboratory. It was therefore common to undertake field trials with less detailed information than is usually available for most comparable work with other insects. The complexity of the field situation made it difficult to interpret the results and, in particular, the importance and difficulty of preventing immigration of tsetse into experimental areas were much underestimated. In addition, experiments were frequently on too small a scale for such a wide ranging insect and it was usually not until governments were prepared to risk thousands instead of scores of pounds that substantial progress was made. Interpretation was also hindered by inadequate post-treatment search for tsetse and especially by discontinuing observations prematurely. It was frequently impossible to decide, on the data available, whether small numbers of tsetse discovered some months after treatment were immigrants or the product of very sparse residual populations; the interpretation of the findings, which was critical for the evaluation of the method, tended to depend on the background of the interpreter—insecticide workers favoured immigration while tsetse ecologists placed greater emphasis on survival.

Experiments with DDT started in East Africa and virtually all the early progress was made in English-speaking territories with their long-established leaning towards vector control as a means of interrupting trypanosome transmission.

Steyn (1949) used DDT dust from an aircraft without success on Lake Victoria in February 1945, but a heavy residual treatment applied in July of the same year was successful. Symes *et al.* (1948) investigated various residual treatments to vegetation in the same area in 1945. In the same year, Vanderplank (1947a) carried out some of the first laboratory trials and assessed the suitability of bait cattle for a field trial that was carried out by Whiteside (1949) early the next year. Du Toit (1954) in Zululand had meanwhile begun the first attempt to eradicate an insect (*G. pallidipes*) by applying insecticide from aircraft, supplemented by smoke canisters and DDT dust from the ground. Smoke canisters were also used in East Africa (*see* EATRO, 1950, p. 24). Morris (1950) in West Africa assessed the value of DDT applied to traps in 1946.

Tests on residual applications to vegetation were successfully concluded by Woodcock (1949) and the process of eliminating *G. fuscipes* from Kenya was commenced in 1951 by Wilson (1953). Dieldrin was first tested in late 1955 (Burnett, Robinson & Le Roux, 1957) and at once replaced DDT in Kenya (Glover, Le Roux & Parker, 1960) and ultimately in all areas where the climate made a single application of DDT inadequate.

Machine-generated fogs were tried in 1949 by the Colonial Insecticide Research Unit (later Tropical Pesticide Research Institute), Arusha, Tanzania, and were used for routine reclamation work in Zambia from 1953 (Steel & Gledhill, 1960). The CIRU started using sprays from aircraft against *G. fuscipes* in Uganda in 1948 and against *G. morsitans* in Tanganyika in 1949. In 1962 they introduced ultra-low-volume aerial treatments. The first reclamation scheme in East Africa using aerial techniques took place in Uganda in 1953, and the first using light aircraft and low volume (but not ultra-low-volume) methods started in Rwanda in 1960 (Buyckx, 1965). Large ground aerosol-dispersing machines were first taken into routine use in Zambia in 1954.

The use of insecticides in West Africa, apart from Morris' traps, started in Nigeria in 1953 and over the next seven years residual treatments were progressively refined and cheapened in large field trials (H. Davies, 1964). Nigerian methods were adopted in French-speaking territories in 1961 (Mouchet, 1963). The first use of residual treatments in diffuse habitats, as opposed to dry season refuges, appears to have been in Uganda in 1960 (Hocking, 1961) where, in 1963, the results were applied on a large scale (Wooff, 1965).

Except in continuous evergreen forest, the application of insecticides is now established practice for the control of all the important species of tsetse. There is most information on their use against *G. palpalis*, *G. fuscipes*, *G. tachinoides*, *G. morsitans*, *G. swynnertoni* and *G. pallidipes*. A little is known of their effect on *G. brevipalpis* and *G. austeni* but virtually nothing concerning other species.

THE USE OF INSECTICIDES: GENERAL CONSIDERATIONS

There are two over-riding considerations governing the strategy and tactics of insecticide application, namely, that the environment remains entirely favourable to the fly, which may re-establish itself if it has the chance, and the life history of the insect. Because 50–75% of any tsetse population is at any given moment in the pupal stage beneath the soil and therefore inaccessible to insecticides, the environment has to be made lethal, either continuously or at intervals, for at least the duration of the maximum pupal period in the climatic conditions prevailing. Failure to do so will permit survivors to larviposit and operations will have to be continued in order to deal with these insects as they eventually emerge. The only way to prevent re-establishment is to exterminate completely and to prevent immigration from elsewhere. Thus operations against tsetse are usually aimed at extermination. This is most exceptional in pest control where the aim is usually to reduce infestation to a sub-economic level and to repeat the attack whenever it rises above it. The reasons for this difference in approach are, firstly, the extreme efficiency of *Glossina* as disease vectors, which makes it difficult, short of extermination, to reduce population density to a level at which they will be innocuous; secondly, the low value and productivity of the land infested is insufficient to support regular expenditure on tsetse control indefinitely; thirdly, the continuance of control measures is such a drain on scarce resources that once these are committed to consolidating the gains made it is impractical to extend the protected area. Thus, if extermination is attainable it is worthwhile because it is progressive and each advance of the tsetse extermination front actually increases the security of the rear areas from reinfestation. The poor return from the land when free of fly requires the use of the cheapest possible methods and the large scale on which the work must be done reinforces this need. Whereas 8s per acre is a very worthwhile price to pay it is not practical to work in terms of acres; a more realistic unit of, say, 10 miles square would cost £25,600, a large item in an annual budget.

The prerequisite of extermination is isolation of the area from reinfestation. The barriers may be natural or artificial, the terrain between the treated woodland and all potential sources of reinfestation being made inhospitable for tsetse at all seasons. This is absolutely essential; it is likely that more experiments and reclamation schemes have been foiled by immigration than for any other reason or combination of reasons.

Personal communications from several workers active in reclamation have shown a tendency for policy to change from direct extermination by insecticides to reduction in numbers by spraying followed by consolidation by settlement, often assisted by chemotherapy. This procedure is favoured for veterinary trypanosomiasis because it is very cheap and can be applied to large areas with the resources available.

A factor of great importance favouring the use of insecticides has been the extreme susceptibility of *Glossina* to some of them. In particular, the group of organochlorines known as the cyclopentadiennes is very lethal to tsetse. This has made it possible to use very low dosage rates with consequent economy and also with considerable selectivity in favour of other animals.

CHOICE OF METHOD: INFORMATION REQUIRED IN PLANNING OPERATIONS

The use of insecticides has come to be the most common method of reducing infestation by *Glossina* in many parts of Africa for two principal reasons—

economy in cash and in manpower. Methods of insecticide treatment are themselves inter-competitive and where there are no special reasons to favour one particular method the cheapest will always be adopted.

The methods of using insecticides described below have all been assessed either experimentally or in reclamation schemes. They fall into two quite distinct groups: (a) those that act by virtue of residual deposits which kill insects contacting them over a period of days or months, and (b) those with no detectable residual effect and which therefore need repeated application to secure more than a transient reduction in tsetse numbers.

Residual treatments applied to:

vegetation
food
traps
pupation sites

Non-residual treatments applied by:

aircraft
chemical smoke generators
ground-based fogging machines.

Choice of the best method to use in any given control scheme depends on a number of factors, which may be interdependent. In particular there is a natural tendency to continue with a tried and tested method because staff is already trained to operate it, or to adopt one found successful in a neighbouring country. Some methods may be discarded at once as inapplicable as, for example, the use of aerosols in dense rain forest. Where there is a choice, the cost of attaining success with an equal degree of probability must be estimated for each available method. There will be a good deal of guesswork in this but the choice has to be made before running pilot schemes, because it is easier and apparently cheaper and safer to modify a method already tried than to start all over again. The more information that is available the better but the following considerations are of general application.

Residual deposits need to be relatively heavy in order to obtain adequate persistence but it is not feasible to apply insecticide on this scale over the whole habitat available to the fly. It is only necessary to treat that part of the habitat which the species concerned is constrained to visit at some time in its life, although such visits may be confined to only part of the year. Within the habitat it may be possible to confine spraying to certain favoured areas and to favoured sites within these areas. In general, the more stringent the climatic conditions or the physiological and behavioural requirements of the species, the more restricted can be the surface treated. It is therefore highly desirable that before even planning a campaign some observations should be made on the resting habits and seasonal movement of the tsetse population in the area concerned. These may vary with the locality and certainly with the climatic zone and it is therefore unwise to rely on observations made elsewhere. If, in the area selected for treatment, the fly is more restricted in requirements than in the area where observations are made, applications will be extravagant and wasteful, but if the reverse, unduly restricted treatment may lead to failure and frequently has done so. Thus, in East Africa, *G.m. morsitans* does not undergo any considerable dry season concentration whereas in Rhodesia it does, so that different treatment patterns are appropriate to the two areas. Especially in diffused habitats, accurate information on resting sites makes it possible to reduce expenditure on insecticide applications to a spectacular degree.

When defining concentration, not only the extent but the degree is important. If tsetse densities are found to be ten times as great in subhabitat A as in the rest of the general habitat, subhabitat B, there is undoubtedly a considerable concentration in A. However, if the total area of B is ten times that of A, the total number of fly in the two zones is equal and treatment of A alone will lead to failure. If, however, it is known that the flies in B will visit A at frequent intervals then treatment of A alone may still be successful. It should always be borne in mind when killing tsetse that males are significant only in that they indicate the presence of breeding females. It is the distribution of the latter that is important since females are considerably more tolerant than males to the most commonly used insecticides (*see* p. 477). Where knowledge of the distribution and habits of a species is based on the behaviour of males only, insecticide applications must be applied with considerably less precision than where there is intimate knowledge of the behaviour of females. It may not be necessary to treat all known resting sites. Where different sites are regularly occupied at different diurnal periods only those favoured at one period need be sprayed. Further selection is possible, especially in restricted habitats, because the tsetse must move to obtain its meals and will thus visit a number of sites, between meals, in any one reproductive cycle. This is fortunate because as the deposit becomes reduced with time those sites originally lightly treated become non-lethal but those heavily treated retain their toxicity; while there are sufficient of the latter the environment as a whole remains lethal. Since one of the major difficulties of insecticide application is to obtain regular and continuous coverage this mobility of the ultimate target is probably important. Knowledge of the daily changes in preferred resting sites may indicate that treatment of leaves and twigs is appropriate for one species but that tree trunks are better for another. It may be noted here that leaves, even of evergreen shrubs, fall rapidly at certain times of the year and at others rapidly expanding leaves, or sprouting herbs, quickly provide a large number of new and uncontaminated resting sites for those species that favour them.

The period which tsetse spend in a restricted habitat is a critical consideration. This period must exceed the maximum pupal period of the species or the fly will survive in the puparial stage outside the adult habitat. The length of the pupal period may be difficult to define since it will vary according to circumstances such as the species of fly, individual variation, prevailing climatic conditions, micro-climates and other unpredictable factors. For these reasons it is unsafe to assume that apparent retreat of adult flies to a favoured habitat for a period approximately equal to the pupal period will be sufficient to ensure success if only this habitat is treated. The period of retreat must exceed the pupal period by at lease 50%, preferably 100%, if reliance is placed on a method based on the treatment of minimum habitats. In order to calculate the minimum or mean pupal period, standard temperature readings are required for the area concerned. From these the period can be calculated (p. 440). This information is, however, of little use if the persistence of the proposed insecticide application is unknown. This can often be gauged on the basis of experience elsewhere but it is strongly influenced by climate, especially rainfall, and if no information is available from areas with a similar climate it will have to be obtained by trial.

When non-persistent applications of aerosols are to be made it is possible to proceed with less detailed information on resting sites, although it is useful to know that the insects will be in exposed places when the insecticide is disseminated. It is essential to know that the whole area inhabited by tsetse is being treated, because a second chance to kill insects which are missed because they are temporarily outside the treated zone will not occur until the next treatment, which will probably be several weeks ahead. If aerosols are being used from ground machines it is useful to have at least a general idea of the preferred resting places of the species under attack so that these can have special attention, or at least not be overlooked; the interior of thickets inhabited by *G. pallidipes* provides an example. A factor to be borne in mind is that to be successful, aerosol applications require suitable meterological conditions; before planning to use aerosols some information is required on the frequency of such conditions in the area concerned and on the time of day (usually between an hour before dusk to two hours after dawn) when they can be expected. If the entire area of bush is not to be treated then it is important to define the limits of tsetse presence at that time of day. The usual direction of the wind at the hour of operations is important in planning the use of aerosols from ground machines.

Before starting on any control scheme it is necessary to ensure that the isolation of the block to be treated is complete. This will require a detailed survey of natural barriers to make certain they are complete and genuinely free from tsetse habitats, or to estimate the cost of making barriers fly-tight.

Apart from necessary biological information operational considerations may be over-riding; some of these are briefly summarized below:

(i) Aerosol treatments must be done on discrete blocks and never piecemeal, whereas residual treatments can advance on a front relying on the barrier of freshly-applied insecticide to prevent re-invasion. On the other hand, with a sufficient number of aircraft, large areas can be covered very rapidly indeed, thus ensuring that most infective flies are destroyed at the first application. Such measures are therefore suited to halting epidemics or fly advances without delay.

(ii) Aircraft require a minimum of preparation on the ground whereas residual treatments or vehicle-based aerosol machines need tracks and roads, accurately laid out paths for treatment, more ground transport and detailed maps. Aircraft however need a local base from which to fly and a system of beacons on which to track.

(iii) Residual treatments are applicable only in situations where the species concerned is confined to a particular limited habitat for a sufficient period or has well defined and restricted resting sites. If preferred habitats are numerous and scattered they may be laborious and expensive to define. An example is given by Gledhill and Caughey (1963) where an elaborate survey was made of the entire treatment area at intervals of 200–300 yards (less in some places). The cost of this preliminary work was of the order of 25% of the total expenditure on the project but it reduced the proportion of sites that were actually treated with a residual spray by some 35%. Since this work was done, the cost of aerial treatment has been reduced and that of ground treatment has increased so that it might now be cheaper to use aircraft without the detailed preliminary survey. This is especially likely where two or more species are present, each with different preferred habitats.

(iv) Aircraft avoid such difficulties as gullies and swamps which hinder ground treatments but they require fairly level terrain. Helicopters have been used successfully in mountainous areas but they are expensive to operate.

(v) Aircraft are most effective when vegetation is leafless at least for the first three applications but they have been used with success over evergreen thickets. This might be because the species concerned, *G. pallidipes*, is active at the time treatment takes place and might not apply to other species. Trees in thick leaf throughout the period available may be better treated from beneath with ground aerosol machines (or residual applications).

(vi) Aerosol techniques as at present developed require repeated operations extending over a period of about eighteen weeks. It is likely that further experience will make it possible to reduce this, possibly by half.

(vii) Wet season operations should be avoided if possible because tsetse are then widely dispersed and operations of any kind are hindered by bad weather.

(viii) The cost of assessing the effectiveness of a scheme is not dependent on the method used.

(ix) Before any method is put into practice, personnel need to be recruited and trained. With aircraft this depends on the availability of experienced pilots. Crop-spraying pilots may need retraining for the different operating conditions involved in applying insecticides against tsetse.

COSTING

It is impossible to make an accurate estimate of the cost of a control scheme without considerable experience in the area concerned, as figures from elsewhere serve only as a general guide and they are rarely complete. Usually the cost of scientific supervision is omitted and frequently also expenditure on operational supervision, capital equipment, depreciation and even transport. Once the method to be used has been selected it is fairly easy to decide upon the insecticide, formulation, application rate and the number of applications required. The extent of the application depends on local information but once decided the expenditure on insecticide, including transport to the site, is fairly easily arrived at and this is likely to be the major cost. The cost of application is fairly easily worked out—number of sprayers, men to operate them, cost of fuel, spares, maintenance, etc., taking into consideration the expected duration of the task. One can now get an idea of the cost of transporting all this both to the site and on the job, and to this must be added the cost of all preliminary work such as cutting access roads, slashing paths for access or spraying, providing beacon roads or fixed beacons for aircraft, constructing or maintaining bush airstrips and the cost of flying from strip to block, etc. Good maps are needed and aerial photography is certainly the quickest and often the cheapest way of getting them, especially if they have already been taken for another purpose. Preliminary survey work, including any detailed mapping of tsetse habitats can be expensive, up to 20% of total costs. Post-treatment surveys need to be even more intensive and may have to be repeated over two or three years. Capital costs include not only spray gear and vehicles but possibly aircraft, radios, boats, housing and tents. Food and other necessities must also be brought to the site.

ASSESSMENT OF RESULTS

No special methods are available for assessing insecticide operations and reliance must be placed on the normal techniques for counting tsetse flies; special efforts must be made after operations are over to find any survivors, using the techniques appropriate to the species concerned and especially those most suitable for the detection of small populations. Pre-treatment surveys are also required not only to establish the level of population, but the trend of any variation with time and its distribution in place. In experimental work it is also necessary to have an index of the expected trend in the absence of treatment and this can only be obtained from similar populations not under attack; in practice, where elimination is the aim, there is only one criterion of success. Natural tsetse populations do not disappear in the few months covered by insecticide operations and when extermination is achieved there is usually no doubt that it is due to the measures employed so that attempts to make a more sensitive assessment of the result would be wasted effort. It has sometimes happened that the intervention of climatic factors has made it impossible to be sure that extermination was due to insecticide but this is only likely where extensive flooding of pupal sites takes place (White, 1963). It is common for catches to show a decrease before actual dissemination of insecticide starts and this is usually attributed to disturbance of the food supply by the activity of preparing for the insecticide treatments.

Since post-treatment surveys must always be thorough and cover all likely pockets of tsetse persistence, pretreatment surveys should be made on a similar scale to establish a basis for comparison. It is sometimes thought desirable to search out localities with high concentration of fly on the assumption that, with an equal proportionate decrease in numbers everywhere, survivors are likely to be most easily detected in these places. In practice, persistence of fly is just as likely to be found in other localities, possibly because they were not given so much care in treatment. Attention should be paid to woodland boundaries through which immigration may be possible, because in the case of failure it is important to decide whether this is due to immigration or failure to kill resident flies.

It is difficult to decide when to discontinue post-treatment searches. Intensive surveys are usually continued for some months after the end of operations and are then reduced or stopped thereby freeing personnel for duty elsewhere.

Searches should be resumed after a year or so and may be repeated annually in order to detect any small residue, or slow immigration, which may have built up to a detectable level in the interval. Such evidence as is available suggests that, in the absence of immigration, no build-up will occur unless fly populations in the whole area are increasing. There appears to be no substitute for making the greatest possible effort to detect the presence of fly by repeated and extensive search, where possible using such specially sensitive methods as cattle patrols. The problem of detection is aggravated by the understandable loss of interest shown by tsetse scouts when they repeatedly fail to discover tsetse. The first few flies caught should be carefully examined for age and, if females, for insemination.

There are many examples of the difficulty of discovering persistent pockets of tsetse. Glover (1963) cites an instance where *G. fuscipes* had eluded discovery for two years and where others in completely atypical habitats had, for this reason, escaped treatment. MacLennan (1965) concluded that it is more profitable to direct the attention of search parties, using special methods, to areas where tsetse are most likely to be present rather than to attempt the impossible task of covering very large areas using orthodox fly-rounds. He found that in order to detect a low density of *G. tachinoides* it may be necessary to spend four to seven days in one restricted locality before a single specimen could be caught.

Care must be taken in the interpretation of attempts to measure the effect of individual insecticide applications on the basis of pre- and post-application catches. In the first three or four days it may be assumed that most teneral flies will have emerged since the application and they can be ignored. On the other hand slow-acting compounds such as dieldrin, isobenzan and endosulfan are not completely lethal in less than 72 hours. Burnett *et al.* (1964) found catches were actually higher immediately after treatment than they were before and they calculated immediate mortalities from catches made two and three days after treatment.

Considerable effort can be saved by delaying post-treatment search until some months after the end of lethal effect because, shortly after treatment, a much smaller than normal proportion of the total population is detectable as adults and any assessment made will grossly underestimate the true population. The reason for this is that the expectation of adult life is drastically reduced by treatment so that a smaller proportion of each individual's total life is spent as an adult, reducing the chances of its capture; the true proportion will not be restored until a maximum adult life-span has passed since the insecticide ceased to kill. In addition, the numbers of pupae present is greater than would be deposited by the number of adults actually emerging because the pupae were deposited by the larger adult population present before reduction by insecticidal action. The number of adults will steadily rise as they emerge from their pupae and attempts to assess the stable population from catches of adults alone will underestimate it. By the end of the first pupal period the number of adults will be the maximum that the stock of pupae can produce but there will not be a normal proportion of adults and pupae in the population until the last of these adults has finished its reproductive career. Thus any attempt to assess the true post-treatment population should be delayed for at least one pupal period after the insecticide has ceased to work. With residual treatment this may be months after it is no longer completely effective. If dispersal from a favoured habitat has meantime taken place a few persistent flies may be completely missed, but, of course, the dispersal might be sufficient to reduce breeding below the threshold for population maintenance so that the insects missed will have no significance. It seems highly probable that the best time for post-treatment assessment in such a habitat is in the next season of retreat to it.

Where applicable, test herds pastured in the treated area provide the most sensitive means of detecting low populations of tsetse, as the animals may develop overt trypanosomiasis when fly cannot be detected by other methods. Absence of captured flies, or infected animals, for two years is usually accepted as indicating tsetse extermination; it is quite common for a few flies to be found in the first year but for these to fail to re-establish themselves permanently.

Immigration may take place across surprising extents of so-called barriers and may defy detection until resident fly populations have been drastically reduced. Attempts to demonstrate this occurrence by marking flies in the suspected source of reinfestation and recapturing them in the treated area are extravagant of effort and of little promise. No method will prove that immigration does not occur but it has been found, with savanna tsetse and especially with *G. pallidipes*, that the most reliable method of detecting immigration is by catching flies from vehicles plying across such barriers. This method has the additional advantage of distinguishing between immigrant flies and those originating in the treated block.

THE FATE OF RESIDUAL TSETSE POPULATIONS

There is no evidence that the low tsetse populations remaining after unsuccessful attempts at extermination will rapidly build up to dangerous proportions, despite extermination of their predators and parasites (Fiedler, Du Toit & Kluge, 1954), unless natural increase is supplemented by immigration. Hocking (1962) reports the results of observations on residual populations over a six-year period following insecticide treatment which effected a 99% reduction of *G. morsitans*. The residual population in the treated area was compared with that on a nearby hillside where the tsetse density was about 300 times greater. The fly population in the two areas showed parallel seasonal and cyclical fluctuations and at the end of the six-year period the numbers in both areas were about 20% of those at the start of the period.

BARRIERS: CHEMICAL AND PHYSICAL

Insecticide operations are valueless unless reinfestation by *Glossina* is prevented by barriers of some sort. These may be natural or man-made or may be belts of vegetation treated with insecticide. The latter are discussed under the heading of residual applications (*see* pp. 500–501); they are only permanent if renewed at intervals and are particularly useful as a temporary holding measure pending further advance of the spray front.

Physical barriers have been used for many years. They are usually found to be inadequate when conditions favour fly advances. Natural barriers are particularly unreliable as they may include unsuspected minor habitats or trees that will not support tsetse permanently but provide refuges as they cross inhospitable cleared country. Gall acacias provide such an opportunity for *G. swynnertoni*. MacLennan (1965) cites an example of an untreated focus in a natural barrier four miles from treated woodland from which reinfestation was facilitated by the movement of cattle along a well-trodden track. Burnett *et al.* (1964), in weekly post-treatment surveys carried out for a year, caught only a single old male *G. morsitans* in each of two blocks, both in the same week, eleven months after treatment ceased. They attributed this occurrence to the incursion of a herd of elephants across three miles of clearing, much of it under cultivation. Both these examples illustrate the importance of animal carriers in reducing the effectiveness of barriers. Barriers three to four miles in width appear to be normally adopted in practice; Wooff (1967) considers a barrier three to four miles wide necessary to restrain *G. morsitans* in Uganda, and in Rhodesia Cockbill (1964) regards a width of three miles as dangerously narrow. Selectively cleared barriers are probably unsuitable for protecting insecticide schemes. Natural barriers must be even more thoroughly surveyed than the treated block if small foci of fly are not to be overlooked.

If more than one species of tsetse is present the barrier must be adequate for each species. *G. tachinoides* will cross barriers that exclude *G. palpalis*. Nash (1948a) found the former moved 2,150 yards through a river clearing while the latter only traversed 810 yards, but he also records that *G. tachinoides* crossed a clearing of 1·75 miles and doubts if two miles would be adequate in the wet season. A barrier nearly three miles long failed to exclude *G. tachinoides* from the Komady Gana scheme (MacLennan & Kirkby, 1958). Nash and Steiner (1957) found *G. palpalis* was excluded by a sheer clearing of 1·5 miles but not by one of only one mile. Glasgow and Duffy (1951) proved migration of *G. fuscipes* across clearings of 2·5 and 3 miles along a permanent river. Some marked flies travelled at least nine miles. On a seasonal river, clearings of only 2·8 miles were adequate. The distances quoted are all measured from end to end of the clearing and take no account of the less direct course followed by the river. In Kenya, sheer-cleared barriers each ten miles wide were originally used to exclude *G. fuscipes* in the Kuja-Migori scheme but these were later replaced by barriers of sprayed vegetation each three miles in width (J. G. Le Roux, personal communication; *see* also pp. 544, 546, 559–560).

THE SUSCEPTIBILITY OF *GLOSSINA* TO INSECTICIDES

When insecticides were first used against tsetse in 1945, DDT and BHC were the only two potent synthetic compounds available. It was known that the powerful natural product pyrethrum was both too unstable in sunlight and too expensive to use in the field. When newer synthetics such as dieldrin became available they were selected for trial because of their known activity against other pests and were assessed against tsetse on a comparative basis, usually cost for cost, with the older products. The first systematic laboratory assessment of a range of insecticidal compounds was reported by Burnett (1961–3). These tests were made with *G. morsitans* and *G. swynnertoni*, the insecticides being applied to the thoraces of the flies in the form of very small drops (0·02 ml.) of oil solutions. Similar tests by Busvine, Abduramen and Mohammed (1967), using dry residual deposits, showed that although the order of toxicities was much the same in both cases the relative magnitudes may be different, and thus tests with oil solutions may be misleading if the results are applied directly to the use of residual deposits in field work. In contrast, when flies have been exposed to tarsal pickup of oil solutions the relative toxicities of DDT and dieldrin have been the same as with topically applied drops, although different species were used (e.g. Challier, 1963a; Riordan, 1966). The differences appear to be due to physical factors and not to the point of application.

Available information is given in Tables 23.1 and 23.2. Minor discrepancies probably due to differences in procedure or subspecies can be ignored. The

TABLE 23.1

The toxicities of insecticides to* Glossina *by topical application in solution.
LD50s in μ.g./fly. In brackets potency relative to DDT (i.e. 1/LD50). Male flies only

Insecticide	*G. morsitans* Burnett, 1961–63	*G.m. submorsitans* Busvine *et al.*, 1967	*G. swynnertoni* Burnett, 1961–63	*G. austeni* Busvine *et al.*, 1967
p.p. DDT	0·0165	0·046	0·0065	0·126
Aldrin	0·0135 (1·2)			
γ BHC	0·0064 (2·6)			
chlorobicyclen	0·0043 (3·8)			
bromocyclen	0·0032 (5·2)			
dieldrin	0·0017 (9·7)	0·0046 (10)	0·00045 (14)	0·0088 (14)
endosulfan	0·0012 (13·7)			
isobenzan	0·006 (27)	0·0039 (12)	0·00018 (36)	0·0056 (23)
malathion	>0·11 (<0·17)	0·231 (0·2)		0·196 (0·6)
fenitrothion }	0·02			
trichlorophon }	to (0·7)			
methylparathion }	0·03			
dimethoate }	0·011			
dichlorvos }	to			
diazinion }	0·013 (1·4)	0·053 (0·87)		0·049 (2·5)
coumaphos	0·005 (3·3)			
fenthion	0·005 (3·3)			
arprocarb	0·0081 (2·1)			0·014 (9·0)
pyrethrins	0·0020 (8·2)			

Burnett (*loc. cit.*) tested a number of other N-methylcarbamates, including carbaryl, all of which were ineffective.

considerable differences between species may also be partly but not entirely due to differences in procedure. The order of toxicities is much the same for different species except for the unusual susceptibility of *G. austeni* to malathion and arprocarb. Tests of this kind need to be extended to other species using both dry deposits and oil solutions. Vanderplank (1947a) attempted this but only DDT was available. He was able to grade twelve species and subspecies, among which he found a fourfold difference between the most susceptible (*G. pallidipes*) and the least susceptible (*G. brevipalpis*, *G. longipennis* and *G. fuscipleuris*). All the available evidence confirms that *Glossina* are exceptionally susceptible to the organochlorine insecticides as compared with other insects tested in a comparable manner. This is particularly so for endosulfan, isobenzan and to a lesser

TABLE 23.2

Lethal doses of insecticides as deposits. Relative toxicity compared with DDT in brackets

Insecticide	As dried suspension mg.a.i./cm.² *G. morsitans* Busvine *et al.* (1967)	*G. austeni* Busvine *et al.* (1967)	% solution in oil (WHO mosquito test kit) *G. palpalis* Challier (1963)
DDT	0·0155	0·014	2·3
dieldrin	0·0070 (2·2)	0·0026 (5·4)	0·07 (33)
isobenzan	0·0070 (2·2)	0·0022 (6·3)	
malathion		0·0042 (3·3)	
diazinon		0·0023 (6·1)	
arprocarb		0·0040 (3·5)	

degree, dieldrin. BHC is unusually ineffective while organophosphates and carbamates are moderately lethal. The level of susceptibility of tsetse is influenced considerably by physiological factors. Burnett (1961–3) found that when *G. morsitans* and *G. swynnertoni* were treated with oil solutions the pregnant females were very much less susceptible to organochlorines than were young flies. Where measured accurately, the LD50 for pregnant flies was five to nine times that for young flies of either sex but for females in the earlier stages of the reproductive cycle the difference was less marked. Males showed no differences with age. These observations have been confirmed for *G. palpalis* and *G. pallidipes* for deposits, both dry and in involatile oil (Challier, 1963a; Baldry, 1963; Bransby-Williams, unpub.). Fenthion (an organophosphate) and arprocarb (a carbamate) are as lethal to pregnant flies as to young ones, after allowing for weight differences. Challier (1963a) has shown that a recent meal can increase the LD50 for *G. palpalis* by three to four times. Thus for all tests on *Glossina*, insects in a standard physiological condition must be used.

THE PROPERTIES OF INSECTICIDES USED TO CONTROL *GLOSSINA*

Only compounds that work by direct contact have so far proved to be effective against *Glossina*, which are protected from stomach poisons by their method of feeding, but the use of poisoned food has not yet been adequately investigated. Only the adult stage is available for insecticidal attack.

Of the wide range of compounds now available only seven have been used against tsetse in practice or experimentally, namely, DDT, BHC, dieldrin, endosulfan, isobenzan, fenthion, and pyrethrum. Chlorbicyclen, bromocyclen and arprocarb may be used in future.

It should be noted that almost all commercially available insecticides are technical grade and are usually mixtures of the principal ingredient with its isomer or other closely related compounds. Where the impurities are markedly less toxic to insects the concentration of a preparation is always given in terms of the toxic principle, conventionally referred to as the active ingredient, abbreviated to a.i. Application rates also should be expressed in terms of a.i. and all references to concentration or quantities should make it quite clear to what they refer.

Chemicals used for tsetse control are listed below under their British Standard names, followed by the American designation if different, and by any other names under which relevant information on the compound has been published. Chemical names and formulae are also given because, on occasions, well-known compounds have been marketed under trade names which imply that the products are new and better.

Organochlorine Compounds

1. DDT (dicophen BP chlorphenophane USP Zerdane (Fr.) Gesarol, Neocid, Dichlorodiphenyl trichloroethane)

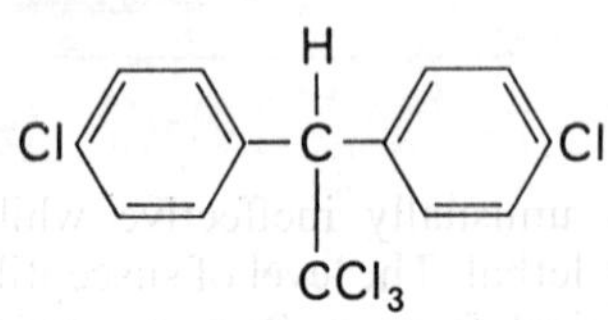

Fig. 23.1 DDT

Technical DDT is a mixture of several isomers of which only the para-pará form given above is usefully insecticidal. The universal specification is for technical DDT to contain at least 70% of the pp′ isomer. Thus, 1 lb./acre of technical DDT is only 0·7 lb./acre of the p-p′ isomer, and 25% technical DDT contains only 17·5% of this isomer.

Pure p-p′ isomer is a fine crystalline powder of m.p. 108·5°C. Vapour pressure 1·9 × 10·7 mm. Hg. at 20°C. The technical product is a waxy solid of indefinite melting point. Practically insoluble in water, moderately soluble in alcohols and kerosene (5–10%), readily soluble in most aromatic and chlorinated solvents. Decomposed by heat and readily dehydrochlorinated in solution by alkalis but not attacked by aqueous acids and alkalis. Persistent contact and stomach poison killing insects mostly within 12–48 hours. Acute LD50 to white rats 113 mg./kg. Little evidence of high chronic toxicity but is stored in body fat and excreted in milk.

Formulations. 5% kerosene solution, 50–75% wettable powders, 25% emulsion concentrates, 1–10% dusts, 10% solution in oil.

2. γBHC (Gammexane, HCH, Lindane, Benzene hexachloride or Hexachloro-cyclohexane)

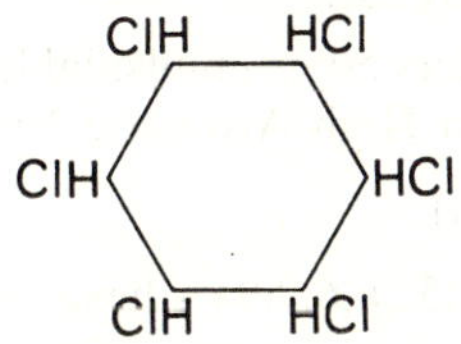

Fig. 23.2 γ BHC

Technical BHC contains only 12–13% of the γ isomer, the remainder being principally the relatively inert α, β and △ isomers. Lindane is a refined technical product containing not less than 99% γ isomer. Thus γBHC or Lindane may be considered eight times as insecticidal as the technical product, which is little used in tsetse control.

γBHC consists of colourless crystals, mp 113°C. Vapour pressure $9{\cdot}4 \times 10^{-6}$ mm. Hg. at 20°C. Practically insoluble in water (10 ppm), slightly soluble in petroleum oils, soluble in acetone, aromatic and chlorinated solvents. Stable to air, light, heat and strong acids. Decomposed by alkali. The technical product is brownish and has a strong musty odour.

Potent contact, fumigant and stomach poison of limited persistence in tropical conditions. Kills rapidly, usually within twenty-four hours. Acute oral LD50 to white rats 125 mg./kg. but is excreted rapidly in urine.

Formulations. Wettable powders, emulsifiable concentrates and dusts with a wide range of concentrations. 4–5% solutions in petroleum oils.

3. DIELDRIN. Hexachloro-epoxy-octahydro-dimethanonaphthalene, (HEOD).

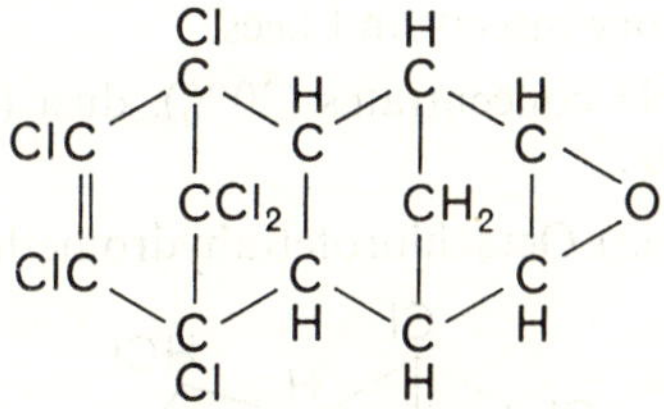

Fig. 23.3 Dieldrin

Dieldrin is the approved name in Great Britain and USA for a material containing not less than 85% of the above compound and in Canada for the pure compound, but in field practice it is assumed that the technical product is as insecticidal as the pure compound and a.i. refers to total technical dieldrin.

Technical dieldrin occurs as buff to light brown flakes, setting point not below 95°C, v.p. 1·8 × 10^{-7} mm. Hg. at 25°C. The recrystallized product is white and odourless, m.p. 175–176°C density 1·75. Insoluble in water, slightly soluble in mineral oils, moderately in acetone and soluble in organic solvents. Stable in alkali, mild acids and light.

Highly persistent and highly toxic stomach and contact poison for many insects, fish, etc. Kills slowly taking 72 hours for complete mortality of tsetse flies. LD50 for white rats 100 mg./kg., relatively high dermal and chronic toxicities. Accumulates in body fat.

Formulations. Wettable powders 50%, emulsifiable concentrates (*c.* 20%), dusts (usually 2%), 20% solution in High Aromatic Naphtha or similar solvents.

4. ENDOSULFAN (Thiodan)

6,7,8,9,10,10 - hexachloro - 1,5,5a,6,9,9a - hexahydro - 6,9 - methano - 2,4,3 - benzodioxathiepin-3-oxide

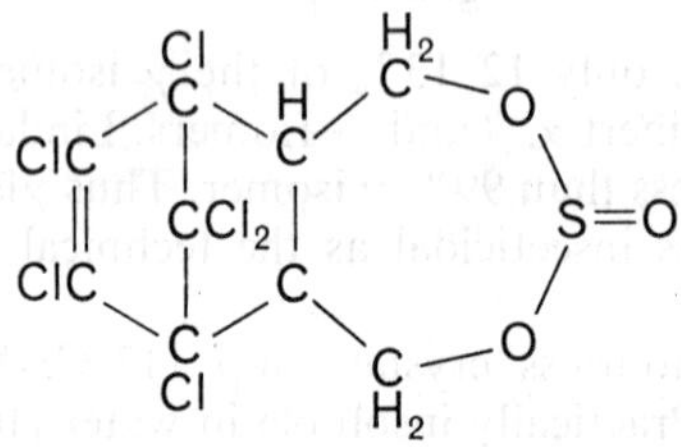

Fig. 23.4 Endosulfan

Endosulfan is a mixture of two isomers, one of m.p. 108°–109°C, the other of m.p. 206°–208°C. Both are insecticidal and technical endosulfan contains up to 90% of the two. This is a brownish crystalline solid of m.p. 70°–100°C and no measurable vapour pressure at 75°C, but it has been found in laboratory and field to be less persistent than dieldrin. Practically insoluble in water but moderately soluble in organic solvents. Acute oral LD50 to white rats about 50 mg./kg. but no evidence of high chronic or cumulative toxicity.

A persistent and powerful contact and stomach poison taking 72 hours to give complete mortality of *Glossina*. Very toxic to fish but claimed to be selective in favour of some predatory insects and bees.

Formulations. Emulsifiable concentrates (20%), dust (3%), 20–35% solutions in High Aromatic solvents.

5. ISOBENZAN (Telodrin) Octachlorotetrahydromethanophthalan

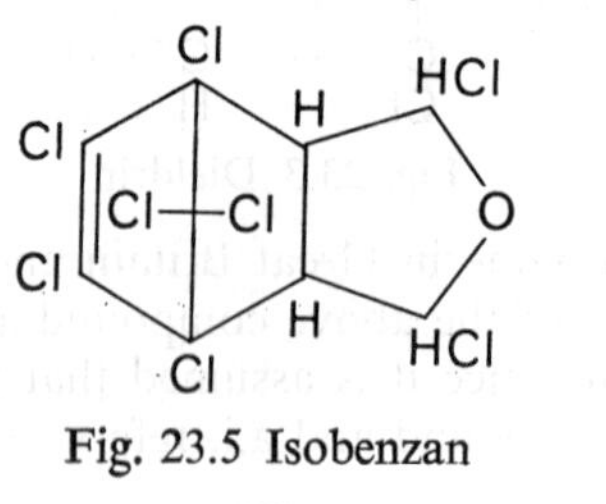

Fig. 23.5 Isobenzan

White solid, m.p. 122°–123°C more volatile than dieldrin but less than aldrin or BHC. Insoluble in water, slightly soluble in kerosene and ethanol. Soluble in acetone, benzene, toluene; decomposed by alkali.

A highly potent moderately persistent contact and stomach poison. Acute oral LD50 to white rats 8·7 mg./kg. High dermal toxicity.

Formulations. Emulsion concentrate (15%), granules (2% and 5%), dust (1·5%). 10% solution to special order.

6. BROMOCYCLEN (bromodan)

7. CHLORBICYCLEN (allodan)

These are chemically related to endosulfan and are of very low mammalian toxicity. They have been used for controlling ectoparasites of stock and might be considered by any worker considering using bait cattle. They are both solids, soluble in the usual organic solvents.

Organophosphates

FENTHION (Baytex, Lebaycid)

O,0,-dimethyl-*O*-4-(methylmercapto)-3-methylphenyl phosphorothioate

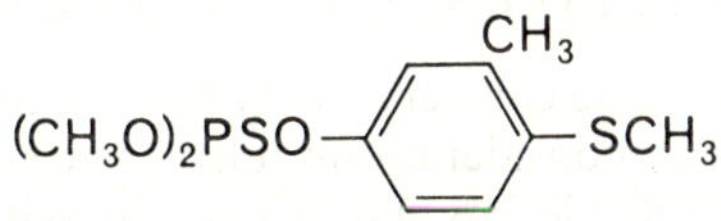

Fig. 23.6 Fenthion

Pure fenthion is a colourless liquid, b.p. 87°C *in vacuo* v.p. 3 × 10^{-5} mm. Hg. at 20°C. The technical compound is a brownish liquid with a weak garlic smell, of 95–98% purity, b.p. 105°C (*in vacuo*) v.p. 2·15 × 10^{-6} mm. Hg. at 20°C, density 1·250. Practically insoluble in water (54–56 mg./l.), soluble in most organic solvents. Stable at 210°C, resistant to light and alkalis. Oxidation products highly toxic to both insects and mammals. Takes 72 hours to complete kill of tsetse flies. Acute LD50 for white rats 190–310 mg./kg., low dermal toxicity. More toxic to birds.

Formulations. Emulsion concentrates. Technical compound (95% pure) has been used experimentally for tsetse control.

N-methyl carbamates

ARPROCARB (Bayer 39007)

2 isopropoxy-phenyl-N-methylcarbamate

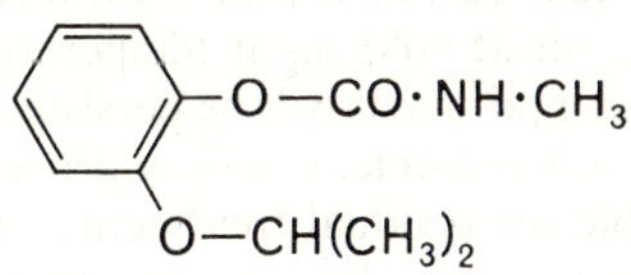

Fig. 23.7 Arprocarb

A white crystalline powder, practically odourless, m.p. 91·5°C v.p. 10^{-2} Torr at 120°C. Soluble in alcohols, about 1% in water. Unstable in highly alkaline media. Insecticide of rapid knockdown. Acute LD50 to white rats 100 mg./kg., low dermal toxicity.

Formulations. 50% wettable powder, 20% emulsion concentrate, granules.

Pyrethrum

A mixture of four esters of chrysanthemum monocarboxylic and dicarboxylic acids with pyrethrolone (pyrethrins I and II) and cinerolone (cinerins I and II), extracted from the flower heads of *Chrysanthemum cineraefolium* as solutions. The esters are unstable to alkali, sunlight and oxygen. Powerful contact insecticides with very rapid knockdown. Relatively harmless to warm blooded animals.

FORMULATIONS. Concentrated extract in oil of *c.* 25%. Kerosene solutions. Aerosols. Much used for mosquito and fly sprays in which synergists are incorporated. These enhance the insecticidal effect and greatly cheapen the product. However, Burnett (1961–3) found that the most commonly used synergist, piperonyl butoxide, did not enhance the lethal action of pyrethrum on *G. morsitans*.

FORMULATION OF INSECTICIDES

The crude technical insecticide can very rarely be used in the form in which it is produced. Apart from other considerations, it has to be extended to an enormous extent in order to contact its victims and this is achieved by dilution either with liquids, with air, or with both in succession. All insecticides so far used against tsetse, except fenthion, are solids. For aerosol production these are best used as solutions, preferably in the cheapest solvent available that has adequate characteristics. For pyrethrum applied by hand sprayers in a de-flying chamber kerosene is adequate but for dissemination in the bush the selection of a correct solvent and concentration depends on the machine and method to be used and requires advice from experts. The literature records recipes used in various successful trials and these should not be varied without expert knowledge. In practice, the choice is confined to common industrial solvents and mineral oils and it is rarely worth while to import special solvents. If the recommended solvent is not available, technical experts employed by local refineries can often give advice on which of their products approximates most closely to the specified liquid and may be prepared to dissolve the insecticide in it, a worthwhile advantage even for plain solutions. The alternative is to purchase equipment and hire staff. The manipulation of fairly toxic chemicals and inflammable liquids which may have to be heated is always hazardous and is best left to experts with the proper equipment. Care must be taken that solutions are not so concentrated that crystals will separate out at cold night temperatures. Should this happen, dosages will be lowered and equipment will be persistently clogged. The redissolving of the crystals, even if it is possible, is a slow process.

Solutions are not suitable for residual treatments and for this purpose emulsions or suspensions of wettable powders are used (these in turn are not suitable for use as aerosols). Emulsions are prepared from emulsion concentrates (frequently abbreviated to e.c.) in which the insecticide is in concentrated solution in an appropriate solvent; toluene or solvent naphtha is frequently used for organochlorines. Suspensions are prepared from wettable (or dispersible) powders (w.p.) for which finely milled solid insecticide is used, often with inert diluent. In both, various surface-acting agents are incorporated whose function is to facilitate the formation and preservation of the emulsion or suspension; stabilizers and stickers may also be added. Formulation of efficient emulsion concentrates and wettable powders is a highly skilled procedure and special machinery is required to prepare wettable powders to meet the WHO specification for suspensibility, etc. Formulation can have a great effect on the lethality and persistence of an insecticide deposit and those designed for the control of agricultural pests or mosquitoes may not be the best for tsetse control. The market for specialized anti-tsetse insecticides is not large enough to make it worth the while of manufacturers to undertake special investigations on the preparation of suitable formulations. The most realistic approach is to try out available preparations and select those which give the best performance. However, the major companies are prepared to apply their current knowledge to the modification of standard preparations. When dieldrin was first used on a large scale for anti-tsetse spraying it was used as a 15% e.c. diluted to give a 5% emulsion. This is far stronger than the normal agricultural spray for which the preparation was designed and the high final concentration of surface-active agents sometimes caused the emulsion to invert, the dispersed oil phase becoming continuous and the water phase dispersed as drops. The inverted emulsion was very thick and jammed the spraying equipment. The company concerned quickly produced a special e.c. with a lower concentration of wetters and this is available, denoted by the suffix 'T', for anti-tsetse spraying.

Wettable powders usually contain 25–75% of active ingredient and emulsions 10–25%, although endosulfan has been marketed at 35%. Care must be taken that when concentration is quoted in pounds per gallon that Imperial (British) or American gallons are specified. Percentages may be quoted as weight/weight or weight/volume, the former giving the lower figure in most cases. The latter is very convenient in the British system in which one gallon of water weighs ten pounds. Thus a nominal 15% w/v e.c. contains 1·5 lb. to the Imperial gallon and dilutions to give required rates of application per acre are readily made.

Most formulations, especially emulsion concentrates, deteriorate with storage in tropical conditions and a few months exposure in metal drums to hot sun may cause the separation of tenacious gummy sludges, or greatly reduce the stability of emulsions or suspensions. Either effect will cause difficulties in use; old stocks of insecticide should be tested before use. When diluting before use clean water should, of course, be used; some waters draining from volcanic soils may contain sufficient ions to reduce the stability of the diluted preparation.

CHOICE OF INSECTICIDE AND FORMULATION

The selection of an insecticide for any particular operation depends on a number of factors of which two, effectiveness and cost (including cost of application), are of prime importance. Effectiveness is partly a matter of formulation, but certain insecticides will always be unsuitable for residual applications because they are too volatile or decompose under the action of sunlight, etc. Thus, for residual application, the choice is restricted to DDT, dieldrin and possibly endosulfan. Should tsetse become resistant to these chlorinated hydrocarbons, fenthion and arprocarb would appear to be the only likely substitutes but neither has been assessed for this purpose. For application as aerosols, DDT, dieldrin, endosulfan, γBHC and isobenzan are all available. Their selection for particular operations will be discussed in the appropriate section but it may be noted here that for aerosol production the relative toxicities from laboratory tests provide a good indication of effectiveness. If from this the relative cost per lethal dose is calculated there is a good basis for comparison. This term can be obtained by the following formula:

$$\text{relative cost per lethal dose of A} = \text{price per unit weight of A} \times \frac{\text{LD50 of A}}{\text{LD50 of B}}$$

where B is the most lethal compound considered and its LD50 and price are both taken as unity. The price per unit weight should be the cost of the appropriate amount of formulation that contains one unit of a.i.

With some insecticides, mortality increases more rapidly as the dose is increased than is the case with others, i.e. the regression lines of mortality on dosage are not parallel. In this case no statistically correct comparison can be made but, for practical purposes, comparison of the values of 95% mortality is more realistic than at 50% mortality. The only compound in use for which this comparison is needed is fenthion.

With residual applications, the ratio of lethal doses is not such a good guide and in any case the information is not available for most species. The choice is very restricted, the data on endosulfan being too inconclusive and scanty to be of much assistance. It is not possible to forecast the performance of a compound in the field from laboratory data alone; dieldrin has been found in practice to kill much more persistently than DDT at the same rate of application (at least where the climate is not extremely dry) although their vapour pressures are very similar. Dieldrin was first assessed in the field (Burnett, Robinson & Le Roux, 1957) by comparing its effect with that of DDT in the same locality for the same cash expenditure on formulated insecticide. It was found to be more persistent and therefore more economical because fewer applications were needed. These observations were made in Kenya where DDT is effective only if used as an emulsion and not a suspension. In Nigeria, MacLennan and Kirkby (1958) found that the much cheaper DDT suspension was effective in the Sudan savanna zone and the more expensive dieldrin was not used. Further south in areas of higher rainfall and less severe dry season, Kernaghan (1961) found that DDT suspensions were ineffective and emulsions had to be used. In these circumstances dieldrin emulsions were competitive and were used successfully by J. B. Davies (1961).

Attempts have been made to control tsetse by the application of insecticides to the external surfaces of bait cattle. So far, only DDT has been used for this purpose but only limited success has been achieved and the method has not been widely used. Dieldrin and isobenzan are too toxic for use on animals while endosulfan is probably too volatile and may also be too toxic. Two little-used compounds, bromocyclen and chlorbicyclen, have very low toxicity for mammals but are highly lethal for tsetse so that they would appear to offer alternatives to DDT for application to bait cattle.

Of the insecticides available for tsetse control, only BHC is marketed in a form designed for application by chemically generated smokes (smoke generators).

SAFETY PRECAUTIONS

Toxic hazards to man and to other animals are not often considered when choosing insecticides for tsetse control. The hazards involved in their use depend largely on the precautions taken in handling them and, for this reason, these will be described in some detail. The LD50 for white rats has been given above for each compound but this serves only as a rough guide to the risks involved; some highly toxic compounds have been extensively used without serious effect.

Concentrates are especially hazardous and should only be handled by persons wearing rubber or plastic gloves and boots, and some sort of impervious apron. Contaminated clothing should be removed at once and the skin beneath washed. Soap and water should always be at hand and drums should be handled in an isolated area, preferably with a hard surface, from which all unprotected people, especially those with bare feet, are excluded. Containers should be frequently checked for leaks and never brought into the same vehicle or store as food stuffs. Drainage from contaminated areas must be rigidly excluded from water and food supplies, rivers and pools. Powders are safer than liquid preparations but when handling either form, even when diluted, the hands should be protected and eating and smoking prohibited. Solutions and emulsion concentrates are commonly highly inflammable.

Of the compounds listed above (pp. 478–482) only iobenzan is highly toxic and it will usually be used in concentrated oil solution. Men handling open containers of this compound should wear, in addition to the protective clothing already recommended, an eyeshield, a mask to cover nose and mouth and an apron to cover the whole front of the body. Transfer of liquids should be done by a pump and as soon as filling is complete any excess liquid should be returned to store. Connecting pipes should be flushed out with kerosene and emptied into a deep soakage pit or burnt.

Contamination with diluted concentrates should also be avoided although it is not so dangerous. Knapsack containers should be taken off for recharging and wiped to remove spilt spraying liquid. Leaking equipment should be repaired or replaced and clothes changed regularly—at once if they are contaminated. DDT has a good safety record but dieldrin is more dangerous and requires greater care in handling than DDT. Endosulfan is probably safer than dieldrin, despite its higher acute toxicity because it does not accumulate in the body fats. All of these insecticides are fish poisons and operatives sometimes deliberately spray streams to obtain fish; this practice should be discouraged.

When movable markers are used in connection with aerial spraying the aircraft may emit while passing over the men carrying them. Contamination can be minimized by starting to spray at the downwind edge of the block, or better still, by locating the beacons a hundred yards or more outside the area actually treated.

RESISTANCE OF TSETSE TO INSECTICIDES

It is well known that insect populations exposed to repeated applications of an insecticide are liable to develop resistant to that insecticide. The explanation for this occurrence is generally believed to be that pre-existing inherited resistance factors in the insect population enable a small proportion to survive and multiply and so replace the susceptible bulk of the population.

Glossina has not yet been shown to acquire resistance to insecticides but it would be extraordinary if it proved to be incapable of doing so. It must be remembered, however, that no thorough pre- and post-treatment studies have so far been made on *Glossina*, presumably because no convenient method has been available. In principle, no campaign to eliminate an insect of importance by the use of insecticides should be initiated without first determining the susceptibility of the insect to the insecticide used as, in the case of failure, it is only in this way that it is possible to ascertain whether or not resistance to the insecticide has been acquired.

A suitable method for this purpose must be simple, sensitive, convenient and capable of yielding reproducible results. It should also bear some relation to the method of control used in the field. The two procedures at present available are described below (pp. 487–488).

In respect of resistance, modern synthetic insecticides fall into three groups, namely, the DDT group, the BHC-cyclodiene group and the organophosphate-carbamate group. The members of each group show some degree of cross-resistance to other members of the same group but not to members of another group.

The acquisition of resistance to insecticides is promoted by (a) the occurrence in the insect population of 'resistant' genes, (b) high but not complete mortalities among populations following the application of the insecticides, (c) repeated applications of the same insecticide or of one belonging to the same resistance group, and (d) repeated attacks on successive generations of the insect.

From consideration of these four factors as they apply to *Glossina* it would appear that this genus might develop resistance but this is likely to be very rare. The low density of *Glossina* populations is unfavourable to the development of resistance since the smaller the numbers the smaller will be the pool of resistant genes. If, for example, resistant genes were present at the high rate of one insect in every thousand, that these occupied a square mile and they they were reduced by 99·9% following the application of insecticide, only a single resistant fly would remain in a large area. Unless this happened to be a pregnant female it is unlikely that it would be able to reproduce. By contrast, 100,000 mosquitoes might emerge from a single pool in one day and if reduced by 99·9% would leave 100 survivors concentrated in a small area.

In the example given above it would not appear that high but incomplete mortality would be favourable to the development of resistance by *Glossina* although something approaching 100% mortality must be assumed in order to account for the permanent collapse of tsetse populations under attack by insecticides. In several reclamation schemes it has been found necessary to re-treat the same area during a second season and success has been achieved even when the same insecticide, or one of the same resistance group, has been used. The extension of a control scheme over a period of years does not usually involve the exposure of the same tsetse population to repeated treatments as the area of attack is constantly changed and in any one place only one or two generations are exposed to insecticide.

METHODS FOR DETERMINING SUSCEPTIBILITY LEVELS

In determining levels of susceptibility to insecticides, topical application is unsuitable for field use and in most cases it will be preferable to use a method which depends on the insect settling on insecticide deposits. The method described by Kernaghan and Johnston (1962) was developed for testing surfaces with dry deposits following spraying in field operations but is equally applicable to deposits prepared in the laboratory. The WHO method (*see* below) utilizes deposits in the form of filter papers soaked in solutions of insecticides in a graded series of concentrations. Riordan (1966) has tested both methods, using the WHO papers cut up for use in the Kernaghan and Johnston apparatus. With the WHO kit and exposures of 60 minutes, and the other method with exposures of 90 seconds, Riordan found the Kernaghan and Johnston method more convenient in practice. The results obtained by these two methods (expressed as the LC50) differ but, provided the same method is aways used, this is of no consequence.

The WHO method utilizes a standard kit supplied by the Vector Control and Biology Unit, Division of Environmental Health, WHO, Geneva. It consists of plastic tubes about 5 cm. in diameter by 10 cm. long. One end is covered with plastic gauze, the other with a sliding cap in which there is a hole large enough for insects to be introduced. The tubes are lined, except for the ends, with filter paper impregnated with insecticide in involatile oil. The flies, five to twelve per tube (but preferably constant in number) are either introduced direct or *via* a clean holding tube which fits onto the end of the exposure tube. Direct introduction minimizes handling of the flies and does not affect the result. After exposure the flies are removed and kept for 24 hours unless control flies, similarly exposed to oiled paper without insecticide, suffer mortalities in excess of about 25% in which event mortalities must be assessed earlier. The experimental mortalities must be corrected for control deaths by Abbott's correction:

$$\text{Corrected mortality } \% = \frac{\text{experimental mortality} - \text{control mortality}}{100 - \text{control mortality}}$$

The results are plotted on log/probit paper and the LC50 read off.

Post-treatment tests may be simplified and economy in insects effected by testing only at the lowest concentration found to give complete mortality with the original insects. More than 5% survival at this dose indicates that acquired resistance may be present.

The Kernaghan and Johnston method exposes individual flies to insecticide in 3 inch × 1 inch specimen tubes. A cork piston is prepared which fits loosely into the tube but which can be held securely in position by passing the stem of the piston through a second cork which fits tightly into the end of the tube. A disc, slightly smaller than the face of the piston, is cut from the surface treated with insecticide and is affixed to the piston face with vaseline in such a way as to ensure that it does not touch and contaminate the walls of the tube. A single fly is then placed in a separate specimen tube which is allowed to stand upright until the fly recovers from the disturbance of handling. The stopper is then removed and a prepared piston is inserted and pushed down to about ½ inch from the botton where it is held in position by the tightly-fitting second cork. The tube containing fly and piston is then inverted so that the fly will settle on the treated disc which now faces upwards. After 90 seconds the tube is again inverted, the piston withdrawn and the tube closed with a gauze cap. The piston with attached disc may then be used for another tubed fly.

Riordan (1966) used five flies per WHO tube and has recorded the following figures for one-day old, unfed *G. fuscipes*. His results may be compared with those of Challier (1963a) which are given in Table 23.2.

Insecticide	*Method*	*Exp. time*	*Sex*	*LC50 %*
DDT	WHO	60 min	F	1·7
	K & J	90 sec	F	6·9
	K & J	90 sec	M	9·0
Dieldrin	WHO	60 min	F	0·18
	K & J	90 sec	F	0·55
	K & J	90 sec	M	0·81

Twenty-four hour mortalities will not be complete with slow-acting compounds such as dieldrin and endosulfan. It is therefore necessary to standardize the procedure as much as possible to obtain consistent results. The physiological state of the insects is also important (*see* above) and the use of males only will at least reduce the inaccuracies due to pregnant insects.

With species that die rapidly in captivity the use of highly concentrated solutions on the test papers and short retention times may give approximate results that would otherwise be unobtainable, but no high degree of accuracy can be expected.

In all tests to determine susceptibility levels great care is needed to exclude contamination of equipment by insecticides; this is much more likely to occur in the tropics than in temperate conditions. Decontamination is difficult to achieve and it is wiser to discard contaminated equipment. Benches, etc., should be well scrubbed with coarse soap and water or painted over. Solvents are sometimes used for cleaning but they tend to spread rather than remove contamination.

EFFECTS OF INSECTICIDES ON OTHER ANIMALS

Few observations have been made on the unwanted side effects of insecticides. The unusual sensitivity of tsetse to insecticides, their well defined habitats and the need for economy have combined to produce some selective and economical methods of control. Residual applications must affect not only other insects but also spiders and lizards though it is unlikely that their habitat preferences will be identical with those of tsetse. Bees are known to escape from aircraft treatments because they are still in their hives when emission takes place. Wooff (1965) kept a careful watch for dead birds, etc., while applying selective residual treatment to large areas but found no evidence of undue mortality. The highly selective type of application is unlikely to give general or mobile predators an opportunity to ingest significant amounts of insecticide in their food although buck have been suspected of picking up a lethal dose from consuming sprayed leaves of shrubs; there was reason to suspect that the species concerned is unusually susceptible as other species in the same area escaped harm. The deliberate poisoning of fish by spraymen has already been mentioned. It is not to be expected that the disappearance of such a relatively rare species as *Glossina* from the fauna will have many direct effects, except on the transmission of disease but Fiedler, Du Toit and Kluge (1954) found that parasites of tsetse pupae were rapidly reduced within eight months of the start of spraying and within another nine months had disappeared completely. This might be explained by the decline in host density apart from direct action on the parasites and may help to account for the persistence of very small residual population of the host, once freed from the controlling effect of its parasites.

Chapter 24

Control by Insecticides (continued): Residual Deposits, Aerial and Ground Application, Pyrethrum Aerosols

G. F. BURNETT

RESIDUAL DEPOSITS ON RESTING SITES

The most firmly established of all methods of insecticide control of tsetse is the application of residual deposits to some part of the insect's habitat. This technique was first used against *G. fuscipes* and a few years later against the closely related *G. palpalis* and *G. tachinoides*. In the places where this was done, the habitats of these species are essentially linear and restricted. The extension of the method to the wider-ranging savanna species awaited detailed information on their resting sites and dry season refuges. The details of application depend very much on the species and the circumstances in which it lives but the principle is the same in all cases, namely, to apply a relatively heavy, and therefore persistent, deposit to selected parts of the fly's habitat. No attempt is made to spray all the places which the fly may visit but only to make a sufficiently high proportion of them lethal. All suitable substrates in a limited part of the habitat may be treated or only a selection of them. If the species moves regularly between branches and leaves, as Jewell (1956) found with *G. swynnertoni*, it is unnecessary to treat both types of resting sites. In this case the branches would be selected for treatment since their total area is smaller and they are not subject to dehiscence. If the fly retreats to dry season refuges then only specified resting sites within these refuges need be treated; if it does not, other methods may be preferable unless it shows preferences for very well-defined and limited sites within a diffuse habitat.

The appropriate resting sites must remain lethal for a sufficiently long period to allow the last pupa that was in the ground at the start of the operation to produce its adult; if the kill has been complete this is sufficient. Residual deposits usually lose effect slowly so that there is a considerable safety margin in the life of the deposit after it is no longer completely effective and this is doubtless capable of eliminating the offspring of any flies that escape shortly after the initial treatment. In fact modern techniques requiring only a single application are very effective at the start and apparently give a complete kill if properly applied. If the initial treatment is not sufficiently persistent it must be repeated until the lethal period exceeds the duration of the pupal period, as was the case in the early use of DDT on Lake Victoria (Woodcock, 1949; Wilson, 1953). Although repeated applications may be necessary in some circumstances, single treatment schedules are now normal practice in most countries.

Available information on current practice is summarized in Table 24.1. The appropriate insecticide and formulation depends on climate. Where the dry season is very prolonged and harsh, DDT wettable powders are adequate. Under less extreme climatic conditions, DDT e.c. may be adequate but dieldrin e.c. is more persistent and reliable and, unless a single treatment with DDT is sufficient, cheaper. No other insecticides have been used on a field scale. Endosulfan may prove to be an alternative to dieldrin but according to Baldry (1964a) isobenzan is inferior.

The early field dosages and schedules originated from semi-laboratory trials designed to measure persistence in the field. The schedules given in Table 24.1 were based on results obtained in actual extermination schemes which, in turn, were based on a previous schedule modified in the light of experience. Wilson (1953), in Kenya, published the first results and his procedure was modified in Nigeria over a period of seven years (H. Davies, 1964) using progressively lighter dosage and more discriminative spraying. This technique was adequate

TABLE 24.1

Satisfactory usage for residual application for tsetse control (from various authors)

Country	Insecticide	Formulation	No. applications	*Glossina* spp.
Nigeria				
N. Sudan				
Savanna	DDT	2·5% susp.	1	*submorsitans*
Zone		5% susp.	1–3 (for barriers)	*tachinoides*
	dieldrin	4% emuls.	1 (annually for barriers)	*palpalis*
Guinea	dieldrin	2% emuls.	1	*tachinoides*
Savanna Zone	DDT	5% emuls.	1	*palpalis*
Cameroon/ Chad	dieldrin	1·8% susp.	1	*palpalis*
Rep. Centr-africaine	dieldrin	1·8% emuls.	1	*fuscipes*
Mali	dieldrin	2% emuls.	1	*palpalis*
		4% emuls.	1 (barriers)	*palpalis*
Kenya	dieldrin	4·6–5% emuls.	1	*fuscipes*
		1·8% emuls.	3–4 4–6 week interval	*pallidipes*
	DDT	5·0% emuls.	4 4 weeks interval (near houses)	*fuscipes*
Tanzania	dieldrin	3% emuls.	1 (2)	*fuscipes martinii* *morsitans* *pallidipes*
	endosulfan	3% emuls.	1 (experimental)	*swynnertoni*
Uganda	dieldrin	3% emuls.	1	*morsitans*
		5% emuls.	1	*palpalis*
Zambia	DDT	5% susp.	1	*morsitans*
	dieldrin	2·9% emuls.	1	*pallidipes* *fuscipes*
Rhodesia	DDT	5% susp.	1	*morsitans*
	dieldrin	3·1% emuls.	1	*pallidipes*

in the Sudan savanna zone of Northern Nigeria. It is possible that progressive reduction in insecticide application proved to be satisfactory because each trial took place in increasingly arid zones and that the treatment finally adopted would not be entirely adequate in less arid areas. In the Southern Guinea savanna where rainfall is higher and the dry season shorter, wettable powders are ineffective but 5% DDT emulsion can be used. A more expensive but more reliable substitute, in that it has a greater persistence, is 2% dieldrin emulsion. Where the Nigerian techniques have been adopted by neighbouring countries, dieldrin has been preferred. In Kenya and Uganda, near Lake Victoria where there is no true dry season, four applications of 5% DDT are required and a better and cheaper alternative is to apply dieldrin emulsion once at 5% a.i., or three or four times at 1·8% a.i. In the drier parts of the east and central African plateau where the dry season is almost rainless but not excessively harsh, a single spray of 3% dieldrin emulsion is the standard control method for all species of *Glossina*, including the three important savanna species. In the harsher conditions of the Zambesi Valley, DDT suspension is effective.

There are some data on the factors affecting the persistence of deposits, although formulation may be as important as any other. Treated foliage may fall and be replaced by clean leaves, especially at the end of the dry season; emulsions may cause leaves to fall and in such cases a reduction in concentration may be tried. Insecticide may be absorbed on bark but normal application rates allow for this. Coarse sprays, giving heavy deposits locally, are more persistent than fine ones and a higher proportion of the insecticide reaches its target. A number of bioassay studies and a few chemical assessments have been made in an attempt to assess loss of deposits. Burnett, Robinson and Le Roux (1957), in Kenya, found that, on leaves, DDT from an emulsion lost some 60% of its original 0·3 gm./m.^{2} in five days and with it most of its lethality. Dieldrin at 0·1 gm./m.^{2} and 0·45 gm./m.^{2} fell by 60% in about fifty days but the heavier deposit remained highly lethal for at least eight weeks. Hocking (1961), in Uganda, reported that, on bark, an initial deposit from 3% dieldrin emulsion lost some 60% of its original 0·80 gm./m.^{2} in twenty-three days and 90% in four months but was still lethal. In Rhodesia, dieldrin deposits on bark lost 50% of their weight in one month (Cockbill, 1964, p. 210). In West Africa, Riordan (1966) found DDT much more persistent on leaves while Baldry (1964a) found dieldrin slightly less persistent. Wooff (1965) has shown that bush fires render dieldrin ineffective, presumably because it is volatilized. Baldry (1963) has produced evidence that, in the dry season, dust may render deposits temporarily harmless but they are restored by heavy rain; 5% DDT w.p. gave some mortality even twelve months after application.

In field practice, the recommended treatment is applied, and its effects assessed, on the basis of information obtained by field surveys. If no tsetse are discovered immediately after the effect of the treatment is expected to be complete—that is after one pupal period—search is intensified in all parts of the treated area in an attempt to find any isolated survivors or immigrant flies. If these are found, a limited second application is usually made in the places where they were discovered. Flies may not be present in detectable numbers until after the next favourable breeding season when the residual tsetse population will have had an opportunity to increase. The locality of stray captures may indicate that they are probably immigrants and action can be taken on this assumption. On occasions, permanent occupation of quite atypical habitats has been revealed. Glover (1963) found *G. fuscipes* in the upper reaches of tributary streams almost bare of woody vegetation, and also a pocket of flies in an area of forest which had escaped attention during the monthly surveys which were continued for two years after spraying. In general, as experience is gained, and also as the area under control is enlarged, the need for repeated treatments diminishes.

Many workers have commented on the spectacular decline in tsetse numbers as soon as insecticide is applied. It is likely to be characteristic of insecticide treatments in general that, where the decline is less than spectacular, the final effect may be unsatisfactory and repeated applications may be needed to achieve success.

Equipment Required for Residual Treatments

Different models of machines have been used by different workers but the reasons for the choice made in each case is not always clear. They can, however, be classified according to types. There is only one report of the use of a large motor-borne machine, an orchard sprayer, designed to give high outputs at pressures over 400 p.s.i., the details of which are given by Gledhill and Caughey (1963). The sprayer is mounted on a four-wheel-drive tractor together with a 180 gal. insecticide tank which is agitated both by fluid return and by two chain driven paddles and which can therefore be used for suspensions of wettable powder. The pump supplies two trigger-operated lances through reinforced hoses. Output can be varied from a very fine spray to a solid jet, the maximum being 5 and 7 pints per minute with disc orifices of 1·5 and 2 mm., respectively; the throw at these outputs is 15 yards in still air but normally only 10 yards of this is employed. The spraymen sit in two swivel seats with footbars fitted on extensions to either side of the rear of the tractor loading platform, each having a backward facing arc of 220° for spraying. Their eyes are about 7 feet above ground and they spray up to this level. The tractor moves at 2–4 m.p.h. and operators treat all trunks and branches of larger trees, or evergreen foliage, according to the species to be controlled and the type of habitat. They treat only that part visible to them—about $\frac{1}{2}$–$\frac{2}{3}$ of the circumference of suitable boles. Expenditure of spray liquid is 35–90 gallons per linear mile, depending on the character of the vegetation. It is used extensively for large scale treatment of level, open dry woodland in which *G. morsitans* and *G. pallidipes* have well-defined dry season retreats. One unit will normally treat 2–5 miles of 'linear habitat' with a single tankful and this can be repeated three times in one day. The use of this machine requires rather elaborate preparations. The area must be carefully surveyed to delimit the parts to be treated, supplies must be deposited in the bush and a supervisor must precede the spraying tractor to ensure that treatment is complete.

All other treatments have been carried out with one-man portable machines of which three types are available, namely, pressure knapsack sprayers, hand-operated knapsack sprayers and portable mist-blowers. These have all been designed for the agricultural sprayer market. The main difference between the first two types is in the way pressure is applied to the spray fluid; both have a container of 1–3 gallons carried on the back by a harness. In the pressure-sprayer, the container is robust and can be made airtight. Air is forced in, to a predetermined pressure, which falls as the liquid is used. In some models air is retained within the container, which is recharged by pumping in spray fluid. Usually a hand pump is incorporated in the container but an external motor pump may be used. When pumps are used, a vehicle is required to transport them and this precludes their use in difficult country. The hand-operated knapsack machines have a diaphragm or a piston pump which is operated by leisurely movements of the left hand. Pressure is equalized to some extent by an air pressure accumulator cylinder and since the container is not airtight it can be of plastic or some other lightweight and cheap material. Spray is discharged through a lance about 30 inches long to which extensions may sometimes be added, and thence from a nozzle. A curved 'swan-neck' between the lance-tip and the nozzle is useful for treating the undersides of low overhanging branches, logs and rocks. Some form of flow control permitting rapid starting and stopping of spraying is necessary and for this purpose pistol-grip controls are probably most convenient. Nozzles are of two types and with some machines there is a choice. The commonest is the swirl plate or hollow cone type. As its name implies, the spray issues in a hollow cone and is deposited in a ringlike pattern on a target. It is inherently uneven and as it is moved over a target the deposit is concentrated at the sides of the sprayed strip, and if the target is narrower than the swath most of the spray misses and is wasted. This is particularly likely in spraying tree trunks. Short-range spraying in an attempt to rectify this is awkward and leads to losses from rebound. The other type of nozzle, the fan nozzle, should give a narrow strip of sprayed surface with equal density except at the edge where it falls off to zero. Unfortunately the pattern is usually irregular but at least it is not inherently bad and the worst specimens among a set of nozzles can be discarded by observing their pattern when spraying. It may be worth measuring throughputs under standard conditions as a routine, when startling variations may be found. Discarding the nozzles giving unusually low or high throughputs will probably get rid of those with the worst patterns as well as assisting regularity of output. All nozzzles, even those of stainless steel and ceramics wear rapidly, especially if suspensions are used. They should be tested from time to time and discarded if throughputs have risen to 20% above normal because the spray pattern will have deteriorated. Aperture plates and fan nozzles of bore about 1/32–3/64 inches will give throughputs of 1·5–2 g.p.m. at 60 p.s.i. and are suitable for most spraying. Too large a throughput leads to hurried and inaccurate spraying. The included angle of the spray cone or fan should not exceed 60°.

Changes in liquid pressure cause variations in throughput, droplet size and spray momentum. A minimum pressure of about 20 p.s.i. is needed to produce a good spray pattern but high pressures produce too many small drops that fall out before reaching the target. Ideally, a constant pressure device should be fitted but, if it is not, pressure should not be raised too high or permitted to fall too low; a range of 30–60 p.s.i. should be maintained.

Filters are sometimes fitted behind nozzles but they cause trouble and should be removed; all liquid should be filtered before pouring into the tank and all foreign matter rigidly excluded. Even so, wettable powders may sediment out and clog the narrow passages of diaphragm pumps.

Lances are sometimes lined with plastic tubing which may deteriorate when exposed to the concentrated emulsions used in tsetse control work, sometimes to such an extent as to occlude the bore; it is essential to wash the tubes thoroughly after use each day and leave them filled with water. Rubber pump diaphragms and washers deteriorate rapidly in contact with strong emulsions under pressure and plastic is preferable. Plastic piping is very vulnerable to thorns, especially in thickets, and needs protection with PVC insulating tape or a similar material.

The knapsack mistblower incorporates a small petrol motor to drive a fan which directs a blast of air down a tube about 4 inches in diameter; the tube can be directed where required. Insecticide as solution, emulsion or suspension is directed into the airblast from a small aperture, shattered by the airflow and carried by it as a spray until it deposits on a surface or falls out as the airblast loses momentum. The spray pattern can only be found by trial but it is usually fairly even and concentrated. The carry may be up to 15 feet and the airblast type of machine is useful for penetrating thickets but has also been used extensively and satisfactorily for tree trunks. It should be possible to cut off the liquid flow easily and quickly to avoid wastage. A serious fault of most models is that the liquid is fed in by gravity and output falls off rapidly as the airblast tube is raised above waist height. A certain amount of liquid is sucked out by the rush of air but delivery and deposit rates may fall by threequarters or more without the operator realizing this. If spraying must be carried out above horizontal, the machine must be fitted with a pump capable of giving a pressure of at least 2 p.s.i. Some manufacturers claim that their 'pressurized' tanks (fed by air bled from the fan housing) provide a positive feed and do not need a liquid pump in the delivery line but all those investigated have been found to produce only negligible pressure and are quite worthless; a liquid line pump is essential for the type of spraying described. Another common weakness is the cock that meters liquid output. Plastic cocks are unsatisfactory as the ports are frequently occluded by fins of material, the drillings may become distorted by pressure or the solvents used in emulsions may cause them to swell.

Choice of knapsack equipment depends on a number of factors that vary in importance according to conditions of work. Lightness may be important in one situation and robustness in another. At least one worker has found that the less powerful of two motorized models was preferable, being lighter and more economical to run. High throughput is not necessarily advantageous as, if the operator is unable to move rapidly, material will be wasted. Simplicity, reliability and robustness appear to be the principal factors affecting the choice of sprayer.

Motorized machines cost about £50–£80 each (in Europe) and hand-operated sprayers approximately £7–£20 each. Motorized mistblowers are useful for penetrating thickets and work fastest for this sort of broadcast treatment. Hand-operated sprayers are lightest and pressure sprayers probably give the best results with unpractised operators. Spare parts and the tools to fit them should be available to all spraygangs in the field.

In Tanzania, a sprayer training centre is operated. All grades of officers of the Tsetse Control Department are required to attend a seven-week course of instruction in servicing, repair and use of all types of spraying equipment. Such a centre is to be recommended to all countries contemplating large-scale tsetse control by insecticides.

Field Operations

The insecticides and rates of application which have been used in various countries are briefly summarized in Table 24.1. The amount of insecticide required varies widely since it depends on the proportion of the total tsetse habitat which is actually treated. The concentration of the spraying fluid used and the amount applied to unit surface also varies though to a lesser extent. Spraying is usually continued until the fluid is about to run down the treated surface. These factors vary greatly in almost all published accounts of field operations so that no routine procedure of general application can be laid down. Some examples of the procedures which have been followed in different localities may serve as a useful guide and will be grouped as 'linear' or 'diffuse' according to the nature of the habitat treated.

Linear Habitats

Linear habitats may be occupied permanently (*G. palpalis, G. fuscipes, G. tachinoides*) or only as dry season refuges (*G. morsitans, G. pallidipes*). *G. tachinoides* is more difficult to eliminate than other species occurring in linear habitats. Some of these habitats, although linear, may have a width of up to ten miles in places.

(1) Nigeria: North Sudan savanna region.

Species: *G. tachinoides* and *G.m. submorsitans*

Treatment: 2·5 % DDT (w.p.) applied to all tree trunks over 9 inches in diameter, to bases of branches (any size) overhanging water, to under-surface of roots projecting from eroded banks and to stems of *Mimosa* along slashed paths. Applications restricted to fringing riverine vegetation, forest islands and some larger thickets. Leaves not sprayed. Where *G.m. submorsitans* is absent or very scarce spraying is restricted to 2 feet above ground level. In the more southerly, moister areas the denser vegetation forming the boundaries of flood plains is also sprayed (H. Davies, 1964).

(2) Nigeria: North Guinea savanna zone.

Species: *G. palpalis, G. tachinoides* and *G.m. submorsitans*

Treatment: For Sudan savanna woodland and complex situations round small lakes comprising swamp woodland, swamp forest, riparian forest and riparian woodland. Against species other than *G.m. submorsitans* spraying with 3·75 % DDT (w.p.) later 2·5 %, to height of 2·5 feet on stems, trunks and exposed roots throughout riparian forest and margins of swamp forest.

G.m. submorsitans only withdrew to riparian forest and woodland at the height of the dry season and against this species spraying was applied, to a height of 5 feet, to shaded tree trunks over 9 inches diameter or, where stands were dense in riparian woodland and forest, to trunks of 5 inches diameter and over. Resprayed to include tree trunks over 5 inches, and branches over 3 inches in diameter up to a height of 12 feet. Persistent tsetse populations in limited areas were eliminated with 3·75 % dieldrin emulsion (MacLennan & Aitchison, 1963).

(3) Nigeria: Southern Guinea savanna zone.

Species: *G. palpalis*

Treatment: Application to leaves and tree trunks throughout riverine vegetation to a height of 4 feet using 4% dieldrin (11·7 gallons of 18% concentrate used per linear mile; J. B. Davies, 1961), to fringing vegetation from stream bed up to 4·5 feet from water with 2% dieldrin, one bank only of small streams (Mahood, 1961). Spraying to a height of only 1 foot above ground level may be sufficient (McDonald, 1961).

(4) Kenya

Species: *G. fuscipes*

Treatment: Insecticide sprayed on riverine vegetation from boat in stream bed or from either side of paths cut as closely as possible to each bank. Where the forest is wider, spray is applied from paths cut at 60 yard intervals. Stems and leaves sprayed to a height of 8 feet (less in more open parts). In 1951, four applications of DDT (Wilson, 1953); in 1956, three applications of 1·8% dieldrin (Glover *et al.*, 1960); in 1960, a single application of 4·6% dieldrin (Glover, 1963). The last method has also been used in Uganda.

(5) Zambia and Rhodesia

Species: *G. morsitans* and *G. pallidipes*

Treatment: In dry deciduous woodland when tsetse are confined by the dry season to lines of thicketed riverine forest, including some evergreen thicket. Only one side of trunks and branches of larger trees, and evergreen foliage, is treated to 7 feet. Either hand sprayers or orchard sprayers are used, details above in section on equipment where use of the latter machine is described. From 1·5 to over 8 linear miles of refuge habitat treated per square mile of woodland. One application of 5% DDT as w.p., or of 2·9% dieldrin emulsion where climate is less harsh (Gledhill & Caughey, 1963; J. A. Gledhill, personal communication).

(6) Tanzania

Species: *G. pallidipes*

Treatment: Insecticide, 3% dieldrin emulsion applied to riverine thicket up to 8 feet on either side of dry river bed using mist blowers. Where thicket is wide the outer edge is also treated. Consumption 3 gallons of 18% e.c. per linear mile (Chadwick *et al.*, 1964).

Diffused Habitats

Where tsetse habitats are diffused treatment is applied to all parts but deposits are concentrated in all, or a proportion, of a particular type of resting site known to be especially favoured by the species which it is desired to eliminate.

(1) Uganda

Species: *G. morsitans* (in open acacia woodland)

Treatment: Application of 3% dieldrin spray to trunks of all trees (except *Acacia hockii*) less than 6 feet in height and to undersides of branches up to a height of 12 feet; to one side only if small trees, to two sides if somewhat larger and to three sides of trees with large boles such as *Euphorbia*. In addition, thickets are lightly sprayed. Operators work in teams of up to 100 with an interval of 25 yards between them. Consumption 40 gallons of 18% e.c. per square mile (Wooff, 1965).

(2) Tanzania

Species: *G. swynnertoni* (in sparse open bush).

Treatment: Insecticide, 3% dieldrin sprayed on undersides of branches having a diameter of 1–4 inches and inclined at less than 35° from the horizontal; spray applied at a height of 4–9 feet above ground level. Consumption 11·1 gallons of 18% e.c. per square mile. (Chadwick *et al.*, 1964).

(3) Kenya

Species: *G. fuscipes* in areas of dense human population where it has invaded peri-domestic vegetation, e.g. overgrown *Euphorbia tirucalli* hedges forming thickets.

Treatment: 4 sprays, at 28-day intervals, of vegetation to height of 8 feet with 5% DDT emulsion. Applied to both sides of undelineated spray lanes made at intervals of 50 yards in dense thicket, or 100 yards in open thicket cultivation (J. G. Le Roux, personal communication).

(4) Kenya

Species: *G. pallidipes* (in evergreen thicket).

Treatment: Application of 1·8% dieldrin, on four occasions, to stems and leaves up to a height of 5 feet. Spraying is done from parallel paths cut through the thicket at intervals of 200 yards. In thickly wooded parts the whole of the outside of the thicket is also treated but in lightly wooded parts it is sufficient to treat 40 yards out of every 100 yards of the perimeter. Consumption 70 gallons of 18% e.c. per square mile (Thompson, Glover & Trump, 1961).

In more recent operations in dense thicket the interval between lanes has been reduced to 50 yards or a grid of 100–200 yards used. Pneumatic or mistblower knapsack sprayers used. (J. G. Le Roux, personal communication).

It is unfortunate that more recent information is not available on controlling the important *G. pallidipes* with residual insecticides. The costs of the last trial could have been reduced considerably by using one treatment of 5% dieldrin. White (1963) reports a large scale trial using the method later successfully applied by Chadwick *et al.* (above), treating only the thicket peripheries, in a large area. The intention was to penetrate the thickets if the limited treatment did not succeed. The first effect was highly successful but heavy rain and floods then made it impossible to determine whether the continued absence of *G. pallidipes* was due to extermination by insecticides or to drowning. It can only be concluded that the method is promising enough to be attempted elsewhere.

Residual Treatments Combined with Other Methods

Residual treatments are sometimes used without intending to achieve complete extermination as, for example, to arrest trypanosomiasis epidemics, to protect specific sites or to permit settlement. It is possible in this way to reduce preliminary surveys and to avoid the need to cut barriers, thereby effecting economies. Kernaghan (1962) reports a rapid method of halting sleeping sickness transmission by *G. palpalis*. Both 5% DDT and 4% dieldrin were used; the dieldrin was more expensive but gave better results against much denser fly. Farrell (1961) arrested an advance of *G. morsitans* in Rhodesia, giving time for a barrier clearing to be cut; 3·6% dieldrin emulsion was applied to parallel swaths 5 to 10 yards wide and 40 yards apart covering an area of 3,000 acres of riverine fringe. This type of application is regular practice in Tanzania (D. Turner, personal communication) where it is expected that planned settlement will complete the elimination of tsetse. The method is also used to halt sleeping sickness outbreaks. Standard procedure is to treat tree trunks over 4 inch diameter and the underside of branches up to 12 feet on parallel swaths 50 yards apart. Trees within 3 yards of each trace are treated, and insides of termitaria thickets. This is done once at a cost of about £150 per square mile, for *G. morsitans* and *G. swynnertoni*. If *G. pallidipes* is also present the edges of thickets between 2 and 10 feet from the ground are also treated. Very promising results have been obtained against *G. austeni* by spraying into thickets with mistblowers along traces 30 yards apart. Cattle grazed in coconut plantations surrounded by thicket or forest have been protected by applying dieldrin every six months to the forest perimeter, to both sides of approach roads and along the fly-round path lying 10 yards inside the forest edge. The species concerned are *G. austeni*, *G. pallidipes* and *G. brevipalpis*.

Chemical Barriers

The use of heavy residual deposits to create a barrier against invasion of reclaimed areas by tsetse has been successful in a number of cases although the width of barrier necessary to prevent reinfestation remains in doubt. Dieldrin is normally used for barriers, usually as 3% or 5% emulsion, even when the cheaper DDT is used for extensive extermination in the same area. The chemical barrier is particularly useful in preventing reinfestation of areas won by insecticidal treatments pending their extension during the next operational season. For this purpose repeated sprayings at intervals of several months may be necessary but, in Nigeria, 4% dieldrin applied to vegetation along 2·3 miles of river bank excluded *G. palpalis* for a year (J. B. Davies, 1961) and *G. tachinoides* for at least 6·5 months (Templeton, 1965). Mahood (1961) excluded *G. tachinoides* from a watershed by treating the headwaters of small streams for about 0·5 mile downstream with 3% dieldrin at 4 to 6 week intervals, for less than one third of the cost of a physical barrier. Glover, Le Roux and Parker (1960) controlled, but did not completely prevent, incursions from a very heavy concentration of *G. fuscipes* across a barrier of riverine vegetation just over one mile long, by spraying with 5% dieldrin emulsion at intervals of three months. Three mile barriers treated monthly with 1·8% dieldrin were effective. In Kenya, *G. fuscipes* and *G. pallidipes* were excluded for eighteen months by a barrier, two miles deep and eight long, maintained by spraying 5% DDT at monthly intervals along lanes 100 yards apart (J. G. Le Roux, personal communication).

Against *G. morsitans* in open woodland, Wooff (1965) records the creation of a completely successful barrier zone, half a mile wide, along the river Katonga. Dieldrin as 3% emulsion was used at 192 gallons per square mile but in denser vegetation this rose to 330 gallons. The barrier treated by Farrell (described in the previous section) was efficient for at least 6·5 months. Although it is known that insecticide barriers have been used in a number of east and central African countries to restrain the movements of populations of savanna species of *Glossina*, very little has been published. In some cases the edges of cleared barriers of inadequate width are treated with insecticide in order to kill those flies which succeed in crossing it. One may assume that insecticide barriers need not be as wide as cleared barriers because, in the latter case, the fly must complete the crossing in one movement or perish. The sprayed barrier, on the other hand, is indistinguishable from the normal habitat so that the fly can settle repeatedly, move in ambits and linger in the treated zone until it picks up a lethal dose. If the barrier is narrower than the extent of an ambit, or if it is broken by treeless drainage lines or pans used by game, then flies may be expected to cross it.

Use of Bait Animals

Bait animals made lethal by treatment with an insecticide may be classed as traps. The principle is exactly the same as the 'catching-out' method used by Symes and Vane (1937) to control *G. palpalis*. This was remarkably successful in small blocks of forest and although baits have not been used against this species they have been tried against the three savanna species, *G. pallidipes*, *G. morsitans* and *G. swynnertoni*.

The first tests with DDT applied to cattle appear to be those of Vanderplank (1947a) who found that all of the thirteen species and forms of *Glossina* investigated were susceptible when applied to deposits on hides. The lethal effect persisted for months in the laboratory but tests in the field using treated oxen showed that the lethal effect persisted for only five days. Using this method, Whiteside (1949) reduced *G. pallidipes* to low levels and Burnett (1954) nearly succeeded in exterminating *G. morsitans* and *G. swynnertoni*.

Both Whiteside and Burnett used DDT emulsions, of 11% and 10% respectively, expending 110–165 c.c. per head. Not all of this was retained on the animals many of which were small. In both cases the cattle had to be sprayed twice a week, which was inconveniently frequent. Burnett found that as the season advanced and the grass grew it not only hid the bait from view but rapidly removed DDT from their bellies and flanks. Both authors found that an insufficient proportion of fly were contacting the cattle, which were herded at 68 per square mile (Whiteside) and 104 per square mile (Burnett); densities of this order are possible only in the rainy season because of lack of forage in the dry season. The cattle, even at these densities, could not compete as tsetse hosts with the game animals permanently available and, in addition, they were brought in too late and taken out too early each day. The numbers of game were either underestimated or the preference of tsetse for small game, especially pig, was greater than expected. There was the added difficulty of ensuring that the cattle were divided up into numerous small herds and kept widely dispersed. Du Toit (1954) had used cattle dipped in DDT at 0·15% p-p′ in an attempt to halt transmission of trypanosomiasis by *G. pallidipes* but this measure was purely ancillary to the main control effort and was carried out only in the dispersal area of the fly; such dilute preparations would have a negligible effect in the true habitat.

There have been no further published results since these experiments although it is believed that the method has been attempted elsewhere, presumably without success. Two prerequisites for the success of this method are more persistent insecticides (or formulations) and better competition with natural hosts. The latter is a matter of organization and may prove to be too expensive. Better formulations may not be easy to devise as a balance must be struck between resistance to attrition and availability of insecticide to the fly. Much of the insecticide is lost by absorption through the animal's skin. Of alternative insecticides, dieldrin, isobenzan and probably endosulfan are too toxic to cattle but bromocyclen and chlorbicyclen are not. BHC is too volatile. Wilson (1948) showed that BHC when fed to cattle made their blood lethal to *Glossina* for several weeks, but the effective and lethal doses were too close for practical application. In recent years systemic compounds, mainly organophosphates have been used with success to kill warble fly larvae (*Hypoderma* spp.) inside cattle. Their use against tsetse might be considered; they have the additional advantage that the meat of the bait animal would not be unsafe for human consumption.

Insecticide-treated Traps and Screens

Morris (1950) attempted to improve the efficiency of box traps by soaking the covering with insecticide on the assumption that many tsetse settling on the outside of the traps would be killed. While this is no doubt true, the method will have little value unless traps can be devised which will attract virtually all the tsetse in their vicinity to settle on them.

Treatment of Pupation Sites

Parr (unpublished) tested the effect of DDT applied to the soil where pupae were buried, but found it had no effect on emerging flies; it is now known that some soils absorb insecticides and render them unavailable. This procedure is distinct from the treatment of logs, branches, rocks, etc., on which females settle in preparation for larviposition and where insecticide is likely to be particularly persistent; the treatment of these along with other favoured resting sites is likely to be useful.

AERIAL APPLICATION OF INSECTICIDES

The use of aircraft for the application of insecticide against tsetse was first tried out by Steyn (1949) on an island in Lake Victoria using a home-made DDT-impregnated dust; this trial was unsuccessful. In the same year, Du Toit (1954) used a 5% solution of DDT in furnace oil dispersed through venturi atomizers. This is stated to have given satisfactory results but it was soon replaced by a 16% DDT solution in diesel oil and toluene, dispersed as a mist generated by injection of the solution into the aircraft exhaust; later, the cheaper 4% γBHC in diesel oil was used. The change to aerosol mist was made because visible traces persisted long enough to facilitate applications on subsequent runs, a distinct advantage over invisible sprays. No physico-chemical assessments were reported but in the light of subsequent experience elsewhere the aerosol certainly penetrated forest and impacted on tsetse more efficiently than the spray. Du Toit later effected economies by using commercially operated light aircraft (Piper Cruisers) in place of medium military aircraft (Ansons). He was also the first to use helicopters successfully for this purpose.

The development in South Africa of aerial applications, combined with other measures, was essentially pragmatic and although highly successful in South Africa the method developed there has not always succeeded elsewhere. In East Africa, the Colonial Insecticide Research Unit (CIRU), later re-designated the Tropical Pesticide Research Institute (TPRI), undertook work on a smaller scale but with a great many attendant physico-chemical and biological assessments, the results of which have been published in a series of some fifteen scientific papers. At first, Anson aircraft of the type discarded in South Africa were used but later (1958) light aircraft were introduced and over the next five years the cost of the method was drastically reduced and its reliability progressively increased. The essential features of the technique ultimately evolved, ultra-low-volume application, may be summarized as follows:

1. Concentrated solutions of insecticides in involatile oils are used.
2. These are dispensed as medium aerosols with as many droplets as possible having diameters in the range 20–50 microns.
3. Insecticides must be highly toxic to *Glossina*. Only dieldrin, isobenzan, and endosulfan meet this requirement, although fenthion is worth investigating because of its high toxicity to pregnant females.
4. Volume dosages per application are of the order 0·012 to 0·025 gallons per acre and of active ingredient 0·2 to 0·5 oz. (6–14 g.) per acre (15–35 g./ha.).
5. The whole area to be treated is covered by successive parallel flights alternately from opposite directions. Swath widths are 50 to 70 yards. The aircraft flies as close as possible to the tops of the trees. There is only a nominal overlap of the areas treated on successive days.
6. Meterological conditions normally restrict treatment to very early morning and late evening.
7. Treatments over any given area ('block') of woodland are repeated at approximately equal intervals up to seven times (eight have been planned but never completed). Experience will probably permit reduction in the number of

treatments. In East Africa the inter-treatment interval is standardized at three weeks.

8. Light but not very light aircraft are the most economical and flexible in operation.

Aerosol Characteristics

The correct droplet size is fundamental to the success of aerosol application. Droplets are characterized by their diameters in microns (1,000 microns (μ) = 1 mm.) and an aerosol is characterized by the range in size of the droplets it contains and by a variety of parameters based on droplet size. Volume median diameter (v.m.d.) is commonly used, that is, the size of droplet at the point where half the liquid is in drops smaller and half larger than the v.m.d. The whole range of data, the drop spectrum, which gives the proportion of droplets in each size range, is the only adequate means of expressing the characteristics of an aerosol but has to be presented in graphic or tabular form. The size range covered by the median 50% of the liquid volume of the cloud (ignoring the very large and very small drops) is a more convenient measure. Except in the laboratory, only very mixed spectra can be produced but the range of sizes is much greater with some methods of dispersion than others.

Each size of droplet has its own characteristics and is most efficiently filtered out of the air by objects of one particular size. Drops of over 50 μ fall rapidly, drift little and are readily removed by twigs and leaves. Smaller droplets remain airborne longer (a drop of 33 μ takes 280 seconds to fall 30 feet) and may be carried in any direction by slow and mildly turbulent air currents. Droplets less than 10 μ in diameter will fail to make contact with an object the size of a tsetse fly.

With droplets in the selected size range of 20–50 μ only the most potent insecticides will carry a lethal dose in a single drop. The diameters of droplets containing the LD95 of 10% and 20% solutions of some common insecticides are given in Table 24.2. Cheap involatile 20% solutions are not available for DDT, γBHC or isobenzan. The only insecticides in which the LD95 is contained in droplets within the preferred size range are dieldrin, endosulfan and isobenzan but in the case of pregnant females none satisfies this requirement. The importance of a single droplet being lethal for a tsetse fly has not been measured but it appears likely that, in protected situations, this would be advantageous. If equal volumes of 10% DDT solution and 20% dieldrin solution are applied as 50 μ drops a young tsetse will receive a LD95 from only one drop of dieldrin as compared with sixteen drops of DDT. In addition, because the volume of a drop varies as the cube root of the diameter, a given volume of solution, when atomized, produces eight times as many 50 μ as 100 μ drops. This gives equal coverage at one eighth the volume expended while each of the smaller droplets has a better chance of reaching the desired target. The introduction of aerosols carrying a lethal dose per drop of 50 μ or less has coincided with noteworthy increases in the efficiency of field applications of insecticides which users have attributed to this characteristic, but there is no direct evidence to support this contention.

TABLE 24.2

Diameter of drops, in microns, containing the LD95 for 10% and 20% solutions of insecticides applied to* Glossina morsitans *(calculated from data in Burnett, 1961–3)

	Males		Pregnant Females	
	10%	20%	10%	20%
DDT (Tech.)	126	100	262	208
γ BHC	69	55	145	115
dieldrin	50	40	100	80
endosulfan	45	36	78	62
isobenzan	34	27	71	56

Insecticides used

Successful extermination of tsetse has been attained with DDT, γBHC, dieldrin, isobenzan and endosulfan sprayed from aircraft. It is not possible to claim that any one of these insecticides is superior to any other. The relative cost (1964) per lethal dose for the formulations which were used successfully was about 5, 7·3, 1·4, 1·2 and 1, respectively; if other factors were equal these insecticides could be used at reciprocal dosage ratios for the same expenditure on toxicant and possibly equal effect. In fact, with DDT and BHC the volume of spray would be increased to such an extent that higher flying costs would outweigh any advantage gained from using high dosages of cheap materials (*see* examples tabulated below). A theoretical addition to the list is fenthion; the relative cost per lethal dose of the technical compound used experimentally is 4·9 for young flies and only 0·54 for pregnant females but it is not yet known what application rates would be needed in practice.

Involatile solvents are required because, with aerosols, any volatile liquid evaporates and reduces the size of the droplet or even converts it to dust, most of which will drift away and be ineffective.

The volume dosage per acre has been determined empirically and depends on the amount of active ingredient required and its solubility in a common cheap solvent. The following formulations have been successfully used at the rates indicated.

Insecticide	Concentration	Solvent	gal./acre	g.a.i./acre
Dieldrin	1·23 lb/gal.	18% e.c. diluted with diesel oil	0·0254	14
	2·0 lb/gal.	High Aromatic Naphtha	0·0156	14
Isobenzan	1·0 lb/gal.	Naphtha	0·0124	6
Endosulfan	2·0 lb/gal.	Naphtha	0·0121	11
DDT	1·1 lb/gal.	Kerosene/diesel oil	0·25	78

The first dieldrin formulation was extemporized to make use of available stocks of emulsion concentrate. This contained volatile solvent and, as dispersed, the actual volume of liquid in the aerosol cloud was certainly less, probably much less, than 0·0254 g.p.a. The second formulation was used before thermal aerosol equipment was available, and dispersal within the aerosol range of drop sizes was obtained by diluting sevenfold with volatile kerosene. After atomization this volatilized and gave the volume quoted as a rather coarse aerosol.

Flying Procedure

When treating an area of woodland, the aircraft must pass over it on parallel runs at regularly spaced intervals, each of which is referred to as a 'swath width'. In practice, this has varied from 25 to 88 yards and in successful field operations from 25 to 70 yards; the wider the swath the cheaper the operation. Limits are set by the regularity of coverage required and the maximum emission rate of the disseminating equipment; the emission rate to obtain a desired mean application rate varies directly as the swath width and the aircraft speed. The aircraft flies at the minimum safe height above the tree canopy and the aerosol cloud drifts with any wind there may be, both before and after passing the canopy, but it is still necessary for the pilot to have a clear indication of the course he must follow. Runs may be several miles in length so that it may be difficult to ensure complete coverage. No difficulty is experienced when markers can be placed at each end of the run so that both are visible to the pilot as he approaches. For longer runs the pilot must fly over a marker placed at the near end of the run and then continue on a compass course. It has been found, in practice, that this can be done with remarkable accuracy and a mean error of only 25 yards has been achieved on a four-mile run. After making several sorties the pilot may be guided by the recognition of local landmarks but this has the disadvantage that his attention is divided between instruments and physical features while flying low over trees.

For short runs reliance can be placed on a single line of beacons along one edge of the block of woodland to be treated, with the machine spraying while flying in one direction only. When the spray run exceeds a mile it is much more economical to spray from alternate directions. This requires that the beacons on each side should be accurately aligned and this may be difficult if accurate maps and surveying equipment are not available. It will be found that a few careful dummy runs by the aircraft on a calm day will give a reasonably good alignment which will improve as the pilot becomes familiar with the run.

A mobile marking party, preferably in touch by radio-telephone, gives close control of the operation and is particularly useful for experimental work or when operators are inexperienced. Such parties can correct errors, check meteorological conditions, ensure that the performance of disseminating equipment is satisfactory and prevent confusion of beacons by the pilot.

It is preferable to have two such parties, one on each side of the block, but both need not be elaborately equipped. The actual beacons used must be portable and should be made from reflecting or otherwise conspicuous material mounted on poles. A disc painted white on one side and black on the other appears to flicker when spun round and thus attracts attention. Markers are more readily visible if not placed too close to the edge of the bush.

When it is possible to run a vehicle along the marker line, other methods may be used. Very early in the morning a signalling lamp, such as the British Aldis lamp, can be seen for miles, even through branches and it is helpful to the pilot if it can be directed towards the aircraft as he starts his run. Vehicle headlights are not suitable for this purpose as they cannot be directed towards the aircraft. As daylight strengthens the usual sort of board or cloth banner can be used or a pale-coloured vehicle may be sufficient. Of greater use is a beacon that will rise above the trees. Hydrogen-filled balloons have been tried but they are difficult to control and are liable to be punctured by twigs. Chemical smoke generators and signal pistol smoke cartridges are useful but expensive; the former give the pilot valuable information on winds and consequent drift to be expected. The best type of marker operated from a vehicle has proved to be smoke ejected from its exhaust. For example, a 30 foot vertical exhaust extension has been fitted to a Land Rover and diesel oil injected into it at 5 p.s.i. pressure generated by a pressure knapsack sprayer tank. The injection point was a nozzle drilled to 0·014 inch inserted in the exhaust manifold. Opening and shutting of the throttle gave a series of puffs that were more conspicuous than a continuous plume. This was visible from at least three miles and was turned on at the pilot's radioed request. Care must be taken to turn off the diesel oil before the vehicle engine to prevent the latter being flooded with oil.

Fixed beacons are an alternative to mobile ones when access is difficult and particularly when a number of discrete blocks, for example, dry season refuges, have to be treated. For such an area, at least two parties would be required for each marker line to avoid the long delays occasioned by parties traversing the often difficult country between blocks. Because repeated applications are required it may be worthwhile to fix permanent markers but as material has to be transported they may cost as much as a mobile party. Beacons must be robust and firmly attached (they must not be made of material, such as cloth, that is of local marketable value). Buyckx (1965) used flat or corrugated reflective material with the run number painted on the panels in large black Roman numerals; these were mounted on trees, or, preferably, on 30 m. eucalyptus poles. When this was done the distant beacon was visible before the aircraft passed the nearer one thus avoiding the need to use a compass. It was found to be unnecessary to mark each run. Experience elsewhere suggests that it is sufficient to mark every third or fifth swath.

For long runs a combination of methods can be employed with advantage, e.g. a run may be started on a compass course and completed when the distant beacon comes into view; the use of an exhaust smoke signal should make accurate tracking over 8–10 miles possible and thereby overcome the principal drawback to the ultra-low-volume method which is the invisibility of the aerosol cloud. The principal reason why Du Toit abandoned spray gear for exhaust smoke was the ease with which aircraft making return runs could keep station on the smoke trail they had already produced. By this means he completely eliminated marking parties. This facility was particularly important when he used helicopters in terrain in which it was very difficult to use mobile markers or to fix beacons; in these situations good coverage depended on the pilot's experience.

Flights into the rising or setting sun should be avoided at all costs. This is more important than having the prevailing wind on the beam (*see* next section). Apart from this, the shape of the spray block is the main consideration. Long runs are efficient in that less time is wasted on non-productive turns, but very long runs are difficult to control and they provide a wide front for reinvasion by fly between treatments on consecutive days, or if spraying is interrupted. If an area can be covered by an aircraft in one day's work the longest practicable run should be used but if it takes several days it is better to fly more or less at right angles to its long axis. Miller and Chadwick (1963) give an excellent account of marking from the pilot's point of view.[1]

Meteorology

The aerosol droplet is small and light and its movement is influenced more by air currents than by gravity. Even the coarse aerosols used in early work on dispersion rarely gave recoveries of over 60% at ground level in open country although collected over a swath of several hundred yards. With the ultra-low-volume method, meterological conditions are particularly important since effectiveness depends on small droplets being kept airborne by slight air currents. The time taken for a droplet to fall a given distance varies inversely as the square of the diameter. A 100 μ droplet of unit density, which might contain an LD95 of 20% DDT (Table 24.2) would fall a probable five feet from aircraft to canopy in 5 seconds and in doing so would drift 5 yards in a 2 m.p.h. wind. Under comparable conditions, a 36 μ droplet containing an LD95 of 20% endosulfan would take 39 seconds and drift 39 yards—more than half a swath width. At canopy level wind speed falls drastically, commonly to about 20% (Thompson, 1953) but if the canopy is 30 feet high, the 100 μ drop will reach the ground in 31 seconds (drifting 6 yards) and the 36 μ will drop in 230 seconds (drifting 46 yards). These figures demonstrate the great influence of atmospheric conditions on the performance of the aerosol cloud.

Airflow over the ground is of two types, laminar and turbulent. In laminar flow each layer of air moves smoothly over the next, more or less parallel to solid surfaces such as the ground or vegetation canopy. The boundary layer next to the surface is stationary but airspeed increases with increasing distance from the surface. In truly laminar flow, particles of solid or liquid fall through the air at their terminal velocities, merely drifting downwind. In turbulent flow, eddies develop that mix the layers of air and in them the vertical component of the air movement may exceed that in the forward direction and also the terminal velocity of small particles, which are whirled into the upper layers and may be carried away. Turbulence is promoted by surface roughness, windspeed over a few miles per hour and thermal convection currents that transport air masses across the lines of the laminar flow. It is marked by gusty winds. Its obverse,

[1] Recent developments using the Decca Navigation system, suggest that this device should be capable of satisfying all requirements and its use should be investigated without delay. [*See* Joyce *et al.* (1968), *Agric. Aviation*, **10,** 118.]

stability, occurs in conditions of laminar flow, in dead calm or particularly in inversions, when the air at some height above the ground is warmer than that at ground level. In these conditions, any parcel of air that tends to rise, sinks back again as it enters levels where the air density is lower than its own. This is well demonstrated on calm evenings or mornings when the smoke of fires, or a dust cloud, spreads in long horizontal drifts beneath the inversion level. The condition is promoted by clear skies that permit loss of heat by radiation from the ground and consequent cooling of the adjacent layer of air until they are colder than the layer above. This condition may be so stable that, as the aircraft passes overhead, a downdraft of warm air is felt but this is at once displaced by the return flow of cold air from the sides.

Atmospheric circulation below the canopy is independent of that above but is generated by winds above, and thermal currents beneath that cause a turnover of air between ground and treetops (Thompson, 1953). The problem is to get the aerosol below canopy level without unacceptable losses and it is this process that has limiting meteorological factors. A moderate amount of drift is an advantage provided conditions are not turbulent. Burnett and Thompson (1956) found that, in conditions of intense inversion and dead calm, kills may be locally very high but tend to be patchy. Clearings may actually reduce kills in surrounding bush by acting as sumps, and the effective swath width is reduced. As the sun rises it warms the tops of the trees and the tree tops warm the air around them, starting thermal circulation that will destroy the inversion. If winds are high these will do the same by mechanical mixing, and inversions are only found after calm intervals without intense insolation—that is just before dusk to just after dawn. Aerosols are probably most effective when air is slightly to moderately stable and the wind is about 2 m.p.h. Such conditions persist only for short periods, most reliably after dawn, and operations should start as early as the light permits and carry on through the decay of the inversion until increasing roughness warns the pilot to finish. The pilot of a light aircraft is very sensitive to turbulence as he passes low over the trees and may detect it in part of the block far from any ground observer; with a little experience he will be the best judge of when treatment should stop. With an unclouded sun on dry ground this may happen in almost calm conditions; under overcast the wind may rise to a mean 8 m.p.h. before work has to stop. If the wind is gusty a stop will have to be made at lower mean speeds. A smoky fire may give some guidance and is also useful to show wind direction to the pilot.

Favourable meteorological conditions persist, in East Africa, for only about 90 minutes after dawn although sometimes for as long as 150 minutes. For about 45 minutes before darkness a suitable but less reliable period may occur but considerable seasonal and local variation is found. Wet soil delays the destruction of an inversion by a hot sun.

The limited amount of suitable flying time available may appear to represent poor aircraft utilization. However, it has been possible to cover over 5 square miles per day with one aircraft when weather is favourable and, when it is not, no form of aerial application should be contemplated. This coverage represents about 2½ hours exacting flying per day which is as much as any pilot can be expected to carry out without risk, and may be compared with commercial agricultural spraying of 110 acres per day. If it were feasible to increase aircraft utilization it would be necessary to employ additional pilots.

Because of the considerable drift of the aerosol, even very light winds tend to close gaps in coverage. It is rarely worth orientating the direction of run to the prevailing wind because when conditions are optimal for the use of aerosols winds tend to be light and very variable and there is no prevailing wind at this time. However, if operations start or finish at the edge of a block, with the wind blowing in the wrong direction, the edge may be underdosed. As this area may be a feeding zone for tsetse it is important to rectify underdosage and this should be done by making an extra run or two upwind of the woodland edge, preferably below the height of its canopy.

In many localities where high winds occur in daylight much of the late night is calm and to take advantage of this Burnett *et al.* (1964) carried out experimental spraying at night, at the full moon. Over flat country no particular difficulty was experienced; because of the deep inversion it was possible to fly much higher than in daylight without wasting insecticide. For routine operations carried out at night it would be necessary to use lights as swath markers and it would assist the pilot to have searchlights fitted to the aircraft; the landing lights are fixed at the wrong angle for work of this kind.

Vegetation

Evergreen rain forest is not amenable to aerial treatment but low dry forest containing a proportion of evergreen trees could probably be sprayed satisfactorily; semi-evergreen thickets have been successfully treated. Excessive canopy height has a diluting effect, the aerosol cloud being dispersed more thinly in the greater enclosed air space. When coarse aerosols were used it was found necessary to operate as much as possible in the leafless season, and the operational advantages of working in the dry season are so great that wet season treatments, which coincide with heavy leaf, should be avoided for this reason alone. The leafless season may not be long enough to cover the usual six to eight treatments but this does not seem to matter provided that some of the applications are made in leafless conditions; when adult populations are high the first three treatments appear to be most critical.

Number of Applications and Inter-treatment Intervals

When aerial treatments were first suggested it was realized that it would be necessary to repeat them at intervals in order to kill those flies that had emerged since the previous treatment. Ideally, if each treatment killed all adult tsetse and the interval between each was less than the interval needed for young females to deposit their first pupa, treatments need continue only until one pupal period, at prevailing temperatures, had passed since the first attack. Because 100% kills were considered very unlikely it was thought necessary to continue for a second pupal period to catch the offspring of those females that escaped the first application.

Eventually, the problem was re-examined by Burnett (1955) and by Yeo and Simpson (1960) by tracing theoretically the fate of the offspring of those females

TABLE 24.3

Theoretical relation between spraying interval and percentage mortality at 24°C. Percentage survival after different numbers of treatments each causing the postulated mean mortality. Inter-treatment interval 21 days

Number of treatments	Percentage Kill				
	95	90	80	70	60
1	39	42	48	55	61
2	14	17	22	30	38
3	1·7	3·7	8·5	14·5	22
4	0·66	1·6	4·4	8·6	14
5	0·20	0·62	1·99	4·6	8·8
6	0·026	0·18	0·84	2·3	5·3
7	0·002	0·04	0·37	1·33	3·4
8		0·006	0·17	0·73	2·12
9			0·07	0·36	1·30
10			0·02	0·17	0·77
11				0·06	0·45
12				0·02	0·26

(From Burnett, 1955)

that escaped death under various assumed levels of mean mortality, life cycle, numbers of applications and interval between them. This led to a reassessment of the assumptions on which current procedure was based. It was found that to obtain a given final reduction in numbers, mean mortality per application and the total number of applications were to a considerable extent interchangeable. Some representative figures are given in Tables 24.3 and 24.4. Yeo and Simpson, using an electronic computer, made a large number of calculations but they give the results for mortalities of 95% and 50% only; Burnett's less accurate figures for five mortality levels are given in illustration. Yeo and Simpson (*loc. cit.*) found that a four-week interval, equal to their postulated pupal period, was the most efficient inter-treatment interval (Table 24.4); this permits the maximum number of fly to emerge and become vulnerable. In much of east Africa, in the season, the interval in fact would be about four weeks. However, since Burnett (1961) has shown that pregnant tsetse are highly tolerant to insecticides, and since by the end of the fourth week 25% or more of the females present will be in this condition, the inter-treatment interval has been cut to three weeks in recent operations. This has been successful, but the exact duration is not critical.

The first experiment utilizing the ultra-low-volume method was designed to employ eight applications, this being based on previous experience with coarse aerosols. However, eight complete treatments have not yet been applied; seven have proved to be sufficient in all cases. It seems probable that this number can be further reduced; Hocking *et al.* (1966) may have eliminated *G. morsitans* and

TABLE 24.4

The effect of inter-treatment interval on the total reduction in population assuming 95% mortality at each application. The final populations expressed as a percentage of the original level after one to eight treatments

Interval in weeks	Number of applications 1	2	3	4	5	6	7	8
1	36·12	25·53	17·25	9·05	0·86	0·06	0·005	0·001
2	36·12	18·14	1·81	0·31	0·13	0·02	0·002	0·0004
3	36·12	10·75	1·30	0·41	0·11	0·02	0·004	0·001
4	36·12	5·07	0·96	0·14	0·03	0·004	0·001	0·0001
5	36·12	6·78	1·17	0·26	0·05	0·009	0·002	0·0003
6	36·12	9·71	2·10	0·50	0·11	0·03	0·006	0·001
⩾6	36·12	13·05	4·71	1·70	0·61	0·22	0·08	0·03

(From Yeo and Simpson, 1960)

G. swynnertoni with only four treatments but the outcome remains in doubt because immigration certainly took place. This result was certainly better than any ever attained with coarse aerosols and was probably due to much higher kills per application.

The total period covered by seven treatments at three-week intervals is slightly over four calendar months so that it is possible to avoid most of the leafy period.

Overlap

It is theoretically possible, when operations have stopped for the day, for tsetse to move from the area to be treated next day into the area already treated where they would be able to survive because the treatment has no residual effect. This appears particularly important where there is a long boundary between daily treatments and a slow rate of forward progress. Much attention was given to this problem in the early experiments conducted by the CIRU (*see* for example, Hocking *et al.*, 1953); much insecticide was expended in attempts to catch escapes by respraying considerable areas each day. Later, it was realized that the whole concept of overlap treatments stemmed from the mistaken attempt to obtain complete kill by each application. The problem was examined in the light of the calculations discussed above and it was found that it would always be better and cheaper not to overlap but to utilize the savings on insecticide and flying for an extra complete application. The earlier procedure is now obsolete but it is still customary to overlap by one swath only, in order to reduce any gap left between the coverage of two consecutive days, due to a reversal of wind direction during the interval or to poor tracking. The single swath overlap also provides an opportunity to line up the compass.

Equipment Required

The only type of equipment capable of producing the correct drop spectra from concentrated solutions is a thermal exhaust aerosol generator utilizing the aircraft engine exhaust. The equipment is simple, does not interfere with the handling of the aircraft and requires little modification to its structure; it must be approved by the relevant air registration and safety authority. The device as used by the TPRI and its development are described by Lee and Miller (1966); that used with success in South Africa on both fixed wing aircraft and helicopters is the same in all essential respects (Du Toit, 1954). Details will vary with the model of aircraft, its engine power and airspeed and with the physical characteristics of the insecticide solution. Here it is only possible to give the general characteristics of the system and the dimensions for the aircraft and formulation used which was 20% endosulfan in High Aromatic Naphtha. The aircraft was a Cessna 182E high wing monoplane with a 235 h.p. engine and twin exhausts to which extension tubes were fitted to carry the outlets outboard of the landing wheels. Insecticide solution was piped from a bellytank by a windmill-driven pump and delivered at 40 p.s.i. through a tube into the centre of the exhaust at a distance of 42 inches from the points of discharge. Delivery was regulated by a $\frac{1}{16}$th inch diameter orifice restrictor. The bore of the restrictor can be varied to give the required emission rate but it must be fitted in the pipe and not at the point of emission in the exhaust extension where it would become clogged by carbonized solution. Exhaust temperature at the injection point was 540°–570°C but fell at once to 340°–420°C during injection. Atomization is accomplished by the rush of hot gases past the nozzle tip. When delivered at 40 p.s.i. at 0·3 gallons per minute per nozzle with a true airspeed of 115 m.p.h., the drop spectrum showed 50% in the range 20–60 μ. Emission was regulated by a pressure release and control valve fitted on the delivery side of the pump and controlled by a gate valve manipulated by the pilot. This may be done by Bowden cable, solenoid or hydraulic line, the last being found most satisfactory. Other aircraft will give different results with these settings and since the whole economics of aerial treatment depend on the capabilities of the aircraft used, the subject will be treated when the type of aircraft is discussed.

It is possible to produce medium aerosols with other equipment if volatile solvents are included in the formulation and this was done before the ultra-low-volume technique was evolved. The concentrate was diluted seven-fold with power kerosene and, on dissemination, evaporation of the latter halved the droplet diameters to give a volume median diameter of 50–60 μ. This was rather high but was successful although relatively extravagant. The diluent is cheap but it reduces the effective load of the aircraft by seven eighths and, being bulky, is particularly extravagant when operating far from railhead (*see* Buyckx, 1965). The best equipment for producing this type of aerosol is the rotary cage such as the Micronair 100A because of its comparatively narrow droplet range. It should be set to give maximum revolutions at the desired flow rate; performance may be improved and large drops eliminated by lining it with four layers of glass fibre tissue. Not more than two cages are needed for the usual emission rates but it is inadvisable to use swath widths of more than 55 yards because of the coarseness of the aerosol produced.

Type of Aircraft

Only fixed wing aircraft are discussed in this section. Four main types of aircraft have been used for aerial treatments of tsetse fly—Anson I, Auster J5G, Cessna 182E and Piper Cruisers. The initial selection of aircraft type will be made on grounds of suitability for the type of operation and cost. Experience has shown that light aircraft are most suitable, being flexible in operation, able to use short bush airstrips and most economical to operate. The only medium aircraft in the four listed is the Anson. It carries 62% greater load than the Cessna but covers the ground no faster and requires a higher standard of facilities, two engines, a crew of two and resident service personnel. On the other hand, the lightest aircraft are no cheaper than the Cessna to operate, cover the ground more slowly and offer no savings in crew. Actual figures from the literature give the cost per flying hour (including pilot's salary) as £10·75 for the Auster (1959), £10 for the Cessna (1962) and £12·5 for the Pipers (1951–2). Efficiency, which may be expressed as area treated at unit cost, depends on available power on which depend useful load, airspeed and emission rate. This last is concerned because energy is required to shatter a liquid insecticide into drops and the specific requirement rises rapidly as the required drop size is reduced. The energy comes from the heat and the kinetic energy of the exhaust gases. Utilization of the heat is restricted by the instability of some insecticides at high temperatures and the kinetic energy of the exhaust varies with the cruising power of the engine. Thus low-powered engines can deal with only a limited emission rate to give a particular drop spectrum. Table 24.5 lists the rate of work experienced using the Anson, Auster and Cessna in actual practice, reduced to a common standard run-length of four miles. Only the Cessna was actually used for ultra-low-volume work but similar figures have been calculated from the known characteristics of the Auster. It has been assumed that the Auster will be able to fly faster than it did with two rotary cages and that its emission rate will be in the same proportion to that of the Cessna as the power of its engine, that is, 65%. This permits an emission rate high enough for the same 55-yard swath covered by the Cessna. The latter is capable of operating at higher emission rates and dealing with greater swath widths but the Auster is not.

With ultra-low-volume applications, deterioration in meteorological conditions invariably cuts short the application before the aircraft empties its tank and it is the rate of work per hour that determines the most economical aircraft to use, provided the costs of operating it are not too high relative to the others. All these aircraft spend the same time making a standard turn so that wide swaths, implying fewer runs and turns, or longer runs requiring fewer turns per acre treated, will favour the faster aircraft, which can cover a greater distance in the time spent actually emitting aerosol. Thus, for really large blocks, the Cessna will be at an even greater advantage than over the standard block. A potential total coverage by a single aircraft of the capacity of the Cessna may be calculated

TABLE 24.5

Operating capacities of different aircraft, over equivalent blocks of bush, assuming a mean run of four miles and a maximum swath width of 55 yards. The first three lines are based on experience, the last is calculated for comparison.

Aircraft	Air speed m.p.h.	Insecticide	gal./acre	single maximum load					No. of sorties per morning
				gals.	acres	time to apply	total time air-borne	acres/hour	
						min.	min.		
1 Anson	100	11% DDT	0·25	130	520	36	80	390	1
2 Auster J5G	70	2½% dieldrin	0·125	52	416	24	34	735	1 to 4
3 Cessna 182E	130	10% isobenzan	0·0124	80	6,460	240	250	1,525	1
4 Auster J5G	80	10% isobenzan	0·0124	52	4,190	208	218	1,153	1

Data derived from: (1) Hocking and Yeo, 1956.
(2) Burnett *et al.*, 1961.
(3) Burnett *et al.*, 1964.

assuming a three-week treatment cycle. Assuming a low operating reliability of fifteen days in this period, a five-day week for the pilot and only one hour's actual spraying per day, one aircraft should be able to cover 1,200 acres per day even when the shape of the block is unfavourable, giving a total of 28 square miles per cycle. In reasonable circumstances of weather and block shape this should be considerably exceeded.

The costs of some schemes to control tsetse populations by aerial application of insecticides are shown in Table 24.6.

Aerial Application in Conjunction with Other Methods

Aircraft operations are quick, cheap and reliable in suitable terrain but they cannot be used in every situation and it is worth considering their combination with other methods. There is no point in doing this unless the combination is either more reliable or cheaper than aerial treatment by itself. The first use of combined methods was in Zululand although most of the supplementary methods were later given up as less efficient. However, it was found useful to dip cattle in the dispersion area to kill the dispersed flies and halt transmission of veterinary trypanosomiasis. It is frequently worthwhile to carry out some felling to tidy up a block and reduce the chance of immigration over a clearing. Extensive patches of very sparse woodland might be cheaper to cut than to spray.

A potential use of the method is in combination with the release of sterile males. This method of extermination depends on outnumbering fertile males and the quickest way to do this and at the same time to remove most of the fertile females is to make one to three applications of non-residual insecticide. The quickest, easiest and cheapest way of doing so is by the use of aircraft; a very high mortality is not essential so that great accuracy in application is not needed and thus much of the expensive preliminary work (surveys, beacons, access paths, etc.) can be omitted, application rates lowered and swath widths increased. The aircraft could subsequently be used to broadcast the sterile males. This combination of methods has the attraction that while the cost of eliminating the last few tsetse with insecticide remains constant as extermination is approached this is not so with sterile males.

So far, the chief adjuvant to aerial treatment has been settlement. If this takes place as soon as spraying has finished tsetse habitats should be so extensively and rapidly altered that it is unnecessary to push spraying to the point of extermination or to take measures to prevent reinfestation from outside. Fewer applications may be needed to achieve satisfactory results and Cockbill *et al.* (1963), who have carried out the most successful combined scheme to date, have taken advantage of this. Hocking *et al.* (1966) have described the earlier phases of a similar scheme but settlement had not taken place at the date of reporting. The use of aerial spraying to initiate the elimination of tsetse is advantageous to the settlers in that they can bring in stock soon after they move, avoid erosion due to deforestation and collect material for housing and fuel. Organized and rapid settlement at an adequate density is, of course, essential for success of this combined method.

TABLE 24.6

Some costs for aerial applications to control tsetse

	Date	Locality	Aircraft	Formulation	Insecticide	Flying	Operation itself[1]	Due to locality	Total	Reference
					Cost per square mile sprayed Stg. £					
1	1948	South Africa	Piper Cruiser	4% γ BHC	186	142	330			Du Toit, 1954
2	1948	South Africa	Helicopter	4% γ BHC	297	450	770			
3	1950	Tanzania	Anson I	11% DDT	352	512			928	Hocking *et al.*, 1953
4	1957	Rhodesia	Anson and Tiger Moth	4% γ BHC	216	238			465	Cockbill *et al.*, 1963
5	1959	Tanzania	Auster J5G	2½% dieldrin	233	55	307	70	377	Burnett *et al.*, 1961
6	1961–2	Rwanda	PA-18A	4% dieldrin	181[2]	149[2]	428[2]	28[2]	456[2]	Buyckx, 1964
7	1962	Tanzania	Cessna 182	12·3% dieldrin	168	40	224	34	258	Burnett *et al.*, 1965
8	1962	Tanzania	Cessna 182	10% isobenzan	123	29	190	30	220	
9	1964	Tanzania	Cessna 182	20% endosulfan	47	19	74	20	94	Hocking *et al.*, 1966

[1] Includes the amounts in the previous two columns.
[2] At exchange rate of 240 Fr. = Stg. £.
Operations 4 and 9 were not intended to exterminate.

GROUND-DISSEMINATED AEROSOLS AND SMOKES

Smoke clouds may be generated either by chemical means or by aerosol generators mounted on vehicles or carried by hand. Both methods produce a cloud which drifts with the wind and has no residual effect and which, in these respects, resembles that produced by aircraft, except that it is already below the canopy and has to be kept airborne. The droplet size should therefore be less than for aerosols disseminated by aircraft. As there is little or no residual effect, applications have to be repeated as described earlier.

The term 'smoke' is properly reserved for a cloud of dry particles which is produced by chemical generators containing insecticide, an oxidizing agent such as a chlorate and combustible material, usually sucrose. About 30% of DDT or BHC is usually lost through thermal decomposition; no other useful insecticide is available in this form. Smoke canisters have been tried in the field in Tanzania (EATRO, 1950, p. 24) and in South Africa (du Toit, 1954), but never with complete success. A critical examination of their use (CIRU, Arusha, unpublished) showed that in conditions of good inversion it was impossible to avoid gaps in the coverage due to variable drift unless a quite uneconomical number of small canisters was used. On slopes, the smoke was invariably channelled down gullies and failed to rise sufficiently to reach all tsetse. Smoke canisters pose considerable operational problems; they are heavy and each has to be deposited individually and lit individually, either when placed or on a later visit, which will probably be at night if a large area has to be treated. Smoke canisters are expensive and at least one half of their contents is burnt up or decomposed by fire; it is difficult to foresee that they will find a useful place in tsetse control.

Two types of ground aerosol generators have been used, small one-man portable machines and a large vehicle-borne type. The only one-man generator reported in use is the Swingfog, a light pulse-jet type of machine. It can disseminate up to 30 litres per hour as a fog of fine droplets. This will treat only about 30 acres with the usual 1–2% dilutions of DDT, γ BHC or, occasionally, dieldrin concentrates that have been used. Dilution is usually with kerosene or diesel oil although the makers claim that the best results are obtainable with the special formulations available. The machine has also been used by de-flying pickets for clearing both railway trains (Fairclough, 1956) and road vehicles. The train or vehicle concerned is halted and usually fogged from two machines, one on each side. Fairclough used 15% DDT + 0·05% pyrethrum but concluded that protection of the cattle at risk by drugs would be cheaper. Swingfog machines have been used for small scale eradication operations in many places, including Kenya, Tanzania, Zambia, Mali, Nigeria and Haute-Volta. They are useful in difficult terrain such as swamps and steep river banks, being light, portable and able to project their fog cloud for some yards. Low output restricts their use to small or linear habitats such as fringing forest on river banks; cutting paths at short intervals through evergreen habitats is more expensive than treating the edges with residual sprays and in more open country larger machines would be more appropriate. As an example of the use of Swingfogs to exterminate tsetse, J. A. Gledhill reports (personal communication) that they have been used on an 800-acre swamp forest on the shores of Lake Tanganyika. This harboured *G. brevipalpis*, which was eliminated, and *G. palpalis* which was also eliminated but returned from the nearby lake shore. Nine treatments with 1% γ BHC in diesoline were made, at intervals of two weeks. *G. brevipalpis* was eliminated by B. Steel (1958) using six applications of 4% γ BHC in diesel oil at 10-day intervals. In contrast, Challier *et al.* (1965) were unsuccessful with 3·3–6·6% γ BHC in diesel oil in a gallery forest in Haute-Volta. They expended 10 litres per kilometre for the last four of six applications which extended over a period of eleven weeks.

A large machine, the Todd Insecticide Fog Applicator, (TIFA), was used experimentally at CIRU in 1949–50 and operationally in Zambia between 1954–60. It is a large, heavy machine which produces fog by spraying an oil solution into a blast of hot air, driven by a pump through a combustion chamber heated to between 450°C and 650°C. It is fairly complex and can be temperamental in use. The method seems to have been given up when the machines wore out. The writer is indebted to Mr J. A. Gledhill for information on this method of exterminating tsetse which supplements information given by Steel and Gledhill (1960) and Steel, Gledhill and Norton (1960). He says that the availability of a really simple fogging device similar in size to the TIFA would extend the usefulness of the technique now to be described. The machine (the larger of two models) was originally mounted on a Landrover trailer, later on a four-wheel-drive tractor (the Mercedes Unimog) together with a 180-gallon insecticide tank. Fogging was done at night in the dry season from parallel paths marked out 200 yards apart, moving at not more than 4 m.p.h., over generally flat terrain bearing open deciduous woodland with short grass. The insecticide was 1·5% γ BHC prepared from 40% γ concentrate, liquid volume dosage about 0·2 gallons per acre, emission rate about two gallons per minute. Suitable meteorological conditions are an inversion with wind speed within the bush 2–8 m.p.h. and direction for preference more or less across the vehicle's track. Above this windspeed (when the inversion would be destroyed) treatment was stopped, below 2 m.p.h. drift was poor and swath width needed to be reduced. With very strong inversions there was rapid drainage of fog into drainage lines. With two supervisors working in shifts for a total of eight hours per night, up to 4 square miles a night and 25 square miles a week were treated. The cycle was normally repeated five times at three-week intervals, being used on diffused habitats that were not restricted during the dry season. Between 1954 and 1960 it was a regular method for exterminating discrete pockets of *G. morsitans* up to 30 square miles in extent and in one place eliminated *G. pallidipes* as well. It is believed that the exposed resting places of these species undoubtedly contributed much to the success of the method.

All fog generators suffer from low output. The drop size regulator is invariably a flow rate control and the maximum output is obtainable only with the largest droplets although this is rarely, if ever, apparent from the manufacturer's instructions. The work in Zambia used droplets of 90–120 μ. This is far too large for effective cover in light winds and it is likely that few of these large drops drifted more than a few yards. The small satellite droplets which are also present would give the impression of a dense advancing cloud but it will contain comparatively little insecticide. It would almost certainly be worth investigating the application of ultra-low-volume techniques to ground disseminated aerosols, using highly insecticidal concentrates.

PYRETHRUM AEROSOLS IN DE-FLYING HOUSES

The only use for pyrethrum in tsetse control is in de-flying houses sited on roads and designed to prevent the carriage of infected tsetse into clean areas where livestock are present. The de-flying house is a more or less light-tight wooden chamber except that windows are provided high up along the two lateral walls. The vehicle or cyclists to be disinfested enter the chamber, the doors are closed and attendants direct blasts of pyrethrum spray from hand sprayers at the infested object. This disturbs the tsetse which make for the windows where they may be captured. Alternatively reliance may be placed on the lethal effect of the spray but this entails exposure to the insecticide for a sufficient length of time for the tsetse to acquire a lethal dose. The spray liquid used is about 0·1% pyrethrum in kerosene. Burnett (1961–3) has shown that there is no advantage in adding the synergist piperonyl butoxide to pyrethrum used to kill tsetse.

Chapter 25

Control by Parasites and Predators of *Glossina*

T. A. M. NASH

The literature on parasites and predators of *Glossina* was reviewed in considerable detail by Buxton (1955). Subsequently Glasgow (1963) discussed the subject in relation to the abundance of tsetse, and Jenkins (1964) produced a valuable list and bibliography of all records of parasites, predators and pathogens of the genus. Hitherto, no attempt has been made to introduce parasites or predators from other continents. Mention will be made of only those indigenous organisms which seem to have an appreciable tsetse control potential or which have been tested in the field.

PATHOGENIC ORGANISMS IN ADULT TSETSE FLIES

Roubaud and Treillard (1935, 1936) isolated *Bacterium mathisi* from one of a batch of adult flies of *G. morsitans* which emerged from puparia sent to Paris from Tanzania. The organism was easily maintained in pure culture, and successfully transmitted to *G. morsitans* and *G. palpalis* by allowing flies to feed on the skin of a guinea-pig which had been smeared with the culture. Such flies died in one to three days with the micro-organisms present in their blood. *G. morsitans* was the more readily infected species. This organism is worthy of further investigation.

In 1930, torrential rains occurred throughout Tanzania. Nash (1933) recorded a remarkable decrease in a population of *G. morsitans* which was under study, and attributed the decrease in part to an entomophagous fungus seen as black spots on the underside of the fly's abdomen. Up to 20% of the flies in a catch were infected. J. D. Scott stated that the fungus was a Phycomycete, and that it was definitely pathogenic for *G. morsitans*. W. H. Potts (personal communication) working at Kikori found that infection with this fungus neither prevented completion of development of larvae nor their deposition. Lester (1934) reported that at the end of the rains in Northern Nigeria, 33% of old female *G. submorsitans* and 11% of female *G. tachinoides* were infected by an unidentified fungus.

There is no evidence that trypanosomes are pathogenic to tsetse flies (*see* also p. 373).

INSECT PARASITES OF TSETSE PUPAE

The proportion of pupae which are dead on collection varies considerably according to site and season, as does further mortality which depends upon the climatic conditions experienced in transit and during subsequent maintenance. Some workers have calculated the proportion of parasitized tsetse pupae on the total number collected while others have based this proportion on the total emergence (tsetse and parasites) giving a figure which excludes dead pupae. When both rates are given, those based on total emergences are shown in brackets; these are higher because the proportion parasitized is calculated on a smaller number. The difference between the two sets of values is greatest when the death rate is highest.

Jenkins (1964) has listed twenty-three species of Hymenoptera belonging to ten families, and ten species of Diptera (all Bombyliids) of the genus *Thyridanthrax*, as parasites of tsetse pupae; but recent work by C. E. Dyte (personal communication) has raised the number of *Thyridanthrax* species to twelve.

Most of the Hymenopterous species listed rarely parasitize tsetse pupae. *Syntomosphyrum glossinae* Waterston[1] (Eulophidae) has received considerable attention since Lamborn (1922) reported very favourably on its longevity, short life cycle, great fecundity, and on the ease with which it could be bred, not only in pupae of *Glossina* but also in pupae of 'flesh' or 'house' flies. Later, he attempted to control *G. morsitans* by liberating this parasite in an area of some 42 square miles on a peninsula in Lake Nyasa, where the natural incidence of the parasite for the first three months of 1922 and 1923 had been 0·22 (0·32)% based on 1,367 pupae (Lamborn, 1925). Parasitized pupae of *Sarcophaga*, protected from predators in bamboo tubes with a small emergence hole for the parasite, were placed in tsetse habitats. Between June and October 1923, an estimated 277,000 parasites were liberated. In the first three months of 1924 the rate of infestation by *S. glossinae* in 516 tsetse pupae was 6·8 (8·7)%. When Lamborn returned from leave eight months later, the percentage of parasitized pupae had dropped to about the original figure (Buxton, 1955).

In 1924, Lamborn sent *S. glossinae* to England where a stock was raised from which consignments of parasitized blow-fly pupae were sent by sea, rail and road

[1] The species formerly known as *S. glossinae* has been divided by Kerrich (1960) into two species, *S. glossinae* and *S. albiclavus*. The former is known from Liberia, Nigeria, Uganda, Tanzania, Kenya and Malawi (from *G. palpalis*, *G. fuscipes*, *G.m. submorsitans*, *G.m. orientalis* and *G. pallidipes* pupae), and the latter from Kenya, Tanzania, Malawi and Zambia (from *G.m. orientalis* and *G. pallidipes* pupae). Early records of *S. glossinae* from Tanzania and Kenya may refer to either species (Saunders 1960). The development stages of *S. albiclavus* have been described by Saunders (1960a).

to Sherifuri, in Northern Nigeria; from the few survivors a large stock was built up by J. W. B. Hanington. Three releases of adults and infected pupae were made at a spot where *G.m. submorsitans* and *G. tachinoides* were breeding actively. Subsequent collections of tsetse pupae from the site failed to yield one that was parasitized (Lloyd, Johnson & Rawson, 1927). *S. glossinae* had not been recorded as occurring in nature in West Africa until Nash (1947) obtained specimens from pupae of *G. palpalis* near Kaduna—a much cooler part of Northern Nigeria than Sherifuri.

Encouraged by Lamborn's (1925) results, Nash (1933a) undertook a similar experiment at Kikori, Tanzania, but on a much larger scale, having first developed specialized techniques for rearing and releasing the parasites. An average yield of seventy parasites from each parasitized *Chrysomya* pupa was achieved; the life cycle ranged from 21–45 days according to season. The releases were made in six miles of woodland along the lower slopes of an escarpment, where the natural incidence of parasitism was either nil or exceedingly low—no *S. glossinae* emerged from 1,500 *G. morsitans* pupae collected in 1928–9. Releases started in March 1931. Tsetse pupae were collected periodically from sites within the release area to determine the parasitization rate. After the elapse of nine months and the release of an estimated 3·5 million parasites, the rate from 254 pupae was 0·8 (1·0)%. In the next month a further two million *S. glossinae* were liberated; the rate from fifty pupae collected on one round was 4·0 (4·4%), and from 171 pupae from another round 9·9 (11·3%). Four months later, and after the release of a further 8·25 million parasites, the respective rates for these two rounds were 0·8 (1·4%) from 124 pupae and 1·6 (2·6%) from 489 pupae. The release of 13·75 million *S. glossinae* had achieved little. Further, there was no evidence that the parasites had spread; during the fourteen-month liberation period, of 777, 462 and 359 pupae collected at distances of about ½, 1½ and 7 miles, respectively, from the liberation area, not one was parasitized by *S. glossinae*.

The failure at Kikori was attributed to the parasites' inability to reach pupae in sandy soils. Experiments by Chorley (1929) had shown that *S. glossinae* was incapable of penetrating light sand to a depth of more than 3–6 mm. Nash (1933a) found that this parasite was virtually incapable of reaching pupae buried under more than 2·5 mm. of dry sand or wet humus, but that it could reach pupae under 15 mm. of dry humus and under 38 mm. of dry leaves; he concluded that *S. glossinae* might be successful in areas where tsetse breed in humus.

In March 1933, H. M. Lloyd transferred the stock of parasites from Kikori to Musoma on Lake Victoria, and started an experiment on Riamugasire Island where *G. palpalis* breeds in humus. After initial difficulties in propagating *S. glossinae*, monthly releases were undertaken but the results were even worse than those at Kikori. For example, in a month when 519,000 parasites emerged on the island only 5% of the tsetse pupae were parasitized. The humus appeared to be too moist for the parasite (Swynnerton, 1936).

Glasgow (1963) has aptly summed up the work mentioned above. 'Looking back, it seems that when it was decided to undertake these experiments, too much weight was given to the ease with which *Syntomosphyrum* can be bred artificially, and too little to the fact that it has never been found abundant in nature.'

On Glasgow's criterion it would seem that the only Hymenopterous parasite of tsetse pupae which might be worthy of investigation is *Mutilla glossinae* Turner; it is an important parasite of *G. morsitans* in Malawi, Zambia and Rhodesia. Rates of parasitization, ranging from 0 to about 10% have been recorded from collections of large numbers of pupae. In smaller samples the rate may be much higher: Buxton (1955) quotes Lamborn, in Malawi, as having obtained 41 *M. glossinae* from 85 pupae of *G. morsitans*, and from another sample 97 *G. morsitans* and 131 *M. glossinae* emerged.

The rate of parasitism may vary greatly from season to season. Chorley (1929) collected pupae of *G. morsitans* from twenty square miles of country around the confluence of two rivers in the Rhodesian Umniati fly-belt. He studied the incidence of parasitism throughout a dry season from weekly samples of at least 300 pupae. Judging from the emergences in his field laboratory, adult *M. glossinae* were rare in the cold dry season, forming only 0–5% of total emergences of tsetse and parasites; frost occurred on several occasions. In the hot dry months the weekly rate was never less than 14% and often over 20%; in one week it was 42·7% based on a total of 344 emergences. Then, coinciding with temperatures up to 40°C and the start of the rains, the rate dropped to 6–12%. At this point the field observations ceased; his parallel observations on *Thyridanthrax* will be discussed shortly. It has recently been confirmed (R. C. Heaversedge, personal communication) that peak parasitization by *M. glossinae* is associated with hot, dry weather.

Mention must be made of certain features in the biology of *M. glossinae* which are relevant to an assessment of its potentialities for use in controlling tsetse. Only one parasite is believed to develop in a tsetse pupa; development may take 2½–4 months. The female is wingless, but may be carried some distance by the male during copulation; however, males are scarce—Chorley recorded only 15% of males from an emergence of 1,176 Mutillids. Lamborn (1925) found that the parasite would breed reluctantly on pupae of *Sarcophaga*; in the example quoted the life cycles of six males ranged from 65–87 days. He considered Mutillids to be unsuitable for exploitation. Chorley (1929) also bred a few Mutillids on pupae of *Sarcophaga*; he suggested that it would be possible to breed a limited number for distribution in fly-belts from which the parasite was absent, but pointed out that the spread of the apterous female would be slow. R. J. Phelps (personal communication) considers that an intensive effort should be made to breed this parasite as it lives well under laboratory conditions. Two other species—*M. auxiliaris* and *M. benefactrix*—have been bred from pupae of *G. morsitans*, in Mozambique and Malawi respectively, but their biology has not been investigated (Buxton, 1955).

Mutillids have never been recorded as parasites of tsetse pupae in West Africa but it might be worth introducing *M. glossinae* to the drier zones where *G. submorsitans* breed in the riverine vegetation in the hotter months, when the tsetse population is at its lowest level (Nash, 1969).

Species of the genus *Thyridanthrax* are the only Diptera which are parasitic on tsetse. Although widely distributed in eastern and central Africa, only one species, *T. argentifrons*[1] has been recorded as parasitizing tsetse pupae in western Africa, and then only from Nigeria. Five species of tsetse are known to be parasitized by flies of this genus. An overall picture of the rate of parasitization by *Thyridanthrax* spp. can be obtained from Table 25.1, based in part on one given by Buxton (1955).

TABLE 25.1

No. of pupae	Tsetse species	Rate %	Locality	Reference
16,887	*G. morsitans*	6·4 (11·1)[1]	Rhodesia	Chorley (1929)
	G. morsitans	(9·7)[2]	Kikori, Tanganyika	Nash (1930)
5,168	*G. morsitans*	5·0 (6·0)	Kikori, Tanganyika	Nash (1933)
2,724	*G. morsitans*	6·2	Kikori, Tanganyika	Potts (1933)
17,300	*G. submorsitans*	0·3	Gadau, Nigeria	Taylor (1932)
106,000	*G. tachinoides*	0·7[3]	Gadau, Nigeria	Taylor (1932)

[1] Chorley's Table 4 and p. 291.
[2] Based on 764 emergences; number of pupae not recorded.
[3] Wrongly quoted by Buxton (1955) as 6·5 instead of 0·65.

There may be a considerable variation in the rate of parasitism in different years. If the figures given by Nash (1933a) collected over 4½ years are divided into the 2 years before and after the torrential rains referred to earlier, the rates of parasitism were as follow: 11·5 (14·2%) from 1,509 pupae in 1928–9 and 2·3 (2·9%) from 3,659 pupae in 1931–2. He also found that in the pre-deluge period parasitism by *Thyridanthrax* varied according to habitat; whereas the incidence for 726 pupae from *Berlinia globiflora* and *Acacia usambarensis* woodland was 15·5 (20·7%), for 783 pupae collected in the hilly *Brachystegia microphylla* woodlands the incidence was 7·8 (9·0%). Three species of *Thyridanthrax* were found at Kikori by Potts (1933)—*T. abruptus* Lw., *T. lineus*[2] Lw.,

[1] The systematics of the genus *Thyridanthrax* are currently being revised by C. E. Dyte (*in litt.*, Feb. 1968) who states that this name as used by Austen and tsetse workers is preoccupied.

[2] C. E. Dyte (*in litt.*, Feb. 1968) writes, 'Hesse (1956) has shown that the tsetse parasites previously regarded as *T. lineus* (Loew) are in fact the males of *T. abruptus*, and that under the name *abruptus* previous workers have included not only the females of the true *T. abruptus*, but also both males and females of a distinct species now recognized as *T. lugens* (Loew). In addition, some tsetse workers have misidentified specimens of other species as *T. abruptus*. It follows that published records of *T. lineus* refer to *T. abruptus*, but that reports of *T. abruptus* other than those of Fiedler and Kluge (1954), Hesse (1956) and Greathead (1967), may refer to other species.'

and *T. argentifrons* Aust.—but they were not differentiated when compiling the rates of parasitism.

Observations on *Thyridanthrax* by Chorley (1929), undertaken concurrently with those already referred to for *Mutilla glossinae*, were made on two species of the genus—one of them probably *T. abruptus*. The emergences from his weekly collections of pupae of *G. morsitans* suggested that, in the field, there was no emergence of *Thyridanthrax* in the cold dry season, a small hatch when the weather started to get warmer, and a great emergence in the hottest weather just before, and at the beginning of, the rains. In the best week, *Thyridanthrax* was responsible for 64%, of a total emergence of 285 tsetse and parasites. Weekly collections made in the hot weather, just before the field investigation closed, were taken back to Salisbury; from one of them, 79% of 362 emergences were *Thyridanthrax*. (Chorley's rate for the whole dry season, based on all species of insect parasites, was 13·6 (23·6%) from 16,887 pupae collected).

In captivity, adult *Thyridanthrax* batter themselves to pieces and die within a few hours (Lamborn, 1925; Chorley, 1929). All laboratory breeding experiments have failed; in consequence the duration of the life cycle is not precisely known. A number of workers have noticed that whereas the majority of parasites emerge within a few weeks of the collection of the tsetse pupae, some individuals do not emerge until four or five months later; this has given rise to the belief that a proportion of the larvae remains dormant inside the pupae of *Glossina* for many months (Chorley, 1929; Buxton, 1955). However, another explanation could be that *Thyridanthrax* has several distinct hatching seasons during the course of the year, as suggested by Chorley's field observations referred to above; if this be so, in any collection of tsetse pupae, there could be a proportion that had been parasitized by *Thyridanthrax* females that had emerged, say, five months before and a proportion parasitized by others that had emerged, say, one month before collection. If the first had been the major emergence it would account for figures such as those obtained by Taylor (1932): from pupae of *G. tachinoides* collected in April, 119 *T. argentifrons* had emerged by early June, after which there was no further emergence until October when seven more parasites emerged. Nash (1930) has recorded the emergence of *T. abruptus* from a batch of *G. morsitans* pupae collected 197 days earlier. The life cycle can be long, and reproductivity is low as only one parasite emerges from one tsetse pupa. Thus apart from the difficulties in breeding *Thyridanthrax* in captivity, this parasite seems unlikely to find a useful place in the control of tsetse.

The species of *Thyridanthrax* which attack *Glossina* were thought to be specific to this genus and therefore impossible to breed in other hosts. However, Dyte (*in litt*., Feb. 1968) states that there is definite evidence that *T. lugens* attack tsetse as well as other insects and believes that the same may be true of *T. abruptus*, *T. transiens* and *T. brevifacies*. He also states that the claim by McDonald (1957) to have found *T. abruptus* in a Calliphorid pupa was based on the faulty identification of the parasite.

In parts of Africa, insect parasites of the pupae undoubtedly contribute appreciably to the natural regulation of tsetse numbers. Thus Chorley (1929), referring to the area under study, wrote 'The combined effect of parasitism and the hot summer sun on deposited puparia is no doubt a contributory cause of the great fall in density that occurs throughout mopane forest at the end of the late dry season after leaf-fall is complete.'

PREDATORS OF PUPARIA TSETSE

Predators probably also play a considerable part in regulating the size of a tsetse population. Many species have been suspected of taking a toll of tsetse puparia because they have been observed burrowing, scratching and feeding in the breeding grounds; thus Swynnerton (1936) strongly suspected the elephant shrew (*Petrodromys tetradactylus*), and others the guinea-fowl (*Numida*, etc.) and the bush-fowl (*Francolinus*, etc.) but Simpson (1918) failed to find positive evidence from examination of the stomach contents of 379 of these birds.

Ants of the genus *Pheidole* have been observed carrying off the full puparia of *G. morsitans*, and empty puparia have been found in their nests. By burying some 1,600 puparia individually, marking the spots with sticks, and looking for them fourteen days later, Ford (1940) obtained results which indicated that losses were twice as great among those buried in unburnt as compared with burnt bush; later studies by E. F. Whiteside and B. Kemp (reported by Potts, 1950, 1950a) showed that increased predation was not necessarily associated with unburnt bush and that when it occurred it was due to a shortage of other sources of food.

Puparia cases of tsetse, obviously damaged by insect predators, are commonly encountered. H. M. Lloyd found that 3·1% of 50,000 cases of *G. palpalis* [*G. fuscipes*] collected on an island in Lake Victoria were damaged (Swynnerton, 1936). On the Uganda shores of the Lake, Fiske (1920) suspected that Carabid and Elaterid beetles and their larvae were mainly responsible for the 7% found damaged among some 9,000 puparia of *G. palpalis* [*G. fuscipes*]; the proportion ranged in different spots from 0–31% and was highest in unusual breeding sites such as tussocks of dried grass.

PREDATORS OF ADULT TSETSE FLIES

Certain birds, either when on the wing or when searching tree trunks and branches, probably catch adult tsetse (Swynnerton, 1936). A number of records has been given by Buxton (1955) of hunting wasps (*Bembix*) and robber-flies (Asilidae) which have been repeatedly observed to catch tsetse either in the air or when about to alight. In six months, 330 Asilids were caught with prey, of which *G. swynnertoni* formed 15% (Southon, 1959a). The dragonfly *Orthetrum chrysostigma* was frequently seen by Lamborn (1915a) to take *G. morsitans* off the backs of Africans.

Fiske (1920) mentioned the large number of big spiders of the genus *Nephila* which spin huge webs between trees on the shores and on some of the islands of Lake Victoria; of 108 insects collected from webs, seven were tsetse flies. The fly population on islands with no *Nephila* appeared to be about four times as great as on islands on which the spiders were very numerous, suggesting that the tsetse population was nearly four times greater in the absence of these spiders. C. W. Chorley agreed with Fiske that spiders do much to control

TABLE 25.2

(W. H. Potts)

***List of parasites and predators of the species of* Glossina**

(+ of adults: * of pupae: (*) of larvae)

	austeni	*brevipalpis*	*fuscipes*	*fuscipleuris*	*longipennis*	*morsitans* (s.l.)	*palpalis* (s.l.)	*pallidipes*	*swynnertoni*	*tachinoides*	*sp. unknown*
PARASITES											
BACTERIA											
Bacterium mathisi						+					
(various other bacteria have been recorded but none is known to be pathogenic)											
FUNGI											
Phycomycetes						+					
Cicadomyces sp.						+	+				
(Various undetermined fungi have also been reported)											
PROTOZOA (other than trypanosomes, for which see pp. 521–522)											
Borrelia glossinae							+				
Hepatozoon pettiti			+				+				
Myxosporidium heibergi			+								
Treponema macfiei							+			+	
NEMATODA											
Mermis sp.			+			+					
Unidentified nematodes			+								
ACARINA											
Trombicula? (2 spp.)						+			+		
INSECTA											
(1) HYMENOPTERA											
Bethylidae											
Prolaelius glossinae						*					
Braconidae											
Coelalysia glossinophaga						*					
Calliceratidae											
Conostigmus rodhaini			*			*					
Chalcididae											
Brachymeria amenocles (= *Chalcis amenocles, C. varipes*)						*				*	
Dirhinus giffardi		*	*			*					
D. inflexus						*					
Dirhinus sp.											*
Haltichella edax						*					
Stomatoceras exaratum						*					
S. micans						*				*	
S. schulthessi						*				*	

TABLE 25.2 (*continued*)

***List of parasites and predators of the species of* Glossina**

(+ of adults: * of pupae: (*) of larvae)

	austeni	*brevipalpis*	*fuscipes*	*fuscipleuris*	*longipennis*	*morsitans* (s.l.)	*palpalis* (s.l.)	*pallidipes*	*swynnertoni*	*tachinoides*	*sp. unknown*
PARASITES (*continued*)											
INSECTA											
(1) HYMENOPTERA											
Diapriidae											
Abothropia lloydi			*								
Trichopria capensis robustior		*						*			
T. lewisi		*		*							
Eulophidae											
Syntomosphyrum albiclavus						*		*			
S. glossinae[1]		*	*			*	*	*			
Eupelmidae											
Anastatus viridiceps						*					
Eupelmella tarsata[1]						*					
Mutillidae											
Mutilla auxiliaris	*	*						*			
M. benefactrix						*					
M. glossinae		*				*					
Perilampidae											
Perilampus ruficornis						*					
P. violaceus						*					
(2) DIPTERA											
Bombyliidae—*see* also Table 25.3	*	*			*	*	*	*	*	*	
Conopidae											
Stylogaster westwood[2]						*					
PREDATORS											
ARACHNIDA											
Hersilia setifrons									+		
Nephele sp.			+								
Plexippus paykulli							+				
INSECTA											
(1) ODONATA											
Cacergates leucosticta			+								
Crocothemis erythraea						+					
Orthetrum brachiale						+					
O. chrysostigma						+					

[1] Also hyperparasitic on *Mutilla glossinae*.

[2] This was recorded as a previously unknown parasite of the puparial stages of *Glossina*, under the name *Stylogaster leonum* Westw., by van den Berghe, Lambrecht and Christiaensen (1956), who obtained a single male that emerged from a puparium of *G. morsitans* collected in the Mutara region of Rwanda; the specimen was subsequently identified as belonging to a hitherto unnamed species by K. G. V. Smith (1967) who described the species under the name *S. westwoodi*, and cited the Rwanda specimen as a paratype.

TABLE 25.2 (*continued*)

***List of parasites and predators of the species of* Glossina**
(+ of adults: * of pupae: (*) of larvae)

PREDATORS (*continued*)	*austeni*	*brevipalpis*	*fuscipes*	*fuscipleuris*	*longipennis*	*morsitans* (s.l.)	*palpalis* (s.l.)	*pallidipes*	*swynnertoni*	*tachinoides*	*sp. unknown*
INSECTA											
(2) DIPTERA											
Asilidae			+			+				+	
(3) HYMENOPTERA											
Formicidae											
Euponera senraarensis[3]						(*)					
Paltothyreus tarsatus[3]			(*)								
Pheidole sp.									*		
SPHECIDAE											
Bembix sp.						+				+	
Sphex sp.			+								
VESPIDAE											
Synagris sp.			+								
(2) COLEOPTERA											
CARABIDAE } considered destructive											
ELATERIDAE } to pupae (Fiske, 1920)											
MELYRIDAE											
Melyris pallidiventris (puparia eaten in laboratory experiments; Nash, 1933a)						*					
VERTEBRATA											
MAMMALS											
Petrodromys tetradactylus	?*										
Mongoose						?*					
BIRDS											
Numida spp. } Presumed to eat											
Francolinus spp. } pupae (Buxton, 1955)											

Swynnerton (1936) who investigated the importance of birds as predators of adult tsetse, showed that the number eaten is a density-dependent factor.

[3] Possibly rare predators on tsetse larvae (Carpenter, 1912; Lamborn, 1915).

TABLE 25.3 (W. H. Potts)

Hosts and Distribution of* Thyridanthrax *spp. recorded as parasites from tsetse pupae

Thyridanthrax spp	Hosts
[1]1 *T. abruptus* (Lw.): Ethiopia, Kenya, Tanzania, Zambia, Malawi, Rhodesia, Mozambique, South Africa, Botswana, South West Africa	*G. brevipalpis, G. longipennis, G. morsitans, G. swynnertoni, G. pallidipes*
2 *T. alliopterus* Hesse: Kenya, Tanzania	*G. austeni, G. brevipalpis, G. longipennis, G. pallidipes, G. swynnertoni*
3 *T. beneficus* Austen: Mozambique, Rhodesia	*G. morsitans*
[1]4 *T. brevifacies* Hesse:	*G. brevipalpis, G. pallidipes, G. austeni*
5 *T. burtti* Hesse: Kenya	*G. austeni*
6 *T. lloydi* (Austen): Rhodesia, Tanzania, Zambia	*G. morsitans*
[1]7 *T. lugens* (Lw.): Kenya, Rhodesia, South Africa, South West Africa, Tanzania	*G. brevipalpis, G. longipennis, G. morsitans, G. pallidipes, G. swynnertoni, G. austeni*
8 *T. salutaris* Austen: Malawi, Rhodesia, Tanzania	*G. morsitans*
[1]9 *T. transiens* Bezzi: Kenya, Malawi, Mozambique, Rhodesia, South Africa, South West Africa	*G. morsitans*
10 *T.* sp. A (= *T. argentifrons* Austen et auct.): Nigeria, Chad, Tanzania	*G. tachinoides, G. morsitans, G. swynnertoni, G. pallidipes*
11 *T.* sp. B: Nigeria	*G. morsitans submorsitans* (and possibly *G. palpalis*, Dyte, *in lit.*, March, 1968)
12 *T.* sp. C: Nigeria	*G. palpalis*

Distribution	*Thyridanthrax* spp.
ETHIOPIA:	*T. abruptus*
KENYA:	*T. abruptus; T. alliopterus; T. burtti; T. lugens; T. transiens*
TANZANIA:	*T. abruptus; T. alliopterus; T. lloydi; T. lugens; T. salutaris;* *T.* sp. A (*T. argentifrons* Austen et auct.—name preoccupied)
MALAWI:	*T. abruptus; T. salutaris; T. transiens*
ZAMBIA:	*T. abruptus; T. lloydi*
RHODESIA:	*T. abruptus; T. beneficus; T. lloydi; T. lugens; T. salutaris; T. transiens*
MOZAMBIQUE:	*T. abruptus; T. beneficus; T. transiens*
BOTSWANA:	*T. abruptus*
SOUTH WEST AFRICA:	*T. abruptus; T. lugens; T. transiens*
SOUTH AFRICA:	*T. abruptus; T. brevifacies; T. lugens; T. transiens*
NIGERIA:	*T.* sp. A (*T. argentifrons* Austen et auct.); *T.* sp. B; *T.* sp. C
CHAD:	*T.* sp. A (*T. argentifrons* Austen et auct.)

[1] Represented by some specimens recorded by Hesse (1956) as collected outside tsetse areas; all the rest are known only from specimens bred from tsetse pupae.

tsetse in this region (Buxton, 1955), a view confirmed by Glasgow (1963) who records that the invasion of Sumba Island by *Nephila* led to the disappearance of *G. palpalis* [*G. fuscipes*].

The observation that jumping spiders (*Plexippus paykulli*), family Attidae, kill a considerable number of *G. palpalis* was made on a boat on the Gambia River by Simpson (1911). The spider *Hersilia setifrons* Lawrence has been studied by Southon (1959a); it lives on the trunks and branches of trees where *G. swynnertoni* rests, and on capturing its prey rapidly envelopes it in a silken shroud and holds it for some hours. During seven months, 100–350 predator meals were examined monthly: *G. swynnertoni* formed 0–3% of these samples. Counts by Southon and his staff indicated that the minimum *Hersilia* population was 384,000 per square mile, Calculations, based on his observations, suggested that the daily mortality due to the spider might be 650 tsetse per square mile.

The only animal, other than man, which has eradicated tsetse from appreciable areas is the elephant. For example, in the Murchison Falls National Park, Uganda, hundreds of square miles of *Terminalia* woodland have been destroyed by an increasing elephant population, with the consequent disappearance of *G. morsitans*. The elephants have de-barked and broken the *Terminalia* trees and grass fires have completed their destruction: forest has been converted to tall *Hyparrhenia* grassland and the elephant from a tree-feeder to a grass-feeder (Ford, 1966).

During the last thirty-five years little work has been done on the subject of parasites and predators of *Glossina*. As pointed out by Buxton, studies on parasitic insects should be undertaken by those experienced in this specialized branch of entomology. The subject of infection of *Glossina* by viruses, bacteria, fungi and protozoa (excluding trypanosomes) has been sadly neglected.

Editor's Note. Tables 25.2 and 25.3 have been compiled by Mr W. H. Potts. Table 25.2 lists the parasites and predators that have been recorded for the adult, larva and pupa of various species of *Glossina*, and is based largely on information given by Jenkins (1964). Table 25.3 lists the species of *Thyridanthrax* parasitic on the pupae of *Glossina* in accordance with a recent revision by Dr C. E. Dyte (*in litt*., 1968) and records the distribution of these species.

Chapter 26

Control by Sterilization of *Glossina*

DAVID A. DAME

INTRODUCTORY

Population control by sexual sterilization is a comparatively recent concept in entomology. The eradication of the screw-worm fly, *Cochliomyia hominivorax*[1] (Coquillett), from the entire south-eastern United States adequately demonstrated the practicality of releasing sterile males for population control (Knipling, 1960). Subsequently, populations of the same fly are being suppressed in the south-western United States where re-establishment in economically damaging numbers is now prevented by a wide barrier zone in which sterile males are continually released. Also, sterile male releases combined with prior population suppression by insecticides eradicated an isolated population of melon flies, *Dacus cucurbitae* Coquillett, from the island of Rota in the Marianas Islands of the Pacific Ocean (Steiner *et al.*, 1965). Other investigations and progress in this field were reviewed by Smith *et al.* (1964), Ascher (1964), LaBrecque and Keller (1965), Campion (1965), Kilgore and Doutt (1967), LaBrecque and Smith (1968) and Binggeli (1963, 1965, 1967), who has compiled an annotated bibliographical series which includes all published reports on the subject up to 1965.

The principal advantage of the sterile male release technique is that the control effort becomes more economical as the natural population declines. This economy results because increasing ratios of sterile to wild males are achieved as the programme proceeds, even when the total number of released flies is reduced (Table 26.1), and control thus becomes increasingly more efficient. In contrast, conventional multiple applications of insecticide become less efficient in terms of the number of insects killed as the population declines because the cost and percentage kill per application remain fixed. In actual practice, a desirable integration of *Glossina* control techniques might make use of insecticides early in a programme when they are most efficient and then

[1] *Callitroga hominivorax* in many publications.—Ed.

introduce sterile males when the population has been reduced to levels where the economic efficiency of sterility can be realized (Knipling, 1964).

Simpson (1958) and Knipling (1963) discussed the application of the sterile male technique to *Glossina* in relation to the biological characteristics of the genus. Knipling estimated that an initial 3:1 overflooding ratio of sterile to wild males, followed by a gradually decreasing release rate could eradicate a low-density population of flies in twelve months (Table 26.1) at a cost of about

TABLE 26.1

Theoretical trend of a low-density population of tsetse flies (average 100 males and 100 females per square mile) subjected to sterile male releases at the rates and periods indicated (after Knipling, 1964)

Period (months)	Natural density at beginning of each period (males plus females)	Number of sterile males released each period	Estimated average ratio of sterile to fertile males	Assumed natural density at the end of each period[1]
0–3	200	900 (300 per month)	3:1	75
4–6	75	450 (150 per month)	4:1	22
7–9	22	225 (75 per month)	7:1	4
10–12	4	112 (37 per month)	16·5:1	1

[1] In calculating the theoretical effect of the sterile male releases, it is assumed that the released males are fully competitive with native males and exert full effect in reducing the reproductive potential of the total population. The assumption is also made that in the absence of control the natural population would increase by 50% from a low level each three months (each generation). Thus, in the absence of sterile male releases, the population trend would be as follows: First period, 200 flies per square mile; Second period, 300 flies per square mile; Third period, 450 flies per square mile; Fourth period, 675 flies per square mile.

£52 per square mile, even if the released males cost as much as 5d each. More extensive populations would require the use of alternate methods to reduce the population density prior to the release of the sterile males. Knipling (1964a) emphasized the economical advantage to be gained, through reductions in the total number of sterile flies required, by preceding a release programme with a single application of a non-residual insecticide to eliminate most of the adult fly population. With dense populations covering wide areas, it might not be feasible to attempt simultaneous control of the entire infested territory. However, such areas might realistically be attacked by systematically expanding smaller control areas along a common front (Table 26.2). In any programme the release patterns would be dictated by the density of local populations and the ecological and behavioural characteristics of the target species.

TABLE 26.2

Estimated number of sterile tsetse fly males needed to eradicate a low density population in a new unit of 1,000 square miles each quarter [1]

Release months	Number of males released per month in 1,000 square mile block					Total number released per month
	Block					
	A	*B*	*C*	*D*	*E*	
1–3	300,000	—	—	—	—	300,000
4–6	150,000	300,000	—	—	—	450,000
7–9	75,000	150,000	300,000	—	—	525,000
10–12	37,000	75,000	150,000	300,000	—	562,000
13–15[2]	—	37,000	75,000	150,000	300,000	562,000

[1] These estimates can be converted directly into estimates for larger or smaller areas.
[2] Programme following similar pattern continues indefinitely.

METHOD OF STERILIZATION

Sterilization of *Glossina* spp. can be accomplished in several ways. Vanderplank (1947) demonstrated that hybrid sterility could be induced by cross-mating species and accumulated evidence that suggested that this phenomenon may be an important limitation on the natural distribution of some species (Glasgow, 1963). Curtis (1968a) has proposed the use of mutant genes in the form of translocation homozygotes for control of *Glossina*; the successful isolation and breeding of such individuals would provide a method of introducing a sterility factor into natural populations. However, the subject of this chapter is primarily concerned with the induction of dominant lethality in the germ cells of *Glossina* by high energy ionizing radiation, e.g. X-rays or gamma rays, or by mutagenic chemicals. Such irradiated and chemosterilized sperm appear normal in their gross external characteristics and in their mobility, but suffer chromosomal damage that prevents normal cell division at some early stage in the life cycle. Thus, embryos resulting from the union of sterile sperm and normal ova usually die before eclosion; occasional death occurs during the larval instars, and infrequently it occurs in the pupal stage.

Radiosterilization of *Glossina* was first attempted by Potts (1958), who achieved a high degree of sterility in pupae of *G. morsitans* exposed to 6,000 or 12,000 r. of gamma irradiation from Cobalt-60. Subsequently, Dean and Wortham (1969) caused complete male sterility by using doses above 4,000 r. when the pupae were less than fourteen days old; 8,000–15,000 r. produced over 95% sterility of older male pupae; and female pupae of all ages were completely sterilized by exposure to 1,000 r. However, the treatment caused pupal mortality ranging from 23 to 64%, with young pupae suffering the higher mortality, though survival among resulting adults was reduced less severely at the lower doses. In contrast, adult males exposed to 8,000–16,000 r. shortly after emergence were 95% sterile and survived as well as untreated flies. Dean, Dame and Birkenmeyer (1969) also found that radiosterilized males were sexually competitive with untreated laboratory-emerged males both in small cages in the laboratory and in larger field cages in the natural habitat. Similar results were obtained in the laboratory with pupae and adults of *G. morsitans* irradiated with Caesium-137 (Itard, 1968), pupae of *G. pallidipes* irradiated with Cobalt-60 (Dean & Clements, 1969) and adult *G. austeni* exposed to Cobalt-60 (Curtis, 1968).

Chemosterilization of *Glossina* was first attempted by Chadwick (1964) who reported that treatment with the alkylating agents apholate and metepa caused excessive mortality of *G. morsitans* at substerilizing doses. Also, Dame and Ford (unpublished data) found that injections of apholate or hempa of as much as 10 and 50 μg., respectively, per fly failed to produce complete sterility in male *G. morsitans*, and the higher doses caused excessive mortality; however, metepa and tepa sterilized male *G. morsitans* without undue mortality when they were injected at doses of 5 and 1 μg. per fly, respectively. In subsequent tests adult males were permanently sterilized by contact with 10 mg. per square foot of tepa or metepa on glass surfaces for 30 or 60 minutes and length of life was not seriously affected. However, flies exposed for shorter periods to 10 mg. tepa per square foot recovered some fertility after an initial sterile period, and exposures of 120 minutes or longer to either tepa or metepa reduced longevity. Also, autosterilization was complete when freshly-emerged flies walked *ad libitum* over a glass surface treated with 10 mg. tepa per square foot while they were *en route* to an exit from the holding chamber. Subsequently, Dame (unpublished data) found that adult males sprayed directly with either tepa or metepa (0·25 ml. of 5% solution in methanol per container of 25–50 flies) were sterilized. Pupae were treated by a 60-second immersion in 5% tepa or metepa in a 50% aqueous methanol solution; flies emerging during the first two weeks after treatment were sterilized by contact with their own puparium, although flies emerging after that period were not completely sterile. In general, freshly-emerged adults are less tolerant to chemosterilization than older flies, but it is usually possible to minimize this effect by reduced exposure of the young flies. Adults sterilized either by contact or exposure to sprays were competitive with other untreated laboratory-emerged flies in small cages in the laboratory, in larger field cages in the natural habitat, and in free flight field releases. Males sterilized by treatment as pupae were competitive in the laboratory, but no field tests have been made.

Pupal sterilization has advantages. Dame, Birkenmeyer and Bursell (1969) found that flies survived well when they actually emerged in the natural habitat. Also, pupal sterilization avoids the problem of handling active adult flies. Irradiation of the pupal stage reduces emergence and often results in some residual fertility unless the pupae are young when they are treated, but the degree of residual fertility (as much as 5%) might not seriously affect a control programme because of the low innate reproductive capacity of the genus. A more serious difficulty would be the diminished sterility which is demonstrable in flies emerging two weeks after chemosterilant treatment in the laboratory. In the field, the effective period would be further reduced by degradation or loss of the water soluble sterilants because of atmospheric conditions. There is at present no completely satisfactory method of separating male and female *Glossina* in the pupal stage but, in the case of pupae of known age, the sexes can be separated with some degree of accuracy by taking advantage of the shorter mean developmental period of the female pupae. Phelps and Burrows (1969a) found that at 26°C, the mean developmental period of puparia for female and male *G. morsitans* was 25 and 27 days, respectively, and Dame (unpublished data) found that when laboratory-reared *G. morsitans* were held at 26°C, 86% and 24% of the female and male emergence, respectively, occurred by the 25th day after larviposition. Thus, at this time, the desired minimum mating ratio of 1 male to each 4 females (Dame and Ford, 1968) was achieved, and the remaining pupae could be used for release with a loss of only 14% of the females. In the absence of an efficient method for their separation, both sexes would probably have to be treated to obtain sterile males. In practice, this method of handling would reduce the number of fertile females available for colony replenishment and could limit a release programme. The degree of such limitation was considered by Jordan and Curtis (personal communication); they calculated that high loss of females in an efficient colony would be relatively unimportant to the maintenance of a fixed rate of pupal production. However, in a less efficient colony only minor losses could be tolerated, and the ability to separate the sexes in the pupal stage might be critical.

Sterilization of adult flies also has advantages. Although the procedure involves much handling, the flies can be immobilized with carbon dioxide or nitrogen gas (Birkenmeyer & Dame, unpublished data) or by using lowered temperatures. Also, complete sterility of adults can be obtained with chemosterilants and 95% sterility with irradiation. A major difficulty of adult treatment is the need to provide a blood meal; survival was reduced when flies that emerged in captivity were released unfed (Dame & Birkenmeyer, unpublished data). The physiological and behavioural effects of holding *Glossina* in captivity are not thoroughly understood, but Langley (1966; *see* also 1967 and Chapter 12) showed that *G. morsitans* held in captivity failed to metabolize the blood meal properly, and Dame, Birkenmeyer and Bursell (1969) demonstrated that captive adults failed to develop normal flight musculature. Furthermore, both sterile and untreated captive adults survived poorly in the field compared with native flies even when they were fed before release (Dame & Birkenmeyer, unpublished data). The possibility of other defects in fly quality resulting from the abnormal environment of emergence and from confinement in the adult stage cannot be disregarded.

Sterilization of native populations of *Glossina* would avoid some of the problems associated with treatment of pupae and adults and would eliminate the necessity of releasing large numbers of sterile males into the environment. In the laboratory, male and female *Glossina* as much as three weeks old have been sterilized without serious side effects, and there is no reason to believe that the sterilization of native males of unknown ages would result in undesirable side effects. Obviously chemosterilization is the most suitable and versatile method for such an approach, but effective chemosterilants are rapidly degraded under field conditions and would have to be reapplied at intervals not exceeding a few days. In addition, a prolonged programme of sterilization in the field might result in the development of resistance to the sterilants. Laboratory exposure of *Aedes aegypti* (L.) to substerilizing doses of apholate for several generations resulted in a substantial degree of resistance (Hazard *et al.*, 1964). Thus, techniques of field sterilization must minimize this possibility by ensuring proper exposure of *Glossina* to adequate levels of sterilant. However, the major difficulty in treating native populations is the mutagenic activity of chemicals currently available; they are potentially capable of affecting any living organism. A field application must therefore be selective to ensure that only the target species would contact the sterilant. Such selectivity could probably be achieved by using an attractant for *Glossina* in combination with a sterilant.

Perhaps the most satisfactory attractant for *Glossina* currently available is the live host animal. Thus control of local populations might be achieved by attracting the individual native flies to bait animals tethered in shelters treated with chemosterilants. Another possibility is the ingestion of chemosterilant by *Glossina* feeding on treated bait animals, e.g. Eddy *et al.* (1965) succeeded in sterilizing *A. aegypti* by introducing chemosterilant into the blood of host mice. The difficulty with such an approach is that the chemicals currently available usually kill the host animal when they are administered in quantities that are sufficient to sterilize ectoparasites and, unfortunately, remain available in the blood for only a few hours. The development of effective chemical or physical attractants for *Glossina* is essential if native populations are to be sterilized directly.

Even with suitable attractant-sterilant devices, sterile males may have to be released to obtain complete eradication. Certainly, sterile males would be needed if behavioural selection resulted in an insufficient proportion of flies in the residual population being responsive to the attractant. Thus, the need for mass production of *Glossina* for work of this kind cannot be dismissed.

POPULATION DYNAMICS AND BEHAVIOUR

Information about the seasonal fluctuations in feeding, dispersal, mating behaviour, reproductive status, birth and death rates, and length of life of the target species, and about the interaction of these and other factors with population density is particularly important when sterilization is to be used for population control. The knowledge is necessary to evaluate the fluctuations in density and reproductive viability of the target population throughout the year and to estimate the relative viability of the released sterile male.

Releases programmed to meet the needs of an entire region would require the widespread distribution of sterile flies that would be expected to migrate successfully into concentrations of the native population. A large proportion of these released sterile flies would therefore be subjected to unusual stresses because of the atypical localities in which they would be released, and from which they would have to migrate to the foci of populations. Moreover, the resident population inhabits suitable niches, but the released fly is likely to be at a disadvantage because it must rapidly find both a suitable habitat and a host animal; those sterile males that were unable to find a host animal would be unlikely to survive long enough to mature sexually and thus might not affect the reproductive capacity of the native population. Thus, maximum ability of the released flies to disperse is essential if they are to obtain a blood meal and to mate. At times when resident fly dispersal is minimum, the released fly would be under maximum stress because its dispersal capabilities would similarly be restricted. Obviously, species behaviour, host dispersal, and environmental conditions would exert pressures that would be apt to affect the released population more than the resident population. Adequate ecological knowledge in such situations would be invaluable in rational planning: it would make it possible to schedule the initial releases at the times most favourable for the survival and dispersal of the sterile males. Also, in unfavourable periods, the rate of release might have to be doubled to compensate for losses and to obtain the desired overflooding ratio. Less favourable seasons should coincide with the later stages of a release programme, if possible, because it is more economical to increase small than large release numbers. These considerations could easily apply to populations of *G. morsitans*. In contrast, with species such as *G. palpalis* whose habitats are normally restricted, these considerations would have minimum influence because releases could be specifically directed at restricted habitats. Indeed, *G. palpalis*, which is known to move over extensive linear distances daily in its riverine habitat, might be an excellent target species because minimum losses and maximum mating potential could be expected as a result of the high rate of dispersal and the restricted habitat.

Estimates of existing population trends before, during, and after the release programme play a major role in any release operation. Female longevity, reproductive status, and mating behaviour can be monitored by determining the physiological age and the proportion of captured specimens that are inseminated (Saunders, 1960b). Also, marking and recapture techniques (Jolly, 1965; Seber, 1965) can provide relatively accurate estimates of birth rates, death rates, longevity, and population density when they are used in conjunction with the existing fly-round techniques in areas of medium to heavy density. Other methods are required when population levels are low. A system of sentinel animals used to detect *Trypanosoma* might be effective in such areas when only one vector exists, but its usefulness would be limited in areas inhabited by more than one species of *Glossina*. As noted, an effective attractant for *Glossina* would be most useful in the detection of low density populations but none is currently available.

Males of *Glossina* are known to inseminate many females under laboratory conditions. Recent studies have demonstrated that females of *G. morsitans* (Dame & Ford, 1968) and *G. austeni* (Curtis, 1968) will accept multiple insemination in the laboratory, the incidence of secondary pairings being about 30%, but this figure may be much lower in the field. Also, females mated by both sterile and fertile males sometimes produced viable offspring and sometimes failed to reproduce. Dame and Ford (1966, 1968) found that sterile sperm were competitive with untreated sperm; the only apparent difference was that dominant lethality had been induced in the treated sperm. Actually, the multiple mating of *Glossina* should not seriously affect control in the field as long as the sterile sperm are competitive with sperm from the native population (von

Borstel, 1960): in a native population overflooded by sterile males, females would have the same mathematical chance of encountering sterile males for second matings as they had for first matings. For example, in a population of three sterile males and one native male, the female has a 3:1 chance of pairing with a sterile male at each mating. Perhaps population control would take slightly longer because of the influence of normal sperm in a female inseminated with both normal and sterile sperm, but control should not be seriously affected. The successful use of sterile melon flies in an eradication programme (Steiner *et al.*, 1965) demonstrated that multiple mating by females is not necessarily a deterrent to the control of native insect populations by the release of sterile males. Indeed, multiple mating may sometimes enhance the rate of control because the reproductive capacity of previously inseminated females may be immediately reduced when these females mate with sterile males (Knipling, 1964). If the females did not accept such second matings, only death would end their reproductive potential, and population control would be limited to sterile matings with virgin females. Multiple mating by males would be detrimental to the technique only if the sterile male behaved abnormally or failed to inseminate as many females as its native counterpart. Laboratory studies indicate that the sterile males mate normally.

If sterile males behave normally in the field as well as in the laboratory will they also act as efficient vectors of trypanosomes? The question has importance because a sterile male release programme might initially treble the number of potential vectors in the control area, although the increase would be transient and could end transmission altogether when eradication was complete. Moreover, it is likely that sterile flies will be used as a supplement to prior suppressive measures, as already noted, and if the natural population destroyed is replaced by fewer reared and sterilized insects, the hazard in the control area at least should not exceed that of the original natural population. Dame and MacKenzie (1968) found that chemosterilized male *G. morsitans* were capable of transmitting *T. congolense* to uninfected hosts, but the incidence of transmission was reduced 50% when the males were sterilized with tepa before they became infected, and 75% when they were sterilized after becoming infected. Thus, liberated chemosterilized males could cause a temporary increase in transmission over that of the suppressed population (though perhaps substantially less than the rate of the uncontrolled population). However, if direct sterilization of native males can eventually be achieved, a lower rate of transmission might be expected because of the immediate effect of the sterilant on the parasite within the vector.

REARING TSETSE FLIES

An efficient system of rearing the target species is a requisite for a sterile male release programme which may require thousands or hundreds of thousands of sterile males per month (Table 26.2), depending upon the scope of control envisaged. Achievement of such numbers might require colonies capable of producing three times as many pupae as the number of sterile males actually required.

As an example, if a colony of *Glossina* produced 332,000 each month, they would probably be used as follows:

	Males	Females
non-viable pupae	16,500	16,500
handling losses	16,500	16,500
colony maintenance	33,000	133,000
release	100,000	—
	166,000	166,000

The figures for nonviable pupae and handling losses are maximum estimates; refinement of methods would be expected to reduce these losses considerably. The 33,000 males listed for maintenance of the colony reflect the ability of male *G. morsitans* to copulate with more than one female. However, after a mean of four matings, both the number and quality of sperm transferred per mating decreases (Dame & Ford, 1968). Thus, the 33,000 males used to inseminate the colony females could not be used for releases because of their mating experience and their advanced age. Then, for releases of 100,000 sterile males, (38% of the total pupal production) overall production would have to approximate 332,000 pupae. At a rate of production of 2·0–2·5 pupae per female per month a self-sustaining colony of 133,000–166,000 females would be necessary.

Means of maintaining self-sustaining colonies of *Glossina* are discussed elsewhere (Chapter 20). Potential rearing systems include the maintenance of individuals or groups in tubes or cages in the laboratory, in larger outdoor cages, or in unenclosed areas of the natural habitat. Although flies have been maintained in outdoor cages with some degree of reproductive success (Harley, personal communication), self-sustaining outdoor colonies have not been achieved (Phelps & Dean, personal communication). The harvesting of pupae from natural breeding areas in which dense populations of *Glossina* exist has been one of the main sources of pupae for general research. If conditions are optimum, these pupae can be hand-collected in the natural environment for approximately 3s 6d per pupa (Dame, unpublished data), an expenditure within the limits given by Knipling as being economically reasonable for the control of low density populations. Also, Phelps *et al.* (1966) harvested over a million pupae in four years from naturally infested areas without any obvious effect on the population of *Glossina*. Even if large numbers of pupae can be collected in the field at reasonable expense, this method of obtaining insects for sterilization may prove to be unsuitable because of seasonal variation in availability and quality of pupae; however, Potts (1965) believes that this method could be successfully exploited.

Because tsetse flies behave erratically in medium to large cages, large scale rearing projects will probably be based on small cage techniques. Successful reproduction has already been achieved by using guinea-pigs, rabbits, goats, sheep, or cattle as hosts for flies held in small containers or cages. The advances made by Southon and Cockings (1963) with membrane feeding may eventually eliminate the need to maintain extensive colonies of small animals. With suitable membrane-feeding techniques, a colony capable of producing 100,000 sterile males per month would need to ingest only 5–6 litres of blood per day.

Langley (1966; *see* also Langley, 1967 and Chapter 12) showed that adult *G. morsitans* held in captivity did not digest the blood meal properly, possibly because of the effects of enforced inactivity; also, this same species may fail to develop the normal flight musculature when it is held in captivity. However, Jordan *et al.* (1967) succeeded in rearing *G. austeni* that equalled the native fly in both size and productivity. Thus, economical large-scale rearing of some species may be possible once the basic requirements for maintaining colonies are established. Of course, an inherent defect in such colonies is the possibility that the behavioural characteristics necessary for survival in nature may be lost while establishing a strain that is suitable for perpetuation indoors. For example, the behaviour of *Anopheles quadrimaculatus* Say changed when maintained in a colony (Dame *et al.*, 1964). Similar detrimental selection could occur in any such artificial conditions and Dame and Azevedo (unpublished data) detected differences in the feeding behaviour of laboratory-reared and wild males of *G. morsitans*. However, laboratory-reared screw-worm flies and fruit flies have been used successfully in sterile male release programmes. The possibility of developing selection procedures and rearing techniques that will preserve or even increase the competitiveness of males when released should be considered as one of the ultimate goals in the development of the sterile insect release procedure.

Whether a laboratory strain of *G. m. orientalis* could be used to control *G. m. morsitans* or *G. m. submorsitans* would depend not only on the adaptation of *G. m. orientalis* to laboratory conditions but also on the behavioural differences between the strains in nature. Glasgow (1963) postulated that hybrid sterility might result with such intraspecific crosses and that this mechanism would prevent coexistence. However, his interpretation does not exclude the possibility of overflooding populations of *G. m. morsitans* or *G. m. submorsitans* with sterile male *G. m. orientalis*. Dame (unpublished data) has shown that sterile male *G. m. orientalis* achieved normal rates of insemination with female *G. m. morsitans* with a resultant 100% reduction in reproduction.

Chapter 27

Control by Clearing of Vegetation

J. FORD, T. A. M. NASH, J. R. WELCH

TOTAL CLEARING

Total, sheer or ruthless clearing means the destruction of all trees and shrubs in the area treated. It is a completely effective method of eliminating *Glossina* and the oldest. The earliest useful statement about tsetse control seems to have been that of Andersson (1856) who hunted along the Taokhe River in Ngamiland. The Taokhe River is usually dry and consists of a wide grass-covered corridor down the southern side of the Okovango swamps kept treeless by periodical flooding. It greatly resembles some of the immense barrier clearings that used to be cut across country in East Africa in the hope of arresting the spread of *Glossina morsitans*. Andersson wrote 'The tsetse is found chiefly in the bush or amongst reeds,[1] but rarely in the open country. Thus cattle may be seen grazing securely on one side of a river, while the opposite bank swarms with the insect.' The classical studies of bush clearing are those of C. F. M. Swynnerton whose enquiries into Ngoni methods of land occupation led him to organize the great tribal turn-outs in the Shinyanga area of Tanzania to halt the spread of *Glossina swynnertoni* (Swynnerton, 1921; 1925), and of other species in other areas (Swynnerton, 1936).

In clearings of this type all trees and shrubs are cut down and, if possible, destroyed by up-rooting and burning of stumps. It is a process made easier and often cheaper by bull-dozing. Arboricides may also be used. The aim is to replace bush or woodland by treeless grassland. Total clearing may be applied over wide areas of country against tsetse of the *morsitans* group or, confined to river banks, against the *palpalis* group. In the latter case it has been criticized

[1] 'Amongst reeds' is very misleading. In the accepted sense of the phrase tsetse do not breed or live amongst reeds, although individuals may be encountered there.

as conducive to bank erosion but the observations of Glasgow and Duffy (1949) and of Nash (1948a) suggest that the grass that replaces the trees and shrubs may be a better protection against 'lateral scour' than is the natural vegetation. Where total clearing is used in savanna country there is much evidence that removal of bush is followed by increased grass growth and improved pasture potential. Experience in Tanzania suggests that removal of trees may be followed by a rise in level of the water table.

During the period of recovery of the East African fly-belts after the recessions induced by rinderpest and, also, of the invasion of land that had become under-occupied from the action of a variety of depopulating agencies (epidemics, famines, colonial wars) between 1890 and 1920, much attention was given to barrier clearings. It was thought that corridors of open grassland, a mile or so in width, cut across the path of the 'advancing' fly-belts might provide barriers to further spread of tsetse. The writer is unable to recall any example of this sort of barrier that was effective in stopping a 'fly advance'. The researches of Lloyd (1935) and of Moggridge (1936) on the crossing of open clearings by *G. swynnertoni* have been discussed by Buxton (1955) and Swynnerton (1936). In certain circumstances clearings of this sort were used to break up fly-belts into smaller components for experimental purposes or to assist programming of control projects over periods of years. Bax (1943–44) gives a good account of past thinking on these lines.

Extensive cleared corridors have also been used to reduce the risk of cattle on stock routes or road users being bitten by tsetse. At Shinyanga very large areas of potential seasonal pasture were cut off from the local cattle population by the *G. swynnertoni* fly-belt. A mile-wide corridor, also serving to reduce movement of tsetse between experimental blocks, allowed cattle to reach these pastures with little risk of infection. During the 1939–45 War a few cases of Rhodesian sleeping sickness were found among troops who had travelled by road through the *G. morsitans* belt between Kondoa and Arusha in Tanzania. A clearing along the Great North Road appeared to have achieved the purpose for which it was intended and trypanosomiasis never became a problem among the troops using this road. In a similar fashion a mile-wide barrier clearing running for thirty miles along the Mbarara-Masaka road in western Uganda, which had failed to stop the spread of *G. morsitans*, was subsequently maintained for many years in order to prevent tsetse from reaching, and being carried by, traffic along the road.

Total clearing may also be used to construct 'defence lines' (Bax, *loc. cit.*). The area between country in which tsetse is excluded by settlement and the fly-bush is usually covered by a zone in which the natural vegetation is only partially destroyed and in which the natural hosts of tsetse are reduced in number but not entirely excluded. People and cattle tend to move into this interzone for various purposes. A defence line consists of a zone, usually about a mile wide, which is cleared and kept clear between a sharply defined bush edge and the fully occupied land. It eliminates the interzone into which game and tsetse may wander. A defence line of this pattern has existed for many years along a thirty mile section of the Rhodesia-Mozambique border. Its construction was claimed to have raised the value of adjacent farmland from 10s to £10 per acre (Thomas, Davey & Potts, 1955). Its maintenance is accepted as a charge against the Government. In some situations defence lines have been supplemented by partial clearing to form a defence in depth (*see* also p. 533).

Where land is to be freed of tsetse in order to assist farm development total clearing has great advantages. It is effective as an anti-tsetse measure; it relieves the future occupiers of the great burden of bush clearing and, provided that subsequent usages follow a properly designed rotation, pasture is greatly improved. Another advantage is that the work of clearing does not require constant expert supervision by entomological staff. It can be carried out by contractors using highly sophisticated machinery or by cooperative effort of peasant farmers using simple hand tools.

PARTIAL CLEARING IN WEST AFRICA

Total or ruthless clearing of riverine vegetation has long been recognized as an effective method of eliminating the tsetse fly. This method was in regular use up to the 1930s when the newer and more refined technique of partial clearing was introduced. Thereafter, ruthless clearing was reserved for the protection of important fords and isolated villages with a bad history of sleeping sickness while the new partial clearing technique was employed for aggressive campaigns designed to eradicate tsetse from whole river systems, starting when possible at the source.

Partial clearing is a method of tsetse control which has proved effective for the eradication of *G. tachinoides* and *G. palpalis* from the streams and rivers of the West African savanna woodlands. In recent years, this method has been largely superseded by the much cheaper technique of spraying insecticides on the riverine vegetation but it would be premature to consider partial clearing as an obsolete method. One great advantage of partial clearing is that it requires nothing more than man-power and a modicum of intelligence. An impoverished country faced by epidemic sleeping sickness could fall back on its man-power, made freely available in an emergency. Residual insecticides are still in their infancy and virtually nothing is yet known about the long-term effects of their use. Instances have been recorded from both West and East Africa of tsetse re-appearing in areas from which they were thought to have been eradicated by the use of insecticides (Kernaghan, 1961; Glover, 1963; Davies, 1964). If repeated applications of insecticides prove to be necessary, a build-up could occur which might have serious effects on the fauna, including man, fishes and pollinating insects.

The earliest record of partial clearing in Nigeria is in a little known paper by Moiser (1912). He removed only the undergrowth from a forest island at Geidam, the most northerly point reached by *G. tachinoides*; a month later only five flies were found in the forest island, and twelve in the adjacent thick bush. He concluded that 'the presence of undergrowth (as well as shady trees) is a necessary condition in the habitation of *G. tachinoides*.' Twenty-one years later, at Gadau which is some 150 miles up-river from Geidam, Buxton and Lewis spent six months investigating *G. submorsitans* and *G. tachinoides*, mainly in the laboratory, and Nash started his ecological studies. From laboratory findings and meteorological data collected in the hottest month, Buxton and Lewis (1934) suggested that the temperature in the late dry season must be close to lethal and that the clearing of undergrowth might kill large numbers of flies.

In the ensuing years studies on the climate and microclimates in relation to the survival, longevity and distribution of both adults and pupae were made at Gadau by Nash (1935, 1936, 1936a, 1937, 1939). The results indicated that in the severe late dry season longevity is minimal, and that even by resting in the heat of the day on the forest floor both *G. tachinoides* and *G. submorsitans* live close to their upper critical temperature zone (39–41°C).

An investigation into the effects of partial clearing on climate and tsetse was begun by Nash in early 1936, when a barrier 330 yards wide was cleared between two forest islands which formed late dry season sanctuaries for the local fly communities; owing to the inadequacy of the barrier, the efficacy of the clearing was assessed by its effect on fly in the hot weather. Data were collected from both islands for a control period of eighteen months; then the peripheral thicket windbreak of *Acacia ataxacantha*[1] was removed from the 10 acre (4 hectare) experimental forest island, so as to allow the entry of the hot dry wind from the savanna; this was followed by a considerable reduction in the size of the *G. tachinoides* population. A year later, clumps of seedling trees, mainly ebony (*Diospyros mespiliformis*) were thinned by hoeing but not a tree over 4 feet in height was destroyed. By the end of the dry season, *G. tachinoides* had been virtually exterminated, probably due to the increased severity of the climate recorded in both adult and pupal environments. Throughout the entire experiment, the *G. tachinoides* population of the control forest island remained high. *G. submorsitans* did not appear to be seriously affected by these measures (Nash, 1940).

Meanwhile, a similar investigation was being undertaken along 200 miles of stream in Anchau District, near Zaria, where the climate was much less severe than at Gadau. Whereas at both Gadau and Geidam the fly population was restricted by climate to a river plain leading to Lake Chad and was still further restricted in the late dry season to the forest islands, at Anchau *G. tachinoides* was ubiquitous along the numerous streams and was only restricted seasonally to the reaches which held water. (On average, there was a linear mile of stream to each square mile of country.)

Under the more equable climatic conditions at Anchau, it was found that a more severe type of partial clearing was required. In addition to cutting out the thicket, all low-branching shade trees had to be felled. By sparing the clean boled trees, many of them huge mahoganies, the clearing costs were halved. Providing no diminutive tributary or tiny thicket was overlooked, this degree of partial clearing resulted in the complete eradication of *G. tachinoides* and *G. palpalis*. Europeans, with no botanical knowledge, and illiterate headmen were easily taught to judge by eye how much they should spare. To prevent wet season reinfestation from the point where the partial clearing stopped, it was essential to construct a ruthless barrier clearing in which every tree was felled. The barrier had to be a straight mile in length, not a mile measured

[1] Misnamed *Dichrostachys platycarpa* in early publications.

round sinuous bends; it therefore paid to site the barrier where the stream ran fairly straight and had no tributaries (Nash, 1940). It was later found that barrier clearings on rivers have to be considerably longer than on streams.

The partial clearing technique devised at Anchau has been described in some detail by Nash (1948a). Briefly, an advance gang of, say, seventy-five men armed with machetes clear the shrubs and undergrowth; behind them come some seventy-five men armed with axes who fell the low-branching trees, and lastly the rearguard of about 150 'pilers' who build bonfires over the stumps which are subsequently ignited. Piling and burning reduces regeneration, and greatly facilitates the annual re-slashing. The costs for 450 linear miles of stream, including barriers, averaged 660 man-days per mile and 46–66 man-days per mile for the annual re-slashing. In fact, most of the re-slashing was undertaken by unpaid communal labour; as sleeping sickness had been rife in the area they maintained their own village clearings. If slashed annually, it takes about seven years for the stumps to become exhausted.

Using the techniques described, the Nigerian Sleeping Sickness Service, between 1938 and 1958, rendered over 6,600 miles of stream and river tsetse-free (Steiner, 1964).

In Ghana the partial clearing concept was approached in a different manner, and was referred to as 'selective' clearing. The veterinary headquarters at Pong Tamale are situated on a ridge three miles above the Naboggo river which annually floods its plain; the floods used to drive *G. tachinoides* inland to form secondary foci in every patch of cover until the tsetse spread right into the veterinary farm. Starting in 1931, Stewart spent six years clearing the river. In the earlier years the clearing was ruthless, but later he appreciated that it was unnecessary to be so severe. Having completed the clearing of streams and rivers, totalling eighty miles, he wrote an account of his campaign which ended with three lists of trees—(a) twenty-five species which must be cleared as they form the fringing forest, (b) thirty-one species growing between the dry season banks and the upper flood level which sometimes have to be cleared, and (c) fourteen species, usually with high clean boles, occurring mainly between the primary and secondary river banks, which rarely need to be felled (Stewart, 1937).

Morris (1944, 1946) introduced to Ghana the principle of clearing vegetation strictly according to species and not according to the growth form of individuals belonging to a species. His Group I consisted of twenty-three species of 'essential fly-belt trees, forming dry-season habitat', which were always cut down; in practice, rarely more than four to nine of these species were found together in any plant association forming a primary fly focus (Morris, 1946). His Group II consisted of twenty-two species which commonly form wet-season dispersal habitats, but are not essential to the formation of the dry-season habitat; species of this group were never destroyed.

After visiting many of Morris' clearings, Nash (1948a) commented on how, owing to the preponderance of Group I trees in the riverine vegetation and insistence that even harmless individuals among the species in this group must be felled, the clearings were far more ruthless than he had expected. He suggested that the method was inelastic; harmless, high-branching individuals of species in Group I had to be destroyed and dangerous low-branching individuals of Group II had to be spared. He instanced the ebony, *Diospyros mespiliformis*, which certainly belongs to Group II when a clean-boled adult, but should be placed in Group I when clumps of its seedlings form thicket. This subject was reviewed in some detail by Buxton (1955) who after visiting the Nigerian and Ghanaian clearings concluded that 'the difference lies in the individual's approach to the subject, and in effect is not great'.

Morris (1946) did not make barrier clearings. He checked regeneration by stumping and burning, and not by annual reslashing. By March 1945, 176 miles of river and stream in Lawra District had been selectively cleared at a cost, excluding stumping, of 600 man-days per mile; in that area there was 0·18 mile of permanently infested stream to each square mile of country rendered fly-free. Rather similar work, in part inspired by Morris, was carried out in savanna areas in what was formerly French West Africa (Buxton, 1955).

PARTIAL CLEARING IN EAST AFRICA

Hocking *et al.* (1963) gave a list of the methods for the control or eradication of tsetse flies and partial clearing, as considered here, covers those methods of indirect action against the flies which involve the removal of part of the vegetation in the fly habitat. These methods were foreshadowed by Swynnerton (1936) and have been used extensively and successfully in Tanzania, so all the examples given below refer to that country. Potts (1930) developed the idea of the fly-round as a method of studying the distribution of tsetse flies and results obtained from fly-rounds have led various authors to the idea that tsetse flies tend to 'concentrate' in certain combinations of woody vegetation. The original fly-rounds were divided subjectively into vegetational sectors but a more objective method was put forward by Ford *et al.* (1959), which enables the 'concentration areas' of the non-teneral male flies to be determined. Partial clearing was based on the modification of the vegetation in these concentration areas and it has achieved a considerable measure of success in Tanzania. Two distinct types of partial clearing are recognized. *Discriminative* clearing involves the removal of all woody vegetation in those plant communities in which fly-rounds and vegetational surveys showed this concentration to exist. *Selective* clearing is the modification of the environment by the removal of certain elements of the plant community. This is discussed in more detail below, but may involve the removal of the upper canopy, the understorey or even particular species of trees.

There was a tendency to make an unrealistic separation of various methods of tsetse and trypanosomiasis control but this is no longer the case in Tanzania. Under present conditions schemes are considered from all angles and a particular scheme may involve a combination of several methods of control of both vector and parasite. Insecticide spraying from the ground or from the air may be combined with discriminative, selective or sheer clearing and with chemotherapy or prophylaxis. In earlier days the aim was complete eradication but the emphasis is now on control. When control has been achieved and transmission cycles have been broken, correct husbandry practices will lead to the final elimination of trypanosomiasis.

Recent work by Pilson and Pilson (1967) and Bursell (1966a) would seem to cast doubt on the underlying principles of partial clearing. It may be that the original theory on which partial clearing was based is incorrect but the fact that this method has been so successful in so many different areas is proof that, in some way not yet known, the concentration areas are parts of the habitat essential to the flies at some period in their life history. The results of one, admittedly biassed, method of sampling cannot be said to be refuted by the results of another biassed method until that has been tested objectively and over a wider range than has yet been done (*see* also p. 298).

Until about fifteen years ago, much of the anti-tsetse work in Tanzania was done by a system of sheer or total clearing, often with its attendant problems of soil erosion. Even when the decision to change to partial clearing was made, the shortage of trained staff meant that, in many urgent cases, sheer clearing was still used. Nevertheless, partial clearing was used whenever possible and sheer clearing has now been almost abandoned. It has been said that partial clearing is an art rather than a science and much of the work done in Tanzania has depended on the subjective judgment of experienced officers. Successes were often achieved by officers with no scientific training, but with the ability to distinguish vegetation types and to use empirical methods to decide on those communities which needed to be removed or modified. The research scientist might be appalled by the paucity of the data collected before schemes were started, but it must be realized that, in many cases, the problems were urgent, there was little time for the collection of data to determine the most economic methods and, provided that the flies were eradicated, there were no criticisms if too much vegetation was cleared. Much of the early work was done by tribal turn-out or by famine relief labour and the main point was to use the plentiful supply of labour to do a useful piece of work. Some schemes failed because of the inexperience of the officers in charge or of insufficient preliminary survey, but the number which succeeded is a tribute to the 'eye for country' possessed by the officers concerned.

Since those days there have been a great many changes. The two most important concern the concept of trypanosomiasis control in place of tsetse eradication, and the necessity for economies in the conduct of this control. Under present conditions it is no longer necessary to remove every tsetse fly. With better case-finding organization and techniques it is now feasible to introduce settlement into a sleeping sickness area whilst some flies still remain. If the numbers of flies can be reduced to a level where the transmission cycle is broken, the people can move in, as a calculated risk, with careful observations being maintained on both flies and people. A similar consideration applies to cattle. Where fly densities are very low it may be justifiable to introduce cattle on curative regimes alone but, where more flies are present, prophylaxis may be necessary. Successful ranching is being practised in areas which are not completely free of flies. Labour is no longer as cheap and plentiful as it used to be. 'Self-help' or 'nation-building' labour, which took the place of the tribal turn-outs, has been shown to be uneconomic as the quality and quantity of effort does not justify the cost of the necessary rations. Paid labour has to be used for any effective hand-clearing operation and labour costs are now three to five times greater than they were ten years ago. Accordingly much more thought has to be given to the economics of any scheme and it has to be decided if the expected benefits will justify the cost of the scheme.

Many schemes which were successful in eradicating testse flies failed in that the land reclaimed was not taken up, the bush regenerated and the flies returned; in some cases this has happened more than once in the same area. However, in a number of cases, a few pioneers took up land and were so successful that other people followed their example and momentum gradually built up, often leading to the position where no more specific reclamation was necessary as the people continued the same methods themselves without supervision.

All the above points are relevant to an appreciation of the present position in Tanzania. Many more trained junior staff are now available and much more detailed survey is possible. There are still difficulties in determining whether a particular scheme is needed and in ensuring that the land will be used properly after anti-tsetse work is complete. Research is still going on in the field to determine the minimum treatments by insecticides and clearing that are needed to control trypanosomiasis in a variety of different environments. The actual methods of reclamation still have to be decided by experienced officers but these officers are becoming fewer and it is hoped that research work at present in progress will lead to more objective decisions being made and to the building up of information which will enable the less experienced officer to decide on which methods he should use.

Selective Clearing

As defined above, selective clearing is the modification of the environment by the removal of certain elements of the plant community. It arose from the observation that concentration areas were often found in plant communities with two or more canopies. Here research has lagged behind practical experience but it is known that flies are often found resting under branches with an uninterrupted downward view but with a canopy of branches at higher levels. There seem to be no publications on the relations between the densities of resting flies and the life-forms of the vegetation and this is a gap in knowledge which needs to be filled.

In most of the schemes in which selective clearing has been used the decision as to the exact method has been dictated more by practical considerations than by any scientific deductions. The felling of the upper canopy is usually the easier method and its effects last longer as it takes a longer time for regeneration to reach the stage where the area can again be occupied by tsetse. This method is useful where the remainder is likely to be cleared by cultivators or where the cleared area is more of a protective zone and is not likely to be occupied. The removal of the understorey is likely to be much more arduous and regeneration may be quicker but it has the advantage of retaining the shade of the clean-boled, tall trees and, since the ground is comparatively clean, it is more likely to encourage the less energetic settlers to move in. It has been found particularly effective for ranching areas. In this case the tall trees are required to provide shade for the cattle and to prevent erosion. All vegetation below five inches diameter at breast height is felled, the trash is piled over the cut stumps, left to dry and then burnt *in situ*. This destroys some of the parts of the woody vegetation likely to regenerate, kills the sticky, fire-resistant herbs and produces a layer of ash on which good grasses can grow. Regeneration can be kept down by the controlled use of fire and grazing, by mechanical means such as the Gyromor or by spot treatment of persistent species by rooting or by herbicides.

Selective clearing does not lend itself to mechanical methods and is usually done by hand labour. Mechanical saws have been tried in Tanzania but it was found that they could only be used effectively by expensive, skilled labour and their rate of deterioration was so rapid that their use had to be discontinued. It was more economical to use unskilled labour with ordinary hand tools.

Few of the partial clearing schemes in Tanzania have been completely documented and the accounts of the various schemes given below are incomplete because of omissions in the records. In some cases there are records of the amounts of land surveyed, cleared or reclaimed, the amount of labour used and the cost but few accounts contain all these items of information for any one particular scheme. Accordingly, none of the details given below is complete in every respect, but it is felt that some account of the schemes which have been successful will be useful. The classification of vegetation used is that given in Pratt *et al.* (1966). Most of the clearing was against *G. morsitans* and *G. swynnertoni*, though some work was also done against *G. pallidipes*.

In the semi-arid *Acacia* woodland and bushed grassland of eastern Irangi in Dodoma Region *G. morsitans* and *G. swynnertoni* were eradicated in country dominated by *Acacia tortilis* (Forsk.) Hayne by cleaning the thicketed parts of the understorey of the bushed grassland, but leaving the woodland untouched. This was part of a large scheme which also included some discriminative clearing. The method was also successfully applied in several other areas, notably in western Mbulu in Arusha Region and a small, similar scheme is now in progress in eastern Mbulu. It failed, however, in *Brachystegia/Julbernadia* woodland, where greater success was achieved by the removal of the upper canopy trees, leaving *Acacia* woodland and the Itigi type of bushland (Swynnerton, 1936; Burtt, 1942) untouched. Even this method failed in some areas and, in once case, *G. morsitans* was eradicated, but its place was taken by *G. swynnertoni*.

In deciduous wooded grassland in the West Lake Region the upper canopy consisted of *Parinari curatellifolia* Planch. ex Benth., *Acacia gerrardii* Benth. and/or *Pericopsis angolensis* (Bak.) van Meeuwen with an understorey dominated by *Acacia holstii* Taub. and *Combretum zeyheri* Sond. Felling of the upper storey species produced a 90% reduction in the density of *G. morsitans*, which was sufficient to break the transmission cycle of human trypanosomiasis.

A successful scheme where only one species was removed involved the cutting down of all *Acacia polyacantha* Willd. trees in *Borassus aethiopum* Mart. woodland, the difficulty here being the phenomenal rate of regeneration of the

A. polyacantha, which probably grows more rapidly than any other tree in Tanzania. In another case success was achieved by the removal of *Acacia nigrescens* Oliv., *A. goetzei* Harms subsp. *microphylla* Brenan, *Bussea massaiensis* (Taub.) Harms and *Commiphora ugogensis* Engl. around sparsely grassed glades on the lower step of the Rift Wall.

In all these cases the concentration areas of the flies were found from fly-round results and then empirical decisions as to how the clearings were to be carried out were made by experienced officers.

Discriminative Clearing

Discriminative clearing is the removal of all woody vegetation from certain plant communities, and this method is the one for which there are hopes of obtaining objective criteria on which to determine the areas to be cleared. The reasons why the clearing of the concentration areas results in the eradication of the flies are still not known, but the successful application of this method over considerable areas ensures that its use will continue. Since the procedure involves the removal of all woody vegetation within certain definable zones, it lends itself to mechanical methods. However, in Tanzania, funds and staff have never been sufficient to develop a mechanical clearing unit and contract clearing has not been completely successful. Where large areas are to be cleared for plantation crops, mechanical clearing is feasible, but the cost of transporting heavy equipment on contract prevents its use for specific anti-tsetse schemes where the financial returns are likely to be small. Mechanical clearing requires the support of a complete maintenance and overhaul organization and efficient control to make the most economic use of the machinery and this necessitates the employment of specialist staff for this purpose only. One instance of successful mechanical clearing is cited below but in all the others described hand clearing was used.

Usually the area to be cleared against *G. morsitans* and *G. swynnertoni* is that on the lower colluvial soils. This zone, which has been called the 'ecotone' or 'interzone' by various authors, is the area where the break occurs between, commonly, woodland or wooded grassland on the eluvial and upper colluvial zones and grassland, with or without trees, on the illuvial soils. It often contains numerous ant-hills, frequently supporting a thicketed bushland vegetation; the removal of the woody vegetation from this zone, leaving a clean edge to the woodland, usually leads to eradication of the flies or to effective reductions in fly density.

There is considerable evidence that *G. pallidipes*, although widespread during the rains, tends to withdraw to semi-evergreen forest and thicketed bushland during the dry season. The removal of this vegetation, mainly in drainage lines, has usually resulted in complete eradication of this species. Where the fly has persisted this has usually been due to immigration during the rains from untreated areas such as inaccessible gorges. In spite of considerable regeneration in some areas, this species takes several years to re-establish itself. There are areas where the clearing of semi-evergreen drainage line vegetation, consisting mainly of *Acacia brevispica* Willd. and *Grewia platyclada* K. Schum., designed to eliminate *G. pallidipes*, also removed *G. swynnertoni* and *G. morsitans* in spite of the presence of large, untouched areas of *Acacia tortilis* thicketed woodland.

Experimental clearing of drainage lines in the Tabora area was not always successful, but success was usually achieved when clearing was extended to include the lower colluvial zones. More experimental work on the subject is still necessary but it is likely that, in wide drainage lines, it is not necessary to clear the lower parts of the valleys to remove *G. morsitans*. In mainland Tanzania the areas of restricted drainage, locally termed 'mbuga' and of illuvial or, less frequently, alluvial origin, carry vegetation of various types, from open grassland to woodland. Lamerton (1962) has described the extreme case of this type, which is known as 'manda'. Even where the central part of the drainage line, which may or may not be on a sand ridge, is covered with woodland, there is usually a narrow grassland fringe. Tsetse flies attack fiercely within the woodland, yet they are effectively eradicated by clearing along the edges of the grassland fringe up to the ant-hill line on the lower colluvial slopes.

In the Tabora and Kigoma Regions early action against human trypanosomiasis was to carry out sheer clearing in restricted areas and to settle the people in these Sleeping Sickness Settlements. Expansion was slow, centrifugal and controlled, to minimize the man-fly contact. However, the soil soon became exhausted in the settlements and there were continual demands for expansion. These demands were met by linking the original settlements by discriminative clearing, a policy which was so successful that large areas of formerly testse-infested land are now safely occupied by the people.

The amounts of clearing necessary vary enormously with the country to be cleared. As stated above, the records are far from complete but such information as is available for a number of schemes has been included in the examples given below. In an area on the Rift Wall, where the upper storey trees were removed by selective clearing, this treatment was only needed over 13 square miles to eradicate the flies from a total area of 150 square miles. In Dodoma and Singida Regions the records show clearings, sheer, discriminative and selective carried out over an area of 610 square miles at a labour cost of three million man-days. Of course, only part of the 610 square miles was cleared and the total area released for settlement was 1,000 square miles. In a scheme of this size a certain amount of land is cleared which is not necessarily usable and this must be taken into account in considering these figures. It was formerly the custom to protect the perimeter of cleared areas by a belt of sheer clearing one mile in width but the practice now usually followed to prevent reinfestation is to continue discriminative clearing for a distance of two to four miles beyond the actual area of the scheme. In eastern Irangi 118 square miles were cleared discriminatively, i.e. only in parts of this area was the woody vegetation felled and this released a total of 260 square miles for the expenditure of 668,861 man-days. At Makatupora in Dodoma Region, 22 square miles of bush were treated by a mixture of discriminative and selective clearing at a cost of £13,000 and released 150 square miles of land. In one mechanical clearing scheme only 6 square miles were cleared by machinery but, with some tidying up by hand clearing, 200 square miles were reclaimed for settlement and largely occupied.

The examples cited above have been selected because at least some relevant data have been recorded but there have been many other successful schemes for which supporting data are not available. In the present state of knowledge, it seems probable that, in general terms, discriminative clearing requires the removal of 5–20% of the vegetation on the rolling country of the plateau of central and western Tanzania but, in the more dissected topography in the eastern part of the country, a greater proportion of the vegetation would have to be removed, perhaps up to 50%. However, there is as yet little experience of the latter area. In all areas it is likely that more precisely planned experimental reclamation would lead to further reductions in the amount of bush which it is necessary to clear.

In each of the areas described above the work took several years to complete and the system in use was often changed when the fall in the density of tsetse was insufficiently rapid. A typical example was one in which work started by felling only *Acacia rovumae* Oliv. in drainage lines. The density of flies decreased slowly and, because of local agitation, the technique had to be modified to the removal of all vegetation in the *Acacia rovumae*-dominated woodland. Reclamation by partial clearing does not have the immediate effects that are seen when insecticides are used. It may take as long as two years after the clearing is completed before fly densities reach their lowest levels, but the results are much more lasting and, even if the land is not developed, it may be anything from five to fifteen years before tsetse become re-established.

Except where reclamation is being carried out for large-scale commercial enterprises sociological considerations may have considerable bearing on the success or otherwise of a scheme. People are often reluctant to move into an area which they know was tsetse-infested and they are even more reluctant to move in their cattle until they are convinced that the methods used are really effective. This is one respect in which clearing is better than insecticide treatment in that, before this confidence has built up, any insecticide-treated area which is not effectively isolated will be reinfested before the people move in. The phenomenal success of the linking up of the Sleeping Sickness Settlements by discriminative clearing in western Tanzania, started in the 1950s, and the opening up of the eastern Irangi plains point the way to effective use of clearing to produce centrifugal enlargement of existing small settlements and to make inroads into the vast areas of infested bush which still exist.

Practical Considerations in Relation to Clearing Projects

Schemes for the control of tsetse by the clearing methods described above require careful planning based on all relevant data available. The greater the amount of information available, the greater will be the chances of success and, usually, the lower the cost. Only too often, valuable records in the form of reports and maps are lost or destroyed and it is sound practice to adopt a system of filing such information, by areas, and to ensure that copies of records are kept in different places as, for example, in district, regional and headquarter offices. Where information has to be acquired afresh it is important to ensure uniformity in coverage and a high standard of recording and reporting. In Tanzania, an attempt has been made to achieve these ends by preparing a

Tsetse Fly Control Manual which is intended to serve as a guide to field workers and a useful handbook for trainees. This Manual (still in course of preparation) covers such subjects as techniques for reconnaissance and survey, mapping, reclamation methods, etc., and recognizes the following sequence of operations in tsetse control schemes:

1. The Demand for Action.
2. The Preliminary Visit.
3. The Preliminary Report.
4. Reconnaissance.
5. The Reconnaissance Report.
6. Survey.
7. Periodic Survey Reports.
8. Decisions on Methods of Reclamation.
9. The Planning of Reclamation.
10. Reclamation.
11. Periodic Reclamation Reports.
12. Observation.
13. Periodic Observation Reports.
14. The Final Field Report.

The first three phases, ordinarily completed within a few weeks, provide a feasibility study from which it will be apparent whether or not the project is economically viable and, if so, the commitments which must be accepted if the scheme is to be successful.

If, on the basis of this feasibility study, the project is found to be viable and acceptable, a reconnaissance of the area to be reclaimed is undertaken. The area is divided into squares the sides of which measure one to five miles. Reconnaissance transects are done around the perimeter of each square and two others are done within each square along specific lines so placed as to be not quite diagonals of the square in order to avoid over-emphasizing data from the corners of the square. These reconnaissance transects fit in with the subsequent survey phase. In making a reconnaissance, the staff are encouraged to make diversions from the standard transect lines to investigate any prominent or unusual features of the area and to note such other important factors as the existence of villages and the availability of water supplies. The time ordinarily taken to reconnoitre and report upon a unit of fifty square miles is about five to six weeks.

Reconnaissance reports should record the itinerary followed and details of the area covered including descriptions of communications, climate, topography, soils, vegetation, game, tsetse flies, sleeping sickness, animal trypanosomiasis, water supplies, local agriculture, etc., together with the estimated cost of any subsequent survey that may be recommended. These reports should be accompanied by maps showing the approximate distribution of vegetation and tsetse flies within the area and accurately plotted vegetational changes along the transects. Exact maps can then be prepared by combining the information recorded on the field maps with that obtained from aerial photographs. Acreages of vegetation types can then be worked out.

The next phase, survey, involves more intensive investigation and is carried out over the whole of smaller areas or in selected parts of larger areas. In the case of *G. morsitans* and *G. swynnertoni*, spiral fly-rounds are fitted to the survey square. The reconnaissance transects provide the access paths to the fly-rounds and one camp near the centre of a 5 × 5 mile square (25 square miles) serves as a base for the operation of the five fly-rounds necessary to cover this square, succeeding spirals being one mile apart. More specialized fly-rounds are necessary for the other species of flies and, as yet, a certain amount of subjectivity cannot be avoided in their disposition. Catches are made on the fly-rounds as often as the staff position will allow. Topographical survey is done along the fly-rounds by the use of the simplest instruments, ranging rods, a steel tape and an Abney level. A survey of woody vegetation is made by the method described by Welch (1960a). From these results profiles can be drawn and, together with the use of air photographs, contoured and more accurate vegetation maps can be produced. Where necessary pasture surveys can be done by a modified step-point method. These observations produce a volume of data on which reclamation methods can be based. Ideally, fly-round catches should continue for at least fifteen months, to determine all the seasonal variations in the distribution of the flies and to ensure that the pattern repeats itself.

Chapter 28

Control by Destruction of the Larger Fauna

J. FORD

The Elimination of the Trypanosome Reservoir

Killing larger African mammals as a means of controlling trypanosomiasis was first advocated by David Bruce. He had demonstrated that *Trypanosoma brucei* was a blood parasite of various antelopes and he believed that this trypanosome and *T. rhodesiense* were identical. He therefore recommended that areas where game–fly–man contact was likely to be frequent should be cleared of the larger wild mammals.

The Report of the Interdepartmental Committee on Sleeping Sickness, under the chairmanship of the Earl of Desart (1914) is one of the most illuminating documents in the history of the tsetse problem. Bruce's proposal aroused powerful opposition and he failed to obtain consent to anything more than a carefully controlled, small scale experiment. Fifteen years later this emerged as a very small game exclusion experiment by Dr Walter Johnson's team in Northern Nigeria and, later still, as a large experiment in Tanzania between 1945 and 1951 (Potts & Jackson, 1952). The main impetus for the latter was Jackson's wish to examine the behaviour of a starving population of *Glossina morsitans*. Buxton (1955) describes both these experiments.

Neither contributed greatly to the problem of how to control tsetse by controlling game, for the effectiveness of the method had already been demonstrated by R. W. Jack in the Gwaai and Shangani River valleys in Southern Rhodesia between 1919 and 1922. Although the appearance of sleeping sickness in Rhodesia in 1912 caused much alarm (*see*, for example, Gelfand, 1961), this would not have prompted the British South Africa Company to embark on a programme that aroused much opposition had it not been thought that the future of cattle farming, a major industry for the growing settler population, was endangered by the spread of *Glossina morsitans*.

The Rinderpest Panzootic in Rhodesia, 1895–6

The use of game destruction in Southern Rhodesia was based, not upon Bruce's thesis, but upon historical evidence that the heavy mortality among game animals caused by the rinderpest panzootic in 1895 and 1896 had been followed by the disappearance of tsetse throughout the Limpopo and Zambesi basins, except in a few, small, widely separated foci. By 1915 it was obvious that the fly was rapidly reoccupying its former territory. It was known that the panzootic had almost exterminated several species of wild mammals, including buffalo (believed by early hunters like Selous to be closely associated with tsetse), warthog, bushbuck, kudu and several other antelopes. (It seems likely that mortality among some of these animals had been on a level with that observed among domestic cattle, namely 90–95%.) Some contemporary observers denied that rinderpest had caused the disappearance of the tsetse, because several animal species were not affected by it and must, so it was thought, have provided an alternative source of blood. Buxton (1955) was sufficiently impressed by these arguments to retain doubts about the causal connection between the rinderpest and the tsetse recession. Since publication of Weitz's evidence on favoured hosts and, especially, of the rejection of certain common species of game as food sources, the problem has been clarified. One hesitates to attribute entirely to coincidence the fact that species markedly susceptible to the very virulent virus of the first rinderpest panzootic included all the favoured hosts of *G. morsitans* and *G. pallidipes*, while those that were little or not at all affected included the rejected species (impala, hartebeest, zebra) and those that, from their habits, are seldom suited for continuous maintenance of *G. morsitans* populations (elephant, rhinoceros, hippopotamus, roan antelope and reedbuck).

The Campaign in Rhodesia

After Jack's demonstrations of the effectiveness of game slaughter as a means of halting the spread of *Glossina morsitans* the method was developed into a large-scale technique by J. K. Chorley. Between about 1930 and 1950 *Glossina morsitans* was removed from about 10,000 square miles of land that had been reinfested following the recovery of the wild mammal population from the effects of the rinderpest panzootic. Tsetse control in Rhodesia is inextricably involved with the politics of land apportionment and it is true to say that, in the conditions of land occupation that prevail there, no other effective method was available. This may still be true of some ecological zones (Cockbill, 1967; Pilson, 1967). Useful accounts of the Rhodesian operations are given by Chorley (1958) and Cockbill (1960).

The history of the controversies that have surrounded the Rhodesian game destruction campaign has little relevance to the control of trypanosomiasis north of the Zambesi. However, it is necessary to affirm that wholesale slaughter of the larger mammal populations is a completely effective method of eliminating *Glossina morsitans* and *G. pallidipes*. There have been failures in Rhodesia, but these have been due to the difficulty of achieving sufficiently intensive killing in certain environments. This point has been greatly illuminated by the physiological studies of Bursell (*see* p. 301) which make it clear that the crucial factor is the time available for the newly emerged teneral fly to find its first meal.

'Game-free–Cattle-free' Defence Corridors in Rhodesia

A Commission set up by the Government of the former Federation of Rhodesia and Nyasaland (Thomas *et al.*, 1955) recommended that game-proof fences should be used to delimit the zones in which animals were killed to control the spread of *G. morsitans*. These so-called 'game-free–cattle-free' barriers were about ten miles wide and they replaced unfenced shooting zones of double this width. Shooting between the fences was intensified and the results confirmed Chorley's contention that he had achieved his results without complete extermination of all animals. On the other hand, the fenced corridors, more empty of animals (though not completely so) than in the past and with crossing points reduced in number, failed in their purpose. In February 1960, two years after the completion of the corridor between them and the fly-belt, the ranches on the Shangani River showed infections for the first time since Jack's reclamation of the area in 1922. The epizootic continued to spread and reached the Gwaai River twenty miles south of the intended 'fly-line'. Evidently the intensively hunted ten-mile zone from which immigrant game was excluded by fencing was not an adequate substitute for the less intensively hunted, but unfenced zone of about twenty miles depth.

The cause of the failure is now understood. The Commission referred to above had been appointed in response to political agitation against continuation of the policy of game slaughter. Because other methods could only be introduced over a period of years it had recommended fencing in order to cut down the numbers of animals killed during the interim. In the further pursuance of this objective the 'game-free–cattle-free' corridors were sited along zones carrying a minimum of wild life. This was a departure from the practices of Chorley who had stated that it was essential to concentrate operations in places, often localized, where tsetse density was greatest and its populations most firmly established (Chorley, 1958).

It was soon evident that the epizootic among the Shangani and Gwaai cattle was caused by flies crossing the barrier from a densely populated *morsitans* focus on the head-waters of the Nagupande River, north of the defence corridor. Although preparations for complete abandonment of shooting were not completed, this failure of the new type of fenced corridor led to a decision to abandon it and to attempt to rectify matters by the use of insecticides on the

Nagupande focus. This operation followed the pattern of the successful use of insecticides on another river system, the Maseme, a year earlier in 1960. However, insecticide treatment of Nagupande was a failure and a partial reduction of apparent density was not long maintained. Meanwhile the epizootic on the Shangani and Gwaai Rivers continued to spread. Reasons for the failure of the insecticide campaign in Nagupande emerge from a recent study of *G. morsitans* behaviour by Pilson and Pilson (1967). The Maseme area, where insecticides had been more successful, although only fifteen miles distant from Nagupande, lies in a more arid, hotter and ecologically distinct zone (Vincent & Thomas *n.d.*) nearer to the floor of the Zambesi valley.

Selective Destruction of Favoured Hosts of Tsetse in Nagupande

The Shangani–Gwaai epizootic was halted and greatly reduced by chemotherapy of the infected cattle, by bush clearing and by the application of insecticides in the infected area and was finally eliminated by the extinction of the parent focus of tsetse infestation on the headwaters of the Nagupande River (Cockbill, 1967). However, it was obvious that if there were to be no repetition, the concentration of *G. morsitans* and *G. pallidipes* on the Nagupande headwaters must be removed in some more permanent manner. It is to be noted that the Nagupande headwaters had been included in the hunting zone of the operations conducted by Chorley. Shooting there had ceased in 1957, in order to allow the fenced corridor to be built. By 1960 the Nagupande basin was abundantly repopulated by game animals of all kinds. It was therefore decided once more to attack the hosts of the tsetse, but to confine shooting to the four species most favoured by the fly and to drive out, beforehand, the elephant, buffalo and rhinoceros which would have interfered with hunting and to some degree themselves provided an alternative diet to the principal host animals, warthog, bushpig, bushbuck and kudu. Earlier analyses had shown that 64% of tsetse feeds in the neighbourhood were derived from Suidae (chiefly warthog) and 25% from Bovidae (mainly bushbuck and kudu).

The Nagupande headwaters occupy an area of 200 square miles. This was first surrounded by a game fence. During its construction harassment of the elephant involving some killing by sportsmen was carried out. (The main opposition to game destruction as an anti-tsetse measure was led by men who were themselves keen hunters. It is always possible to reduce public indignation by allowing sportsmen to share in the killing.)

Shooting of the selected species was begun inside the fenced area in October 1962, and resulted in an immediate rise in the catch on the Nagupande fly-rounds which reached its peak in December. This may be attributed to the prolongation of Phase 2 sexual appetitive behaviour towards the human bait, now more numerous in relation to the density of favoured hosts and also to increased hunger leading to a greater proportion of tsetse approaching man for the purposes of feeding. (A similar peak in apparent density of tsetse after commencement of shooting had been noted some years earlier by Moggridge during the Uganda game destruction operations.) It was followed by an increase in the numbers of infections recorded in cattle south of the defence zone that reached a peak in February 1963 and then declined to zero in June 1964.

As has so often been the case in tsetse control operations lack of time and staff have prevented the collection of all the data desirable for an accurate assessment of the results. It is known that game animals, other than the selected species, are still present inside the Nagupande fence and include zebra, impala, reedbuck, eland, duiker, roan, sable, grysbok and baboons. The densities of these species before shooting began, and of those destroyed, are not known (Cockbill, 1967).

The success of the selective shooting in Nagupande, coupled with the difficulty of maintaining adequate control by the alternatives of bush clearing and insecticides has led to its introduction (supplemented by local application of other methods) throughout the Rhodesian tsetse defence zone.

Game Destruction in Uganda

This was described by Robertson and Bernacca (1958). Uganda had been subject to extensive invasion and spread of *Glossina* (chiefly *G. morsitans* and *G. pallidipes*) from the mid-1930s. In Central Uganda, this is attributed to two factors: firstly, the restriction of movement and reduction in numbers of elephants and secondly, the introduction of early grass burning as an anti-erosion measure. Both these factors led to the invasion of formerly open grassland by bush. Peripherally a third factor was also important, namely, the evacuation as a prophylactic measure against sleeping sickness of large populations along the floor of the western Rift Valley and near the shores of Lake Victoria, especially in Busoga. Most of these depopulations were over by 1920. During the decade ending in the early 1940s, about 8,000 square miles of former cattle pasture were invaded by the two species named.

With very small (war-time) resources, T. W. Chorley organized an operation in the Buruli district of Buganda which involved shooting of buffaloes (and later of other game animals); organization of fierce, late, grass fires; encouragement of hunting of wild pigs by local inhabitants and, finally, the control and deflying of road traffic. This work came under the Entomological Section of the Medical Department, but in 1947 a Tsetse Control Department was formed. This was taken over by J. Y. Moggridge in 1948 and a tsetse eradication programme to cost £1 million was inaugurated as part of a ten-year Development Programme (Worthington & Harris, 1949). Moggridge's principal innovation was to dispose groups of hunters so that destruction of animals was intensified in foci of high tsetse density. A similar principle enunciated by J. K. Chorley for the Rhodesian method has already been mentioned. It is not clear to whom the original statement of this principle was due but it does not seem to have influenced the conduct of the Shinyanga experiment conducted by Potts and Jackson (1952). Since the most likely explanation of the effectiveness of certain types of partial clearing, especially against flies of the *morsitans* group, is that it interferes with feeding, this principle as applied to shooting has some theoretical importance. In Uganda, in rather less than ten years, reclamation or near reclamation of some 7,500 square miles of country (mostly invaded during the previous fifteen years) was achieved, chiefly by shooting. Some discriminative bush clearing was undertaken and insecticides were also used in certain areas.

Organization of Game Slaughter Techniques in Rhodesia and Uganda

The operations conducted by J. K. Chorley in Rhodesia employed hunters, using ·303 rifles, at a mean density of one per ten square miles. In areas of high density of tsetse and host populations, hunter density was one in five square miles. In 1954, when 36,910 head of game were shot, 750 hunters were employed over an operations area of 6,000 square miles (Chorley, 1958). This included not only the 20-mile wide defence zone, but also an additional reclamation area (Urungwe) of about 500 square miles.

During the phase of shooting between fences to create 'game-free–cattle-free' corridors the same density of hunters with ·303 rifles was used. In the Sebungwe defence corridor, through which the passage of tsetse from the Nagupande focus has been described, 120 rifle hunters were supplemented by fifty hunters with shotguns operating at night with torches. This operation has been described by Lovemore (1963), especially with regard to the game populations in the untouched, tsetse infested, fly-belt to its north.

In the Nagupande area, sixty hunters were used inside the fenced area of 200 square miles. The object of this was to achieve a very rapid reduction of density of the four selected hosts, as it was considered possible that their too gradual removal, especially in a fenced area, would allow the tsetse to become adapted to other host species.

In Uganda the operations initiated by T. W. Chorley in 1944 were first conceived as an attempt to stop the spread of *G. pallidipes* associated with annual migration of buffaloes. Hunters, armed with ·303 rifles, worked in pairs under a supervisor (to ten pairs) who was armed with a more powerful weapon. Later, when other, less dangerous animals were also shot, hunters worked separately. In 1954, a decade after the first introduction of the method and at the height of the reclamation campaign, 250 hunters were employed. It is not possible to compare this figure with that for Rhodesia because the circumstances in the two countries are so different.

The problems associated with control of firearms and ammunition and of supervision of large numbers of employees over great areas of undeveloped bush are formidable and differ from country to country. The publications listed as well as annual reports of the organizations concerned may be consulted for further details.

Disadvantages of the Game Destruction Method

One disadvantage that needs to be mentioned, but need not be discussed here, is that use of this method provokes powerful opposition that may become politically embarrassing.

Local destruction of the hosts of *Glossina* has a disadvantage shared with insecticides, namely, that recovery after application of the technique, except where isolation is complete, takes place very quickly. The extremely rapid multiplication of the survivors of the great rinderpest pandemic was described by Percival (1918). The beginning of infection in the Rhodesian Shangani–Gwaai epizootic in February 1960 indicated that in three years the host population of the Nagupande basin in Rhodesia had recovered sufficiently to permit the build-up of an associated testse population to the extent that emigrant tsetse were producing infection in cattle at least ten miles distant, across country in which the wild mammal population was certainly very sparse.

The Urungwe Reserve in Rhodesia had been reclaimed from *G. morsitans* by 1944, in which year 4,000 head of cattle entered it. These had increased to 8,000 by 1951. Trypanosomiasis was first observed among them in 1950 and re-invasion by tsetse was confirmed in 1952. The growth of the tsetse population was rapid and mortality among the cattle reached 300 per month until they were removed (Chorley, 1954). Some years later Pilson and Harley (1959) showed that domestic cattle could become favoured hosts of *G. morsitans*. In the absence of drug protection cattle should only be brought into reclaimed land that is not fully isolated from the parent fly-belt, after cultivation has proceeded far enough to destroy the natural vegetation. This had not happened in Urungwe by 1950.

Of a somewhat different nature are the failures to obtain sufficient reduction in the host population to eliminate *Glossina*. The extensive reclamation successes in Rhodesia were all achieved in country closely adjacent to areas in which *G. morsitans* populations could not maintain themselves indefinitely because of the effects of prolonged winters on puparial metabolism. Bursell (1960b) suggested that a limit would be set by areas in which winters extend to ninety or more days with mean temperature at 16°C or below. The consumption of nutritional reserves during a puparial life of ninety days results in the emergence of teneral flies unable to survive long enough to obtain the first blood meal. When shooting operations were introduced into the Sabi valley, some 3,000 feet below the level at which successful reclamation had been achieved and with much shorter winters, it proved impossible to stop the spread of *G. morsitans*. This does not imply any intrinsic failure of the method, but indicates only that to achieve control much more intensive killing would have been required.

It is significant that the breakdown of control of the *G. morsitans* front in Rhodesia should have occurred in the place where the spread of tsetse had been most rapid between 1910 and 1920. Similarly, in Uganda the principal failure in the ten-year reclamation programme occurred in the Maruzi area of Lango district. This had been an isolated focus of *G. pallidipes* and *G. morsitans* infestation before the great spread of these two species began between 1930 and 1935. This infestation survived several successive attacks by shooting, bush clearing and insecticides. Persistence with these techniques has now, after many years, led to its elimination. Among the reasons for its survival for so long were its inaccessibility between two arms of Lake Kioga, its cover of heavy thicket and a population of mosquitoes so dense as to make it virtually uninhabitable. Until quite recently, the research approach to the problem of tsetse control by game destruction has been negligible, principally because of the lack of research, again until the last decade, on the wild mammal fauna in general. The examples quoted—Shangani–Gwaai in Rhodesia and Maruzi in Uganda—suggest that an approach to the problem along the lines developed by the Russian school of epidemiologists for the description of the 'natural foci of infection' or 'nidality' of, especially, zoonoses, might be very fruitful.

Chapter 29

An Appraisal of Methods for the Control of *Glossina*

W. H. POTTS

The various methods available for the control of tsetse populations have been described in detail in the preceding chapters. In some, indeed in many, campaigns against the tsetse fly it has been found necessary or expedient to employ two or more of these methods. The selection of the method, or methods, to be used in a given situation may present some difficulty and it may be helpful to those responsible for the planning of control programmes to have at their disposal a brief appraisal of the available measures, with some indication of the lines of approach likely to offer the best prospects of success.

The control measures which have been described fall into two main categories, namely, those which involve a *direct* attack on the tsetse fly itself and those which depend on *indirect* action by rendering the environment unfavourable to the fly. Direct methods of control comprise hand-catching, catching by means of traps, the use of predators and parasites, the application of chemical insecticides and the still unproved expedient of interfering with tsetse reproduction either by the release of sterilized male flies or by the use of chemosterilants against wild individuals of both sexes. Indirect methods aim to alter the fly's environment by some means or other, such as the clearance (complete or partial) of vegetation, or by interference with the fly's food supply, as by the elimination of the larger mammalian fauna.

Hand-catching (Chapter 22), the oldest means of insect control, has, in special circumstances, achieved complete extermination of tsetse flies over limited areas. This method is tedious and time-consuming and is obviously inapplicable to the control of tsetse which are prevalent and widely dispersed over extensive areas. The method may, however, prove useful for the elimination of tsetse from limited areas, as when flies are confined to riverine habitats; results will not be permanent unless the area can be completely isolated by natural or artificial means. Hand-catching has now been largely superseded by the new powerful insecticides.

The use of traps to control tsetse populations has been investigated in widely divergent circumstances in East, Central and West Africa (Chapter 22). Although the original use of the Harris trap in Zululand appeared to have achieved success, the method was subsequently shown to have failed. Elsewhere, the use of traps has, at times, appeared to be of some value but the conclusion is inescapable that traps are too erratic in performance to be relied upon as a means of tsetse control. If and when reliable and effective attractants are developed, their use in conjunction with traps may prove of value not only for investigatory purposes but also for control (*see* also pp. 460, 462–3).

Predators and parasites (Chapter 25) undoubtedly play a significant role in controlling tsetse populations under natural conditions, as is clear from many observations made in the field. Determined efforts have been made to exploit parasites of tsetse as a means of control and the quite extensive researches on this subject have been reviewed in Chapter 25; up to the present, no practical and effective control of tsetse populations has been achieved in this way. This approach has received little attention in recent years and whereas, in our present state of knowledge, the use of predators and parasites is unlikely to find a place in practical control programmes, it would be unwise to conclude that further research in this neglected field would be unrewarding.

Interference with reproduction by the release of sterilized males is a method which has achieved conspicuous success in other spheres, notably in the control of the screw-worm fly in the southern United States of America. The application of this principle to the control of tsetse flies has received considerable attention; this and related work is described in Chapter 26. It is as yet too early to assess the practical value of this method but it is one which may find a useful place among control measures in the future. As in the case of traps, the availability of effective attractants would enhance the prospects of success by this means. The latest variation of this concept envisages the production and introduction of lethal mutants induced by exposure to sub-sterilant doses of radiation or chemosterilants (Curtis, 1968, 1968a, b; Curtis & Hill, 1968), but the work is still at an early experimental stage. Should either of these methods of tsetse control eventually necessitate the availability of a plentiful supply of laboratory-reared tsetse flies, this is now a practical possibility, for some species at least (*see* Chapter 20).

The powerful chemical insecticides now available and the means of applying them in tsetse control programmes have been described at length in Chapters 23 and 24. At the present time, the application of insecticides is probably the most widely practised method of tsetse control and one which seems likely, with further refinement, to find a continuing place in reclamation projects. The first extensive use of insecticides for the control of tsetse populations was the ambitious campaign carried out in Zululand and adjacent areas in Swaziland during the period 1945–54. The flies concerned were mainly *G. pallidipes* but *G. brevipalpis* and *G. austeni* were also present in some parts. The investigations which preceded this campaign and the principles on which it was based and the methods employed, have been described (up to the end of 1952) by Du Toit (1954); the results achieved (up to January 1954, when application of insecticides ceased) have been recorded by Du Toit, Kluge and Fiedler (1954). At first, the insecticide used was DDT but this was later replaced by BHC which was found to be cheaper and more rapid in action. Applications of insecticide were made mainly from fixed-wing aircraft but helicopters were also used for difficult mountainous country. In particularly difficult terrain, insecticides were applied from the ground by means of smoke generators or from hand- or power-operated machines. In addition to the use of insecticides, some discriminative and thicket clearing was carried out against *G. pallidipes* in regions where it was difficult to apply insecticides; some barrier clearings were also made. Game animals were eradicated from some areas. These combined operations carried out over an area of less than 200 square miles freed some 7,000 square miles from trypanosomiasis and removed a serious threat to the cattle industry. The results of this campaign, which was pursued with great vigour and persistence, are said to have justified the trouble and high expenditure involved. Later, many other campaigns for the elimination or control of tsetse flies by the use of insecticides have been undertaken, often on a considerable scale. As experience in the use of insecticides has been gained, the tendency has been to restrict their application to limited parts of the fly's habitat (*see* below) thereby simplifying and reducing the cost of this method.

Indirect methods of attack on the tsetse fly must now be considered. Total, sheer or ruthless clearing of vegetation means the complete destruction of all trees and shrubs. This method is completely effective in eliminating tsetse but, if the results are to be permanent, regrowth of the vegetation must be prevented. Although total clearing has frequently been used to reclaim land from tsetse, it is obvious that the wholesale destruction of trees and shrubs over the vast areas of tropical Africa infested by tsetse flies is neither practicable nor acceptable. The method has been successfully applied to the control of both woodland and riverine species of tsetse, often to create barriers against re-infestation of areas freed from tsetse by other means such as insecticides. Its use to halt widespread 'advances' of tsetse has not always been successful, generally because the advance has been so rapid that tsetse have become established beyond the barrier before there has been time to complete the clearings. So far, there is no clear indication of the actual width of clearing necessary to make certain that tsetse will be unable to cross the barrier (*see* also pp. 475, 543, 544, 546–7, 575, and discussions in Buxton, 1955).

Partial clearing involves the destruction of sufficient vegetation to render the environment unsuitable for the survival of tsetse; it is a more refined and cheaper method than ruthless clearing. Partial clearing is capable of exploitation on a large scale and is particularly applicable to the control of riverine tsetse, especially where the species is dependent on the protection afforded by dense vegetation to survive the rigours of a hot, dry climate. It has, however, also been used on a large scale against the woodland species, *G. morsitans*, in Tanzania.

Fire exclusion is another potential method of rendering the environment unfavourable for certain species of tsetse but because of almost insuperable practical difficulties it has not found a permanent place among control methods; for this reason it has not been described above along with other methods of indirect control. Nevertheless, fire exclusion cannot be disregarded in any appraisal of control measures. The concept of fire exclusion was based on an observation first made by Swedi Abdulla, KM[1] a senior African Assistant in the Tanganyika Tsetse Research Department. In 1924, Swedi Abdulla drew Swynnerton's attention to the absence of tsetse (*G. morsitans*) from the extensive areas of thicket in the Itigi region of central Tanganyika, although the flies

[1] Swedi Abdulla was also the actual discoverer of the species now known as *G. swynnertoni*. An exceptionally acute observer, he noticed that the tsetse of the thorn-bush area south of Lake Victoria differed from those of the Tabora area. Up to that time, flies from both these areas were regarded as *G. morsitans*. Swynnerton sent specimens to the British Museum of Natural History, where Major Austen recognized them as belonging to a species new to science and he lost no time in describing it under the name *G. swynnertoni*. Swynnerton was disturbed that this haste precluded him from suggesting that it be named *G. swedii* after the discoverer.

were numerous in the woodlands immediately abutting on the thicket and often exceptionally abundant along the thicket edges. Swynnerton was quick to realize the possibilities opened up by this observation.

He had long been aware of the destruction of thickets by the annual grass fires that sweep through the grassed woodlands of Africa and he argued that, were grass fires to be prevented, the tsetse-infested woodlands might well be transformed into fly-free thicket. One of the writer's first assignments, on arrival in Tanganyika in 1925, was to verify this observation. Its correctness was duly confirmed, and experimental fire exclusion was attempted in the *Acacia* woodlands of Shinyanga as a possible means of eradicating the closely related species, *G. swynnertoni*. The surprising outcome of this experiment was that it was found to be unnecessary to wait for a period of years to allow the vegetation to thicken to a point where the flies were affected; some reduction in their numbers was evident in the year following the initiation of the experiment and continued progressively in each subsequent year. The possible reasons for these findings are discussed in a brief but excellent account of this measure and its subsequent history by Glasgow (1960a), but the ways in which fire exclusion effects this reduction in fly numbers have never been fully explained. In one small patch of country, the general woodland became so thick after a considerable number of years that *G. swynnertoni* disappeared from it, but in another larger area (of some 60 square miles) parts of the woodland, the short-grassed 'hard pans', remained comparatively open and in these the fly persisted. It was evident that fire exclusion alone would not result in the complete disappearance of tsetse from country of this type within a reasonable period of time. The observed concentration of tsetse flies in the hard pan areas re-focused attention on the concept of fly foci first suggested by Shircore (1914); this led to the development of partial clearing as a method of attack on tsetse of the woodland savannas. The idea of using fire exclusion as a practical means of fly control was abandoned, partly for the reasons stated above and partly because of the elaborate and expensive organization needed to carry it out.

Of all the control measures mentioned above, the only one, other than total clearing, that has resulted in consistent and complete freeing of land from tsetse infestation is interference with the fly's food supply by elimination of the larger fauna (Chapter 28). The serious disadvantages of, and objections to, this method have already been described but, thanks to newer knowledge of the feeding habits of various species of *Glossina* (*see* Chapter 13) there is some prospect that this measure may prove equally effective when only selected mammalian hosts are eliminated. An attempt to apply this modified technique on a field scale is currently being made in Rhodesia (Cockbill, 1967; *see* also p. 560).

When the various methods available for the control of tsetse populations are examined, it is apparent that all have been based on a knowledge of the ecology of the fly. As this has increased so has it been possible to refine existing techniques and to evolve better and more sophisticated methods of control. This holds true also of other diseases which are transmitted by insects or other intermediate hosts. Hope for the future lies, therefore, in the acquisition of further intimate knowledge of the behaviour and essential requirement of the vector. This subject deserves further consideration.

Only half a century ago, Swynnerton, an ardent naturalist, made his first acquaintance with trypanosomiasis and tsetse flies in Portuguese East Africa. His description of these experiences (Swynnerton, 1921) was hailed by Townsend (1923) as 'by all odds the best contribution to tsetse environment and bionomics' that had then appeared and, even today, will repay careful study. Swynnerton was convinced that attack on the vector *Glossina* was the best means of controlling trypanosomiasis. He was equally convinced that the essential prerequisite to the achievement of success by this means was the thorough study of the ecology of the fly. Only this would give the needed comprehensive knowledge of the nature of its habitat, the relations between the fly and its environment (living and non-living) and, in short, an intimate knowledge of how the fly lives and moves. These convictions led him to make an early attempt to apply what was then the new science of ecology to practical measures of tsetse control. This early work was carried out under the aegis of the Tsetse Advisory Committee of the British Colonial Office, with the strong and continued support of that powerful personality, Dr (later Sir Guy) Marshall, the founder of the Imperial Bureau (now Commonwealth Institute) of Entomology. To this end Swynnerton gathered a team of workers who presently formed the staff of the Tsetse Research Department of Tanganyika Territory, and this was later expanded to form the East African Tsetse and Trypanosomiasis Research and Reclamation Organization, now known by the shorter title of the East African Trypanosomiasis Research Organization (EATRO), with headquarters at Tororo, Uganda. More or less concurrently, an ecological approach to the problem was developed in West Africa, inspired by the pioneer work of Buxton and other early investigators of the relation of tsetse to climate. This work was energetically pursued for many years by Nash, whose apprenticeship had been served under Swynnerton in Tanganyika, and later by Nash and his co-workers on the staff of the West African (now Nigerian) Institute for Trypanosomiasis Research, with headquarters at Kaduna, Nigeria. In describing the development of this work in West Africa, Buxton (1955a) emphasized the value of alternating research between the laboratory and the field, each approach contributing to the other.

These lines of investigation, in both East and West Africa, led to the concept of tsetse control by making a partial (discriminative or selective) attack on the vector. At first, this took the form of altering, by clearing vegetation, those limited portions of the environment that seemed to be essential to the survival of the tsetse fly during the rigours of the late dry season. Later, with the advent of the powerful and sometimes persistent insecticides developed during and after the second World War, the concept of partial attack has increasingly taken the form of restricted application of insecticides to limited portions of the general habitat of the fly, often to only those resting sites most frequented by the fly.

Restricted application of insecticides has been fully described in Chapter 24. A recent instance of the use of this method is afforded by the arrest of an advance of *G. morsitans orientalis* in south-eastern Rhodesia, an account of which is given by Robertson and Kluge (1968). Insecticide was applied, by mechanized spraying from the ground, to the putative principal resting places of *Glossina* in areas regarded as breeding grounds of the fly; the determination of the situation and limits of these sites was greatly facilitated by the use of aerial photographs. Examples of attack by alteration of parts of the fly's habitat have been cited (Chapter 27) from the extensive work carried out in Tanzania. Other examples are given in the account by Ford (1954) of the use of discriminative clearing in the Abercorn area of Northern Rhodesia (*see* also Glover *et al.*, 1955), in south-eastern Uganda (*see* also Harley & Pilson, 1961) and in the earlier work in the Songea (*see* also Bursell, 1955a), Tabora and Urambo areas of Tanzania. The situation in Urambo (infested with *G. m. morsitans*) has been described in rather more detail by Glasgow (1961e). It is of interest because here the clearing of 64% of the woodland for the mechanized cultivation of groundnuts left the fly untouched; the areas unsuitable for the crop were left uncleared as wind-breaks and these uncleared areas contained the drainage lines which provided favourable habitats for the fly. This persistence of *Glossina* placed a considerable labour force at risk by bringing it into close contact with tsetse in an area not far removed from one in which sleeping sickness was endemic. Danger was, however, averted and a safe situation eventually established by instituting a combination of control measures; these comprised a protective barrier of sheer clearing, aerial application of insecticide to the uncleared parts of the area and the creation of a two-mile wide defence zone in the surrounding infested woodland by partial clearing (i.e. clearing of the drainage lines). This provides another excellent example of the use of a number of different methods of control to meet a particular situation.

It is worthwhile to record here a situation in Tanzania (Shinyanga and Sukumaland generally) which was precisely the reverse of that obtaining in the Urambo area of groundnut cultivation. In Sukumaland, the areas believed to be particularly favourable to the fly (*G. swynnertoni*) are the short-grassed 'hard pans' (Burtt, B. D., 1942, pp. 87–9, pls. 10 (photo 17) and 11; *see* also Buxton, 1955, pls. 21 and 27, fig. B). By clearing these hard pans (Bax, 1943–4) tsetse were finally eradicated from an experimental area of bush, some 50 square miles in extent, in the neighbourhood of Shinyanga (Buxton, 1955, p. 572; *see* also Glasgow, 1960a). Traditional methods of land usage in Sukumaland facilitate the type of agricultural occupation that consolidates such clearings, although the actual soils of the hard pans themselves are not cultivated. The hard pans lie in the drainage lines but the ridges between them, which are comparatively unimportant to the fly, are left largely untouched. Thus, human occupation renders the effects of partial clearing on the fly operative for considerable periods of time. Even in the absence of human settlement, the arid conditions prevailing in the region and the nature of the soil in the hard pans mitigate against regeneration of the bush so that it can remain unfavourable to the fly for quite a long time. This is in striking contrast to the situation pertaining in riverine tsetse habitats in areas of high rainfall and rich soil where rapid regeneration of woody growth presents a serious problem. Buxton (*loc. cit.*) has recorded an earlier use of partial clearing against *G. swynnertoni* for the arrest of an epidemic of sleeping sickness on the Ukerewe mainland near Lake Victoria, again in Sukumaland (*see* also Bax, 1943–4). Goodier

(1961) has also described the partial clearing of bush, against *G. morsitans orientalis*, in south-eastern Rhodesia.

Before leaving the subject of tsetse control by attack on those parts of the fly's habitat that are considered to be of particular importance to it, reference must be made to the views of Pilson and Pilson (1967) and of Bursell (1966), based on their recent investigations in Rhodesia, of which an account has been given on pp. 386–388. In this it is suggested that the concept of restricted parts of the habitat being essential to *Glossina* may be an illusion arising from faulty sampling. Bursell (1968) has ably discoursed on the great independence of its physical environment achieved by *Glossina* by virtue of its peculiar method of reproduction and of the various delicate adaptations of the adult stage to life in an arid environment. At the same time he points out that *Glossina* has not achieved a similar degree of independence of its food supply and that this is the most vulnerable point in the life-cycle of the fly, a contention supported by the successes achieved by attack at this point. He suggests that this independence of its physical environment does not augur well for the complete success of attempts to control the fly by partial alteration of its habitat, and may well account for the failures recorded from time to time (e.g. Harley & Pilson, 1961), as well as for the doubts that have been entertained as to the reality of some of the successes that have been claimed (*see*, for example, Kernaghan, 1961). It must be admitted that the basis of the claims for success have seldom if ever been so fully and unequivocally established as to make it certain that the results achieved could be attributed solely to partial attack, without any intervention by other contributory factors. If the views of the Pilsons and Bursell are well-founded, similar successes might well be achieved by indiscriminate and random alteration of an equal proportion of the environment; such an experiment would be of great value and is, the writer believes, under way in Rhodesia. The uncertainties raised by this work of the Pilsons and Bursell call for the extension of similar investigations to a wider range of situations and, until this has been done, final judgement must be reserved.

Buxton (1955, pp. 585–90) has presented an able summary of the vast amount of information then available on methods of control and he has also discussed (pp. 575–83) the place of human settlement in control programmes. In the writer's view, the only sound approach to tsetse control lies in incorporating measures directed against the fly into a general scheme of land utilization, planned in such a way as to ensure that the area freed from tsetse is maintained in a condition in which the flies cannot survive. The selection of the measures directed against the fly would be made from those described in these pages, having regard to particular circumstances of the situation. The incorporation of tsetse control measures in a scheme of land-management is facilitated by the availability of powerful chemotherapeutic and chemoprophylactic agents by the skilful use of which man and livestock may now be protected when in contact with light or even moderate infestations of *Glossina* (*see* Chapters 37 and 43; also Whiteside, 1962). The ability to introduce human settlement and livestock at an early stage of development schemes is important also from the financial point of view since cattle maintained on the unusually rich virgin pastures would be highly profitable.

Nevertheless, the writer has sometimes doubted whether intensive and permanent human occupation of the land, such as that envisaged above, is ultimately practicable in much of the arid country inhabited by *Glossina* or, even if practicable, whether this is necessarily the best means of utilizing such country for man's benefit. There can be little doubt but that, were it possible to eradicate tsetse permanently without recourse to intensive and permanent occupation of the land, much of the arid grassed woodlands could be used for ranching, thereby providing the animal protein so badly needed in Africa and other parts of the world. It is even possible that, without eradicating tsetse, the cropping of the game animals supported by the pastures and foliage of these arid lands might serve to provide much of this protein; Ford (1963a) discusses these possibilities. It must, however, be realized that the adoption of a policy of land utilization that would leave *Glossina* in occupation would involve a continuing risk of outbreaks of sleeping sickness; this, in turn, would necessitate unceasing vigilance, with the consequent high recurring expenditure on surveillance, to detect outbreaks at any early stage and on measures to bring them under prompt control. The writer would therefore re-echo the words of Jackson (1950a) that we cannot 'abandon attempts to find methods of dealing with the tsetse itself; and if these methods are to be really successful they must aim at removing the last fly, where necessary without the aid of dense human settlement'.

Chapter 30

Administrative and Organizational Aspects of Control Programmes

K. C. WILLETT

ADMINISTRATIVE ASPECTS

The administration of programmes for the control of trypanosomiasis is frequently complicated by the fact that it is difficult, if not impossible, to separate the interests of human and animal trypanosomiasis. The difficulty is least in control by attack on the parasite which, in the absence of any effective immunological weapon, must be by curative or prophylactic drugs, since these will necessarily be administered by the medical or veterinary authorities, acting under their respective ministries. However, whether in research aimed at improving control methods or in control by attack on the insect vector, the interests of human and animal trypanosomiasis overlap so greatly that it is often impossible to separate them entirely.

This fact is well illustrated by the way in which the British anti-trypanosomiasis effort was formerly administered. The Secretary of State for the Colonies was advised on medical matters by one body (Tropical Medical Research Board) and on agricultural and veterinary matters by another (Tropical Agricultural Research Board). This division of responsibility did not prove satisfactory and a more diversified advisory body was set up, the Tsetse Fly and Trypanosomiasis Committee, later designated the Trypanosomiasis Panel of the Ministry of Overseas Development.

The same type of difficulty was encountered in many of the previous colonies.

In Tanganyika Territory, for example, a Department of Tsetse Research was set up in 1927 as an offshoot of the Game Department while, at the same time, a Sleeping Sickness Service was established by the Medical Department and was responsible in the following years for extensive re-settlement of population in the west of the country as Rhodesian sleeping sickness spread (Fairbairn, 1948).

In Tanzania today the Sleeping Sickness Service continues to function under the Ministry of Health but resettlement has long since become the responsibility of Settlement Officers under the Administration. In 1949, tsetse control in Tanganyika became the responsibility of a Department of Tsetse Survey and Reclamation which, in recent years, has been amalgamated with the veterinary services of the Ministry of Agriculture.

In both Kenya and Uganda special tsetse control organizations were set up but in Kenya the Tsetse Survey and Control Unit has always been an integral part of the Veterinary Department. Kenya's example has now been followed by Tanzania, as mentioned above, and by Uganda, where the Tsetse Control Department has now been made part of the Ministry of Animal Industry, Game and Fisheries.

In Northern Nigeria control of human trypanosomiasis is the responsibility of the Sleeping Sickness Service, a part of the Rural Health Services of the Ministry of Health; control of animal trypanosomiasis is vested in the Veterinary Tsetse and Trypanosomiasis Unit of the Ministry of Animal and Forest Resources. Both these organizations undertake tsetse control programmes which, inevitably, have an effect upon both human and animal trypanosomiasis. Necessarily, therefore, their programmes must be co-ordinated and this is achieved through a Standing Committee on Tsetse Control on which are represented not only the two ministries directly concerned but also the Nigerian (lately West African) Institute for Trypanosomiasis Research, and the Ministries of Agriculture and Finance.

Where substantial schemes of trypanosomiasis (including tsetse) control or eradication are under consideration many varying interests may be involved and should be given every opportunity to take their full part in the resulting development from an early stage. It is a well-known fact that trypanosomiasis is exceptional amongst diseases in that it has held back, and is still holding back, the economic development of very large areas of Africa. Many African countries have, apart from the Ministry responsible for finance, a separate Ministry dealing with economic development. These two Ministries therefore, in addition to those for human health and agriculture or veterinary services, will be intimately involved. The same is true of forestry interests.

Some African countries have invaluable assets of vast numbers and many varieties of wild animals which, quite apart from their immense intrinsic and scientific value, are nowadays an ever increasing attraction to tourists and so bring substantial amounts of foreign exchange to support the local economy. Since tsetse areas coincide to a great extent with the areas where game animals are still to be seen, the authorities responsible for wild life and tourism will often be intimately concerned with anti-trypanosomiasis projects, quite apart from tsetse control by game elimination which is nowadays contemplated in only very few countries.

Since the ultimate object of trypanosomiasis or tsetse control is to make land available for development, plans may have to be made at a very early stage for the expected influx of population and these will require the additional attention of the Ministries concerned with health, education, communications and water resources.

ORGANIZATIONAL ASPECTS

The problems encountered in the organization of control programmes differ greatly according to whether the method of control is directed against the parasite or the insect vector.[1]

Control of the Parasite

The only point at which the parasite can be attacked is in the infection of the vertebrate host and this attack can only be made by use of curative or prophylactic drugs; nothing is yet known about means of controlling the infection in the vector tsetse.

The primary requirement for such campaigns, whether they be against human or animal trypanosomiasis, is either the effective control, or the adequate co-operation, of the human population. This is an obvious necessity in anti-sleeping sickness campaigns but for control of trypanosomiasis in domestic stock it is equally necessary to have either effective control over, or the confidence of, the stock owners.

In the ex-British territories, in general, it has not been considered justifiable to exercise the degree of compulsion necessary to ensure the success of mass campaigns using prophylactic drugs. However, when outbreaks occur the co-operation of the people is more easily obtained and widespread prophylaxis can be, and has been, used to control epidemics. Other groups of people may, from the nature of their employment, be under sufficiently strict control to enable regular drug prophylaxis to be given; examples of these are tin-mining and railway labour in Northern Nigeria, and the staff of Tsetse Fly Control in Bechuanaland (now Botswana).

However complete the control of any group of people, the success of drug prophylaxis depends upon the drug being effective for a sufficiently long time. In Bechuanaland the staff of the Tsetse Fly Control organization were, at first, given prophylactic pentamidine at six-monthly intervals. It was soon found that this drug did not provide effective protection against the local strains of *Trypanosoma rhodesiense* for six months and the interval between injections was reduced first to three and then to two months. Finally pentamidine prophylaxis was abandoned as even the two-monthly injections did not provide adequate protection. Further, with a parasite that invades the central nervous system as rapidly as does *T. rhodesiense*—usually within four to six weeks of infection—an ineffective dose of drug may merely suppress the clinical manifestations of infection without delaying involvement of the central nervous

[1] For details of methods of control the reader is referred to Chapters 21 to 29, 36, 37, 42 and 43.

system. It is chiefly because of this risk that pentamidine prophylaxis against *T. rhodesiense* has never been used in Tanzania.

Another situation in which the co-operation of the people is essential in control of human trypanosomiasis arises when the method employed aims to eliminate contact between man and tsetse. Beginning in 1924, an epidemic caused by *T. rhodesiense* swept up the western side of Tanganyika Territory (Fairbairn, 1948). In the absence of any effective prophylactic drug, and also of any drug which could effect a cure once the central nervous system became involved, the main recourse was to re-settlement of the people in large, cleared, sleeping sickness settlements thus preventing contact with the fly. This policy was, in general, extremely successful and must have saved many thousands of lives, but, as Apted (1962) remarked, such compulsory and large-scale movements of populations 'are no longer acceptable, but something as effective is still needed in their place'.

Another, lesser, problem of control campaigns using drugs—which are expensive—is whether to attempt to recover some, or all, of the cost by charging for the treatment. This problem rarely arises in the treatment of human trypanosomiasis which is nearly always provided free by the medical authorities, but it does arise in treatment of domestic stock which may cost hundreds of thousands of pounds annually. The fundamental problem is to balance the possible deterrent effect of cost to owners of large numbers of stock against the all too common suspicion that anything provided free can hardly be worth having.

Control of the Vector

Campaigns directed against the insect vector are much more a matter of straightforward organization, logistics and costing, the primary consideration usually being whether the economic return from development after tsetse eradication will be sufficient to justify the cost of the operation.

When, however, the primary objective is the control or eradication of epidemic or endemic human trypanosomiasis, the cost of the operation becomes a secondary consideration. Examples of such campaigns in which insecticide has been used, sometimes economically but sometimes only at considerable expense, have been:

(i) the eradication of *Glossina fuscipes* from the Nyando River and Kuja-Migori basins in Nyanza Province, Kenya, which has eliminated endemic foci of *T. gambiense* previously responsible for hundreds of cases per year;

(ii) the KKZ (Kano-Katsina-Zaria) scheme in Northern Nigeria, also directed at a large and widespread endemic focus of *T. gambiense*;

(iii) the spraying of the Aswa River, Lango, Uganda, in 1957–8 which eliminated a sharp epidemic of *T. gambiense* causing hundreds of cases in a year, and

(iv) the elimination in 1965–6 of the *G. fuscipes* infestation in the Alego and surrounding locations of Central Nyanza, Kenya, which rapidly terminated an explosive epidemic of *T. rhodesiense*.

Insecticidal attack on the vector has been increasingly used in recent years, partly because the cost of hand-clearing of bush has increased sharply with rising wages and partly because improved formulations of insecticides have become available and more refined techniques for their application have been devised. Such refinements have become possible as more precise knowledge of the resting sites of various tsetse species has been obtained and costs have been correspondingly reduced. Most of the present operations for control or eradication of tsetse depend on the application of residual insecticides by knapsack sprayers from the ground. Great advances have been made in the application of insecticide from the air but this has so far been limited to the use of 'knock down' insecticide in aerosols and has not included the use of residual insecticides because of the difficulty of getting an adequate deposit of such chemicals at the required, relatively low, levels on the vegetation. Therefore, in this section, most attention will be paid to the organizational aspects of ground-applied, residual insecticide operations.

How such campaigns are to be organized depends on many factors, such as:

The Extent of the Operation

Increasing the scale of operations often brings entirely new factors into play; the requirements for a small scheme covering a limited area cannot simply be multiplied by a factor of 10, 100 or 1,000 to cover a correspondingly larger area. Mere increase in size calls for proportionately more organization.

The Habitat of the Species of Tsetse Attacked

In general, tsetse of the *palpalis* group have a restricted, linear, waterside distribution while those of the *morsitans* group are widely scattered throughout their savanna habitats. Exceptions to this broad division may be found; in Northern Nigeria, towards the northern limit of the distribution of *G. m. submorsitans*, the fly habitat at the height of the dry season becomes linear along water courses and flood-plains and in Central Nyanza, Kenya, *G. fuscipes* may spread to occupy large tracts of vegetation away from its normal riverine habitat.

This difference between these two groups also has, commonly, another bearing on the organization of control and acceptable cost since attack on the *palpalis* group is often for medical reasons with their acceptably higher costs, and that on the *morsitans* group for agricultural or veterinary reasons, normally requiring more stringent economic justification.

Climatic Factors and Insecticide Persistence

It is obvious that a residual insecticide deposit must remain effective, or be renewed, for long enough to kill every fly in the adult population and every fly that will emerge from the puparia already deposited before the first application. The length of persistence, and hence the number of applications necessary, is greatly affected by the length of the dry season and the amount of rainfall.

Climatic conditions may further affect the organization of spray campaigns by determining that at certain seasons of the year only very limited parts of the vegetation provide resting sites within the limits of temperature and desiccation that the fly can withstand. In such circumstances it may be possible to be extremely selective in the use of insecticide and still achieve eradication.

Delimitation of the Fly-Belt

This factor is extremely important because insecticidal treatment, as opposed to bush clearing, leaves the fly-habitat unaltered when the effect of the insecticide has worn off. Therefore, the delimitation and isolation of the fly-belt must be certain and completely proof against re-invasion or the whole effort will be wasted. Another problem is the difficulty of detecting tsetse at low density. Repeated careful searches may sometimes fail to reveal tsetse at densities which are very low but from which they can not only survive but also multiply. This problem is particularly acute when a control operation is planned to begin at the fringe of the fly distribution and work inwards. There have been instances where such operations, intended to start several miles beyond the tsetse limit, have failed because the tsetse were already established, in undetected low density, some distance behind the starting-line.

DETAILED ORGANIZATION AND COSTS

Insecticidal Campaigns

In order to make clear the type of detailed organization on which tsetse control schemes may be based and how costs can be built up, some examples will now be given of spraying team arrangement, their capabilities of coverage (in linear distance or area per day) and the consumption and cost of insecticide. These figures were originally obtained in 1966 and take no account of subsequent devaluation of the pound sterling; that is, twenty shillings are taken as equivalent to one pound.

KENYA—Linear Spraying against Riverine Tsetse (*G. fuscipes*).

Before spraying a path is cut as close as possible to (within a few feet of) the water's edge, on lake shore or on both banks of a river. A team for spraying both sides of a river, and their costs, are as follows:

STAFF	Total cost in shillings per month
6 path cutters (3 each side)	450
5 pump operators (2 each side spraying alternately and one in reserve)	500
4 porters (2 each side)	300
2 spray mixers (1 each side)	200
1 task demarcator	100
1 supervisor	350
1/3 Assistant Field Officer (responsible for 3 teams)	412
1/6 Field Zoologist (responsible for 6 teams)	500
Total	2,812

Standard task—3 miles per day
Insecticide Consumption—(5% Dieldrin)—3·5 gallons per mile for both sides (= 10·5 gallons per day)
Costs and Coverage per month of 20 working days:

210 gallons insecticide at 36s per gallon	= 7,560 Shs.
Total cost per month per application	10,372 Shs.

Standard task per month = 60 miles of river:

Cost per mile per application	= 173 Shs.
Cost per mile per 4 applications	= 692 Shs.
	= £35 (approx.)

KENYA—Block Spraying against *G. pallidipes*.

Ten pump operators are employed advancing in parallel on a front of 400 yards. The organization of the team and their costs are as follows:

	Total cost in shillings per month
Pre-cut paths (up to 30 cutters, average 15)	1,125
Pump operators (10 operators and 1 in reserve)	1,100
Filler porters (5)	400
Porters (3 forward, 4 rear)	525
Mechanic (1)	160
Flank demarcator (1)	100
Supervisor (2)	350
½ Assistant Field Officer (responsible for 2 teams)	625
1/6 Field Zoologist (responsible for 6 teams)	500
Standard task—1¼ square miles per day per team	
Insecticide consumption—12·5 gallons DDT concentrate per square mile per application	
Insecticidal cost per month of 20 working days at 20s per gallon	6,250
Total cost per month, staff and insecticide	11,135 Shs.
Approx. cost per square mile per application	450 Shs.
Cost per square mile for 4 applications	1,800 Shs. = £90
Approximate cost per acre for 4 applications	2·8 Shs.

In addition to the above costs there will be those of transport and of setting up and maintaining base camps for the staff. For riverine (linear) spraying three or four teams may operate from one camp but for block spraying only two. The transport allocated to one camp is normally three long-wheel-base Land Rovers and nine 3 to 5-ton lorries.

An example of total costs for an eradication scheme begun some ten years ago is given by Glover, le Roux and Parker (1960) in which the total costs of eradication of *G. fuscipes* in the Kuja-Migori river system, South Nyanza,

Kenya, were £120 per river mile, but these were total costs, including those of barrier clearing (varying from £150–£300 per mile), wages, insecticides and transport.

It is of interest to compare the above costs with those reported by Mahood (1961) in an experiment on the control of *G. palpalis* in the Guinea Savanna Zone of Northern Nigeria by single applications of various concentrations of Dieldrin to one or both banks of rivers. He found that the minimum cost for sprayers, labour and insecticide for a technique which was effective for any size of river was £8 per mile, which is very close to the £35 per mile for four applications quoted from Kenya, and the comparison only serves to accentuate the vast saving that can be achieved if climatic conditions permit reduction of the number of applications of insecticide.

UGANDA—Block spraying for eradication of *G. morsitans* is undertaken with the following spray teams:

10 Spray operators
10 Porters (insecticides)
1 Ganger (supply of insecticides)
1 Mechanic
1 Reserve Spray Operator
1 'Slasher-man'
1 Tsetse Assistant

Three teams constitute one Spraying Unit which not only has a Tsetse Officer in charge but also has at its base:

1 Insecticide Mixer
1 Storeman
1 Nightwatchman
Drivers and Van Boys for

Transport
1 Land Rover for Office i/c.
3 3-ton lorries
1 500-gallon tanker

Using such an organization, costs, including preliminary trials and capital equipment, worked out at Shs. 8/50 per acre (or approximately £275 per square mile).

However, as an example of the decrease in costs that can be achieved with experience and refinement, the operating costs of two well-trained and experienced teams fell to Shs. 3/68 per acre, or, with a 20% allowance for capital costs Shs. 4/42 per acre or £141 per square mile.

NIGERIA—Interesting examples of costs are given in 1963–64 and 1965–66 reports of the Tsetse and Trypanosomiasis Division (also referred to above as the Veterinary Tsetse and Trypanosomiasis Unit) of the Ministry of Animal and Forest Resources of Northern Nigeria. A schedule of these is given below;

Locality	Total cost of Insecticides, Vehicle Maintenance and Labour	Extent		Cost	
		Area sq. miles	Length miles	per sq. mile	per linear mile
1963–4	£				
Zonkwa	2,909	195	263	?	?
Shika	6,758	177·5	—	£38	—
Katagum	5,721	165	—	£35	—
Kiyawa	6,042	125	—	£48	—
Fika	7,341	190	—	£39	—
Yedsaram	2,931	954	—	£3[1]	—
Wikki (10.4.63)	25	—	1	—	£25
Wikki (20–23.11.63)	140	—	1	—	£140
1965–6					
Zonkwa	7,210	—	400	—	£18
Shika	7,360	281	—	£26	—
Komadugu Yobe	4,961	110	—	£45	—
Mayo Ine	611	—	143	—	£4·3
Jilli	233	—	22	—	£10·5

[1] Spraying of isolated and scattered habitats of *G. tachinoides* only, in the Sudan Zone vegetation.

Glover (*in press*) has pointed out that exact calculation of costs of tsetse eradication schemes is very difficult; it varies not only with the criteria used for extraction of costs from vote books, and with the method of measurement of the area reclaimed, but also with the relationship of the area actually sprayed to the area reclaimed and with the distribution of the sprayed areas—whether scattered or concentrated—and gives some overall figures for block and linear single application spraying schemes in Northern Nigeria not including senior staff salaries, capital expenditure or depreciation of equipment.[1]

'(a) *Against* G. morsitans [submorsitans] *in the Northern Guinea zone on the Shika scheme in Zaria Province.*

The actual square miles treated were 44;
the cost per square mile actually treated was £465;
the size of the scheme was 418 square miles;
the average cost per square mile was £51.

'(b) *Against* G. morsitans [submorsitans] *and* G. tachinoides *in the Sudan zone in a river flood plain on the Komadugu Gana–Katagum scheme over ten years.*

The actual square miles sprayed were 1,468;
the actual cost per square mile was £77;

[1] The writer is indebted to Dr P. E. Glover for permission to quote the following passages from his unpublished work.

the number of square miles freed of fly was 7,800;
the average expenditure per square mile over the whole area was £15.

'(c) *Against* G. morsitans [submorsitans], G. tachinoides *and* G. palpalis *in the sub-Sudan zone in a river flood plain on the Matyoro scheme.*

The number of square miles actually sprayed was 16;
the actual cost per square mile sprayed was £128;
the number of square miles freed of fly was 250;
the average expenditure per square mile over the whole area was £8;
the number of miles of river sprayed was 34;
the cost per river mile was £58.

In similar country the Fika scheme with the same three species of fly involved:
'the number of square miles sprayed was 190;
the cost per square mile was £50.

'(d) *Against* G. tachinoides *in the Sudan and sub-Sudan zones on the Mayo Ine Scheme.*

The number of river miles sprayed is difficult to calculate because of wide meandering flood plains;
The average expenditure per river mile was £20.

On the Yedseram scheme in the Sudan zone.
The number of square miles sprayed was 1,247;
The average cost per square mile over the whole area was £5 10s 0d.

'(e) *Against* G. palpalis *in the Northern Guinea zone on the Zonkwa scheme.*

The number of river miles sprayed was 1,846;
the number of square miles treated was 1,264;
the cost per river mile was £15;
the cost per square mile was £25.

'(f) *Against* G. palpalis *in the sub-Sudan zone on the Biu scheme.*

The number of river miles sprayed was 1,400;
the number of square miles sprayed was 644;
the cost per river mile was £2.
the cost per square mile was about £4.

'It must be noted here, however, that on neither of these schemes was *G. palpalis* completely exterminated nor on any of the schemes mentioned above was the cost of initial survey, follow-up checks or off-season expenses taken into account.

'It is therefore estimated that a realistic average price per square mile actually sprayed in the northern Guinea zones of Northern Nigeria would be £110 and the cost per river mile actually sprayed, about £50, taking everything into account—capital expenditure, depreciation of equipment, surveys, the creation of insecticidal and cleared barriers, etc. (Glover & Aitchison, 1966).'

Hand-clearing of Vegetation

The costs of hand-clearing of bush have risen so sharply with increasing labour costs that this method is now little used and consequently up-to-date figures are difficult to obtain.

Glover, le Roux and Parker (1960) mentioned that from 1948 to 1950 the cost of total clearing of some rivers in South Nyanza 'proved to be prohibitive, i.e. £200–£300 per river mile'.

More recent figures were made available to the writer in 1966 by Dr W. R. Wooff, Chief Tsetse Officer, Uganda, for clearing light *Acacia* bush and secondary forest; for light *Acacia* bush 4 man-days per acre were required, at a cost of Shs. 21 per acre or £670 per square mile, and for secondary forest 20 man-days per acre, costing Shs. 105 per acre or £3,360 per square mile. These costs did not include supervisory and demarcation expenses or the cost of re-slashing after eighteen months growth. The former were put at 5% of the above costs and the latter at 40%. The total costs therefore for the original clearing plus re-slashing would be £970 per square mile in light *Acacia* and £4,860 per square mile in secondary forest if only one re-slashing were needed.

Mechanical Clearing of Vegetation

Glover, Trump and Williams (1959) gave costs for both 'blade' and 'chain' clearing with various types of tractor.

Blade clearing is straightforward bull-dozing of the bush but in chain clearing a heavy naval anchor-chain is attached to two heavy tractors normally operating 60–80 yards apart with 220–250 yards of chain between them. Very heavy chain is used, that used in Kenya having links of 10·5 × 7·25 inches constructed of 2 inch diameter steel. Formerly, heavy steel balls were attached to the chain to prevent it riding over vegetation but with very heavy chain this has been found unnecessary.

The costs quoted by Glover *et al.* (1959) may be summarized as follows:

Tractor	Hire cost per hour shillings	Acres per hour	Cost: Shs. per acre
BLADE CLEARING			
International T.D.18A	74	1·20–1·6	61·66–46·25
Caterpillar D8	93–100	1·00–2·3	100–43·47
Caterpillar D7	90	2·0	45
CHAIN CLEARING			
International T.D.18A	74	3·0	24·67
Caterpillar D8	97–100	2·48–5·4	40·32–18·51
Caterpillar D7	90	5·0	18

Mixed blade and chain clearing in the Lambwe Valley, South Nyanza, Kenya, cost Shs. 38·70 per acre.

More recent figures (1966) from Dr Wooff in Uganda for chain clearing are based on an acceptable hire cost of a Caterpillar D8 tractor of Shs. 120 per hour—though rates as high as Shs. 135 per hour had been asked. The Caterpillar

D8 was chosen as the only machine heavy enough for some of the work and its capabilities in chain clearing were given as follows:

Type of Vegetation	Acres per tractor hour	Cost in Shs. per acre
Open *Acacia*	9	13·33
Terminalia—Combretum—Albizzia in Bunyoro, Western Uganda	3·6	33·33
Secondary forest	2·5	48·00

However, if 'wind-rowing' (clearing of the felled vegetation into wind-rows) is necessary the cost is greatly increased as this process is four to five times as expensive as the original chain clearing.

Part III

HUMAN TRYPANOSOMIASIS (SLEEPING SICKNESS)

Chapter 31

Pathogenesis and Pathology of Trypanosomiasis in Man

W. E. ORMEROD

INTRODUCTORY

The variation in pathological types of sleeping sickness which has occurred in different parts of Africa and at different times since it was first identified, shows that the relationship between parasite and host is not static. This variation covers a wide range, from the fleeting parasitaemia of a strain derived from animals (van Hoof, 1947), through the heavy parasitaemia of virulent Rhodesian disease, the insidious Gambian disease which can exterminate a whole population, to the balanced situation noted in Nigeria (Macfie, 1913; Duggan, 1962) and in Sierra Leone (Harding & Hutchinson, 1948) where high rates of infection are associated with mild symptoms and a normal death rate.

Although the geographical distribution of the different types of sleeping sickness has in the past justified the use of the specific terms *Trypanosoma gambiense* and *T. rhodesiense*, the basic pathological process and morbid anatomical findings are similar throughout, and such differences of detail as do occur, do not conform to, but cut across, the usual division into two species. For instance, perivascular cuffing, described in a later section of this chapter, is almost absent in acute epidemic Rhodesian disease and is at its densest in chronic Gambian disease, but almost equal density is also found in the disease from the Zambesi basin usually classified as of Rhodesian type. Similarly, the swelling of glands in the posterior triangle of the neck, Winterbottom's sign noted by the slave traders of the West African coast as denoting the onset of the fatal 'Negro lethargy,' occurs frequently in some, but not all, areas in West Africa and also in occasional foci of epidemic Rhodesian disease; Kunert (1939) noted that although he had seen swollen glands in all patients in Tanzania in 1927–8, he could find none in the same area ten years later.

Normally, an infectious disease changes its natural history as parasite and host establish a genetic balance based on the invasiveness of the one and the resistance of the other but, where reservoir hosts and insect-transmitting agents are also involved, the scope for variation is greatly increased; for example, the strains giving rise to epidemic Rhodesian disease increase in virulence when the infection is being transmitted from man to man by *Glossina morsitans* but, when an animal reservoir intervenes, the organism, by adapting to the new host, decreases its virulence and changes its pathogenicity for man. This would explain the findings of Kunert and others in Tanzania (Ormerod, 1961), and this and similar processes would account for the diversity of different forms of the disease occurring at different times and places throughout Africa.

THE INITIAL INFECTION

Number of Trypanosomes required to Infect

A factor which may be important in determining whether or not man develops an infection is the number of metacyclic form sinjected by the insect vector. By an indirect method, using the 'probing technique' (*see* pp. 87–88), Fairbairn & Burtt (1946) concluded that the minimum infective dose for man was 300–450 metacyclic trypanosomes. However, the number injected may vary widely and

Harley *et al.* (1966) have shown, by a different technique involving titration in mice, that *Glossina morsitans* can inject from 0–40,000 (mean 3,200) infective doses for mice on the ID63 scale (one infective does for a mouse being presumed to be equivalent to one metacyclic trypanosome).

It might be expected that the greater the number of trypanosomes injected the higher would be the parasitaemia and the more rapid the progress of the infection but this is not always the case. Baker (1960) demonstrated a clear-cut inverse logarithmic relationship between the number of trypanosomes injected and the pre-patent period with a strain of *T. brucei* of animal origin from south-east Uganda. On the other hand Ormerod (1963) compared three human strains from Botswana, Tanzania and south-east Uganda and showed that only the strain from south-east Uganda produced a higher parasitaemia and a more rapidly developing infection at the high dose level; the others gave approximately the same pattern of infection whatever the initial dose of trypanosomes. Both workers used trypanosomes derived from blood but different methods of assay. It will be necessary to repeat this work using metacyclic trypanosomes before firm conclusions can be drawn.

The Tsetse Bite

Of the means of injection, more information is available. Gordon *et al.* (1956) in studying the method of feeding of the tsetse fly, have shown that it is possible for metacyclic trypanosomes to be injected either directly into the blood stream or to gain access to the tissues from the pool of blood from which the tsetse feeds. If injected directly into the blood, the trypanosomes remain infective as found by Willett and Gordon (1957) who were able to demonstrate that trypanosomes injected directly into the blood of rabbits were recoverable by sub-inoculation from the moment of the initial injection to the time that the infection became fully patent; thus in the strict sense there is no 'pre-patent' period and no cryptic form of the disease analogous to the exoerythrocytic phase of malaria.

Distinction between Human and Experimental Infections

In human trypanosomiasis, parasites appear in the circulating blood in relatively small numbers and the growth of the trypanosomes occurs mainly in other tissues. In laboratory rodents, on the other hand, infections are associated with a high prevalence of trypanosomes in the blood where they are easy to detect and to estimate quantitatively. There has been a tendency in the past to apply the results of investigations on laboratory rodents to the human disease thus giving rise to an unbalanced view of the pathogenesis of the disease in man.

The Trypanosome 'Chancre'

When the tsetse probes the subcutaneous tissues, trypanosomes become lodged and give rise to a 'trypanosomal chancre'. In four to ten days a hard, painful, red nodule appears in the skin and heat and swelling spread to the surrounding tissues; the appearance is similar to the cellulitis surrounding a staphylococcal boil as it begins to localize but differs in that on puncture no pus is withdrawn but clear fluid containing trypanosomes. The histopathology of a chancre excised ten days after the feeding of a fly infected with a strain from Botswana was studied by Fairbairn and Godfrey (1957). Long-thin trypanosomes were seen both within and below the dermis and, in both sites, there was an exudation of lymph and round cell infiltration, consisting mainly of lymphocytes, which extended along the vessels into subcutaneous fatty tissue. Within two weeks most chancres have resolved sometimes leaving slight scarring but often no visible trace. Few patients give a history of trypanosomal chancre but Fairbairn and Godfrey (1958) report that 239 out of 257 volunteers showed chancres when experimentally infected; it is possible that chancres are rare in some areas, but it is more probable that the patient forgets that he has had one, there being little apparent connection between the 'boil' and the subsequent disease.

Trypanosomes in the chancre develop from the short metacyclic form into the long-thin form which also invades the blood. In man, penetration of the lymph vessels occurs and it is by this route rather than by the blood that the lymphatic glands are invaded and the stage of acute generalized trypanosomiasis is initiated.

Typical chancre also occurs when blood forms are injected under the skin (Manson-Bahr, 1959) so that neither metacyclic trypanosomes nor tsetse saliva are essential to its development.

Sensitivity to Tsetse Bite

Severe reaction of an anaphylactic type is often observed to tsetse bite. This may take the form of an Arthus type reaction with, in extreme cases, sloughing at the site, or the severe constitutional changes typical of anaphylactic shock may be observed. Such reactions may occur following the bites of infected or uninfected flies. Fairbairn and Williamson (1956) have shown that the proteins of tsetse saliva are greatly diminished when the salivary glands of the fly are infected so that it is possible that the bite of an infected fly may be less liable than that of an uninfected fly to produce a reaction in a sensitized subject. Cases reported by Graf (1929) indicate that infection may follow bites that have produced severe reaction. Further work on this subject is required. Some Europeans continue to suffer anaphylactic reactions from tsetse bites whilst others rapidly become desensitized.

Transmission by means other than Tsetse Bite

Biting flies other than tsetse probably transmit infection at the height of an epidemic although there is no definite proof that this occurs. When it has been suspected, as in the Mazwa epidemic recorded by Swynnerton (1923), virulence has been exalted in much the same way as by syringe passage in the laboratory.

Congenital infection has been described on a number of occasions (Capponi, 1953; Darré *et al.*, 1937; David & Pape, 1942; Pinto, 1960) and experimental observations on the reason for its occurrence have been reported by Werner and Kunert (1958). Lanfranchi (1915) has claimed that infection can also be transmitted from mother to offspring through the milk but this is denied by Werner (1954).

MORPHOLOGICAL CHANGES IN THE TRYPANOSOME AS RELATED TO THE COURSE OF THE INFECTION

Metacyclic trypanosomes develop into long-thin forms during the first three to five days of the infection; thereafter, short-stumpy forms and a complete range of intermediate forms appear. This development may occur either in the blood or in the chancre but it is only under experimental conditions and with certain strains that a 'synchronous' infection can be observed, that is, an infection where all trypanosomes are transformed from one form to the other at approximately the same time.

Fine Structure

The long-thin forms undergo rapid division and are characterized by frequent reduplication of kinetoplast, nucleus and flagellum; under electron microscopy the cytoplasm is shown to contain free ribosomes which are grouped into polysomes as in other rapidly dividing cells. The short-stumpy trypanosome which does not divide, shows, on the other hand, the accumulation of loculae and of material inside a swollen rough endoplasmic reticulum giving the parasite the characteristic appearance of a secretory cell (Bird *et al.*, 1966). These loculae can also be seen as refractile granules under phase microscopy and their appearance precedes the removal of trypanosomes from the blood (*see* also p. 601).

Relation of Virulence to Rate of Growth and to Immune Response of the Host

The degree of virulence of an infection can be determined either by the rate of growth of the trypanosome or by the extent to which its rate of growth is checked by the host. It is widely recognized that strains which have undergone laboratory passage become virulent by the selection of organisms which grow rapidly; thus, a laboratory animal infected by a strain of exalted virulence develops intense parasitaemia and dies before any inhibition reaction occurs. But in strains which have not undergone this selection those which produce the more chronic infections in man are not necessarily those which grow more slowly but those in which growth is checked by the defensive mechanism of the host. Moreover, it can be shown by assay methods in experimental animals (Ormerod, 1963) that the difference in the type of infection is as much a property of the strain of parasite as of the host.

Relation of Virulence to the Morphology of the Trypanosome

The virulence of sleeping sickness trypanosomes is closely related to their morphology. It is well known that in strains which have undergone prolonged laboratory passage only the long-thin form of the parasite is to be seen; the short-stumpy form is absent and hence the loculae of the endoplasmic reticulum are so small and infrequent as rarely to be seen under phase contrast. But with Rhodesian strains that have not been passaged in the laboratory the frequency and size of the loculae (here clearly visible under phase contrast) are related to virulence; strains with large loculae cause a chronic form of the disease in man and an infection in rats in which a marked crisis occurs, whereas those with smaller loculae cause a disease in man which is relatively acute and an infection in rats which tends to be progressive (Ormerod, 1963).

MORPHOLOGICAL CHANGES IN THE INFECTED HOST

Acute Generalized Trypanosomiasis

The chancre has already been described in relation to the bite of the fly and it has been pointed out that there is evidence of direct lymphatic spread of the disease in man as well as of spread by the blood which is such an obvious feature in experimental animals. The fact that infection in man is disseminated mainly through the lymphatic system prompted earlier workers (Schuberg & Böing, 1913; Reichenow, 1921) to draw an analogy between sleeping sickness and syphilis based on (a) the occurrence of chancre, (b) the subsequent swelling of glands both in local drainage of chancre and in the body as a whole, and (c) subsequent involvement of the central nervous system.

Mott (1906) pointed out that although the initial effects on the central nervous system were similar, the demyelinization and neurone damage which are characteristic of the tertiary leutic lesion were not, in his experience, important features of sleeping sickness.

Lymph Glands

Swollen lymphatic glands, an important diagnostic feature in the epidemiological situations in which it occurs, can be studied either by biopsy or aspiration. There are, however, no records of biopsy having been performed, and our outline of knowledge of lymph gland pathology is derived from *post mortem* material. Sections of lymphatic glands, taken during the acute phase of the disease, show that the lymphoid germinal centres, normally composed of clusters of small lymphocytes, have changed into cells of the lymphocyte—plasma cell series; macrophages are also present especially in the early stages of the disease. The same appearances can be produced in experimental rats (Castro *et al.*, 1967) using the technique developed by Nossal (1962) of injecting antigenic material—in this case live trypanosomes—into the foot pad of the rat and studying the cellular reaction in the popliteal gland; by this means it can be shown that there is no demonstrable difference between the cellular reaction stimulated by trypanosomes and that stimulated by, say, pneumococcal antigen.

Aspiration of swollen glands is one of the most effective methods of isolating trypanosomes from suspected cases. Theoretically, the cellular reaction could also be studied by this means but this has not been reported.

Blood and Bone Marrow

The blood changes which occur in the early stages of sleeping sickness are not of much diagnostic help; they consist of gradual fall of both red and white cell elements, the differential white count showing a relative fall in granulocytes and a rise in mononuclears. No information is available on the state of the marrow in human trypanosomiasis and it is not known whether the anaemia and granulopenia is caused by inhibition of growth, by replacement of these elements in the marrow space by lymphocyte or macrophage elements, or by some other factor such as haemolysis which has no relation to the marrow. Polymorphonuclear leucocytes appear to play very little part in the reaction of man to trypanosome infection.

Spleen

The spleen increases in size roughly in proportion to the anaemia, the texture of the organ is firm and cellular and there is little fibrosis at any but the latest stages. The sinusoids in the early stages of the disease contain active macrophages, and since Levaditi and Mutermilch (1910) and Delanöe (1912), it has been generally believed that these cells, both in the spleen and to a lesser extent elsewhere, are the main source of phagocytic activity against trypanosomes; it has also been assumed that in early sleeping sickness haemolysis occurred in the sinusoids and that this was the cause of the anaemia. There is, however, little evidence that destruction of red cells occurs on any abnormal scale. Increase in the Malpignian corpuscles is the most important change; their structure is analogous to that of the lymph glands and the transformation of cells, from inactive small lymphocytes through to plasma cells, occurs in the same manner. The spleen thus appears to be the main source of plasma cells but the lymph glands are also important in some cases; the importance of the bone marrow in this respect is still unknown.

Globulin Production

The production of globulins is shown dramatically by the rising erythrocyte sedimentation rates (Gall *et al.*, 1957) which in advanced cases rise to 114 mm./hr. Westergren. In infectious diseases generally there is an initial rise in high molecular weight globulin IgM and this is succeeded in a few days by a rise in the IgG which normally contains the main antibody activity; but sleeping sickness does not follow the usual pattern in that no significant secondary IgG response occurs (Mattern, 1962) and the amounts of IgM in the blood continue to accumulate. Although it is uncertain how much of the large accumulation of globulin represents specific antibody, immune electrophoresis against trypanosomal antigen demonstrates the presence of antibody in the IgM but only to a negligible extent in the IgG.

If, as seems probable, antibody is largely, if not wholly, linked with the larger IgM molecule which is unable to pass across membranes with the comparative ease of IgG, an explanation is provided for some of the pathological changes which have been observed in trypanosomiasis. Clapier (1921) found a surprisingly large number of trypanosomes in hydrocoel fluid and Heisch and Killick-Kendrick (personal communication) have recently observed prolific growth of both Gambian and Rhodesian strains in the testes of rabbits. Failure of IgM to reach these sites would account for these observations and, for the same reason, it would seem to be unlikely that antibodies occur in milk or colostrum although there is no factual evidence that this is so.

It is well known that immunity to sleeping sickness does not persist for long after infection has been eradicated and that patients recovered from the disease are susceptible to subsequent re-infection on one or more occasions. This is what might be expected from present knowledge of the behaviour of IgM.

The Heart

In the early stages of infection with Rhodesian disease, the heart is generally considered to be the organ most at risk and myocarditis was said to be the main cause of mortality in the Uganda epidemic of the 1940s, where death sometimes occurred in as little as four to six weeks. Peruzzi (1928) and Regendanz and Hoeppli (1929) obtained convincing evidence of myocarditis in *post mortem* material taken from monkeys suffering from acute trypanosomiasis but comparable evidence for the human disease is curiously lacking. Hawking and Greenfield (1941) described a severe myocarditis in Rhodesian infection but this may not have been specific, whilst Mott (1906) in studying cases of Gambian disease ascribed the myocardial changes that he observed to secondary infection. Of the two cases of myocardial lesion in sleeping sickness described by Mackie (1935) one was clearly the result of secondary bacterial infection and the other, a massive haemorrhagic lesion, was ascribed to arsenic treatment because of its similarity to lesions in the brain under such circumstances (*see* below). Two cases of Gambian disease (Lavier & Leroux, 1939) showed intense lesions consisting of sclerotic endocarditis and periarterial myocarditis with arteritis of branches of the coronary vessel. There is little doubt, however, that the heart is affected functionally either through vagal stimulation which may result in severe bradycardia (Lagane, 1913), the liberation of kinins such as those described by Goodwin and Boreham (1966) or the other general effects of the disease which, whatever their nature, are sufficient to cause electrocardiographic abnormalities as described by Bertrand *et al.* (1965) and by Manson-Bahr and Charters (1963) who described congestive heart failure which returned to normal after trypanocidal therapy.

Skin Rash

Little is known of the pathology of the rash which is seen only in white-skinned patients but the fact that it is a fleeting erythema suggests that it is more likely to be connected with the liberation of histamine rather than with cellular infiltration of the skin.

Hyperaethesia

The deep hyperaethesia known as Kérandel's sign (Martin & Darré, 1908) is transitory. This symptom is often supposed to be due to periostitis but there is no positive evidence for this hypothesis and much to suggest that it is of nervous origin, being the equivalent in the sensory nervous system of the motor changes considered in a later section.

Kidney and Liver

Changes in the kidney are not known to be a feature of untreated sleeping sickness, but the liver is probably affected to some extent in most cases but in only two cases (Gelfand & Friedlander, 1963) has jaundice been described as a symptom. It is difficult to assess how much of the cloudy swelling and centrilobular necrosis found at autopsy is a result of the primary disease process and how much is due to secondary infection and the terminal state. Robertson and Jenkins (1959) have shown that there is indeed disfunction of the liver during life.

Early Meningeal Reaction

The meninges and the brain probably begin to be affected early in the infection although it is not possible to say at what stage this occurs; many observers think that the severe headache which accompanies the early stages of the disease cannot be explained in terms of the general constitutional disturbance of a severe infection with high pyrexia. Perivascular cuffing (*see* below) does not seem to occur until three months at the earliest but it is accompanied and, no doubt, preceded by adventitious small round cells in the brain substance, and the appearance of cells, protein and immune globulins in the cerebrospinal fluid, suggesting that the meninges may be affected quite early in the disease. The fact that meningeal infection is described here only in the final stage of sleeping sickness must not be taken to indicate that the process does not begin, or even develop substantially, at an earlier stage; it is this possibility of early involvement of the meninges that gave rise to the penetrating, but ill-documented, study by Le Port (1935) who produced evidence that headache and mental changes may be due to ventricular hypertension causing compression of the floor of the third and fourth ventricles. This occurs, he says, as a result of swelling of the choroid plexus with consequent blockage of the lateral apertures of the fourth ventricle and of the interventricular foramen. This plausible hypothesis needs further investigation but indicates the practical possibility that spinal or cisternal decompression might exacerbate symptoms, and that restitution of fluid should in these circumstances be considered so as not to increase the blockage of ventricular apertures.

Toxicity of Trypanocidal Drugs

The effect of arsenical drugs on the nervous system of some sleeping sickness patients appears to be more profound than the effects of either drug or disease alone. Optic atrophy is probably rare or absent in untreated cases of sleeping sickness but very common in those treated with tryparsamide; similarly, cerebral disasters occur unexpectedly in patients treated with either tryparsamide or melarsoprol. These disasters have seldom been investigated in detail, but the clinical histories suggest a resemblance to the case of Mackie (1935) which showed sudden and unexpected deterioration on arsenical therapy; at autopsy, large haemorrhagic areas were found in the brain and myocardium. Mackie suggests that the mechanism of production of this lesion may be similar to the Jarisch-Herxheimer reaction in which similar lesions are occasionally produced during the treatment of syphilis; it is believed that, in this reaction, antigen to which the host has already been sensitized is suddenly liberated from the parasite, with resulting tissue destruction due to anaphylaxis. A more familiar analogy today would be the severe reaction which frequently follows treatment of onchocerciasis with Banocide.

Although little has been recorded and nothing further published about these disasters, it is the writer's subjective impression, based on one personal case treated with melarsoprol and on discussions with other workers with more experience, that it is not the most severe cases of sleeping sickness that are liable to this accident; consequently, it is necessary to assess carefully whether it is necessary to treat individual patients with arsenicals, or whether suramin treatment would suffice, remembering also that arsenic is itself highly toxic to the brain (Pentschew, 1958).

Suramin is normally a non-toxic drug but is well known to produce urinary casts because it is absorbed in large amounts by the epithelial cells of the proximal tubules of the kidney (Janscó & Janscó-Gabor, 1952). Suramin has an action on the foetus in experimental animals (Whitten, 1956); this is not fully understood and has not been observed in man.

Advanced Sleeping Sickness

Depending on the type of disease, cerebral lesions can be expected to appear from about three to eighteen months from the beginning of symptoms. Clinically, there is no precise time when cerebral symptoms may be said to have begun; the intense headache of the earlier stage often decreases but a general increase in drowsiness in the daytime and insomnia at night indicate the advance of cerebral lesions. The progress of the disease is characterized by increasing anaemia, leucopoenia and great wasting of limb, abdominal and thoracic muscles. Wasting may be associated with pigmentation, suggesting the possibility of suprarenal involvement, and although no lesions of the suprarenal have yet been described in man, Chaterji and Sen Gupta (1962) have observed them in experimental rats infected with *T. evansi*.

Fibrosis of the lymph vessels is a characteristic change at this stage and glands which presumably were highly cellular during earlier phases of the disease later become small and sometimes hard and shotty; during this transition they may contain morular cells (Low & Mott, 1904).

In many late cases the level of globulins in the blood remains high but despite this there may be evidence of immunological failure as shown by the absence of complement, the occurrence of pseudo-positive Wassermann reactions and the presence of heterophile antibodies (Henderson-Begg, 1946). Mott (1906) states that in 80% of the cases of the Gambian disease examined *post mortem* there was infiltration of the organs with *cocci* and that this was the usual cause of death.

Several descriptions of the cerebral lesions in sleeping sickness, in gross anatomical terms, were published during the nineteenth century, the best being that of Clark (1840) who, in a series of *post mortem* examinations, observed inflammation of the brain associated with swelling and adhesion of the dura to arachnoid mater.

Meningo-encephalitis was first observed by Mott (1899). The same author (Mott, 1906) and Van Bogaert (1958) published descriptions of the cerebral lesions in Gambian sleeping sickness and these two accounts provide most of the information available on this subject.

Late Meningeal Reaction

Most workers believe that the brain becomes infected by the transference of trypanosomes from blood to cerebrospinal fluid across a hypothetical 'barrier' which normally prevents the passage of large molecules, including drugs and proteins. Mott's original hypothesis that the infection penetrates by way of lymph connections along nerves entering the skull is probably a more satisfactory explanation; thus he considers that infection of the base of the brain may arise directly from glands of the neck. Just as the earlier phase of the disease can be considered a chronic lymph-borne inflammation of glands and vessels, so the disease in the nervous system can be considered as similar infection of the meninges carried by the cerebrospinal fluid. The lesion is most marked where the spinal fluid is most abundant, i.e. the lateral cisternae and the base of the brain; the more chronic the infection, the more intense the inflammatory process and the more widespread its occurrence. Thus, Neujean (1950), as a result of a study of 312 patients, states that the fluid obtained by cisternal puncture gives a better indication of the pathological process than that obtained by lumbar puncture.

The inflammation affects mainly the pia-arachnoid mater which becomes thickened and 'felted' onto the surface of the brain; its cellularity is increased by infiltration of cells of the lymphocyte series; thus, all stages of lymphocytes, plasma cell and morular cell are found, and in very chronic cases morular cells are the most characteristic finding. In addition, there is an increase in numbers of microglial cells in the subarachnoid space.

As the disease progresses the more remote parts of the subarachnoid space are affected, thus, only in advanced cases are morular cells obtained at lumbar puncture; but the most characteristic lesion which results from this spreading of the disease process is a cellular infiltration which invades the spaces surrounding the blood vessels as they penetrate the brain substance, carrying with them a layer of pia mater. The vessels then become surrounded by the same types of cell as are found in the affected meninges in a lesion known as 'perivascular cuffing': this may consist of a single layer of cells or in advanced cases of a sheath, 20–30 cells deep, surrounding the vessel. The appearance of morular cells in perivascular cuffing is considered to be pathognomonic of sleeping sickness.

The areas of perivascular cuffing are also infiltrated with microglial cells and there is a great general increase of these cells in the brain substance. This increase precedes the appearance of cuffing and may be well advanced in cases of Rhodesian disease where cuffing is absent or minimal.

Brain Damage

Despite the observation (Mott, 1906) that the main difference between sleeping sickness and general paralysis of the insane lies in the relative absence of brain damage in sleeping sickness, some damage does occur in advanced cases and is responsible for a degree of mental deterioration. Mott (1906) pointed out that, in chronic cases, chromatolysis of neurones occurred around the cuffed vessels and may proceed to Wallerian degeneration of nerve tracts. Where this occurs swollen masses of macroglial cells may be seen; these, however, are comparatively rare. This type of degeneration probably does not occur in Rhodesian disease as it appears to be associated solely with advanced perivascular cuffing.

Functional Studies of the Nervous System

Recent studies of the sequelae of sleeping sickness by electro- and pneumo-encephalography have produced divergent results. Gallais *et al.* (1956) found that in Gambian disease severe destruction of cortical tissue could be demonstrated by pneumo-encephalography and that these patients, even after cure of the parasitic disease, were left with a degree of dementia. Collomb and Miletto (1957) found that their patients either died or made a complete recovery as estimated by electro- and pneumo-encephalography; neither of these findings is incompatible with the general conclusion of Mott that, whereas syphilis causes a primary cerebral degeneration, the degeneration in sleeping sickness is secondary to the perivascular infiltration; it may be added, however, that these degenerations are equally irreversible once they have begun to occur.

Differential Diagnosis at *Post Mortem* Examination

The differential diagnosis of cerebral sleeping sickness from other meningo-encephalitides rarely offers difficulty except where death has preceded the development of perivascular cuffing in which case death may fairly be ascribed to extracerebral causes. Superficially, syphilis may be similar, but as stated previously, can be distinguished by greater cerebral degeneration; septic meningitis may be distinguished by the prevalence of polymorphonuclear leucocytes which are inconspicuous or absent in uncomplicated sleeping sickness. It must be remembered, however, that sepsis is a frequent sequel of sleeping sickness.

Virus encephalitides sometimes cause dense perivascular cuffing but this occurs as a result of relatively acute illness and it is unlikely that similar densities would be produced in sleeping sickness in under a year's illness; the presence of the morular cell in the cuffing is a sign that the disease is very chronic.

Cerebral malaria is not a meningo-encephalitis and can easily be distinguished by the presence of pigmented schizonts in the capillaries of the brain which are frequently completely blocked. When rupture of capillaries occurs, petechial haemorrhages can be seen. Similar petechial haemorrhages are observed in acute sleeping sickness, but thrombosis rarely occurs (Ormerod, unpublished observation) and is probably due to some unrelated disease process.

Cerebral Localization and Peripheral Nervous Disorders

Localization of the disease process in the brain is generally absent and neurological signs of the disease, although frequent, are fleeting and seldom localized. Abnormal hunger, said to be due to pressure on the floor of the fourth ventricle, is sometimes noted. Christy (1903) states 'by a cruel irony, one of the most conspicuous symptoms of this mysterious disease in a large number of cases, is an inordinate appetite, 'til the last, the patient continually waking up and asking for food, when he is so weak he cannot raise himself upon his elbows'. This is not a constant feature of the disease but in the cases which occur it may persist after recovery and produce obesity in previously cachectic patients.

In some outbreaks, however, neurological signs may occasionally feature. Sensory symptoms have been noted above. Van Bogaert and Janssen (1957), in Ruanda-Urundi, observed extra-pyramidal and cerebellar signs. Evidence of polyneuritis has been observed but the signs are fleeting and changeable; Gelfand (1947) observed a case from Zambia and Janssen *et al.* (1956), in a series of seven autopsies, noted peripheral nerve involvement in all although clinical evidence was apparent in only one of these cases.

PROBLEMS OF SLEEPING SICKNESS PATHOLOGY

The study of the histo-pathology of sleeping sickness has developed surprisingly little since the classical studies of Mott (1906) which are as valid today as they were sixty years ago; but more information is needed especially on the detailed histology of the brain lesions which could probably be redefined in terms of modern concepts of brain histology if supplies of suitable autopsy material could be obtained. But sleeping sickness is usually treated in the bush and not in clinics and fatal cases are not often examined *post mortem*; in the absence of refrigeration the tissues rarely come to a neuro-pathologist in a condition fit for examination. Consequently, much of our pathological knowledge is in outline only and will have to be filled in before any clear picture can emerge; in the meantime it is worthwhile to consider several aspects of the pathogenesis since much experimental work has been done, especially in the immunological field, which it will be profitable to discuss in pathological terms.

The Plasma Cell and Immune Globulins

Nossal (1962) showed that individual plasma cells were capable of producing both IgM and IgG, the latter being the more important source of antibody in most infectious diseases. In sleeping sickness, however, despite the large numbers of plasma cells available, only IgM is produced in significant amount and it seems likely that this unusual occurrence may be related to other unusual features of the pathogenesis of sleeping sickness.

As has been mentioned above (p. 593) the large IgM molecule is probably too large to pass readily through membranes. Several workers (Reichenow, 1921; Lucasse, 1964) have observed that, in the early stages of the disease, trypanosomes appear in the cerebrospinal fluid in greater numbers than in the blood and have suggested that this invasion of the cerebrospinal fluid occurs at a time when antibodies begin to accumulate in the blood but are not yet present in the cerebrospinal fluid. But this state of affairs does not persist throughout the infection and, at a later stage, immune globulins appear in the cerebrospinal fluid probably as the result of secretion *in situ* by cells of the lymphocyte-plasma cell series, infiltrations of which are a prominent feature of meningeal involvement in sleeping sickness. Whatever the source of these immune globulins, Mattern *et al.* (1965) have shown that there is a progressive accumulation of IgM in the cerebrospinal fluid as the disease advances and, in the late stages of the disease, this may account for the fact that trypanosomes in the cerebrospinal fluid become almost as scarce as in other parts of the body.

It is not known why, in sleeping sickness, IgG fails to appear in significant amounts although large quantities of IgM are poured into the blood. A similar failure in IgG formation occurs in Waldenstrom's macroglobulinaemia despite an increase in plasma cells and there may be a basic similarity between these two conditions. In the case of sleeping sickness, a possible explanation is that the rapid antigenic variations which have been shown to occur (Gray, 1965) may allow sufficient time for the formation of IgM but not for the delayed IgG response. Alternatively, there may be direct interference with the synthesis of IgG by some factor such as a hypothetical trypanosome toxin but there is no positive evidence for this.

The Nature of Morular Cells

Although an abundance of lymphocytes and plasma cells is a feature of all stages of the disease the later stages are also characterized by the presence of morular cells. These were first recognized by Christy (1904) who saw them in cerebrospinal fluid. Mott (1906) recognized them as being derived from the 'plasma cells of Marshalko' but others (notably Peruzzi, 1928) have supposed them to be neuroglial in origin; Mott also stated that they were the same as the 'Kornshenzellen of Alzheimer'. Recent studies of the secretion of globulins by plasma cells (White, 1960) have shown, by using fluorescent antibody technique, that spherical globules in active plasma cells (Russell bodies) consist of immune globulins, that these bodies are produced in plasma cells in the lymph glands in many chronic infections and, so far as studies have been carried out, that they have the same appearance and staining properties as the spherical bodies in morular cells. There seems little doubt that morular cells represent the end point in the development of the lymphocyte-plasma cell series but it is not known whether the globules contain active immune globulin or whether the morular cells themselves are moribund.

Possible Cause of an Anaphylactic Reaction

The most characteristic feature of the late stage of the disease in man is a very severe meningo-encephalitis associated with such a scarcity of trypanosomes that diagnosis by microscopy may be very difficult. The more advanced this pathological progress becomes the smaller the number of detectable trypanosomes yet, after successful treatment, the lesion undergoes almost complete regression. This strongly suggests that the pathological changes observed are the result of the immune response of the host, and that they are not produced by direct toxic or mechanical damage caused by the organism, as appears to be the case in some experimentally infected animals.

It is possible that, in man, these late changes may be associated with an auto-immune reaction. Kosma (1962) has shown that, in infection with *Trypanosoma cruzi*, anti-heart antibody may be produced and the possibility should be borne in mind that, in sleeping sickness, anti-nerve cell antibody may be formed although, as has been discussed, the degree of destruction of nerve cells is not of such magnitude as to make this likely.

An alternative explanation may be that man produces more antibody than other animals so that a severe anaphylactic reaction may follow the continuing destruction of the small numbers of trypanosomes present. Such a reaction could be regarded as analogous, albeit on a smaller scale, to that which occurs when trypanosomes are rapidly destroyed following administration of an arsenical trypanocide to a subject with plentiful antibodies. It is, however, difficult to understand how the trypanosome can survive, let alone reproduce, in a host in which antibodies are present at a very high level unless, at some stage of its development, the trypanosome is not antigenic. The generally accepted concept is that the major determining antigens are liberated from the intact trypanosome into the surrounding medium as 'exo-antigen' (Weitz, 1960a). However, it has now been demonstrated that the short-stumpy form possesses the apparatus of an active secretory cell while the long-thin form is not so equipped. If, as seems possible, exo-antigen is secreted by the short-stumpy form but not by the long-thin form, an explanation would be provided for the survival of the infection in man in the presence of abundant antibody, for only the long-thin form would reproduce and only the short-stumpy form would cause anaphylaxis.

Possible Causes of the Lesions of Sleeping Sickness

Goodwin and Boreham (1966) have demonstrated the liberation of kinins in infections with pathogenic trypanosomes; such kinins and possibly other reaction products are known to be produced as a result of anaphylactic reactions and may account for the morphological changes which occur in the tissues in sleeping sickness. So far their studies have been confined to experimental animals in which relatively large numbers of trypanosomes were present, but different morphological changes may result if the balance of trypanosomes and immune globulins is equivalent to that occurring in man.

Although it is difficult to produce perivascular cuffing in laboratory animals this has been successfully accomplished on several occasions (Roubaud *et al.*, 1944; Stefanopoulo *et al.*, 1945; Peruzzi, 1928; Van Bogaert & Dubois, 1956). These few observations have not provided sufficient information to indicate the cause of the lesion, but the fact that it can be produced experimentally offers hope that the basic pharmacology of the lesion will be investigated along the lines indicated by Goodwin and Boreham (1966), and extended to include the action of inhibitors on the formation of the lesion.

So little certain information is available about the pathogenesis, or even the basic histo-pathology, of sleeping sickness that it has seemed worthwhile to postulate these various theories of pathogenesis at a time when work in this and related fields is receiving much attention. These tentative hypotheses will doubtless require modification as new knowledge becomes available, but this is a healthy situation for an aspect of the study of trypanosomiasis which has been neglected for so long.

Chapter 32

The Ecology of the West African Riverine Species of Tsetse in Relation to Man-fly Contact

T. A. M. NASH

Only two species of tsetse fly, *G. palpalis* and *G. tachinoides*, are of importance in the transmission of human trypanosomiasis in West Africa; their systematics and geographical distribution have already been described in Chapters 9 and10, respectively.

An account of the ecology of these two riverine species of tsetse is an essential prelude to a proper understanding of the epidemiology of human trypanosomiasis in West Africa. The importance of these vectors of sleeping sickness is associated with their ability to tolerate man-made changes in their environment, an ability which often leads to intimate contact between man and fly.

Climate and vegetation, themselves intimately inter-related, are factors of great importance in determining the distribution and behaviour of *G. palpalis* and *G. tachinoides* in West Africa. In general, as one proceeds northwards from the sea-board towards the desert areas of the Sahara, the rainfall decreases, the duration of the dry season increases and the vegetation becomes gradually drier and more open (Nash, 1948a; Keay, 1953 and 1959).

G. palpalis extends inland from the coast through mangrove swamp and/or rain forest to reach the savanna woodland; thence, as it penetrates further inland along the streams, it becomes progressively more dependent upon the presence of water within the riverine vegetation. When the annual rainfall becomes less than 45 inches, when the last oil palm is seen and when *Uapaca somon* ceases to occur in the savanna, *G. palpalis* usually disappears, although the presence of a large river may enable it to penetrate even further into arid regions.

G. tachinoides does not occur along the coastal belt or in dense rain forest but it may be found in the Derived Savanna with its many islands of vestigeal forest. It commonly occurs along the rivers and streams of the drier woodland savanna where it is often found together with *G. palpalis*, but when the riverine vegetation ceases to be darkly evergreen *G. palpalis* disappears while *G. tachinoides* may still be present along water courses penetrating far into the arid Sudan vegetation zone. In some places *G. tachinoides* survives the climatic severities of the late dry season in clumps of feathery-leaved *Mimosa asperata* or *Salix ledermannii* which grow in sandy river beds; here, subsoil moisture provides the cooler and more humid environment essential to this species' survival (Nash, 1937, 1939).

Attention will be confined mainly to the savanna woodland region where most cases of human trypanosomiasis are found. There is a great area of overlap in the distribution of the two riverine species, but *G. tachinoides* by its ability to survive in more arid zones carries sleeping sickness considerably further northwards.

The distribution of *G. tachinoides* is probably influenced by the very low height at which it flies. If, when lying flat on the ground, one looks through woody stems the vegetation is suitable for this species, but if the flight line is blocked by a mass of evergreen leaves it is unsuitable. A low flight level, combined with a low level of attack, probably enables this tsetse to utilize favourable micro-climates and so penetrate far northwards, but prevents its colonization of the forest belt. In an investigation carried out in the late dry season in a stream where both the riverine species were present, it was found that 79% of *G. tachinoides* attacked man below the knee, as against only 15% of *G. palpalis*; *G. tachinoides* was also found to be operating in a cooler and more humid environment (Nash, 1948a). In northern Ghana it was noted that fly catchers took advantage of the low flight level of *G. tachinoides*; they would sit comfortably on the ground with their bare legs exposed, waiting for flies to alight, rather than stand and catch the flies off their ankles.

G. tachinoides is extremely skilful in obtaining blood meals from man. With its small size and silent approach it frequently succeeds in engorging without provoking any host reaction; its low level of attack enables it to find an exposed area of skin below the hem of an African's gown. In contrast, *G. palpalis*, if thwarted by clothing, will attack the head or neck where its audible flight will provoke host reaction.

G. tachinoides has a greater ability than *G. palpalis* to spread out from its riverine habitat in the wet season and to colonize small thickets, or clumps of trees around ponds, where it may linger well into the dry season. This was exemplified at Pong Tamale in Ghana, before the banks of the local river were cleared of vegetation; the wet season floods would drive the tsetse inland to form secondary foci in every patch of cover, including the farms of the veterinary station situated on a ridge three miles from the river (Stewart, 1937). Under such conditions transmission of sleeping sickness by *G. tachinoides* could occur well away from any obvious watercourse or forest island, a situation which is unlikely to arise with *G. palpalis* which does not usually establish isolated secondary foci in the wet season.

Both these species have been recorded as living in villages during the rains. In the case of *G. palpalis* this is unusual, except in areas of heavy rainfall and heavy vegetation. At Ganawuri, on the western escarpment of the Jos Plateau in Northern Nigeria, fly distribution became almost continuous in the wet season and tsetse were commonly found in the villages (Taylor, 1930); at this season in the Rukuba country, some twenty miles further north, *G. palpalis* would follow sunken footpaths, running through tunnels of euphorbia, from the evergreen vegetation of the rocky gorges up into the villages (Nash, 1948a). With *G. tachinoides* a mere clump of low-branching mango trees within the settlement, or an inconspicuous low thicket growing in the moat of the town wall, may be all that is needed to provide this tsetse with a base from which it can batten on the populace. Breeding beneath the overhanging roofs of huts within a village has been recorded (Glover, 1961).

Mention must also be made of the 'sacred groves' which are common in many parts of West Africa. These are small islands of forest, rarely more than an acre in extent, which can be found in densely-populated, heavily-cultivated areas from which all the woodland has long since been cleared. The groves commonly consist of a few evergreen trees, shading a shrubbery and surrounded by thicket; they often encircle the village water supply and provide a place of worship, sometimes a cemetery and a permanent habitat for the tsetse. In Ghana they may contain several pools with several sacred crocodiles—a source of food much favoured by *G. palpalis* (Morris & Morris, 1949). Before the advent of modern insecticides, these groves presented a problem, since the felling of each sacred tree or even the removal of undergrowth was strenuously opposed by the village elders.

The vegetation which fringes the streams forms the major permanent habitat of the riverine tsetse. The term 'riverine' is misleading because it suggests 'rivers' which, although important, form only a fraction of the total habitat; in the Northern Guinea Savanna of Nigeria there may be one linear mile of stream to each square mile of country (Nash, 1948a).

In the more humid Derived Savanna, the riverine vegetation may consist of strips of forest 50 yards or more in width on each bank, but through much of the drier savanna the width may be only a few yards. This specialized vegetation can only exist in the drier savanna because of the edaphic conditions found along water courses; it is protected from the annual fires by the greener grass and often by a curtain of creepers, billowing down from the taller trees. Shaded tunnels or galleries are formed along the stream-beds where the climate is appreciably less severe than in the adjacent woodland; riverine tsetse take advantage of these more favourable conditions to penetrate the savanna.

Most species of tsetse tend to disappear when the human population has increased to such an extent that the fly's environment has been extensively changed by the conversion of natural vegetation into farmland and by the reduction or elimination of its hosts by hunting; but in the case of riverine tsetse the requirements of man and fly are not incompatible.

Man rarely clears the riverine vegetation right up to the banks, and so spares the tsetse's life-line; the higher ground is best suited to the cultivation of staple crops, the woodland is easier to clear, the soil is lighter to hoe and there is no risk of flooding. Even in heavily populated, intensively cultivated regions the river systems, as seen from the air, are sharply delineated by a dark green fringe set against a dry season background of seemingly barren farmland. Man may even create a perfect habitat for tsetse as happened along the banks of the Chalawa river, south of Kano City and just beyond the northern limit for *G. tachinoides*: the river was treeless and fly-free until mango trees and vegetable gardens were planted along the banks; then fly got in, even entering the city, and hundreds of donkeys contracted trypanosomiasis, but man could have been the victim of these circumstances.[1]

In the dry season, the requirements of man and fly are similar; man sites his village near a stream at a point where he knows that water will be available

[1] In 1953 the mango trees were pruned and sprayed with insecticide; in 1968 Dr K. D. B. Thomson recorded the re-invasion of the mango plantations by fly and the finding of fifty cases of human trypanosomiasis.

even in the driest year. Such places are vital to the survival of the riverine tsetse, which vacate long stretches of waterless stream-bed and concentrate at the permanent pools where they obtain the benefit of suitable microclimates and of a steady food supply (Nash, 1948b; Nash & Page, 1953). Since man, his stock and wild animals are dependent on the same pools for water, the hosts have to come to the riverine tsetse whose dry season behaviour resembles that of the spider in its web.

The establishment of a sizeable village near a permanent pool will drive away most of the tsetse's normal hosts, but this is of no account to *G. palpalis* and *G. tachinoides* which having catholic tastes will feed readily on man, his domestic animals and any remaining reptiles such as the *Varanus* lizard. By destroying and driving away the game, and by sharing the same water-hole with the tsetse, man has created conditions of close man–fly contact. The secret of the success of these two species of tsetse as vectors of human trypanosomiasis lies in their adaptability to changing circumstance.

In the wet season man–fly contact usually lessens; the fly tends to recolonize vacated reaches of stream, whilst the villager needs less water and tends to take it from the replenished village wells or from borrow pits around the compound (Nash & Page, 1953).

In 1935 the writer undertook a tsetse survey of Kudaru District in Northern Nigeria, some months after a sleeping sickness survey of the area had been completed; *G. palpalis* was the vector. The district was interesting and unusual in that certain hamlets had permanent wells and were situated as much as a mile from the nearest stream; others which had to rely on a stream for water were situated much closer to it. Among these hamlets, there was a direct relationship between the incidence of sleeping sickness and the distance from the nearest stream. On the same survey it was observed that a very high incidence of sleeping sickness could be associated with an extremely low density of tsetse flies.[1] The earlier survey had revealed that over two-thirds of the forty-three inhabitants of Sambo hamlet had sleeping sickness. The subsequent fly survey, made in the late dry season, showed that for some miles on either side of Sambo the village stream was dry and completely fly-free. However, in the stream-bed immediately below the hamlet a two feet deep hole had been dug in damp sand into which water slowly seeped; at this spot four *G. palpalis* were found. It took each woman about 15 minutes to fill her water pot, using a curved section of calabash to raise a cupful of water at a time. The very small tsetse population could feed off a queue of waiting women without the expenditure of appreciable energy. Man-fly contact was very close (Nash, 1944a).

At Sambo, and elsewhere in the savanna woodland streams, one often finds close *personal* man–fly contact. A few individual tsetse, confined by the severity of the late dry season climate to a permanent pool, attack the villagers who water there; if one person is infected, he may infect several of the local flies, and through them his fellow-villagers.

In other circumstances man–fly contact may be close but quite *impersonal*. Nash (1948a) found that on the River Gambia and its wider creeks, swarms

[1] On Lake Victoria, Fiske (1920) concluded that a density of 15–20 *G. palpalis* [*G. fuscipes*] per man hour was dangerous, but that a figure of six was normally safe.

of *G. palpalis* viciously attacked canoe travellers; here, man–fly contact was close but completely impersonal. Few people live in the vicinity of the river because of the extensive swamps and annual floods; the people do not indulge in fishing. Since in these circumstances man is an unimportant and irregular source of food, the chances of a fly becoming infected and later transmitting the disease are very small. Conditions of close personal man–fly contact were found in some small freshwater creeks up-river. Hutchinson (1953) subsequently made a sleeping sickness survey of this territory and related the incidence of the disease to the fly distribution and the type of man–fly contact.

As one proceeds northwards in West Africa the climate becomes more arid, permanent pools in the streams become scarcer and both man and fly become more dependent on water. Hence on ecological grounds, personal man-fly contact should be greatest near the northern limit of a species' range and sleeping sickness should achieve epidemic proportions more readily near that limit. There is evidence to support this hypothesis. In central northern Ghana *G. tachinoides* is ubiquitous, but the distribution of *G. palpalis*, which is at its northern limit, is patchy; both species are often found together. It has been convincingly demonstrated by Scott (1961) and La Croix (1961), that the distribution of human trypanosomiasis in nothern Ghana is closely associated with the distribution of *G. palpalis* and not with that of *G. tachinoides*; yet it is known that towards the northern limit of *G. tachinoides*, which is some 150 miles further north in Upper Volta, this species has been responsible for much sleeping sickness (Morris, 1946).

Over a period of six years, Nash and Page (1953) studied a population of *G. palpalis* in great detail along 5,217 yards of stream, situated near the northern limit of this species' range in Nigeria; *G. tachinoides* also occurred but at very low density. Some of their more relevant findings are given in the succeeding paragraphs.

The advantage to *G. palpalis* of living in the fringing forest and the added advantage of the microclimate near water were established; for example, the highest maximum temperatures recorded in three meteorological stations over six years were as follows:

	Height above ground level	Temperature
Open woodland	4 feet	103·0°F (39·4°C)
Fringing forest	4 feet	97·3°F (36·3°C)
(In vicinity of water)	4 feet	90·0°F (32·2°C)

Judging from a population kept in the stream-bed the fly was sometimes living at a temperature which was close to the danger level: over ten-day periods, average maximum temperatures of 88°F (31·1°C) were associated with abnormally high mortality.

The amount of water which persisted in the stream each dry season varied greatly and was related to the rainfall of the preceding year or years as well as to the severity of the current dry season. When a season of abnormally low rainfall is followed by a very severe dry season, the extent of the favourable microclimate is minimal, fly concentration is maximal and personal man-fly contact is closest. In dry seasons when water is abundant, as well as in every wet season, flies continue to travel up and down the streams, man-fly contact is impersonal and transmission of sleeping sickness is likely to be on a much smaller scale.

During the course of the investigation nearly 7,000 marked flies were recaptured. A study of the monthly proportion which had travelled over 1,000 yards indicated that both sexes travelled most in the heavy rains (21–31%), less in the early dry season (18–21%) and least in the last, and hottest, month of the dry season and in the first two months of the wet season (5–8%). The proportion for the last period would have been much lower in severe dry seasons but owing to the small number of flies at that time of year it was necessary to group by months all the data collected over six years. The longest distance travelled by a marked fly was 3 miles; a distance of 2,000 yards within 24 hours of marking was not uncommon.

Female flies live much longer than males and are therefore the more dangerous sex when infected. For both sexes, life-expectation is minimal in the cold, mid-dry season, because the attainment of old age is rendered impossible by the rigours of the late dry season which discriminate against the older flies; however, at the start of the rains the expectation of life is greatest because the surviving population is young and has some months of very favourable conditions ahead. The onset of the rainy season is gradual and it is some two months before fly dispersal begins, and even longer before man ceases to be entirely dependent on the water-hole. Hence close, personal man-fly contact persists for a considerable period at a time when the flies have the greatest expectation of life; these flies would have originated from pupae deposited in the hottest month in the year, when the mean soil temperature at half an inch depth in a severe season was found to be 76·2°F (24·5°C) and the mean maximum 86·6°F (30·3°C).

Burtt (1946) showed that *G. morsitans* adults, bred from pupae incubated at a high temperature, are more readily infected with *T. rhodesiense* than flies bred from pupae kept at a lower temperature. Fairbairn and Culwick (1950) confirmed Burtt's observation and also showed that the temperature of adult fly maintenance is important, as did Taylor (1932a) working with *G. tachinoides* and *T. gambiense*. Should the findings of these workers be equally applicable to wild *G. palpalis* and *T. gambiense*, flies should become most readily infected when concentrated in the hottest weather at the water-hole, more especially if flies hatching in such weather are exceptionally willing to take their first meal within 24 hours of emergence when Wijers (1958) showed that *G. palpalis* is much more readily infected.

Nash and Page (*loc. cit.*) found that the fly population decreased gradually throughout the dry season becoming minimal at the beginning of the rains; in the early rains it started to increase, at first slowly and then very rapidly, to reach a peak in the heavy rains.

When the findings described above are considered in relation to the habits and customs of the peasants in the drier zones of West Africa an interesting picture emerges. After the crops are harvested many villagers go on long journeys, either to trade, seek dry season employment or visit distant relatives. They return in good time to prepare their farms before the planting season; a few will have contracted sleeping sickness on their journeys, and will get home at the season when there is the closest personal man–fly contact at their village water-hole where people sit in the shade and gossip in hot weather. With high temperature, conditions are probably optimal for a newly hatched fly to take its first meal within a day of emergence. Should a fly become infected, there is still ample time for it to transmit the disease to a number of villagers before the season of long travel and impersonal man–fly contact begins; it will then travel and encounter numerous farmers weeding the minor crops which are grown along the edge of the riverine vegetation and may even reach the lands and water-hole of the next village since such a fly, if female, has an estimated average life expectation of 3½ months.

Even though *G. palpalis* is present, sleeping sickness is very rare in all but the driest parts of the West African forest belt. A satisfactory explanation for this previously perplexing situation was found by Page and McDonald (1959). Page, working at the edge of the humid forest belt in the south of Nigeria, and McDonald in sleeping sickness country in the arid savanna in the north, undertook two similar fly-marking experiments at stream-bed watering places. Any fly marked and released at the water-hole which was recaptured there eighteen days or longer after marking was considered to be a potential transmitter, because sufficient time would have elapsed for it to have become infective; in the dry season the proportion of such flies in the north was nine times greater, and in the wet season about seven times greater, than in the south. In the north the proportion of such 'transmitters' was nearly twice as great in the dry season as in the wet, reflecting concentration at the water-hole, but in the south the proportions were similar at both seasons. The experiment in the north was undertaken in a mild dry season, following rains which were some 13 inches above average and which lasted for a month longer than usual, otherwise the proportions for this season might have been considerably greater. In Page's humid southern area, *G. palpalis* is widespread and barely riverine in habit; whereas man is dependent on the stream the fly is not (Page, 1959), yet it feeds readily on man (Jordan, Lee-Jones & Weitz, 1961). Foster (1963a) undertook a similar experiment at a village watering place on a permanently flowing, 20 feet wide, stream in the north-western corner of Liberia, which adjoins the Kissi sleeping sickness area of Sierra Leone (Hutchinson, 1954). The watering place was only 15 miles north of the forest belt. Foster found no appreciable difference between the dry and wet season proportions of marked flies recaptured at the watering place eighteen days or longer after marking, which agreed with Page's finding in Southern Nigeria. However, whereas Page's proportions for such flies ranged from 0·55–0·80%, Foster's proportions ranged from 2·73–3·06%. The writer suggests that the difference was due to the fact that whereas Page's site was just within the forest, enabling flies to disperse in all directions through shaded vegetation and cocoa farms, Foster's stream ran through open grass lands compelling the fly to remain strictly riverine in habit. In Page's area, unlike Foster's, there was no history of sleeping sickness. Whereas Foster's proportion of about 3% was comparable to McDonald's wet season figure of about 4% in the arid north, it was not comparable to McDonald's dry season proportion of about 7%. To summarize:

Distribution linear and seasonally contracted (McDonald)—most dangerous.
Distribution linear but not seasonally contracted (Foster)—dangerous.
Distribution barely linear and not seasonally contracted (Page)—safe.

No investigation similar to that of Nash and Page (1953) has been undertaken on *G. tachinoides*, but observations on many streams, at many times of year, suggest that the general picture given above for drier regions is applicable to this fly. For example, Morris (1946, 1949) has described the conditions in the Mossi country, over 100 miles north of Ghana, which lies between the Red and White Volta rivers near the northern limit for *G. tachinoides*. A 20-inch rainfall is precipitated in three months of the year; such a poor rainfall so restricts the amount of water available and the extent of the flies' habitat, that the closest possible man–fly contact is maintained almost continuously throughout the year. A high human population, mostly agricultural, still further restricts the tsetse's habitat and ensures man–fly contact wherever a fly-infested river exists; in addition there is close contact at the village water-hole. High rates of infection (above 5%) occurred right up to the nothern limit of *G. tachinoides*.

When important trade routes cross streams at a point where there is a permanent pool, conditions are similar to those described above for the village water-hole, with the important difference that the fly is not in close contact with a village community but with individuals many of whom are travelling long distances; such fords must be of major importance in disseminating sleeping sickness over a wide front. Where well-frequented paths, used only by the local inhabitants, cross streams at permanent pools, the danger is much more localized.

Certain streams, or parts of a stream, are choked with the *Raphia* palm whose mid-ribs provide long, straight poles which are invaluable in a country where small straight timber for roofing is unprocurable. In areas where the palms grow to a good height there is a local pole-cutting industry which brings those engaged in it into close contact with riverine tsetse during the dry season when house building takes place. Since people working in this trade come from neighbouring villages, suitable conditions occur for the local spread of sleeping sickness (Nash, 1944). A far more dangerous industry to the country as a whole used to be alluvial tin mining in streams flowing from the Jos Plateau of Nigeria, an industry which still attracts itinerant labourers from long distances. Here, man–fly contact is close and personal, and before appropriate control measures were instituted, many labourers contracted sleeping sickness and carried the infection back to their homes (Lester, 1938).

The type of man–fly contact occurring on large permanent rivers has never been established by fly-marking experiments. Certainly, both *G. palpalis* and *G. tachinoides* can traverse much greater lengths of barrier clearing on permanently flowing rivers than on streams (Nash 1948a), which suggests that both species may travel much further when freed from the restrictions imposed by the vegetational obstructions and adverse climatic conditions encountered on narrow streams which cease to flow in the dry season. If this be so, man–fly contact along the actual banks of large rivers is probably largely impersonal.

Morris (1949) has described an interesting sequence of events on the Black Volta. In 1899 there was sleeping sickness in many Volta-side villages and by 1907 many were being abandoned, the survivors moving to new sites in the savanna a mile or more from the river banks; the disease was still confined to the vicinity of the river and was being spread by canoe traffic. By 1920, sleeping sickness had spread up the larger tributaries and by 1938 up many of the smaller streams. The country within three miles of the river was depopulated, except for a few heavily-infected villages, invariably situated on side streams infested with *G. tachinoides* and *G. palpalis*. The disease had largely shifted inland and up into the headwaters of the tributaries. In 1949, Morris (*loc. cit.*) recorded that the incidence of sleeping sickness was usually much lower in Volta fishing camps than in neighbouring farming villages, despite greater man–fly contact on the river; he attributed this low incidence in the fishing camps to a lack of continuity of contact between tsetse and the same sections of the population, brought about by the camps being vacated during the rains. An alternative explanation may be that, on a depopulated and unfrequented river, the source of infection was greatly reduced.

These observations on the Volta suggest that on rivers where there has been no such marked depopulation the disease may be 'incubated' in villages situated on side streams where there is close personal man–fly contact and is then spread up and down the river by long-ranging flies. Along permanently flowing rivers, it is probable that man-fly contact is impersonal so long as the banks are lined with continuous vegetation providing suitable fly habitats. Under severe climatic conditions with strictly limited fly-habitats in the vicinity of riverside communities, as found up-river on the Benue, epidemic foci of sleeping sickness occur which suggest personal man–fly contact.

The type of man-fly contact described above, with its emphasis on the dangers of the late dry season and early rains, does not hold good when the fly is entirely dependent on man and his domestic animals for food. In these circumstances, if the fly is to survive, it must continue to feed on man and his beasts in the rains so that theoretically transmission should take place throughout the year, and might be greatest in the rains when *G. palpalis* is most numerous.

An excellent practical illustration that this theory is well-founded is provided by the observations of Taylor (1930) who studied sleeping sickness among the Ganawuri pagans living along the escarpment of the Jos Plateau in Northern Nigeria. Formerly a warrior race constantly engaged in tribal warfare and the hunting of game animals, the Ganawuri, under the Pax Britannica, continued to hunt game until it was exterminated and then became cultivators. In 1930, the incidence of sleeping sickness among them lay between 50 and 75%. Most of their villages had been sited for defensive purposes in the hills near springs and streams. The hills, where not precipitous, were well wooded with occasional patches of forest. At the foot of the hills some of the streams flowed for a short distance through deep ravines choked with heavy fringing forest, but further out in the plains the streams flowed between shadeless banks through intensively cultivated land. In the dry season *G. palpalis* were found mainly at the foot of the escarpment but in the wet season they dispersed up the streams into the villages. In the early dry season Taylor (*loc. cit.*) collected 236 flies, most of them from two important watering places at the foot of the escarpment; of these seventy-eight contained recognizable blood, none of reptilian origin but all mammalian. He estimated, on the basis of erythrocyte size, that just under one half of the blood feeds were from man and the remainder from sheep and goats. Of the 236 flies dissected eight showed immature trypanosome infection of the gut and one a mature infection of the salivary glands. Taylor concluded that all these infections were *T. gambiense* because of the absence of proboscis infections and his failure to find trypanosomes in the sheep and goats in this game-free locality.

Some years later, a very severe epidemic occurred amongst the Rukuba tribe living on the face of the escarpment some 20 miles north of Ganawuri. The conditions were similar except that here there was no question of the flies spreading up from the foot of the hills in the rains; they survived in the adequately thicketed streams running down the face of the escarpment, concentrating at the watering places and path crossings, and in the rains moving up the euphorbia-enclosed paths into the villages. There were also a number of sacred groves and forested cemeteries. Man–fly contact was close and personal throughout the year, as in the complete absence of game the fly were permanently dependent on man and his domestic animals. Many villages were depopulated and fell into ruins (Nash, 1948a; Duggan, 1962a).

In any heavily populated area where man has destroyed all wild hosts including the aquatic reptiles, he has removed all buffers between himself, his domestic animals and the fly; the contact is perennial. The fewer the number of domestic animals kept, the more personal is this perennial contact between man and fly. These conditions are exemplified in villages sited within forest islands in the Derived Savanna.

Unfortunately, collections of tsetse for the indentification of their blood meals, using the serological technique devised by Weitz (1956), have never been made for *G. tachinoides* and *G. palpalis* occurring in the same streams, and only once for riverine tsetse collected on a river system during the course of an outbreak of sleeping sickness. Nevertheless, some informative data from Northern Nigeria are given below which are supported by figures for reptilian feeds from other localities, based on microscopic identification by earlier workers.

G. palpalis.

For 266 blood meals, collected in Zaria Province from three areas which have had a history of sleeping sickness, the proportion of feeds for different groups ranged as follows:

Reptiles. From 33–46% (Jordan, Lee-Jones & Weitz, (1962). *cf.* 22% of ninety-six meals from various localities (Johnson & Lloyd, 1923).

Primates. From 21–32%, almost all man (Jordan *et al.*, 1962).

Bovids. From 16–24%, mainly cattle and bush buck (Jordan *et al.*, 1962).

G. tachinoides.

For 668 blood meals, collected in five scattered areas in Northern Nigeria which have had a history of sleeping sickness, the proportion of feeds for different groups ranged as follows:

Reptiles. From 0–60% (Jordan *et al*., 1962; Leach, 1965). *cf*. 41% of 550 meals from Sherifuri (Lloyd, Johnson, Young & Morrison, 1924).

Primates. From 14–72%, almost all man (Jordan *et al*., 1962; Leach, 1965).

Bovids. From 14–65%, mainly cattle (Jordan *et al*., 1962; Leach, 1965).

Eighty-seven of these blood meals were collected by Baldry in villages and hamlets on the Kano river system at the time of the 1963 outbreak of sleeping sickness; 60% of the feeds were from primates, almost certainly all man (Leach, 1965). Of twenty-seven *G. tachinoides* blood meals, collected by Baldry from an uninhabited game reserve, half were from bovids—all game animals, one quarter from hippopotamus and porcupine, and only two from reptiles (Leach, 1964).

The above figures, although inadequate for *G. palpalis* and collected from too few areas, illustrate that both species of riverine tsetse have catholic tastes which enable them to adapt themselves readily to disturbances which drive out the game.

Baldry has recently shown that the feeding behaviour of *G. tachinoides* in the heavily populated south-eastern region of Nigeria is entirely different from its known behaviour elsewhere in West Africa. It lives within and around the villages, provided suitable domestic animals are kept, and virtually ignores man; there is no history of sleeping sickness. In the Nsukka area it takes three-quarters of its meals from domestic pigs; in the Awka area, where very few pigs are kept, it virtually feeds entirely on cattle. Of a total of 379 meals from these areas, only 1·8% were from primates (Baldry, 1964; Leach, 1965). One wonders whether the very different diet of the south-eastern Nigerian, which includes palm oil, could make him unattractive to *G. tachinoides*? Under these most exceptional conditions this tsetse would appear to be a highly selective, rather than an opportunist, feeder.

It has been shown that on ecological grounds *G. palpalis* and *G. tachinoides*, both as individual species and as a pair of species, are perfectly adapted to the transmission of human trypanosomiasis. Between them their distribution covers most of West Africa from the sea to the northern limit for *Glossina*. They can both withstand much curtailment of their vegetational environment by man. In the drier months, in the drier regions the riverine tsetse and man are dependent on water and share the same source of supply. Finally, if man destroys all wild hosts, these tsetse adapt themselves to such conditions and are able to survive on man and his domestic animals.

Mention must be made of *G. caliginea* because Ford (1963b), acting on a personal communication from Mouchet, has stated that at Douala this tsetse has been confirmed as a vector of sleeping sickness. The writer, having corresponded with Mouchet and studied the literature, suggests that it would be wiser to consider this species as highly suspect. *G. caliginea* has an intermittent distribution between western Ghana and Cape Lopez. Little is known about its ecology: it can be numerous in mangrove swamps and may penetrate inland for some distance along rivers and streams bordered by swamp forest: it feeds on man with avidity. In 1933 there was an outbreak of sleeping sickness in Ahoada Division in the Niger delta: of 16,000 people examined, 29% were infected: of 142 tsetse sent for identification seventy-two were *G. caliginea* and seventy *G. palpalis* (Nash, 1960). In 1950, 223 *G. caliginea* collected from mangrove swamps around Douala were maintained in Paris and dissected during the course of the next two months; eight-four were infected, but only one with polymorphic trypanosomes (Roubaud, Maillot & Rageau, 1951): at that time sleeping sickness was relatively rare in the area and the authors concluded that there was no reason to deduce that *G. caliginea* plays a part in the transmission of this disease. Mouchet (personal communication) states that around Douala *G. caliginea* were about nine times more numerous than *G. palpalis* and would even enter native huts; further, that in the 1955 survey, fifty cases, mainly new, were found among 2,000 people examined for the disease.

Chapter 33

The Epidemiology of Gambian Sleeping Sickness

D. SCOTT

INTRODUCTION

Almost immediately after sleeping sickness was first shown to be due to a trypanosomal infection, in 1903, it was demonstrated that it is transmitted by the tsetse fly. At first it was thought that this was a simple mechanical process but further work showed that it is necessary for the parasite to undergo a period of cyclical development in the fly before transmission can be effected.

It soon appeared that in areas infested by the riverine tsetse man was the only important reservoir of infection, the disease being spread in a man-fly-man cycle. Thus, at an early stage in the experience with the West African form of sleeping sickness, the basic epidemiological facts seemed to be unequivocal, and consequently there was little stimulus to investigation in this field. This was not the case in Central and in parts of East Africa where the disease was associated only with game tsetse and where, from early times, there was strong presumptive evidence that some infections were being acquired from the larger game animals; however, this was not established as a fact until 1958. Partly for these reasons interest in the epidemiology of human trypanosomiasis was, for several years, greatest on the eastern side of the continent, an interest which was mainly channelled into endeavours to distinguish between *T. rhodesiense* and *T. brucei.*

Almost fifty years ago a series of epidemics of Gambian sleeping sickness began in West Africa and spanned three decades. At this time, when the collection and study of epidemiological information would have been most rewarding, opportunities to undertake this work were generally lacking. The limited field resources of the various medical authorities were wholly engaged in the urgent task of detecting and treating thousands of cases annually and with the need to undertake other forms of control. It was not until after the Second World War that detailed attention could be given to this discipline but by then the prevalence of the disease was falling to low levels and significant data could only be obtained from field investigations made on an increasing scale.

Simultaneously, it was becoming evident that the methods of mass control, which had been employed with such success during the epidemic period, were less effective in dealing with the hard core of endemic infection which remained. The need for a new approach to control has been dictated by the experience of recent years and it is now clear that solutions will be found only by acquiring a much more detailed knowledge of the epidemiology of the disease. In the last twenty years workers in Africa have responded to this challenge, both in the laboratory and in the field, and investigations into various epidemiological aspects of the disease have been made on a greater scale than previously. Nevertheless, facilities and resources have hardly been adequate to enable field studies of the natural history of the behaviour of trypanosomiasis in whole populations to be carried out on the scale, and with the sense of purpose and the degree of continuity, which the present *impasse* in progress towards eradication demands.

Definition and Purpose

Epidemiology is the study of the factors which determine the distribution of the disease, its patterns of prevalence within the endemic area and the variations in these prevalences which may occur from time to time. The understanding which accrues from such studies, made in a particular locality, often leads to the development of methods of control especially suited to the area, which might not otherwise have emerged.

Three fundamental methods for the control of human trypanosomiasis are available: the elimination of the reservoir of infection in man, usually by mass survey of whole populations and the treatment of the cases discovered; mass administration of chemoprophylaxis to the communities at risk; and eradication of the tsetse vector. Where, however, infection rates are low, as in many *T. gambiense* zones today, the general, widespread and almost indiscriminate application of any of these methods over a vast endemic area sooner or later meets with some insuperable difficulty. The community, understandably, tires of repeated surveys and fails to give the co-operation necessary for the success of mass treatment, or declines the regular injections which are essential for the maintenance of effective prophylaxis; or tsetse eradication over a wide area is economically unacceptable. Indeed, in areas of low endemicity, and certainly in those of very low endemicity, the control of trypanosomiasis in very large populations either by indefinitely repeated *ad hoc* examination, or by pentamidinization, is already largely outmoded. What is required now is progress to more refined applications of these three basic methods. Control measures must, in future, be applied in a selective manner based on more detailed knowledge of the residual infection in the community and more accurate identification of the points of transmission. Such methods would make more intelligent use of the resources available and would be cheaper, faster and more acceptable to the public than a continuation of the mass approach.

The primary objective of epidemiological investigations is to improve on existing methods of control and to adapt them to deal more appropriately with the contemporary problem of widespread infection at low rates of incidence. These studies must be directed towards revealing the factors which promote the spread of the disease, for once these are sufficiently understood specific counter-action may be possible. A thorough appreciation of the *local* epidemiology is, therefore, a prerequisite for sound planning and only after this has been gained is it possible to decide where, when, and by what means control can be logically and economically applied. The expression 'local epidemiology' is emphasized, since factors which influence the spread of the disease in one community may be quite different from those in another.

From time to time sleeping sickness breaks out in epidemic form, a tendency which remains even today. Such epidemics have, in the past, occurred on a vast scale and at present their occurrence is unpredictable. A better understanding of the epidemiology of the disease may well enable future epidemics to be forestalled or at least countered at an early stage. The study of past records and continuous surveillance in the field enable the contemporary behaviour of the disease to be intelligently interpreted on the basis of data relayed from the field.

The Nature of Epidemiological Studies

The epidemiology of *T. gambiense* infection is complex, for it is determined by the inter-relationships of the three biological elements concerned, the host, the vector and the parasite. All are susceptible in their own ways to a wide range of influences and even simple changes may result in a variation in the behaviour of one of them, affecting its association with the others. Very many factors may have a bearing on the potential for transmission. The role of some has been proved; with others there are varying degrees of presumptive evidence of their involvement, while some epidemiological factors may still be unsuspected.

Much detailed scientific information, both from the laboratory and from the field, is available regarding the effect of varying environments on the tsetse. In recent years the importance of the nature of the contact between man and the fly has been recognized and investigated. Studies of the role of the parasite and its relationships with the host and the vector have, in terms of applied epidemiology, been less fruitful.

Essentially, however, epidemiological study requires the collection of data on the distribution of the disease in endemic areas and their presentation in such a way as to demonstrate the detailed natural history of the disease in the community; it is essential to determine which groups of people are at risk, where the infection occurs and, if the investigation is sufficiently prolonged, its behaviour in time and its trends in prevalence. These three patterns, demographical, geographical and chronological can best be presented in tables, histograms, graphs and maps. Their epidemiological interpretation, in the light of a knowledge of local sociological conditions and of the distribution and bionomics of the tsetse, is then undertaken. Much of the evidence regarding the factors which promote the spread of the disease is presumptive, but it leads inevitably to further specific and more searching enquiries in an attempt to establish the facts more precisely.

If the best use is to be made of field surveys, certain basic information must be recorded from each person examined; in practice the amount of information obtained will be strictly limited hence very careful consideration must be given to its selection. It is essential to record sex and age groups and valuable to note the ethnic group as this often has a close bearing on occupation and social customs. It may also be desirable to record some specific occupations, noting all persons engaged in a particular line of work irrespective of whether or not they are infected. The period of local residence may also be usefully recorded in limited areas. Only by collecting identical information from every person in the community is it possible to define the size of the different groups and so obtain specific infection rates. By making comparisons between the behaviour of the disease in one group with that in another, as measured by the incidence of the infection, social and geographical factors influencing the spread of the disease may be revealed. Depending on the wealth of data collected, these comparisons can be made between different groups at different times and in different places. The acquisition of detailed information about infection rates is a *sine qua non* in epidemiological work.

Sources of Data: Some Limitations of Field Investigations into the Distribution of the Disease

There are two sources of evidence regarding the epidemiology of sleeping sickness. The first is from experimental work, carried out either in the laboratory or in the field, into the influences of specific factors on the potential for disease transmission. Evidence established in this manner and relating to the entomological and parasitological facets is considered elsewhere and its epidemiological significance is discussed in later sections of this chapter.

The second source is in field surveys which provide information on the distribution patterns of the disease among the people. From these, by a process of deductive reasoning, the factors associated with the spread of the infection begin to emerge. Inevitably, deductive reasoning has sometimes been replaced by speculation and not infrequently this has been based on impressions of the patterns of the disease, rather than on facts, where the facts might have been ascertained.

In the absence of field surveys, information may be obtained from the records of cases attending voluntarily at hospitals and other centres of treatment in the endemic area. But data from these sources may be of only limited value. It is fortunate, therefore, that in most countries with a *T. gambiense* problem it has been the custom, from the earliest days, to set up mobile field units, part of whose duties has been to examine every person in a community for evidence of infection, often over very large areas. From the facts recorded during these surveys epidemiological analyses of varying usefulness have been made.

One advantage of field surveys over the use of clinic records is that they give a fairly precise indication of the number of cases occurring and enable calculations to be made of the incidence in different sex, age and other groups with some confidence; from clinic records the incidence of the disease for the whole population can only be surmised and detailed analyses cannot be undertaken. Surveys also enable cases to be marked accurately on a map, and this may suggest some localization of transmission and so lead to further investigation; moreover, seeing the cases in their homes may reveal some particular association between one and another and so prompt additional inquiry.

Despite the fact that it is a fundamental concept of epidemiological study that the information obtained during case finding surveys should be presented in terms of the three patterns mentioned above, the amount of relevant detailed statistical data which has been published has not been great. This is surprising when it is remembered that surveys for *T. gambiense* infection have been continuously in progress, on a large scale and over vast areas, for several decades. The presentation from some surveys has been little more than a statement of the overall prevalence of the disease in a large population. Occasionally, a comparison may be made between the activity of the disease in the male and female elements of the community but frequently this is only implied by recording the number of cases for each sex. Detailed infection rates, by sex, age and other groups, are rarely given. It is true that a considerable amount of sociological detail is often presented on individual cases and that frequently the number belonging to a particular group is stated; but this is of much less value than the recording of infection rates which allows comparisons to be made, identifies those for whom the risk is greatest and provides a measurement of that risk. The present dearth of exact information has generally been due to failure to record simple standard details about each person examined in a community and the restriction of this routine to identified cases only.

The detailed geographical pattern has likewise been masked by presenting the results of a survey as a single prevalence relating to hundreds, or even thousands, of square miles.

There are several reasons why the contribution to the epidemiology of *T. gambiense* infection, made from studies of its patterns, has been less scientific than the researches in the related entomological and parasitological fields. Government medical authorities have been primarily concerned to control the spread of the infection, generally by using mobile teams of auxiliaries working under medical supervision; the main function of these teams has been to diagnose and treat cases. Apart from noting the persons infected, few demands have been made regarding the collection and assessment of epidemiological data which might readily have been obtained from each member of the community in the course of the survey. As this work takes a little extra time and does not immediately contribute to the principal objective, the provision of a public service, it has been left to the individual doctor working with the teams to develop his own interests in epidemiological investigation and to exploit for himself the considerable possibilities which rapid surveys of large populations can offer. Although these diagnostic and treatment teams have been the main, if not the only, source of epidemiological data they have not always been staffed or otherwise equipped for this role; they have rarely been regarded as research units as in the case of parallel entomological and parasitological work.

EPIDEMIOLOGICAL FACTORS OF KNOWN SIGNIFICANCE

The Transmission Cycle

T. gambiense is transmitted from man to man by the bite of an infected tsetse fly and whilst, under laboratory conditions, most species of *Glossina* will transmit this infection, it is evident from the distribution of the disease in nature that it is almost exclusively carried by tsetse of the *palpalis* group. After a fly has fed on a person with trypanosomes in the blood, the parasite undergoes a period of cyclical development and it is not until 18–35 days later that the infective forms appear in the salivary glands and the tsetse fly becomes capable of transmitting the disease. The interval required to complete this development depends on several factors among which temperature is particularly important. A tsetse fly once infected remains so for the rest of its life.

In addition to cyclical transmission, the disease may perhaps be passed mechanically from man to man. A tsetse disturbed whilst feeding on an infected person may continue its meal on someone nearby, before the blood has dried on its mouthparts, and thus directly inoculate trypanosomes into the second host. Instances of direct transmission of this kind are not uncommonly suspected in the field but are always impossible to prove. As few wild flies are infected with polymorphic trypanosomes (some of which could be *T. gambiense*), even in the presence of sleeping sickness, it may be that, as suggested by Duke (1923), direct transmission may have been responsible, in part at least, for the very high prevalence of the disease encountered in some areas in the past. Opportunities for direct transmission are greatest where people are closely bunched together in the presence of tsetse, as on ferries and in canoes, or at much-frequented water holes. It is possible that other biting insects may also serve as mechanical vectors and on occasion the occurrence of multiple infections among persons sharing the same room has suggested spread in this way. However, the fact that Gambian sleeping sickness is so exactly confined within the limits of the waterside tsetse indicates that even if mechanical transmission by other insects does occur it is of little significance.

Congenital transmission of *T. gambiense* has sometimes been recorded (*see* Chapter 35) but it is of rare occurrence and of negligible epidemiological significance.

The Reservoir of Infection

The Possibility of a Non-human Host

Man is the only important reservoir of infection of *T. gambiense*. Although there are sometimes grounds for suspecting that there may be an alternative host, no irrefutable evidence of its existence has yet been put forward.

Many experimental infections of domestic sheep, goats and pigs with strains of *T. gambiense* have been recorded. These animals are not very suitable hosts and either because the infections are light, or are of short duration, or because the trypanosome loses its power to infect the tsetse, their maintenance in these animals and their onward cyclical transmission is often difficult and sometimes impossible. On this account it is generally accepted that they are unlikely to play any major part in maintaining the disease in man. The possible role of the domestic pig attracted attention after Van Hoof (1947) had transmitted *T. gambiense* cyclically through these animals and human volunteers were cyclically infected from this source. Interest in the pig was renewed when Watson (1963) demonstrated that *G. palpalis* could be infected from experimentally infected animals and when, in conjunction with this work, it was found that in certain areas of Nigeria the domestic black pig, sometimes carrying a polymorphic trypanosome, is a preferred host of *G. tachinoides*.

Whenever infection with polymorphic trypanosomes is found in domestic animals it appears to be generally assumed that the infection is *T. brucei* and not *T. gambiense*. As these two organisms are distinguishable only by the ability of *T. gambiense* alone to infect man, it would require the inoculation of a large number of human volunteers with polymorphic trypanosomes obtained from a considerable range of domestic animals to determine whether or not *T. gambiense* occurs naturally among them. As such experiments have not been undertaken in Gambian sleeping sickness areas, the question of a reservoir of *T. gambiense* infection, occurring perhaps in some of the more susceptible of these animals, must remain open.

Certain species of game can be infected with *T. gambiense* in the laboratory but in the main the parasite is not well adapted to them. Transmission back to man from such experimental infections has not been achieved and, in the single instance where a natural infection in game with polymorphic trypanosomes was successfully inoculated into a human volunteer, it proved to be *T. rhodesiense* and not *T. gambiense* (Heisch *et al.*, 1958). Although the role of game is not clear it certainly appears, from the evidence of the distribution of the disease, that it is unlikely to be of much significance. Human infections can usually be traced to areas where at least the larger game animals are not found while colonies of riverine tsetse in constant contact with man may have little opportunity to feed on game.

Small mammals such as rats, mice, guinea-pigs and monkeys may be found peridomestically, or otherwise in association with man, and must be considered as possible reservoirs of infection. All have been repeatedly infected with *T. gambiense* in the laboratory; the giant African rat (*Cricetomys gambianus*) may be a particularly good host. Cyclical transmission from animal to animal through *G. palpalis* has been achieved, but not always readily. Transmission back to man from these experimental infections has not been reported, possibly because of the difficulties surrounding work with human volunteers. Natural infection with polymorphic trypanosomes has not been recorded in these animals but this may only indicate that a sufficiently wide and persistent search has not yet been made. However, the results of identification of blood meals of the riverine tsetse fly show that they are little attracted to these animals and this evidence alone is a fair indication that they cannot be an important reservoir of the infection.

Where the prevalence of Gambian sleeping sickness is high, the distribution of the disease supports the view that man is the only host of the infection; cases are grouped together and some mutual point of contact with tsetse can be found between one case and another. Moreover, the results obtained from mass survey and treatment are generally so satisfactory that the question of an alternative reservoir of infection cannot reasonably be raised. Where the incidence is very low, a different pattern of the disease is often revealed, but even in such circumstances careful investigation may reveal social and geographical concentration of the infection suggestive of spread from man to man only (Morris, 1960). During the course of extensive field surveys it is not uncommon to discover an exceedingly low prevalence (less than one case per 1,000 persons examined) and widely scattered infections, sometimes in a population of relatively low density. Such findings would be compatible with a situation in which the disease was dying out but this is not always the case. A survey undertaken some years later may show that the *status quo* of a low and scattered prevalence has been maintained. As the requirements both for infection to be achieved in the tsetse in the first place, and its subsequent transmission are, in any event, exacting, it is difficult to understand how the disease can continue to survive in this manner, unless it were supported from a non-human reservoir.

Even in areas of moderate endemicity, with many of the infections acquired on the patients' farms a mile or two from the village, a pattern which is commonly found, there sometimes appears to be no possible line of transmission between one infection and the others. The farms are often in relatively isolated clearings, visited by only the few engaged there, a picture which is seen so frequently that it inevitably raises the question of how the tsetse became infected in the first place. It is true that cases may be missed during surveys, perhaps by as much as 20 or 30% (Lotte, 1951a; Hutchinson, 1954), or that unsuspected healthy carriers may be present (*see* Chapter 35). It is true also that casual visits from infected persons may have been responsible in some instances, or that transmission may have occurred on a common footpath, but such a consistent pattern of infection, apparently acquired in areas at some distance from dwellings, suggests, as with sylvatic plague and jungle yellow fever, that there is another host besides man.

Man as the Host

The initial stages of Gambian sleeping sickness are generally relatively mild and the victim may continue at work for many months, or even for years, before he is eventually driven by increasing illness to seek treatment or to retire to his home. During this time he is a constant source of infection to tsetse so that the very nature of the illness provides great opportunities for its spread. It also permits a dangerous increase in prevalence to occur silently and unobserved, for even in areas where the disease is well known and where there are efficient, long-established and popular *ad hoc* sleeping sickness clinics, many patients may fail to come early for treatment. Epidemics have reached considerable proportions in the near vicinity of medical centres before being suspected (Kleine, 1919; Hutchinson, 1954; Scott, 1961). In passing, the point must be made that only by surveillance, by making field checks in some manner, can the behaviour of the disease in a particular locality be known at any time; figures of cases attending voluntarily at treatment centres may reflect changes only months after they have taken place. Sleeping sickness occurs in rural areas where the people, constantly harassed by various infections, tend to accept minor ill-health as their normal lot, and with medical posts widely scattered it is understandable that cases do not always seek treatment early. The response of the public to illness, the accessibility of treatment, the degree of confidence in the services provided as well as the initial mildness of the disease, all have a considerable bearing on the spread of the infection.

Another factor which might conceivably influence the pattern of the disease is the possible existence of an undetected and perhaps unsuspected reservoir of infection in the form of human 'healthy carriers' of *T. gambiense*. The evidence that healthy carriers may occur has been reviewed elsewhere (Chapter 35) and although their existence is strongly suspected there is as yet no definite proof of the occurrence of a significant number of individuals who remain infected for indefinite periods without showing any symptoms or other evidence of disease. On the other hand, it is certainly true that many cases of early

Gambian disease approximate closely to the healthy carrier state so that the differentiation of true healthy carriers becomes a matter of minor epidemiological significance.

Man–fly Contact

For a detailed account of the ecology of the West African species of riverine tsetse in relation to man–fly contact the reader is referred to Chapter 32.

The Concept

It is perhaps surprising that it is only about twenty-five years ago that particular attention was first turned to the epidemiological importance of the nature of the contact between man and the tsetse fly.

A tsetse which bites man only once in its life cannot transmit *T. gambiense*. If it feeds twice on humans it could carry the disease provided that the first host was infected and that the second was bitten more than eighteen days later. As the number of times an individual fly returns to man increases so are the chances of transmission enhanced. The most intimate degree of contact possible is where the fly population, severely restricted in its movement, must feed exclusively on man. Whilst to ensure maximal spread of the disease, the same flies must be involved in their repeated association with man, it is not a requirement that the human population should be unchanging; in fact, the chances of a fly becoming infected may be increased where every feed is taken from a different person. A colony of tsetse located at some busy place, such as at the approaches to a ferry, is more liable to become infected, and to transmit the disease, than a colony at a water point serving only half a dozen folk. Where a small group of persons is in constant contact with fly, infection, once introduced, will result in a small but obvious outbreak—few cases but high prevalence. Where the fly are feeding on a constantly changing population cases will occur over a wide area but the rise in the prevalence will not be so dramatic as in a strictly localized and static population.

The expressions 'personal' and 'impersonal' man–fly contact were introduced by Nash (1948a) and later developed by Hutchinson (1953). Personal contact describes those circumstances where a particular group of tsetse is repeatedly feeding on man; impersonal contact refers to the situation where the fly has no more than casual association with humans, and is not dependent on them as hosts. It must be appreciated that the degree of man–fly contact bears no relationship to the number of tsetse involved. It may happen that fly abound and man is being freely bitten yet, because they are able to roam widely and use other hosts, their degree of dependence on humans is very slight and contact is is impersonal. Conversely, a small group of tsetse, hardly noticeable, or even difficult to find, may be severely restricted in its habitat and utterly dependent on man with a resultant high degree of personal contact which may be extremely dangerous. Nash (1944a) cities an example where a few *G. palpalis*, marooned during the dry season at a water point in Northern Nigeria, were responsible for an infection rate of 70% in a population of forty-three. Obviously, the greater the number of fly in personal contact with man the greater will be the risk; but as conditions adverse to the tsetse are those which promote close association with man, it often happens that only a few fly are involved in the rapid spread of the disease.

The importance of repeated contact applies only where man is the sole host of *T. gambiense*. Should there be an alternative reservoir of infection then transmission from this source could be effected by the most casual association between man and the vector.

Factors Influencing the Degree of Man–fly Contact

The epidemiological significance of the distribution and behaviour of the tsetse

The characteristic feature of the distributions of *G. palpalis* and *G. tachinoides* is their continued limitation within certain broad areas of tropical Africa and their complete absence from others. As far as is known, this has been determined primarily by the macro-climate, through its influence on vegetation.

Within these vast belts neither the distribution nor the behaviour of the fly, in terms of its potential for repeated contact with man, are uniform. Here, it is the suitability of the micro-climate provided by the vegetation which is the deciding factor.

In the more humid areas of its distribution, in forest and coastal zones, *G. palpalis* enjoys minimal restriction of habitat. It is not closely confined to the vicinity of surface water, but is widely distributed and, being free to roam, has a considerable choice of hosts. In these circumstances contact with man is impersonal. By contrast, in the harsher climate of woodland savanna the fly is only found close to rivers and streams. Its distribution and its movement are strictly linear and there may be many miles of fly-free country between one drainage system and another. During the prolonged dry season, which is characteristic of the area, when streams have dried up and fires have destroyed much of the wet season habitat, the fly may be closely confined to isolated pools or to other areas of localized moisture. In such circumstances, if contact occurs with man, it is likely to be personal for there may be few alternative hosts available within the limited fly focus. In transitional vegetation zones, which lie between forest and woodland savanna, the small islands of evergreen vegetation provide ideal habitats for the fly, and the surrounding open country allows easy sighting of hosts. As the transitional zones are often favoured areas for farming, a dangerous degree of man–fly contact not infrequently develops here also (Hutchinson, 1954; Scott, 1957).

The effect of increasing severity of climate on localization of the fly is similar with both species of the waterside tsetse; but in the case of *G. tachinoides*, except at the western part of its distribution, this occurs at more northerly latitudes than with *G. palpalis*. Thus, where they co-exist, and more particularly in areas where *G. palpalis* is nearing the limit of its distribution, it is this fly, rather than *G. tachinoides*, which is forced into the closest association with man and is mainly responsible for the local spread of the infection (La Croix, 1961).

Tsetse distribution maps show the edge of the fly-belt as a distinct line but it is only along the seaboard that this line accurately delimits distribution. In other places, where the limit of distribution is imposed by gradually increasing adverse climatic conditions, the line is discontinuous. Islands of tsetse survive at varying distances outside the main belt and although these change from season to season, and perhaps from year to year, in general they will cover a relatively fixed band of country, represented on the map as the edge of the fly-belt. The significant point is that it is at the limit of the distribution where, in general terms, confinement of the fly within a small area is most likely to occur and where, in consequence, the potential for a dangerous degree of personal contact with man will be greatest.

Where the host preferences of riverine tsetse are for man and his domestic animals, their distribution and behaviour may be determined by host availability as well as by suitable microclimates. Examination of blood from engorged *G. palpalis* shows that where the opportunity offers about one third of the feeds have been taken from man and his stock, mainy bovids (WAITR, 1956, 1957, 1958, 1959, 1960, 1961). Riverine tsetse are known to survive readily in unpopulated areas, where their hosts are reptiles, smaller game and perhaps even birds, but there is little precise information about the influence of the distribution of human populations on that of the fly. Morris (1946) considers that *G. palpalis*, at least in parts of West Africa, tends to live only in association with man, possibly on account of the ready source of food which human communities provide.

The role of man in promoting intimate contact with tsetse

If population densities are sufficiently great, local tsetse habitats are inevitably destroyed by farming and in the search for firewood and building material. Man–fly contact does not occur and the disease is absent where, with fewer people, it would have been endemic. Densities greater than 200 persons to the square mile will probably be inimical to the fly, but no firm figure can be given since the size of the population, as well as its density, influences the amount of vegetation which will be cleared.

Personal man–fly contact can occur as readily with very light densities of population as with any other, but because in such circumstances very few people are involved, the chances of a fly becoming infected, and the opportunities for it to transmit the disease, are severely limited. Consequently a significant incidence of sleeping sickness is less liable to be found in areas in which the population density is extremely light.

The denser the human population, within the limits compatible with the survival of the tsetse, the more intimate will be man–fly contact; the fly depends increasingly on man when alternative hosts are destroyed or are driven away. In savanna zones, agricultural and domestic activities may reduce suitable fly habitats to isolated foci which may be conducive to more personal contact. In heavier vegetation, man-made clearings produce conditions which may offer considerable possibilities for close association with tsetse, and here, also, the number of *G. palpalis* will increase. During the 1939–43 epidemic in Sierra Leone, higher infection rates were discovered in the Kissi than in the Kono people; the respective population densities per square mile were 100–127 and 50–70. Although other factors were probably involved, it was thought that the difference in the densities of the population *per se* was particularly important (Hutchinson, 1954). Duggan (1962) mentions increasing population as favourable to the spread of the disease in Northern Nigeria, as does Morris (1959) in Uganda.

Man's role in determining the nature of his contact with tsetse may be inferred from the varying degrees of risk of acquiring the infection associated with his diverse occupational and social habits. As tsetse are virtually absent from towns and often from their immediate environs, only those who work in, or visit, the countryside are exposed. Sleeping sickness is a disease of the rural areas. Under endemic conditions it is generally most prevalent among adult males, suggesting that infection is contracted at some distance from the home as, for example, when they are at work on the farm or engaged in some other largely masculine activity. Women, and less frequently children, are liable to become infected when the family visits the farms or when they are exposed during ordinary domestic and social activities such as washing clothes, bathing, collecting water, gathering firewood, going to market, visiting friends and attending funerals, marriages or traditional celebrations. Here and there the disease is more prevalent in women but this is usually quite localized and is associated with some activity, such as visiting the village water-point, which involves exposure to infected tsetse.

The siting of villages and hamlets is a further important sociological influence. Where the potential for personal man–fly contact is considerable, the risk to the community will vary inversely with the distance between the dwellings and the permanent fly habitat. Close proximity to a tortuous fly-infested stream is particularly dangerous; for example, a village lying within a loop of such a stream would be surrounded on three sides by tsetse (Morris, 1959). In Gambia, Hutchinson (1953) recorded rates of infection ranging from 0·3–1·2% when 200 villages were allocated to one of four tribal groups; he considered that the differences in incidence were due to the siting, size and permanence of the villages rather than to variations in occupation of the people.

The Relationship of *T. gambiense* to *T. rhodesiense*: the Association between Vector and Parasite

The more acute and severe cases of sleeping sickness are ascribed to infection with *T. rhodesiense* and are found in areas where only game (woodland) species of tsetse occur. In contrast, the mild and chronic form of the disease is ascribed to *T. gambiense*, the distribution of which coincides with that of the riverine tsetse. However, as the consistent difference between these trypanosomes appears to be only one of virulence (Ashcroft, 1963), it is becoming increasingly accepted that the classical clinical descriptions of these two infections represent only the extremes of the range of the behaviour of a single species of trypanosome. As variations in virulence occur naturally, the constant association of the more virulent strains with transmission by the *morsitans* group of tsetse and of the less virulent strains by the *palpalis* group requires some explanation. It was formerly held that virulence of the trypanosome was, in some way, dependent on the species of the fly by which it was carried but a more rational view has been put forward by Ashcroft (1959a).

In country where only flies of the *morsitans* group are found the usual hosts of the fly are game animals. In these, the milder strains of the human trypanosomes are inevitably destroyed so that, by a process of natural selection, only the more virulent will survive and when man is, by chance, involved in the game-*morsitans* cycle of transmission it is the relatively acute form of the disease, described as *T. rhodesiense* infection, which he acquires. By contrast, in zones of riverine tsetse the milder strains of trypanosomes are selected out for survival; here man is a favoured host of the fly. A strain which causes a relatively asymptomatic infection in man, allowing him to continue his normal activities for many months, or even for years, will have a greater opportunity for onward transmission than a virulent strain which, by quickly disabling its host, is exposed to tsetse for a shorter time. Ashcroft sums up this theory by stating that the strains of trypanosomes which endure are those which are so well adapted to the major hosts of the local vectors that contact between the fly and the trypanosome is maintained.

A further point requires examination. In East and Central Africa the savanna tsetse transmit the infection, albeit to produce, in general, only low incidences of the disease; but where these species co-exist with the riverine group of fly, as in West Africa, their role as possible vectors has been generally discounted. This may be because the number of infections which might arise in this way would be negligible in comparison with those carried by the *palpalis* group. In terms of planning the control of the disease they would have little significance. There is yet no definite evidence to incriminate *G. morsitans* in these areas for it is notoriously difficult to determine where an individual infection has been acquired and, if *G. palpalis* or *G. tachinoides* are found in the neighbourhood, it would be illogical to consider transmission to have been by *G. morsitans*. There have, however, been reports, particularly from Northern Nigeria (Lester, 1933; Duggan, 1962), of the disease in a whole community showing unusually severe features which Lester considered to be more akin to *T. rhodesiense* than to *T. gambiense*. Duggan suggested that the strain might have been introduced from game animals, either through *G. tachinoides* or *G. morsitans*.

It is possible that isolated cases of a *T. rhodesiense*-like infection may have been overlooked in areas regarded as endemic zones of *T. gambiense* only; it would require a most careful taking of case histories over a very large area, and over a considerable period, to reveal such infections at the low incidence at which they might be expected to occur. Even if this were done, the evidence would probably be inconclusive for if severe infections were occasionally discovered it would be very difficult to prove that they had been carried by *G. morsitans*.

It is not suggested that *G. morsitans*-acquired infections present a significant problem on the western side of Africa but that they may occur at an extremely low prevalence (often typical of *T. rhodesiense*) and are masked by the overwhelming preponderance of the milder form of the disease transmitted either through *G. palpalis* or *G. tachinoides*. This question is not entirely academic for, should control of transmission through the riverine tsetse be effected over a large area, a low incidence of a *T. rhodesiense*-like infection might remain, or even be found to be more common than is at present apparent.

The introduction of *T. rhodesiense* into a *T. gambiense* area, under endemic conditions, would be expected to have only very limited opportunities to spread and, according to Ashcroft's theory (*see* p. 627), it would eventually die out. On the other hand, the introduction of *T. rhodesiense*, under conditions suitable for epidemic spread, might be fraught with the danger of a severe outbreak of *T. rhodesiense* infection transmitted by *G. palpalis*, since the process of natural selection suggested by Ashcroft would not become effective immediately. This was, in fact, the experience at Alego in Kenya (Willett, 1965).

EPIDEMIOLOGICAL FACTORS OF DOUBTFUL SIGNIFICANCE

The epidemiological factors so far considered are of fundamental importance and their significance is fairly well understood. There are, however, other factors of potential importance which have not been so clearly defined but which it is necessary to consider before describing the contemporary pattern of Gambian sleeping sickness. Some of these are suggested by studies made on the distribution and behaviour of the natural disease, and some by the results of experimental work.

Relationships between Man and Parasite

The behaviour of Gambian sleeping sickness in parts of the total area in which the diseases is endemic suggests that, as a result of long continued exposure to trypanosome infection, communities may develop a degree of tolerance or resistance to the disease. It is, however, difficult to determine whether the comparative mildness of the infection is attributable to heightened resistance on the part of the human host, or to reduced virulence of the infective agent, or to interplay of both these factors.

Population Susceptibility

It has been suggested that malnutrition may render populations more susceptible to trypanosome infection (Duke, 1923) but it has not been the general experience that a sudden and marked lowering of the physical state of a community influences the prevalence of sleeping sickness. The remarkable and widespread debilitation which followed the influenza pandemic of 1918–19 was not, apparently, associated with increased incidence of human trypanosomiasis, though this may, perhaps, have been overlooked. On the other hand, Hutchinson (1954) recorded that the serious epidemic of sleeping sickness which occurred among the Kissi people in Sierra Leone in the early 1940s had shortly been preceded by near famine conditions, and in the West Nile district of Uganda the epidemic which occurred there in 1927–8 followed within a few months of famine. In the latter instance, as Morris (1962a) has pointed out, abnormal population migration caused by the famine may have been a more important factor than malnutrition resulting from it.

It is generally believed that human trypanosomiasis was unknown in East Africa prior to the serious epidemic which broke out in 1901 and that the epidemic followed the recent introduction of infection by travellers. This epidemic was characterized by a very high incidence of the disease and by unusually virulent infections, a pattern which is compatible with complete absence of any protection which might have been conferred by previous exposure to the disease. Similarly, workers in West Africa observed that the epidemics which occurred in the 1920s and 1930s were associated with exceptionally severe infections as compared with those seen in the permanent endemic foci from which the disease had spread along rapidly expanding communications (Duggan, 1962). The more recent epidemic in Sierra Leone may also be attributable, in part at least, to the introduction of the disease to areas in which conditions were favourable for its spread but which had hitherto been free from infection (Hutchinson, 1954).

As with some other diseases, the periodicity of epidemics of sleeping sickness may be associated with the growing up of new generations of people with no previous experience of the disease.

Strain Variations of *T. gambiense*

Considerable variations have been observed between one wild strain of *T. gambiense* and another; these differences may be manifested in diverse ways. Apart from variations in virulence, which are discussed below, the ratio of blood to lymph gland infections may vary. As a rule, trypanosomes are much more readily detected in lymph gland juice than in blood films but sometimes, in quite circumscribed communities, this pattern is reversed, perhaps in association with some other unusual features of the disease (Akwei, 1952; Hutchinson, 1954). Strains of *T. gambiense* can also be induced to develop varying degrees of drug-resistance.

Variation in virulence

Gambian sleeping sickness is normally a mild disease, in its early stages at least, but there are exceptions to this general rule. Lester (1933) observed that some strains in Northern Nigeria showed unusual virulence and in this respect resembled *T. rhodesiense* more closely than *T. gambiense*. Hutchinson (1954) reported significant differences in the mortality rates from sleeping sickness in two separate areas in Sierra Leone, and Harding (1940) made a similar observation in Northern Nigeria. Duggan (1962) noted that, in Northern Nigeria, a more severe type of disease occurred in the Lake Chad basin than in the Niger-Benue valley. An exceptionally mild form of the disease was reported during an outbreak at Eket in southern Nigeria by Macfie and Gallacher (1914).

Strains of enhanced virulence could, theoretically, arise from existing strains by mutation or selection. Alternatively, strains of increased virulence may be derived from hosts other than man. In the parts of Northern Nigeria in which the more acute form of the disease has been most frequently observed the usual man to man transmission of *T. gambiense* may be supplemented by the more complicated man–game–man cycle thereby narrowing the gap, epidemiologically as well as clinically, between the classical forms of *T. rhodesiense* and *T. gambiense*.

The possible existence of epidemic strains

Gambian sleeping sickness is particularly liable to occur in epidemic form but this tendency has not been adequately explained. Since, as has been shown, several of the characteristics of *T. gambiense* are prone to variation it must be considered whether the power of a strain to spread in a given community is also a variable characteristic. In doing so, it must be remembered that virulence and infectivity for man are quite distinct characters and that they do not, as is sometimes implied, increase or decrease in unison; indeed, the disease may show a tendency to exceptional mildness during its epidemic phases (McLetchie, 1953).

There is at least a suspicion, based on field observations, that strains of *T. gambiense* introduced into fresh localities may exhibit an enhanced ability to spread through the community. Scott (1961) has reported two instances in which the introduction of infected persons from an established epidemic area resulted in sharp outbreaks of the disease in endemic localities far removed from the original focus of infection. There are other similar observations suggesting that the severe local outbreaks which quickly follow the introduction of infected persons to fresh localities are in some way connected with enhanced ability of the strain to spread.

The Number of Trypanosomes Inoculated

The number of trypanosomes inoculated into the mammalian host by an infected tsetse fly varies greatly even among flies infected from the same host and in the same fly at different times.

Fairbairn and Burtt (1946) estimated that the minimal infective dose of *T. rhodesiense* for man is of the order of 350 trypanosomes and it is probable that a similar number would be required to establish infection with *T. gambiense*. If, as seems probable, strains vary in their infectivity, the size of the minimal infective dose may be an important factor in the transmission of the disease.

Relationships between Vector and Parasite

In terms of applied epidemiology, remarkably little is known of the influence on the distribution of the disease of the variations in the relationships between vector and parasite which may occur under field conditions. It is probable that many factors are involved and, as Willett (1963) has pointed out, their complexity and the difficulties in investigating them have severely restricted progress in this field. However, such of these factors as have been investigated contribute to a better understanding of the epidemiology of the disease.

It has been shown that, under laboratory conditions, pupae of *G. palpalis* incubated at 25°–26°C yield adult flies that are more readily infected with *T. gambiense* than flies emerging from pupae incubated at 20°C (WAITR, 1959). It has also been observed that, in the laboratory, the highest infection rates in the fly are attained when an infective feed is taken early in the life of the fly. Wijers (1958) observed that infection rates were highest in flies taking an infective blood meal on the day on which they emerged, somewhat lower on the second day after emergence, and did not occur thereafter. If the reasonable assumption is made that flies emerging during the hot season are likely to feed early in their adult life, the probability is that infection rates in the fly would be maximal when desiccation and heat are greatest.

It is known that, under experimental conditions, infection rates in the fly vary with the strain of trypanosome concerned. Duke (1930) believed that recently-acquired infections in man were more readily transmissible than older infections but no such difference was found by Taylor (1932a) when working with *T. gambiense* and *G. tachinoides*. Strain variation in the trypanosome in relation to infection rates in the fly is a factor of obvious potential significance in the transmission of the disease but its epidemiological significance has not yet been elucidated.

Flies emerging at the end of the hot, dry season are particularly receptive to trypanosome infection since they will feed early in adult life. With the onset of the rainy season the expectation of life of *G. palpalis* is maximal (Nash & Page, 1953) so that a combination of these factors produces a situation in which infected flies are liable to survive for protracted periods. While exceptional longevity *per se* is unlikely to influence the infection rate in the fly population, it greatly enhances the potential for infected flies to transmit the disease, though it is possible that this potential may be reduced by other consequences of seasonal change such as reduced man–fly contact.

THE INFLUENCE OF CLIMATE ON EPIDEMIOLOGY

Climatic conditions exert a profound effect on the epidemiology of sleeping sickness. It becomes immediately obvious from an examination of national records describing the distribution of the disease that, in all areas of West Africa infested by *G. palpalis*, sleeping sickness has, in general, been much more prevalent in the hotter and drier savanna regions than in the more equable climate of the forest and coastal zones from which it is often completely absent. All of the major epidemics in West Africa have occurred in the savanna regions.

As has been mentioned above, temperature plays an important part in determining infectivity rates in the fly and the duration of the developmental cycle of the parasite in the insect host. Climate is also a factor of prime importance in relation to the degree of contact between man and fly. These factors have been described in some detail elsewhere (Chapter 32) and only a brief summary of the salient points will be given here.

Under the hot, dry conditions prevailing typically in savanna regions during the dry season, several known factors combine to promote the spread of the disease. When exposed to severe degrees of heat and desiccation the fly can survive only in very restricted habitats to which man is also compelled to resort in search of shade and water. Contact between man and fly is therefore very close and personal. The same severe climatic conditions also induce the fly to feed soon after emergence, increase the liability of the fly to become infected and accelerate the rate at which the development of the parasite in the fly occurs. All of these factors are conducive to the spread of the disease and, under natural conditions, operate to their maximal extent in the savanna zones, at or near the limit of the fly's distribution and at the season of the year when movement of the fly is restricted to the greatest extent. At other seasons, even in the same locality, the fly enjoys greater freedom of movement and its contact with man becomes correspondingly less personal and intimate; in zones in which climatic conditions are less exacting, movement of the fly is comparatively unrestricted and its contact with man is reduced to more or less casual encounter.

THE BROAD EPIDEMIOLOGICAL PATTERNS OF SLEEPING SICKNESS

Trends in Prevalence

Tendency for Periodic Epidemics to Occur

One of the most notable characteristics of Gambian sleeping sickness is a tendency to break out in epidemic form. Before the present century epidemics occurred in West Africa (Morris, 1951), but their histories are fragmentary and the pattern of their behaviour is not revealed.

Two major epidemics have occurred since 1901. The first of these was observed in Uganda in Eastern Africa between 1902 and 1905 and the second in central and West Africa between 1915 and 1940. The latter made its appearance in the Congo basin whence it spread as a slow, continuous wave until, twenty-five years later, it reached the conjunction of the frontiers of Liberia, Guinea and Sierra Leone some 2,000 miles to the north-west of the original focus (Scott, 1957). The experience of the countries which lay in the path of this epidemic cannot be considered in isolation but must be regarded as part of a single manifestation. In localized areas the outbreak covered a period of about ten years but in the larger countries such as Nigeria it lasted almost twenty years. It is probable that this great epidemic wave covered a much larger area, lasted longer and was responsible for many more cases than any previous episode since it occurred at a time when social and economic development facilitated the movement of people into and through the areas affected on an unprecedented scale, thereby providing exceptionally favourable conditions for the dissemination of the disease.

In the last two decades the epidemic tendency has reappeared. In a number of West African countries, Ghana and Nigeria among others, small and quite localized outbreaks have been noted but because of long-continued control and the ready means of its intensification, they have not developed their full potential. The impression is that, in the absence of control, they would have attained the proportions of previous epidemics, with which they showed certain features in common, including selection of the same locations and the same direction of spread (Scott, 1961).

The time during which sleeping sickness has been observed is too short to allow any long-term trend in the periodicity of epidemics to be recognized with assurance, particularly where the natural behaviour of the disease has been modified by control; there does, however, seem to be a suggestion that sleeping sickness is most apparent at intervals of about twenty-five years in parts of West Africa (Duggan, 1962) and perhaps more frequently in East Africa (Morris, 1960).

There are several possible explanations to account for this tendency for epidemics to recur. It has been suggested (Duggan, *loc. cit.*) that an epidemic compels people to leave the stricken area but after some years they return and the stage is then set for a repetition. This may have been so in some instances, but it does not provide an explanation of general application. Duggan also suggested that at the end of an epidemic the number of susceptibles remaining in a community is reduced but with the growth of a new generation of susceptibles the liability of a further outbreak becomes greater. Another possible explanation is that some cyclical change in the climate may occur which cannot be observed from normal meteorological records but which may cause a periodical intensification of man–fly contact. Alternatively, trypanosomes may, like other organisms, exhibit periods of activity and decline, of growth and decay (Morris, 1962a), and that epidemics are manifestations of a dynamic phase caused, perhaps, by the periodic development of a strain of parasite with enchanced ability to spread.

Of these possible explanations for the occurrence of epidemics and their periodicity only the last is compatible with the behaviour of the disease in the vast epidemic which swept over the western side of tropical Africa thirty to forty years ago. Had this great event been due solely to increasing man–fly contact resulting from more settled conditions, or to the spread of the infection along expanding communications into areas where it had previously been almost unknown, then it would be necessary to postulate that social progress in the many countries affected by this epidemic wave had also developed in the same orderly east–west manner. This was certainly not the case. As with periodicity so in regard to the great epidemic, a possible explanation lies in the emergence of a strain of trypanosome with enhanced power to spread, its appearance in the south-eastern part of the area, and its slow movement in a succession of infected persons towards the north-west.

The Apparent Absence of Seasonal Variations in Prevalence

In woodland savanna areas, the various factors which combine to promote the spread of human trypanosomiasis during the late dry and early wet seasons have already been discussed. At this time of the year man–fly contact is most intimate and sustained; the likelihood of an infection developing in the fly is greatest and, at the beginning of the rains, the longevity of the vector is maximal. Yet seasonal variation in the prevalence of sleeping sickness is not recorded. That it is not seen at clinics is probably due to several factors. In the initial stages the disease is mild, patients are often unwilling to make the journey to seek treatment on account of only minor symptoms to which, indeed, they are constantly subjected from one cause or another. More particularly will they be disinclined to do so when work on the land is becoming urgent, as is the case just at this time. Thus an increase in the number of cases occurring in an area in the course of a few weeks would not be discernible from clinic records but might be spread over several months. Even frank outbreaks are not reflected in the attendances until they are well established. The prevalences discovered by survey teams are of no value in making comparisons of seasonal variations for these units are constantly on the move and variations in incidence which might be discovered could be as readily attributed to differences between localities as to a seasonal effect.

Current Trends

At present, the incidence of Gambian sleeping sickness is generally low except in Congo Kinshasa where, due to cessation of a vast programme of chemoprohylaxis, the prevalence of the disease has increased considerably in recent years, and in certain other countries where small localized outbreaks have been occurring here and there. But the rate of decline has lessened and there is now revealed an obstinate core of residual infection.

Considered in terms of the total number of cases occurring in a country during a year, the figure today is about one tenth of what it was during the epidemic period. Field surveys show that among all persons examined for trypanosomiasis current prevalence rates are of the order of less than one case per thousand persons.

Some examples of the incidence revealed by recent surveys are given in Table 33.1.

TABLE 33.1

Country	Year	No. persons examined in thousands	No. cases	Incidence %
[1]Ivory Coast	1965	2,159	394	0·018
[1]Mali	1965	636	432	0·067
Nigeria	1965	1,118	752	0·08
[1]Guinea	1965	1,476	471	0·03

[1] WHO, 1967.

For comparison; in Nigeria in 1935, 84,364 cases were found in a surveyed population of 407,203 (McLetchie, 1948); in Guinea in 1940, 4,086 cases were found among 123,472 persons examined.

The figures cited above represent the current trend of prevalence in most countries (with the notable exception of Congo Kinshasa) when they are considered from the national level. The results of surveys, presented on a country-wide basis, show very clearly that there has been a remarkable decline of sleeping sickness during the last thirty years but they do not reveal the manner in which the disease survives to produce persistent, intractable infection at a low level; the local behaviour of the disease in those small but active foci which remain a source of danger to the community is completely masked. A true assessment of the problem will be possible only when more detailed information becomes available.

The waning of epidemics is generally ascribed to the application of control measures. But just as the origins of the epidemic may have lain in the trypanosome itself, rather than in the physical environment in which it encountered man, so may its decline be accountable, in part at least, to reversion of the trypanosome to an earlier status. Hutchinson (1953) records that, in Gambia, there was evidence that the prevalence of the disease began to decline before special control measures, in the form of increased diagnostic and treatment services, were introduced. Certainly control holds down the incidence during the epidemic and limits its spread but, as with other epidemic diseases, a natural decline may eventually occur. Persistence in the application of control has clearly reduced the endemic level far below the figures that would otherwise have been found but there is a danger that, if control is relaxed before eradication is achieved, an epidemic might break out before the equilibrium of an endemic period was re-established.

The Geographical Pattern

Residual Endemic Foci of the Disease

Distribution

Gambian sleeping sickness is not uniformly distributed throughout those parts of Africa which are infested by the riverine tsetse fly but presents a mottled pattern of varying prevalences. The disease is absent from some areas and present in others at incidences perhaps up to 2% in endemic periods. Although the pattern of prevalence is uneven it is not haphazard, ever-changing and entirely unpredictable. It has two characteristics of stability which immediately help in its rationalization. Firstly, it is relatively fixed from year to year, and even from decade to decade. Surveys repeated at intervals demonstrate that within tsetse infested zones the same localities are constantly infected, whilst others always remain free of the disease. This is seen in a broad fashion in the long absence of sleeping sickness from most of the southern parts of the countries in West Africa—from Ivory Coast to Nigeria—in contrast to its constant predominence in the north. Not only is the pattern fixed in respect of those areas which are infected and those which are not but, in the truly endemic zones, so is the distribution of the relative prevalences. In successive surveys it is found that it is always the same communities which tend to show the highest prevalences of the time, others constantly experience moderate rates whilst some communities are always least involved.

The second characteristic is that the distribution of the higher prevalences is usually localized and well-defined. These are the true foci of the infection and typically, because they lie embedded in areas where the disease occurs much less frequently, they stand out clearly. Some may involve no more than one or two neighbouring villages or hamlets but their close grouping, which may often be apparent, allows a larger area of relatively high prevalence to be defined, and so the pattern builds up. Thus, whilst many of the foci are small, others which have been recognized are vast, covering some hundreds of square miles, as in the case of the Niger-Benue focus in Northern Nigeria.

As the epidemic wave of human trypanosomiasis receded from West Africa in the last twenty-five years these foci, which are the permanent home of the disease in endemic times, have become more apparent, just as pools remain to mark an unevenness in the ground when flood waters dry up. In Northern Nigeria, Duggan (1962) has described two primordial sleeping sickness foci, one related to the Lake Chad basin in the north and the other to the Niger-Benue valley in the south. Between these lie others, smaller and more recently established, in which the disease has been particularly persistent since the great epidemic passed; the Pitti locality on the western edge of the Jos Plateau is an example. Hutchinson *et al.* (1964) gave an account of the present foci in the bordering areas of Guinea, Sierra Leone and Liberia, all of which are long-established. In spite of repeated Lomidine prophylaxis over several years two small foci remain in Guinea, one in the region of Guekedou and the other near N'Zerekóre. Likewise, in Liberia, two foci remain—a small pocket in the Kissi area and a larger focus near Gbarnga in Central Province to which attention was first directed when the disease was discovered in the country in 1927. In Sierra Leone, Sherbro Island is an old though low-grade focus. The foci in Ghana have been described by Scott (1961).

A persistent focus has been recognized at Abengourou, Ivory Coast, for some years. There is evidence that residual endemic foci also persist in other French-speaking countries as, for example, at Bamako in Mali and on the upper reaches of the River Oti in Togo and Dahomey. Lotte (1951a), describing the pattern of the disease in the countries of the former French Equatorial Africa, defined two types of focus, one being small and surrounded by uninfected country, the other much larger with the disease showing virulent endo-epidemic behaviour. In East Africa where features of the vegetation found at the limit of the fly's distribution may be similar to those in West Africa, a comparable pattern is also shown; in Kenya and Uganda the persistence of endemic foci over many years has been described by Morris (1959, 1960, 1960a, 1962a).

Many of the endemic foci are found near the limit of the distribution of the vector. Associated in this way with *G. palpalis* are the Niger-Benue focus, the River Oti foci and all those in northern Ghana. The Lake Chad basin focus lies at the upper limit of the *G. tachinoides* belt. In East Africa the foci are found, in general, in islands of *G. fuscipes* (*see* Map 10.3) separated from the main belt of *palpalis* group distribution, around the great lakes of Kenya and Uganda and along the lower reaches of the rivers which feed them. The old foci of Sudan are also at the limit of the distribution of the tsetse. The reason for this relationship is clear. At the limit of its range the movement of fly may be severely restricted by climatic conditions and if, at this point, contact occurs with man it is most likely to be personal. It is here that infection, once introduced, is most likely to be transmitted. A few foci are found dispersed in the transitional vegetation zones which lie between forest and woodland savanna and also provide conditions favourable for personal contact. More exceptionally a focus is found in forest, sometimes where it abuts onto a transitional type of vegetation. In general, however, the distribution of the foci within the fly belt is centrifugal; their absence from the centre is notable.

The nature and epidemiological importance of residual endemic foci

There is considerable evidence that epidemics originate in the residual foci of the disease (Morris, 1960, 1960a, 1962a; Scott, 1961). This is to be expected for, whatever the underlying cause of an epidemic, it is not unreasonable to suppose that opportunities for its appearance would be most likely to occur first in those places where transmission is already taking place most readily.

It is here that an epidemic tendency would most easily find expression. In practice, however, and particularly where the influence of the smaller foci is being sought, the increased prevalence will have spread beyond their limits by the time that attention is drawn to the outbreak, and frequently the data presented from the field is insufficiently detailed to yield information on this point. During epidemics the highest rates of infection may be found at the centre of the affected area and progressively declining rates as the periphery is reached (Morris, 1960; Scott, 1961).

The occurrence of an epidemic in one locality tends to promote increased prevalence in other areas, the infection being carried by travellers. During endemic periods there are grounds for believing that the movement of people from areas of residual infection maintains the incidence of the disease in other less heavily infected parts of the country; the mechanism by which this is effected is discussed below.

The nature of the residual foci of the disease in Ghana has been described by Scott (1959, 1961) and an example from that country will serve to illustrate the principal characteristics of these foci, their persistence and unchanging location, often towards the limit of the fly belt, and their role in the early stages of an epidemic and in producing zonation of prevalence. During the great West Africa epidemic two areas in the north of Ghana were mainly affected, each covering about 2,000 square miles. One of these lay in the east, in the district of South-East Mamprussi. Here a large island of *G. palpalis* is projected from the main belt, the tsetse being able to survive the normally harsher climate of that latitude on account of the area being at a higher altitude. From surveys made in this district in the early 1950s, when endemic conditions had been re-established for some years, three residual foci of the disease could be readily defined. In 1957 a new series of outbreaks began in northern Ghana. Although they were on a much smaller scale than the epidemic of twenty-five years previously, the pattern of behaviour was, in some respects, very similar and it could be regarded as a repetition of the previous event but with full development modified by the early application of control measures. In March, 1957, it was noticed that among the few cases attending the sleeping sickness clinic in South-East Mamprussi, three came from a single village (Timpella) which lay at the centre of one of the defined foci. An immediate survey showed that 33% of the inhabitants were infected (59 cases in a population of 183), an unusually high incidence for these times. In the following months the whole district was examined and 659 cases were discovered; 300 others were diagnosed either on resurveys made in selected areas or by voluntary attendance at local treatment centres. Table 33.2 compares the findings of the endemic period (surveys 1951–2) with those of the new epidemic episode (1957–9) and illustrates the persistence of the foci over the years, during both phases of the disease.

Accurate maps made of the Sameme focus and the immediate surrounding country showed that there was a definite concentric pattern of prevalence with the centre based on the village of Timpella. The incidence of the disease within a radius of 1 mile of Timpella was 30·7%, at a distance of 1–2 miles it was 11·75%, at 3–5 miles 3·6% and beyond 5 miles only 1·53%. The number of villages within the limits stated was 2, 3, 12 and 28 respectively. It is unlikely that this progressive diminution of incidence was fortuitous and the explanation would seem to be either that conditions for spread were optimal at the centre and diminished peripherally, or that the outbreak first appeared at the centre and spread outwards.

The other two foci, situated 20 and 40 miles respectively from Sameme, were involved to a lesser extent. It seems probable that they were sufficiently close to the primary focus to permit the eventual introduction of the new strain of trypanosome and that, once this had occurred, the favourable conditions for transmission which already existed facilitated the spread of the disease locally.

Sleeping sickness has occasionally been observed to disappear naturally from small foci situated at, or near, the limit of the fly's distribution. In such cases

TABLE 33.2

Area	Endemic period Surveys 1951–52			Epidemic period Surveys 1957–59		
	Pop.	Cases	% Inf.	Pop.	Cases	% Inf.
Sameme focus	8,331	21	0·25	9,095	293	3·22
Sakoga focus	8,488	39	0·46	10,685	166	1·55
Bumbuna focus	3,269	7	0·21	3,657	71	1·94
Total for the 3 foci	20,088	67	0·33	23,437	530	2·26
Rest of S.E. Mamprussi	22,961	19	0·08	33,041	129	0·39

the probable explanation is that tsetse have retreated either because of human activities or as a result of marginal climatic changes in areas in which it was already difficult for the fly to survive.

Linear Distribution of Increased Prevalence: the Importance of Lines of Communication

In addition to the fairly even geographical distribution of residual and endemic foci of infection, the disease sometimes shows a marked linear distribution related to river and stream systems and to lines of communication. In the savanna areas both man and fly are closely tied to the vicinity of water courses and the distribution of the disease is characteristically linear. In the wetter and more humid forest regions, on the other hand, human settlements are not restricted to the vicinity of rivers and streams and the vector, *G. palpalis*, is widely dispersed so that the linear pattern of distribution is not seen.

It has been repeatedly observed that movement of people is an important factor in the spread and ultimate distribution of sleeping sickness (Todd, 1912; Kleine, 1919; Lester, 1933a, 1938, 1945; McLetchie, 1953; Hutchinson, 1954; Scott, 1957; Morris, 1951, 1959, 1962a; Duggan, 1962). The nature of the disease promotes its wide dissemination since, in its initial stages, it is so mild that infected individuals are often able to travel great distances, even on foot. Improved communications and means of transport have increasingly encouraged the inherent desire of indigenous people to travel and this is reflected in the greater dissemination of the disease during the last three or four decades.

The spread of the disease over long distances is accountable mainly to the movement of man; the insect vector's role is insignificant in that its flight range and life-span are short and infection rates in the fly are very low. The accidental transportation of tsetse in vehicles seldom occurs on a sufficiently large scale to be a factor of importance.

Human migration may introduce trypanosome infections into areas which, although suitable for their further spread, have previously been free from the disease. The extent to which this has happened in the past cannot now be assessed but there are several instances of its undoubted occurrence including the epidemics observed in the island of Principe during last century, in Uganda in 1902 and in Northern Nigeria (Duggan, 1962) a quarter of a century later.

Of greater practical significance is the consequence of frequent movements of people within areas where the disease is already endemic. The effect of introducing infected immigrants may be merely to increase the local incidence by the number of imported cases; no spread of the disease from the infected immigrants may take place. It is, however, dangerous to assume that a high incidence of trypanosomiasis in a non-indigenous group is due to the arrival of infected persons because newcomers may, by reason of their occupation, be subject to exceptional risk in their new environment.

Infection introduced by immigrants may spread locally and in some cases may cause sharp outbreaks. Several factors may be involved. The number of imported cases may be sufficiently large greatly to augment the reservoir of infection available to the insect vector and so, in a quantitative manner, promote transmission. An imported strain may also show qualitative differences such as enhanced virulence or ability to spread, or may be one to which the indigenous population has not previously been exposed and to which no resistance has been acquired.

Movement of cases through the country appears to be responsible for maintaining a higher level of endemicity in the areas visited by infected persons than would otherwise be expected. This effect is more apparent among populations concentrated around lines of communication along which migrants pass than in the scattered destinations to which they proceed. It cannot be assumed that traffic routes promote the spread of the disease simply because most cases are found in a 'sleeve' distribution around roads since the population itself is frequently distributed in this way. It is necessary, therefore, to compare incidences of infection in different elements of the population which have varying relationships with roads.

Such an investigation was undertaken in 1952–4 in a large area of northern Ashanti, in Ghana, through which many thousands of migrants travel annually. All the villages of the area were classified into five groups: (1) those lying on the major roads; (2) those within 5 miles of the major roads; (3) those on secondary roads; (4) those within 5 miles of the secondary roads; (5) those more than 5 miles from any motorable road or track. In Table 33.3 the incidence per cent of the disease is given for each of these localities and separately for each of three elements of the population:

A. The total population of 157,000 persons.
B. Ashanti males in the age group 15–44.

C. Moshie males aged 15–44, a non-indigenous group temporarily resident in the locality.

Table 33.3 shows clearly that the risk of infection varies directly with proximity to, and importance of, roads and for this there are several possible

TABLE 33.3

Location	Prevalence rate % of trypanosomiasis in population group		
	A	*B*	*C*
1 On major roads	0·35	0·72	1·5
2 Within 5 miles of major roads	0·27	0·42	1·2
3 On secondary roads	0·16	0·23	0·75
4 Within 5 miles of secondary roads	0·12	0·10	0·36
5 Beyond these limits	0·0	0·0	0·0

explanations. For many reasons roads attract settlement and the higher population density in their neighbourhood is more favourable for transmission of trypanosomiasis than in the remoter areas. By providing easy access to markets for cash crops roads stimulate farming and thereby promote more continuous contact with tsetse. The distribution of *G. palpalis* may also be influenced by that of man, being most attracted to areas where human hosts are readily available. A high rate of infection in migrants moving along roads would necessarily increase the local reservoir of infection; however, in the Ashanti investigation this factor did not operate since surveys over several years had shown that infection rates among immigrants were lower than among indigenous people of comparable age and sex groups.

The intermingling of peoples from widely separated parts of the West African endemic zone, which occurs along the main traffic routes, may bring together strains of trypanosomes which present an unusual challenge to local populations and so be responsible for higher rates of infection. Harding (1940) described two areas in Northern Nigeria, one relatively isolated and the other crossed by several major roads. In the latter the mortality rate from all causes was considerably greater than in the former, a finding which was ascribed to the greater severity of sleeping sickness caused by the continual introduction of fresh strains of trypanosomes.

While it may be accepted that lines of communication undoubtedly promote the transmission of Gambian sleeping sickness, the various factors involved have not yet been precisely determined.

The Demographical Pattern

Age and Sex Distribution of the Infection

In general Gambian sleeping sickness is a disease of males rather than of females, and of the working age group of men in particular, although this is by no means invariably so. Under endemic conditions the ratio of the prevalence in males to that in females is of the order of 2:1 or 3:1, applying equally between boys and girls as between men and women. In over 1½ million persons examined during field surveys in Ghana between 1949 and 1956 the infection rate in males was precisely twice that in females. Rates in children are usually about one third to one fifth of those in the respective adult sex group. These figures reflect the different degrees of exposure to fly in the course of the daily activities of each group. Instances of the highest rates occurring in women are frequently found over relatively small areas, generally indicating that transmission is localized to village water points where the women may spend much of their time. In parts of Gambia, rice farming along the side creeks of the river, where tsetse may be severely restricted in its habitat, is the prerogative of the women and Hutchinson (1953) has described how, in one such group, this resulted in a 23% incidence of the disease.

During epidemic episodes it is often found that as the incidence rises so the gap between male and female prevalences narrows, until eventually the women may be the more heavily infected. The explanation for this is that whereas in endemic periods transmission is generally taking place at some distance from the village, and men are consequently at greater risk, the enhanced transmission of epidemics takes place closer to, and, even in some instances, in the immediate vicinity of the homes. All age and sex groups are then more evenly at risk.

Multiple infections in a family are sometimes seen, husband and wife being the most common relationship. They are less frequently encountered when the prevalence is low. During outbreaks the chance of more than one case occurring in the same home is obviously increased but, in addition, transmission may be taking place at some part of the periphery of the village, or even in the compounds, and in these instances some dwellings may be particularly involved. Occasions have been recorded where 'hut' infections were such a feature that mechanical transmission by mosquitoes was suggested as the cause. It appears fairly certain, however, that all instances of family infections can be explained by a shared exposure to infected tsetse.

Macfie and Gallacher (1914) recorded an outbreak of sleeping sickness at Eket in Southern Nigeria in which over 56% of the 222 cases were children. The high incidence among boys was attributed to the fact that they did most of the water carrying and collection of firewood in this area.

The Influence of Occupation

Fundamentally, the demographic pattern is determined by exposure to infected tsetse fly. As this in turn is largely dependent on the daily activities of the individual (and since in the circumstances of a rural economy the daily round of most men appears to be very similar) there has been a tendency to overlook the need for specific investigations into occupational hazards but, occasionally, examples of unusual risk have been recorded.

In Northern Nigeria labourers employed in open-cast tin mining showed prevalences of up to 2–5% new cases every six weeks until pentamidine prophylaxis was initiated in 1946. In Ghana, the infection rate among nearly 2,000 licensed palm wine tappers was 0·75% and among 1,200 wood sawyers it was

0·4%, whereas in the 80,000 other adult males of the same population, who were employed almost exclusively in peasant agriculture, it was only 0·17%. Labourers working on road construction and maintenance are also at unusual risk; in the same area in a labour force of more than 1,000 the infection rate was more than four times that in farmers. Formerly, men operating ferries were at unusual risk but with chemoprophylaxis, which is well suited for use with organized and stable labour, they are now less frequently infected.

The disease may also be associated with fishing. In some areas, on the shores of Lake Victoria for example, this may be a full-time occupation. In other places it is only an occasional pursuit but, even so, infection can sometimes be traced to this source with confidence. The *Raphia* trade of Northern Nigeria has also involved exceptional risks and Nash (1944) recommended that the cutters should be licensed to operate only during the first fortnight of each quarter, so that fly infected in one period would be dead before the next.

Rates of infection may show marked variations between peoples of different ethnic groups living in the same area. This is more likely to be due to differences in occupation or social customs than to variations in resistance to the local strains of trypanosomes. The Moshie immigrants in the Ashanti and Brong-Ahafo regions of Ghana provide an example. Several thousands of these young men emigrate annually from their homes in Upper Volta for a season's employment in general agricultural work, some returning on a number of occasions, a few settling permanently. In the late 1930s a high prevalence of infection was found in a small sample survey made among these men and it was assumed that they were importing the infection from Upper Volta where, at that time, the disease was prevalent. However, by the 1950s, when the infection rates in Upper Volta had been very much reduced by chemoprophylaxis, the number of Moshie cases found in these two regions of Ghana, both during field surveys and at voluntary attendance at clinics, remained disproportionately high. Special investigations into the distribution of the disease in this group confirmed that the infection rate among them was considerably higher than in the local adult male population. In those who had settled, this increase was most marked in the early years of their residence, thereafter gradually declining, but always being well above the local figure. That this high prevalence was not due to the group having arrived in the country already heavily infected was shown from investigations made over several years. Among those making their first visit, the prevalence was less than in the local population but it was much higher in those returning home; clearly they had been at exceptional risk during their employment. Those coming on second and later visits showed a higher rate than the newcomers, indicating that a number of them had gone home with the disease and were returning to work without having taken treatment. These findings are summarized in Table 33.4.

The Moshies are representative of immigrant labour as a whole, which plays such an important role in the economy of the more prosperous areas of West Africa. The hired man spends more time on the farm than his employer; his exposure to tsetse is thus proportionately greater and this factor may be largely responsible for the higher incidence of the disease in the group.

It is well known that population movements are liable to precipitate epidemics.

Refugees displaced as the result of war, famine, earthquakes and other similar occurrences are notoriously prone to disease in epidemic form as are also immigrant labour forces recruited for large-scale construction work (tropical aggregation of labour) and pilgrims attending major religious festivals.

In respect of its epidemiology, perhaps the closest parallel to human trypanosomiasis is malaria, another insect-borne protozoal disease. It has been conclusively demonstrated that a static community in which malaria is endemic acquires a considerable degree of resistance or tolerance to the species and

TABLE 33.4

Surveys among the static population	
Infection rates per cent among Moshie adult males	
During the first year of residence in the regions	0·89
During residence of 1 to 10 years in the regions	1·44
After 10 years' residence	1·15
Infection rates per cent in indigenous adult males	0·35
Surveys among migrants entering and leaving the regions	
Infection rates per cent in Moshie adult males	
Entering the regions for the first time	0·14
On leaving	0·89
On re-entry	0·25

(The Moshie population involved in these investigations was over 15,000).

strains of Plasmodium which prevail locally but that this resistance becomes largely inoperative when fresh strains of parasites are introduced or when the community is translated to a new environment where the disease is endemic. The intermingling of species and strains of Plasmodium in the ways indicated gives rise to enhanced prevalence and virulence of the infection.

The degree to which the behaviour of human sleeping sickness is influenced by similar factors has not yet been clearly elucidated but there is considerable evidence to suggest that such factors as population movement, strain variations of the trypanosome and communal susceptibility to infection may play an important part in determining the spread, distribution, severity and epidemic potential of sleeping sickness. There is an obvious need for further investigation on these aspects of the epidemiology of the disease.

THE PRESENT POSITION AND FUTURE PROSPECTS

In most of the countries in Africa in which human trypanosomiasis is endemic, great efforts have been made during recent decades to control the disease and, if possible, to achieve its ultimate eradication. During this time the overall incidence of sleeping sickness has been greatly reduced, but a hard core of residual infection persists and the danger of recrudescence remains.

If epidemics are to be forestalled or at least detected before they reach serious proportions, it is imperative that control measures be maintained at an effective level and that adequate surveillance be continued for an indefinite period. Persistence of the present low level of incidence carries the danger that responsible authorities will be lulled into a state of apathy and that, as time passes, the devastating epidemics of the past will be forgotten. There will then be the temptation to curtail expenditure on the services responsible for control and surveillance which, if yielded to, will inevitably result in the forfeit of the gains already made at great cost in effort and expenditure.

The contemporary problem is to ensure that the progress made is consolidated and that, by further investigation, means are evolved to deal effectively with obstinate residual foci of infection. It is not too much to expect that, as new knowledge is acquired, eventual eradication will be achieved.

It seems to be a characteristic of the disease that as former high prevalences have declined, circumscribed residual foci of infection have emerged. The distribution of these residual foci has not yet been accurately mapped and it may well be that the larger of those already identified may represent an aggregation of a number of smaller discrete foci. The exact role of these residual foci in maintaining the disease throughout the whole endemic area and in initiating epidemics has not yet been determined and calls for urgent investigation.

Further information is also required about the various factors suspected of influencing the severity and distribution of the disease and of initiating epidemics, to which reference has been made above.

There is need also to ascertain whether or not an animal reservoir of *T. gambiense* exists and, if so, its importance in determining the severity of the disease and in perpetuating its transmission.

There are other epidemiological problems which will be solved only by carefully planned and executed investigations. Such investigations should be undertaken in a large area, or areas, over a long period of time and should ensure that social and geographical data are recorded in sufficient detail, and in a form suitable for subsequent analyses by statistical and other means.

Chapter 34

The Epidemiology of Rhodesian Sleeping Sickness

F. I. C. APTED

DISTRIBUTION AND PREVALENCE OF RHODESIAN SLEEPING SICKNESS

Rhodesian sleeping sickness extends from southern Uganda and the Central and South Nyanza Provinces of Kenya through Rwanda and Burundi, Tanzania, Mozambique, Zambia, Malawi and Rhodesia to N'gamiland in northern Botswana and to eastern Angola. This whole area of some 1,700,000 square miles is inhabited by 50 million people, but in contrast to the thousands of cases of Gambian sleeping sickness still diagnosed every year in West Africa, the total number of new cases of the Rhodesian disease rarely exceeds 2,000 in a single year and is usually between 1,000 and 1,500. These figures may come as a surprise to those who have heard of the serious nature of the disease and of the fear with which it is regarded throughout much of eastern Africa, but this fear is nevertheless well justified. The figures themselves give no indication of the past epidemics, or of the ever present threat of new outbreaks necessitating constant vigilance and extensive measures of control, nor do they reflect the economic loss to the countries involved.

The tsetse fly infests areas far greater than those actually affected by sleeping sickness; two-thirds of Tanzania, for example, are covered by fly, but the threat that the disease may break out anywhere at any time enforces control and prohibition of settlement over much land which would otherwise be open for development. Furthermore the presence of the tsetse fly restricts cattle and cattle owners to the relatively small areas of fly-free country in many of which there is overpopulation and soil erosion.

The origin of Rhodesian sleeping sickness has been the subject of much discussion. In 1910 Stephens and Fantham described *Trypanosoma rhodesiense* which differed from the Gambian trypanosome in its resistance to Atoxyl, and in its greater virulence for laboratory animals, with a high proportion of posterior nuclear forms. This trypanosome had been isolated from one of the first twelve patients with sleeping sickness to be diagnosed in Nyasaland and Northern Rhodesia between 1908 and 1909. Ormerod (1961) mentions an early report which indicated that sleeping sickness may have existed in the Luangwa valley in Northern Rhodesia for many years before it was discovered, for the inhabitants gave the name *chilotera* (= dreaming sickness) to a disease with very similar features which had been known for 'as long as their fathers and grandfathers remember'. There were like suspicions of a long-standing disease in N'gamiland, in northern Bechuanaland, which was known as *gotsello* or *kotsela* (= drowsiness), although a survey in 1909 failed to verify its existence and it was not until some thirty years later that the first definite diagnosis was made.

There is another early account, mentioned by Ormerod, of a focus in the Sebungwe area of Southern Rhodesia which appeared to him to have been long established by the time it was discovered in 1912, and indeed he believes that it was in the Zambesi river system that Rhodesian sleeping sickness arose, as a zoonotic infection derived from *Trypanosoma brucei*. In contrast, Willett (1965) holds the view that the Rhodesian type of infection resulted from the introduction of a virulent strain of trypanosome into a *Glossina morsitans* area by travellers from the Congo, and he gives much interesting historical detail in support of this belief. Further discussion of this subject is not possible here, but much food for thought and many useful references to the literature will be found in these two papers.

Whatever its origin, the subsequent history of Rhodesian sleeping sickness after the discovery of the first cases is for the most part well documented. In brief, it was known to be present in the Rovuma river area between Tanganyika and Mozambique in 1911. From what was probably a separate focus in south-western Tanganyika it spread northwards in epidemic form throughout the greater part of western Tanganyika in the 1920s and 1930s. South-east Uganda was affected by a severe outbreak in late 1940 which spread towards the Kenya border and entered Kenya in 1942. The last major extension was from Tanganyika into Ruanda-Urundi in 1954. Some of the main events and the present position in each country are summarized below.

Botswana

The early rumour of a sleeping sickness-like disease in N'gamiland has been mentioned above but the first proved infections were discovered in 1934, when two cases were found and some evidence was obtained that there had been a small outbreak. The disease is confined to the north of the country, in the Okovango swamp area and around Chobe in the north-east. With the exception of an epidemic in 1942–3 about which there is insufficient information (it may or may not have been sleeping sickness) only some 5–20 cases were recorded annually until 1957. From 1958 onwards the number rose to between 50 and 100 each year until 1967, when it fell to 41.

The Caprivi Strip

There was an outbreak in 1959 along the Kwando river in the Eastern Caprivi Strip, between Botswana and Zambia. This was probably an extension of the infection from N'gamiland.

Angola

Rhodesian sleeping sickness occurs in two areas in the south-east of the country. Some fifty cases were diagnosed in 1965 and a similar number in 1966.

Rhodesia

The first cases were reported in 1909. Within recent years some 1–5 cases have been reported annually, all the infections being contracted in the north of the country, in the Zambesi valley, often by people who visited the area on hunting trips. There were ten such infections in 1966.

Zambia

The Luangwa valley in the east, where the first cases were reported in 1908–9, remains one of the areas chiefly affected. Cases are now reported from all over the country, the main areas involved, apart from the Luangwa valley, being around Kasempa in the North-Western Province, and Mpika in the Northern Province. In 1965 there were small outbreaks in two areas in the Southern Province, at Mazubuka and at Choma, but these appear to have subsided. For the four years 1964–7 inclusive the reported cases totalled 155, 99, 128 and 96 respectively.

Malawi

The first case of sleeping sickness in this country was reported in the Nkata Bay area in 1908, but after a relatively high prevalence in the first few years only occasional cases were diagnosed until recently when there appears to have been an increase. Ten cases were reported in 1964, one in 1965, twenty in 1966 and six in 1967. The infections were sporadic and were contracted in the Nkhota-Kota and Nsanje areas and in the lower Shire valley.

Mozambique

Two distinct areas are affected, one in the north and north-east towards the Rovuma river and the Tanzania border, and the other in the south-west along the Zambesi. The first case was diagnosed in 1909, and a patient is known to have been infected in the north of the country in 1912. From 1942 to 1958 the number of cases reported annually was between about 150 and 300, but during the next seven years, up to 1965, only some 30–80 cases were recorded each year.

Tanzania

From the Rovuma river, where it was known that the disease existed about 1911, there was a slow diffusion northwards through the Eastern *morsitans* fly belt to involve the Eastern Province in the late 1920s, but in the western fly belt there was a severe epidemic which started in the south-west of the territory about 1920, or possibly some years earlier, and which had involved the greater part of the Western Province by the early 1930s. Some 11,000 cases had been reported by 1932, 3,000 of them in one year, and over 2,000 in a single district. It is not surprising that there was what Maclean (1926) described as 'a stampede' of the population from the affected areas which must have aided the spread of the infection, but his very successful policy of resettlement of the population rapidly brought the situation under control (Maclean, 1930). There was another outbreak which started at about the same time, in 1922, in the *swynnertoni* fly belt to the east of Lake Victoria but this remained localized and had come to an end by 1935. Subsequent outbreaks occurred in the Ukerewe peninsula to the south-east of Lake Victoria in 1939, and towards the north-east of the territory, at Mkalama and at Babati in 1932 and 1943. The next, and the last major extension of the infection, was in 1954, when a severe outbreak involved Ngara district in the extreme north-west of the country, together with the neighbouring territory of Ruanda-Urundi. For some years, apart from small local outbreaks, the position has remained fairly stable, but it is now such that the greater part of the vast tsetse-infested area in the country has been, or is at present, affected by sleeping sickness.

The number of cases of sleeping sickness reported each year is between about 500 and 900, with some tendency towards a peak incidence every 9–10 years. For each of the four years 1964–7 the total number of cases was 616, 473, 800 and 560. Most of the infections occur in the west of the country, in the West Lake and Kigoma regions.

A small outbreak of Gambian sleeping sickness occurred on Lake Tanganyika to the north of Kigoma in 1952, but this was controlled over the next few years and there have been no recent cases.

Uganda

In 1932 several cases of a very acute form of sleeping sickness were found near Kampala and it was thought that the infection had been introduced from across the Tanganyika border. Nothing further was heard of this form of the disease until late 1940 when it was discovered near Jinja. By the middle of 1943 2,432 cases with 274 deaths had been recorded and the disease had spread eastwards towards the Kenya border.

The great interest of this epidemic lies in the fact that *Glossina pallidipes* was shown to be the vector responsible (MacKichan, 1944) and it has been suggested by Ford (1965) that this was a zoonotic infection which followed the spread of *G. pallidipes* in Busoga and the introduction of *T. rhodesiense* into a situation in which there was man-fly-man transmission. This point is referred to later (p. 659) in the discussion on the epidemiology of the disease. At the time of the epidemic the opinion was that, as in the first outbreak, the infection had spread up the west side of the lake from across the Tanganyika border.

The Rhodesian disease has persisted in the Busoga area around the north-east of Lake Victoria, but the numbers are now comparatively low. In 1964, 1965, 1966 and 1967, there were 82, 91, 130, and 64 cases, respectively. Thirty cases of the Gambian form of the disease were reported during these four years.

Kenya

The sleeping sickness situation in Kenya is complex. The Gambian disease which affected the shores of Lake Victoria and the associated rivers at the time of the great Uganda outbreak at the beginning of the century persisted in suitable foci; its prevalence was reduced only within comparatively recent years by anti-tsetse measures which included the spraying of the Nyando and the Kuja-Migori river systems.

The Rhodesian infection entered the territory in about 1942, by extension from Uganda, and also appeared in the south-west in 1947. In South Nyanza the spraying of the rivers had reduced the incidence of Gambian sleeping sickness from 100–150 cases a year to about fifteen cases, but in 1960–1 an outbreak of Rhodesian sleeping sickness started in the Lambwe valley where there had been new settlement in a *pallidipes* area, and this resulted in some 260 cases over the next four years.

In Central Nyanza, where *G. palpalis* [*G. fuscipes*] had been eradicated in the many foci of Gambian sleeping sickness, the incidence of the disease had fallen almost to nil by 1964, and the number of cases of the Rhodesian infection in the *pallidipes* areas ranged from about 5 to 30 annually. However, in 1963–4 there was an explosive outbreak of the Rhodesian disease in Alego location, with over 300 cases, the interest of which lay in the fact that the fly responsible was *G. fuscipes*. This is the first instance of the Rhodesian infection being transmitted in epidemic form by a fly of the *palpalis* group. Further reference to this is made in the discussion on epidemiology (p. 659).

The number of cases of sleeping sickness notified in Kenya in 1964 totalled 408, and in 1965 there were 279, nearly all from the Alego outbreak. In 1966 only ninety cases were reported.

EPIDEMIOLOGY OF RHODESIAN SLEEPING SICKNESS

The epidemiology of Rhodesian sleeping sickness is a subject which has fascinated many people and the number of observations and deductions made, some of them conflicting, has produced a considerable literature. In the account which follows few references to this literature are given, but it has been fully reviewed and discussed by Fairbairn (1948), Ashcroft (1959b), and Nash (1960a).

There are four main characters in the story—the trypanosome, the tsetse fly, game animals and man. It is proposed first to delineate these characters, or those features of them which appear to be most relevant, and then to discuss their many interrelationships in an attempt to show how Rhodesian sleeping sickness is acquired, transmitted and spread.

The Trypanosome

Mention has already been made of the uncertain origin of the strain of trypanosome which gave rise to the Rhodesian form of infection, although it does seem very likely that it began as a zoonotic infection derived from *Trypanosoma brucei*. The most recent opinion with regard to '*Trypanosoma rhodesiense*' (Ormerod, 1967) is that this trypanosome and also '*T. gambiense*' are but strains or demes of *T. brucei*, different only in the epidemiology and geographical distribution of the infections they produce. Mutation and selection of strains in the '*brucei-rhodesiense*' complex is undoubtedly one of the important factors in the epidemiology of Rhodesian sleeping sickness; for example, there is some indication that the virulence of the trypanosome for laboratory animals and for man increases from the southern part of eastern Africa, where the infection is often relatively mild, towards the north where, in Uganda, it is usually acute and severe. Ormerod (1960) has shown that trypanosomes from Botswana have large dense inclusion bodies, whereas these inclusions in trypanosomes from Uganda take the form of small granules.

The Tsetse Fly

In Africa, human trypanosomiasis, in contrast to the disease in domestic animals, is contracted only in areas where tsetse-flies exist. Only certain species of the genus *Glossina* transmit the disease and their ability to do so is profoundly influenced by a host of factors—behavioural and environmental—which vary considerably with different species of tsetse. For the details essential to a proper understanding of the role of the insect vector in the epidemiology of the disease reference should be made to the relevant Chapters in this book and to the standard work, *The Natural History of Tsetse Flies*, by Buxton (1955). The factors involved are so numerous and so complex that it is not possible to summarize them here but it will be advantageous to mention some of the more important ways in which they may influence the transmission of sleeping sickness.

Rhodesian sleeping sickness is ordinarily transmitted by certain species of the *morsitans* group—*Glossina morsitans*, *G. pallidipes* and *G. swynnertoni*—and until recently it was thought that these were the only vectors of the infection in nature. In 1961, Southon and Robertson reported the isolation of *T. rhodesiense* from wild *G. palpalis* [*G. fuscipes*] and in 1964 there was a sharp outbreak of Rhodesian sleeping sickness in Kenya in which *G. fuscipes* was the vector (Willett, 1965). *G. fuscipes* is not found south of Tanzania, and in Tanzania itself it is confined to the shores of Lake Tanganyika so that its importance as a vector is severely restricted.

The habits of the tsetse flies of the *morsitans* group which are important in the epidemiology of Rhodesian sleeping sickness include those which concern their sources of food, their range and their preference for various types of vegetation—those habits, in fact, which determine their association with man. None of these flies prefers to feed on man, but the species of game animal on which they usually feed, and the behaviour of trypanosome infections in these animals, are closely connected with the zoonotic infection in man. This is discussed more fully in Chapters 13 and 28.

G. morsitans is found throughout the *miombo* and similar woodland which covers the greater part of eastern Africa, although it will also inhabit other types of vegetation. During the rainy season the fly is widely distributed, but often in the harsh conditions of the dry season it retreats into the most favourable areas available. Observations made in the heat of the day may suggest that an area has been vacated, when in fact the flies are sheltering in tree rot-holes and the like. *G. morsitans* is always far more numerous at the edges of drainage lines (*mbuga*) than it is in the open woodland, a fact which is closely brought home to anyone who drives along a road through such woodland, for a cloud of flies will attack the car as it approaches the edge of an *mbuga* and will leave it as the road continues.

G. swynnertoni is found only in the area immediately to the south and south-east of Lake Victoria, but within this area its habits are somewhat similar to those of *G. morsitans*, although the country it occupies is more arid and it inhabits thorn bush rather than miombo.

G. pallidipes needs thicket in which to live, but provided that suitable thicket is available it is found widely distributed throughout eastern Africa, often together with *G. morsitans*. This association of *G. pallidipes* with thicket is important epidemiologically, for the bushbuck also lives in thicket, often near human habitation, and this animal is almost certainly the most important reservoir host of the trypanosome which causes Rhodesian sleeping sickness. In south-east Uganda, and in Kenya, *G. pallidipes* is the main vector of the infection, and elsewhere its probable importance is becoming increasingly recognized.

Tsetse flies do not ordinarily travel far from their place of origin but they may be passively transported for greater distances—sometimes many miles—on vehicles, on pedestrians and cyclists or on cattle, an occurrence of potential importance in the spread of infection. The flies themselves tend to travel longer distances during the rainy season than during the drier and hotter seasons. In places with a severe hot, dry season some species of tsetse concentrate at the restricted number of water sources where they come into close contact with man and game animals.

Temperature is also important in that it influences the infection rate in the tsetse fly. Burtt (1946) found that infection rates with *T. rhodesiense* were higher in flies which had emerged from pupae maintained at high temperatures and field observations show that in areas where the mean annual temperature is high the infection rate is higher than in places where the mean temperature is low. The type of food host may also influence the infection rate in tsetse. Jordan (1964, 1965), working in Nigeria, showed that where tsetse depend largely on Suidae for their food, infection rates tend to be lower than where Bovidae are the main source of blood meals; locally, this effect completely obscured correlation of infection rate with temperature. Temperature in relation to the epidemiology of sleeping sickness in different parts of eastern Africa is discussed by Ford (1965).

Temperature, together with light, is also important in determining the time of activity of the fly which is ordinarily greatest in sunlight, although when the temperature is very high the fly tends to seek shade; flies are less active on dull days and when it is cold. Most species of tsetse are diurnal in behaviour but a few show some degree of nocturnal activity.

It is possible that sleeping sickness could be spread by mechanical (non-cyclical) transmission of trypanosomes, either by tsetse or other biting flies. It is unlikely that this form of transmission is of any real epidemiological significance in human trypanosomiasis though it is known to occur in animal trypanosomiasis in some places.

Game Animals

Almost from the time of discovery of the Rhodesian strain of trypanosome in 1910, epidemiological evidence had suggested that game animals are an important reservoir of the human infection, but only comparatively recently was *T. rhodesiense* actually isolated from a wild animal, the bushbuck, by Heisch *et al.* (1958). The examples often quoted in support of the existence of a game reservoir are 'Jackson's fly-boys' who contracted sleeping sickness in a part of Tanganyika where there was no human habitation and which was closed to all ordinary foot and other traffic; the fishermen on the Ugalla river in Tanganyika among whom infections occurred regularly every year, although for the greater part of the year the area was uninhabited; and the remote area also in Tanganyika where salt was produced and which was similarly a focus of seasonal infection. These examples are discussed in the reviews by Fairbairn, Ashcroft and Nash already mentioned.

This epidemiological evidence is supported by the classical experiments initiated by Corson at the Tinde Laboratory (Ashcroft, 1959a) which showed that *T. rhodesiense* which had been passed through sheep and antelopes for twenty-three years still retained its infectivity for man.

For an animal to play an effective part as a reservoir host of the human infection it must be one with which man comes into sufficiently frequent contact, or which lives near his home. It must also be one in which a *T. rhodesiense* infection is not so virulent that it quickly kills the animal (there is no evidence that such infections occur in nature) or so sparse or fleeting that the chance of a fly becoming infected is remote. In many areas, for example, the warthog is known to provide the fly with a high proportion of its meals but in this animal *T. rhodesiense* produces only a low and short-lived parasitaemia. Some animals, including monkeys and Thomson's gazelle, succumb rapidly to experimental infections, and only those in a third group in which there is a sufficiently high and long-lasting parasitaemia are potentially important reservoirs. The animals in this third group include the common duiker, eland, impala and bushbuck, but of these the bushbuck, which lives in thicket near habitations, is likely to be the most important, for contact between man and the other animals in this group is far less close. Such animals may play their part in maintaining the infection in a fly-game-fly cycle into which man may enter to contract a chance infection (Ashcroft *et al.*, 1959; Nash, 1960a).

The dependence of the more important species of the *morsitans* group on game has been demonstrated in nature by the disappearance of the fly from vast areas after the animals had died in rinderpest outbreaks. Game destruction is known to be a successful method of tsetse control in certain special circumstances, and further evidence is available from the planned experiment at Shinyanga, Tanganyika, where elimination of the game by controlled shooting resulted in the eradication of *G. morsitans* and *G. swynnertoni* and probably also of *G. pallidipes* (Potts & Jackson, 1952).

This dependence of the *morsitans* group on game means essentially that they are confined to country away from human habitation, although the bushbuck in its thicket is to some extent an exception, but even this animal is discouraged by anything approaching full development of the land. In general, man runs the risk of infection with *T. rhodesiense* only when he travels into or through fly country, or when he builds his houses or farms in or too near the edge of such country, or when the fly belt advances to invade his villages, as it may do when these are small and scattered. Full occupation or use of the land, the presence of game and the presence of the tsetse fly are not compatible.

Man

Rhodesian sleeping sickness is an occupational hazard. Age, sex and to a great extent race have no influence on the risk of contracting the infection except in so far as they are related to occupation or custom, as illustrated by the examples given below.

Women, young children, and the very elderly are not often infected because they spend much of their time in or near their homes, and these are usually free or relatively free from the tsetse fly. An increase in the number of cases among women and children is, in fact, often an indication that an outbreak situation is developing, that there has been settlement in fly country or a tsetse invasion of the villages. In some parts, the nature of the country and also tribal custom may play their part. Among the Waha in western Tanzania, for example, some of the villages are in treeless open country, and it is the women, sometimes accompanied by young children, who go into the forest to collect firewood and so become infected. The search for mushrooms is another occupation in which women run the risk of infection, particularly in western Tanzania. It is also the custom among the Waha to hold regular weekly markets, and within quite a small area there will be a market somewhere on nearly every day of the week. The amount of travelling between home and market in this part of the country is considerable, and much of it is through fly-infested country, so that again the women, who attend these markets in great numbers, provide a high proportion of the cases, but this is not typical of the greater part of eastern Africa.

Men become infected when they travel, hunt, fish, or collect honey, or when they have to work in fly-bush, as do many who are employed on the roads and railways. Fishing and 'honey hunting' are particularly hazardous occupations. While they are fishing in riverine pools surrounded by thicket the men may be in close contact with tsetse fly for many days at a time, a situation in which the association between man, bushbuck and *Glossina pallidipes* is likely to be significant. Fishing is of prime importance in the epidemiology of Rhodesian sleeping sickness in south-east Uganda where, on Sigulu Island in Lake Victoria, Robertson and Baker (1958) found that 60% of the patients were directly concerned with fishing, and nearly all were men. Nearby in Lugala, on the mainland, however, nearly a third of the patients were women, and many of the men were farmers rather than fishermen—here was a situation such as has already been noted, in which the people were being infected in their villages.

The hives of the 'honey hunters' are often many days walk from the villages, sometimes in the ancestral family home. Not only are the men exposed to infection on their journey through the woodland, but during the main season for the collection of beeswax and honey, camps are established in the woodland which provide ideal conditions for close and prolonged contact between man and the tsetse fly. With the exception of America, Tanzania is the world's greatest producer of beeswax, and nearly every man, in some parts of the country at least, owns his own hives. Again, there is some difference according to area and tribe. The keeping of bee hives is general and widespread, but among some tribes fishing, for example, is restricted to certain persons. Hunting is the preoccupation of the men in some areas, while in others agriculture is the main pursuit. Properly organized, agriculture gives protection against the risk of sleeping sickness, for the clearing of the land drives back the fly, and the game on which the fly depends tends to leave the area—this, indeed, was the basis for Maclean's (1930) settlement policy in Tanzania which so successfully controlled the spread of the disease. There is, however, a continuous desire for new land and this involves encroachment on the fly bush and farming either within it or very near its edge; the edges of clearings, where man is very liable to be bitten by tsetse, are particularly dangerous.

The question of race deserves further consideration. Occupation largely determines the likelihood of infection, for persons of all races are susceptible. Sleeping sickness is uncommon in Asians for most of them live in the towns and only a relatively small proportion of the European population is regularly exposed to risk. In this connection, however, there is a point of some interest. Among those Europeans who are regularly exposed (district officers, game and tsetse control officers and the like), infection is uncommon, but Europeans who are new to the country not infrequently contract sleeping sickness, particularly those who are members of hunting parties. This observation has been made not only in east Africa but also in Botswana and infection among European members of hunting parties in the Zambesi valley is not unusual. It has been suggested that an immunological factor may be operating here, the person who is exposed fairly regularly perhaps receiving some degree of protection from frequent inoculation with non-pathogenic strains of trypanosome. This appears possible, but it is probably not the whole story. Probably the type of exposure and its duration are important. Members of hunting parties, camped perhaps near water for several days, may experience just the sustained close contact with tsetse fly and a game reservoir as is believed to be particularly significant, and which is discussed below. Gelfand (1966) has described the occurrence of sleeping sickness in three European boys camped with their father for two weeks on the Zambesi. All became ill within two weeks of leaving the camp. The regular field worker, on the other hand, unless he is one of the very few game or tsetse officers, is usually exposed only for brief periods or while travelling, and will not ordinarily camp in fly bush.

THE INTERRELATIONSHIP BETWEEN THE TRYPANOSOME, THE TSETSE FLY, GAME ANIMALS AND MAN

From the preceding account it will already have been realized that infection with *Trypanosoma rhodesiense* is essentially a zoonosis, a disease primarily of animals but one which may be contracted by man if he exposes himself to risk or if the risk intrudes upon him. It now remains to consider and to attempt to explain why the disease in man behaves as it does in different areas, and the ways in which it is contracted and spread.

Ford (1965) has discussed the interrelationships of populations—populations of human beings, tsetse flies and game animals. In a correlation of many previously observed facts, the significance of some of which had not before been appreciated, he has related the expansion of the fly belts throughout eastern Africa to the epidemic of sleeping sickness in Tanganyika in the 1920s and 1930s, and to the different pattern of endemicity in the eastern fly belt compared with the epidemics in the western belt. For the writer, at least, this paper has so clarified a complicated situation that he hopes that it will be read by everyone who seeks an understanding of the problem. The following account is based very largely upon Ford's work.

The death of the game animals during the rinderpest panzootics of the 1890s caused a marked recession of the fly belts and for up to some twenty-five years afterwards man and his cattle were separated from the tsetse fly and the game animals. As the fly belts expanded so did the cattle population and the area occupied by man, and when the inevitable meeting came, conditions for the epidemic spread of Rhodesian sleeping sickness were ideal, with the possibility of close man-fly-man transmission and a susceptible population. This is the picture typical of the western *morsitans* fly belt—a sharp outbreak on the periphery of the belt resulting either from man's encroachment on the fly territory, or from his being overtaken by an advance of the fly. Under natural conditions, with a virulent infection, deaths, and the panic evacuation such as is described so well by Maclean (1926) in his account of the early epidemic in Tanganyika, these outbreaks would be self-limiting. In the conditions in Tanganyika in the 1920s, with an advance of fly over a wide front the outbreaks were also many and extensive, and such conditions are unlikely to be repeated, but the pattern of each isolated outbreak is still the same—sudden, even explosive, and often in an area previously untouched, or uninvolved for many years. Nowadays such outbreaks are controlled by case-finding, treatment and other measures, but the tendency is for the infection to persist in the area at a low endemicity, possibly owing to the selection of the less virulent strains of trypanosome which these measures would tend to encourage.

Ford contrasted events as they occur in the western fly belt with those in the eastern *morsitans* belt. This eastern fly belt is continuous northwards from the Zambesi valley into the southern and eastern regions of Tanzania; much of it is climatically more favourable to human settlement than is the drier western belt, population density is on the whole therefore correspondingly greater, with a greater possibility of man-fly-man contact. In addition, over much of this eastern belt the high mean temperature favours a high trypanosome infection rate in the tsetse fly. The contrast is that whereas in the western fly-belt contact at the periphery with a susceptible human population gives rise to acute epidemic outbreaks, in the eastern belt greater numbers of people have been living with the fly for much longer, and probably the process of selection has given rise to a strain of trypanosome more adapted to the human being. As Ford points out, this suggestion is supported by observed facts. Human infections in the eastern belt are on the whole milder than those in the west, and the disease is sporadically endemic, rather than epidemic. Such mild infections are characteristic of the whole of the eastern fly belt, from the Zambesi basin northwards, and it will be remembered that it is within this area that most of the instances of 'healthy carriers' have been reported. It will be recalled that Ormerod (1960) demonstrated morphological differences between trypanosomes from the south of the sleeping sickness area in eastern Africa and those from the north, and it would seem that this is compatible with the observations brought out by Ford's ecological approach.

The relative importance of man-fly-man and game-fly-man transmission in Rhodesian sleeping sickness is a subject which has given rise to much discussion. Many of the early observers, men of long experience, in particular Dye, Maclean, Swynnerton, and Fairbairn in Tanganyika, were convinced of the importance of man-fly-man transmission and of the role which man was thought to play in the spread of the infection from one area to another. Reference to the writings of these experts has been made by Apted (1962), among others, and the details and arguments will not be expanded here but the combined experience of such men should not be lightly set aside, even though recent concepts of the relationship between '*T. brucei*' and '*T. rhodesiense*', and the part this may play in the zoonotic origin of human infection have introduced factors of which the earlier workers were unaware.

Ford has pointed out that the acceptance of Rhodesian sleeping sickness as a zoonotic infection means that it is not essential to bring man into the picture as the cause of an outbreak in a new area. A zoonotic origin of the infection in man, indeed, supplies the only satisfactory explanation of the typically 'Rhodesian' strains of trypanosome which have been found from time to time well outside the ordinary limits of the disease—for example in the Sudan and in western Uganda. It is of interest to note that Maclean (1926), in spite of his conviction of the important role played by man, could not always establish a link between the appearance of the disease in a village and the arrival of a person from an infected area, although he usually managed to do so.

The writer (Apted, 1962) believes that man-fly-man transmission is important in an epidemic situation, although there is no direct evidence for this. Ordinarily, when the infection is contracted by man as he travels in the bush, these are chance single infections. Sometimes two people in the same party will be infected at the same time, but this will probably be from the bite of a single fly, itself infected from a game animal. Hunters who wait at water holes, or, even more, fishermen who stay at their pools for several days or longer, provide opportunity for the 'sustained triple contact' between man, tsetse fly and game animal (notably *G. pallidipes* and the bushbuck) which is believed to be of great significance (Apted *et al.*, 1963). The woman going to fetch water may be at a similar risk, although her contact with the fly will be frequent rather than sustained. This 'triple contact' is probably important in the maintenance of endemic foci such as are found in all areas, but particularly in the eastern fly belt. Here, especially, the picture is often one of a rise in the number of infections within a limited area over one or two successive years, but usually gradual rather than sudden, and not amounting to an epidemic. Sometimes it is possible to lay suspicion on one place, perhaps quite a small area of bush, as a focus of infection.

However the infection in the bush is contracted, there is the possibility that it will be transmitted to others when the infected person returns to his village, if this village is fly-infested. In such a village, most of the men, if they are not being bitten continually on their farms, will be away in the bush for the greater part of the day, cutting poles for their houses, collecting honey or beeswax, fishing and so forth, and over a period of time there is the probability that more than one of them will be infected. A gradual rise in the number of such persons in close contact with fly within the village would seem to give increasing opportunity for man-fly-man transmission and a build up of infections towards the start of an epidemic.

A similar situation exists if man attempts to enter or to encroach on the fly bush in order to farm; an outbreak of sleeping sickness which followed such an attempt is described by Apted *et al.* (1963). These risks are not confined to the individual farmer or to small villages; one of the main centres of the Groundnut Scheme in the Western Province of Tanganyika was in danger of being closed down because sufficient attention had not been given to the threat of sleeping sickness.

It may appear from this account that the risk of contracting sleeping sickness is high but in fact it is high only in certain circumstances. For the ordinary traveller in tsetse country the chance of being infected is very low. This can be appreciated when it is realized that trypanosome infection rates in the salivary glands of tsetse flies range from about 0·1–0·6% according to the area; that is to say on the average about three to four flies in every thousand carry trypanosomes and of these trypanosomes only a very small proportion will be strains infective for man. Furthermore the tsetse fly, even if carrying an infective strain, has to inject a certain number of trypanosomes before the infection will 'take'. This explains why many people live and work for years or for their whole lives in fly country without contracting sleeping sickness. In Tanzania, for example, hundreds of men are employed in road and railway maintenance gangs; they are constantly exposed to tsetse bites and their camps are often in remote areas in the middle of the forest, yet only a few are infected—there were twenty-four infections among such men in Tanzania in 1959, and a further six among tsetse control staff, another group at special risk, and these may be regarded as high rather than average figures. Infections at road and railway camps often tend to cluster, one or two particular camps providing an unusual proportion of the cases—perhaps another example of sustained triple contact between man, fly and a game reservoir, or perhaps of man-fly-man transmission. Similarly, other workers who might be supposed to be at special risk, for example, those employed in game control, or as messengers constantly travelling through the bush, are rarely infected. It would be misleading to generalize, however. Information from Botswana suggests that tsetse control workers there provide a significant proportion of the annual total of cases of sleeping sickness, and undoubtedly elsewhere, including Tanzania, there are places where the risk is comparatively high, although this may be only in a particular area in a particular year. Some regard must be given to the conditions under which these workers at special risk are exposed. Road and railway workers in maintenance gangs are often living in the fly bush, and tsetse control workers may also be housed for some weeks in temporary camps. On the other hand, game control staff and messengers travel through but do not usually live in tsetse bush so that the risk of their receiving an infected bite is so much the less. Yet chance infections do occur and the risk for anyone in tsetse country, although very low, is not negligible. One of the first instances the writer met with in Tanzania was that of a European who was infected while travelling in a train, and it is by no means unknown, as has already been noted, for members of hunting parties to be infected although they may have been in Africa for only a few days.

The risk of infection is high if men in any number attempt to settle or to farm in tsetse bush, and numerous examples could be given, apart from the one already cited (Apted *et al.*, 1963), of outbreaks of sleeping sickness which have followed such an intrusion into the fly habitat. Uncontrolled settlement in tsetse bush is almost certain to provoke an outbreak unless it is at such a density that the fly is driven back.

Associated with this matter of the risk of infection is a feature of the epidemiology of Rhodesian sleeping sickness which has puzzled many people, namely, the question of why the disease is present in certain areas yet absent from other areas in which conditions appear to be equally suitable for transmission. In fact no tsetse area can be regarded as free from the possibility of infection, and there are constant examples of sleeping sickness being contracted in places where previously it was unknown. The zoonotic origin of the human infection explains such occurrences, but Ashcroft (1959b) has made a suggestion which provides further understanding. A tsetse fly feeding on a number of animals and possibly also on man may become infected with many different strains of trypanosome. Most of these strains will be non-pathogenic for man and even if a strain of '*T. rhodesiense*' is acquired by the fly the tendency will be for it to be so diluted by the non-pathogenic strains that it will not be passed on in a number sufficient to cause an infection. This is linked with the feeding habits of the tsetse fly and with the behaviour of the infection in different game animals, already noted. In areas, for example, where warthog provide most of the meals for the fly a reservoir of '*T. rhodesiense*', i.e. of strains pathogenic for man, is unlikely to be established because this animal is relatively resistant to infection. Where there are bushbuck and reedbuck a significant reservoir of pathogenic strains may be built up, and in or near areas where sleeping sickness is endemic this reservoir is likely to be recharged by pathogenic strains acquired directly from man.

There remains for consideration the atypical behaviour of Rhodesian strains of trypanosome in their relationship with man and the tsetse fly towards the northern limits of the *morsitans* group in Uganda and Kenya. Here *G. pallidipes* is the main vector, at least of the sporadic infection; there is close man-fly contact (as described by Robertson and Baker, 1958) among the fishermen on Lake Victoria and in the nearby villages in Busoga, and *G. palpalis* [*G. fuscipes*] has recently been recognized as playing an important part. In the Alego outbreak in Kenya described by Willett (1965), *G. fuscipes* was the only vector; there was intimate contact between man and the fly which was living in the hedges of vegetation surrounding the houses and compounds in that area. A most interesting observation made during the Alego outbreak was the isolation of *T. rhodesiense* from domestic cattle (Onyango *et al.*, 1966). These cattle are kept within the compounds at night and during the day they are taken for watering to streams and water holes frequented by *G. fuscipes* which are used also by the people as sources of water and for washing and bathing. The possibility that these cattle could have acted as a reservoir of the infection and also assisted in its spread, is obvious.

Ford has suggested that Rhodesian sleeping sickness in south-east Uganda arose as a zoonotic infection transmitted by *G. pallidipes* which had invaded this area; here it found ideal conditions in the secondary vegetation which had replaced former dense cultivation after the population was evacuated in the great sleeping sickness epidemic at the beginning of the century. The sporadic Rhodesian infections which occur in this area are characteristic of such a zoonotic origin, but there is too, as we now know, the probability that *G. fuscipes* is responsible for much man-fly-man transmission. The entry of the zoonotic *T. rhodesiense* infection into a man-fly-man cycle such as existed at Alego would cause just such a sharp outbreak as did in fact happen.

In these complex relationships between man, game and the tsetse fly there is one factor—climate—which appears to be of more than ordinary importance. Mention has been made of the increased salivary gland infection rate in tsetse flies at higher temperatures, but in addition to this direct effect there are many ways in which the climate influences a closer association between man and fly.

In Kenya a succession of heavy rains provided *G. fuscipes* with suitable conditions well outside its usual riverine habitat so that it was able to live and breed in the vegetation surrounding the homesteads—conditions which gave rise to the Alego outbreak.

In Botswana the marked rise in the number of cases of sleeping sickness coincided with a period of five to six years of drought and with an advance of the tsetse fly. The failure of crops almost certainly encouraged deeper penetration into the fly-infested swamp in search of better land, and there was probably also an increase in hunting owing to the shortage of food. In Botswana there is, in addition, the seasonal influence of climate, for many of the people move during the wet season to farming land nearer the swamp and nearer the fly.

Experience in Tanzania is similar. A period of drought always means an increase in the number of infections. The few sources of water are shared by man, fly and game animals in close association; there is also more hunting and more searching for wild forest products at times when crops are bad. Possibly there is a long-term climatic effect associated with the tendency for the incidence of sleeping sickness in Tanzania to rise to a peak about every ten years and then to fall away, but this is uncertain.

Fairbairn (1948) studied the incidence of the disease in Tanganyika in relation to seasonal variation in temperature and found that there was a significant correlation between the monthly mean maximum temperature and the number of cases diagnosed during the next one or two months, high temperatures being related to high incidence. Probably several factors were involved, in particular those which brought about a closer contact between man and fly such as have been mentioned above. There is, too, the influence of climate in determining where people choose to live, and the population density of both flies and human beings, as discussed by Ford, and this is relevant to the proper use and planned full development of land which is the ideal at which to aim in the eradication of the tsetse fly and of trypanosomiasis.

Chapter 35

Clinical Manifestations and Diagnosis of Sleeping Sickness

F. I. C. APTED

SIGNS AND SYMPTOMS OF SLEEPING SICKNESS

African trypanosomiasis in the human being is a disease in which the effect of trypanosome invasion is shown mainly in the reticulo-endothelial (lymphoid-macrophage), cardiac and nervous systems by physical and, in many cases, mental deterioration over a period of months or years. The chronic form of the disease, classical 'sleeping sickness', is found in West Africa, the Congo and Angola while the more acute form is seen in East and Central Africa as far south as Botswana. Although the trypanosomes responsible for these two forms of the disease have been named *Trypanosoma gambiense* and *Trypanosoma rhodesiense*, the view now generally held is that the differences between them, and between the illnesses they cause, are not such as to justify separate specific status. The relationship between these trypanosomes is dealt with elsewhere (p. 39 *et seq.*) and the point is mentioned here only because in the account which follows reference is made to the Gambian and the Rhodesian forms of sleeping sickness. The use of these terms is necessary because for the physician there are important differences, in the clinical picture and in the response to treatment, between the disease as it is seen in West and in East Africa. These differences, however, are not absolute; acute Rhodesian-like infections occur in what are ordinarily 'Gambian' areas, and more chronic, mild infections, though unusual, are found in East and Central Africa, especially towards the south, with every gradation between the two extremes.

Onset

The first sign of trypanosome infection may be the development of a lesion at the site of the tsetse bite, often within five to fifteen days, usually about eight to ten days, after the bite, although shorter and also much longer periods have been reported. Graf (1929a, 1937) whose name is associated with this lesion (also commonly called the trypanosome chancre) described it in its typical form as seen in one of his patients as a round inflamed area about 3 cm. in diameter with a red spot in the middle surrounded by a waxen zone 3–4 cm. in breadth which appeared to be a mass of minute vesicles. This area was surrounded by a red zone and the tissue around it was swollen. The lesion itself was hard and painful and felt like a button embedded in the tissues. Graf also noted that this typical appearance was not constant; there might be little more than a small blue-red indurated and slightly raised area, a fact which has perhaps led to its being overlooked or not remarked upon in some patients. Willett (1966a) has given a description of the development of this lesion based on many observations in volunteers in East Africa. He notes its progress over 48 hours from a small subcutaneous nodule to a tender visible swelling which rapidly increases in size, commonly to 3 or 4 inches in diameter. After it has reached its full development the chancre gradually subsides over a period of about two weeks to leave an area of scaly desquamation. In the African, residual pigmentation may remain for some time.

The frequency with which this lesion occurs has been the subject of some discussion. It is certainly more commonly seen in Europeans than in Africans and has been more often reported in Europeans in East Africa than in West Africa. Duggan and Hutchinson (1966) in a review of published cases of sleeping sickness in Europeans, found it mentioned in eleven out of twenty-four cases in East Africa but in only eleven of eighty-four cases from other parts. Gelfand (1966) states that in his experience in Rhodesia 70% of his European patients with sleeping sickness had this lesion. In contrast, the chancre is seen only rarely in the African in endemic areas in West Africa and the writer never saw an undoubted chancre in an African patient in Tanzania, during some ten years experience there, although admittedly he saw personally only a few patients during the first few days of the illness. On the other hand Robertson and Baker (1958) frequently saw chancres in African patients in south-east Uganda, mainly on the legs, the site of attack favoured by the local vector, *Glossina pallidipes*. It is perhaps significant that Willett (1966a) found that the number of trypanosomes inoculated influenced the development of the chancre and that *G. pallidipes* is known to be a particularly efficient vector. In the well-known series of volunteer trials at Tinde in Tanzania, which lasted for many years, it was rare for one of the volunteers not to develop a chancre.

Sometimes within a few hours of the appearance of the chancre, or a few days later, or, if there is no chancre, some one to three weeks (commonly about ten days) after the infective tsetse bite, there is an attack of fever in response to the invasion of the bloodstream by the trypanosomes. This initial fever usually lasts from one to seven days, is often high, and is accompanied by headache, usually temporal or frontal, and perhaps also by rigors and vomiting. The European patient, in both Gambian and Rhodesian infections, nearly always suffers this sudden and severe onset, the fever is often hyperpyrexial and the general constitutional upset more marked than is usual in most other acute tropical fevers. Sleeping sickness is a disease of exceptions, however, and there are accounts of mild or even asymptomatic infections in Europeans, although these are unusual. In the African, especially in West Africa, the onset is usually more gradual and may even be overlooked; in East Africa, with the Rhodesian type of infection, the African patient may be quite ill, particularly in areas where the disease is gaining new ground and where the infections tend to be more acute. This type of onset, with high fever and rigors, was a feature of many of the early accounts from Nyasaland and Tanganyika when sleeping sickness was a new disease there some fifty to sixty years ago. It has become somewhat modified with time but is still often a severe illness.

The pattern which follows the first febrile attack, or which the disease takes if there has been no marked initial illness, is one of bouts of fever separated by remissions which may last from a few days to a month or more, these intervals tending to become longer as the disease progresses. In the Gambian form, this 'blood-lymphatic' stage, before there are marked signs of involvement of the nervous system, may last for several weeks, for months, or even for two or more years. There is great clinical variation but often at this stage, during long apyrexial periods, the affected person appears and feels in at least reasonable health, although there may be some tiredness or lassitude and headache may become constant. Many patients in this stage seem to be unaware of any illness. The picture in the Rhodesian disease is quite different; the cerebrospinal fluid shows evidence of nervous system involvement a mere three to four weeks after the onset of the illness and within two months or less there are obvious outward signs of a well-advanced disease. In this form, there may be no apyrexial period, although often there are short intervals between recurrent bouts of fever. Weakness or tiredness are prominent features, and headache, which is sometimes occipital, is almost constant. In some Rhodesian infections the course is that of an acute toxaemia with death within a week or two of onset. At the other extreme, there are patients with this infection who have little general upset and a few who maintain that they feel perfectly well.

Irritability, insomnia and changes in personality or mood are characteristic early signs, especially in the European, in both Gambian and Rhodesian sleeping sickness. These personality changes may be too readily ascribed to 'tropical neurasthenia' or to the effects of alcohol or isolation. Occasionally somnolence may be marked, even in the very early phase of the illness, long before there are detectable changes in the cerebrospinal fluid.

Other features of the first weeks of the illness are anaemia, moderate splenomegaly, tachycardia, enlargement of the lymph glands, local oedema (especially of the face and eyelids), the appearance of a rash (visible only on light skins) and deep hyperaesthesia (Kérandel's sign). Both the rash and Kérandel's sign, although almost pathognomonic, are by no means always present. There may be some manifestations of endocrine dysfunction (for example, sterility or abortion in women) and occasionally the eyes may be involved as evidenced by conjunctivitis or keratitis. Some of these features are considered here in more detail.

The Lymph Glands

Especially if there is a chancre, the local glands draining the site of the infective bite will enlarge, but in nearly every case a general glandular enlargement follows, although this appears to be less frequent in European patients. In the Gambian disease the glands most characteristically enlarged are those in the posterior cervical and supraclavicular groups. Sometimes the enlarged glands in the neck are easily visible (Winterbottom's sign) but usually it is necessary to palpate the neck to discover them; they have a typically rubbery feel and are discrete and freely movable. Palpation of the neck is an important part of the diagnostic procedure in Gambian areas but in the Rhodesian infection the neck glands are often not enlarged to any degree. In the latter, the axillary and particularly the epitrochlear glands are those most commonly involved. In both East and West Africa the degree of glandular involvement varies in different areas and in different outbreaks. In a recent atypical outbreak in Nigeria there was gross enlargement of the cervical, axillary, inguinal and other glands. Cervical glandular enlargement has sometimes been noticed in the Rhodesian infection, especially in the acute phase of an epidemic (Kunert, 1939). In general, glandular enlargement tends to be more pronounced in areas where the disease is invading new ground. In the individual patient the glands become smaller and harder as the disease progresses and may eventually disappear. They never suppurate, unless secondarily infected.

The Rash

This is seen only in light-skinned peoples; if it does occur in the African it is invisible on his dark skin and even in the European it is evanescent and may be difficult to find. The rash often fades and reappears several times over a period of weeks, a feature which may account for its being noted in only a proportion of cases—it was seen in about half the patients in the series analysed by Duggan and Hutchinson (1966). The rash may appear early but is commonly seen some six to eight weeks after the onset of the illness when it takes the form of scattered large erythematous circinate patches, often 3–4 inches in diameter, which occur mainly on the trunk and shoulders. The rings formed by the rash may have internal borders which are sharply defined while the external edges are less well marked. The rash may be accentuated by cold, heat or sweating and there may be a sensation of formication but no true itching. In African patients, rashes of various types, mainly finely papular, have been described but these are too inconstant and non-specific in nature to be of much diagnostic value.

Kérandel's Sign

Kérandel described a sensation of deep hyperaesthesia as he himself experienced it. His description is contained in a paper by Martin and Darré (1908). The sensation occurs when soft tissues are compressed, for example, by a sharp squeeze, or by a blow, as when a limb knocks against furniture. The pain caused is out of all proportion to the force and Kérandel found that the fear of hurting himself became a real obsession. The characteristic feature of this pain is that it does not follow the blow immediately but is felt one or two seconds later, rapidly becomes severe, lasts some seconds, then fades and disappears within a few minutes. When present in its classical form this peculiar deep hyperaesthesia is almost diagnostic but it does not occur very often—it was reported in only 29 of the 109 European patients in the series reviewed by Duggan and Hutchinson (1966) and it appears to be uncommon, or at least to be rarely reported, in African patients.

The Heart

A pulse rate faster than expected from the height of the temperature may be one of the earliest signs suggestive of a trypanosome infection and in a proportion of patients indicates some degree of damage to the heart almost from the onset of the illness. The frequency with which the heart is affected is difficult to estimate. Buchanan (1929), when the Rhodesian disease was invading southern Tanganyika and when a number of acute infections were occurring, found tachycardia in 70% of his patients in the first month of the illness and it was almost constantly present in the later stages. Some twenty to thirty years later, however, tachycardia was not a marked feature among patients under observation in hospital in Tanganyika. Buchanan also noted all degrees of cardiac disorder, including heart failure, but the writer cannot recall having seen a single case of heart failure in Tanganyika between 1950 and 1960 but he saw only a very small proportion of the total number of patients and most of them were under treatment in hospital. That cardiac failure still occurs in the Rhodesian form of the disease is shown in a report by Manson-Bahr and Charters (1963) who give the case histories of two patients in Kenya, both with many trypanosomes in the blood and both with severe congestive heart failure. The notable feature in both these cases was the rapidity with which the condition returned to normal after the start of treatment. The hearts were clinically enlarged initially and the very rapid reduction in size probably indicated the presence of pericardial effusions. These authors suggest that the condition was analogous to the diffuse myocarditis with pericardial effusion which is seen in Chagas' disease. Hawking and Greenfield (1941) performed autopsies on two patients who had died from Rhodesian sleeping sickness and found subacute inflammation of the heart, especially of the myocardium and epicardium, and trypanosomes in inflammatory effusions in the pleura, pericardium and peritoneum; there have been similar autopsy reports on patients with the Gambian infection. Bertrand *et al.* (1965) found abnormal electrocardiographic tracings in one third of sixty patients with the Gambian form of the disease, mainly flattening or inversion of the T waves, but in a few patients there was evidence of conduction defect and of cardiac ischaemia. In this connection it should be noted that other observers have found abnormal tracings in apparently healthy Africans, but in Bertrand's patients, again, the signs of heart damage disappeared after specific treatment. In a later paper Bertrand *et al.* (1967) reported the finding of a slow pulse rate in 53% of patients with the Gambian disease and a fast pulse in 31%. In one third of their patients there were radiological abnormalities, the heart frequently being enlarged, sometimes grossly.

Local Oedema

An oedematous swelling of the lower eyelids is sometimes seen and also a puffy, swollen appearance of the face which gives an expression of dullness or sadness even at a fairly early stage of the disease. As with nearly every other sign, however, this facial oedema is not constant and many, if not most, persons seem in the early phases of the illness to be quite unaffected; this is true for both forms of the disease and is one of the reasons why diagnosis at this stage may so easily be missed. Later in the disease the facial expression—'a certain intangible, swollen, stupid look' as Kellersberger (1933) describes it—becomes a more characteristic feature, partly endocrinal and possibly partly nervous in origin, since a degree of ptosis may be present. This expression has defied description, for 'intangible' it is, and yet once seen it is unmistakable. It is perhaps sad rather than stupid and there is a certain look about the eyes, an alertness or a stare, which contrasts oddly with the stillness of the face. Transient local oedema of other parts of the body may occur in the early stage. The peripheral oedema of the later stages, seen especially in the legs, is associated with anaemia.

The Spleen

is often moderately enlarged and soft, but this is so common in other tropical diseases, especially malaria, that it is not of great help in diagnosis.

The Liver

A recent report by Gelfand and Friedlander (1963) described the occurrence of jaundice as the presenting symptom in two Europeans who had been infected in the Zambesi valley. Both patients were seriously ill and in one, although the correct diagnosis was suspected, trypanosomes could not be found on repeated blood examination. A tentative diagnosis of infective hepatitis was considered but the isolation of trypanosomes by animal inoculation confirmed the original suspicion. These cases are unusual but they indicate the possibility of serious liver damage in Rhodesian sleeping sickness. This subject had been studied previously by Robertson and Jenkins (1959) in African patients in south-east Uganda. They found that although visible jaundice, as detected in the sclera, was rare (3·8 % of cases), nearly half the patients in the early stage of the disease had liver tenderness and there was palpable enlargement in about one quarter. Excess urinary urobilinogen was present in 83 % of the patients in the early stage and nearly all had a raised serum bilirubin. These abnormalities were less frequent in patients with more advanced illness and specific treatment brought about a return to normal. In some respects, for example the frequent occurrence of chancres in African patients and the tendency for the illness to be more acute, this part of Uganda is not a 'typical' Rhodesian sleeping sickness area and it may be that these findings are not applicable everywhere. In Tanzania, hepatic tenderness was not a marked feature and visible jaundice was rare, as it was in Uganda, but no special study was made. Further investigations in other areas are obviously desirable.

Endocrine Dysfunction

shows itself, in women, by the occurrence of sterility, menstrual disorders and a high abortion rate. Menstruation may be arrested even soon after the onset of the disease although this becomes more common later—in one reported series menstruation had ceased in one quarter of the women examined. There is often a return to normal function after treatment of the infection. Abortion has been shown to be associated with a uterine hypoplasia secondary to defective hormonal secretions. Figures quoted from one sleeping sickness area in the early days before any effective treatment was known, show an abortion rate of 32 % of total births compared with a rate of 7 % in an uninfected control area. In addition, premature births, stillbirths and perinatal deaths are frequent accompaniments of trypanosomiasis in women.

In men, there may be impotence and, in the later stages of the disease, a small proportion develop gynaecomastia; a feminine distribution of fat may be seen in a few cases or there may be a myxoedematous infiltration of the subcutaneous tissues which gives rise to the appearance known as the 'forme bouffie''. These people may appear well-nourished at first sight, except for such tell-tale signs as the dullness of the skin and the facial expression. Orchitis has been recorded and was seen frequently in the first years of the Rhodesian outbreak in Nyasaland some sixty years ago but it does not appear to have been reported in recent years.

The Eyes

There has been much discussion on the eye lesions which have been reported in association with sleeping sickness and on their specific or non-specific nature. Interstitial keratitis seems to have been seen not infrequently in patients in the early days of the Rhodesian disease in Central Africa. Daniels (1916) mentions a toxic iridocyclitis with variable degrees of keratitis, circumcorneal injection, conjunctivitis and photophobia, such lesions being seen in five out of six patients in Rhodesia. Other reports refer to conjunctivitis as being seen only as a secondary infection and to interstitial keratitis as rare. Bilateral keratitis has been reported in a European patient in Rhodesia and iridocyclitis in a European with a Gambian type infection. Choroiditis and choroidoretinitis have been seen but all authors appear to agree that posterior lesions are very rare and some believe that, even if they are seen, trypanosomiasis plays no part in the causation. Papilloedema may occur but is secondary to the general meningeal reaction. Optic atrophy unfortunately was at one time common after the use of Atoxyl or tryparsamide in treatment but probably never occurs as the result of the infection itself. Diplopia or paralytic strabismus may be among the many manifestations of nervous system involvement but are rarely seen. It is perhaps of interest that the reports of keratitis came mostly from Rhodesia when the disease was new and in its invasive phase; recent reports make no mention of this complication. Presumably a change in the nature of the trypanosome strains is responsible for the difference. Readers interested in ocular troubles in trypanosomiasis are referred to the publications of Daniels (1916), Hissette (1932), Van den Branden and Appelmans (1934), Ridley (1945) Toulant (1950) and Pieraerts (1952).

The Nervous System

Although the effects of trypanosome infection on the nervous system cannot usually be detected in the cerebrospinal fluid for some time after infection—about three to four weeks in the Rhodesian form and some months in the Gambian form of the disease—there is evidence to suggest that the brain is one of the first parts of the body to be affected. Mention has already been made of the various clinical signs and symptoms of early nervous system involvement—headache, irritability, insomnia, changes in mood and the like. Collomb (1957), in the course of electroencephalographic studies found alterations in the tracings during the initial febrile period, only eight to ten days after infection. Radermecker (1954) claims to have detected even earlier changes. Le Port (1935) has suggested that the early headache and also the somnolence which is occasionally present at the onset of the illness may be accounted for by a plexo-choroiditis involving the fourth ventricle and causing a partial obstruction to the flow of cerebrospinal fluid.

As the disease progresses, the outward signs of nervous system involvement become more obvious. These may take almost any form, the actual manifestations being dependent on the part of the system affected; in general they are those which are associated with a diffuse meningoencephalitis with predominant involvement of the base of the brain. Commonly there are signs of extrapyramidal damage—tremors of the hand; fasciculation of the muscles of the limbs, face, lips and tongue; choreiform, athetoid or oscillatory movements of the arms, head, neck or trunk, especially in children; and an increase in tonicity or muscular rigidity. The picture may sometimes approach that of Parkinsonism, although the walk is stiff, shuffling and unsteady, rather than festinating, the tremors are coarser and there is not the fixed facial mask which is so characteristic of true Parkinson's disease. There is usually a considerable element of cerebellar ataxia, the subject being able to walk only with sticks or with the help of friends—a sight which in itself arouses the suspicion of sleeping sickness.

Focal lesions, or the effects of pressure, may cause paralysis of one or more groups of muscles, occasionally transient but more usually permanent, and various forms of neuritis or polyneuritis may develop. These and other manifestations of nervous system involvement have been studied particularly by French and Belgian workers, notably by Gallais *et al.* (1956), Van Bogaert (1956) and Van Bogaert and Janssen (1957).

Epileptiform convulsions may occur but, as with so much in sleeping sickness, there seems to be considerable geographical variation; while in some areas such fits appear to be common, in other parts they are rarely seen or are associated only with the terminal stage of the disease. This variation similarly applies to the focal lesions, paralysis being a rare phenomenon in some parts of Africa.

Involvement of the sensory system shows itself in hyperaesthesia, of which Kérandel's sign, already mentioned, is one example, or there may be a general hypersensitivity to all stimuli, paraesthesiae, or a variety of cramps or muscle or bone pains. Formication and pruritus are other sensory disorders which are often associated with the later stages of the illness but which sometimes occur earlier. Variable responses are obtained to the testing of the superficial and deep reflexes, as is only to be expected in a disease which can affect the nervous system in so many ways.

The most characteristic of all the signs of nervous system involvement is the daytime somnolence which gives the disease its name. From a tendency to 'nod off', the drowsiness gradually becomes more pronounced until sleep is continuous, although the subject can usually be roused and can even be induced to walk if physically capable. At this stage headache is usually persistent although it may be dull rather than intense, speech is slow and indistinct and the sufferer becomes more and more helpless until he spends the whole day asleep, often seeking the warmth of the sun. In the earlier months of the illness wasting is usually not marked but when the late nervous stage is reached, with its continuous sleep, there may be pronounced wasting or even emaciation, partly through the effects of the disease and partly through neglect. The pruritus mentioned above, which often accompanies this later stage, gives rise to constant scratching, the marks of which are almost diagnostic especially when seen together with the dull expression and other signs of the disease which will be present by this time. In the final weeks the somnolence deepens to coma, sphincter control is lost and death follows, often from pneumonia or other inter-current infection before the terminal stage is reached.

In the Rhodesian infection, with its natural duration of only six to nine months instead of the two years or more of the Gambian disease, the somnolence and other signs of late-stage nervous damage are not seen, or are seen only rarely, although there may be drowsiness or coma in the terminal illness. Tremors of the hands and tongue appear from about the second or third month of the illness and also unsteadiness and difficulty in walking, although this is possibly due more to general weakness than to specific nervous lesions. In Rhodesian infections which have been unsuccessfully treated, for example with tryparsamide before the advent of the newer drugs, a Gambian-like picture is sometimes seen, as if the disease process had been prolonged, so allowing the development of the endocrinal disturbances and late nervous manifestations which are not ordinarily seen.

Mental Changes

The appearance of temporary mental change, in personality or mood, in the initial phase of both Gambian and Rhodesian infections has already been noted. Even in the earlier months of the Gambian disease some mental dullness is often present but later nearly every sufferer will exhibit a marked apathy, lethargy and indifference to his surroundings. Sometimes the mental deterioration is more noticeable, often taking the form of 'simple-mindedness'. Emotional lability is common; laughter, crying or outbursts of rage are frequent occurrences and there may be episodes of manic or confusional behaviour, sometimes with hallucinations, persons so affected often running off into the bush. Almost any type of mental illness may result, including the schizoid pattern, as seen in general paralysis of the insane but these fully developed forms are not common. It has to be remembered that the person's behaviour, especially as it is often irrational, irresponsible or aggressive, may bring him into conflict with the law. In an endemic sleeping sickness area any unusual or anti-social behaviour should arouse the suspicion that sleeping sickness may be the underlying cause. A good description of the mental changes associated with Gambian sleeping sickness, as observed by a psychiatrist, is given by Tooth (1950). He draws attention to the similarity between these changes and those seen in cerebral syphilis and schizophrenia and gives many illustrative case histories.

In the Rhodesian disease mental disturbances of the types found in the later stages of the Gambian infection are rare although mental slowness or dullness is not uncommon. In the acute early stage there may be delirium or mania and confusional or hallucinatory states but these are usually temporary and subside when the temperature falls or soon after the start of treatment.

CLINICAL VARIATIONS

So many are the variations that it is difficult to describe a 'typical' case of sleeping sickness but in so far as this can be attempted the natural course of the Gambian disease is as follows. In the African, after an onset which is usually mild, and may go unnoticed, there is a period of several months during which there may be little general upset apart, perhaps, from an increase in headache and occasional bouts of fever. In the European the onset is nearly always acute and severe but, when this has passed, the same relatively asymptomatic period may follow and may last for weeks or months. After the initial onset the course of the disease is similar in both races. Gradually, somnolence develops and increases and evidence of nervous damage appears, mainly in the form of tremors, unsteadiness and other signs of extrapyramidal lesions. The skin is dull and the body, usually at first fairly well covered, begins to waste. The final downhill progress is often rapid with death in from 1 to 3 years after the onset although shorter and longer periods are not uncommon. Often the course is cut short by an intercurrent terminal infection such as pneumonia.

In the Rhodesian infection the onset is almost invariably acute and severe in the European and often severe enough in the African to confine him to his bed. Once the acute phase is over both Europeans and Africans may go through a relatively asymptomatic and apyrexial period although headache may be constant and may be accompanied by other cerebral signs such as insomnia or irritability. Weakness and tiredness are common in the early stage but may not prevent the subject from going about his ordinary work and he may appear, for the first few weeks at least, to be in reasonable health. Between the fourth and sixth weeks after the onset of the disease, sometimes sooner but rarely later, signs of the advancing illness become more noticeable. Weakness becomes more pronounced, anaemia is marked and there is often peripheral oedema, especially in the legs. Tremors of the hands and tongue become obvious, the sufferer is nearly always thin or wasted, his gait is unsteady and often he can walk only with the aid of sticks or with the help of friends. Somnolence is rare but there is often some mental slowness and the face has a fixed expression which has been well described as a 'fishy stare'. This is not quite the same as the dull sleepy look of the advanced Gambian disease but is equally characteristic. Within the next weeks the disease progresses rapidly and, if it is untreated, death will occur in from six to nine months after the onset of the illness, sometimes sooner. As in the Gambian disease, other infections may supervene or cardiac failure may bring an earlier death.

From these two 'typical' forms there are wide variations. In the Gambian disease these are usually towards mildness or chronicity, with a prolonged latent period between infection and the appearance of symptoms. The most reliable information on such cases is provided by patients who have remained in good health in Europe for between two and three years after leaving Africa or, occasionally, for even longer periods. Lapeyssonnie (1960) described the case of a woman in Togoland in whom an infection had persisted for twenty-one years in spite of treatment but she had remained in good health. In this instance, however, the strain of trypanosome (the Féo strain) appeared to be atypical morphologically and in other respects.

The onset of the Gambian infection may, rarely, be mild or unnoticed even in the European. Cooke *et al.* (1937) found such infections in three men from the Gold Coast and Nigeria in whom trypanosomes were discovered only at routine examinations; similar avirulent infections have been reported from the Congo and the Ivory Coast. An early paper by Horn (1910) describes sleeping sickness as being well known to the Africans in the Gold Coast but little feared as there was 'no large mortality'. Earlier, Dutton and Todd (1903) in their survey in Senegambia thought the disease 'a peculiarly mild one' and stated that some of those infected 'believed themselves to be perfectly healthy'. Gambian infections of low pathogenicity have been observed in exceptionally well-nourished and healthy populations and this has suggested a parallel between the disease in man and in cattle which may tolerate trypanosome infections well if their nutritional state is good. In human infections, differences in the strain of trypanosome are probably more important in relation to virulence than the state of health. On the other hand, stresses such as famine, childbirth or another illness may bring to light or aggravate a trypanosome infection and in the less well-nourished the disease may take a more rapid course.

Another example of a very mild Gambian infection has been reported by Harding and Hutchinson (1948) from Fuero, Sierra Leone. In this outbreak some of the patients who were examined regularly for up to nine months before being treated, showed no symptoms and no signs of physical impairment. Trypanosomes appeared in the blood at irregular intervals and in some patients were very numerous, an unusual finding in avirulent infections.

In contrast, the Gambian disease may be exceptionally virulent; infections have occurred in Eastern Nigeria in which the nervous system has been involved within two months of the onset of the illness. Duggan (1962) has given an account of the well-known Rhodesian-like infections in the Lake Chad area where virulent epidemics occur and where the strains of trypanosome behave similarly to those isolated from Rhodesian infections in East Africa.

In the Rhodesian disease also, some infections are seen which are more virulent than usual and some which are less virulent. In the former there may be an overwhelming toxaemia, with death within one or two weeks; such cases are uncommon and occur not in any one area, but apparently sporadically, while other infections occurring in the same area at the same time run a normal course. There is also a tendency for infections at the beginning of an outbreak to be more virulent than those which are seen in the same area later, in the sense that the patients are more ill and often have a higher parasitaemia than those who come from places where the disease has been endemic for some time. A similar increase in virulence when the disease reaches communities which have previously been untouched is seen in Gambian areas, and is referred to, for example, by Duggan (1962).

Again, over a long period of time, the Rhodesian disease appears to have changed its nature. The frequent references to acute and severe illness, with rigors and hyperpyrexia, in the early days of this infection in Nyasaland and Tanganyika have already been noted. Today the disease is certainly, in general, less acute and such severe illnesses are uncommon.

The occurrence of mild, chronic or asymptomatic Rhodesian infections is one of the many puzzling features of this disease, for it is not fully understood why an infection which is usually moderately virulent should occasionally manifest itself in this way. This subject is discussed more fully, however, in connection with the epidemiology of this disease (Chapter 34) and it is necessary here only to refer to some of the cases. Lamborn and Howat (1936) and Davey (1936) record the finding of asymptomatic infections in two Africans in Nyasaland, both of whom remained in apparently good health. Davey stated that there were 'good grounds for believing that one of them actually recovered, for her blood, inoculated into a monkey one year after diagnosis, proved to be non-infective', and the second patient showed no signs of infection when examined 8½ months after the diagnosis was made. Blair (1939) recorded two instances of this 'healthy carrier' state in Southern Rhodesia and it is of interest to note that the strain of trypanosome isolated from one of the patients was initially only of moderate virulence in laboratory animals and in some respects was intermediate in character between '*Trypanosoma gambiense*' and '*T. rhodesiense*'. Conran (1921) reported the case of a child in Nyasaland whose parents refused treatment for him. He seemed to remain in good health and his blood was examined at intervals, with negative results, until one year after diagnosis when trypanosomes were again found. This child, however, died soon afterwards with a heavy infection. More recently Apted *et al.* (1963) reported the discovery of two possibly healthy carriers in Ngamiland, but in this area the infection tends to be more chronic and to resemble the Gambian disease in some respects. Further to the north the evidence for the existence of this carrier state is scanty and although such cases undoubtedly occur they are probably rare. In this connection, though, it must be remembered that the infection, once diagnosed, is invariably treated immediately and often without too searching an enquiry into symptoms or the lack of them. Dye (1927) reported one such case in southern Tanganyika, but Buchanan (1929), also working in Tanganyika but further to the west, found only three persons among many thousands examined who might have been regarded as carriers. Laufer (1955) made a survey in north-west Tanganyika, one of the purposes of which was to determine the prevalence of the carrier state, but he found not a single instance of it in nearly 9,000 persons examined. One possible case has been recorded in south-east Uganda by Robertson and Baker (1958).

It will have been noticed that nearly all these 'healthy carriers' have been reported from the southern part of the Rhodesian sleeping sickness area, a finding which is probably related to the observation that, in general, there is a trend towards an increase in virulence of the infection from south to north (Ormerod, 1961a).

SLEEPING SICKNESS IN CHILDREN

Children are not commonly infected because, under ordinary circumstances, they are less often exposed to risk than are adults; young babies are sometimes infected while being carried on their mothers' backs. Children have little or no immunity and the course of the illness is usually rapid, sometimes fulminating, with early involvement of the nervous system.

Congenital Sleeping Sickness

Placental transmission of the infection can occur but reported and well-documented instances are few. These include two cases reported by David and Pape (1942) in which both mothers appeared healthy but trypanosomes were present in routine blood slides taken immediately after birth and were also found in slides from the babies and from the cord blood. In another case recorded by Darré *et al.* (1937) a child aged two years was seen in France suffering from hydrocephalus. The cell and protein content of the cerebrospinal fluid were raised and trypanosomes were present. The child had been born in Marseilles of a mother who had left the Chad district for France when she was five months pregnant.

DIAGNOSIS OF HUMAN TRYPANOSOMIASIS

Clinical Signs and Symptoms

In the early weeks of the disease there are three signs which can be regarded as pathognomonic—the trypanosome chancre, Kérandel's deep hyperaesthesia and the rash; none of these is constant. The rash is seen only on light skins and even then in only a proportion of patients; Kérandel's sign is not a common feature; the chancre is, in general, rarely seen in the African and is not always present in the European.

Of the other signs and symptoms in the early stage, fever and headache are common accompaniments of many illnesses, and splenic enlargement from other causes is frequent in any sleeping sickness area. The usual severity of the onset in the European and the nature of the fever—an initial bout followed by an apyrexial period which is succeeded at intervals by further bouts of fever—may be suggestive, especially if accompanied by insomnia, irritability or changes in mood. Localized oedema, especially around the eyes and a puffiness of the face itself are suspicious signs and so, particularly, are the enlarged glands which appear as the disease progresses, although these are not present so often in the European as in the African. Persistent headache, lassitude or weakness are additional symptoms but in themselves merely indicate a need for further investigation. In the early weeks of the illness many patients show no outward signs and have few or no symptoms and it may not be until the later stage, with the appearance of tremors, unsteadiness, somnolence and other signs of nervous involvement, that it becomes apparent.

Detection of Trypanosomes in Blood and Other Tissues

The technical methods available for the detection of trypanosome infections are described in detail in Chapter 4.

The diagnostic methods used in laboratory and field practice are here considered in two groups: firstly, those by means of which a positive diagnosis can be established by demonstrating the presence of the trypanosome itself and, secondly, those serological and other methods which may give valuable suggestive or supportive evidence of trypanosome infection but which, by themselves, do not provide unequivocal proof of infection.

Trypanosomes may be found in the initial chancre, in the blood, the lymph glands, the cerebrospinal fluid or the bone marrow; they may also be isolated by cultural methods or after animal inoculation. Trypanosomes may be present in other body fluids, for example, in the pericardium or in the peritoneum, but they are not sought for in such sites in ordinary diagnostic procedures.

The Chancre

If a chancre is present it provides the earliest means of making a definite diagnosis, for trypanosomes may be demonstrated in the lesion up to two days before they can be found in the blood. The chancre is punctured and a drop of the serous fluid which exudes is examined under a cover-slip as a wet preparation.

The Blood

A heavy blood infection may be detected by the examinination of a fresh drop under a cover-slip but heavy infections are not usual and this step is ordinarily omitted. A thick drop preparation is made, stained by Giemsa's method, and examined with the $\frac{1}{12}$ inch objective. A prolonged search should be made before a negative result is declared. Trypanosomes appear in, and disappear from, the blood with disturbing fickleness—present one day they may be absent the next so that repeated blood slides should be taken over a period of several days in suspected infections. The chance of finding the parasites is greater if the slide is taken during a pyrexial period, preferably at the beginning of the rise in temperature. In general, trypanosomes can be demonstrated in the blood fairly easily in Rhodesian infections but they are usually scanty in the Gambian disease, although there are variations in different areas and in different outbreaks. If trypanosomes cannot be found in smears taken directly from the patient their presence may be detected after triple centrifugation of the blood and examination of the stained deposit.

The Lymph Glands

In Gambian areas, the examination of a drop of fluid taken from one of the enlarged cervical glands is the standard method. This fluid should always be examined as a wet preparation under the $\frac{1}{6}$ inch objective when the trypanosomes, if present, can be detected by their movements among the mass of cells. A long search may be needed and experience in the technique brings added success. In suspected Rhodesian infections gland puncture is rarely used, for even if suitably enlarged glands are present which is not usual in these infections, the trypanosomes are found more easily in the blood.

The Cerebrospinal Fluid

Occasionally, trypanosomes may be present in the cerebrospinal fluid in the early stages of the infection but this is very unusual; ordinarily, they are not seen until a rise in the cell and protein content of the fluid provides definite evidence of nervous system involvement. The examination of the fluid is usually undertaken to determine the stage which the disease has reached, or its progress under treatment, and not primarily as a diagnostic measure except in suspected infections in which trypanosomes are not demonstrable in blood or glands, as is often the case in the later phases of the disease. Trypanosomes may be seen by direct examination of a drop of the fluid, but they are more likely to be found if a centrifuged deposit is searched.

The Bone Marrow

Trypanosomes may be found in the bone marrow, taken by sternal puncture, on occasions when they cannot be demonstrated in blood, glands or cerebrospinal fluid but this method is not suitable for use in the field, is not without its dangers and in fact is rarely used. It has been suggested that puncture of the iliac crest or the great trochanter—or the tibia in young children—are safer procedures than sternal puncture.

Demonstration of Trypanosomes by Other Means

Cultural Methods

In a review of various laboratory techniques for the diagnosis of sleeping sickness Weinman (1963) discusses the superiority of cultural methods; for example, in one series of fifty-three isolations by culture from the blood or cerebrospinal fluid, conventional methods gave negative results on nineteen occasions and, furthermore, culture proved positive in four persons in whom there was no reason to suspect the infection. With cerebrospinal fluid, the comparison is even more in favour of the culture method. Other points worth noting are that the result may be obtained within five to thirty days; positive cultures have been obtained from long-standing infections and also from persons who have suffered a relapse of the infection; non-specific therapy, for example treatment for malaria or typhoid, does not interfere with the result. Both Gambian and Rhodesian strains are equally easy to cultivate. In spite of these apparent advantages cultural methods have not been widely used, even though they have been adapted for field use. This is possibly because the excellent results reported have been obtained by workers experienced in techniques which others have not found it easy to reproduce. It is necessary also to have a ready supply of culture media and this may explain why laboratories in many sleeping sickness areas have not taken up this development.

Pinto *et al.* (1953) have described the successful culture of trypanosomes from the bone marrow but this would appear to have little, if any, advantage over the use of blood or cerebrospinal fluid.

Animal Inoculation

This procedure can be a very valuable diagnostic aid especially in suspected cases in which ordinary methods have failed to reveal the presence of trypanosomes. It is a wise precaution to take blood for animal inoculation from any patient in or from a sleeping sickness area who is suffering from 'pyrexia of unknown origin'. A point of importance is that Rhodesian strains of trypanosome will easily infect small laboratory animals—rats are ordinarily used—but Gambian strains infect these animals only with difficulty or not at all. In patients from a Gambian area, blood should be inoculated into a monkey in the first instance and when infection develops in the monkey its blood will usually be infective for the rat. This difference in infectivity for laboratory animals is, indeed, one of the procedures used to distinguish between Gambian and Rhodesian strains of trypanosome.

After intraperitoneal inoculation of infected blood Rhodesian infections often become patent in the rat in four to seven days and nearly always within two weeks.

Indirect Laboratory Tests

Methods of laboratory diagnosis which do not aim at the demonstration of the trypanosome but which nevertheless may give extremely valuable information are, firstly, non-specific tests including investigation of changes in the cerebrospinal fluid, the erythrocyte sedimentation rate and the formol-gel reaction; secondly, specific tests such as the complement-fixation, agglutination, precipitin and fluorescent-antibody tests; and, thirdly, the estimation of immunoglobulin levels.

Changes in the Cerebrospinal Fluid

Examination of the cerebrospinal fluid may yield information of great value in the diagnosis and prognosis of the disease. Apart from the possibility of finding trypanosomes in the fluid, estimations of the protein content and of the number of cells present provide information which is not only of value as a diagnostic aid but which is essential in determining the degree of involvement of the central nervous system and in assessing the response to specific treatment.

A rise in the cell count—mainly small lymphocytes with occasional large lymphocytes and macrophages—is the first indication which the fluid will give of a possible trypanosome infection of the nervous system. Different authorities vary in their standard; some regard three cells and other five cells per cmm. as the upper limit of normal but certainly any increase over five is suspicious.

Together with the cell count an estimation of the total protein content of the fluid is usually made. A rise in the protein level cannot ordinarily be detected as early as a rise in the cell count but it is a more stable feature and does not tend to fluctuate, as may the cell count, with changes in the activity of the disease.

The examination of the cerebrospinal fluid is usually limited to the estimation of the protein level and the cell count—and a search for trypanosomes, by centrifugation if necessary, if diagnosis is the purpose. Further investigations may include the Lange gold curve, which is usually tabetic in type, but a paretic curve is occasionally seen in advanced infections and indicates a poor prognosis. Sugar and chloride levels are diminished in the late stage of the disease. Janssens *et al.* (1961) in a study of the protein fractions in the fluid noted a rise in gamma globulins in all the fractions, and a relative increase of β–2 (IgM) globulins relative to the β–1 fraction. This is a ratio that is rarely disturbed in other neurological diseases.

Cerebrospinal fluid for cell and protein studies is usually removed by lumbar puncture, but the changes may be detected earlier in fluid taken by cisternal puncture. Neujean (1950) in an extensive study of the changes in the cerebrospinal fluid, especially in relation to the influence of treatment, found that the cephalic fluid had a higher cell count and a lower albumin content than the spinal fluid. The early change in cell count in the cephalic fluid was of particular value in the detection of a relapsing infection, a rise in the count indicating an actively progressive disease.

The Erythrocyte Sedimentation Rate

In untreated sleeping sickness the sedimentation rate is very markedly increased. By the Westergren method, which is the technique preferred, rates of fall of over 100 mm. in the first hour are common; there are few other conditions which give sedimentation rates as high as this. The rate tends to be high in early infections, becomes lower as the disease advances and, after successful treatment, drops to within normal limits. A point of considerable interest is that in patients who relapse after treatment the sedimentation rate usually does not again increase. Among those who have studied this test in relation to sleeping sickness are Hollins and Lewis-Faning (1947), Gall *et al.* (1957) and Franco (1960).

The Formol-Gel or Serum Formalin Reaction

This test, details of which are given in Chapter 4, is usually strongly positive in untreated sleeping sickness infections. Dye (1926) found that in patients with sleeping sickness the gel was usually solid after five hours. Patients with leprosy gave a very strongly positive reaction, with solidification within one hour, but this was rare in sleeping sickness. To distinguish further between these two conditions, Dye added a very small quantity of suramin (0·25 grain) to the serum one hour before the formalin was added and found that this retarded the reaction in sleeping sickness for forty-eight hours but there was no such retardation if the serum was from a patient with leprosy. Hope-Gill (1938) considered that if the reaction was completely negative after one hour this was strong evidence against a sleeping sickness infection, and that if the reaction was still negative after twenty-four hours it was almost certain that the patient was not suffering from sleeping sickness. It is possibly best to regard this test as a very useful supplementary diagnostic measure which is simple to perform but on which too much reliance should not be placed. As with the erythrocyte sedimentation rate the results depend on the high serum gamma globulin levels which are commonly, but not exclusively, found in sleeping sickness. Kala azar is another disease in which a strongly positive serum formalin reaction is obtained. Not every patient with an early sleeping sickness infection gives a positive formol-gel test and in those with more advanced disease the test may be negative. The reaction becomes slight or negative after treatment.

Complement-Fixation Test

The application of this test to the diagnosis of sleeping sickness has been studied by a number of workers, for example, Schoenaers *et al.* (1953), Evens *et al.* (1963) and Pautrizel *et al.* (1959, 1960). This test, which is discussed more fully in Chapter 4, is sensitive and highly specific and is positive in nearly all patients in the early stage of the infection. However, the most intense reactions are obtained in persons in whom parasites are demonstrable by other means; they become less strong as the disease progresses and particularly when the nervous system becomes involved. In patients who have been cured the test is negative. In spite of its apparent value the complement-fixation test has not found general favour, probably because of the technical difficulties involved. Similarly, precipitation, agglutination and neutralization tests have been investigated but have not been widely used in clinical or field practice.

Fluorescent Antibody Test

Lucasse (1964) has applied the fluorescent antibody test to cerebrospinal fluid in the diagnosis of sleeping sickness and has found it to be sensitive, specific and of value for the early detection of nervous system involvement. Mattern *et al.* (1965) also studied the immunofluorescence test in patients with trypanosomiasis affecting the nervous system and concluded that this test applied to the cerebrospinal fluid was a valuable method of diagnosis. More recently Bailey *et al.* (1967) have successfully applied the indirect fluorescent antibody technique to samples of blood dried on filter paper; 92% of patients known to be suffering from sleeping sickness showed positive immunofluorescence (nearly all strongly positive) compared with 6% of healthy control subjects (nearly all the 6% only weakly positive). The fact that a large number of samples can be examined by a small staff in one day suggests that this may become a very useful screening test.

The Immunoglobulin Reaction

This is perhaps the most important development in the diagnosis of sleeping sickness in recent years. Investigations into the globulin fractions of the serum protein have revealed a complicated pattern involving changes in the different fractions, and in the proportions between them, in different diseases. In sleeping sickness the significant finding is a great (8- to 16-fold or more) increase in the macroglobulin (IgM) fraction above the normal value. An increase in IgM is found in other diseases including leprosy, kala azar, malaria and syphilis but it is rarely as marked as it is in sleeping sickness. McKelvey and Fahey (1965) in a study of immunoglobulin levels in a wide variety of diseases showed that in most of these conditions, including kala azar, the IgG was higher than the IgM value, but in trypanosomiasis the ratio IgM:IgG was 3:1. The immunoglobulins are still the subject of intensive study and there is a growing literature; much of the work in connection with sleeping sickness has been done by Bentz and Mattern and their colleagues (Mattern *et al.*, 1961; Mattern, 1962, 1962a; Bentz and Diallo, 1963; Mattern, 1964; Mattern *et al.*, 1965). Mattern, in Dakar, found an increase of IgM in 97% of 234 patients who were known to have sleeping sickness but in only 6·3% of persons in whom no trypanosomes could be demonstrated and similar results have been reported by others in field trials elsewhere.

The importance of the immunoglobulin reaction lies in its application as a screening test. A raised IgM level, although it may be due to causes other than sleeping sickness, is a clear indication that further efforts must be made to prove or disprove this diagnosis. Courtois and Bideau (1966) have suggested that the fluorescent antibody test is of use in differentiating trypanosome from other infections; if the fluorescent antibody test is negative, a raised IgM is probably due to some other infection. In field trials some results have emerged which are both valuable and disturbing, for the immunoglobulin test reveals the presence of trypanosome infections in persons who appear to be quite free from any illness. In one series, repeated examinations succeeded in proving the presence of trypanosomes in one fifth of a group of subjects with a raised IgM titre in whom there was no other reason to suspect the infection and in most of the others the effect of specific treatment was to lower the titre. It has long been known that some trypanosome infections are missed by the conventional field methods of blood and gland examination, even when the technique is as perfect as it can be made, but the results of these immunoglobulin tests suggest that the number of missed cases may be much higher than was suspected. This is confirmed also by the findings of Weinman, already mentioned, who showed the superiority of cultural techniques over conventional methods.

A raised IgM titre in the blood may be found even in very early infections, within the first two weeks, and in the cerebrospinal fluid a rise in titre is a sensitive indication of nervous involvement. Micro-techniques have been evolved for which the blood from a finger prick is sufficient and by such means it is possible to examine very large numbers of persons in the course of one day (Mattern, 1964). A recent further development by Cunningham *et al.* (1967) is the use of samples of dried blood on filter paper, a procedure which eases the problem of the transport of specimens from the field to a central laboratory.

In connection with the work on immunoglobulins an interesting report by Houba and Allison (1966) on the rheumatoid factor-like globulins in parasitic infections showed that these globulins (M anti-globulins) were present in high titre in 12% of patients with Gambian infections and in 25% of patients with the Rhodesian disease. Furthermore, tests for heterophile antibodies in an agglutination reaction showed these to be present in high titre in 85% of sera from patients with Rhodesian infections while patients with the Gambian infection gave only low titres in this test. Further investigation may show this reaction to be useful in differentiating between these two infections and so of value in epidemiological studies.

DIFFERENTIAL DIAGNOSIS

In the early stage of the disease, diagnosis on clinical grounds alone can be made with any degree of certainty in only a small proportion of patients. It is true that the typical trypanosome chancre is unique but there may be a problem if it is fading or if a less typical lesion is present; boils and infected bites from insects other than tsetse flies may also cause confusion. Again, the typical circinate erythematous rash is pathognomonic but urticarial and drug rashes, and even leprosy, may give cause for doubt. Kérandel's sign, if present in its classical form, is also diagnostic but it may be difficult to decide on the significance of lesser degrees of hypersensitivity.

Among the many causes of fever in patients in or from a sleeping sickness area are malaria, relapsing fever, typhoid and kala azar. Hodgkin's disease, with adenopathy and characteristic temperature chart, is clearly an alternative diagnosis while infectious mononucleosis and brucellosis are other causes of prolonged pyrexia. The possibility of a double infection—malaria and trypanosomiasis for example—has to be borne in mind.

The enlarged glands may be thought to be due to tuberculosis, Hodgkin's disease or the glandular form of mononucleosis but it has also to be remembered that, in the African patient particularly, the glands may be chronically enlarged from ever-present minor skin lesions, scabies, pediculosis and the like.

Later in the disease, nervous manifestations give rise to multiple possibilities but syphilis of the nervous system and tuberculous meningitis may cause real difficulty and there may be the usual problems in connection with the differential diagnosis of the causes of coma. A recent paper by Kagwa (1967) describes cases of 'viral encephalitis' in Uganda in which some of the signs and symptoms could well have been those of sleeping sickness including tremors and other involuntary movements, coma, Parkinsonism, mental clouding and lethargy. In Kagwa's cases the cerebrospinal fluid was normal, or showed only a slight lymphocytosis, and one of the three patients described recovered spontaneously within a month. No causative agent was isolated and no post-mortem studies were made on two patients who died but this report, incomplete though it is, illustrates the liability to encounter conditions other than sleeping sickness which give rise to a very similar syndrome. Sleeping sickness must also be remembered as a possible cause of mental illness.

Finally, there is the wasting which is so often associated with the later stages of the Gambian infection and with even the early stages of the Rhodesian disease. Tuberculosis may be thought of as a cause but does not usually present a diagnostic problem, especially in the African in whom this disease is so often acute. Hookworm infection—not necessarily hookworm disease—presents a more important problem. Assistants in rural dispensaries and outpatient clinics who have been taught to recognize the classical picture of hookworm disease, with its anaemia, wasting and peripheral oedema, tend to search first for hookworm ova in any patient with even a minor degree of this syndrome; naturally, the ova are often found and the patient is treated for hookworm and sent away. It is often not sufficiently well recognized that sleeping sickness may present just such a picture or that trypanosome and hookworm infections may coexist.

In Africa, especially in the sleeping sickness areas where blood slides or gland punctures are made as a routine and where lumbar puncture, although performed with caution, is not regarded as a major procedure, differential diagnosis is not usually a great problem. The constant suspicion that almost any condition may be due to or may be associated with a trypanosome infection leads almost automatically to the performance of additional tests where these seem desirable. In other countries, however, the diagnosis of sleeping sickness is often difficult and delayed, for it is natural to think first of the familiar conditions—tuberculous glands, Hodgkin's disease, infectious mononucleosis, brucellosis, typhoid and so forth. The insidious nature of the Gambian disease and the often long latent period of several years, during which reasonable health may be maintained and trypanosomes may be absent or difficult to find, make delay in diagnosis understandable. Collomb *et al.* (1956) studied twenty-seven Africans in France who had left endemic sleeping sickness areas some years previously. In fourteen of these patients three to four years had elapsed between their departure from Africa and the appearance of symptoms and signs which resulted in the diagnosis of sleeping sickness being made, and in only five was the interval one year or less. It must be noted that in all but four of these twenty-seven patients examination of the cerebrospinal fluid revealed the presence of trypanosomes or of changes which indicated the advanced stage which the disease had reached by the time it was diagnosed. There are many reports, some of them tragic, of patients in whom the diagnosis has been delayed or made only after death, and of others who have been subjected to extensive neurological investigations and even to operation for cerebral tumour. Very rarely the disease may remain completely silent until far advanced, but far more often there are signs and symptoms in the earlier stages which could lead to a diagnosis. Much time and some lives would be saved if only the words *Unde venis* (Maegraith, 1963) were kept in mind. If patients were always asked where they had come from, and if the answer were tropical Africa, then sleeping sickness should be among the first of the possible conditions to be considered. Once thought of, it is not usually a difficult diagnosis to confirm.

APPLICATION OF DIAGNOSTIC TECHNIQUES

In a Rhodesian sleeping sickness area the taking of a thick blood film is the first routine procedure in any person who complains of fever, headache or weakness, or whose history or appearance is suggestive of a trypanosome infection. Throughout West Africa and the Congo, the first procedure will be palpation of the neck and the examination of the fluid from an enlarged gland if such is found. In an individual patient a blood slide will probably be taken at the time the gland is punctured and this will be necessary also in any area where the two forms of sleeping sickness coexist, for example, in parts of Uganda. When large numbers of people are being examined in a mass survey the same procedures are followed in the respective areas but when the search is for the Gambian disease a blood slide is not usually taken from every person in whom a gland puncture is made; this will depend upon local experience or the result of a pilot survey in the area. The relative scarcity of trypanosomes in the blood in most Gambian infections has already been noted.

If the initial blood slide or gland puncture is negative, these examinations may be repeated on one or more occasions and, at the same time, further tests may be made the nature of which will depend on the degree of suspicion and on the facilities available. In nearly every hospital it will be possible to determine the erythrocyte sedimentation rate and to do the serum formalin test; these may give valuable help. A markedly raised sedimentation rate or a solid gel in the formalin test are sufficient indications of the need to proceed further if the results of repeated blood or gland examinations are still negative. Where suitable facilities exist determination of the immunoglobulin level in the serum may replace the sedimentation rate or the serum formalin test as part of the routine at the initial examination. Complement-fixation or fluorescent antibody tests may be applied at this stage at centres where these tests are practicable.

The further measures which will be necessary if positive results in any of these tests indicate the probability or even the possibility of a trypanosome infection, include lumbar puncture, inoculation of blood from the patient into a susceptible animal, or the taking of blood or cerebrospinal fluid for culture. It has already been suggested that animal inoculation should be performed on every occasion when attempts to demonstrate the presence of the trypanosome more directly have failed and when the patient has a suspicious history, a persistent headache or a puzzling 'pyrexia of unknown origin'. It may not be possible to follow this practice everywhere but often a patient can be referred to a laboratory centre where facilities for animal inoculation are available or animals can be sent from the centre to the patient. It is in fact not often that these facilities are called for, but it is useful to have such arrangements in readiness in case of need.

In Rhodesian sleeping sickness lumbar puncture is invariably performed at diagnosis or as soon as possible afterwards so that the stage which the disease has reached can be ascertained and the appropriate treatment given. Lumbar puncture is often part of the diagnostic procedure in hospitals and special sleeping sickness clinics. It has to be remembered that, in acute Rhodesian infection, evidence of nervous system involvement may be found in the cerebrospinal fluid within three to four weeks of the onset of illness. Also, treatment which is effective in the early stage of this infection is of no value once the nervous system is invaded and other drugs have to be used, hence the vital importance of examining the cerebrospinal fluid in the Rhodesian disease. In the Gambian infection, lumbar puncture is of little diagnostic value in the early weeks when the nervous system is unlikely to be affected but it may be of great help later. As the disease advances it often becomes difficult to demonstrate trypanosomes in the blood or glands and in such cases a rise in the cell count or protein level in the cerebrospinal fluid should be regarded as indicative of a trypanosome infection in any person who has been exposed to risk.

If all attempts to confirm a suspected diagnosis fail and if the grounds for suspicion remain strong it is justifiable to treat the patient for sleeping sickness and, where possible, to assess the effect of treatment on the immunoglobulin level, sedimentation rate and other values. A fall in the levels is a very strong indication that the original suspicion was correct.

Chapter 36

Treatment of Human Trypanosomiasis

F. I. C. APTED

INTRODUCTORY

A review of the drugs which have been used for the curative and prophylactic treatment of the African trypanosomiases has been given in Chapter 7. In this Chapter attention will be confined to those drugs which are currently in use, or are under investigation, for the treatment of Gambian and Rhodesian sleeping sickness and to the clinical aspects of their administration.

Many drugs, mainly arsenicals and antimonials, have been used in the treatment of sleeping sickness. Atoxyl, one of the first to show promise, was introduced in 1905, but unfortunately its use was sometimes followed by optic atrophy. Tartar emetic was tried a few years later and was effective, but relapses after its use were frequent. Tryparsamide became available in 1919, and suramin (Bayer 205), developed some years earlier, was first used in sleeping sickness in 1922. Other drugs in great variety have been tried, but of the early drugs only suramin and tryparsamide have survived in common use, although tartar emetic may occasionally still be of value in an emergency if other drugs are not available. The present tendency is for tryparsamide to be superseded by the newer melaminyl compounds, the first of which was introduced in 1939, but in certain areas with special problems tryparsamide still has its uses.

The drugs discussed here are divided into two groups: (1) those which are of value only in the early stages of the disease before the nervous system becomes involved, and (2) those which are effective in advanced infections.

DRUGS EFFECTIVE ONLY IN THE EARLY STAGES OF INFECTION

These are suramin, pentamidine, Berenil and tartar emetic, although the last named is no longer in general use.

Suramin (Sodium suramin, Antrypol, Bayer 205, Belganyl, Fourneau 309, Germanin, Moranyl, Naganin, Naganol, Naphuride).

Suramin is the symmetrical 3-urea of the sodium salt of 8-(3-benzamido-4-methylbenzamido) naphthalene -1,3,5,-trisulphonic acid. It is a white or faintly pink or cream-coloured odourless hygroscopic powder with a slightly bitter alkaline taste, easily soluble in water to form a solution which is given by intravenous injection. This solution deteriorates on keeping in contact with air and must be used immediately it is prepared. The drug is available either in powder form or as an aqueous solution in ampoules ready for injection.

Trypanosomes disappear from the blood and glands a few hours after the injection of suramin and the drug will cure nearly every patient in whom there is no involvement of the nervous system detectable by changes in the cerebrospinal fluid. It is equally effective in both Gambian and Rhodesian forms of the disease. In a very few persons, as was shown by Hawking (1940), suramin fails to accumulate in the blood to a curative level so that a relapse of the infection occurs even within a few days of the last of a course of injections. Hawking quotes a number of such instances, from his own experience and that of others; although in one early series the failure rate from this cause was about 10% it does not appear to be a serious problem nowadays, but the possibility must be kept in mind. For practical purposes the cure rate with suramin in the early stage of the disease may be regarded as nearly 100%.

Suramin will not pass from the blood into the cerebrospinal fluid and therefore will have no effect on the course of the infection once this has reached the nervous system, although it will still clear the blood of trypanosomes and so render the patient non-infective. There is some clinical evidence that in spite of the theoretical impossibility of suramin reaching the cerebrospinal fluid it does in fact have some effect on early nervous system infections. Keevill (1934), for example, showed that patients who had trypanosomes in their cerebrospinal fluid and a cell count which was raised in some instances to 80–90 cells per cmm., and who were treated only with suramin, were in good health with a normal cerebrospinal fluid several years afterwards. Later experience bears this out and certainly suramin appears to allow a certain degree of latitude such as is not the case with the other early-stage drugs, pentamidine and Berenil. This has its value, although once it has been ascertained that the nervous system is involved, treatment with a drug known to be effective in the late stage should be started immediately.

Dosage

The suramin powder is dissolved in sterile distilled water to give a 10% solution (1 g.–10 ml. water). The injection is given intravenously. Intramuscular injection is irritant and painful and is not advised, although the drug may be given by this route on the rare occasion when a vein is difficult to find.

The dose for a single injection is 20 mg./kg. of body weight, the usual, and maximum, adult dose being 1 g., but an initial test dose of 0·2 g. is often given before the start of the full course in case the patient is one of the very few who show an indiosyncrasy to the drug (*see* below). The injections are repeated, usually at intervals of five to seven days, the course ordinarily being completed in five injections, or when the total dose has reached 5 g. The exact interval between injections is not important, but it should not exceed seven days—local circumstances will often dictate the choice of a particular schedule. In Tanzania, a course which has proved satisfactory and effective for many years comprises five injections given on days 1, 3, 7, 14 and 21, so that the treatment is completed in three weeks. This course has the additional advantage that the first three injections are given within a week, which allows a high concentration to build up quickly in the blood.

When it is possible for the drug to be given on a body weight basis, and under experienced supervision, there should be few difficulties, but in rural dispensary practice it may be wise to rule that the full dose of 1 gm. should be given only to patients of good weight and in a reasonable state of health. Thin persons, and especially women, who are often small or underweight, and anyone who is markedly anaemic or acutely ill, should receive only 0·25 g. initially, followed by 0·5 g., perhaps on the 3rd day, and then, if all is well, by 1 g. on the 8th, 14th, 21st and 28th days. A dose rather higher than one calculated on the body weight will normally be well tolerated by children but, again, similar precautions should be taken in those whose general condition is poor.

Toxicity

Although not a true toxic reaction, a febrile response to the first one or two injections of suramin is almost invariable, and it may be quite severe. The reaction to the second injection is usually less than to the first, and subsequent injections are often without incident.

In a few persons who appear to have an idiosyncrasy to the drug the injection is followed immediately by vomiting, shock and collapse. This may be transient, but has proved fatal. The incidence of this untoward reaction has been estimated at between 1 in 2,000 and 1 in 4,500 treated cases but despite this low level the administration of a test dose of 0·2 g. is advised. After many years' experience in Tanganyika, Fairbairn considered these reactions to be of such extreme rarity in that territory that the administration of a test dose was omitted from the routine; this may well have been due to local variation. Unless reliable local experience indicates otherwise, it is advisable to give a test dose.

Other early toxic reactions include pruritus, urticaria, a papular eruption, conjunctivitis, photophobia, palpebral oedema and stomatitis. Cutaneous hyperaesthesia may be noted and particularly pain in the soles of the feet which may be so severe as to cause difficulty in walking. This pain in the feet is one of many features of sleeping sickness and its treatment which are seen in some areas and in some outbreaks and not in others. It was quite common among the Kissi people in Sierra Leone, but must be rare, if it occurs at all, in Tanzania. Whether this is due to some local racial variation or to diet or the nutritional state, or perhaps to variations between different batches of the drug, has not been explained. Desquamation of the skin may occur and may be extensive but it is liable to affect particularly the skin of the palms and the soles of the feet. It is not an immediate reaction but is seen occasionally about a week after a single injection, or later in the course.

Finally, the most common toxic effect of suramin is some degree of damage to the kidneys. Usually this causes no more than a mild albuminuria and is no indication for the suspension of treatment, but if there is much albumin or if casts or red cells are seen in the urinary deposit treatment should be continued, if necessary, with some other drug such as pentamidine. It follows that the urine should be tested before each injection and suramin should not be given to a patient who shows evidence of severe kidney damage.

It may appear, from this rather formidable list of possible reactions, that suramin is a dangerously toxic drug. It is in fact one of the most widely used and one of the safest. With the exception of kidney damage, usually mild, none of these reactions is common. The drug has remained in constant use for some forty-five years and it is still usually the choice in early infections in spite of the advent of newer drugs.

There is some evidence, mainly from workers who have used the drug in the treatment of onchocerciasis (Rodger, 1958; Nnochiri, 1964), that storage in the tropics may affect potency and that toxic reactions may be more frequent after one batch than after another.

Suramin may be given together with pentamidine and also together with and in various combinations in courses with tryparsamide. Its use in this way is discussed on pp. 705 and 706.

The prophylactic action of suramin

Suramin forms a combination with plasma protein and is excreted very slowly so that a single injection of 1 g. will maintain a concentration in the blood sufficient to prevent overt infection for some weeks, usually about three months. The use of suramin as a prophylactic is discussed elsewhere (*see* Chapter 37).

Pentamidine

Pentamidine is one of the aromatic diamidines (4:4′-diamidino-1,5-diphenoxypentane). It is an odourless, white, hygroscopic powder with a solubility in water of 1 in 10. The solution deteriorates in contact with air and it should be prepared immediately before use. The drug is available as the powder, in ampoules or bottles, or in solution in ampoules ready for injection. Formerly, it was given intravenously (as pentamidine hydrochloride) but severe hypotensive reactions and collapse were frequent; now the intramuscular route is used.

There are two forms of the drug in present use, pentamidine isethionate and the closely related methanesulphonate (Lomidine). The doses, actions and effects of these two compounds are so similar that they are considered together under the single name pentamidine.

Pentamidine is very effective in the treatment of Gambian sleeping sickness in the early stage, provided that there is no indication in the cerebrospinal fluid of even the slightest degree of nervous system involvement. As with suramin, it will clear trypanosomes from the blood and glands even in the later stages, but it will not influence the course of the disease if the nervous system is affected.

There is some suggestion that pentamidine is less certain in its effects in the Rhodesian disease, for occasionally some of these infections appear to be resistant. In spite of this, it is regularly used in some areas for the treatment of early Rhodesian sleeping sickness, and with success. The present writer prefers the use of suramin in these infections, with pentamidine as a valuable second drug for the treatment of patients in whom suramin is not appropriate, such as those with kidney damage or those who develop a severe albuminuria in the course of treatment with suramin. This preference is based on experience in Tanzania but what is judged to be the best procedure in one part of Africa is not necessarily the best elsewhere. In this connection, a point of some importance is that in patients in Tanzania who have relapsed after treatment with pentamidine the deterioration has been rapid and the illness has been far more severe than was usual in persons who had not received the drug. This has also been the experience in West Africa (Hutchinson & Watson, 1962).

Dosage

One of the main advantages of pentamidine over suramin is the shortness of the course, a mere seven to ten days instead of three to four weeks. The dose, for each injection, is 3–4 mg./kg. of body weight, calculated on the pentamidine *base*, the usual adult dose of the isethionate or of Lomidine being 300–400 mg. (dosage of pentamidine = 1·74 × dosage of pentamidine base; dosage of Lomidine = 1·5 × dosage of pentamidine base). The drug is made up to a 10% solution in sterile distilled water and given intramuscularly, one injection every day for seven to ten days, preferably for ten days, at least in Rhodesian infections, unless local experience dictates otherwise.

Toxicity

When pentamidine is given intramuscularly there are few ill effects. Histamine is liberated, with consequent hypotension, and sometimes a feeling of faintness, and occasionally collapse. These symptoms respond rapidly to adrenaline, which should always be available when pentamidine is used. Patients should lie down immediately after the injection has been given and should rest for a short time.

The drug also causes hypoglycaemia; Collomb *et al.* (1956) have reported the onset of diabetes in association with its use.

Pentamidine may be given together with suramin, with which it forms a complex, and in this way the side reactions of both drugs are reduced and the tolerated doses increased. Its use in this way is mentioned in the section on the choice of drugs (p. 705).

The prophylactic action of pentamidine

Pentamidine is a valuable prophylactic and a single injection will give protection against the Gambian infection for at least six months. Its prophylactic action against Rhodesian strains is less certain. This subject is discussed in detail in Chapter 37.

Berenil (diminazene aceturate)

Berenil, like pentamidine, is an aromatic diamidine (*pp'*-diamidinodiazoamino-benzene diaceturate tetrahydrate). It is a yellow powder soluble in water 1 in 14.

Berenil is a useful drug in veterinary trypanosomiasis, curing *Trypanosoma congolense* and *T. vivax* infections and it has been shown more recently to be effective in sleeping sickness both in the Gambian form (Hutchinson & Watson, 1962) and in the Rhodesian infection (Apted, unpublished). As with pentamidine, its use is limited to the treatment of the early infection, and it is essential that there should be no sign of involvement of the nervous system.

Dosage

The powder is dissolved in 5% glucose to give a 2% solution and is given by intramuscular injection. For each injection the dose is 2 mg./kg. of body weight, and injections are given every day for seven to ten days. Patients with the Gambian disease, and also those with the Rhodesian disease, have responded rapidly to such a course and the cure rate has been high; sixteen of seventeen patients in the series reported by Hutchinson and Watson (1962) were alive and well thirty-nine months after treatment. Experience has been limited, however, as the drug appears to offer no advantages over the well-tried pentamidine.

A recent development of interest has been the use of oral Berenil before the start of a course of melarsoprol for the same purpose as suramin is sometimes used to control fever and to prepare the patient for the action of the more toxic drug. Berenil may perhaps have some advantage over suramin in this respect owing to its more gradual action when given orally. These studies are still in their early stages and further comment must be deferred (Bailey, 1968).

Toxicity

From the very limited experience so far available toxic effects appear to be rare, apart from a tendency to cause a slight but persistent albuminuria.

Antimony Potassium Tartrate (Tartar emetic) and Antimony Sodium Tartrate

These are trivalent antimony compounds which are mentioned only because they may be used in the treatment of early infections if another more suitable drug such as suramin, pentamidine or Berenil is not immediately available. They will clear trypanosomes from the blood very rapidly, but relapses after their use are frequent. Even so, they may occasionally be of value, in association with other drugs, in the management of a patient whose infection persistently relapses; although they cannot cure such an infection they may help to prolong life.

Dosage

This is the same for both the sodium and potassium salt but the sodium salt is to be preferred as it is more easily soluble in water and the solution is less irritant and more suitable for injection. Both drugs have similar properties and effects.

The colourless crystals or the white powder are dissolved in water, normal saline or 5% glucose to make a 1% solution. This solution may be sterilized by boiling and is given by intravenous injection. The injection should be made slowly to lessen the risk of toxic effects.

The initial dose, for an adult, should not be more than 30 mg. A second injection is given after forty-eight hours, and subsequent injections usually on alternate days, but sometimes daily, the dose at each injection gradually being increased over a total of ten injections to a maximum single dose of 120 mg. For children the dosage should be based on body weight, with a similar gradual increase from an initial dose of 0·5 mg./kg.

Toxic reactions

These may be immediate and severe, and can be fatal—they include coughing, vomiting, colic and cardiovascular collapse which may be associated with a toxic myocarditis.

The decision whether to use such potentially toxic drugs in the treatment of an infection which is not usually rapidly fatal must obviously be based on circumstances.

DRUGS WHICH ARE EFFECTIVE IN THE LATER STAGES OF THE INFECTION, WHEN THE NERVOUS SYSTEM IS INVOLVED

These are tryparsamide, the melaminyl drugs (Melarsen, melarsoprol and melarsonyl potassium) and the nitrofurans (nitrofurazone and furaltadone).

Tryparsamide (Sodium hydrogen *p*-carbamoylmethylamino-phenylarsonate hemihydrate).

Orsanine (Fourneau 270) is a closely related compound with similar action and effects.

Tryparsamide is a white crystalline powder, easily soluble in water. Solutions deteriorate and must be freshly prepared. *Cold* water must be used and the solution must not be heated. The powder also deteriorates slowly on storage; any which has been in stock for three years should be discarded.

For very many years tryparsamide was the most useful drug available for the treatment of Gambian sleeping sickness. The increasing number of strains of trypanosome resistant to the drug, the long course of treatment required and its tendency to cause optic atrophy have led to tryparsamide being largely superseded by the newer melaminyl compounds, but it is still of value in certain circumstances. It is particularly useful in remote areas, such as parts of Nigeria where treatment has to be given without close medical supervision, but where there is a long tradition of such treatment and the rural staff is experienced in its use.

Tryparsamide will cure early Gambian infections but its action is slower than that of suramin, pentamidine or Berenil and it has no advantage over these drugs at this stage. The great virtue of tryparsamide lies in its ability, through its content of pentavalent arsenic, to penetrate into the cerebrospinal fluid and to cure the disease in its late stage.

Tryparsamide is of no value in the Rhodesian disease; indeed one of the characteristics of Rhodesian strains of trypanosome is that they are resistant to this drug. Before the advent of the melaminyl drugs, all patients with a Rhodesian infection in whom the disease had advanced to the stage where the protein level in the cerebrospinal fluid, as estimated by the Sicard-Cantaloube method, was 40 mg./100 ml. or more were regarded as incurable.

Dosage

(The powder is dissolved in sterile distilled water to give a 20% solution 2 g.–10 ml. water), which is given by intravenous injection. It may be given intramuscularly if it is impracticable to use the intravenous route.

The dosage is 30 mg./kg. of body weight, up to a maximum single dose of 2 g. This dose is given at intervals of five to seven days, usually for a total of ten to twelve injections, although up to fourteen injections may sometimes be advised. The course may be repeated but an interval of at least one month should elapse between one course and the next.

Tryparsamide may be given together with suramin, and in courses in which the tryparsamide is preceded by a series of suramin injections. Further mention of these combinations is made on p. 706.

Toxicity

Nausea, vomiting, diarrhoea and cramps may occur, sometimes immediately after the injection, but more usually one to four hours later. There may be sweating, pallor, tingling and flushing of the skin, accompanied by a fall in blood pressure leading to the shock syndrome—the nitritoid crisis. Occasionally a Jarisch-Herxheimer reaction is seen, with hyperpyrexia, convulsions and coma, and this is invariably fatal, confluent punctate haemorrhages being found throughout the brain. Both the nitritoid crisis and the Herxheimer reaction appear to have been more common in the early days when a course of a trivalent arsenical such as arsphenamine had often preceded the tryparsamide, and both reactions were seen more often in patients who had received a large amount of tryparsamide over a long period.

Status epilepticus has been described in a patient after a single injection of 2 g. tryparsamide.

As with other arsenical drugs there may be skin reactions, including severe exfoliative dermatitis. Urticaria may involve particularly the face and the lips, or there may be acute oedema of the tongue and larynx, with respiratory obstruction.

Jaundice has been noted, but is not common and usually is not severe.

The greatest risk associated with the use of tryparsamide is that of damage to the optic nerve. Rarely, this may occur suddenly, and even after the first injection, but there is usually some warning so that treatment can be stopped and the risk of permanent and total optic atrophy lessened. The first sensation noticed by the patient may be one of shimmering vision—'like looking through waving smoke' as Ridley (1945) has described it. Within a few days this may be followed by a general depression of vision with loss of the peripheral fields and then by a decrease in central acuity. After the drug has been stopped the vision will usually recover slowly, over a period of three to six months, but occasionally permanent blindness will result. There seems to be a special risk of damage to the optic nerve in patients in whom the nervous system is seriously affected, with marked changes in the cerebrospinal fluid.

It is essential that note be taken before each injection of any subjective sensation experienced by the patient and that a test be made for decrease in peripheral and central vision. A simple but practical test is to ask the patient to pick up a pin. Should there be any hint of visual damage, or should any other toxic manifestation develop, the drug must be stopped immediately and completely, and dimercaprol (BAL) should be given in maximum dosage (3 mg./kg. body weight intramuscularly at intervals of four hours throughout the first forty-eight hours, followed by four similar doses on the third day and two doses on each of the next ten days).

Tryparsamide has been in use for so long that accounts of its use and toxic effects are too numerous to mention individually. The description by Ridley of ocular damage has already been noted and another good account of the more general untoward reactions has been given by Kopp and Solomon (1940), based on their experience of over 40,000 injections.

The Melaminyl Drugs

The development of this group of drugs was the greatest advance in the treatment of sleeping sickness since the introduction of suramin and tryparsamide in the early 1920s. Friedheim, to whom all credit for this is due, made a field trial with the first of these drugs, Melarsen, in French West Africa in 1939 (Friedheim, 1941) with results which were so promising that he continued his investigations in spite of conflicting reports on the toxicity of these compounds. Melarsen was followed by Melarsen oxide, melarsoprol (Mel B), melarsonyl potassium (Mel W) and by the antimony derivatives MSb and MSbB. Of these, melarsoprol has become firmly and widely established among the drugs of real value in the treatment of sleeping sickness and Melarsen and melarsonyl potassium have proved themselves of benefit in some areas in West Africa.

By 1947 it had been shown both in the field and experimentally that Melarsen oxide was active against tryparsamide-resistant strains of *T. gambiense* (Van Hoof, 1947; Williamson & Lourie, 1948), a discovery which came at the right time, for resistance to tryparsamide was becoming a serious problem in West Africa. Friedheim (1949) quotes an estimate that in the Congo at that time 80% of all second-stage infections were resistant to tryparsamide. This discovery was followed by a trial of melarsoprol in Tanganyika (Apted, 1953) where the tryparsamide-resistant Rhodesian disease was incurable in the late stage. Almost miraculously, it seemed, melarsoprol proved to be effective in these hitherto fatal infections and the whole picture was changed. Before its introduction, over a third of all persons who contracted sleeping sickness in Tanganyika had died but within a few years melarsoprol had reduced the death rate to about 10% (Apted, 1957).

As will be seen from the description of the drugs in this group, they are not without their dangers but when they are used with care the risks are low. A certain risk is justified if otherwise a cure is impossible—and this was the situation with all late-stage tryparsamide-resistant infections before the advent of Friedheim's melaminyl drugs.

Melarsoprol (Mel B, Melarsen oxide-BAL, Arsobal, 2-[*p*-(4,6-diamino-1,3,5-triazin-2-ylamino phenyl]-4-hydroxymethyl-1,3,2-dithiarsolan).

Although not the first of the melaminyl drugs to be developed, melarsoprol has been by far the most widely used, both in West and in East Africa, and a description of its properties and effects, based on this extensive experience, forms a useful introduction to a consideration of the other members of the group.

Melarsoprol was formed from Melarsen oxide, the trivalent equivalent of Melarsen, by the incorporation of dimercaprol (BAL), after Melarsen oxide itself had proved to be too toxic. Melarsoprol, which contains 18·8% arsenic, will cure both the Rhodesian and the Gambian disease at all stages, even the very advanced. Early infections, before the nervous system is affected, may be cured by a single injection but its use for this purpose is not generally advised because for this stage other less toxic drugs such as suramin and pentamidine are effective. Once the nervous system is demonstrably involved a course of injections over a period of two to four weeks is necessary and such a course will cure all but the few infections resistant to the drug. Even in areas where it is still possible to use tryparsamide, the much shorter course of treatment gives melarsoprol a great advantage, provided that adequate supervision is possible. In areas where tryparsamide resistance is a problem the use of melarsoprol, or of one of the other melaminyl drugs is essential and in the Rhodesian disease it is the only drug in regular use, with the exception of nitrofurazone, which will give a cure in the late stage; melarsonyl potassium has proved unreliable in Rhodesian infections and there is only very limited experience of Melarsen itself in this form of the disease.

Dosage

Monnet and Baylet (1951, 1951a) and Hawking (1962a) have shown that melarsoprol is rapidly excreted in the urine, but that if it is given on three successive days a certain concentration in the plasma is achieved. The drug cannot be detected in the cerebrospinal fluid until after the third or fourth injection and even then in only very small amounts, but further injections do not increase the chance of penetration into the nervous system and lead to the risk of a dangerous degree of arsenic retention. The dosage schemes outlined below are based on these findings. It is usually advised that the drug should be given only to patients who are in hospital and under experienced supervision, although in French-speaking West Africa where Arsobal is widely given, its use is no longer confined to hospitals. In Tanzania it is used in selected rural dispensaries where the staff has been specially trained and where there are hostel facilities.

Melarsoprol is presented ready for use in ampoules as a 3·6% solution in propylene glycol, for which a dry syringe and needle are essential. This solution is intensely irritant and care has to be taken to see that the injections are given strictly intravenously. The solution is somewhat viscous, but if a large-bore needle is used to withdraw it from the ampoule, a change to a small needle may be made for the injection, thus ensuring a slow delivery and lessening the chance of perivenous leakage.

Most authorities give the dose for each injection as 3·6 mg. per kg. body weight, with a maximum single dose of 5 ml. (180 mg.); a course often recommended is one of four such injections on consecutive days, repeated after an interval of a week. In some circumstances such a dosage *may well be far too high*—it is certainly too high for general use in East Africa, and although experience in West Africa indicates that such a course is well tolerated in some areas, it has been found too dangerous in others (Ceccaldi *et al.*, 1950). It is best to adopt a much more cautious approach in any area in which experience has not already shown such an intensive course at maximum dosage to be safe. This approach might follow the lines suggested below and evolved as the result of some years' experience in East Africa. For nearly all patients the following course is suitable:

On the 1st, 3rd and 5th days (or the 1st, 2nd and 3rd days), 0·5, 1·0 and 1·5 ml. respectively. This is followed by a rest period without treatment of five to seven days, and then by injections of 2·5 ml. on each of the next three consecutive days. After a further rest period of seven days, injections of 3·0, 3·5–4·0 or 5·0 ml. are given on each of the next three days, and finally, after another week's rest, three injections each of 5 ml. on consecutive days. In this course a total of 36·0–37·5 ml. is given over a period of about one month.

This course is suggested as a guide only—the exact dose, whether it be 2·5 or 3·0 ml., or 4·0 or 5·0 ml. on a particular day is of no great significance. What is important is the low initial dosage which is gradually increased according to the patient's response. It is the patient's condition which must be studied rather than strict adherence to a schedule. If it is thought wise to withhold an injection for two or three days, then this should be done; on the other hand, it may be considered safe to increase the dosage rather more rapidly.

A course which was in regular use for a long time and which gave very satisfactory results was as follows: injections of 2·0, 2·5, 3·0 ml. on the first three days, respectively, followed by a rest period of one week. Injections of 3·5, 4·0, 5·0 ml. on the next three days, and a further rest period of one week, after which the final three injections, each of 5·0 ml. were given on the next three days. In this course a total of 35·0 ml. was given in just over three weeks.

As experience was gained there was a tendency to adopt the more gradual dosage first outlined and to reserve the second or similar dosage schemes for patients who appeared to be in good condition and in whom the spinal fluid was not grossly abnormal.

For children, and for patients who are underweight, the dosage is calculated on the basis of the body weight, with a similar low initial dose and a gradual increase, i.e. from one tenth of the calculated maximum dose for the body weight (at 3·6 mg./kg.) up to the full calculated maximum dose in the third week of treatment.

It is not intended that these dosage schedules should be rigidly followed; they are given merely to illustrate the type of scheme which has proved successful in areas where tolerance to melarsoprol is not as good as it may be elsewhere. There is no reason why shorter and more intensive courses should not be used where it is known that they are safe.

The response to treatment with melarsoprol

The improvement is usually rapid, even dramatic, and is often marked by a sense of well-being noticeable within the first few days. In particular, patients who are dull or mentally confused, as they often are in the advanced stage of the Rhodesian disease, lose this dullness and become alert and cheerful soon after the start of treatment. Occasionally a patient, particularly one who is in an advanced stage of the disease, may fail to respond to melarsoprol.

Cure, relapse and death rates

Comparison between the results reported by different authors is difficult because of variations in dosage and in the selection of cases. In the Rhodesian infection, Robertson (1963a) obtained a cure rate of 90% in 52 patients, 31 of whom were in the 'late' stage of the disease. In an earlier series reported by Apted (1957) the cure rate was up to 73% in patients all of whom were in the 'late' stage, and the relapse rate was 10%. It was shown that some of the patients who relapsed could be cured by a second course of melarsoprol but in persistent relapses further courses were largely ineffective. Relapses occurred usually within a year, and often between four and seven months after treatment, but occasionally the interval between treatment and relapse has been as long as two years.

In the Gambian disease, rates of cure have varied from between 50 and 60% in patients in the advanced stage (Ceccaldi, 1952; Richet *et al.*, 1959), to 88% (Richet, *et al., loc. cit.*) and 97% (Friedheim, 1951) in early infections.

Death rates are equally difficult to assess and compare. In Rhodesian infections they have ranged between 4·5% (Robertson, 1963a), 8% (De Andrade Silva, 1957), 10% (Apted, 1957) and 17–18% (Marneffe, 1955; Adriaenssens, 1961).

These differences are accounted for in part by the selection of cases, and also by the dosage, with a notable improvement (e.g. Robertson, 1963a) as experience was gained. In the Gambian disease, death rates have on the whole been lower; for example, Richet *et al.* (1959) reported only nineteen deaths in 795 patients treated over a period of ten years (2·4%), and with rigorous case selection the death rate was reduced to nil. It is, of course, often possible in Gambian infections to use an alternative treatment such as tryparsamide, or a combination of suramin and tryparsamide, for patients for whom melarsoprol is not thought suitable, but in the Rhodesian disease there is no alternative other than nitrofurazone which has its own serious disadvantages.

The value of a preliminary course of suramin

Suramin, in addition to its ability to clear trypanosomes from the blood and to control the fever, has a marked tonic effect and this property has been used to improve the condition of the patient so that he may be the better able to stand a course of the more toxic melarsoprol (Apted, 1957). Suramin is not given as a routine before every course of melarsoprol, but it is of value if the patient is acutely ill, febrile, or has a high parasitaemia. In such a patient two to four injections of suramin, 0·25–0·5 g. on alternate days, before the start of the melarsoprol course, are usually of benefit, but should there not be an immediate improvement treatment with melarsoprol should be started without further delay.

Recent work indicates that Berenil, given by mouth, may be of similar value and may even have some advantage over suramin, but this is still in the investigational stage (Bailey, 1968).

Toxicity

Reactions which may occur immediately or very soon after an injection of melarsoprol include fever, pains in the chest, griping abdominal pains and subjective sensations of heat and disturbances of smell. With the exception of the febrile response, which frequently follows the first injection, especially if there is parasitaemia, none of these reactions is common. Local thrombophlebitis of the vein used for the injection may occur and a tender induration of the arm is a sign of a leak of the solution into the tissues.

The most important and serious of the toxic effects of melarsoprol, or of any of the other melaminyl drugs, are those which involve the nervous system. Robertson (1963) has given an excellent account of these reactions which he divides into two main groups—*reactive encephalopathy*, relatively common (about 13% in his own series of cases), but from which the patients often recover, and *haemorrhagic encephalopathy*, rare but almost invariably fatal. These untoward reactions usually occur during treatment, often after the completion of the first course of injections, but death has followed a single injection. There appears to be no way of predicting which patients are likely to suffer, although they are usually in the later stages of nervous system involvement; however, most late-stage patients are treated and recover without incident. The general condition of the patient is no guide, for an encephalopathy may develop in a patient who seems to be in reasonable health and yet those in a very advanced stage of the disease—emaciated or semi-comatose—may escape. For this reason, a cautious approach to dosage is advisable whatever the apparent condition of the patient.

Reactive encephalopathy shows itself in a variety of ways and often, fortunately, with warning signs. Increased mental excitement, twitching, choreic movements, or picking at the bedclothes are early signs of nervous damage, or there may be a deepening instead of the looked-for lessening of an initial somnolence. Sometimes the reaction may be extremely violent; Robertson has described one such patient who recovered but who was difficult to control even with full doses of chlorpromazine and paraldehyde.

This reactive encephalopathy appears to result from the effect of the drug on the diseased brain. It is not strictly a toxic drug reaction, for if the patient recovers, as he usually does, he is able to tolerate further melarsoprol in increased dosage, and the course may be completed without further trouble. After a few days have been allowed for the patient to recover from his reaction, during which time sedation or other appropriate treatment is given, the melarsoprol course is cautiously started again, the dosage being increased very gradually. Robertson advises that large doses of ascorbic acid should be given to patients before and during treatment with melarsoprol, a recommendation which is based on experimental work by Hurst (1959) in monkeys. It is of interest to note that Hurst also showed that small initial doses of melarsoprol were of benefit, for monkeys which had received a series of small doses were later able to tolerate doses which would have been fatal initially. Although this work was in monkeys, it does perhaps tend to confirm an early conviction (Apted, 1957) that an initial low dosage is the key to successful treatment with melarsoprol in man. Robertson (1963) also discusses the use of corticosteroids in the management of these toxic hypersensitivity reactions, but experience is limited.

Haemorrhagic encephalopathy, in which the signs in the brain are typical of those found in fatal reactions to other arsenical drugs, is a direct toxic reaction, probably due to overdosage; this may be only relative as a fatal reaction may follow a very small dose. Typically, there is sudden loss of consciousness with the stertorous breathing and hyperpyrexia which accompany acute cerebral accidents. Fortunately this reaction, which by its nature is almost always, if not invariably, fatal, is uncommon. In Robertson's series of 110 patients it occurred once, and in another series (Apted, 1957) it was diagnosed with certainty only once in 176 cases.

Dimercaprol

The use of dimercaprol (BAL) in melarsoprol encephalopathy is debatable. Patients have recovered without it, and it is difficult to be sure in any patient to whom it is given that it is of any real benefit. Some workers believe that it is of no value, but even so it is not easy to withhold a drug which may contribute to recovery. Neujean and Evens (1958) considered it was beneficial. On theoretical grounds it is unlikely that dimercaprol will help in reactive encephalopathy, for it is probably not a true drug toxicity which is responsible, but if there is any possibility of a relative overdosage of melarsoprol it would seem desirable to use dimercaprol. (For the dosage of dimercaprol see under tryparsamide).

Virus infections in relation to sleeping sickness and melarsoprol

Richet *et al.* (1958) reported that during an influenza epidemic, influenzal encephalitis was particularly severe in patients suffering from sleeping sickness who had been treated with melarsoprol—in fact, out of eighteen patients involved, all the ten who had received melarsoprol died. In the same epidemic, encephalitis ran a benign course in patients who were not suffering from sleeping sickness. It also appears, from observations by Bezon and Ducasse (1958), that influenza has the effect of activating trypanosomiasis, whether the patient is under treatment for sleeping sickness or not. Janssens *et al.* (1960) have reported the case of a patient who developed severe headache, convulsions and coma during a course of melarsoprol. He improved, but his condition later worsened and he was shown to be infected with Coxsackie B virus.

It is clear from these reports that as far as is practicable it would be wise to suspend the use of melaminyl drugs during an outbreak of influenza or other virus infection.

Other toxic and side effects of melarsoprol

These include pains in the muscles and limbs, albuminuria (sometimes with casts in the urine), erythematous or papular rashes, angioneurotic and hypersensitivity reactions, desquamation of the skin of the legs and hyperkeratosis of the feet. Robertson (1963), who has given a full description of these effects and discusses their causation, has also observed an instance of agranulocytosis and the occurrence of erythema nodosum leprosum in a patient who was suffering from both leprosy and sleeping sickness. Robertson notes the desirability of investigating the possible use of corticosteroids in the prevention or management of some of these reactions.

Resistance to melarsoprol

There is remarkably little evidence on drug resistance when it is considered that melarsoprol has been in use for some twenty years. Rollo and Williamson (1951) have shown experimentally that trypanosomes which have been maintained in contact with Melarsen develop resistance not only to Melarsen but also to tryparsamide and to pentamidine. In early trials in Tanganyika it was noticed that an occasional patient was resistant to treatment with melarsoprol, but this was before the drug came into general use and it seems unlikely that the resistance was drug-induced. At the same time there was also a suggestion that under-dosage might produce drug resistance (Apted, 1953). Because of this, and also of the fact that relapses are more frequent after a low total dosage, it is recommended that this dosage should not be less than 30–35 ml. even though individual patients may be cured by doses considerably less than this. Robertson (1963b) has described the case of a man who proved to be resistant to both melarsoprol and melarsonyl potassium. Strains of the infecting trypanosome isolated at different periods showed an increasing resistance to melarsoprol when tested in mice and in the thirty-second month of the illness the highly resistant strain isolated was shown to be transmissible by *Glossina morsitans*. Fortunately, in practice, resistance to the melaminyl drugs has not yet become a serious problem.

Melarsonyl Potassium (Mel W, Trimelarsan, melarsenoxide potassium dimercaptosuccinate, pentylthiarsphenylmelamine).

This is a water-soluble analogue of melarsoprol over which it has an advantage in that it is given by intramuscular or subcutaneous injection. In other respects, and particularly with regard to its toxicity, it is similar to melarsoprol and can be used only under supervision and with strict precautions. Some workers have found it to be effective in Gambian infections (*see* below) but the results in the treatment of the Rhodesian disease have been disappointing.

Melarsonyl potassium is a white powder presented in ampoules of 200 mg. which is prepared for use by dissolving it in distilled water, normal saline or 5% glucose to give a 5% solution (50 mg. per ml.).

Dosage

The dosage usually employed has been 3–4 mg./kg. with a maximum single dose of 200 mg., given on three or four consecutive days, this course being repeated after an interval of two weeks. Some authors, e.g. Schneider *et al.* (1961) have preferred to use a graduated dosage for patients in the later stages of the disease, for example, 1, 2, 3 and 4 mg./kg. respectively in the first four days of the course.

Response to treatment

Reports, even in West Africa, have been somewhat conflicting. De Jongh and Friedheim (1959) obtained excellent results in a small series of eleven patients, with no toxic effects apart from a morbilliform eruption in a young child. Nodenot *et al.* (1960) considered Mel W to be much less toxic than melarsoprol. Schneider *et al.* (*loc. cit.*) thought it suitable for the ambulant treatment of patients with early-stage infections, in view of its lack of toxicity, but experienced a relapse rate of 13–20% in the late stage. They noted that the rapid restoration of the cerebrospinal fluid to normal did not preclude a subsequent relapse. Collomb *et al.* (1963, 1964a, 1964b), in a series of patients carefully observed over a period of years, reported that of 78 patients treated, 14 had died and 10 of the remaining 31 who had continued under supervision had relapsed. The toxic effects included hemiplegia, cardiovascular collapse, hyperpyrexia, and meningo-encephalitic involvement. They remarked that in a course which consisted of a single series of four or five injections each of 5 mg./kg. the mortality rate was lower than it was in a double-series course with an interval of two weeks, although the incidence of toxic effects was similar. Watson (1962, 1965) found the drug to be well tolerated and considered the toxicity to be less than would be expected from melarsoprol. Excellent results were obtained with a single-series course in patients in the early and intermediate stages of the disease, but in late-stage infections there was persistence of an abnormal cerebrospinal fluid in some patients, and in others there was a rise in the cerebrospinal fluid protein content two years after treatment.

In the treatment of the Rhodesian disease, Robertson (1963b) used a course of three series, each of four injections separated by intervals of seven days, but this was unsuccessful in at least nine of the sixteen patients treated. In three of these patients parasites were isolated from the cerebrospinal fluid immediately after treatment, by inoculation into rats. Initially there was a marked clinical improvement but the incidence of serious toxic effects was high and included psychomotor disturbances, hallucinations, manic excitement, epileptiform convulsions and stupor. Subsequent treatment with melarsoprol in those in whom Mel W had failed was disturbingly unsatisfactory, for four of the nine patients died although the remaining five were well a year later. Apted (unpublished) also tried melarsonyl potassium in a few patients with Rhodesian infections but the initial results were so poor that the trial was abandoned.

It seems clear that melarsonyl potassium has no place in the treatment of Rhodesian sleeping sickness. In the Gambian disease the drug, with its ease of administration, may be of value in certain circumstances where it can be given under supervision and where a short course of treatment is of advantage, but in view of the tendency towards late relapses it should be used only when a periodical follow-up for at least two years, and preferably for three years or more, can be guaranteed.

Melarsen (Melarsen sodium. Disodium-*p*-melaminyl phenylarsonate).

This pentavalent compound, containing 20·2% arsenic, was the first of the melaminyl drugs to be introduced (Friedheim, 1941). The long course of treatment of up to twelve injections at intervals of a week, and also its greater cost, caused it to be overshadowed by melarsoprol in spite of its early promise. Later studies have confirmed its value in certain areas in West Africa for, as with tryparsamide, it may be given by trained staff in the field without direct medical supervision. Its toxicity is little greater than that of tryparsamide and there is not the same risk of ocular complications.

Dosage

The white powder, in ampoules of 1 g. is dissolved in sterile distilled water to make a 10% solution which is given by intravenous injection. In different trials the dosage for each single injection has ranged from 15–40 mg./kg. and courses of eight to twelve injections have been given at intervals of five to seven days. Butler *et al.* (1957) obtained a cure rate of 56% in patients in the advanced stage who were given 25 mg./kg. and of 71% with 30 mg./kg. The incidence of toxic reactions is greater at the higher dosage and it is recommended that for use in the field the dose should not exceed 20 mg./kg. At this level the incidence of significant toxic effects is only about 1% and the cure rate is considerably better than would be expected from tryparsamide in similar circumstances. In Nigeria it is used widely, some 600–700 patients being treated with this drug each year.

Melarsen has been found to be of particular value in patients who have relapsed after treatment with tryparsamide.

There is little experience of the use of Melarsen in the treatment of Rhodesian infections. A few patients were treated with results which were regarded as comparable with those obtained with melarsoprol (Apted, unpublished) but at the time melarsoprol was proving so successful that trials with Melarsen were discontinued so that no true comparison is possible. On theoretical grounds it seems that the pentavalent Melarsen, with its ability to penetrate the blood-brain barrier more easily than melarsoprol, may prove to be a better, and possibly a less toxic drug than melarsoprol (Hawking, 1962a).

MSb and MSb B

These antimony analogues of Melarsen and melarsoprol are of great interest, expecially as MSb showed promise as a prophylactic (Le Rouzic, 1949), but there appears to have been no recorded development or further study of their potentialities since the report of a trial by Friedheim (1953). Briefly, both drugs were shown to be effective in the treatment of Gambian sleeping sickness and they combined the advantages of a short course of treatment and of freedom from the risks of arsenical encephalopathy, but there was tendency towards later relapse. In preliminary trials which started shortly before the writer left Tanzania both MSb and MSb B showed evidence of having some effect in late-stage Rhodesian sleeping sickness, although, as with the Gambian infection, there was a tendency towards relapse after initial improvement. Only a few patients were treated as it was not considered justifiable to continue the trials. In one patient who had relapsed repeatedly after all other forms of treatment, MSb B also failed. MSb given prophylactically to rats protected them against heavy (syringe) challenge with *Trypanosoma rhodesiense* for at least three months.

The Nitrofuran Drugs

Two of these drugs, nitrofurazone and Furaltadone, have been used in the treatment of sleeping sickness.

Nitrofurazone Furacin, 5-nitrofurfuraldehydesemicarbazone).

After experimental work had demonstrated that nitrofurazone possessed curative properties against *T. gambiense* infections in mice, the compound was subjected to trial in patients suffering from the Gambian disease (Evens *et al.*, 1957) and favourable results were reported. Even better results were obtained after a 'cocktail' course in which nitrofurazone was given together with suramin, pentamidine and melarsoprol. Although nitrofurazone was found to be less effective against *T. rhodesiense* infections in mice, it was nevertheless thought to be worthy of trial in patients with the Rhodesian disease since no alternative drug was available for the treatment of the few patients whose infections had proved resistant to melarsoprol. Apted (1960) treated nine patients with various dosages of nitrofurazone and cured four who would otherwise certainly have died, and Robertson (1960) cured four out of eight patients. Here, therefore, in spite of the high failure rate, was a drug of great promise, although further experience was to show that it had severe limitations, in particular a tendency to cause polyneuropathy and acute haemolytic anaemia.

Dosage

Nitrofurazone, a stable yellow powder, is given orally in tablet form, usually 0·5 g. three or four times a day for five to seven days. The course may be repeated after a rest period of one week and in some patients has been repeated on two further occasions, again after similar rest periods. It is advisable to use small initial doses, e.g. 0·5 g. daily, to test the patient's sensitivity and response to the drug. It should not be given to patients who are febrile.

Toxicity

The most prominent of the toxic effects of nitrofurazone is a polyneuropathy, which is associated with a disturbance of pyruvate metabolism in which the biochemical and neurological changes are similar to those which occur in beriberi. This neuropathy takes a variety of forms which have been fully investigated and described by Robertson (1960) and Robertson and Knight (1964). There may be paraesthesia, hyperaesthesia, loss of sensation, disorders of sweating, disordered reflexes, ataxia, and motor nerve involvement with muscular wasting and paralysis. Pain in the limbs, especially in the balls of the feet, is often a marked feature, and Robertson distinguishes this pain, which is relieved temporarily by amyl nitrite and more permanently by calcium pantothenate, from a more persistent chronic ache which is not relieved by these drugs. These untoward effects may persist for many weeks or months even though the trypanosome infection may have responded favourably, and sometimes they may develop later, after the patient has been discharged from hospital. Polyneuropathy is unfortunately a common complication; in Robertson's (1960) series of eight patients, six developed it in a severe form, as did four out of the nine patients in the series reported by Apted (1960).

The heart is also involved, as in beriberi, and an increase in the pulse rate is one of the first signs of toxicity. There is often a fall in blood pressure, but this may be succeeded by hypertension.

The second serious toxic effect of nitrofurazone is the haemolysis which it causes in persons with the haemolytic trait, such as those who are sensitive to primaquine. Again, this has been fully investigated by Robertson (1961, 1961a). In Africa this problem may be serious, for it has been shown that 15–28% of people in different tribes in East Africa carry this trait and in Nigeria the figure is 10%. It is recommended that, if possible, Beutler's Heinz-body formation test, or preferably Motulsky's test for glucose-6-phosphate dehydrogenase deficiency, should be performed to detect persons who are drug-sensitive before treatment is commenced. If the trait is present and if there is no alternative to the use of nitrofurazone, haemoglobin estimations should be done daily and the level should not be allowed to fall below 8 g./100 ml. Haematocrit readings should be taken likewise and should not fall below 25%. In all patients, treatment should not be continued for more than seven days on any one occasion, and there should be an interval of at least seven days between each course. All these points are discussed by Robertson in the papers mentioned and anyone who contemplates the use of a nitrofuran drug in the treatment of sleeping sickness should read them in the original.

Other toxic effects of nitrofurazone are headache, gastrointestinal upset with vomiting, which may be severe, urticarial skin reactions, desquamation, hyperpigmentation, mental excitement and loss of weight. The drug also causes a degeneration of the seminiferous tubules of the testis and although this is likely to be of secondary consideration if it is a matter of attempting to cure an otherwise fatal infection, it is yet another reason for the restriction of this drug to the treatment of patients for whom there is no other hope; it should be given only to persons whose infections have proved resistant to melarsoprol. If a patient has relapsed after a first course of melarsoprol a second course should be tried, for this may well succeed. Only if there is a further relapse should nitrofurazone be used.

Another point of importance, already mentioned, is that nitrofurazone should not be given to patients who are febrile for it is known that such patients may already have a high concentration of pyruvate in the blood. The fever should be controlled with suramin before the start of the nitrofurazone course.

Patients should be at rest in bed during treatment and should receive a high protein diet. Thiamine should be given together with the nitrofurazone in the hope that polyneuropathy may be prevented or its severity lessened, but such prophylactic thiamine is by no means always successful.

It is important that the drug be withdrawn immediately should there be any sign of toxicity such as a steady increase in the pulse rate.

Furaltadone (Altafur. N-(5, nitro-2-furfurylidene)-3-amino-5-(N′-morpholinyl-methyl)-2-oxazolidone).

This drug, and a laevo form of the hydrochloride, have been used by Adriaenssens (1960, 1962) in the treatment of Rhodesian sleeping sickness. It was at first thought that the incidence of polyneuropathy was likely to be lower than it was with nitrofurazone, but the later study showed that it had few, if any, advantages. In 34 patients treated, toxic effects included diplopia in 15, amblyopia in 4, and severe neurotoxic reactions in 6, with 3 deaths. Several different dosage schemes were tested and the drug was given both orally and intravenously. Adriaenssens concluded that a dose of 60 mg./kg. daily for twenty days was curative in moderately severe Rhodesian sleeping sickness, but that the drug was not suitable for the treatment of patients in an advanced stage of the disease. Apted tried the drug in a few patients but the results (unpublished) were so disappointing that it was soon discontinued. It is nevertheless mentioned because this, or similar drugs, may be worthy of further investigation by those who are concerned with the treatment of patients resistant to the melaminyl drugs.

CASE MANAGEMENT: THE CHOICE OF TREATMENT

If there were drugs of low toxicity which would cure sleeping sickness in both its forms and in all stages, treatment would be simple. Unfortunately, although the drugs which are effective in the later stages will also cure early infections, all are toxic and it is unjustifiable to use them in the treatment of early-stage infections which can be cured with other drugs at much less risk to the patient. These other drugs, however, will not affect the course of the disease once the nervous system has been demonstrably involved and it is necessary, therefore, first to determine by examination of the cerebrospinal fluid whether there is any evidence of infection of the nervous system.

Different authorities vary in slight detail in the criteria they adopt for 'early', 'late', and in some instances 'intermediate' infections, but for the present purpose an 'early' infection is regarded as one in which the protein content of the cerebrospinal fluid as measured by the Sicard-Cantaloube method is 25 mg./100 ml. or less and the cell count is 5 cell/cmm. or less.

In the examination of the cerebrospinal fluid it is preferable to estimate both the protein content and the cell count, although often only the former is used. The cell count is a sensitive indicator of nervous system infection and may give valuable information—for example, there may be two patients with CSF protein values of 25 mg./100 ml., one with a cell count of 3/cmm. and the other with a count of 15/cmm.; the first may be said to have a normal fluid, with no evidence of nervous system infection but in the second the raised cell count is suspicious and a cure with, say, pentamidine or Berenil would be proportionately less likely.

Only by examination of the spinal fluid can a proper assessment of the situation be made, but under rural conditions it will often be impossible to arrange for a lumbar puncture to be performed before the start of treatment. In these circumstances treatment may be begun—with suramin in the Rhodesian disease, and with suramin, tryparsamide or Melarsen (*see* below) in Gambian infections—before a proper assessment of the patient's needs can be made. In Rhodesian infections this must not be delayed for more than three or four weeks at the most, and it should be made much earlier if possible, for once the nervous system becomes involved the prognosis worsens with every week that passes. In Gambian infections more latitude is allowable. In some remote areas in West Africa it may be necessary to dispense with lumbar puncture and to adopt a scheme of treatment with suramin plus tryparsamide, tryparsamide, or Melarsen which will cure most of the patients irrespective of the stage of their disease. This is not ideal as it will mean that some patients in the early stage will receive more treatment than is necessary, but it may be unavoidable.

Although there is much that is similar in the treatment of Gambian and Rhodesian sleeping sickness there are also important differences and it is best to consider the two forms separately:

Rhodesian infections, early stage

Suramin is the drug of choice. Over much of East Africa pentamidine is less certainly effective, although where experience has proved its value it may of course be used in routine treatment and elsewhere it is useful for the occasional patient in whom suramin is contraindicated. These remarks in respect of pentamidine probably apply also to Berenil of which there is as yet little experience.

Rhodesian infections, intermediate and late stage

Patients in whom the nervous system is slightly involved, i.e. those with a CSF protein content of 25–30 mg./100 ml. *may* be cured with suramin alone, and this can be tried provided that there is reasonable certainty that the patient will be seen again at intervals of one to two months for the next few months. If follow-up is uncertain, or is not possible, then melarsoprol should be given instead of suramin. Some would recommend that melarsoprol should be used for every patient in whom there is evidence of even slight infection of the nervous system; however, it seems justifiable to try the less toxic suramin if follow-up can be guaranteed.

In all other patients with involvement of the nervous system, melarsoprol is the only drug of proved value (with the exception of nitrofurazone), although, as was mentioned above, there are good theoretical grounds for an extended trial of Melarsen under controlled conditions. Results with melarsonyl potassium (Mel W) have been disappointing, and it is considered that this drug has no place in the treatment of the Rhodesian infection.

Rhodesian infections—Relapses

A relapse after suramin or pentamidine should be treated with melarsoprol. A patient whose infection has relapsed after one course of melarsoprol should be given another, but after a second relapse nitrofurazone should be used, preferably together with melarsoprol. There appears to be some suggestion that a combination of the two drugs is more effective in the treatment of relapses than is nitrofurazone alone.

Gambian infections—early stage

There is a choice of suramin or pentamidine, or possibly Berenil, and local circumstances will often dictate which should be used. For example, patients may be more willing to come from a distance once a week for four to five weeks than to make the same journey every day for seven to ten days, but if in-patient or hostel facilities are available the shorter course with pentamidine has obvious advantages.

A combination of suramin and pentamidine has been found to be very effective, and by this means a higher dose of each drug can be given with a lower incidence of toxic effects. Neujean and Evens (1958) in an analysis of their experience at Leopoldville over a period of ten years, considered that this combination was the treatment of choice. Suramin, 1–2 g., intravenously, was given at the same time as pentamidine, 4 mg./kg. intramuscularly, on three occasions on alternate days, and up to a further three such courses could be given at intervals of two weeks. In spite of the lower incidence of side effects this course has not been widely used, partly no doubt because of the need for two injections instead of one (attempts to prepare a complex suitable for use in a single injection have been unsuccessful), and partly because in rural practice it is usually desirable to keep treatment as simple as possible.

Gambian infections—intermediate and late stages

The drug of choice is melarsoprol, although Melarsen, in spite of its much greater cost and longer course, may be preferred in special circumstances when treatment has to be given in rural areas and to out-patients without direct medical supervision. As has been mentioned above, Melarsen is widely used, and with great success, in Nigeria.

In general, the melaminyl drugs appear to be better tolerated in West Africa than they are in East Africa, and there is probably no good reason for the use of suramin in patients with intermediate-stage infections (CSF protein up to 30 mg./100 ml.), unless local experience suggests otherwise. Also, in conditions in West Africa, frequent follow-up facilities are often not easy to arrange.

The other melaminyl drug, Mel W, must still be regarded as one for use in restricted circumstances, although where it has proved its value and relative safety it has great advantages.

Tryparsamide is still of value in certain areas where resistance to the drug has not become a problem and where treatment has to be given by rural staff with only occasional medical supervision. Nowadays it is unlikely that tryparsamide would be given to any patient under direct medical care unless there appeared to be some contraindication to the use of melarsoprol.

Combinations of suramin and tryparsamide have proved of value in Northern Nigeria, both when given together and in courses in which suramin is followed by tryparsamide. When given together, suramin 0·5 g. is dissolved in 10 ml. water with tryparsamide 1·5 g. and this (maximum adult dose) is given weekly for eight weeks, followed by tryparsamide 2 g. weekly for a further six weeks. These courses of suramin and tryparsamide, and of tryparsamide alone, are also useful when circumstances do not permit of a preliminary examination of the cerebrospinal fluid. The patient, in any stage of the disease, can be started on such a course, and the assessment can be made later.

The use of suramin followed by tryparsamide may sometimes allow the total dosage of tryparsamide to be reduced. Thus, in Sierra Leone, Harding (1945) showed that an effective course could consist of 3 injections of suramin followed by 5 of tryparsamide, 2 of suramin and 6 of tryparsamide, or 1 of suramin and 7 of tryparsamide. However, toxicity was related to the rest interval which it was possible to allow between the courses of suramin and tryparsamide; if this was three weeks or more, the first of the above courses was suitable, but if the interval had to be less than two weeks the last of the three courses (S1 + T7) was the best. It should be noted also that in Sierra Leone fewer injections of tryparsamide were given than would have been used in Nigeria; in fact, the standard Nigerian course, when first applied in Sierra Leone, proved far too toxic. This provides yet another example of regional variation in this disease and its treatment, and of the need for caution in any area where there is no firm experience by which to be guided. Regional variation is also one of the factors which make it so difficult to compare experience—in drug trials for example—in different areas.

Neujean and Evens (1958) found that pentamidine followed by tryparsamide produced dangerous toxic effects.

Gambian infections—Relapses

Management should be as outlined for the treatment of relapses of Rhodesian infections, but with the addition that if the infection is not resistant to tryparsamide this drug may prove of value, particularly if nitrofurazone is contra-indicated or has failed. Unfortunately, infections which have been treated with melarsoprol may be tryparsamide-resistant, but even so life may be prolonged.

ASSESSMENT OF CURE

Unless the treatment is obviously going to fail, there is usually a rapid and marked improvement in the patient's condition, but to determine whether it has been really effective, and to see that progress is maintained, it is essential to examine the cerebrospinal fluid periodically. If it was known before the start of treatment that the infection was an early one, and if a full course of suramin, pentamidine, or Berenil has been given, a single cerebrospinal fluid examination one to two months after treatment should suffice, but the patient should be seen at intervals thereafter. Provided that his health remains good there is no need for further lumbar punctures, but if there is any doubt—any complaint of fever or headache, for example—the spinal fluid should be re-examined. If the patient had a 'borderline' infection, say a CSF protein of 30 mg./100 ml. and a cell count of 15–20 per cmm., it may be desirable to examine the fluid at intervals of two to three months for the first six to nine months in order to detect a possible relapse without any delay.

If the patient's nervous system was at all seriously involved, the follow-up should be correspondingly more thorough. Ideally, a lumbar puncture should be done at intervals of two to three months for the first six months, and then every four to six months until eighteen months have elapsed since treatment, but this may not always be possible. The patient's general condition, too, has to be taken into account. It may not be justifiable to perform a lumbar puncture on every occasion on a patient who appears to be in good health, but examinations at six months, and again at twelve months after treatment should not be omitted. It is desirable to see patients periodically thereafter until two to three years have elapsed and for even longer in Gambian infections. In the Rhodesian disease, if a relapse is going to occur it usually does so within six to nine months, and in the Gambian disease within a year, but relapses of Rhodesian infections have occurred two years or so after treatment, and in the Gambian disease the interval may be much longer.

In these periodical examinations of the spinal fluid, a steady decrease in the protein level and the cell count, ultimately reaching normal in most cases, is a favourable sign, but a cure cannot be presumed until at least two years have elapsed in Rhodesian infections, and in Gambian infections the period should be three to four years, or even longer.

The first signs of a relapse will usually be an increase in the cell count in the cerebrospinal fluid followed by a rise in the protein level. These signs may or may not be accompanied by subjective or objective changes in the patient's condition, but complaints of headache, fever, tiredness, weakness and the like in any patient who has been treated for sleeping sickness should always arouse suspicion. Occasionally trypanosomes may be seen but time should not be wasted in searching for them; a rise in the CSF cell count or protein is alone sufficient to indicate the need for further treatment.

Two further points are of importance. Firstly, an examination of the spinal fluid immediately after treatment, particularly after melarsoprol, may show an actual rise in both cell count and protein level, and not until two to three months have elapsed can a true picture be obtained. Secondly, a high cerebrospinal protein level may occasionally persist in spite of an obvious and maintained improvement in the patient's condition. This is not in itself an indication for further treatment, which need be given only if the patient's health deteriorates or if a rise in the cell count indicates that the infection is still active.

PROGNOSIS

In both Gambian and Rhodesian infections the prognosis is excellent provided that the nervous system has not been infected. With appropriate treatment the cure rate is nearly 100% in patients in whom the cerebrospinal fluid is strictly normal. As the disease advances, demonstrated by a progressive increase in the protein content of the spinal fluid, the outlook becomes progressively less favourable, but in the individual patient it is never hopeless as even those who are almost moribund may sometimes be cured. Under hospital conditions, with expert attention, remarkably good results may be obtained even in the late stage of the disease. For example, in the patients treated by Robertson (1963a) eighteen out of twenty with an initial CSF protein level of 40 mg./100 ml. or more were cured, one relapsed and only one died; these were Rhodesian infections which are in general more difficult to cure than Gambian infections. In the same series, seven out of seven patients with late-stage Gambian infections were cured. Unfortunately, ideal conditions for treatment are not always available and in Tanzania, for example, where some 500–800 new cases are diagnosed annually and where most of the treatment is given in rural dispensaries and small district hospitals, the death rate, when all grades of severity are taken into account, is still about 10%.

Patients who have suffered a single relapse have a good prospect of an eventual cure. A relapse after suramin or pentamidine will nearly always respond to melarsoprol and cure is usually permanent. A relapse after melarsoprol will usually be cured by a second course of melarsoprol, but subsequent relapses carry a much less favourable prognosis.

In West Africa, as has already been mentioned, there are areas in which the disease is exceptionally mild and the mortality is very low, and there are others where it is more acute, resembling the Rhodesian disease, with a correspondingly high mortality. In both Rhodesian and Gambian areas the disease tends to be more acute and more lethal in places where it is invading new ground, and occasional fulminating infections occur from which the patient may die in spite of treatment and before there is any evidence in the spinal fluid of involvement of the nervous system.

The Cause of Death

Few patients who die from sleeping sickness are examined at autopsy and there is little firm information on which to base an opinion. Collomb *et al.* (1964)

reported a series of 20 deaths, 6 of which were directly due to the toxic effects of treatment (Mel W), 3 to cardiovascular collapse or pericarditis, 2 to intercurrent infections, 1 to pulmonary oedema, 3 to cachexia and 5 to coma, but these findings should not be applied generally. Heart failure is probably an important cause of death, more so than has been generally realized, but deaths attributable directly to drug toxicity are much less common than this series would suggest (*see* above, under melarsoprol). Intercurrent infection probably still accounts for some deaths, but now that effective treatment for sleeping sickness is generally available this is probably no longer an important cause. Most of the deaths, apart from those due to heart failure, almost certainly occur directly as a result of the infection itself, in patients in whom treatment has failed. Coma, from extensive cerebral involvement is the usual terminal state, and this may sometimes be accompanied by an overwhelming trypanosome invasion of the blood, spinal fluid and other tissues.

Spontaneous Recovery

It is difficult to answer the question, often asked, whether a patient with sleeping sickness can recover in the absence of specific treatment. Examples have been given elsewhere (Chapter 33) of exceptionally mild or asymptomatic infections and of patients who have remained in good health for many years without treatment. In some of these cases trypanosomes have been found during periodic examinations on some occasions but not on others. Yorke (1921) records a number of patients diagnosed as suffering from sleeping sickness who received no treatment but who remained in good health and were seemingly free from infection three to eight years later. McLetchie (1948) reported instances of patients in Nigeria with a history of sleeping sickness for five to eight years in whom symptoms appeared to be abating although no treatment had been given. Macfie (1913) described a very mild form of the disease in Eket in Southern Nigeria and believed that many of the persons infected recovered in the early stages of the disease. Dyleff (1932) described three European patients in the Congo all of whom showed trypanosomes in their blood but who were found to be negative at all subsequent examinations. All of the above instances relate to the Gambian disease in which it would appear that spontaneous cure may occasionally occur but it is clear that this can be accepted only after prolonged and exhaustive investigations have been made.

In the more acute Rhodesian infection, spontaneous recovery, if it ever takes place, must be very exceptional. Maclean and Corson, both men with long and intimate experience of the disease in Tanganyika, knew of no such occurrence. Davey (1936) described a patient from Nyasaland who remained in good health and whose blood failed to cause infection when inoculated into a monkey a year after the diagnosis was made. Ormerod (in a paper by Apted *et al.*, 1963) mentions a strain of trypanosome from Ngamiland which caused infection in a rat from which recovery was spontaneous and refers to the possible occurrence of spontaneous recovery in one, if not two, persons in the Bumi river area in Rhodesia but there was no proof of this in either case. The mild nature of some of the infections in the southern part of eastern Africa has already been noted and it seems possible that in these, as in the milder Gambian infections, an occasional spontaneous cure may occur, but it is unlikely that this ever happens in the more virulent form of the disease which is seen further north.

The Sequelae of Trypanosomiasis

Sleeping sickness, when properly treated, ordinarily leaves no sequelae. Patients with some degree of mental or intellectual impairment usually show marked improvement after treatment although when impairment has been severe, irreversible damage to the brain is likely to have occurred and recovery may not be complete. Field (1968) mentions that trypanosomiasis which has been treated too late to avert permanent brain damage may leave the patient 'complainingly paranoid like the burnt-out psychotic, but with a warmer, more resentful demeanour'. Collomb and Miletto (1957), who made a special study of this subject, described a number of patients, all 'cured' parasitologically who several years later suffered from irritability, insomnia, attacks of violent or hypomanic behaviour, expansiveness, paranoia, and endocrinal dysfunction. Electroencephalographic and pneumoencephalographic studies showed permanent abnormalities in the tracings and evidence of subcortical cerebral atrophy. Gallais *et al.* (1956) in a similar investigation in twenty specially selected subjects, all of whom had been 'cured', showed by pneumoencephalography that there was an organic basis for the residual neuro-psychic changes in sixteen of the patients, and in the remaining four, who died, histological study revealed evidence of leucoencephalitis with demyelination. It appears to be generally agreed, however, that such sequelae are rare, and Collomb and Miletto (*loc. cit.*) state that major psychoses and focal epilepsy are not seen. In any event, mental changes of this type occur only in persons with a considerable degree of nervous system involvement before the start of treatment. The patient who is treated in the early stage of the illness may be assured with confidence that there is no likelihood of future mental disturbance as a direct result of the disease. This is important because some patients have a not unnatural fear of the consequences of a disease bearing the name 'sleeping sickness'.

The few reports of mental change relate to Gambian sleeping sickness in which there is likely to be greater damage to the brain than in the Rhodesian infection. The writer, when working in Tanganyika, was impressed by the frequency with which melarsoprol restored to normal persons who were formerly mentally dull or confused; it is probable that in these Rhodesian infections there is little or no permanent damage to the brain.

Apart from the brain, the other organ likely to suffer damage is the heart, but as has been mentioned elsewhere (p. 655) treatment brings a rapid return to normality which is reflected in electrocardiographic tracings. Although the few post-mortem studies which have been made have shown that the myocardium is involved, which suggests that sometimes there may be permanent damage, this cannot be common for the great majority of patients who recover are able to do a full day's hard work with no apparent ill effects. Terminal heart failure occurs, but chronic failure must be rare and certainly heart disease does not figure prominently as one of the sequelae of sleeping sickness.

Although the liver may be involved there is no suggestion that the damage is permanent, but this subject has been little studied. Signs of endocrine dysfunction such as menstrual disturbance and sterility tend to disappear with treatment,

Chapter 37

Chemoprophylaxis of Human Trypanosomiasis

B. B. WADDY

INTRODUCTORY

The chemoprophylaxis of trypanosomiasis, or indeed of any disease, may be considered in relation to individuals, or small groups whose subsequent health is under some degree of supervision, or whole communities in large areas. For a drug to be suitable for use in large-scale chemoprophylaxis in rural areas of tropical Africa, it must be cheap, free from serious toxic hazards and capable of giving protection from infection for a period measurable in months rather than weeks. Of the drugs that have been considered for chemoprophylaxis of trypanosomiasis, namely suramin and diamidine compounds, the last named meet all the requirements particularly well and are the only ones used in practice.

Suramin, which was introduced in 1920, is eliminated from the body very slowly, due to its fixation on the serum proteins and its chemical stability. It was therefore the first drug to offer the possibility of chemoprophylactic action against human trypanosomiasis. The dose recommended varied from 4 milligrams per kilogram of body weight (4 mg./kg.) to as much as 2 grammes (Duke, 1936). It is given intravenously, intramuscular injection being too painful for routine use. With the lower doses, protection against infection with *Trypanosoma gambiense* for two to three months was claimed. According to Duke the high dose gave protection against both *T. gambiense* and *T. rhodesiense* for at least three months. A schedule involving the giving of the drug intravenously every three months would give rise to great administrative difficulties for large scale use in rural Africa. In addition, suramin causes damage to the kidneys with some frequency and should not be given without a preliminary urine test; it occasionally gives rise to exfoliative dermatitis and even (very occasionally, but dramatically) to sudden death. These hazards can be anticipated and guarded against for individual patients, but not for whole communities.

Harding and Hutchinson (1948) gave prophylactic suramin, in a dose of 1–2 g., to 3,572 persons in Sierra Leone of whom 0·95% had 'immediate reactions' (vomiting, mild syncope, colic, pyrexia, urticaria) compared with 0·59% of those given pentamidine in the same project. There were no serious ill effects in those given suramin, but pentamidine was much easier to administer and appeared to give more complete and prolonged protection. Suramin was used to some extent in the (then) Belgian Congo, but its use was discontinued as soon as diamidines became available.

Suramin was revived for a period in the 1950s, as a synergist of pentamidine and an antidote to the toxic effects of the latter (Masseguin *et al.*, 1955); a preparation combining the two drugs was marketed by a French pharmaceutical firm. This practice has been abandoned completely.

The arsenical Trimelarsan and the antimonial MSb are mentioned in a few French reports as having been tried as prophylactic drugs.

Throughout the great epidemics of Gambian sleeping sickness that occurred in West and Central Africa in the 1920s and 1930s chemoprophylaxis was not available as a method of control.

King, Lourie and Yorke (1937) announced the trypanocidal action of diamidine compounds. The train of reasoning that prompted their investigations is interesting in relation to the principal hazard involved in administering diamidines to human beings, namely the inducement of hypoglycaemia. It had been noted earlier that trypanosome metabolism requires large quantities of carbohydrate; experiments with decamethylenediguanidine (Synthalin) were undertaken primarily because it induces hypoglycaemia and might for this reason interfere with trypanosomal metabolism. It was found that this drug had a trypanocidal action out of proportion to its effect on the blood sugar and the investigation developed around quite different chemical characteristics, namely 'a central inert carbon chain with terminal polar groups of strongly basic nature' (Lourie & Yorke, 1939). The investigation was continued by Dr A. J. Ewins of May and Baker, Ltd., until pentamidine[1] (variously described as 4:4′- or 1:5′-diamidino diphenoxy pentane) was evolved. Pentamidine is usually marketed as the diisethionate (M & B 800), the dimethyl sulphonate (Lomidine, commonly used in the French-speaking African countries), and dihydrochloride. Like suramin, pentamidine and its salts become bound to serum proteins and are excreted from the body very slowly. Another diamidine, Berenil, in contrast, is excreted rapidly. So far, Berenil has been used exclusively in treatment of diagnosed (mainly animal) trypanosomiasis, but it has been suggested that it might act as a prophylactic in man if taken daily by mouth.

There has been some confusion over the dosage of pentamidine and its salts.

[1] The word 'pentamidine' is a convenient colloquial expression for this compound. The British Pharmacopoeia recognizes pentamidine isethionate and 'pentamidine injection', which is also pentamidine isethionate.

Unless otherwise stated, dosage mentioned here refers to dose of base; 1 g. of base is equivalent to 1·74 g. of the diisethionate, 1·56 g. of the dimethyl sulphonate and 1·21 g. of the dihydrochloride.

Launoy and Lagodsky (1940) first recorded the prophylactic effect of pentamidine diisethionate against *Trypanosoma brucei* in mice. Van Hoof, Henrard and Peel (1944) described successful prophylactic experiments carried out on guinea pigs and on two human volunteers. The latter received single doses of 2 and 3 mg./kg. and were protected from repeated challenge by tsetse infected with *T. gambiense* for 364 and 295 days, respectively. In December 1942, Van Hoof and his co-workers began a field trial of the prophylaxis of *T. gambiense* with pentamidine, involving a population of about a thousand including controls. They reported complete protection for at least six months (Van Hoof *et al.*, 1946).

The first dose, given to 721 subjects, was 3 mg./kg. apparently of the hydrochloride. Seven months later, 360 of these were given a dose of 4 mg./kg. of 'isethionic acid pentamidine salt,' presumably M & B 800. Those who received only one injection acted as controls.

From this time, pentamidine was employed on rapidly increasing scales in the (then) French and Belgian colonies, in Nigeria and for a time in Sierra Leone, for the chemoprophylaxis of *T. gambiense* infection. The total number of injections given must be numbered in millions. The standard dose accepted by the World Health Organization's Expert Committee on Trypanosomiasis (*Report*, 1962) and other authorities is 4 mg./kg. base, up to a maximum of 300 mg. In persons not infected before the drug is administered, protection appears to be virtually complete for at least six months. Gall (1954) estimates the failure rate as of the order of 0·1% up to a year after injection. The toxic hazards are slight, and those that cannot be averted by simple precautions (described below) are readily treatable. Examination to exclude an already existing infection must always precede administration of a prophylactic drug. This will be discussed later. The means exist, therefore; what are the ends?

The first, and simplest, aim of prophylaxis is the protection of individuals or organized groups whose work exposes them to the risk of infection. Surprisingly, those who work professionally on sleeping sickness or tsetse control seldom demand or receive prophylactic pentamidine and very rarely become infected. Among the first groups to be protected regularly by chemoprophylaxis were tin mining labourers around the Jos Plateau in Nigeria whose occupation placed them at serious risk of infection.

'In 1946 mines managements were encouraged to adopt universal protection for their mining labourers, and legislation was prepared to make such protection compulsory. Even without legislation the response was good and the results have fully justified the measure. Pentamidine was given as the diisethionate in doses of 200–250 mg. to each labourer on engagement and thereafter at four to six months' intervals.

'During two years' protection of several thousands of labourers, the only overt cases were found among those who had not received an injection. In 1948, 3,243 miners who had received prophylaxis were closely questioned, and lumbar punctures were performed on 105. Of six cases showing altered cerebrospinal fluid, four proved to have had sleeping sickness two to three years previously, and two appeared to be true cryptic infections' (Gall, 1954).

The same precaution can and should be applied to gangs of labourers working on road, railway or similar works in areas of high risk. It should be borne in mind that the risk may be only a potential one, before a labour force is brought into being. The fact that trypanosomiasis is not reported, or does not exist, in a tsetse infested area may be due merely to a low human population density. The inception of a public works project in Africa invariably attracts large numbers of itinerant unskilled labourers, many of whom travel long distances to seek work. Almost inevitably some of them come from or through endemic foci and are infected on arrival. The creation of a relatively high population density therafter facilitates the cycle of infection.

In contrast, it has not been necessary to use chemoprophylaxis to protect the large labour forces at major dam sites in Africa, such as the Volta Dam in Ghana, the Kainji Dam in Nigeria and the Kariba Dam in Rhodesia. The existence of multiple subcontractors, each with its own labour force, in such a project means that health control of labour is far from straightforward. On the Niger and Volta Dam projects tsetse control in the working area was a fairly simple operation and effectively removed the risk of *T. gambiense* infection spreading. In the Kariba area a more extensive and complicated tsetse control operation was undertaken, the cost of which was justified because it enabled the labour township to be sited on the heights and not in the torrid valley.

A possible use of chemoprophylaxis is to enable closed communities such as leper settlements to be set up on good agricultural land which is not used by its legal owners because of the risk of sleeping sickness. Such controlled groups can be protected without difficulty.

CHEMOPROPHYLAXIS FOR COMMUNITIES

Gambian Sleeping Sickness

An exclusively human infection should be capable of eradication by the protection of a high proportion, not necessarily 100%, of the community. The possible existence of animal reservoirs of *T. gambiense* is considered in Chapter 33 but, in relation to the maintenance of Gambian sleeping sickness, the very prolonged symptomless incubation period in man and the African's propensity for travel are factors of greater importance. There is also the phenomenon (which must be experienced to be believed) of the existence of villages in epidemic areas, undiscovered by survey teams for years.

According to Vaucel (1952), Robert Koch envisaged a mass treatment campaign, aimed at eradication, as early as 1909, but as Atoxyl was the only drug then available this was not practicable. With the development of suramin (which clears trypanosomes from the blood very rapidly) and tryparsamide, mass survey followed by treatment of diagnosed cases was capable of reducing the annual incidence of sleeping sickness in savanna foci to something of the order of 0·1%. In certain forest foci incidence did not fall below 2–3%. Because of the slow development of the disease, mortality was extremely low provided that surveys were regular and comprehensive.

When pentamidine was introduced, Belgian and French workers again considered the possibility of eradicating Gambian sleeping sickness by chemoprophylaxis, given for a limited period. The procedure has been adopted in most of the endemic areas of West and Equatorial Africa, but nowhere has the hope of eradication been fulfilled even after pentamidine has been given twice yearly for many years. In the Congo (Kinshasa) where annual incidence in endemic foci was reduced from 0·21% in 1948 to 0·02% in 1958, sleeping sickness has reappeared on an epidemic scale since control was interrupted by political disturbances.

Some examples of the use of chemoprophylaxis in savanna areas are described below. Most of these projects were undertaken before tsetse control by the use of insecticides (which seems to the writer to offer far better prospects of permanent results) was developed.

In Nigeria, 'In 1950 a local increase in sleeping sickness was reported from a group of villages in the Lere District of Zaria Province, and it was decided to make use of pentamidine prophylaxis. The area was divided into two: Juran Kari, consisting of the few villages which suffered most from the exacerbation, with about 600 population; and Lere, comprising the remainder, about 3,500 population. It proved possible to clear the streams in the immediate neighbourhood of Juran Kari village, and the area was therefore at first excluded from the pentamidine campaign. On the second visit it was included at the inhabitants' own request. The results are shown in Table 37.1 below.

TABLE 37.1

Table showing the incidence of sleeping sickness in two areas of Lere District, Zaria Province, Nigeria, before and after mass prophylaxis with pentamidine

Date	Lere area		Juran Kari area	
	No. examined	Incidence %	No. examined	Incidence %
1948–52 (average)	—	1·49	—	2·33
Jan. 1952	2,485	1·32	399	2·25
Oct. 1952	2,628	0·34[1]	483	1·02
April 1953	2,429	0·12[2]	406	0·00[1]
Jan. 1954	1,807	0·11[3]	292	0·00[2]

[1] After first mass prophylaxis.
[2] After second mass prophylaxis.
[3] After third mass prophylaxis.

'At the preliminary survey in January 1952, 42 new cases were diagnosed. Since then, among those who received prophylactic injections, 2 cases, in which trypanosomes could not be found, have been diagnosed on clinical grounds,

1 in April 1953, and 1 in January 1954, and 1 case, showing scanty blood trypanosomes only, was detected in January 1954. Of these three cases, at least one was probably infected before receiving pentamidine.

'Among the unprotected population 16 new cases have been detected, 14 in October 1952, 2 in April 1953, and none in January 1954. The unprotected population probably constitutes 20–30% of the total, but in spite of this high proportion the incidence of sleeping sickness amongst the unprotected has dwindled to nil.

'This strongly suggests that the reservoir of circulating trypanosomes has been reduced to a level where transmission is approaching extinction' (Gall, 1954).

In 1963, however, survey and treatment appears to have been re-established in this area, with local incidences ranging from 0·03–0·26% (*Report*, 1964).

In the (then) Belgian Congo, attempts to implement Van Hoof's conception of a campaign of limited duration are described in the annual reports of FORÉAMI, notably that for 1958. Usually two to four doses were given at six-monthly intervals, with the hope of reducing incidence to sporadic cases, or even achieving permanent eradication of the disease. In the Lufimi- Basse-Sele sub-sector a prophylactic campaign along the left bank of the Congo was started in 1948, while the French treated the community along the right bank. Annual incidence in the population of approximately 5,000, before prophylaxis was initiated, was 0·85%. Thereafter successive surveys reported incidences as follows:

	1949	1950		1951		1952	
Incidence New cases, per cent	July 0·85	Jan. 0·14	Oct. 0·04	March 0·04	Oct. 0·00	March 0·01	Oct. 0·05

Results were excellent at first, but in 1952 cases began to appear in disturbing numbers outside the area in which prophylaxis was given. The area protected had to be increased greatly, and chemoprophylaxis became an annual event in a population of nearly a million. In 1958, 788,628 persons were examined and dosed, the incidence of new cases being 0·024%. The report states that an unspecified number ('relativement restraint') of cryptic infections (*see* below) was found in the re-surveys following the first prophylactic rounds, and that these were probably persons who were already infected at the time they received their first dose.

Lotte (1951) reported in optimistic terms on the results of four years' chemoprophylaxis in countries of French Equatorial Africa, now Congo (Brazzaville), and in Central African Republic. Survey and Lomidine injection were carried out twice yearly from 1947–1951 in foci ranging from one of the highest epidemic potential down to some with consistent but low endemicity. He concluded that if prophylaxis is applied to areas sufficiently large to contain a homogeneous population, and if absenteeism can be reduced to a minimum, it should be possible to end transmission and eradicate *T. gambiense* infection.

Richet (1954) reported more cautiously on this campaign. Up to the end of 1953, 1,306,860 injections of Lomidine were given, but so far from admitting defeat the trypanosome 'is attempting to hide, and . . . is becoming more difficult to detect under the microscope'. Suspected cases, in which the probable diagnosis was difficult or impossible to confirm by microscopic examinations, were becoming increasingly frequent and cryptic infections were also increasing. There was a marked improvement between 1946, with 2,691 cases of trypanosomiasis diagnosed out of 386,031 persons examined (0·72%) and 1951 with 1,911 cases diagnosed out of 1,110,697 persons examined (0·18%); of the latter, 531 cases came from a district not included in the Lomidine campaign.

Congo (Brazzaville), Central African Republic, Cameroun, Chad and Gabon now join together in the Organisation de Coordination pour la Lutte contre les Endémies en Afrique Central (OCEAC). At the 1967 technical conference of OCEAC it was stated that sleeping sickness incidence had ceased to regress, and some doubt was expressed about the advisability of continuing the practice of mass chemoprophylaxis (OCEAC, 1967).

Early results in the French speaking countries of West Africa were reviewed by Jonchère (1951) and Diallo (1951). As elsewhere, in epidemic foci the effect in reducing the incidence of new cases was dramatic. In three villages in the Casamance and the Guinea Forest, in which previous surveys had revealed an annual incidence of 5%, 1,002 persons were given an injection of pentamidine and 901 were left as controls. Six months later no cases were found in those protected but nineteen new cases occurred among the controls. At the second re-survey, undertaken partly eleven and partly fourteen months later, three cases were found in the protected persons and twenty-eight among the controls. With Lomidine instead of M & B 800 the campaign was then extended to all areas with an annual incidence of more than 1%. The dose was standardized at 4 mg./kg. of 'Lomidine-base' (either prepared on the spot from ampoules of 1 g. or taken from 5 ml. ampoules of 2·5% Lomidine. Lomidine is now issued in 4% solution). In surveys in 1949, undertaken at intervals of from six to twelve months after first injections, incidence of *T. gambiense* infection was 0·06% and 0·45% in protected and unprotected groups, respectively. Cryptic infections, characterized by grossly altered cerebrospinal fluid with no trypanosomes in blood or glands, were seen, but the numbers were not given by either author.

In the independent French language States of West Africa (the OCCGE States) until 1960 chemoprophylaxis, which is onerous, unpopular and not free from accidents, was used only when prevalence ('IVC') in a focus exceeded 1%. It became extremely rare to find such a prevalence. None the less, a number of residual foci remained, maintaining a low endemic state and capable of epidemic exacerbations on the least slackening of vigilance. In 1961, the principle of using chemoprophylaxis in any area where a genuinely autochthonous case was discovered was suggested. However attractive this might sound in theory, offering the prospect of a rapid eradication of the disease, it was not easy to apply in practice. The unpopularity of the procedure gave rise to a serious risk of concealment of cases. Therefore, although the principle remains, of using chemoprophylaxis at the first sign of danger, in practice its application is left to the discretion of the Sector Medical Chiefs, who base their decisions on the picture presented by past years and the repeated appearance of isolated autochthonous cases. If an actual focus of infection, however small, is discovered, chemoprophylaxis should be applied automatically.

Chemoprophylaxis must always be preceded by a thorough diagnostic survey, including both blood and gland juice examination, and followed up after six months. Diagnosis by more refined methods such as IgM estimation is theoretically desirable, but at the time of writing this is being practised in only two foci (Richet, personal communication).

The annual incidence of trypanosomiasis in the OCCGE States has declined steadily year by year and, in 1965, it fell to only 0·021% among 981,524 persons examined. This is a splendid achievement, which closely parallels that in the Congo (Kinshasa) before it became independent. The need for vigilance remains.

It seems to the writer that too little consideration has been given to the precise objectives in applying chemoprophylaxis to different types of sleeping sickness focus. The only objective stated in publications appears to be the actual or near extinction of Gambian sleeping sickness, which events in the Congo have proved dramatically to be no more than temporary, at the best.

In the savanna type of focus, of high epidemic potential, the mobility of the male population is tremendous. Mansell-Prothero (1965) estimates that in some areas 25–50% of the men may leave their homes annually to seek work as seasonal labourers in more developed areas. In doing so, they may carry infection with them, and give rise to a 'sleeve' of endemicity in suitable places along the road. An example of this is given by the relation of the disease in the Wenchi District of Ghana (a forest area) to the savanna epidemic area of Wa-Lawra. In the Wenchi District simple mass survey, with treatment of diagnosed cases, was carried out in 1940–3 and again in 1950–1. No other control measure was undertaken locally, but a serious epidemic in Wa-Lawra was controlled between 1939 and 1943. Table 37.2 (Waddy, 1956) shows the effect on trypanosomiasis in Wenchi.

TABLE 37.2

	On the main road		Away from the main road		S.E. of the difference in the two percentages
	No. examined	Infection rate	No. examined	Infection rate	
1940–43	28,848	0·87%	8,374	0·47%	0·092
1950–51	39,693	0·08%	14,990	0·05%	0·023
S.E. of difference between two percentages		0·056		0·077	

Experience indicates that sleeping sickness will not be eradicated from a natural endemic focus by means of chemoprophylaxis alone, but that in the savanna, tsetse control by insecticides offers good prospects of permanent eradication from a campaign of limited duration. While a savanna focus continues in being, clearly the resulting danger of sleeve endemicity on roads leading away from it can be minimized by thorough surveys followed by chemoprophylaxis. But this is true only if the operation is undertaken at a suitable time of year, namely before the beginning of the dry season. Since mass surveys are unlikely to be well attended during the harvest weeks of late August to October, the period for an effective campaign seems to be confined to the period extending approximately from mid-June to mid-August.

In forest foci, tsetse control is (or has hitherto been) impracticable. A forest focus may be of the sleeve type, at least partly kept in being by travellers from distant foci, or may be a true natural endemic focus. If it is the latter, Scott (1957) has pointed out that only those in certain occupations are at serious risk and not the entire population. Trades that take those who follow them into the bush, such as that of palm wine tapper, carry an occupational hazard of infection, but the farm labourer from savanna-dwelling tribes, regardless of whether he has arrived recently or has lived in the forest for a long time, is the main sufferer. The seasonal labourer returns to his home in the savanna eventually and may carry infection back to a quiescent epidemic focus. The strategy of applying chemoprophylaxis selectively to those in certain occupations, in forest foci, might be worth considering. In 'sleeve' foci, the relative risks to which different elements of the population may be exposed do not appear to have been investigated and analysed. Such an investigation might be worth undertaking since lack of co-operation by the community would probably make universal chemoprophylaxis impracticable.

Rhodesian Sleeping Sickness

The epidemiology of Rhodesian sleeping sickness is very different from that of the Gambian disease. Although in one area *T. rhodesiense* has become adapted to a man-fly cycle with a member of the *palpalis* group (*G. fuscipes*) as vector, it is normally a zoonosis the reservoir hosts of which are wild mammals. Man is infected sporadically in areas with human population densities sufficiently low to allow large numbers of wild animals to exist.

The administration of chemoprophylactic drugs to scattered communities in areas where the animal reservoir greatly exceeds the human one could not have any effect in reducing transmission of the infection; all that could be offered would be individual protection.

In practice, the only area in which regular injections of pentamidine have been given for prophylactic purposes is Botswana where tsetse control staff suffered very high infection rates. In 1947, it was decided to give them pentamipine at six-month intervals, but as six of the ten cases diagnosed among the staff during the next year had been given pentamidine, the interval between injections was shortened to three months and later to two months, during the working season. This practice was continued until 1957, but no statistical records of the results appear to exist (Scott, personal communication).

Silva and Caseiro (1957) describe the use of pentamidine to control an epidemic that occurred in an area close to the Tanzania frontier. In the years 1951, 1952 and 1953, diagnosed cases numbered 32, 75 and 104 respectively, and when a further 59 cases were found in the first quarter of 1954 it was decided to give the whole population four injections of pentamidine at intervals of six months. A census of the area revealed 16,946 persons of whom 11,869 were given the first injection; the remaining 5,077, who comprised infants, young children and old persons, were not injected and thus acted as controls. The first injection was very popular, but attendance for the second, third and fourth dropped to 7,952, 5,165 and 4,092, respectively. From April 1954 to April 1956, 53 further cases were diagnosed of whom only 6 had received pentamidine; of these 2 had been regarded as suspects at the time of their first injection. For the other 4, the intervals between the last injection and the date when a positive diagnosis was made were seven, four, four and five months.

Duke (1936) reported an experiment with suramin as a prophylactic of *T. gambiense* and *T. rhodesiense* infection. This drug was apparently more effective against *T. rhodesiense* than *T. gambiense* infection and the recommended dose, 2 g., protected human volunteers deliberately exposed to flies known to be infective, for at least three months and possibly longer. However, if infection did occur later it tended to be of a cryptic type.

Suramin does not appear to have been used anywhere on a large scale for the chemoprophylaxis of Rhodesian trypanosomiasis.

CHEMOPROPHYLAXIS FOR INDIVIDUALS

The question is often asked, whether or not to recommend the use of a chemoprophylactic drug for persons visiting areas in which sleeping sickness is endemic. The general consensus is that chemoprophylaxis is not advisable for visitors to Rhodesian sleeping sickness areas, but that reliance should be placed on rapid diagnosis and treatment if infection should occur.

For visitors to areas in which Gambian sleeping sickness is endemic opinion is not unanimous. Some authorities consulted by the writer say that they have recommended an injection of pentamidine to individuals about to pay a short visit (six weeks or less) to certain areas, but in general the risk of infection is not great enough to justify adding this to the formidable list of prophylactic procedures recommended to the traveller.

It must not be forgotten, however, that visitors to tropical Africa are occasionally infected, and they should be advised to insist on having the opinion of a tropical diseases consultant in the event of their suffering from any febrile or nervous illness within at least two years after leaving.

TOXIC HAZARDS AND OTHER ILL-EFFECTS

Pentamidine has the effects of lowering the blood sugar and the blood pressure. Its administration therefore may be followed immediately by hypoglycaemic symptoms and syncope. Richet (personal communication) found an average lowering of the blood sugar of 15 to 20%, at its maximum fifteen to thirty minutes after injection, and apparently accentuated during the hot hours of the day. More common are transitory discomfort, nausea and sweating. The occurrence of these symptoms can be reduced greatly by giving the drug on an empty stomach (in particular free from alcohol) and making the patient rest in the shade afterwards (*see* below for details). Hypoglycaemia can be prevented by administration of sugar by mouth or even intravenously, and syncope is relieved by adrenaline, or, according to some French workers (e.g. Beaudiment *et al.*, 1954), by intravenous suramin, a dose of which puts a patient with syncope 'back on his feet in a few seconds'.

Collomb *et al.* (1956) described three cases of diabetes occurring after pentamidine treatment (not prophylaxis). One developed after fifty days and lasted for two months; another appeared after four to six months and lasted for five to six months; the third appeared after sixty days and was still active, though improving, two years later.

Gas gangrene has followed prophylactic injection of pentamidine, the worst reported episode having been in Gabon where fourteen cases occurred in 685 persons injected (Richet, 1954).

Richet (1954) also reported fifteen cases of poliomyelitis, thirteen of whom had received Lomidine during the previous month; all these had paralysis exclusively in the lower limbs. Gall (1954) observed motor paresis of the injected limb within a few days of a pentamidine injection and suspected that this could have been poliomyelitis.

As might be expected, abortion or miscarriage following pentamidine injection has been ascribed to the drug. The general consensus is that it is not actually an abortifacient; nevertheless, it is wise to withhold it from pregnant women in places where abortion is common, in order to avoid opprobrium.

The most disquieting hazard connected with large scale pentamidine prophylaxis is the subsequent appearance of 'cryptic cases' in whom trypanosomes cannot be found in the blood or glands but who, when eventually diagnosed, show evidence of serious involvement of the central nervous system, with considerably raised protein and cell count in the cerebrospinal fluid. Trypanosomes may or may not be found in the cerebrospinal fluid. Every worker, French, Belgian and British, who has reported on the chemoprophylaxis of Gambian sleeping sickness has described these cases but figures of incidence are not usually given. Harding and Hutchinson (1948) found cerebrospinal fluid changes, but no trypanosomes, in 9 out of 1,061 persons seven months after their pentamidine injections and concluded that 'some new infections had occurred after prophylaxis but had remained cryptic'. Others believe that cryptic infections usually result from chemoprophylaxis being given to persons already infected. The problem is still unresolved. An ordinary, well-conducted mass survey in which gland juice whenever possible and one stained thick blood film are examined for everyone, misses between 20 and 35% of early cases. If blood film examinations are repeated twice on later days, a large proportion, but not all, of the missed cases will be detected. The IgM test is more sensitive but has not yet come into general use.

It is hardly practicable in a large scale survey to repeat stained blood film examination three times. Infections are certain to be missed in any survey, and cryptic infections are certain to follow chemoprophylaxis. From the preventive viewpoint, they are of little importance, being in all probability uninfective to tsetse. But regarded as sick individuals their plight is serious, and every effort must be made to detect as many infections as possible on initial survey and to diagnose the cryptic infections at re-surveys—not a very easy matter unless experienced men are looking out for them.

In the mining areas of Northern Nigeria, where chemoprophylaxis has been practised for twenty years, cryptic infections have not presented a serious problem.

LOGISTICS OF CHEMOPROPHYLAXIS

The avoidance of toxic effects and, as far as possible, of cryptic infections, and the need for good public relations are the main factors setting the pattern of procedure.

Every authority is agreed that a census, as complete as possible, must be part of each round of survey and dosing, that every effort is made to attain 100% diagnosis and that either prophylaxis or treatment is administered to everyone. Injection must be strictly intramuscular: the syringe should be withdrawn to make sure that the needle is not in a vein, before the actual injection is given.

The strictest regimen employed at present appears to be that of the OCEAC States, Central African Republic, Cameroon, Chad, Congo (Brazzaville) and Gabon (OCEAC, 1967).

The dose is 1 ml. of 4% Lomidine solution per 10 kg. body weight, to a maximum of 7·5 ml., equivalent to 300 mg. of drug.

The population to be treated is assembled on the eve of the day for injection and ordered to attend in the morning, fasting, and having refrained from drinking alcohol. To avoid hypoglycaemic and hypotensive incidents, nausea, etc., patients are given their injections lying down in the shade, each having been weighed and given a paper indicating the individual dose. They then rest for an hour. Anyone who complains of malaise receives a lump of sugar to which five drops of adrenaline solution have been added.

Very rarely syncope ensues, mostly in persons who have taken alcohol or food. The materials to effect rapid resuscitation should be ready to hand, namely 30% glucose solution for intravenous injection (20 ml.) and adrenaline for subcutaneous injection. It is essential, to keep up public morale, that this treatment should be given immediately and in public view. To avoid the probable accusation of having caused abortions, Lomidine should not be given to pregnant women.

Lotte (1951) at first excluded from prophylaxis children under 15 kg. in weight, the aged, pregnant women, those in general ill-health and patients previously cured of sleeping sickness. Later, he included young children, pregnant women and cured cases.

The OCCGE States of West Africa[1] the procedure is that a census is made,

[1] Organisation de Coordination et de Cooperation pour la Lutte Contre les Grandes Endémies (OCCGE) was founded in 1960 with the following African member states: Ivory Coast, Dahomey, Upper Volta, Mali, Mauritania, Niger, Senegal (Richet, 1965).

by families, immediately before the diagnostic survey. The IgM test is used only in a few hard core residual foci. Persons should receive their injections fasting, but some doctors give a lump of sugar before the injection. A warning is given about refraining from alcohol but teams have few illusions about the observance of this. Persons injected rest in the shade for an hour or two. Infants on the breast and pregnant women are excluded but weaned children included. The exclusion of those in bad general health is left to the discretion of the man in charge of the team. Treatment of malaise and syncope are similar to those in the OCEAC instructions.

In Nigeria, emphasis is placed mainly on strictly intramuscular injection and on keeping adrenaline ready for use.

A mass survey, including universal blood examination, is a slow affair, costly in terms of the salaries and transport of those concerned. It can be combined advantageously with other diagnostic and even curative procedures, provided that the time rhythms of these are all strictly compatible. The basic team method employed in sleeping sickness surveys in Ghana has stood the test of time and always depended on, and obtained, the voluntary co-operation of the community.

The team consists of a leader promoted from the ranks through character and initiative, a variable number of microscopists, two men capable of doubling the roles of diagnostician and clerk and one or two labourer-cleaners. Even the last should be impressed with the undoubted fact that human lives depend on their conscientiousness.

Each microscopist can examine a certain number of slides daily. The number can be set high or low, but if it is set too high, standards must suffer. In Ghana 20 to 25 slides daily, for about 300 days a year, was the standard. The number of persons to be seen daily is calculated simply by multiplying the number of microscopists available by the number of slides each man can examine satisfactorily in a day. On the evening before work starts, the leader and clerk go from house to house taking down and numbering names in their survey book, cross-examining house-owners assiduously in order to discover forgotten grandparents, concealed lepers and the like. Those written in the book are asked to attend at dawn.

At dawn each one is called in turn, has a blood film and if necessary a gland juice specimen taken, is weighed and is then free to go. Blood films are left to stain slowly in Giemsa, and the day's round of examining them starts after breakfast. Cases of sleeping sickness must be referred to a treatment centre, but the prophylactic injections of those found negative can simply be given on the following morning, while the next day's survey is being done. The virtue of this method is that it wastes extremely little of the time of those examined. Survey teams have never been unpopular in Ghana. For the chemoprophylactic team the man in charge, who is unlikely to be a doctor, must be a senior and highly responsible auxiliary. The principles of mass production and time and motion study should be invoked to ensure the maximum speed and efficiency in getting through, say, 250 injections in a morning. The man actually giving the injection should merely have to turn half around in order to hand over his used syringe and take a freshly charged one. Equally, as he turns back again, a freshly iodined buttock, and the appropriate dose, should present themselves before him. Finally, the persons injected must be rubbed, led away to rest, and supervised. For all this, the team must consist of 1 dispenser, 1 injector, 1 man charging syringes, 1 man sterilizing syringes, 1 man preparing buttocks, 1 man doing aftercare on buttocks and setting patients at rest. All except the dispenser, the injector and the man responsible for surveillance of persons resting after injection can be intelligent labourers, even illiterates.

Pentamidine diisethionate is marketed by Messrs May and Baker in bottles of 200 mg. or of 25 g. It is readily soluble in water and is generally used as a 5% solution. It is highly hygroscopic and according to Pille (1953) tends to hydrolyze in the presence of water with the production of a toxic amide. Therefore, precautions must be taken to keep stocks dry. Opened bottles that show signs of deliquescence must be rejected, and solutions when prepared should be used immediately.

Lotte (1954) described in detail the logistics of a prophylactic campaign in aquatic regions of Equatorial Africa. These areas had been depopulated almost to extinction by sleeping sickness and the costly effort to save the remaining population was thoroughly justifiable. His team consisted, essentially, of a boat load of eight men—a doctor, a boatman trained to do clinical cleaning work, and six nurses, all of whom must be interchangeable and all trained microscopists. Lotte claimed to be able to do 200 to 250 examinations in a day with this team, in which all secretarial work devolved on the doctor.

The Abengourou Focus

Abengourou, in the forest country of the Ivory Coast, is of interest in several ways. It is a persistent forest endemic focus. It has also some of the characteristics of a 'sleeve' focus, because a little-considered side branch of the road leading north from the endemic foci of the Ghana forest passes across to it.

From 1956–62 the area was subjected to systematic survey and Lomidine chemoprophylaxis regularly every six months, but the results were mediocre and transmission continued to occur. The endemic diseases organization of Ivory Coast is particularly efficient, and its lack of success is a fair indication of the probable result of campaigning against sleeping sickness in such a focus, by this method. It is true that infected travellers from Ghana must have been reintroducing infection constantly, but this is significant less in terms of international non-cooperation than as a reminder that infected travellers are liable to turn up anywhere in West Africa.

In 1963, it was decided to mount a campaign against trypanosomiasis in the Abengourou area by every known method; survey (including IgM estimation) and treatment, chemoprophylaxis, and tsetse control. Mobile teams were to examine travellers on roads leading to the area. At the same time, campaigns against tuberculosis (tuberculin test, mass X-ray, and BCG examination) and yaws (Kline test followed by curative or prophylactic penicillin), and smallpox vaccination, were to be undertaken.

The preliminary preparations for this campaign, in particular investigation of the tsetse population, the general logistical preparations and the training of auxiliary staff, took one year.

The survey team consisted of four groups travelling together, but the timing of all the operations turned out to be completely harmonious. The entire team consisted of 27 men, comprising 1 doctor, 1 entomologist, 3 auxiliaries with special biological training, 11 nurses of whom one was trained in radiography, 6 technicians and 5 auxiliary nurses.

The general survey group, consisting of 8 nurses and 4 auxiliary nurses, did blood and other microscope examinations, tuberculin testing, BCG and smallpox vaccinations and the prophylactic injection of penicillin to yaws contacts. A laboratory group of 4 men did IgM serum testing and some examinations for trypanosomes. The mass X-ray group consisted of the radiographer and 2 nurses, and the entomologist had 6 technicians.

Everyone was seen twice, at four-day intervals. The first visit, conducted in the morning, comprised:

1. Census taking and provision of 'carte sanitaire'.
2. Clinical survey, and selection of suspects to be sent to the laboratory.
3. Tuberculin test.
4. Smallpox vaccination.
5. Venepuncture, for IgM and Kline tests.

The second visit, conducted in the afternoon, comprised:

1. Penicillin treatment according to the results of the Kline test.
2. Those with raised IgM referred to the laboratory for further search for trypanosomes, lumbar puncture and treatment.
   Positive cases referred to hospitals for full treatment.
3. Those negative to *T. gambiense* infection given prophylactic Lomidine or Trimelarsan.
4. Those with negative tuberculin test given BCG.
5. Universal chest X-ray.

These arrangements (OCCGE, 1966) are given in detail mainly to indicate the amount of organization and of staff required to mount such an operation. The number of persons dealt with daily by this considerable team averaged 150. At the time of writing the project has not been completed. The number of new cases of sleeping sickness diagnosed, by most scrupulous survey, dropped from 79 in 1964 to 28 in 1965.

Part IV

THE ANIMAL TRYPANOSOMIASES OF AFRICA

Chapter 38

Pathogenesis and Pathology of Animal Trypanosomiases

R. N. T.-W.-FIENNES

INTRODUCTORY

The species of trypanosomes which are capable of infecting domestic animals in Africa have been described in detail in Chapters 1 and 2; they fall into three main groups. The widely distributed megatrypanosomes are of little or no importance as they are virtually non-pathogenic. The *brucei* group of polymorphic trypanosomes is of great medical importance because it includes the causative agents of human trypanosomiasis and may also infect wild and domesticated ungulates in silent or active form. In veterinary pathology, the group of monomorphic trypanosomes is by far the most important, including as it does two species, *T. congolense* and *T. vivax*, which are widely distributed and which are responsible for great economic losses of domestic stock. The monomorphic group also includes two species—*T. uniforme* and *T. dimorphon*—which have been accorded specific rank but which will not receive special attention in considering the pathology of the disease; *T. uniforme* is believed to be non-pathogenic while *T. dimorphon* has not been distinguished from *T. congolense* in most of the pathological studies which have been reported. *T. evansi* has some local importance in the Sudan where it is pathogenic for camels and horses but is of little or no importance elsewhere in Africa.

The disease processes of animal trypanosomiasis are complex and variable depending upon the nature and stage of the infection studied. Infections with *T. congolense* and *T. vivax* vary greatly in severity, duration and eventual outcome. Sometimes they run an acute course causing the death of the host in about ten days; alternatively, they may cause a more protracted illness from which the infected animal may ultimately make a complete recovery. Again, the infection may run a course intermediate between these two extremes. These striking variations are determined by a variety of factors which include the host's powers of resistance to the infection, the consequences of this on the infecting agents themselves, and the inherent virulence or 'invasiveness' of the causative organism.

The susceptibility of domestic stock to the pathogenic effects of certain species of trypanosomes contrasts strongly with the complete absence of symptoms in wild ungulates which inhabit the tsetse belts of Africa and which normally harbour trypanosomes pathogenic to other species. This mutual tolerance between host and parasite has probably been evolved over many millennia. It seems likely that in domestic stock in which trypanosomes cause disease the host-parasite relationship is of relatively recent origin.

A characteristic feature of trypanosomiasis in domestic animals is its tendency to relapse. A fatal termination is indicative of failure of the host's defensive mechanism while complete recovery denotes the host's ability to overcome the infection. An intermediate condition commonly occurs in which equilibrium is reached between host and parasite, i.e. the host is infected but remains in good health. In this latter state, often known as premunity, the host is refractory to fresh infection with the same species and strain of trypanosome. The premune host is, however, in a vulnerable condition since recrudescences of the disease are liable to occur if the animal is subjected to conditions of stress or physical strain.

Relatively little work has been published on the pathology of animal trypanosomiasis apart from the writer's own studies on the clinical pathology, morbid anatomy and histology of infections with *T. congolense* in cattle. In general, *T. congolense* causes a more acute form of the disease than does *T. vivax* but this is not always the case. No essential differences in the pathological picture as between these two infections are apparent and indeed the fundamental pathological processes in all forms of animal trypanosomiasis are probably similar. For descriptive purposes infection with *T. congolense*, on which most work has been done, will be taken as a model.

The course of infection with *T. congolense* and the associated pathological changes which occur will be described under the following circumstances:

1. in fully susceptible adult cattle
2. in calves of susceptible cattle infected early in life, and
3. in relatively resistant breeds of cattle and in animals which have acquired resistance either through exposure to low grade infection in early life or through the control of the infection by drugs.

CLINICAL ASPECTS OF PATHOLOGY

The relapsing nature of trypanosomiasis was first demonstrated by Ritz (1914, 1916) and of *T. congolense* disease in cattle, both adults and calves, by Fiennes, Jones and Laws (1946). Typical temperature curves are reproduced in Fig. 38.1. Temperatures in both normal and infected animals are subject to erratic fluctuations but the febrile changes which occur in trypanosomiasis can be seen clearly by plotting three-day averages. Peaks are then seen to occur at regular twelve-day intervals, each lasting for two to three days. These peaks are associated with an increase in the number of trypanosomes in the circulating blood. After three to four such peak periods a prolonged period of temperature elevation occurs lasting some thirty days. Up to this point, the pattern of disease is typically that of a relapsing fever, febrile episodes being followed by parasite destruction and an afebrile period. The end of the parasitaemic period is the 'crisis' and appears to correspond to the 'trypanolytic' crisis described by Ritz (1914, 1916), and by Mütermilch and Salamon (1928) who believe that the crisis is associated with antibody formation. Death commonly coincides with one of these crises, that is, when the temperature falls and the number of trypanosomes in the circulating blood diminishes. Thus, the crisis is the period following a temperature peak when trypanosomes are being destroyed in very large numbers.

A prolonged period of temperature elevation following the three initial crises is associated with the development of profound anaemic changes. In the acute disease death most commonly occurs at the termination of this prolonged period of fever, anaemia and parasitaemia. At this stage a 'haemolytic crisis' develops which is associated with massive destruction of trypanosomes and frequently equally massive destruction of red blood cells.

If the affected animal survives this crisis, it does so with greatly strengthened anti-trypanosomal defences, as a result of which parasites rarely reappear in the blood in such large numbers. Nevertheless, the animal suffers from a form of chronic wasting disease during which further episodes of the acute type of disease may occur. In animals which survive, gradual improvement may occur, particularly with *T. vivax* infections and more commonly in calves than in adult cattle. The end-point may be complete recovery with temporary immunity to the infecting strain of trypanosome or, alternatively, the development of the premune state.

In fully susceptible adult cattle, the infection usually causes death which is associated with extreme anaemia, cachexia and hypoproteinaemia. It is preceded by a period of twenty-four hours or more of recumbency, when the animal is

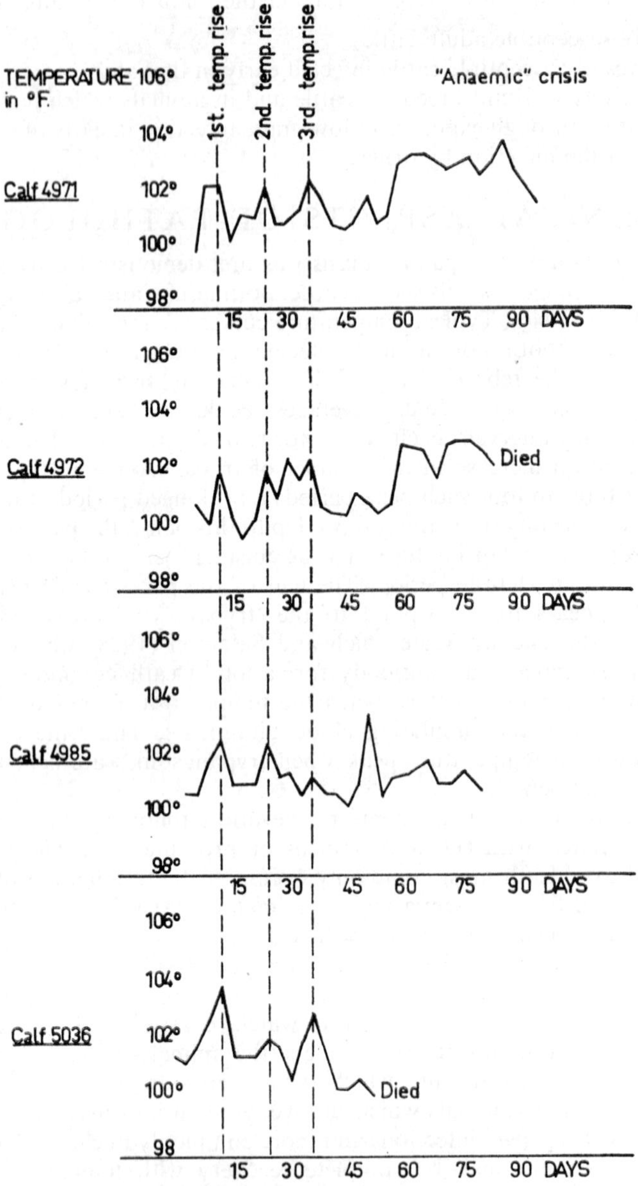

Fig. 38.1 'Smoothed' temperature curves of calves infected with *T. congolense*. (After Fiennes, Jones & Laws, 1946)

unable to rise to its feet, although paraplegia is not present and reflexes are not impaired. The affected animal is in a state of extreme emaciation, but the eye is bright. A feature of the chronic disease is the voracious appetite which continues until death; often affected animals are found dead with grass still in their mouths.

During the relapsing stages of trypanosomiasis the most severe symptoms occur at the time of crisis although at other times the temperature may still be elevated. At the critical period, appetite is lost, the eye becomes dull, and the animal is weak and lags behind the herd. The superficial lymphatic glands are invariably enlarged during all stages of the disease; the prescapular and precrural glands are not only palpable but may be seen to be enlarged from some distance away. Chronically infected cattle have the typical 'fly-struck' appearance well known to those acquainted with these diseases but somewhat difficult to describe. The animals are thin and emaciated and the hair has a characteristic rough, upstanding appearance. The skin is drawn tightly over the ribs and pelvis and lacks the healthy looseness found in normal animals. Muscular wasting is evident over the ilium. During the course of the chronic infection, supernumerary haemolymph glands of variable size develop in numerous sites in the body. Enlarged subcutaneous glands may be palpated at almost any site, particularly over the ribs and along the flanks. During the course of the disease weight loss is marked in adult cattle, while calves do not gain weight as quickly as uninfected ones. In experimental animals weight charts are a useful guide to the progress of the disease, since weight gain occurs when the animal is on the road to recovery (Fig. 38.2).

MORBID ANATOMY

The gross morbid anatomy of cattle dying from trypanosomiasis varies with the stage of the disease. Diagnosis, if not made from blood or lymph examination before death, may be difficult to establish from examination of the carcase *post-mortem*, particularly if it is not fresh. Trypanosomes quickly disappear from blood and organs once death has occurred and so may be difficult to demonstrate. Nevertheless, smears of blood should be taken for examination and smears should be made also from such organs as the lymphatic glands, spleen, lungs, heart, liver, kidneys, adrenal glands and, if feasible, brain and bone marrow.

In the early stages of the disease the spleen is grossly enlarged, the cut surface bulges around the capsule and the Malpighian follicles are very prominent. The lymphatic glands throughout the body are grossly enlarged and the cut surface is pale and watery; sometimes the medullary cells contain dark pigment which gives the medulla a blackish appearance.

In the chronic stage the spleen is small and atrophic but the lymphatic glands have the same appearance as in the acute stage. Fatty tissues throughout the body, especially around the heart and kidneys, become myxomatous. The lungs are oedematous; if incised and held up fluid will drip from them and there is some 'marbling' due to dilation of the lymphatic vessels.

Whereas during the acute stage of the disease red marrow is present throughout

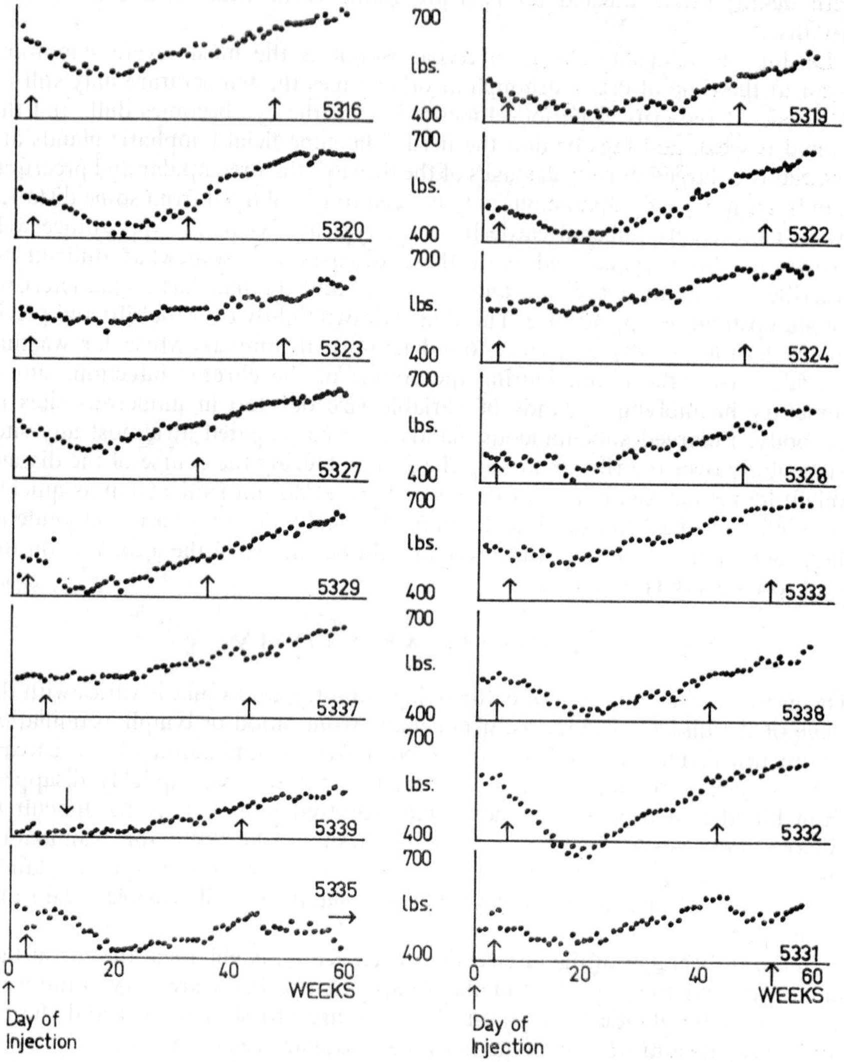

Fig. 38.2 Weight curves of adult bovines infected with *T. congolense*. Arrows indicate the days on which trypanosomes were detected in the blood for the first, and last, time. (After Fiennes, 1947)

Fig. 38.3

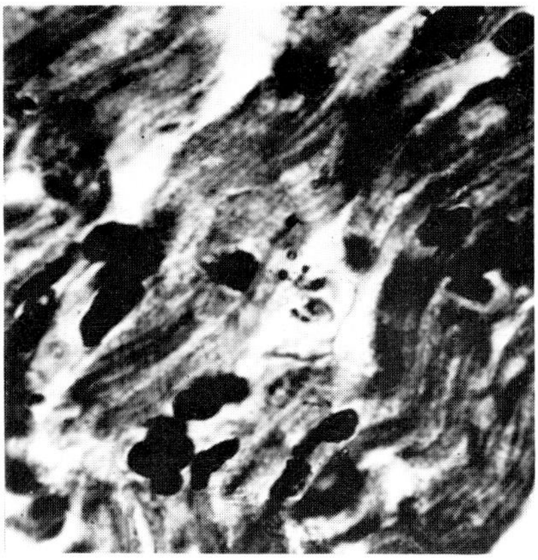

(1) Heart of Ox ×1,500. Trypanosomal embolus in a capillary.

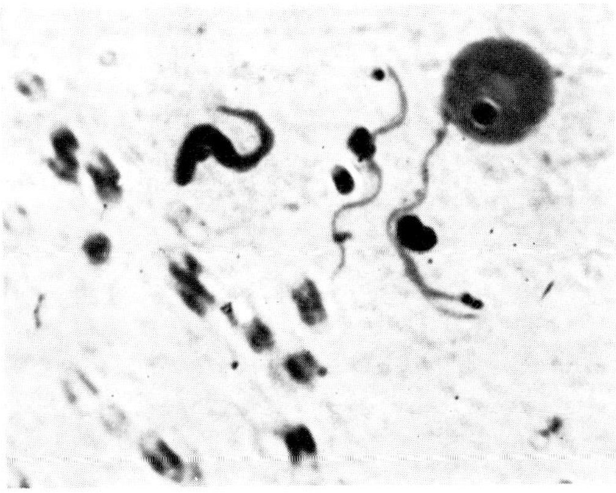

(2) Smear from Heart of Ox ×2,250, showing *Trypanosoma congolense* in early stage of lysis.

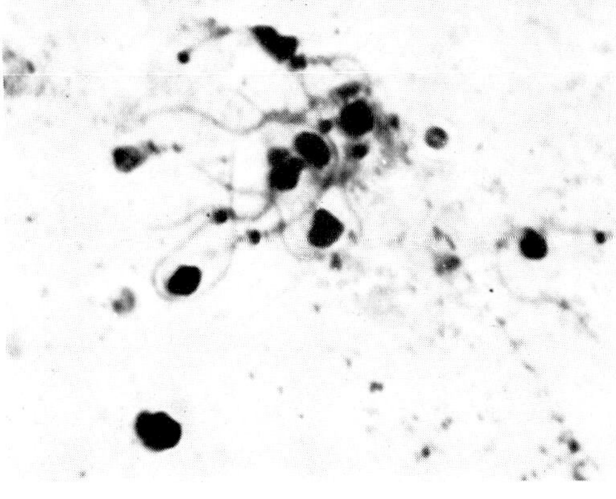

(3) Smear from Heart of Ox ×2,250, showing agglutinated *T. congolense* in second stage of lysis.

Fig. 38.3

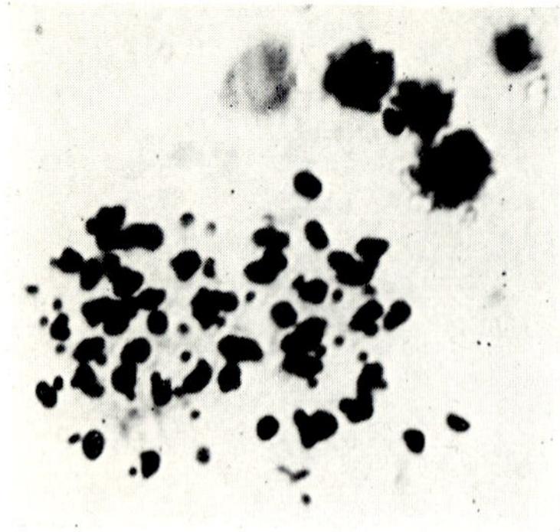

(4) Smear from Heart of Ox ×2,250, showing agglutinated *T. congolense* in final rounded stage ('Trypanosomes en boule' of Laveran)

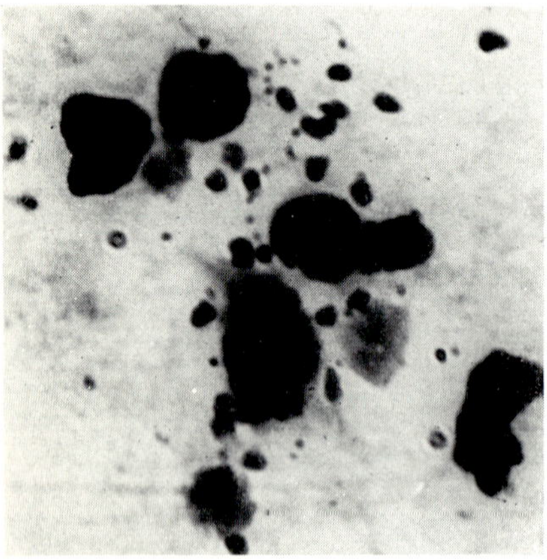

(5) Smear from Heart of Ox ×2,250, showing final stage of lysis of *T. congolense* and phagocytosis of debris.

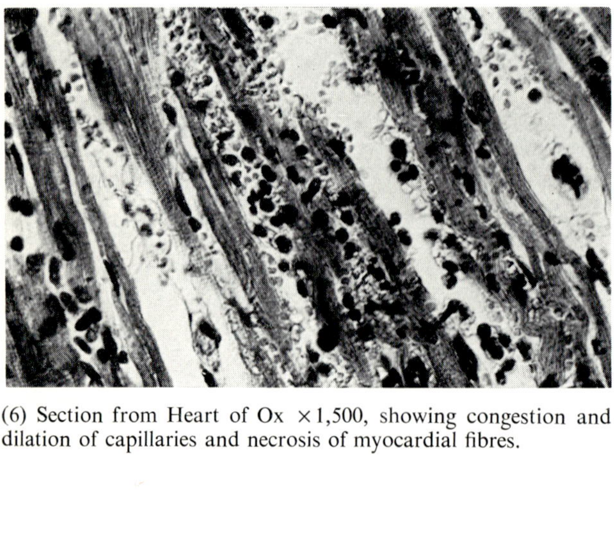

(6) Section from Heart of Ox ×1,500, showing congestion and dilation of capillaries and necrosis of myocardial fibres.

the shafts of the long bones, in the chronic disease red marrow disappears from the long bones but not from the ribs and vertebrae.

The presence of numerous haemolymph glands in many different sites is a further aid to diagnosis; these may be widespread in the subcutaneous tissue or may be attached to organs such as the thyroid or adrenal or may be embedded in the lymphatic glands.

In blood and tissue smears intact trypanosomes may not be found but the experienced observer may be able to identify degenerating forms such as those described by Laveran (1911) as 'trypanosomes en boule' and by Fiennes (1952b) in his studies on cryptic trypanosomiasis (Fig. 38.3, 2–4). Trypanosomes undergoing disintegration first lose their cytoplasm and give rise to 'ghost' forms consisting of ectoplast, kinetoplast and flagellum; subsequently they curl into rounded balls (the 'boules' of Laveran) which may be found singly or more often in agglutinated masses.

If trypanosomes cannot be found, a definite diagnosis cannot be established either from gross morbid or histological changes. Red-water fever (*Babesia bigemina*) is most likely to be confused with the early febrile stages of trypanosomiasis which it closely resembles. East Coast Fever (*Theileria parva*) in adult cattle frequently shows changes not present in trypanosomiasis, such as gastric ulceration and pseudo-infarcts of the kidneys. Other changes seen in trypanosome infections are signs of chronic anaemia with pale watery blood which does not clot well and the anaemic appearance of all organs. The right heart is dilated in chronic cases and the cardiac muscle is flabby and oedematous. The kidneys are nephritic and the liver is usually swollen, congested and dark in colour. Blood-tinged fluid is often present in the pericardial sac and in the thoracic and peritoneal cavities.

The lymphatic glands show progressive changes leading eventually to fibrosis. The germinal centres are depleted of adult cells and show Flemming's centres. The lymph sinuses are blocked by cellular debris. The medulla shows hypertrophy of the reticulum, the cells of which are often found to contain granules of dark brown or black pigment (Fiennes, 1952). Extensive deposits of haemosiderin are often present.

The parenchyma of the liver shows varying degrees of central lobular necrosis. The central veins and sinusoids are dilated and the Kupffer cells are very much enlarged. Periportal round cell infiltration is invariably present, consisting mainly of lymphocytes and occasional plasma cells.

The kidneys show severe tubular necrosis and round cell infiltrations frequently extend throughout the organ. In some kidneys extensive fibrosis is encountered. The glomeruli may be unaffected but many are found in a state of glomerular retraction. Pigment granules are often present in the tubular epithelium, particularly of the medulla (Fiennes, 1952).

In the acute disease, the histology of the heart may appear to be normal. In chronic cases, the cardiac muscle fibres are thin and appear to be atrophic; they are widely separated by dilated capillaries (Fig. 38.3, 6). Trypanosomes are often found in these capillaries but are difficult to recognize in sections unless by experienced observers. Small focal necroses are often associated with the presence of trypanosomes.

Fiennes, Jones and Laws (1946) described colloid cysts in the anterior lobe of the pituitary gland in three cases; these appeared to arise from disintegration of the oxyphil cells. There was in addition some round cell infiltration and cellular degeneration in this same lobe. It is, however, possible that these changes were not associated with the trypanosome infection because similar degenerations may occur as the result of previous infection with foot-and-mouth-disease.

The thyroid glands in trypanosomiasis cases are invariably affected. The acini become greatly distended with colloid and eventually disintegrate, after which round cell infiltrations occur and ultimately fibrosis.

The adrenal glands are constantly and severely affected. Round cell infiltrations occur below the capsule and sometimes extend between the bundles of the *zona fascicularis*. The whole cortex tends to become necrotic and sometimes necrosis and fibrosis extend into the medulla.

Appearances in sections of bone marrow vary according to the stage of the disease. In the acute stages, there are infiltrations with islets of lymphoblastic tissue; the haemopoietic tissue is abundant and contains an excess of normoblasts. In chronic cases, as recorded by Fiennes (1953a), marrow in the long bones is virtually destroyed but is still present in the ribs and vertebrae. The histology of the bone marrow at this stage of the disease has not been described.

The histological picture of the lungs is variable. In chronic cases, death often results from superimposed pneumonia and in such cases pneumonic lesions will be found. When such lesions are absent, some alveoli are found to be grossly dilated and sometimes ruptured; other alveoli contain fluid and the septa are greatly distended. The alveolar cells are enlarged and swollen.

HAEMATOLOGY

Hornby (1933) claimed that *T. congolense* was essentially a parasite of the blood, a view not seriously challenged prior to the writer's studies on prophylactic drugs. Fiennes (1950b) showed that this concept could not be reconciled with the known clinical pathology of chronic *T. congolense* and *T. vivax* infection of cattle, and he was able (Fiennes, 1952a) to demonstrate cryptic locations of parasites. Even in the acute stages of the disease, the distribution of trypanosomes in the blood is irregular; Fiennes (1946) observed that trypanosomes were more numerous in superficial capillary blood than in blood drawn from the jugular vein.

It is common practice in field work to examine wet blood preparations to detect the presence of trypanosomes but, if the parasites are inactive, their presence is easily missed since they are detected by their motility. It is, therefore, necessary to make blood smears for subsequent staining and examination in the laboratory.

In the past, much work has been vitiated because thin instead of thick blood smears have been used in diagnosis. Thin blood smears, fixed immediately in methyl alcohol, are excellent for differentiating trypanosome species, and, if fixed initially in osmic acid vapour, for the study of trypanosome morphology. It was, however, shown by Fiennes (1952a) that approximately 120 times more blood was scanned in thick smears, in which the red cells were haemolysed, than in thin. In his laboratory, it was standard practice to examine 600 fields of thick smear preparations but in some cases trypanosomes were only detected after weeks or even months of daily searching.

Where trypanosomes cannot be detected in blood smears, they may often be found—particularly with *T. vivax*—in smears made from lymphatic gland juice. These are easily prepared by aspiration of fluid from the much enlarged prescapular lymphatic glands by means of a hypodermic syringe. In cases in which trypanosomes still cannot be detected blood may be inoculated into susceptible laboratory animals but this procedure also often fails to reveal the presence of parasites.

Fiennes (1953a) described the results of autopsies on cattle dying from cryptic trypanosomiasis at an experimental station at Kiboko in Kenya. These cattle had been protected by injections of Antrycide and Dimidium and had developed cryptic infections such as have been described. Surprisingly, autopsy revealed lesions suggestive of the primary, rather than the secondary, stage of trypanosomiasis. Spleens were always grossly enlarged as in the primary stage of infection and never small and atrophic as in the secondary stage. This response, typical of the primary stage of disease, was probably evoked by repeated, short-lived episodes of high parasitaemia.

The haematological changes found in cattle during the various stages of infection with *T. congolense* have been described in detail by Fiennes (1954). Early haematological studies showed surprising discrepancies which suggested that there might be diurnal variations in the blood picture of normal cattle such as were used in these experiments; it was found that the total red cell count, haemoglobin percentage, mean corpuscular volume, mean corpuscular haemoglobin and mean corpuscular haemoglobin concentration varied quite considerably during the course of a single day and that such variations coincided with a rise or fall of the specific gravity of the blood plasma. Similar changes could be provoked by adrenalin injections and it became plain that they were due to variations of circulating blood volume and haemodilution. Thus, an ox might at 8 a.m., when still inactive, have a total red cell count of 8·0 million per c.mm. and a plasma specific gravity of 1·030. An hour later the red cell count might be reduced to 6·0 million and the plasma specific gravity to 1·028. Circulating blood volume estimations showed that the later readings were associated with an increased volume of circulating blood and, in spite of the lower erythrocyte count, the numbers of circulating red cells were in fact increased. It was also found both by the writer and independently by Unsworth (1949) that over a 52-week period, cyclical changes occurred in the blood picture of normal cattle so that the haematological findings varied within quite wide limits. It is important that investigators interested in the haematology of cattle should be aware of these physiological variations.

The haematological changes which occur in the course of *T. congolense* infections of cattle have been described by Fiennes (1954). In infections with *T. congolense* or *T. vivax* two clearly defined stages occur:

1. an acute stage with pre-critical and critical phases, and,
2. a chronic stage which is post-critical.

Macrocytic anaemia is found during the acute stage while, during the chronic stage, the anaemia is microcytic and is due to changes affecting both the red blood cells and the blood plasma. These changes operating in different proportion, determine four different courses of the disease:

1. THE HYPERACUTE COURSE. The hyperacute form of the disease (Fig. 38.4)

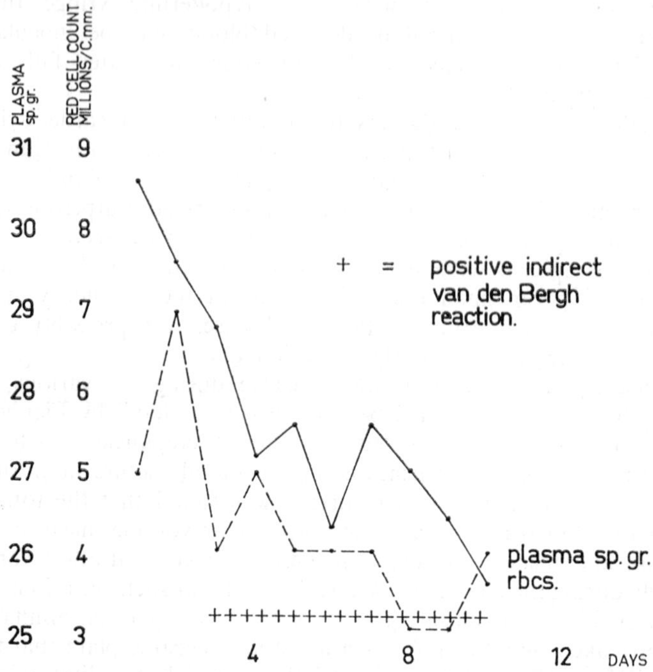

Fig. 38.4 Total red blood cell counts (rbcs), plasma specific gravity estimations (sp. gr.), and indirect van den Bergh reactions (+) during the course of a hyperacute infection with *T. vivax* in an adult bovine. (After Fiennes, 1954)

is characterized by severe haemolysis accompanied by hydraemia and is rapidly fatal.

2. THE ACUTE COURSE. In the acute course (Fig. 38.5) haemolysis is less severe in the early stages. There is an initial hydraemia, which is followed by dehydration. The end point is death at the time of a haemolytic crisis.

3. THE CHRONIC COURSE. The early stages of the chronic course are similar to those of the acute but hydraemia persists without dehydration. The haemolytic crisis, when it comes, does not prove fatal; the animal enters upon a chronic wasting disease which may persist for months and may eventually prove fatal.

4. THE RECOVERY COURSE. Recovery without treatment occurs exceptionally after several months of infection. In this form of the disease, the hydraemic factor is either absent or of rare occurrence.

The haemolytic nature of the blood changes during the relapsing stage of the disease is clearly shown (Figs. 38.4, 38.5) by the periodical positive indirect Van den Bergh reaction and by the demonstration that haemolysin is intermittently present. The presence of haemolysin in the sera of infected cattle is not easily demonstrated, probably because it is transitory and occurs only at the rare intervals of active trypanolysis. The test was done by separating the infected plasma and mixing it with normal ox red cells; normal plasma

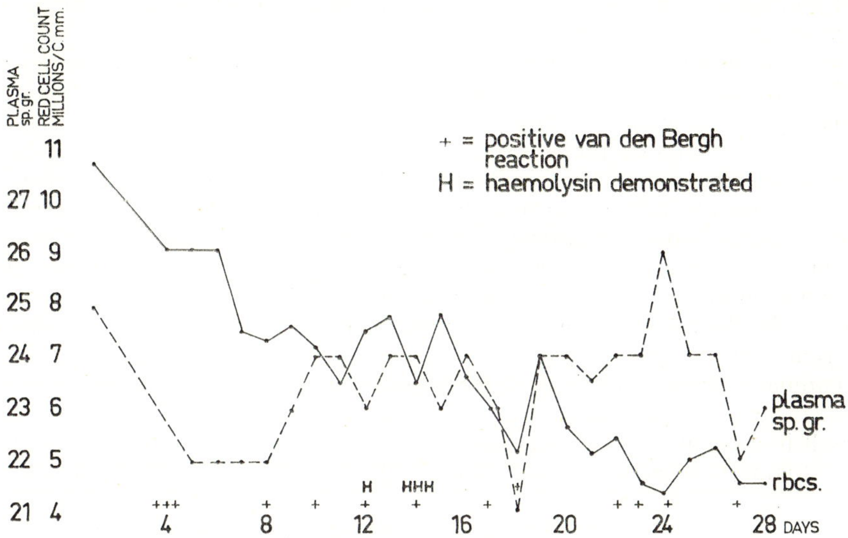

Fig. 38.5 Total red blood cell counts (rbcs), plasma specific gravity estimations (sp. gr.), and indirect van den Bergh reactions (+) during the course of an acute infection with *T. congolense* in an adult bovine. (After Fiennes, 1954)

was mixed with red cells from the infected animals. The mixture of cells and plasma was incubated at 37°C for half an hour and compared for colour changes with the original plasma. When positive, the test plasma haemolysed red cells from normal oxen, although the red cells from the infected animals were not usually haemolysed when transferred to normal plasma. Haemolysis did not occur when the plasma was inactivated at 56°C in the water bath for half an hour. In one case, however, red cells derived from an animal in the terminal stages of *T. congolense* infection were subject to continued haemolysis even in normal ox plasma.

The anaemia in the chronic and cryptic types of disease is microcytic and associated with low red cell count, haematocrit and haemoglobin. There is thus a continuous anaemia of varying severity but inadequate to account for the chronic wasting condition and the generalized parenchymatous degenerations which are features of the disease. During this stage, hydraemia is the distinguishing feature and in the writer's experience natural recovery occurs only in the absence of diminished plasma specific gravity. This hydraemic form of the disease is accompanied by (a) loss of plasma solids, (b) loss of water, and (c) changes of osmotic pressure resulting from plasma dilution. In addition, two other important vascular and circulatory changes occur, namely, generalized vasodilatation and greatly reduced circulation time. It would appear that the cachectic condition of affected animals depends more on changes in the composition of the plasma than of the red cells.

Plasma failure is evidently as important as red cell failure in the anaemia of chronic trypanosomiasis. The tissue degenerations which are common to the disease are typical of those arising from amino-acid deprivation and the centrilobular degeneration of the liver is similar to that of methionine starvation. This conclusion is supported by the observations of French (1935) who showed that trypanosome-infected cattle were in negative nitrogen balance.

Studies on plasma proteins in human sleeping sickness (Gall, 1956) have shown that the albumin levels of the plasma become seriously diminished whereas beta-globulin is increased. The important factor, both in the haemolytic stage of the disease and in the chronic, is the presence of dead, and not living, trypanosomes in the circulation. In the chronic stages of the disease living trypanosomes are present in the cardiac capillaries where they are apparently protected against attack by the body's defences. These are continually replenishing the animal's system with daughter trypanosomes which are destroyed, thereby imposing a continuous drain on the body defences and contributing to capillary dilatation and increased permeability. There is thus a continuous protein leak which reveals itself in a condition of hypoproteinaemia, this being, with the hydraemia, the most important haematological change in the secondary stage of the disease.

CHEMICAL PATHOLOGY

Several workers have investigated different aspects of the chemical changes which occur in the blood during the course of trypanosomiasis infections but the only studies in which anything approaching a full range of estimations has been made are those of E. R. Jones recorded in Fiennes, Jones and Laws (1946).

No significant changes have been reported in the blood or plasma levels of glucose (except for terminal hypoglycaemia), uric acid, creatine and amino nitrogen in either adult cattle or calves suffering from trypanosomiasis. Blood cholesterol levels closely follow red cell counts, both in adult cattle and calves. Very infrequently high levels of non-protein nitrogen have been found. Total protein estimations have shown low values.

At the time of relapse, blood chloride values in both adult cattle and calves may reach high levels and tend to remain high in adult cattle but gradually return to normal in calves (Fig. 38.6). The maximum increase occurs from the sixth week of infection in calves and from the eighth to tenth week in adults.

Calcium levels tend to be low at times of relapse but are otherwise normal in both adult and young animals. Inorganic phosphorus levels fall gradually in adult cattle but remain within the normal range in calves. Magnesium levels may be slightly decreased in adult cattle and calves at times of relapse but thereafter return to normal.

A significant reduction in the calcium/phosphorus ratio may occur in adult

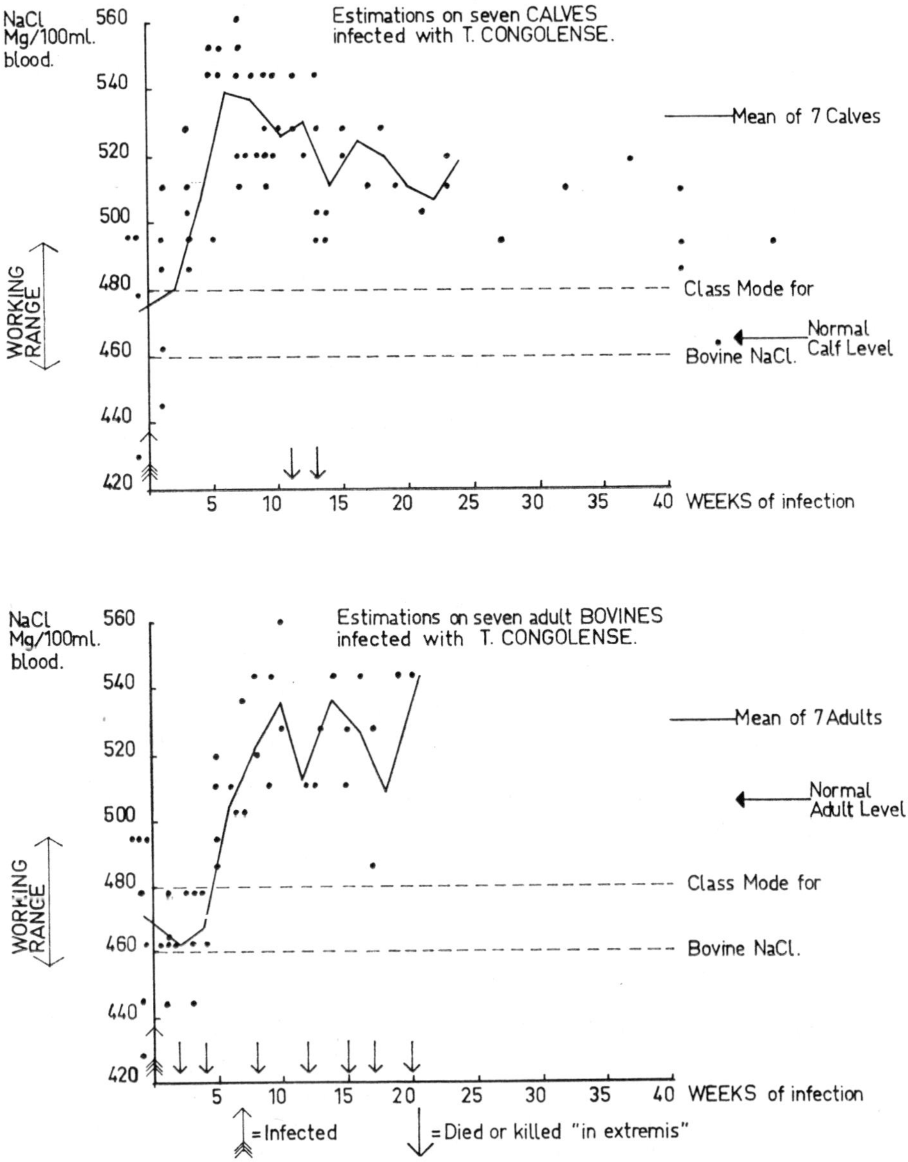

Fig. 38.6 Blood chloride estimations (NaCl) in seven calves and seven adult bovines during the course of infection with *T. congolense*. (After Fiennes, Jones & Laws, 1946)

cattle but not in calves (Fig. 38.7). Henderson (1931) and Le Roux (1933) found that the feeding of minerals to cattle suffering from trypanosomiasis helped to prevent geophagia.

It would seem to be important to obtain estimations of total protein levels and of albumin and alpha- and beta-globulins in the three types of disease under consideration, namely the acute relapsing stage, the chronic stage and the disease in calves.

Unfortunately, in earlier work only a few estimations of protein values were made and for evidence on this point reliance must be placed on the later work of Fiennes (1954) and of other observers such as Gall (1956). The work of the former relates to haematological studies and a fall of protein values in the serum is inferred from the reduction of plasma specific gravity; plasma specific gravity estimations are, of course, accepted as a field method for rough and ready estimation of serum protein values so that this inference has some validity.

Fluctuation in almost all blood chemicals indicates a profound disturbance of physiological mechanisms generally associated with morbid changes and no doubt impaired function of many organs. It was suggested by Fiennes, Jones and Laws (1946) that the changes of calcium and phosphorus values might be associated with the severe damage seen in the thyroid gland. These aberrations occurred only in adults and not in the less severely affected calves.

Evidently during the course of the disease there is profound electrolyte disturbance shown not only in the calcium and phosphorus variations but also in changes in the levels of magnesium and sodium chloride. The latter may possibly be associated with the pathological condition found to be present in the adreno-cortical glands.

Reference has already been made to the finding of positive indirect Van den Bergh reactions at times of crisis. The indirect test was invariably positive in moribund animals. No direct Van den Bergh positives were ever found and the blood chemistry does not suggest gross functional impairment of the liver. Very little has been done in the way of urinalysis; Fiennes (1954) found urobilin in the urine on rare occasions but only when the animal was *in extremis*.

CELLULAR PATHOLOGY

The commonest and most characteristic pathological change in chronic trypanosomiasis is the extensive involvement of lymphoid and reticular tissues especially those commonly known as the reticulo-endothelial or lymphoid-macrophage system. The lining endothelium of the blood vessels may also be hypertrophied and severely denuded (Fiennes, 1946). The writer has suggested that this is not due to agonal stripping but is a result of the intense mobilization of macrophage reserves. Where the endothelial lining of the blood vessels is deficient thrombosis may occur.

The widespread round cell infiltrations found in many organs, almost entirely of lymphoid type, are of the same order as those which occur in protein deficiency states like Kwashiorkor, but the generalized lymphoplasia is probably also a response to parasite attack and may be associated with antibody production. These and other factors will be discussed in greater detail later. It is here wished

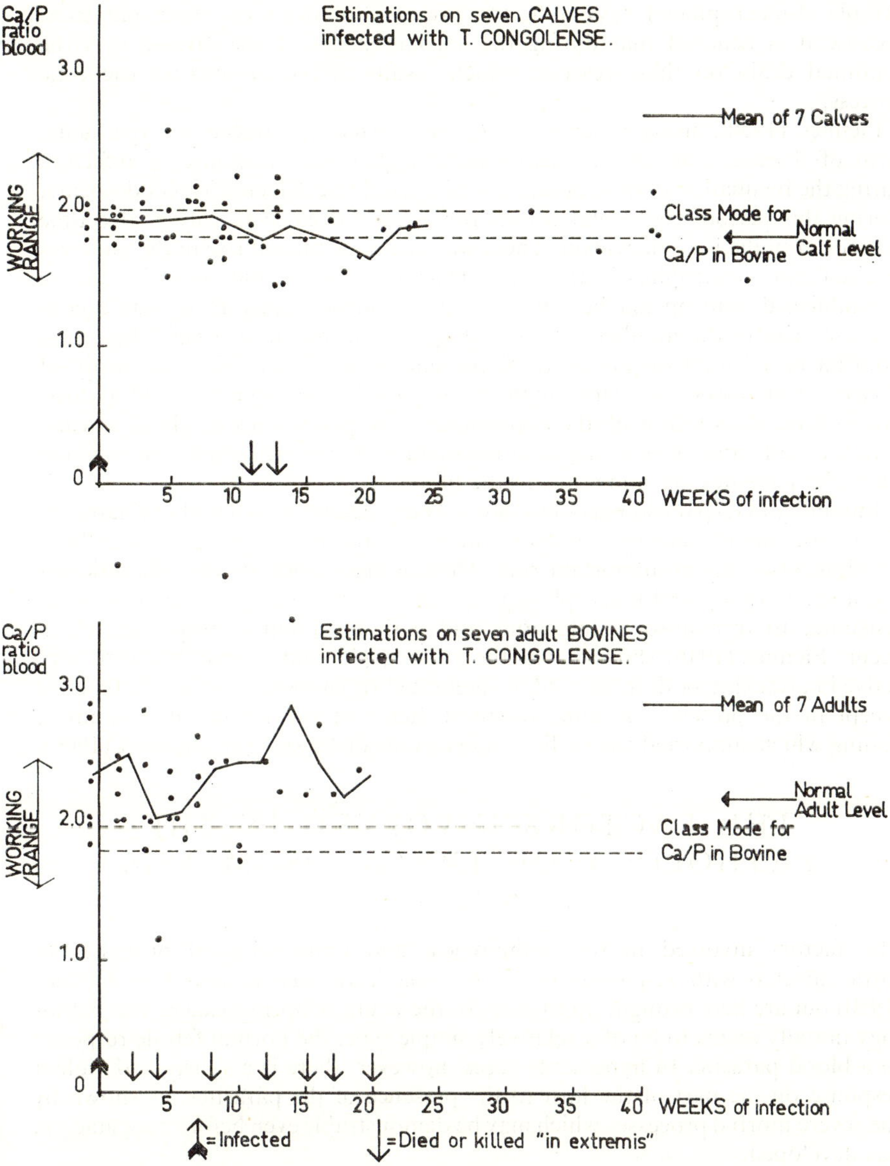

Fig. 38.7 Calcium/phosphorus (Ca/P) ratios estimated in seven calves and seven adult bovines during the course of infection with *T. congolense*. (After Fiennes, Jones & Laws, 1946)

to consider the problem of the more direct response of the reticulo-endothelial (lymphoid-macrophage) system to the presence of dead or living parasites, because it is believed that during the chronic stages of the disease it is the continual drain on these reserves which results in the progressive cachectic process.

Fiennes (1950), using a strain of *T. vivax* which produced a hyper-acute form of disease, was able to demonstrate a profound response to infection during the incubation period, before parasites could be detected in blood smears. During this period, eosinophil counts rose, and indeed, it is only at this time that eosinophilia is at all evident. There was also a significant rise in the numbers of circulating neutrophils in the early stages of infection but once the disease is established neutropenia becomes a feature. Subsequently there was a considerable rise in the numbers of circulating monocytes; in one case these rose from an initial level of 360 to 1,200 per c.mm. of blood. With this strain of *T. vivax*, death associated with a high level of parasitaemia occurred in adult cattle two to three days following the appearance of trypanosomes in blood smears.

In the acute and chronic stages of the disease, monocyte counts become high whenever parasites are numerous in the blood.

Immunity in trypanosomiasis has already been described in detail in Chapter 6. While one line of defence is humoral in nature (antibody production) cellular reactions also play an important role. There is clear evidence that the reticulo-endothelial (lymphoid-macrophage) system is intimately concerned with resistance to trypanosome infections and with the immune responses which occur. Fiennes (1946) showed that the polymorphs and monocytes were very active in attacking both intact and disintegrated trypanosomes but were inactive except in the presence of some humoral factor of the nature of opsonin, a finding which supported the earlier observations of Mesnil and Brimont (1909).

THE FACTORS INVOLVED IN THE PATHOLOGY OF TRYPANOSOMIASIS IN CATTLE

The factors involved in the pathological and immunological processes in cattle infected with *T. congolense* or *T. vivax* have been reviewed by Fiennes (1950) but are here brought up to date. In the acute relapsing stages, the pathology initially seems to be of a relatively simple type, the normal febrile response to a blood parasite. In hyperacute cases, however, there is an early and violent response on the part of the host to the presence of the parasites, as shown by the severe morbid processes which may be demonstrable even before parasitaemia has developed.

The chronic stage of trypanosomiasis is characterized by increasing cachexia usually terminating in the death of the animal. It is difficult to account for this progressive decline at a time when the numbers of trypanosomes present are steadily diminishing. Some possible reasons for this perplexing sequence of events have been mentioned above, namely, excessive stimulation of the reticulo-endothelial system and the mobilization of other endothelial reserves to an extent where the lining of the blood vessels becomes denuded with consequent thrombosis, hydraemia, serum electrolyte disturbance and hypoproteinaemia. Other possible contributory factors are considered below.

Direct Intervention of the Parasite

Neither *T. congolense* nor *T. vivax*, so far as is known, ever acts as a true tissue parasite either in the sense of being present sporadically in tissues or in forming the nests and islets found in infections with *T. gambiense* and *T. rhodesiense*. Trypanosomes may be found in an apparently resting stage in some organs, notably in the heart but in such cases they are always present in capillaries and not in the tissues themselves. Many workers, including the writer, have at one time or another believed that they had found developmental forms of *T. congolense* and *T. vivax* but no unequivocal evidence of their existence has so far been adduced. Schwetz (1928) and Schwetz and Fornara (1929) described leishmanoid forms of *T. congolense* from the brains and hearts of cattle, but these were almost certainly the 'trypanosomes en boule' of Laveran (1911), also described by the writer in his work on cryptic locations of *T. congolense*. There is thus no evidence that any form of tissue development takes place in the vertebrate body, analogous to that which occurs with *T. cruzi*.

The Anaemic Factor

During the course of both acute and chronic stages of *T. congolense* and *T. vivax* infections, anaemia may be severe. Red cell counts may fall as low as 2·5–3·0 millions per c.mm., haematocrit below 30%, and haemoglobin 40% to 50% of the normal human level.[1] Often, however, cattle which show a severe degree of anaemia are far less sick and survive much longer than others with less marked anaemia. It is difficult, therefore, to reconcile the anaemic changes with the clinical course of the disease. It has been suggested, particularly by Maegraith (1948), that tissue anoxia is the prime cause of the widespread tissue degenerations present in malaria which closely resemble those occurring in trypanosomiasis. It seems improbable that widespread tissue degeneration of the severity observed in cattle suffering from trypanosomiasis is accountable solely to the reduced oxygen-carrying capacity of the blood when it is remembered that the severity of symptoms is not directly related to the degree of anaemia present and that in other anoxic states, such as the 'blue baby', tissue degenerations of the same magnitude do not occur. It is unlikely that anaemia would have any profound influence on the course of the disease in experimental animals maintained in an inactive state from which most data have been obtained but might have a more pronounced effect on herds of cattle obliged to cover long distances to graze and to water. If, however, thrombosis of the smaller blood vessels in trypanosomiasis (as originally suggested by the writer) is eventually found to be widespread then anoxia would prove to be a factor of greater significance.

Intoxication

Many early workers attempted to demonstrate the presence of trypanotoxin by injection of massive doses of dead trypanosomes into laboratory animals.

[1] Normal values for cattle correspond with 80% of human values.

No conclusive evidence for the existence of a toxin was obtained, except that produced by the writer in relation to production of haemolysin from disintegrating trypanosome material. Fiennes (1950) reviewed the literature and repeated much of the work but was unable to demonstrate any deleterious effects from the injection of massive doses of dead trypanosomes into calves whether by the intravenous, the subcutaneous or the intradermal routes.

Anaphylactic States

Factors favourable to the development of anaphylactic states are present in trypanosomiasis. At each crisis, trypanosomes are destroyed in the blood in very large numbers and the system is permeated with dead trypanosome protein. At peak temperature periods trypanosome counts may be as high as 78,000 per c.mm. of blood; within a few hours the numbers may be reduced to a few hundreds. The animal may, therefore, become sensitized to trypanosome protein at each crisis so that at any crisis, except the first, anaphylactic shock might be induced. In hyperacute cases autopsy shows the mucous and serous membranes and the subcutaneous tissues to be splashed with haemorrhages. Death follows collapse and usually occurs after the temperature curve has fallen and after trypanosomes have to a large degree been eliminated from the blood. The picture is suggestive of anaphylactic shock.

Experimental evidence that protein, including trypanosome protein, can act as anaphylactogen is given by Novy, de Kruif and Novy (1917) using *T. evansi*, *T. equiperdum*, *T. lewisi* and *T. brucei*. Dead trypanosomes, obtained from rat blood, were washed and incubated with guinea pig serum (the sensitizing dose) both fresh and inactivated at 56°C for half an hour. The mixture when injected into healthy guinea-pigs (activating dose), caused acute anaphylactic shock in every case and usually death in two to four minutes, but only provided that all traces of trypanosome debris were not removed from the mixture by centrifugation at 88,000 revolutions per minute. The same trypanosome protein could be used repeatedly to sensitize sera for the passive transference of anaphylactic sensitivity. Neither the dead trypanosomes alone nor guinea-pig serum alone was able to reproduce this result. When the experiments were repeated with agar, peptone, normal serum and egg albumin as anaphylactogen, the results were identical, showing that the anaphylactic state was dependent on the inert trypanosome protein.

It is therefore evident that anaphylactic processes may contribute to the pathology of trypanosomiasis and reasonably certain that in the hyperacute type of disease death results from anaphylaxis.

Protein Deficiency States

The evidence adduced above suggests that serum dilution and hypoproteinaemia are the factors mainly responsible for the progressive decline of animals during the chronic stages of trypanosome infections. Fiennes (1954) found that cattle in which there was a demonstrable fall in the specific gravity of the plasma sooner or later succumbed during the chronic stages of the disease and that only those in which the specific gravity was maintained at, or near, normal levels recovered. In further (unpublished) work on the course and pathology of trypanosomiasis in 'resistant' breeds of cattle in Ghana additional evidence on this point was obtained. These 'resistant' breeds of cattle could be readily infected either experimentally or by natural exposure to tsetse-flies during calfhood. The course of the disease was similar to that in 'non-resistant' breeds of cattle except in one important respect, namely, that a fall in the specific gravity of the plasma did not occur.

The reasons for a reduction in the level of circulating protein in chronic trypanosomiasis are not fully understood. It has been shown that, as a result of trypanosome infection, the capillaries are dilated and their endothelial lining damaged so that loss of protein may occur through leakage or seepage. Boreham and Goodwin (1967) have demonstrated increased vascular permeability in chronic trypanosomiasis in rabbits which may be due to the presence of kinins as shown by Holdstock, Mathias and Schachter (1957). Boreham (1968) has shown that these pharmacologically active peptides occur in rabbit, cattle and man suffering from chronic infections with trypanosomes of the *brucei* group. Goodwin and Richards (1960) observed a progressive increase in the amount of kinin present in the urine of mice with acute trypanosome infections and Richards (1965) showed increases of kinin in the blood, ears, skin and feet of rabbits similarly infected. Kinins are not released in rats infected with *T. lewisi* even with heavy parasitaemia (Boreham, 1966; Goodwin & Boreham, 1966) suggesting that, since *T. lewisi* is non-pathogenic for rats, the production of kinin may be associated with pathogenicity. Kinins are believed to be produced during the antigen-antibody reaction.

THE PATHOLOGY OF TRYPANOSOMIASIS IN CALVES, RESISTANT BREEDS AND DRUG-PROTECTED CATTLE

The greater powers of resistance possessed by very young calves to the common disease o *f ica*e present in tsetse infested country was first noticed by that shrewd obfrsre Dr David Livingstone and recorded in his *Missionary Travels in South* cattlev (1857). Van Saceghem (1934, 1936, 1938), Schilling (1933, 1935, 1935a, 1936, 1936a, b), Schilling *et al.* (1933, 1934, 1934a, 1935, 1936, 1936a), Bevan (1928, 1936), Hornby and Bailey (1932) and Hornby (1941) recognized the greater resistance of calves to trypanosomiasis and foresaw the possibility of exploiting this resistance to develop cattle with a useful degree of tolerance to the disease. Fiennes, Jones and Laws (1946) studied in detail the differences in the clinical pathology, haematology and morbid anatomy, in calves as compared with adult cattle. These workers demonstrated that adult cattle infected with their strains of *T. congolense* invariably died after a febrile course of the disease lasting five to seven months. In adult cattle, at the 8th–12th week of infection a prolonged period of haemolytic symptoms leading to crisis occurred; thereafter, the acute stage gave way to the chronic. The adult cattle then went gradually downhill, whereas the calves began to recover. Throughout the course of the disease the calves had a bright appearance and their condition only became poor during times of crisis, when the coat was harsh and staring and the appetite lost. After the crises, appetite was regained and appearance was restored to something surprisingly like normal despite severe and persistent anaemia but weight increase was less than in normal calves. Nevertheless, the general trend of the chronic disease in most calves was towards recovery and by about the 26th week the blood picture approached normality. During the course of infection the calves did not show the neutropenia which is a feature of the disease in the adults and lymphocyte counts were relatively higher. Whereas infected adult cattle showed a tendency to hypoglycaemia at the time of the haemolytic crisis, the values in infected calves followed the same age curve as in uninfected calves. The high blood chloride figures of infected adults were present also in calves and serum magnesium showed some decrease as with the adults. Calcium/phosphorus ratios in the blood were normal in the calves whereas there was profound disturbance in the adult cattle.

Fiennes (1953b) pursued his work on calf infections in the course of experiments on the maintenance of cattle protected with Antrycide prosalt kept in country infested with *Glossina austeni*. In this series of experiments, all the Antrycide-treated cows produced normal healthy calves and returned to the bull. The second parturitions also proceeded normally. Haemoglobin levels were normal in the calves at birth. The heifer calves received treatment with Antrycide but no treatment was given to the bull calves until infection was demonstrated by positive blood smears. The results showed that the calves remained more or less refractory to infection since positive blood smears with *T. vivax* were not found until 73–224 days and with *T. congolense* from 47–279 days, the averages in each case being 129 and 120. These experiments confirmed that young stock are much more resistant than adults and showed that when treatment was given there was a progressive increase of resistance to trypanosomiasis resulting in a lengthening of the interval between treatments. Factors beyond the writer's control prevented the completion of these experiments.

In the writer's opinion there is little doubt that the greater resistance of very young animals to trypanosome infections, which is similar to that seen with redwater and anaplasmosis, is the key to finding a regime by which cattle can be raised in contact with tsetse flies. It is known that offspring of game animals of species which thrive in tsetse country succumb to trypanosomiasis if exposed to infection for the first time when they are adult. Adults of 'resistant' breeds of cattle, Muturu and N'dama, succumb to trypanosomiasis if they have not been exposed to infection when very young, and their calves—as shown above—are not resistant to infection but pass through the disease and some succumb to it. Adults of these breeds when transferred from the tsetse belt in which they are reared to another tsetse belt also succumb to trypanosomiasis. The differences between the pathology of very young animals and adult cattle is, therefore, a crucial point for investigation since greater understanding could lead to the development of methods to assist their resistant properties. In many parts of Africa, both in East and West, the native herdsmen deliberately take their cattle at certain periods and for a limited length of time into lightly infested tsetse country thus exposing them to infection. As a result, in numerous places, there exist herds, whether of resistant breeds or not, which are able to withstand intermittent exposure to infection where the tsetse challenge is not too high (*see* also Chapter 43).

In this connection the following account (hitherto unpublished) of the history of a European-owned herd of cattle maintained in light 'fly' country in Kenya is of particular interest.

An elderly and experienced European farmer of limited means obtained a lease of an uninhabited tract of country of two to three thousand acres some 90 miles from Nairobi. The area was regarded as unsuitable for stock-raising because animals previously introduced had died from trypanosomiasis. However, the new lessee believed that, with the promised co-operation of the Veterinary Department, he would be able to raise stock successfully. Veterinary advice and assistance were provided over a period of seven years in all and by the writer himself for some four years. The project became of such interest that a small experimental station was installed on the farm.

The land was developed by the provision of roads, fences, watering-places and roughly prepared pastures so that stock did not travel far to obtain fodder and water. Zebu cattle were introduced and, to improve this stock, Sahiwal bulls were imported from India. The objective was to raise cattle for beef; milking of cows was forbidden. Cattle were routinely dipped to protect them against tick-borne diseases and latterly, when the dips contained gammexane, some protection against tsetse-flies may have been afforded.

Although no tsetse breeding-places were discovered on the farm or its nearby environs, flies were present in considerable numbers, having been brought into the area by rolling stock on the railway which passed close to the farm. Regular fly counts revealed that tsetse were constantly present and that they attacked cattle. Wet blood films from all cattle were regularly examined and any infected animals detected were treated with Dimidium.

During the first and second years of the project losses from trypanosomiasis amounted to 20% or more of the herd and had this continued the business would undoubtedly have failed. During the third year the situation improved; cattle regained condition and the death rate fell. In the fourth year the cattle began to thrive, calves were being produced, the incidence of trypanosomiasis was markedly reduced and the death rate fell to a low level. In subsequent years very few cases of trypanosomiasis occurred and in any detected by blood examination the animals did not appear to be in ill-health. An especially careful watch was kept on the calves and it was found that they were becoming infected early in life but recovered without treatment and without overt signs of illness. One calf was found to be infected with *T. congolense* at birth but the infection disappeared after eight months, only to be replaced by infection with *T. vivax*. This calf was never treated and never appeared to be sick from either infection.

These interesting observations were discontinued after the death of the farmer but they had continued long enough to illustrate the ability of calves, born of dams with experience of trypanosomiasis resulting from light exposure to tsetse, to resist or tolerate infection with pathogenic trypanosomes.

TRYPANOSOME INFECTIONS OF RESISTANT BREEDS AND DRUG-PROTECTED CATTLE

The term 'resistant' in relation to breeds of cattle is plainly a misnomer, because they suffer from trypanosomiasis in early life and their ability to withstand trypanosome infections when adult depends on infection during calfhood and constant exposure thereafter. It is probable that these breeds have some genetical factor which enables them to resist a higher intensity of tsetse attack than would 'salted' Zebus. Nevertheless, it appears that the dwarf characteristics of these cattle and a tendency to delayed puberty are associated with calfhood infection. Often the calves have a stunted, unthrifty appearance similar to that seen in calves which have been infected with East Coast Fever. Moreover, it would appear that a number of calves, perhaps 25%, die from trypanosomiasis and never reach the resistant adult stage. It is plain that their resistance depends initially on acclimatization to trypanosome infections.

It has been shown that subcurative drug therapy acts to eliminate the acute stage of the disease, so that infected cattle pass to the chronic stage; they are then difficult to cure both because the chronic stage of the disease is always more difficult to cure than the acute and because the trypanosomes may be drug resistant. However, Fiennes (1953) confirming the observations of Calver (1945) in mice, has shown that both in mice and cattle infection with drug-fast trypanosomes can be cured by daily sub-curative dosage with trypanocidal drugs continued over some weeks. The pathology of this is not known, but one may suggest that the resistant powers of the trypanosomes are gradually weakened, so that the body's own defences are enabled to overcome them.

Fiennes (1953a) has given a detailed account of the autopsies of cattle exposed to natural infection from tsetse while under the protection of drugs. In these cases, cattle were ostensibly suffering from chronic or from cryptic trypanosomiasis in which the outstanding feature of the disease was splenomegaly, a finding in marked contrast to the small spleen seen in the chronic stage of untreated trypanosomiasis. These findings suggest that, under conditions of inadequate drug prophylaxis, cattle exposed to the continuing risk of infection from tsetse suffer from recurrences of modified acute attacks. Fiennes (1953) reviewed the work done on the therapeutic and prophylactic use of Antrycide in cattle and concluded that the effectiveness of the drug depended mainly on its ability to suppress infection to a point where the animal's own defence mechanisms were able to gain control. Although the cattle appeared to be in good health while under drug protection there was evidence that most, if not all, of them remained infected as shown by their lowered haemoglobin values and by the re-appearance of trypanosomes in the blood after exposure to undue fatigue or when subjected to artificial stimuli such as injection of adrenalin and TAB vaccine or rinderpest vaccination; serum antibodies could also be demonstrated by mouse protection tests.

Chapter 39

The Epizootiology of Trypanosomiasis in Livestock in West Africa

K. J. R. MACLENNAN

INTRODUCTORY

Many of the factors concerned with the occurrence and spread of trypanosomiasis have been described in detail in previous chapters and in considering the epizootiology of the disease in livestock in West Africa the reader will be referred to the relevant section for details of the processes involved.

Although, in West Africa, trypanosomiasis of livestock may be encountered in localities where tsetse flies cannot be found, the incidence and severity of the disease is usually closely related to the presence and prevalence of species of *Glossina*. The latter vary in their efficacy as vectors of pathogenic trypanosomes.

As has been described previously, the distribution and density of certain species of *Glossina* in West Africa are closely linked with climatic, vegetational and other environmental factors and, in most parts, seasonal changes occur which markedly influence the epidemiology of the disease in man and its epizootiology in livestock. Where the vector is one or other of the *palpalis* group (riverine tsetse) the same factors may influence the spread of the disease in man and in his domestic animals. For a description of the ecology of the riverine tsetse of West Africa the reader is referred to Chapter 32.

Where the vector belongs to the *morsitans* group (woodland tsetse) there is no such close parallelism between human and animal trypanosomiasis. The woodland species play little, if any, part in the transmission of the human disease in West Africa (*see* Chapter 33) but are of prime importance in relation to trypanosomiasis in livestock. Major changes in their distribution, usually of a non-seasonal and more permanent nature, are often associated with large scale epizootics. Conversely, regressions result in diminished incidence of the disease.

The trypanosome itself shows a remarkable capacity for variation as is evidenced by the differences observed in virulence, immunogenicity and response to chemotherapeutic agents. The animal host also differs in its response to trypanosome infection depending upon species, breed, strain or even the individual animal. The level of animal husbandry practised may have a marked influence on the epizootiology of the disease, particularly such factors as the nutritional state of the animals, the work load imposed upon them and the extent to which they are exposed to stress and strain. The type of husbandry adopted is often a reflection of general economic factors so that these may have an indirect bearing on the epizootiology of trypanosomiasis in livestock.

TRYPANOSOMIASIS IN THE ABSENCE OF *GLOSSINA*

Animal husbandry in West Africa is practised under a wide variety of environmental conditions ranging from the rain forests of the coastal belt through the sparser woodland savanna zones and the even scantier vegetational areas of the Sahel to the true desert of the Sahara.

As one proceeds from the coastal rain forests towards the desert areas of the interior, the localities in which livestock are exposed to the risk of contracting tsetse-borne trypanosomiasis become increasingly restricted to areas in which the fly can survive. The true desert is tsetse-free. The Sahel is almost entirely free from tsetse infestation except for specialized isolated foci of limited extent as seen, for example, along the river Komadugu Yobe north-east of Geidam in Northern Nigeria. In the Sudan zone, tsetse infest much more extensive areas of riparian vegetation lying between substantial areas of tsetse-free upland vegetation and farm land but there is sometimes dispersal into, and even permanent infestation of, non-riparian habitats. Through the increasingly moister vegetation of the Northern and Southern Guinea zones and the forests nearer the coast, permanent habitats become less restricted and the occurrence of tsetse becomes progressively more widespread.

Trypanosomiasis caused by *T. vivax* and *T. congolense* may occur outside the known range of *Glossina*. The seasonal migrations of nomadic stockowners in search of water and grazing often expose livestock to the risk of contracting trypanosomiasis in tsetse-infested localities; the resultant infections may be seen in animals far (sometimes hundreds of miles) removed from the area in which the infection was acquired and may spread to members of the herd which were not exposed to risk from *Glossina.* Such infections are more often due to *T. vivax* than to *T. congolense.* It is an observed fact that the further the herd is removed from areas infested with tsetse the higher the proportion of infections caused by *T. vivax.*

Infections with both *T. vivax* and *T. congolense* are not infrequently the cause of considerable ill-health among static groups of cattle in localities in which no *Glossina* can be found but which are within the geographical limits of tsetse distribution. The means by which such infections are transmitted has not been definitely established. It is unlikely that the incidence could be wholly accounted for by non-cyclical ('mechanical') transmission by biting flies other than tsetse though these may play a part in maintaining or augmenting the disease.

It is certainly true that a serious incidence of trypanosomiasis may occur among cattle maintained under static conditions when the nearest known primary focus of tsetse is ten or more miles distant and where no habitats capable of sustaining self-supporting colonies of tsetse are to be found in the intervening territory. While, even after several searches, it may not be possible to detect the presence of *Glossina* on or immediately adjacent to the land grazed by the cattle, this does not preclude the possibility of their presence as persistent searching may eventually reveal occasional individuals. In such circumstances contact between vector and host would be very close (analogous to the close man–fly contact referred to in Chapters 32 and 33) and the presence of tsetse below a detectable level would account, in part at least, for the incidence of the disease although 'mechanical' transmission may also play a part. It has, however, been shown that removal of the distant primary focus of *Glossina* combined with the effective administration of mass treatment may reduce the infection rate in cattle to zero. Furthermore, in such situations, the re-introduction of infected cattle is not followed by the further spread of the disease despite the continued presence of potential 'mechanical' vectors (Kirkby, 1963; Folkers & Mohammed, 1965). Although there is strong circumstantial evidence that infections with *T. simiae* in pigs, initiated by tsetse, may be maintained by non-cyclical transmission, this has not yet been confirmed by experiment.

Where trypanosomiasis recurs in a herd of cattle in which apparently effective chemotherapy has been administered to those animals showing patent infections, but not to those with possible occult infections, it is not justifiable to assume that, in the absence of tsetse, fresh transmission has taken place. Likewise, where the disease persists in a group of cattle, even after *all* animals have received mass therapy, it is not a warrantable assumption that this is due to the persistence of tsetse infestation, albeit below detectable level, when development of a degree of resistance to the drug employed would provide an alternative explanation.

Trypanosomiasis in camels caused by *T. evansi* is not linked to the distribution of *Glossina* but may occur, sometimes in a high proportion of these animals, in areas remote from tsetse. Infection rates of 27·6% (Godfrey & Killick-Kendrick, 1962) and of 5·3% (NITR, 1965) have been reported in camels infected with *T. evansi* but little information is available about the pathogenicity of this disease in West Africa.

Infections with *T. evansi* have not been reported as a cause of significant disease in equines, bovines or canines in West Africa although *T. evansi* is known to cause serious disease in other parts of Africa and in southern Asia.

T. theileri is frequently observed in blood films taken from cattle. The parasitaemia is usually sparse but is occasionally heavy. Infection rates ranging from 62% to 100% have been detected by *in vitro* culture of blood from young and mature stock whilst 12% of calves have shown infections (NITR, 1964). This trypanosome has only rarely been recorded as being pathogenic as a complication following, for example, rinderpest immunization.

TRYPANOSOMIASIS TRANSMITTED BY *GLOSSINA*

In livestock, the incidence of trypanosomiasis transmitted by *Glossina* is the product of the risk to which stock is exposed. The degree of risk depends on a number of factors including the species and density of the tsetse present; the infection rate in the tsetse; the species and strains of trypanosomes present; the sources of these infections (whether predominantly from feral or domestic animals); the feeding preferences of the flies and the extent to which the flies transmitting the disease are dependent on particular species of livestock as their source of food. The severity of the disease is also influenced by other factors including the breed and strain of the livestock at risk and the type of husbandry practised.

Factors Involving the Insect Vector

Species, Density and Infection Rate

The pattern of disease incidence in livestock is closely linked to the species and density of the tsetse which are responsible for transmitting it, but not always in a manner which can be clearly defined or predicted.

The savanna species, *G. morsitans* and *G. longipalpis*, and the forest species of the *fusca* group exhibit higher rates of infection than the riverine species and are much more efficient vectors. Larger livestock, with the special exception of slaughter cattle, are not taken in substantial numbers into the habitats of forest species because of the scarcity of suitable grazing. Of the savanna species, *G. morsitans* is the more important cause of disease but *G. longipalpis* can be responsible for very high infection rates in Zebu cattle which inadvisedly venture into localities infested by this species. The common riverine species, *G. palpalis* and *G. tachinoides*, show lower infection rates and mammalian livestock can exist in much closer association with these flies than with the savanna or forest species. The trypanosomiasis transmitted by riverine tsetse is frequently less acutely pathogenic and it is not unusual to find substantial numbers of stock surviving, with varying degrees of loss, where exposure to risk from riverine tsetse is present but not severe; in such circumstances livestock may develop a degree of tolerance to the disease.

It is difficult to assess the relative importance of these species of tsetse in the epizootiology of trypanosomiasis in livestock. Areas of savanna known to be infested with *G. morsitans* tend to be avoided by stockowners but livestock owned by nomadic pastoralists are often briefly exposed to severe risk during annual seasonal migrations. Contact between riverine tsetse and livestock may sometimes be close and even prolonged and, although these species are less efficient vectors, they are probably responsible for a significant proportion of the trypanosomiasis occurring in livestock in West Africa.

Very little information is available about the types of infection which result from exposure to different species of tsetse. Godfrey (1961), using *G. palpalis* in the laboratory, failed to transmit *T. congolense* (including *intermediate* and *dimorphon* types) to cattle, sheep or dogs. However, in the field, infections with trypanosomes of the *congolense* group occur, and may predominate, in cattle which are apparently exposed exclusively to *G. palpalis*, but in such circumstances it is virtually impossible to rule out the occasional presence of some other vector species such as *G. tachinoides*, dispersed *G. morsitans* or even *G. longipalpis*.

The density of *Glossina* may also be an important factor in determining the severity of the disease. A high density of an efficient vector may result in frequent transmission of fresh strains of trypanosomes which may overwhelm the hosts' defence mechanism. On the other hand, close animal–fly contact (analogous to the close man–fly contact described in Chapter 32) may, even at low fly density, lead to serious disease incidence. When a small group of tsetse, not necessarily self-contained but perhaps constantly replenished from a distant primary focus, become based on static livestock the incidence of trypanosomiasis may be serious; such circumstances are very favourable to the development of drug-resistant strains of trypanosomes unless the use of drugs is carefully planned and executed.

Distribution and Changes in Distribution of *Glossina*

The pattern of *G. morsitans* distribution (and possibly also that of *G. longipalpis* about which much less is known) is subject to very substantial fluctuations in West Africa. Particularly is this so where the activities of man, principally cultivation and hunting are, as in northern Nigeria, important factors in determining tsetse distribution. There have been large scale advances in some areas and regressions in others. When a livestock population is overtaken by an advance of *G. morsitans*, a high incidence of trypanosomiasis results and is usually apparent before the presence of tsetse is detected. Such epizootics are of dramatic intensity and may lead to substantial mortality in spite of curative therapy. If the stockowners are basically pastoralists they evacuate the area. Where this has happened in the past the following historical sequence of events is often discernible. Many years previously a large farming community may have died out as the result of some epidemic or may have abandoned their farms because the soil was impoverished or for some other reason such as war or slaving. With the passage of time the savanna woodland regenerates in the evacuated area and since such areas are often adjacent to populous country, pastoralists find them well suited to their needs. In due course tree cover and wild animals become re-established and the area again becomes a suitable habitat for *G. morsitans* though it may remain uninfested until conditions favourable for the spread of the fly from a more distant focus have been established. The creation of substantial forest reserves, routes for migratory cattle or further regression in the pattern of human settlement may provide the necessary bridge for the re-invasion of the area by tsetse from some pre-existing and perhaps distant habitats.

Influxes of human population have caused large scale shrinkages in the areas infested by savanna tsetse but usually have less effect on the riverine species. In such localities the incidence of trypanosomiasis may be sufficiently low to permit seasonal or even all-season use for rearing livestock. However, the intensive cultivation of such trees as mango, guava and banana and of tall crops such as sugar-cane can provide suitable habitats for tsetse thereby causing a serious incidence of trypanosomiasis in susceptible livestock.

Influence of Seasonal Fluctuations on Livestock Distribution

Seasonal climatic changes, which throughout West Africa are pronounced, fundamentally affect the epizootiology of trypanosomiasis of livestock because they oblige pastoralists to migrate in search of water and grazing in the dry season and also because of their influence on the distribution and density of tsetse. Streams shrink or dry out progressively during the dry season and fire makes inroads into the vegetation which provides suitable microclimates in which riverine tsetse are able to survive when the ambient climate becomes unfavourable (*see* Chapter 32). Savanna species also become more restricted during the hot dry season, though this tendency is less marked in southerly zones of higher humidity. The result is that exposure to the bites of *Glossina* becomes progressively less general as the hot season advances. The risk of contracting trypanosomiasis may however become more intense where tsetse are concentrated, as at watering places and seasonal swamps favoured for grazing, but the general risk is sufficiently reduced to make possible the massive seasonal migration of Zebu cattle which is such a prominent feature of stock management in much of West Africa. The stock move in very large numbers into areas of risk from riverine tsetse, and often pass through areas infested by savanna species on their journeys to the fairly closely delineated areas in the south where risk from savanna tsetse is minimal or non-existent, but which are usually infested by riverine tsetse. The cattle then remain at some risk until sufficient rain has fallen in their wet-season homes in the north to enable them to return. In northern Nigeria, for example, the five provinces which have substantial areas uninfested by *Glossina* cover 44% of the country but hold 76% of the counted cattle population during the rains. South of these provinces are the tsetse-free Jos and Mambilla plateaux. If these are excluded, 54% of the country is seen to hold only 14% of the total counted cattle population, trypanosomiasis being the most important cause of failure to exploit to a greater extent this very large grazing potential (MacLennan, 1963). The dry season regression in tsetse density and distribution facilitates the dry season exploitation of southerly grazing areas not infested by savanna tsetse. Such cattle experience a degree of trypanosomiasis but can usually avoid severe consequences by leaving infested areas when the advent of rain again makes possible their return to safer areas. Nevertheless, severe outbreaks of trypanosomiasis result from injudicious exposures to risk. This movement accounts for the occurrence of trypanosomiasis well outside the infested area. But as will be seen later, there are circumstances which enable livestock to survive with varying degrees of economic loss in areas of light risk.

Host Preferences

Host preference of *Glossina* is a factor which may be expected to influence the pattern of disease in domestic stock. The frequency with which tsetse feed on livestock has an important influence on the degree of risk to which the animals are exposed and the fact that they are seldom fed upon may account for the presence of certain classes of susceptible mammalian livestock in apparently good health in some areas of risk. This could also account for the presence of apparently healthy sheep and goats under certain circumstances. However, where tsetse density is high, even stock which are not ordinarily favoured as sources of food may be fed upon sufficiently often to cause severe trypanosomiasis. In both East and West Africa it has been shown that as the proportion of feeds derived from bovids increases so does the infection rate among tsetse. In the largely 'artificial' conditions prevailing along the cattle trade routes in Nigeria, exceptionally high infection rates have been observed among the associated tsetse populations. Food sources evidently have an important influence on degree of risk.

Factors Involving the Parasite

Species and Strain of Trypanosome

The clinical significance of different species and types of trypanosomes in livestock is described in Chapter 41.

The species and strain of trypanosome involved affect the disease pattern and one aspect has been alluded to earlier (p. 755) when considering *T. vivax* and *T. congolense* in relation to *Glossina* distribution. The subject will be discussed again when considering the epizootiology in different species of livestock. Pigs, for example, may exist in reasonable health, although exposed to some risk, until a strain of *T. simiae* of appropriate virulence is introduced, when a startling mortality may result. Under some circumstances, horses and donkeys may do reasonably well until a virulent strain of *T. brucei* appears. Cattle previously exposed to some risk, but nevertheless thriving, may be taken into a new area where a particularly virulent strain of *T. vivax* may cause a severe epizootic with such rapid fatalities that considerable losses may be sustained before treatment can be made available. It is suspected that *G. longipalpis* is prone to transmit this type of disease.

Differences in the course of infection caused by *T. congolense* and by its *intermediate* and *dimorphon* types have been noted by Godfrey (1961). He has shown that in cyclically transmitted infections in oxen and sheep *congolense* and *intermediate* types were less pathogenic than *dimorphon* types. A *dimorphon* type was also more pathogenic for the dog than a *congolense* type which caused only a low parasitaemia and did not kill. 'In general the *congolense* type was characterized by low infection, low pathogenicity, and low parasitaemia; the *intermediate* type by high infectivity and high parasitaemia but low pathogenicity; and the *dimorphon* type by high infectivity, high parasitaemia and high pathogenicity' (Godfrey, 1961). Certainly in the field in northern Nigeria the longer types occur much more frequently in blood slides taken from cattle presented for treatment for trypanosomiasis than the classical small *congolense* types. The longer *dimorphon* types also tend to become drug resistant and this may be a factor leading to their predominance.

Variations in pathogenicity are also a feature of *T. vivax* strains. Fairbairn (1953) suggests that the longer strains of *T. vivax* give rise to a less acute type of disease than do the shorter strains.

Folkers and Jones Davies (1966) have shown that in Zebu cattle infected with trypanosomes but removed from areas where cyclical transmission is occurring, *T. vivax* progressively becomes the predominant infection, whereas the ratio between infections with *T. vivax* and *T. congolense* is not affected in this way when the cattle remain in a tsetse-infested area, an experience confirmed by workers in Zambia.

There is no doubt that epizootics of bovine trypanosomiasis are most frequently caused by infection with *T. vivax* and *T. congolense*. Infections with *T. brucei* are seldom seen in routine blood examinations and then only when cattle are maintained in close contact with tsetse. Godfrey and Killick-Kendrick (1961), examining Zebu cattle in an area where the risk of contracting trypanosomiasis was regarded as moderate, were unable to detect infections with *T. brucei* by thick and thin blood film examinations although the combined infection rate by *T. congolense* and *T. vivax* was 16·1% for thick smears and 14·6% for thin smears. However, by sub-inoculation of blood from the cattle into susceptible rats they succeeded in showing that *T. brucei* was in fact present in 6·4% of the cattle examined. In two other localities where the risk to which the Zebu cattle were exposed was of a different type, the overall infection rates revealed by the combined examination of thick and thin blood films and rat inoculation were found to be 42% and 50%, respectively, but the infection rate with *T. brucei* was 0% and 6%, respectively. Among Zebu cattle exposed to severe risk along a stock route for slaughter cattle, the infection rate with *T. brucei* was found to be 1·6% whereas 24% were infected with *T. vivax* and 7% with *T. congolense* (NITR, 1964). Even though the actual infection rate with *T. brucei* may be much higher than is indicated by routine blood film examinations, it cannot be regarded as an important cause of acute clinical trypanosomiasis in cattle in West Africa as compared with *T. vivax* and *T. congolense*. *T. brucei* is, however, often the cause of serious disease in equines and canines. Whether it may play a part in chronic bovine trypanosomiasis has not been fully studied.

When susceptible cattle are freshly exposed to the risk of contracting trypanosomiasis in the field, they are liable to become infected with one or more species of pathogenic trypanosomes. In West Africa when infections first appear, *T. vivax* is the predominant species and often causes acute illness and death;

occasionally, the onset and history are suggestive of anthrax. In the animals which survive, either naturally or with the aid of drugs, *T. congolense* tends to become the dominant infection seen in blood films, even though its presence may have escaped detection in the early stages of the outbreak. The pathogenicity of both *T. vivax* and *T. congolense* varies within wide limits.

T. simiae is a most important pathogen of pigs and may also cause acute illness in susceptible goats exposed to *G. morsitans* in areas where this trypanosome is present. Infections with *T. simiae* provide an interesting illustration of the effect on the virulence of the disease which may be determined by the species of animal from which the infecting strain is derived. Bruce *et al.* (1913) as quoted by Stephen (1966a), recorded that 'if goats are infected with *T. simiae* directly by the bite of the fly most of them will die, whereas if the parasite is passed for a generation or two through goats, monkeys or the wart-hog the rate of mortality for the goat will fall. It may also be remembered that the matter is of little practical importance as under natural conditions goats will always be infected by the bite of the fly; but it is interesting in showing the fallacy of judging from the action of laboratory strains as to what will occur in nature'.

Although trypanosomes resembling *T. simiae* are occasionally seen in blood films from cattle in West Africa, Stephen (1966) draws attention to the 'universal failure of research workers to infect cattle by sub-inoculation and fly challenge'.

Therapy and the Source of Trypanosomes

The incidence of the species of trypanosomes causing disease may be influenced by long-term curative and prophylactic therapy; this subject is considered further in Chapter 43. There is some evidence (Folkers & Jones-Davies, 1966) to suggest that the widespread use of homidium over a period of years leads to a decrease in the incidence of *T. vivax* infections as compared to those caused by *T. congolense* in cattle in northern Nigeria. The extent to which this influence affects the type of infection will depend on the extent to which infections in tsetse are themselves derived from feral or domestic animals, and on the relative effectiveness of the treatment for the two species of trypanosome.

Factors Involving the Mammalian Host

Species and Breed of Host

The most significant factors involving the host are susceptibility to trypansome infection and ability to tolerate the effects of infection. These factors have already been discussed in Chapter 6 and the pathological processes involved have been described in Chapter 38.

Livestock vary greatly in their reaction to trypanosome infection, depending upon breed, strain or even the individual animal. Much also depends on the conditions under which livestock have been raised and maintained. The ability of animals to survive, and even to thrive, in tsetse-infested localities is dependent on the acquisition of a degree of tolerance or immunity resulting from earlier exposure to infection, and this in turn is influenced by the degree of risk to which they were previously exposed. Even the so-called 'resistant' breeds may succumb to severe trypanosomiasis when exposed to infection for the first time, or to new risks, or are worked for draught purposes, unless protected by maternal antibodies or by therapy. In animals without previous experience of the disease, the outcome of infection depends largely on the severity of the risk to which they are exposed, whereas those which have been previously exposed, and which possess the potential to respond, will have acquired a partial tolerance and may therefore be able to withstand a more severe challenge. In the latter case, indirect influences, such as the occurrence of other infectious diseases, parasitism or malnutrition, may be of greater importance than the severity of the trypanosome challenge. Because of these influences, it is often difficult to assess the true significance of the degree of parasitaemia observed in blood films taken from tolerant livestock, and this probably explains the conflict of opinions which have been expressed on this subject.

It has been reported that wild animals, normally thought to be tolerant or resistant, may become ill from trypanosomiasis when subjected to stress factors associated with capture.

BOVINES. Certain aspects of the epizootiology of trypanosomiasis in bovines have been described above and will not be repeated.

Various breeds of cattle are encountered in West Africa, including freshly imported exotic stock, Zebu cattle of remote or recent Asiatic origin, and aboriginal breeds such as N'dama (Hamitic longhorn) and Muturu (dwarf shorthorn). The two latter breeds, which are dwarf and humpless, are able to adapt themselves to a degree of risk from trypanosomiasis which the other breeds are unable to withstand. The nature of this adaptation has been discussed in Chapter 6. Imported exotic breeds are highly susceptible to the effects of trypanosome infection while the various types of indigenous Zebu stock occupy an intermediate position. The latter, in turn, show distinct differences in their susceptibility to trypanosomiasis, varying from the 'White Fulani' type which withstands exposure to continuous slight or periodic risk to the larger 'Bororo' or 'Red Fulani' cattle of the drier zone which are more vulnerable. The reaction to trypanosome infection is only one, but sometimes the most important, of a complexity of factors which determine breed suitability for different localities.

Crosses between Zebu (usually 'White Fulani') and indigenous dwarf breeds provide a group of cattle types in West Africa which are less susceptible to trypanosomiasis than the larger Zebu, but more susceptible than the indigenous dwarfs. Zebu cattle are preferred by pastoralists because of their larger size, higher milk yields and better herd instinct but, where the trypanosomiasis risk is sufficiently great, cross-breeding may be practised in an endeavour to rear resistant stock; as much Zebu blood is introduced as the trypanosome risk will permit. This method of livestock husbandry is adopted in several parts of West Africa and is well exemplified by the Kateku Fulani of Borgu in the Ilorin Province of Nigeria, where stock are maintained under relatively static conditions in close contact with *G. morsitans* and riverine tsetse. Outbreaks of trypanosomiasis are liable to occur in times of drought when stock-owners are obliged to move their animals into fresh territory in search of water and grazing, thus exposing them to infection with different strains of trypanosomes. In such circumstances, even dwarf cattle are liable to contract acute trypanosomiasis particularly if, when living in association with tsetse, they are exposed to other adverse influences such as malnutrition, intercurrent disease, or the earlier types of anti-rinderpest inoculation. Several observers have recorded trypanosomiasis breakdown in dwarf cattle which are worked.

In Zebu cattle in Nigeria, the more severe reactions associated with the older type of anti-rinderpest vaccination were not infrequently accompanied by serious clinical trypanosomiasis due to the exacerbation of latent or mild infections. The occurrence of clinical trypanosomiasis can also be a serious problem in animals with occult or mild infections which are being broken in for draught purposes.

EQUINES. Horses do not thrive, even if they do not soon succumb to trypanosomiasis, in tsetse-infested areas. Where the risk is slight, they may survive and be useful for a time, but sooner or later they succumb to the disease in the absence of treatment. Horses die out rapidly when exposed to infection with *T. brucei* even when the risk appears to be only moderate. While they cannot be maintained in areas of high risk, horses are often observed to pass through such areas during the dry season; some individuals may be able to adjust themselves to risks of this kind, and so become 'salted' and consequently of enhanced value. There is little documented evidence either on this subject or on the ability of indigenous dwarf breeds such as the Pagan pony to withstand trypanosome infection better than animals of Barb or Bahr el Gazal (Dongola) extraction. Baker (1958) recorded the existence of a thriving group of the latter in the apparently tsetse-infested Central Province of Liberia.

Donkeys may show a definite tolerance to trypanosome infections and are commonly used as beasts of burden on routes traversing areas where exposure to both savanna and riverine tsetse constitutes substantial risk.

The trade in natural soda (kanwa) between the Bilma Oasis and the Bamenda highlands provides a notable example of the use of donkeys to carry loads through areas where the risk is sufficiently great to decimate herds of Zebu cattle. These donkeys survive when exposure is periodic and when it is not a new experience for them. Donkeys may die from acute trypanosomiasis in substantial numbers when first exposed to infection with *T. brucei*, as happened some years ago among animals carrying produce into Kano City from neighbouring fruit and vegetable farms (*see* Chapter 32).

T. brucei causes serious disease in both horses and donkeys. Infections with *T. vivax* and *T. congolense* are not uncommon. Infections with *T. congolense* are secondary only to *T. brucei* in severity but infections with *T. vivax* are comparatively mild.

SHEEP AND GOATS. The epizootiology of trypanosomiasis in sheep and goats in West Africa is similar in some respects to that in bovines. Susceptibility to the effects of trypanosome infection varies according to breed and strain and, as a general rule, dwarf types are more resistant than larger animals. As with cattle, sheep and goats are often subject to seasonal migrations. The larger types owned by pastoralists migrate into tsetse-infested areas in huge flocks during the dry season. Sheep penetrate further into these areas than goats, but it is questionable whether this is related solely to the risk of contracting trypanosomiasis, since goats are known to be more susceptible than sheep to other influences.

The smaller, more tolerant types of sheep and goats, and even some intermediate types, may be maintained in tsetse-infested areas as village livestock, the smaller types being the more adaptable to these conditions. In the main savanna areas, the types of sheep and goats kept as village livestock, while capable of withstanding slight to moderate risks, do not survive in the face of greater risks. When advances of *G. morsitans* occur it is usual to be told that the sheep and goats have died.

Little information is available on the relative importance of the different species of trypanosomes which infect sheep and goats in West Africa. Edwards, Judd and Squire (1956) studied the disease caused by *T. vivax*, *T. congolense* and *T. brucei*, in different types of sheep and goats in Ghana. The strain of *T. brucei* used in these experiments originated from a pig and was found to be pathogenic for both dwarf and long-legged sheep and goats. The course of the disease observed followed a general pattern irrespective of the species of trypanosome causing the infection. The cases which occurred fell into four categories, namely, acute, sub-acute, chronic and cryptic.

On occasions *T. simiae* has been noted as an important pathogen in goats.

PIGS. The epizootiology of trypanosomiasis in pigs has been described by Stephen (1966a) in his admirable review of pig trypanosomiasis in West Africa.

According to circumstances, the disease in pigs may be mild or even clinically occult, may be the cause of chronic ill-health, or may be so severe as to cause sudden death.

The severity of the disease in pigs varies with the species and strain of the infecting trypanosome and with the susceptibility of the animal. Variations in breed susceptibility are evident; exotic breeds are highly susceptible to virulent trypanosome infections while indigenous breeds often show a degree of tolerance or resistance to the disease (Birkett, 1958).

Infections caused by *T. congolense* and *T. brucei* are usually associated with a relatively mild type of disease during which the animal may harbour trypanosomes for up to 200 days; some animals remain in apparently good health while others show signs of chronic ill-health. *T. vivax* has not been observed to cause trypanosomiasis in pigs maintained under natural conditions in West Africa.

T. simiae is by far the most important cause of trypanosomiasis in pigs in West Africa and may give rise to acute or peracute outbreaks with severe symptoms and high mortality. The outbreaks may be of such severity as to simulate anthrax. The prepatent period is usually 4–6 days and death is usual within five days but often within twenty-four hours of detectable parasitaemia.

Pigs may live and thrive reasonably well in areas of light risk in West Africa until a virulent strain of *T. simiae* is introduced. Such risk is evidently greater in the presence of woodland than of riverine tsetse though, under field conditions, it is often difficult to exclude the possible presence of the savanna species as the cause of an outbreak. According to Stephen (1966a) the warthog is the principal, and possibly the only, reservoir of *T. simiae* though other species of wild pig may also harbour this species of trypanosome. It is known that marked changes in the virulence of *T. simiae* may follow syringe passage in different animals, but since natural infections in pigs always originate from tsetse this observation probably has no epizootiological significance.

Some interesting observations have been made by Killick-Kendrick and Godfrey (1963) and by Baldry (1964) on populations of *G. tachinoides* living in substantial numbers in close association with domestic pigs. This provides an interesting example of tsetse living largely on domestic animals and finding a suitable habitat divorced from the riverine vegetation previously thought to be necessary for their survival. Several other points of epizootiological significance emerge from these studies. Unfortunately, the incidence of *T. simiae* among the pigs was not determined, but a high (86%) incidence of *T. congolense* and *T. brucei* was observed. Out of 274 tsetse flies dissected, 11 showed infection with trypanosomes of the *vivax* group, 3 of the *congolense* group and 4 of the *brucei* group. Analysis of tsetse blood meals showed that 54·7% were derived from pigs during the wet season and 94·5% during the dry season. Although goats were amongst the livestock kept they were not observed to be fed upon. Incidentally, it is also evident from these studies that, if measures for the control or extermination of tsetse are to be successfully applied, the ecology of the vector must be fully elucidated.

DOGS AND CATS. Little information is available on the epizootiology of trypanosomiasis of dogs and cats in West Africa. The disease is uncommon in cats and is usually encountered in dogs on an individual basis. *T. brucei* causes the most severe infections in dogs but infections with *T. congolense* are not infrequently seen. Both dogs and cats are stated to be refractory to infection with *T. vivax*. Dogs may not survive in areas of high risk but small indigenous dogs are encountered in areas in which the risk is light to moderate. Dogs of exotic extraction kept in towns may be infected by stray or transported tsetse.

CAMELS. Camels are susceptible to infection with *T. brucei*, *T. vivax*, *T. congolense* and *T. simiae*, but little is known of the epizootiology of cyclically transmitted trypanosomiasis in these animals in West Africa. Elsewhere in Africa, *T. brucei* and *T. simiae* have been reported as the cause of serious illness in camels.

Livestock Husbandry

The epizootiology of trypanosomiasis in livestock may be greatly influenced by the methods of animal husbandry adopted. Under intensive systems of husbandry it may be possible to avoid infection by maintaining stock in fly-proof accommodation, but range and migrant stock are often exposed, seasonally or continuously, to varying degrees of risk with the consequences already described.

Nutrition and other management factors

The level of nutrition in stock may be an important factor in determining the effects of trypanosome infection in animals which possess some degree of tolerance or resistance to the disease. In times of drought, the lower nutritional state of the stock and the need to move into areas of enhanced risk to find water and grazing, not only increase the liability to contract infection but render the animals less capable of withstanding the effects of infection. Thus, animals which would otherwise suffer from only mild or occult infections, and which would ordinarily recover when removed from risk of infection, become less productive in times of drought and may even die in considerable numbers from trypanosomiasis.

Trypanosomiasis is responsible for impaired productiveness for other reasons such as failure of infected stock to utilize available food as efficiently as healthy animals, loss of carcase quality and weight, loss of milk yield and, not infrequently, loss of productivity through abortion.

Exacerbations of trypanosomiasis are liable to be associated with parturition and with the use of animals for draught purposes. These factors have frequently frustrated attempts by the small arable farmer to maintain cattle in circumstances in which the pastoralist is able to achieve limited success in raising stock. The latter, despite losses, may be able to maintain his herd as a profitable venture.

In practice, the extent to which the effects of trypanosomiasis in livestock can be ameliorated by better methods of husbandry is often determined by economic factors, but there is a critical degree of risk beyond which animals will not respond to improved methods of husbandry.

A striking example of the effect of husbandry on epizootiology is provided by a herd of Zebu (White Fulani) cattle maintained at Ibadan University in Nigeria. These cattle are more or less continuously exposed to a relatively light risk from *G. palpalis*, but the standard of husbandry is so good that the herd thrives, and clinical symptoms of trypanosomiasis are only occasionally seen, whereas similar cattle maintained in a similar locality on lower standards of husbandry would suffer more severely. But these animals experience trypanosomiasis breakdowns when worked, or at parturition, and may then require chemotherapeutic support (Hill, 1956).

Livestock which possess some degree of tolerance to trypanosomiasis, but which are exposed to adverse influences such as undue stress or movement to a new 'climate' of risk, may be protected against the consequences by the judicious use of chemotherapy. The use of drugs must, however, be very carefully controlled where animals are bred for qualities of tolerance, owing to the risk of obscuring the criteria on which selective breeding is based, or of creating reservoirs of drug-resistant strains of trypanosomes.

Trade routes for slaughter cattle

In West Africa, there is an important trade in slaughter cattle which are moved on the hoof from the stock-raising areas of the interior to the meat-starved markets nearer the coast. The trade routes used for this purpose are distinct from those followed by stockowners during their seasonal migrations and the traffic along them is unidirectional. Conditions for the transmission of trypanosomiasis along these trade routes are such as to expose livestock to exceptional risk of contracting trypanosomiasis.

Animals already infected with trypanosomes, including those which have failed to respond to therapy, are unthrifty and are the first to be offered for sale, so that at the outset of their journey the incidence of trypanosomiasis among them is above average. The routes followed harbour communities of tsetse, particularly *G. morsitans*, which tend to concentrate along them and often extend beyond the usual limits of infestation. By the time the cattle reach their destination, after several weeks in transit, they are usually very heavily infected. The chance of infecting strains being drug-resistant must be high. Several studies have been made on trade cattle arriving at Ilorin in northern Nigeria, after two to three weeks exposure to risk on the trade route. The cattle remain at Ilorin for short periods while herds change hands and are broken up into new groups before continuing the journey south. Some are sold for slaughter locally. At the Ilorin cattle control post, the animals live in close contact with colonies of *G. morsitans*, *G. palpalis* and *G. tachinoides*, so the risk of contracting trypanosomiasis is further intensified. *G. morsitans* here exhibit *T. vivax* and *T. congolense* type infections approximating 45% (WAITR, 1963). The studies have shown that trypanosomiasis is the principal cause of losses and early slaughter of trade cattle. Ferguson (1964) recorded trypanosomiasis infection rates of 17·9% to 40·8% in a sample of 805 cattle arriving at Ilorin, randomly, over a period of two years, and 31·7% to 57·7% in 3,321 cattle slaughtered at Ilorin over the same period, the rate of infection varying according to the season of the year. An earlier investigation by Unsworth and Birkett (1952) indicated that if, during transit, the cattle were moved in easy stages and were protected at the outset by quinapyramine prophylactic,[1] many of the animals actually gained weight. More recently Jones-Davies (1967b) reported the results of a small trial carried out with immature stock at an adverse season of the year. Before commencing their journey the animals were divided into four groups, three of which received treatment with isometamidium chloride[2] at different dose levels (0·25, 0·5 and 0·75 mg./kg.) while the fourth group served as untreated controls. All groups were held at Ilorin after completion of their trek along the trade route. Four out of five of the untreated animals survived the journey to Ilorin but all died of trypanosomiasis after an average survival period of 56 days and after exhibiting patent parasitaemia. Among the group which was treated at the lowest (0·25) dose level, four out of five animals died at Ilorin after an average survival period of 72 days and one survived the experiment. Three animals in the two groups treated at the higher (0·5 and 0·75) dose levels died in transit from causes other than trypanosomiasis. The survivors to reach Ilorin were observed for 57 days before being treated with diminazene-aceturate[3] and sold for slaughter. The animals in the two latter groups all showed massive parasitaemia with *T. vivax* or *T. congolense*, or both, but despite this the physical condition of some improved greatly, though one died of babesiasis. The prepatent periods in these two groups averaged 70 and 72 days, respectively.

[1] Antrycide prosalt (ICI).
[2] Samorin (M & B).
[3] Berenil (Hoechst).

Chapter 40

Epizootiology of Trypanosomiasis in Livestock in East and Central Africa

K. C. WILLETT

INTRODUCTORY

It is a well-known fact that some four million square miles of Africa, wholly within the tropics except for small areas on the south-east coast, are infested with tsetse (Buxton, 1955) and that within almost the whole of that area productive cattle cannot be kept because of the threat of trypanosomiasis.

This threat, and that of human trypanosomiasis, are major obstacles to the economic development of the continent and are also responsible for an incalculable toll in human ill-health. It is a debatable point whether animal trypanosomiasis, through the vast extent of malnutrition and protein shortage for which it is largely to blame, is not now a greater problem, even on purely medical grounds, than human trypanosomiasis itself.

RESERVOIR OF INFECTION

There can be no doubt that the main reservoir of trypanosomiasis is in the wild animals. Ashcroft (1959) has summarized many surveys of trypanosomiasis in African wild animals, going back to 1913, some of which revealed remarkably high infection rates. Examples of high incidences of all forms of trypanosomiasis (*Trypanosoma vivax*, *T. congolense*, and *T. brucei*) in some species were: 52% in waterbuck (*Kobus* spp.); 45% in kudu (*Strepsiceros* spp.); 44% in reedbuck (*Redunca* spp.); 37% in giraffe (*Giraffa* sp.); 31% in bushbuck (*Tragelaphus* sp.); and 29% in eland (*Taurotragus* sp.). In buffalo (*Syncerus* sp.), duiker (*Sylvicapra* spp.), hartebeeste (*Alcelaphus* spp.), impala (*Aepyceros* sp.), oribi (*Ourebia* spp.), puku (*Adenota* spp.), roan antelope (*Hippotragus* sp.), topi (*Damaliscus* spp.), bushpig (*Potamochoerus* sp.) and warthog (*Phacochoerus* sp.) infection rates were found between 10 and 16%.

Santos Dias (1961) recorded 16 out of 394 suni antelope (*Neostragus livingstonianus*) in Mozambique infected with trypanosomes of the three main pathogenic groups, the only record known to the author of this very small antelope having been examined, and remarked that 'it is the more important trypanosome carrier which may be due to the similarity of this animal's habitat with that of *G. austeni*'.

These figures have been derived mainly from the examination of blood-slides but Godfrey and Killick-Kendrick (1961), examining cattle in Nigeria using blood-slide examination and rat-inoculation, found that 6·4% of the cattle examined (and 20·4% of the cattle found infected) harboured *T. brucei* sub-group organisms; these infections were demonstrated only by inoculation of rats and were not seen in the blood-slides, thin or thick.

A similar result was obtained by Baker (1967) who examined sixty-one wild animals in an area of Tanzania just north of the Serengeti National Park, also by blood-slides and rat-inoculation. He found *T. brucei* sub-group organisms in eight animals (13%), mainly by rat-inoculation, *T. congolense* in nine and *T. vivax* in five.

It therefore seems highly probable that infections with trypanosomes of the *T. brucei* sub-group are much commoner than figures derived solely from blood-slide examination would indicate, and in investigations in which the infection rates with this sub-group are important or of interest rat- or mouse-inoculation should never be omitted. In addition, this technique will reveal some sub-patent *T. congolense* infections but there is unfortunately still no laboratory animal that can conveniently be used to reveal sub-patent *T. vivax* infections. The incidence of *T. vivax* is therefore liable to be underestimated.

In addition to the evidence from natural sources there is much laboratory evidence that wild animals can act as reservoirs of infection, a great deal of which comes from Tinde Laboratory during the long-term experiment of the transmission of *T. rhodesiense* through animals or from the work of H. Lyndhurst Duke at Entebbe, Uganda. The evidence from Tinde has been assembled in a valuable paper by Ashcroft, Burtt and Fairbairn (1959). Some of the more striking examples of periods for which infections were shown to persist in some species of animals are given in Table 40.1.

Duke (1935a, 1937), at Entebbe, also obtained from a bushbuck (*Tragelaphus scriptus*) a successful fly transmission of *T. rhodesiense* 594 days after it was first infected, and from a spotted hyena (*Crocuta crocuta*) a successful sub-inoculation to a monkey after nearly nineteen months.

THE EPIZOOTIOLOGY OF *VIVAX* GROUP INFECTIONS

The *T. vivax* group, classified by Hoare (p. 18) as subgenus *Duttonella*, comprises the two species, *T.* (*D.*) *vivax* and *T.* (*D.*) *uniforme* and the latter is distinguishable only by its shorter length. *T. vivax* is common throughout all tsetse belts and infection rates in flies are normally much higher with this species than with those of any other group; *T. uniforme* has been recorded in east and central Africa mostly from around the Uganda lakes in areas infested with *Glossina fuscipes*. However, the fact that it can so easily be mistaken for *T. vivax* led Hoare and Broom (1938) to suggest that: 'the sporadic nature of the records of *T. uniforme* is due not so much to its rareness, as to failure on the part of observers to recognize and differentiate this species'.

The domestic animals chiefly affected by *T. vivax* are cattle, sheep and goats and in east and central Africa the resulting disease tends to be less severe than

TABLE 40.1

Showing the periods, in months, for which some species of trypanosomes—* (R) = T. rhodesiense: (B) = T. brucei (sensu stricto); (C) = T. congolense—*were demonstrated at Tinde Laboratory by various methods to have persisted in certain wild animals

Species of animal	Species of infecting trypanosome, in brackets, and period from infection to last:		
	successful fly-transmission	positive blood-slide	successful sub-inoculation
Bush-pig (*Potamochoerus koiropotamus*)	9 (R)	—	11 (R)
Duiker (*Sylvicapra grimmia*)	7 (B)	—	16 (R)
Eland (*Taurotragus oryx*)	4½ (R)[1]	4 (R)	11 (R)
Impala (*Aepyceros melampus*)	—	3½ (R)	7 (R)
Bohor reedbuck (*Redunca redunca*)	10 (R)	20 (R)	6 (R)
	14 (B)	20 (B)	—
	—	12 (C)	—
Steinbok (*Raphicephalus campestris*)	—	10 (C)	—

[1] Author's personal observation at Tinde, not recorded in the paper cited.

infections with *T. congolense*. Nevertheless, occasional instances of extremely severe and rapidly fatal *T. vivax* infections have been recorded.

One of the most remarkable features of *T. vivax* is its ability to become established in the absence of tsetse. It is well known that it has spread to Central and South America and to Mauritius but another aspect of the same ability of *T. vivax* to spread has recently been described by Ford (1964). From records of the geographical distribution of trypanosome infections in cattle in Rhodesia he pointed out that as the distance from the recognized edge of a tsetse belt increased so also did the proportion of infections diagnosed as due to *T. vivax*. Ford continued: 'Provisionally, therefore, the hypothesis of Ziemann (1905), the discoverer of *T. vivax* is, in part, revived. Ziemann, studying the changes in seasonal incidence of *T. vivax* in the Cameroons, concluded that the principal vectors were not tsetse-flies but other haematophagous Diptera.'

THE EPIZOOTIOLOGY OF *CONGOLENSE* GROUP INFECTIONS

The *T. congolense* group, classified by Hoare (p. 18) as subgenus *Nannomonas* comprises the species *T. congolense* and *T. simiae*, and their developmental cycle in tsetse, taking place in the mid-gut and proboscis, is more complex than that of *T. vivax* but much less so than that of the *T. brucei* sub-group trypanosomes. Naturally occurring infection rates in tsetse—and also infection rates than can be obtained in the laboratory—conform to the general pattern that the simpler the cycle of development in the fly the higher the infection rate. Thus in areas where the pattern has not been affected by extensive drug treatment, the proportion of tsetse infected with *T. congolense* is usually substantially less than that infected with *T. vivax*.

Nevertheless, infection with *T. congolense* is very common in cattle in contact with tsetse, with one possible exception which will be mentioned below. Further, as stated by Hornby (1952) after vast experience of trypanosomiasis over large areas of Africa: 'This is the most important animal trypanosomiasis in Africa. There is no tsetse-fly belt where it does not occur, and every kind of domestic mammal is susceptible to grievous infection. This ubiquity gives a sameness to the syndrome of whatever animal is affected; only in the pig is there a resistance to infection markedly higher than that shown by other species.'

Despite the close association of *T. congolense* with tsetse and the consequent presumption that transmission is predominantly cyclical, mechanical transmission can take place—as was shown by Lucas (1955)—but most authorities would probably agree that it plays only a minor part in the spread of this infection.

Two points in connection with the general epizootiology of *T. congolense* infections, in East and Central Africa as well as elsewhere, are perhaps of particular interest and importance.

The first is that, within the species as generally recognized, there are wide variations in both morphology and pathogenicity. Thus, Belgian workers regarded some strains of *T. congolense* from Rwandi-Burundi as distinct species (*T. urundiense*, *T. berghei*, *T. mossoense*), while workers in West Africa recognized the existence there of strains showing a gradation of characters. According to Godfrey (1960) *T. congolense* comprises 'a complex of types, ranging from the short *congolense* type, through an intermediate and *dimorphon* type, to the longest, which corresponds to the *T. dimorphon* of Laveran and Mesnil (1904)' (*see* also Chapter 2).

These morphological distinctions are not merely of taxonomic interest but also have a bearing on the epizootiology of *T. congolense* infections. Working in West Africa with various strains in cattle, sheep, dogs and laboratory rats, Godfrey (1961) found that: 'In general, the *congolense* type was characterized by low infectivity, low pathogenicity and low parasitaemia; the intermediate type by high infectivity and high parasitaemia but low pathogenicity; and the *dimorphon* type by high infectivity, high pathogenicity and high parasitaemia.' These findings are in agreement with the general experience of the writer with strains of *T. congolense* isolated in East Africa, though his impressions were not based on detailed study of the problem as were Godfrey's conclusions.

The second point of interest is that there appears to be a marked difference in the risk of domestic stock contracting infections with *T. congolense* according to whether the animals are in contact with tsetse of the *palpalis* or of the *morsitans* group. It has been noticed that cattle can sometimes be kept safely in contact with *G. fuscipes* around Lake Victoria but not in contact with *G. pallidipes*, even in low density, and this may be because there is a much greater risk of contracting *T. congolense* infections from flies of the *morsitans* group. Willett *et al.* (1964), by feeding batches of approximately fifty flies on rats, isolated forty strains of *T. congolense* from 6,953 *G. pallidipes* but not a single strain from 9,441 *G. fuscipes* (described in the paper as *G. palpalis*). The contrast between these two species in the transmission of *T. congolense* may be a consequence of the fact that *G. pallidipes* tends to feed on animals which may carry the infection whereas *G. fuscipes* feeds mainly on man and reptiles, both insusceptible to *T. congolense*. On the other hand, *palpalis* group tsetse may be genuinely less susceptible to infection with this trypanosome. Godfrey (1961), in his work mentioned above on *T. congolense* strains, stated that: 'The isolations were transmitted through *G. morsitans* (*submorsitans*): all attempts to transmit them through *G. palpalis* were unsuccessful.' The writer is well aware that Godfrey made many such attempts. Godfrey's experience lends support to the possibility that flies of the *palpalis* group, generally, are relatively insusceptible to infection with *T. congolense*. Godfrey's result is also of particular interest as it is perhaps the only recorded instance in which persistent attempts to transmit any species of the African pathogenic trypanosomes by any species of tsetse have failed. Whatever the cause of the reduced chance of contracting *T. congolense* infections from flies of the *palpalis* group, which are so widespread, it is of great epizootiological importance.

Trypanosoma simiae is well known for the very rapidly fatal, fulminating infection it causes in domestic pigs. It also normally causes fulminating infections in monkeys, though there may be exceptions to this rule as will be mentioned below. According to Pellegrini (1948) camels are also highly susceptible, but it is known that passage through a goat may drastically reduce the pathogenicity of this trypanosome. As Hornby (1952) remarked: '*T. simiae* differs from all other pathogenic trypanosomes by its excessively variable character; both morphologically and in pathogenicity it shows amazing transformations. . . . Nobody could fail to recognize *T. simiae* in . . . fulminating infections, but let it be seen in its quiescent state in any animal, and one perceives what could be, and very often is, mistaken for a rather long *T. congolense*.'

These remarks of Hornby's carry the implication that *T. simiae* may be far more common than is suspected and that many animals may be infected without causing easily recognizable fulminating infections. Culwick and Fairbairn (1947) isolated *T. simiae* from a horse and also claimed to have found a naturally-infected bovine, but Pellegrini (1948) failed to infect any of six cattle from his heavily infected camels and stated: 'Absence of pathogenicity in the bovine is the crucial biological characteristic. Of all the pathogenic trypanosomes found here (Somalia) *T. simiae* is the only one not even experimentally transmissible to bovines.' Peel and Chardome (1954d) criticized the work of Culwick and Fairbairn on the grounds that they had not proved the identity of their *T. simiae* by infecting a pig. The present writer had the opportunity to see the fulminating infections in monkeys caused by the Culwick and Fairbairn equine strain and they were typical of classical *T. simiae*. In contrast, Peel and Chardome reported that their strain would not infect monkeys at all, and Pellegrini also failed to infect any of two *Cercopithecus* and one *Macaca* monkeys.

There appear to be many unresolved difficulties presented by *T. simiae*. The whole subject has recently been admirably reviewed in all its aspects by Stephen (1966a).

In short, it seems that much remains to be learned of the epizootiology of the whole *T. congolense* group, of the wide range of trypanosomes currently labelled *T. congolense*, and of *T. simiae*.

A brief mention should be made of *T. suis*, classified by Hoare (p. 19) as the sole representative of the subgenus *Pycnomonas*. This trypanosome is unusual in two respects, the first the great infrequency with which it has been reported and the second that, though monomorphic and morphologically bearing some resemblance to *T. congolense* (though perhaps more to short-stumpy forms of *T. brucei*), its cycle of development in tsetse, as described in *brevipalpalis* by Peel and Chardome (1953, 1954, 1954e) resembles that of the *brucei* sub-group in that it reaches completion in the salivary glands.

The pig is the only animal known to be susceptible to infection with *T.* (*P.*) *suis* and Peel and Chardome found that their strain caused chronic infection in adults but more acute infections in young pigs, usually fatal within two months. The reservoir hosts of *T. suis* are probably wild pigs. Present knowledge of the species is again well reviewed by Stephen (1966a).

THE EPIZOOTIOLOGY OF *BRUCEI* SUB-GROUP INFECTIONS

Hoare (*see* pp. 18–19) classifies this subgroup as sub-genus *Trypanozoon* which comprises the species *T.* (*T.*) *brucei*, *T.* (*T.*) *gambiense*, *T.* (*T.*) *rhodesiense*, *T.* (*T.*) *evansi* and *T.* (*T.*) *equiperdum*. An account of *T.* (*T.*) *equiperdum* is given at pp. 54–56 but, as this species does not occur in East or Central Africa, it will not be considered further here.

T. evansi is the causative agent of surra, which in Africa affects mainly camels but horses, donkeys, dogs and cattle are also susceptible. The disease is usually acute in camels, horses and dogs, more chronic in donkeys and commonly mild or transient in cattle. Hoare (1956), after twenty years' work on many aspects of *T. evansi*, published a revision of the species and concluded from a substantial body of evidence that it was derived from *T. brucei* which had become adapted to mechanical transmission by Tabanid (and sometimes other) biting flies and had lost its polymorphism as a result of long-term blood-passage, exactly as happens with *T. brucei* passaged in the laboratory. Hornby (1952) held the same opinion.

The epizootiology of *T. evansi* infections in Africa is therefore dominated by three main facts. The first is that it is essentially a disease of camels, the second that it is found only at and beyond the fringe of the tsetse distribution (though it extends all over the north of Africa and far beyond, to south-east Asia and the Phillipines), and the third that its incidence is related to the prevalence of Tabanids, in particular, which is seasonally very variable.

T. gambiense need hardly be considered in the epizootiology of *brucei* sub-group infections in eastern Africa since it is now almost non-existent in this part of the continent and also because there is little evidence that any animal, other than perhaps the domestic pig, suffers from the infection.

The epizootiology of *T. brucei* infections is greatly complicated by the fact that there is still no means whatever of distinguishing *T. brucei* from *T. rhodesiense* except by a direct test of a given strain's infectivity to man. Hence, if a strain is isolated from an animal or from tsetse and has the characteristics of *T. brucei* it cannot be so labelled with certainty until it has been proved non-infective to man. This difficulty has given rise to the valuable device of describing strains which have been tested and proved non-infective to man as *T. brucei* (*sensu stricto*). The general convention has been to describe any unknown strain isolated from an animal as *T. brucei* but there have been rare instances when such strains have been proved, either by accident or by deliberate test, to be infective to man and therefore, by definition, *T. rhodesiense*.

The specific status of isolates from tsetse, particularly in an area where sleeping sickness has been known or still exists, is even more uncertain. Strains of *T. brucei* (*sensu stricto*) may be expected to be in the great majority, but there can be no certainty. For example, Willett *et al.* (1964) isolated fifteen strains of *brucei* sub-group trypanosomes from *G. palpalis* (*G. fuscipes*) and *G. pallidipes* in Sakwa, Kenya, and were able to test the infectivity to man of eleven of the strains, only one of which proved to be *T. rhodesiense*. Only if a *brucei* sub-group trypanosome were isolated from an area in which there never had been any human sleeping sickness would it be reasonable to assume that it was *T. brucei* (*sensu stricto*), but it should always be clearly stated whether the specific status has been assumed or definitely established.

It has sometimes been objected that a single test on one human volunteer might be regarded as inconclusive, but the author is of the opinion, based on a substantial number of volunteer tests at Tinde Laboratory, that a strain which has the characteristic virulence to laboratory animals of *T. brucei* or *T. rhodesiense* is most unlikely to fail to infect man if it is *T. rhodesiense* and a subcutaneous inoculation is given of one to two million trypanosomes freshly taken from a laboratory rodent. One experiment (Willett, 1956) was done with a single strain in which the smallest dose that infected a man was 80,000 blood-forms from a rat, but the strain used was unusual in several respects. It had been blood-passaged for several years and since it would be reasonable to assume that a freshly isolated strain of *T. rhodesiense* would be no less infective to man, the administration of a million trypanosomes should provide a reliable test. Much larger inocula are only likely to result in a more acute and severe onset of infection if the strain under test proves to be *T. rhodesiense*. Certainly, in the writer's experience, the administration of this number of *T. brucei* (*sensu stricto*), or even much larger doses, produces no reaction.

With the above provisos it can be stated that *T. brucei* is ubiquitous in all tsetse belts, but as mentioned above, may not be readily found in blood-films from infected animals; sub-inoculation of small laboratory rodents is much more reliable for detecting this species. Laboratory and field evidence has long pointed to the conclusion that wild animals acted as a reservoir of *T. rhodesiense* where that species has once become established, but it was only in 1958 that Heisch, McMahon and Manson-Bahr successfully isolated a strain from a wild bushbuck (*Tragelaphus scriptus*) and proved its infectivity to man.

Even more recently has it been proved in the field that cattle can, and do, act as a reservoir of *T. rhodesiense*. Although Wilde and French demonstrated as far back as 1945 that Zebu cattle could carry the infection for at least six months, it was not until 1966 that Onyango *et al.* obtained the first isolation from naturally infected cattle.

Chapter 41

Clinical Manifestations of the Trypanosomiases in Livestock and Other Domestic Animals

L. E. STEPHEN

INTRODUCTORY

The mammalian trypanosomes of Africa have been fully described in Chapters 1 and 2. In the present context, attention will be directed to the clinical manifestations of the diseases caused by different species of trypanosomes in various domestic animals. The species of trypanosome considered here include *T. brucei*, *T. congolense*, *T. vivax*, *T. uniforme*, *T. simiae*, *T. suis*, *T. evansi*, *T. equiperdum* and *T. theileri*.

There are as many trypanosomiases as there are specific trypanosomes, and since each species of trypanosome may infect several species of animals, with different effects and degrees of severity (Table 41.1), the clinical signs vary in different mammalian species. For example, trypanosomiasis in the domestic pig, caused by *T. simiae*, is a fulminating disease characterized by massive parasitaemia and ending in death often within a period of twenty-four hours. The same trypanosome in the sheep causes a mild disease from which the animal may recover spontaneously while cattle are resistant even to a severe challenge.

The pathogenicity of strains (demes) within a species is another variable character which may affect the clinical signs, and such differences in biological characters, in morphologically identical trypanosomes, have sometimes resulted in their being accorded independent species status; for example, *T. gambiense*, *T. rhodesiense* and *T. brucei* have long been regarded as separate species because of differences in their ability to infect man, in their clinical manifestations and in their geographical distribution.

Further work, especially in the fields of immunological and biochemical research, may show that trypanosomes which are at present regarded as belonging to a single species are in fact deserving of their own species status. Anyone who has worked with *T. congolense* is soon impressed with the small morphological differences, as seen in blood films from different animals, such as the presence or absence of a short free flagellum, the size and position of the kinetoplast and the variation in width and length. Individual infections with various isolates of *T. congolense* show considerable variation in pathogenicity for different mammalian species and even for animals of the same breed, suggesting that what are loosely called *T. congolense* infections may in fact be infections due to several different species.

Another very important factor which must be considered is the relative susceptibility of different breeds of animals. This is particularly evident in cattle where great variation in the susceptibility of breeds is observed. For example, the Zebu cattle of West Africa are much more seriously affected by trypanosomiasis than the dwarf breeds such as the N'dama and Muturu; and in East Africa pure-bred and grade animals react to trypanosome infections quite differently from indigenous cattle.

The clinical manifestations of trypanosomiasis in animals may be greatly influenced by a number of other factors such as the state of nutrition, the occurrence of intercurrent bacterial, viral and helminthic infections and stress due to vaccination regimens, trekking, thirst and temperature changes.

Although it is possible to cause an infection in an animal by the bite of a single tsetse fly, and, experimentally, to establish a clonal infection from a single organism, there is no doubt that the severity of challenge, i.e. the numbers

TABLE 41.1

Showing susceptibility of animals to trypanosomes pathogenic for domestic animals

Trypanosome	Equines	Cattle	Sheep	Goats	Camels	Pigs	Dogs	Rats	Mice	Rabbit	Guinea Pig	Monkey
T. brucei	+++	+	+	++	+++	±	+++	+++	+++	++	+	++
T. congolense	++	+++	++	++	++	±	+++ or ±	+++ or ±	++ or ±	+	+	+
T. equiperdum	+++	+	+	+	?	±	+	±	±	±	±	?
T. evansi	++	++	+	+	+++	±	++	++	+	+	+	+
T. simiae	–	–	+	++	+++	+++	–	–	–	[1]±	–	+++ or –
T. suis	–	–	–	–	–	++	–	–	–	–	–	–
T. uniforme	++	++	++	++	?	–	–	–	–	–	–	–
T. vivax	+++ or +	+++	++	++	+	–	–	–	–	–	–	–

[1] Only splenectomized rabbits.

of metacyclic trypanosomes introduced into the animal body in any unit of time, is an important factor in the character of the resultant infection.

The writer has, on many occasions, been impressed by the apparent reduction in pathogenicity of trypanosomes appearing in the peripheral blood at the end of a period of chemoprophylaxis, or those re-appearing in relapses due to inadequate treatment or to the use of a drug that was not completely trypanocidal. Such infections are often characterized by a very scanty and sporadic parasitaemia and the animals may show little clinical evidence of trypanosomiasis. The parasite may, however, retain its virulence for clean untreated animals.

Relatively few descriptions exist in the literature of the clinical course of trypanosome infections when caused by a particular species of trypanosome and transmitted by the bites of infective *Glossina*. The literature, however, abounds in descriptions of infections caused by syringe inoculation of trypanosomes, often by the inoculation of blood from one species of animal into a completely different species as, for example, from rat to sheep or goat to cattle. Such reports must be viewed with circumspection. It is well-known that trypanosomes that have been syringe-passaged in, say, rats for a period of time may show changes in their morphology, in their reaction to chemotherapeutic agents, in their pathogenicity for a more natural host and in their ability to develop cyclically in *Glossina*. In other words, the trypanosome may bear very little resemblance to its former self.

Bruce *et al.* (1914) were well aware of this capacity for transformation (transmutation); they wrote:

'The rapidity with which the virulence of *T. simiae* becomes modified is also remarkable. When a cage containing wild *Glossina morsitans* is placed on a monkey and a goat, both animals take the disease, and the monkey in such an acute form that the average duration of life is only a few days. But if it is attempted to pass *T. simiae* from an infected goat to a healthy monkey by the inoculation of goat's blood the experiment usually fails, showing that a short sojourn in the blood of the goat has almost nullified the virulence of the parasite for the monkey.'

These workers also demonstrated the interesting fact that the virulence of this trypanosome is considerably exalted by cyclical passage through tsetse fly. When blood from warthogs was injected into goats the mortality was zero but when infection was induced by the bite of wild *G. morsitans* the mortality was 86% to 90%; yet presumably the fly had acquired its infection by feeding on wild warthog!

Bruce *et al.* (*loc. cit.*) end by saying:

'It may also be remembered that the matter is of little practical importance, as under natural conditions goats will always be infected by the bite of the "fly"; *but it is interesting as showing the fallacy of judging from the action of laboratory strains as to what will occur in nature.*' [the writer's italics].

Much time, money and effort have been wasted in trypanosomiasis research because these early observations were unknown, forgotten or ignored.

Furthermore, there is reason to believe that cyclical development in different species of *Glossina* may affect the virulence of trypanosomes to a considerable extent, and that what we have considered to be nosodemes are, in fact, ecodemes (Hoare, 1955). Or, in other words, that the pathogenicity of an organism may vary under ecological influences.

The student of trypanosomiasis should keep the above-mentioned variables in mind when studying individual accounts of trypanosome infections.

Trypanosomiasis may be described as it occurs in groups of related animals; for example, the disease in horses, donkeys and mules may be described as equine trypanosomiasis. Similarly, sheep and goats form another natural class. Cats and dogs may also be grouped but as cats are seldom naturally infected, and in any case have no commercial value, they will receive very little attention in this account. Some authors group animals as above and then give consecutive descriptions of the disease caused by each trypanosome species. Here, for ease of reference, a description will be given of the disease caused by each species of trypanosome as it occurs in equines, bovines (i.e. cattle, because there are no domestic buffaloes in tropical Africa), sheep and goats, camels, pigs, and dogs.

Although the descriptions given will be for 'pure' infections it must be remembered that, in the field, infections will frequently be 'mixed'. Examination of a blood film from an infected animal may show only one species of trypanosome to be present; however, if the blood is examined daily over a period of time, or if selective chemotherapy is given, or if various types of susceptible animals are sub-inoculated, other species may be revealed.

Certain species appear to be able to suppress the appearance of less dominant species in the peripheral blood; for example, *T. vivax* in cattle—at least in West Africa—may be the only species seen in serial blood films taken over a period of weeks, but if the animal is treated with a trypanocidal drug that is particularly active against *vivax* infections, *T. congolense* or *T. brucei* may appear later.

On one occasion, the writer infected a sheep using a batch of wild-caught *Glossina morsitans submorsitans* and nine days later the animal developed what appeared to be a 'pure' *T. vivax* infection, as seen in stained thin blood films. However, sub-inoculations of blood into rats and pigs caused infection with *T. brucei* in the rats and a virulent infection with *T. simiae* in the pigs. When this sheep was treated with homidium at a low dose rate, *T. congolense* later appeared in its blood. Thus, an animal that appeared to be parasitized by only *one* species of trypanosome was actually harbouring *four* different species.

A warning should perhaps be given regarding the use of anthelmintics in animals suffering from trypanosomiasis, especially the use of phenothiazine. The writer and other workers in West Africa have killed cattle by administering this drug even when the infecting organism was *T. brucei* which is usually considered to be non-pathogenic for the bovine. The reason for this enhanced toxicity of the drug or increased virulence of the trypanosome has not been investigated, but it suggests an interesting line of research.

TRYPANOSOMIASIS CAUSED BY *T. BRUCEI*

Disease of Equines

Horses, donkeys and mules are very susceptible to infection with this trypanosome and death occurs within a fortnight to three months in untreated animals.

Transmission studies using infective *Glossina* do not appear to have been made, but earlier records indicate that the prepatent period is about six to ten days.

The disease, if untreated, may be acute, subacute or chronic. Locomotor ataxia is usually one of the earliest signs of the disease and is manifested by a stumbling or weaving gait when walking or trotting and a tendency to fall when turning or when a hoof is lifted for examination. The animal has a dejected look; the ears tend to droop, the eyes become sunken and the hair coat loses its lustre and becomes harsh and stary. There is a tendency for the penis to extend from the prepuce. Closer clinical examination will reveal the sporadic appearance of urticarial plaques on the body measuring up to 10 centimetres in diameter, or even more. Oedema is a prominent sign and usually affects the ventral parts such as the sternum, belly, prepuce and legs, any or all of which may be involved at the same time. The head region is seldom oedematous. The mucous membranes of the eye become progressively paler as anaemia progresses, but in acute cases, they may be injected and icteric indicating rapid destruction of erythrocytes. Similar signs may be seen on the gums and on the mucous membrane of the vagina. Lymphadenitis is usually present but in the horse the superficial lymph nodes are not prominent and careful palpation is required to detect glandular enlargement.

Serial temperature readings reveal a remittent fever with peaks of up to 107°F and intervals of normal or even subnormal readings. It bears a close relationship to the degree of parasitaemia, being highest when trypanosomes are most numerous in the peripheral blood. The pulse and respirations show a correlation with the pyrexial periods, but as the anaemia becomes greater there is usually a continuous tachycardia and polypnoea.

Acute cases may terminate fatally in a week or two and the animal may show very little loss of condition; chronic cases may continue for two or three months and the animal will be severely emaciated. In the terminal stages the animal is recumbent and sometimes comatose. This is probably due more to muscular weakness and anaemia than to lesions of the central nervous system. Untreated cases almost invariably end fatally.

Disease of Cattle

Cattle in all regions of tropical Africa exhibit a high degree of resistance to *T. brucei*. Infections are readily established in these animals but clinical signs of disease are seldom observed, even when there is high parasitaemia. Exotic breeds, however, are much more susceptible.

Disease of Sheep and Goats

Sheep and goats are not often found infected with trypanosomes under natural conditions. Recent studies have shown that tsetse seldom feed on these animals (*see* Chapter 13) and this may indicate that they find the blood of these hosts unpalatable or that it is difficult for them to penetrate the hosts' dense coats of wool or hair. Sheep and goats are, however, readily infected with a number of trypanosome species experimentally, and serve as very useful laboratory animals.

Clinically, *T. brucei* infections in sheep and goats are usually chronic, with low to medium parasitaemias and the disease may end in spontaneous cure. The chief signs are progressive anaemia, moderate pyrexia and loss of body condition; oedema and ocular lesions are seldom seen. Reports of lachrymation, salivation, nasal discharge and facial oedema are probably due to intercurrent infections such as *Oestrus ovis* causing nasal discharge, and 'bottle jaw' due to haemonchosis or chronic fascioliasis.

Acute *brucei* infections have been reported in laboratory experiments.

Disease of Camels

Camels are highly susceptible to infection with *T. brucei.* This is readily understandable since surra is well documented as a serious disease of camels. The cause of surra is *T. evansi*, a trypanosome species that undoubtedly arose from *T. brucei* but which now shows a high degree of monomorphism and is not cyclically transmissible by tsetse, presumably because it has for long been transmitted mechanically by other biting insects.

Wenyon (1926) reported that a convoy of over seventy camels taken into the Bahr el Ghazal province of the Sudan all died of infection with *T. brucei* within a period of two months.

The clinical manifestations of *T. brucei* infections in camels are the same as those seen in acute cases of surra (*see* below).

Disease of Pigs

There are very few reports of natural infections in pigs due to *T. brucei.* Most observers regard infections in pigs with this species as the cause of a mild, chronic disease, although intercurrent helminthosis may increase the pathogenicity considerably.

Despite its low pathogenicity for the pig *T. brucei* appears to have a special predilection for that animal. It has been observed that when pigs are challenged by tsetse flies known to be infected with *T. vivax*, *T. congolense* and *T. brucei* they usually develop an infection by the polymorphic trypanosome.

The signs most often seen in trypanosomiasis of pigs caused by *T. brucei* are cachexia, anaemia, weakness in the hind-quarters seen as a swaying gait (locomotor ataxia) and even paraplegia. Pregnant sows may abort and die on the same, or the following, day.

Disease of Dogs

This is usually an acute disease and, if untreated, almost invariably ends fatally.

Fever develops with the appearance of trypanosomes in the peripheral blood and continues with only slight remissions until death. Anaemia develops rapidly as may be seen by examining the conjunctivae and gums, and there is accompanying muscular weakness, depression, anorexia, oedema of the limbs and severe weight loss. Terminally, movements are incoordinated and there is evidence of paralysis. A common and notable feature of this disease in dogs is corneal opacity, blepharitis, conjunctivitis and keratitis caused apparently by the invasion of these tissues by the trypanosome. Death usually occurs within two months.

Cats are also highly susceptible to infection with *T. brucei.*

TRYPANOSOMIASIS CAUSED BY *T. CONGOLENSE*

Disease of Equines

There are very few reports in the literature on the effects of *T. congolense* in equines. Stephen (1962) described an experimental fly-transmitted infection in the horse; parasites were never seen in large numbers in the peripheral blood. The clinical manifestations were described thus: 'Appetite, faeces and urine were unchanged throughout the infection. The mucous membranes of the mouth and eye became progressively paler as the animal became anaemic, but no jaundice or other evidence of pathological pigmentation was observed. The horse did not lose weight or condition during the infection and, in fact, it gained 15 kg. during the first two months. Curiously, the early parasitaemia did not induce a pyrexial reaction. However, on the 18th day of the infection the temperature rose sharply to 104·4°F in association with quite a high level of parasitaemia (70 trypanosomes per 60 microscopic fields) on the *previous* day. Thereafter, the temperature rose above 100°F on only three occasions which were each associated with larger numbers of trypanosomes in the blood.'

'Oedematous plaques developed in the saddle area of the back, i.e. in the area to which flies were applied during the challenge, six days before trypanosomes were found in wet blood films. These plaques, which measured up to 9 inches by 5·5 inches decreased in size after the appearance of parasites in the blood but others appeared in different areas of the back 10–14 days later. From the 14th day there was some oedema of the legs below the carpus and hock joints and a moderate hydrocoele.'

The infection caused by *T. congolense* in this horse was very mild and although the anaemia was moderately severe, the animal remained alert and lively. By the 45th day the horse had practically recovered spontaneously.

Disease of Cattle

T. congolense is undoubtedly the most important trypanosome affecting cattle in Africa. It should be remembered, however, that there are many different strains of this organism and that they vary considerably in their virulence. In West Africa, *congolense* trypanosomiasis in cattle is generally regarded as being a relatively mild, chronic infection whereas in East Africa it may be seen as an acute, subacute or mild chronic infection.

There is a distinct pyrexial reaction with the appearance of trypanosomes in the peripheral blood; the temperature rises to 103°–104°F, seldom higher. Throughout the infection the temperature rises and falls with peaks of parasitaemia, except in the terminal stages when it is usually sub-normal. Appetite is usually good except during periods of high pyrexia when the animal standing at pasture has a dejected look. Urine and faeces are unchanged. There are few distinctive signs of trypanosomiasis in cattle and none that is pathognomonic. As the disease progresses they develop a marked anaemia, the hair coat becomes lustreless and stary and there is severe loss of bodily condition seen as sunken eyes, prominent vertebrae and ribs and wasted gluteal and crural muscles. This is the so-called 'fly-struck' appearance. In chronic cases, there may be loss of libido and interference with reproduction, and infected calves fail to reach sexual maturity.

In the terminal stages the animal is too weak to rise or eat. Respirations are laboured and accompanied by grunts and a jugular pulse may be observed; these signs are due to the severe anaemia. The writer has seen cattle in which the erythrocyte count dropped to as low as one and a half million cells per cubic millimetre before death supervened. Death may occur within a few weeks but usually takes several months to a year. Spontaneous cures sometimes occur.

Disease of Sheep and Goats

As mentioned earlier, sheep and goats are seldom found naturally infected.

In an experiment involving fifteen sheep the writer found that the prepatent period was 7–26 (average 13·2) days. Parasitaemia is rarely high.

There are no pathognomonic signs of trypanosomiasis in sheep and goats. Fever, anaemia and wasting are the principal manifestations. Animals die in a state of complete exhaustion and their carcases may show extreme emaciation.

Disease of Camels

There are a few reports of *T. congolense* infections in camels although they are known to be susceptible to this species.

The disease probably shows similar clinical manifestations to those seen in cattle, their severity depending on the virulence of the infecting strain.

Disease of Pigs

Pigs are susceptible to *T. congolense* infections, but parasitaemia is usually low and the course of the infection is normally mild. However, it is not true to say that the trypanosome causes no ill effects. Close observation of pigs with chronic infections will reveal progressive anaemia, loss of condition, muscular weakness and incoordination. Pathogenicity may be increased if intercurrent helminthiasis exists.

Since pigs are raised for meat, chronic infection in a herd could cause serious losses. This was well illustrated in an experiment conducted by the writer. A pig infected with *T. congolense* showed no clinical signs of ill health but it did not thrive. By the end of the second month of infection it weighed 1 kg. less than before infection, while control pigs had gained an average of 28 kg. during the same period.

Most pigs probably recover spontaneously after a variable period of infection.

Disease of Dogs

Depending on the strain, European and local breeds of dogs may be highly susceptible to *T. congolense* infections. Kafir or 'pie-dogs' reared in the vicinity of tsetse country, however, may show a high degree of resistance. Virulent strains cause a high and sustained parasitaemia and dogs may die within one to four weeks.

The usual clinical manifestations are anaemia indicated by increasing pallor of the gums, loss of bodily condition, dejection, weakness and patchy alopecia. Appetite is reduced and pyrexia accompanies the peaks of parasitaemia.

Oedema is not observed, and ocular lesions, as seen in *T. brucei* infections, are seldom noticed. Avirulent strains result in a scanty and sporadic parasitaemia, with very little evidence of illness and the dog recovers spontaneously.

Cats are susceptible to infection with *T. congolense* but are said to be more resistant than European breeds of dogs.

TRYPANOSOMIASIS CAUSED BY *T. EQUIPERDUM*

Natural infection with this trypanosome occurs only in equines in which it causes a disease known as dourine. Transmission occurs from stallion to mare or *vice versa* by direct contact of the mucous membranes of the genitalia during the act of coitus. Thus the disease is mainly one of breeding animals and may be classified as a venereal infection.

The trypanosome is not transmissible by tsetse or so far as is known by any other insect vector and is consequently the only trypanosomiasis of domestic animals that is not transmitted by a blood-sucking insect.

The virulence of the infection varies with the strain; Canadian and South African strains cause relatively mild, chronic and insidious disease while the European strain is much more pathogenic.

For descriptive purposes the clinical manifestations of this disease can be divided into two forms: the *vascular* form in which the genital organs and local subcutaneous tissues are affected and the *nervous* form in which locomotor disturbances appear. Excellent descriptions of the clinical manifestations of this disease have been provided by Watson (1920) and by Theiler (1918) in Canada and South Africa, respectively.

Parasitaemia is almost always very scanty and it is generally very difficult or impossible to demonstrate the organism in the blood.

The Vascular Form

In the mare, the first sign of the disease is usually the presence of a mucous discharge from the vagina which may be copious, especially on movement, and which causes the tail and hind-quarters to be soiled. The tail may be raised away from the vulva which is swollen and inflamed. On palpation, the swelling of the vulva may be felt to extend into the perineum and down to the udder and even to the posterior abdomen. There is hyperaemia of the mucous membrane of the vagina which may be associated with nodules and ulcers and areas of depigmentation may be seen in the area of the vulva and anus. The irritation causes frequent micturition or attempts to urinate and some animals show an increase in libido.

Abortions or the birth of weak foals may be seen. There may be some rise in body temperature, but pyrexial reactions are not a common feature. Examination of vaginal washings may reveal large numbers of motile trypanosomes in some cases, but in others they may be scanty or absent.

In the stallion the initial signs may be so slight that they are not noticed, or the first sign of illness may be locomotor disturbances. Otherwise, vascular signs consist of oedema of the prepuce and glans penis and the urethral process may be quite prominent. Paraphimosis is common and there may be ulceration of the penis. Cutaneous plaques have often been described and there may be frequent urination and increased libido.

In both sexes, there is loss of condition and the hair coat becomes rough and stary.

The Nervous Form

Signs of nervous disorder may appear soon after the vascular signs or the two forms may be separated by a distinct though variable interval.

Affected animals are often hyperaesthetic and restless at first and then locomotor disturbances gradually appear. This is usually seen as a hind-limb lameness, usually commencing in one leg but later extending to both; the lesion seems to be located between the coxo-femoral and stifle joints. The gait becomes straddled, the lame leg being swung outwards from the median line when the animal walks. Frequently the animal knuckles over and stumbles when forced to move. In the later stages the animal lies down and can only rise with difficulty and finally it may fall down and be unable to get up.

Some writers report facial paralysis and ocular lesions, but these are not commonly seen. A progressive anaemia may be seen by the increasing pallor of the mucous membranes of the eyes and mouth. The good general condition and lack of clinical signs in some animals makes control difficult especially as these cases may be carriers of the parasite. Mortality is generally high especially in animals imported into an area where the disease is enzootic.

Small laboratory animals, dogs, sheep and goats and even cattle may be infected experimentally, but the natural disease is confined to equines.

TRYPANOSOMIASIS CAUSED BY *T. EVANSI*

As mentioned earlier, *T. evansi* undoubtedly arose from *T. brucei* and it is conceivable that caravans entering even lightly infested tsetse belts acquired the infection which was then propagated in tsetse-free areas by other biting flies. For centuries, the camel has been the chief means of long-range transport in North Africa, the Middle East and western Asia, and infections acquired in tropical Africa were probably gradually disseminated to the areas of the Middle East and Asia where it now exists.

Trypanosomiasis caused by *T. evansi*, commonly known as surra, is essentially a disease of camels but it may also have serious effects on a variety of domestic and wild animals including horses, donkeys, cattle, dogs, elephants and Asiatic buffaloes.

In Africa, surra is mainly a disease of camels and to a lesser extent of equines so that only the clinical manifestations observed in these animals will be described here.

Disease of Camels

As stated by Hornby (1952), 'Almost all that is necessary for the clinician to know about surra in camels is contained in two papers by Bennett (1933).'

One of the best brief descriptions of the clinical manifestations of surra in camels is Hornby's translation of page 99 of *Tropenkrankheiten der Haustiere* by Knuth and Du Toit:

'Trypanosomes make their first appearance in the blood about one week after infection and before there is any clinical evidence of illness. Only after a month or longer are progressive weakness and loss of condition noticeable. The coat becomes rough and staring, and the animal tends to stumble. After even a short journey it lies down and only with difficulty is persuaded to stand up again. Pregnant camels abort, and even if calves are full-term, they are weak and cachectic, and generally die within a few months. The appetite, at first unaffected, later declines. The body temperature, in the chronic form of the disease, is usually between 38·5°C and 39°C. Loss of condition is progressive. There are recurrent bouts of fever; and there may be petechiae on the visible mucous membranes. The disease may be fatal within a few months, but it can also last for one or two years before it causes death. In Egypt, it is usual for an affected camel to live for three or four years. Cases of spontaneous recovery, though rare, do occur, and such naturally immunized animals acquire thereby an enhanced value.'

Disease of Equines

The writer had an opportunity in Nigeria to observe a horse infected experimentally with *T. evansi* and recorded the following (unpublished) description of the disease.

The site of the inoculation showed a swelling 4 inches by 2 inches on the following morning and was painful when palpated. The swelling had disappeared by the 5th day. On the 4th day, when trypanosomes were first seen in the peripheral blood, a line of oedematous swelling was observed along the ventral aspect of the belly. Later this swelling increased in extent and occupied the region from the prepuce to the xiphoid cartilage. At its maximum size it measured 2 inches in width in the region immediately anterior to the prepuce and it was hot and painful when touched. The scrotal sac was distended, more or less, throughout the infection and increased coincident with peaks of temperature. This distension is thought to indicate ascites, more than an oedema of the scrotum. As the disease progressed, evidence of anaemia was revealed by the increasing pallor of the mucous membranes of the eye, gums and nares, but icterus was never pronounced. By the 12th day an ecchymotic haemorrhage appeared in the right eye; similar lesions were observed on three occasions and appeared to be associated with a drop in body temperature and reduction in parasitaemia; at the same time, petechiae were seen in the nares. Small (8 mm.) urticarial plaques appeared on the body on the 13th day of the infection and lasted for three days, then disappeared, but returned a week later. These plaques recurred periodically throughout the infection and appeared to coincide with parasitaemic and temperature rises. Oedema of the legs did not occur. Very early in the infection the coat had a stary, dry appearance. By the 25th day muscular weakness was evident; the horse was reluctant to walk and when it did it walked with a swaying, unsteady gait, the fore-legs moving in a circular manner and the hind legs overreaching the fore-leg with a tendency to cross over. At the end of a month the horse was observed to be eating earth and this geophagia continued until the animal died. Appetite was variable throughout the infection, but ceased only when the horse was *in extremis*. Faeces were usually normal, but at times there was evidence of slight constipation. Body weight dropped by 25 kg. during the first month, but thereafter it remained more or less constant. Body temperature ranged from 99°–106·6°F and pyrexial peaks coincided with high parasitaemia. Frequently, the evening temperature was considerably higher than the morning temperature possibly indicating that parasitaemia rose towards evening. In the terminal stages of the infection the horse developed a purulent conjunctivitis. Death occurred after 110 days of infection.

In summary, the principal clinical signs of infection with *T. evansi* in this horse were pyrexia associated with peaks in parasitaemia, ecchymoses and petechiae in the visible mucous membranes, sporadic occurrence of urticarial plaques on the body surface and hydrocoele, oedema of the belly but not of the limbs, anaemia and muscular weakness.

T. evansi is notorious for its variable pathogenicity in different areas but where it causes clinical signs of disease it appears to affect the host-species in the same way as *T. brucei*.

TRYPANOSOMIASIS CAUSED BY *T. SIMIAE*

Cattle and equines are highly resistant to infection by *T. simiae* and no cases of *proved* infection with this trypanosome have been reported in these animals.

Disease of Sheep and Goats

Sheep and goats have shown variable susceptibility to infection with *T. simiae*. Frequently goats infected by the bites of wild-caught *Glossina* develop an acute or subacute infection resulting in death within one and a half months. However, infections caused by the sub-inoculation of blood may be chronic and even end in self-cure. Sheep are readily infected by infective tsetse but the disease is more chronic than that usually seen in goats. Parasitaemias may be moderately high in goats, but are generally lower in sheep. At *post-mortem* examination the carcases are seen to be very anaemic and wasted. There are no pathognomonic signs of *simiae* trypanosomiasis in these animals.

Disease of Camels

Camels are highly susceptible to infection by *T. simiae* and workers in Italian Somaliland have described the disease in the dromedary as being hyperacute and have stated that, after the pig, it is the most susceptible animal to this trypanosome.

No distinctive signs of trypanosomiasis are seen; the animal dies as if infected by a severe septicaemia.

Disease of Pigs

Bruce, *et al.* (1912), the discoverers of *T. simiae*, aptly described it as 'the lightening destroyer of the domestic pig', and added the fitting remark that: 'In the whole range of trypanosome diseases in animals there is surely nothing so striking as the rapidly fatal action of *T. simiae* on the domestic pig.' Other investigators have described the rapidly fatal course of the disease as 'sturmisch' and 'prèsque foudroyante'.

Death frequently occurs so soon after the appearance of the first trypanosome in the peripheral blood of the infected pig that the clinician will seldom have the opportunity of observing a sick living animal.

The clinical signs of illness are pyrexia (up to 106°F or 41·1°C), dullness, inappetence and sometimes anorexia, decreased activity varying from slight stiffness and disinclination to rise to an unsteady gait, respiratory distress seen as accelerated and 'thumping' breathing, and coldness of the extremities. Some workers have reported hyperaemia of the skin, salivation, frothing at the mouth, diarrhoea, oedema of the prepuce and heavy cough. It is likely that some of these signs were caused or aggravated by intercurrent infections such as helminthiasis due to lungworms (*Metastrongylus apri*), ascarids, strongyles and hookworms. The prepatent period in tsetse-transmitted infections is four to six days, and the parasitaemia when the animal is *in extremis* is massive: the blood is literally swarming with trypanosomes. For a complete description of trypanosomiasis in pigs in tropical Africa, the reader should consult the monograph by Stephen (1966a).

Disease of Dogs

The dog is refractory to infection with *T. simiae*.

TRYPANOSOMIASIS CAUSED BY *T. SUIS*

T. suis is almost certainly the least known and most infrequently reported pathogenic mammalian trypanosome. It has been seen only three times: in Dar-es-Salaam in 1905, in Tanganyika in 1912 and at Mosso in Burundi in 1953. The following information is derived from Peel and Chardome (1954).

Only the pig is susceptible to infection. The prepatent period in tsetse transmitted infections is six days. The disease runs a chronic course in adult pigs but is pathogenic in young pigs, causing death in less than two months.

Goats, sheep, donkey, dog, calves and small laboratory animals are all refractory.

TRYPANOSOMIASIS CAUSED BY *T. THEILERI*

It is generally conceded that *T. theileri* is non-pathogenic in cattle except perhaps in animals exposed to episodes of severe stress.

Most adult cattle in tropical Africa are probably exposed to infection with *T. theileri* since the biting tabanid flies by which it is transmitted are as ubiquitous as the cattle themselves. The principal reason for mentioning it here is to encourage workers to look for an alternative pathogen in cases of disease which might appear to be due to *T. theileri*.

Other species of animals are frequently infected with trypanosomes resembling *T. theileri*, such as *T. melophagium* in sheep.

TRYPANOSOMIASIS CAUSED BY *T. UNIFORME*

Infections with this trypanosome occur mainly in east and south Central Africa; *T. uniforme* has not been reported from West Africa. The literature contains conflicting reports on the pathogenicity of this organism for domestic animals and it appears that although some strains are virulent, the majority of infections run a relatively mild course.

The parasite closely resembles *T. vivax*, except for its smaller size, and it affects the same range of animals. Cattle, sheep and goats are the usual domestic animals infected; the writer is not aware of any *bona fide* reports of infections in horses, pigs and dogs. Laboratory animals are resistant.

The clinical manifestations caused by infection with *T. uniforme* bear such a close resemblance to those caused by *T. vivax* (*see* below) that a separate description of them need not be given.

TRYPANOSOMIASIS CAUSED BY *T. VIVAX*

Disease of Equines

Several observers of clinical trypanosomiasis in the horse have indicated that *T. vivax* infection is a relatively innocuous disease in both West and East Africa. However, Stephen and MacKenzie (1959) infected a horse by exposure to tsetse infected with a recently isolated, cyclically passaged strain of *T. vivax* in Nigeria and found that *T. vivax*, or at least the organism causing the infection in this instance, was pathogenic for the horse. Trypanosomes were found in the peripheral blood sixteen days after the first fly-challenge. During the sixteen days that the patent infection was allowed to run, there were four distinct peaks of parasitaemia, followed by periods when trypanosomes were present at only a low level or were not detectable. These crises were accompanied by pyrexia and fluctuations in the pulse and respiration rates.

Urticarial swellings appeared in the saddle area of the horse's back ten days after the first challenge and recurred periodically during the infection, coinciding with the interval between parasitaemic and temperature crises. On the latter occasions they appeared also on the face, neck and body.

The conjunctivae were distinctly congested three days before trypanosomes were detected and definite icterus was present on the day on which they were first seen in wet films. The icterus was pronounced until two days after treatment, although the conjunctivae and gums became increasingly paler as the disease progressed. Undoubtedly the presence or absence of icterus, in the horse, is related to the rate of destruction of erythrocytes.

The scrotal sac was distended, more or less, throughout the period of infection but the greatest distension coincided with the peaks of parasitaemia and temperature. This scrotal distension is thought to indicate an ascites rather than an oedema of the scrotal sac or testicles. Return to normal was rapid following treatment.

Oedema of the legs began with the onset of parasitaemia and was pronounced; the oedema was first seen at the fetlock and gradually rose to the level of the carpus and hock. Once again, however, the swelling was most clearly evident during the peak periods of parasitaemia.

The horse developed muscle tremors three days before trypanosomes appeared; these tremors were first noticed in the triceps muscles but were later observed to affect the latissimus dorsi and other superficial muscles of the thorax, abdomen and neck. As the animal became progressively weaker a distinct knee tremor was seen.

By the 5th day of infection the horse began to walk with a swaying gait which became progressively worse until, at seven days, the animal was only able to rise and to maintain its balance with great difficulty.

Throughout most of the period of infection appetite varied between good and poor, but towards the 15th day was definitely poor. During the week before trypanosomes appeared in the peripheral blood the horse lost 33 lbs. in weight and a further 42 lbs. during the period of infection.

On the 16th day of the infection the horse was walked to the balance for weighing prior to treatment. It was then very weak and walked with difficulty, swaying and dragging its feet. When standing it placed the legs wide apart to avoid falling down. The walk to the balance, a distance of 30 yards, caused great fatigue, polynoea and a pulse rate of 120 per minute.

Disease of Cattle

In East Africa, *T. vivax* infections in cattle are commonly encountered but the disease is usually regarded as mild. There are exceptions, however, and a number of reports mention acute, fatal disease due to this parasite.

The position in West Africa is quite different. *T. vivax* is widespread and infections in cattle usually run a rapidly fatal course.

Of the seventeen cattle challenged by wild-caught *Glossina morsitans submorsitans* in Nigeria, the writer found that in *T. vivax* infections, the prepatent period averaged eleven days (range 7–18 days) and the average duration of the infection until death occurred was 41·3 days (range 5–92 days).

In the acute form the disease may resemble a septicaemia and the animal may die within about a week. The body temperature rises to 104°–106°F, the animal looks dejected and frequently stands at pasture with the head hanging down. Appetite may be unimpaired but it usually reduced. Respirations are rapid and laboured and a jugular pulse may be seen. Faeces and urine are normal in most cases. Death occurs before the body looses condition although weight loss is frequently severe in animals in good condition at the beginning of infection. Parasitaemia is often massive and sustained.

In less severe cases there is progressive anaemia and loss of condition. The hair coat loses its lustre and becomes stary and the body loses its rounded contours and appears bony and angular. The superficial lymph nodes, especially the prescapulars and prefemorals are swollen and prominent. In other words, the animal develops the characteristic ‘fly-struck’ appearance. In the terminal stages the animal is unable to rise and dies in a state of exhaustion. Rises in body temperature accompany peaks in parasitaemia but oedema and ocular lesions are seldom observed. In cattle purchased from Nigerian traders for experimental purposes, the writer has, on rare occasions, encountered animals harbouring very scanty infections with *T. vivax* which did not appear to cause clinical symptoms.

Disease of Sheep and Goats

Sheep and goats are readily infected with *T. vivax* and are excellent laboratory animals for maintaining strains of the organism. Most infections end fatally, although a few sheep may develop chronic infections and survive for prolonged periods. Massive parasitaemia is sometimes observed, especially in goats. Intercurrent helminthic infections enhance the pathogenicity of the trypanosome.

The only clinical signs of any consequence are anaemia and loss of bodily condition.

Disease of Camels

Hornby (1952) states that camels are susceptible to infection with *T. vivax* and that although the disease may run an acute and fatal course, it is usually less severe than the disease caused by *T. congolense*.

Disease of Pigs

There are no reports of natural *T. vivax* infection in pigs. The writer has challenged pigs with wild tsetse in which the ratio of *T. vivax* to *T. congolense*-type infections in the fly was 2:1, but in no case was *T. vivax* ever seen in the blood of the pigs. There is no doubt that the pig is extremely resistant to infection with *T. vivax* and it may be completely refractory.

Disease of Dogs

The dog cannot be infected with *T. vivax*.

DIAGNOSIS AND DIFFERENTIAL DIAGNOSIS

Blood Examination

The only means by which a diagnosis of trypanosomiasis in domestic animals can be made with certainty is by demonstrating the presence of the infecting organism. This is ordinarily done by microscopical examination of a sample of blood or, in certain circumstances, of other body fluids or tissues. The techniques available for the detection of trypanosome infections have been described in detail in Chapter 4 and it is only necessary here to consider points of practical importance in the application of these techniques to domestic animals.

Samples of the peripheral blood for microscropical examination may be obtained quite simply by making and staining thin or thick blood films or by placing a drop of blood on a slide and covering it with a coverslip ('wet' blood film).

In domestic animals blood can usually be obtained from a small ear vein. The selected area should be prepared by clipping the hair with a pair of curved scissors, cleaning with alcohol and drying; a vein is then punctured with a needle of the Hagedoorn type or the edge of the ear may be snipped with scissors. The animal should be suitably restrained to avoid accidents.

The 'wet' film method provides a quick and convenient means of detecting the presence of trypanosomes but their specific identity cannot be determined with certainty although an experienced observer may be able to make a reasonable guess.

Examination of thin blood films affords the best means of identifying the species of trypanosome but has the disadvantage that scanty infections may be overlooked in the very small quantity of blood available for examination. This difficulty can be overcome, to some extent, by examining thick blood films but the morphological characters of the trypanosomes are not so easily distinguished as in thin films. The method of making and staining thick films described by MacLennan (1957) facilitates the identification of *T. vivax*, *T. congolense* and *T. brucei.*

Animal Inoculation as a Diagnostic Aid

The main disadvantage of blood film techniques is that only minute quantities of blood can be examined. Larger quantities can be inoculated into susceptible animals in which infections may be expected to develop. Godfrey and Killick-Kendrick (1961) have described a technique for the detection of trypanosome infections which involves the intra-peritoneal inoculation of 3 ml. of heparinized blood into laboratory-bred white rats. This method increases the likelihood of detecting infections with *T. congolense* and, especially, *T. brucei* but cannot be relied upon to detect *T. vivax* since this species usually fails to infect rats or produces only a scanty and transitory infection. The blood of inoculated rats should be examined for up to sixty days before a negative result is reported.

Ideally, several different species of animal should be inoculated with blood from a suspected case of trypanosomiasis because of the predilection of different species of trypanosome for various animals but the expense involved limits the use of this practice. It should be remembered that 'mixed' infections frequently occur in the field.

A technique (unpublished) employed by a Nigerian technical assistant in the writer's laboratory merits further examination. Heparinized blood (2–3 ml.) is injected intraperitoneally into a laboratory-bred white rat and 10–15 minutes later a splenic puncture is made through the thin body wall and examined as a wet and stained film. The spleen is readily observed if the hair over the region has been previously shaved off. The originator of this method frequently discovered trypanosomes by this means when other rapid tests were negative.

Lymph Node Puncture

Some workers have reported finding trypanosomes in lymph juice when the blood was negative. The technique of lymph gland puncture is useful in the diagnosis of *T. gambiense* infections in man but, in the writer's experience, it is of doubtful value in domestic animals. The procedure has the disadvantage that animals, especially cattle, resist it strenuously so that the operator is placed at considerable risk of injury.

Xenodiagnosis

If clean laboratory-reared *Glossina* are available they can be fed on the suspect animal on several occasions and subsequently on a clean animal in which an infection may later develop; alternatively, the flies can be dissected and examined for infection at the end of the period of cyclical development of the trypanosome. Although this method is commonly used to detect infections with *T. cruzi* in South and Central America, it is not a practicable method for the routine diagnosis of animal trypanosomiasis in Africa.

It is, however, a useful research tool for separating trypanosome species in mixed infections or for establishing 'pure' infections. For example, *Glossina palpalis* is seldom (perhaps never in West Africa) infected with *T. congolense* but is readily infected with *T. vivax*; small numbers may become infected with *T. brucei*. Thus, if a batch of *G. palpalis* is fed on a sheep with a mixed infection of *T. vivax*, *T. congolense* and *T. brucei*, *T. congolense* will not develop and infection with *T. vivax* will develop more rapidly than *T. brucei*. If the flies are fed on, say, a goat during the ensuing two weeks and thereafter on a dog, the goat will become infected with *T. vivax* and the dog, being refractory to *T. vivax*, will become infected with *T. brucei*.

Serological Tests

A variety of serological tests (*see* Chapter 6) have been used for the detection of trypanosome infections such as the red cell adhesion test, agglutination reaction, trypanolytic reaction, precipitin test, immunoconglutinin level, immunodiffusion reaction, complement fixation test and fluorescent antibody test. However, none is useful for species diagnosis.

The complement-fixation test has been widely used to detect dourine in horses but is of value only where no trypanosome infections other than *T. equiperdum* are present because other species would also give a positive reaction. A detailed description of the complement fixation test as applied to the diagnosis of dourine is given by Watson (1920). The test has also been used to detect trypanosomiasis in camels in regions where only *T. evansi* exists.

Chemical Tests

The only chemical test for animal trypanosomiasis that has had wide application is the mercuric chloride test for surra in camels. It is not specific for *T. evansi* infections, however, since it simply indicates a rise in globulin levels.

Culture

The African trypanosomes which are pathogenic for domestic animals have not been successfully propagated in artificial culture media. *T. theileri* has been successfully cultured but this is of little practical significance.

PROGNOSIS

The progress and outcome of untreated trypanosome infections in domestic animals depend on a variety of factors such as age, condition of the animal, presence of intercurrent infections, stress factors, whether the infection was due to cyclical or mechanical transmission, species and strain of the infecting organism, previous exposure to infection and so on. The host-parasite relationships of the various species of African mammalian trypanosomes have been described in Chapter 2. The course of various trypanosome infections in different groups of domestic animals is described below in general terms but it must be remembered that exceptions to these generalizations can, and do, occur.

Equines

Animals in this group are high susceptible to *T. brucei* and death is the general expectation; spontaneous recoveries are rare. Infections with *T. equiperdum* result in a high mortality but some animals acquire a mild infection and may be carriers for long periods before they show signs of infection; some cases undoubtedly recover. *T. evansi* infections vary from area to area; for example, in the Sudan, horses are said to be highly resistant while in some other countries the disease is disastrous. Reports of *T. vivax* infections are conflicting but when parasitaemias are high the disease will often end fatally within a short period of time. The same may be said about *T. congolense* but cognizance must be taken of the wide variety of strains seen in this species. The horse is highly resistant to *T. simiae* and may be refractory to it.

Cattle

Here one must recall the possibility of breed susceptibility, e.g. the Muturu and N'dama breeds of West Africa exist in areas where Zebu and exotic breeds would rapidly succumb to trypanosome infections. The area where the infection occurs is also very important. In West Africa, animals infected with *T. vivax* rarely recover and usually die within two months whereas in East Africa the disease is usually mild and many animals show few ill effects and may recover spontaneously, but acute and rapidly fatal cases may sometimes occur. *T. brucei* infections only rarely cause overt ill health in cattle.

In East Africa, the majority of infections with *T. congolense* terminate in death although the disease is seldom as rapidly fatal as that caused by *T. vivax* in West Africa.

T. uniforme has only been reported from east and south Central Africa where it usually causes a mild disease in cattle.

T. evansi is probably of little consequence as a pathogenic trypanosome in African cattle except in parts of the Republic of Sudan.

T. simiae and *T. suis* do not infect cattle.

Sheep and Goats

Natural trypanosome infection in sheep and goats are relatively uncommon but may be found in areas where it would be impossible to keep cattle. These animals are, however, readily infected with *T. vivax* and *T. congolense* experimentally. Sheep generally develop more chronic infections than goats. Some strains of *T. vivax* in West Africa are capable of causing death regularly in goats but only the long forms of *T. congolense* appear to be pathogenic.

Natural infections with *T. simiae* in sheep usually run a chronic course but fly-transmitted infections in goats may be rapidly fatal.

Other species of trypanosomes in sheep and goats are only laboratory curiosities.

Camels

Infections due to *T. evansi* will be the ones usually met by the clinician and a high mortality can be expected in untreated animals. If there is a possibility that camels have been in contact with tsetse then infections due to *T. brucei*, *T. vivax*, *T. congolense* and *T. simiae* may be encountered and specific treatment will be required if the animals are to survive. *T. brucei* infections are especially severe and *T. simiae* is so pathogenic that animals may be found dead before any significant signs of illness are noticed.

Pigs

Only *T. simiae* in the pig will be of particular concern to the clinician: other species produce chronic infections from which the animal may recover. Since tsetse-transmitted infections are often propagated by mechanical vectors such as Tabanid flies or *Stomoxys*, a high mortality rate, frequently decimating entire herds, can be expected in unprotected animals.

In areas where it occurs, *T. suis* causes death in young pigs and chronic infections in mature animals. Because of its extreme rarity, this organism will be of little or no concern to farmers or clinicians.

Dogs

T. brucei infections in dogs usually end fatally within a month if untreated, and *T. congolense* may cause fatal infections, especially those due to the long or *dimorphon*-type organism.

Chapter 42

Care and Treatment of Animals Suffering from Trypanosomiasis

L. E. STEPHEN

Probably the most important effect of trypanosomiasis in domestic animals is the severe anaemia. Although specific chemotherapy will usually result in destruction of the parasite and a halt to the progression of the anaemia, thought must be given to supportive therapy. An adequate diet should be provided and should include green feeds. Rest is essential, otherwise a severe strain is placed on the heart. The administration of a tonic containing haematinics such as iron salts and arsenical compounds helps to speed recovery. Shelter from inclement weather should be provided during the rainy season because debilitated animals are frequently predisposed to other diseases.

In the treatment of animal trypanosomiasis with specific chemotherapeutic agents, the practical procedures described below are of prime importance and the need for their strict observance cannot be too strongly emphasized. Undoubtedly, many drug-resistant strains have arisen because field workers (admittedly working under difficult conditions) have failed to realize the great importance of administering adequate dosages of freshly prepared drugs.

Many chemotherapeutic agents, once they are in solution, do not keep well and it is therefore wise to make them up freshly before they are administered. Some are readily soluble in water while others are much less so and may have to be dissolved in hot or warm water. Because many trypanocidal compounds are highly coloured it is important to make certain that all the powder has gone into solution, otherwise under-dosing will result.

Sterile distilled water should normally be used as diluent but this may not be readily available in the field and ordinary *boiled* water may have to be used.

The recommended route of administration should be followed, since many trypanocidal drugs cause severe local reactions if given by an alternative route. If the drug has been injected subcutaneously the site should be well massaged to disperse the inoculum. In meat animals, intramuscular injections should be made into muscles that have low sale value because of the possibility of discoloration or tissue damage.

Trypanosomes are notoriously liable to develop resistance to the therapeutic activity of drugs and since the chemical structures of many of the compounds in current use are closely related, resistance to one drug often results in a degree of resistance to others. It is essential therefore that freshly prepared drug in adequate dosage should be given. Most trypanocidal drugs are administered on a live weight basis so that it is important to estimate body weight as accurately as possible and to use a calibrated syringe for the injection.

While under-dosage may result in the production of drug-resistant trypanosomes, over-dosage can easily result in the death or serious illness of the animal because the therapeutic index for some trypanocidal drugs is very narrow.

In seriously debilitated animals, or when a drug has a narrow therapeutic index, it may be wise to give the drug in a divided dose.

After treatment, animals should always be kept under observation for at least an hour so that toxic signs can be observed and unnecessary exertion prevented. The usual signs of toxicity in animals are salivation and chewing movements, lachrymation, sweating, muscle tremors and sometimes temporary collapse.

Most of the drugs used in chemoprophylactic regimens are also active therapeutically but they should be reserved for preventive, and not curative, use because of the possibility of producing drug-resistant strains of trypanosomes.

The drugs available for the treatment of the trypanosomiases of animals have been described in detail in Chapter 7.

T. brucei Infections

Horses and dogs develop serious infections with this organism. The most satisfactory chemotherapeutic agent is quinapyramine sulphate injected subcutaneously at a dose rate of 5 mg./kg. employing a 10% aqueous solution. As toxic reactions are not unusual the total dose should be divided into two or three equal parts and injected at six-hourly intervals.

The next most useful drug in these animals is suramin (*BP*) at a dose rate of 7–10 mg./kg. given as a 10% aqueous solution by the intravenous route. This treatment should be repeated one week later. It should be remembered that suramin is a hygroscopic material and may absorb up to 35% moisture if left exposed to tropical atmospheric conditions; it is therefore wise to dry it at 130°C for 24 hours before use. Toxic reactions may occur following treatment with suramin.

If it is necessary to treat cattle or camels, quinapyramine sulphate at the same dose rate as for horses should be chosen. The same may be said about infections in pigs, sheep and goats.

T. congolense Infections

Cattle infected with *T. congolense* may usually be treated successfully with any one of the following trypanocidal drug preparations:

(a) Homidium bromide, *B. vet. C.* (Ethidium bromide) or homidium chloride, *B. vet. C.* (Novidium) at a dose rate of 1·0 mg./kg. given as a 1 or 2% w/v aqueous solution intramuscularly (usually the triceps or crural muscles). Subcutaneous injections may cause severe swelling but intramuscular administration is seldom followed by toxic sequelae. The chloride salt is more soluble than the bromide, and concentration may be varied to make the injection volume of suitable size.

(b) Isometamidium chloride (Samorin) at a dose rate of 0·25 mg./kg. given as a 2% aqueous solution intramuscularly. Subcutaneous injections of this compound, even in the dewlap, cause large oedematous swellings. The dosage should be increased if drug-resistance is suspected.

(c) N-1, 3-diamidinophenyl-triazene diaceturate (Berenil) at a dose rate of 3·5 mg./kg. given by intramuscular or subcutaneous injection of a 7% aqueous solution. It is important to remember that, though stable when dry, Berenil in aqueous solutions remains stable for only two or three days. This drug will frequently cure infections by trypanosomes that are resistant to other drugs.

Homidium and isometamidium have some prophylactic activity but Berenil is degraded metabolically and excreted rapidly, usually within twenty-four hours, and this probably explains its lack of prophylactic activity and its only slight tendency to give rise to resistant trypanosome strains.

Should treatment be required, sheep and goats may be treated as recommended for cattle using the same body weight calculations.

Equines may be treated with homidium, quinapyramine or Berenil but as toxic reactions sometimes occur the dose should be divided.

Berenil at 7·0 mg./kg. in camels can cause toxic signs but is probably safe at 3·5 mg./kg. Experience in this animal with the other 'cattle' drugs is limited.

T. evansi Infections

Suramin at 7–10 mg./kg. by intravenous injection of a 10% aqueous solution is the drug of choice for *T. evansi* infections in camels. Recent reports from Asia suggest that quinapyramine sulphate at 5 mg./kg. in 10% aqueous solution given subcutaneously is effective in horses, cattle and buffaloes. Untoward reactions have been reported more commonly in horses than in other species and in certain areas suramin may be the better drug to employ.

T. equiperdum Infections

Suramin and quinapyramine have been reported as having a beneficial effect on dourine infections at the usual dose rates, but control by test and slaughter methods are probably the most useful in countries where total eradication of the disease is the objective.

T. simiae Infections

Infections due to this trypanosome are highly resistant to most of the drugs generally used in veterinary medicine. In the pig, various quinapyramine preparations have been shown to have quite a high degree of therapeutic activity against *T. simiae*. However, infections in this animal are fulminating and there will seldom be an opportunity to use drugs therapeutically before death supervenes. Furthermore, the most useful drug therapeutically (quinapyramine) is also the most useful chemoprophylactic agent and because of the danger of producing drug resistance it cannot be over-emphasized that, in this case especially, *prevention is better than cure*. For the same reason, the treatment of sheep and goats with quinapyramine is not recommended.

T. suis Infection

Chemotherapeutic studies have not been made on this trypanosome, but because of its biological resemblances to those of the *brucei*-group, agents effective against the latter should be tried if necessary.

T. vivax and *T. uniforme* Infections

Infections with *T. vivax* in cattle, sheep, goats and horses are readily cured by homidium bromide or chloride *B. vet. C.* at a dose rate of 1·0 mg./kg. administered as a 2% aqueous solution by intramuscular injection. The subcutaneous route should not be used as local oedematous swellings of varying severity usually result.

In horses it is advisable to divide the dose equally and to give the second dose six hours after the first.

Isometamidium chloride and Berenil are also effective against *T. vivax* and should be used at the same dose rate and concentration as suggested for *T. congolense* infections.

Treated animals should be closely watched to detect the occurrence of relapses, preferably by blood examination. It should also be recalled that relapse infections are often characterized by a low, sporadic parasitaemia and an apparent reduction in pathogenicity for the original host. The animal may, however, constitute a serious focus of infection from which other animals in the area may be infected by mechanical or cyclical transmission—possibly with a drug-resistant trypanosome. Relapse infections should always be treated with an entirely different drug.

Chapter 43

Practical Application of Measures for the Control of Tsetse-borne Trypanosomiases of Livestock

K. J. R. MACLENNAN

INTRODUCTORY

Methods of controlling or eliminating losses in livestock husbandry from vector-borne trypanosomiasis may be aimed directly or indirectly at the insect vectors or at the parasites in the domestic animal concerned. The alternative approaches of eliminating the trypanosome infection in flies or in feral reservoir hosts are impracticable in *Glossina*-borne trypanosomiasis because of the existence of uncontrollable mammalian sources of infection, and because of movement of the livestock and wild animals or dispersal of *Glossina* from other localities. But elimination of the source of infection carried by the insect vector is the only practicable method of preventing infections from non-cyclical transmission which are dependent on the existence of infection and close contact between individuals within the affected herd or flock. There are practical possibilities of controlling or exterminating *Glossina* over substantial areas but this approach is usually inapplicable to the potential non-cyclical vectors of the disease which are widespread, and sometimes exceedingly numerous, in the environment in which most livestock are raised.

The eradication of *Glossina* will eliminate, or reduce to comparatively insignificant proportions, the incidence of vector-borne trypanosomiasis in livestock; in fact, this has been the outcome where extermination of *Glossina* has been achieved. However, this is not the case with *T. evansi* infections or in the rather exceptional circumstances where strains or species of trypanosomes completely adapted to the absence of *Glossina* are prevalent. The elimination of *Glossina* also ends the transmission of human trypanosomiasis. Substantial progress in controlling *T. gambiense* infections has been made by treating the human host, thereby reducing the liability of *Glossina* to become infected, but in many cases residual foci of the disease persist at an irreducible level. So long as the appropriate tsetse are present trypanosomiasis remains a continuous problem in livestock and, at best, a potential and grave threat to the human population. *Glossina*-borne trypanosomiasis cannot at present be completely eliminated by use of trypanocidal drugs in the human or animal host, but drugs, despite imperfections, are valuable and essential palliatives. The administration of adequate quantities of therapeutic agents to man and his domestic animals, amounts to a very heavy financial, administrative and technical burden which may prove difficult to sustain continuously, but over much of Africa, with or without vector control measures, it is currently the only practicable measure for checking the ravages of the disease. The control of *Glossina* may also be a repetitive commitment which may be difficult to sustain but, where permanent extermination can be attained and where the land is needed and is capable of sound exploitation, substantial expenditure on this objective is clearly justified.

METHODS OF GENERAL APPLICATION

The Selection of Healthy Areas

Glossina-borne trypanosomiasis may be avoided by selecting localities where tsetse flies are absent. Outside the geographical limits of tsetse infestation this is a comparatively simple matter provided these limits have been accurately defined; however, even under these circumstances, trypanosomiasis may be transmitted by tsetse which have been transported by vehicles over substantial distances. In areas where such flies cannot establish self-sustaining colonies they may live long enough to transmit disease. In many places, knowledge of the extent of tsetse infestation is not precise and sometimes these flies may be discovered in areas well outside previously defined limits.

Within the geographical limits of *Glossina* distribution there may be substantial areas from which tsetse are absent or where density may be low or limited to certain species. Local circumstances are so diverse and so variable that it is impossible to generalize but the following points should always be borne in mind. Firstly, the situation cannot be assessed without experience and knowledge of the ecology of the species of tsetse involved in the particular locality; secondly, the introduction of livestock into the locality can sometimes encourage the extension of infestation; and, thirdly, the distribution and density of *Glossina* in the surrounding country, particularly of the savanna species, are subject to significant alteration and this has, not infrequently, led to a serious trypanosomiasis problem in areas which had previously been suitable for stock raising. For the reasons discussed elsewhere (*see* Chapter 39), the presence of semi-nomadic stock cannot be taken as an indication that an area is necessarily suited to a more settled and advanced form of stock-raising, although it may sometimes indicate that the risk may be moderate rather than severe. It does not follow that the risk is sufficiently low to ensure the economic success of a more static form of husbandry. It should also be borne in mind that changes in the riparian and upland vegetation are inevitable in areas reserved for stock raising, cultivation or forestry. Depending on the nature of these changes, they may encourage or discourage tsetse infestations. A cadre of trained, experienced and reliable personnel is required for assessment of actual or potential tsetse infestations. Reliable maps are an essential prerequisite and good aerial photographs can be of very great assistance. It is also very helpful to view localities from a low-flying light aircraft. Because of seasonal changes, assessments may take some time to complete and in conditions of low tsetse density, or with species which are difficult to detect, surveys must be repeated. Indicator herds of susceptible livestock should be used to confirm field survey findings unless these are decisive.

Seldom has it proved practicable in West Africa to select routes for seasonal migration or for slaughter stock which significantly ameliorate the risk from tsetse. The migratory routes are multiple and have evolved over a period of time to meet the constantly changing pattern of cultivation and human population. They already avoid, when this is feasible, the more important tsetse infestations. The trade cattle routes may change according to season, avoiding waterless upland infested by *G. morsitans* in the dry season to follow more low lying areas which would be impassable in the rains. The problem of trypanosomiasis on stock routes certainly merits the most careful attention but diversion of these to localities of lighter risk seldom seems to be a practicable procedure in West Africa.

The Selection of Suitable Livestock

In many classes of livestock there exist breeds and strains which have a well developed capacity to tolerate or resist infection with pathogenic trypanosomes (*see* Chapters 6 and 39). The fuller utilization of such stock is not a straightforward problem and the concept of large herds and flocks of tolerant or resistant stock utilizing the huge empty spaces of the more heavily infested savanna areas, in the same manner as less tolerant stock are used to exploit the less heavily infested areas, has proved difficult to realize. Whatever the reasons, it seems to be true that when even highly tolerant cattle are maintained under continuous risk and are managed on a herd basis by pastoralists dedicated to the welfare of their stock, as with the Kateku Fulani of Borgu, these animals are neither as productive nor as numerous as the larger stock maintained in more lightly infested areas. The extreme susceptibility of the dwarf cattle breeds to rinderpest is a factor in limiting their numbers. There is, therefore, a tendency to up-grade trypanosome-tolerant breeds by introducing as much Zebu blood as possible, but the extent to which this expedient can be safely exploited is limited by a variety of complex factors including not only trypanosomiasis but also other forms of parasitism. But it is also evident that where tsetse have been eliminated or greatly reduced in previously infested areas, Zebu cattle introduced by pastoralists may thrive where previously only a few dwarf cattle had been kept by the indigenous arable farmers; this was clearly demonstrated in parts of the Tiv country in northern Nigeria but, unfortunately, the owners of the Zebu stock were reluctantly compelled to vacate the area for socio-political reasons.

In many communities in West Africa, strains of sheep and goats exist which have become adapted to local conditions. Indeed, over much of West Africa, strains of stock exist which can adapt themselves to a considerable degree of exposure to trypanosome infection but, for a great variety of reasons, their numbers fall far short of the potential maximum. The introduction or development of further tolerant or resistant types seems unlikely to have much impact unless the numerous other factors involved can be identified and suitably met.

Game cropping and game farming are potential methods of deriving animal products—notably meat, hides and skins—from grazing areas infested by *Glossina*. The suitability of these methods and the type of animal used will vary considerably according to circumstances. Assessment of the value of some types of game animal in making productive use of certain areas indicates that they may have worthwhile potential but much further work remains to be done.[1] Not only are some wild animals able to tolerate a substantial trypanosomiasis risk but they may be able to thrive in areas where water is scarce and where pasturage is barely sufficient for domestic stock.

Pearsall (1959) has pointed out that domestic breeds of animals are unlikely to be found which are as well attuned to their habitat as wild animals (Glover, 1965). There are several practical disadvantages in the adoption of methods of this kind but their ultimate potential cannot be disregarded.

Land Utilization

It is of fundamental importance that land resources made available by tsetse reclamation projects are utilized in such a way as to ensure optimal productivity and, at the same time, minimize the risk of re-infestation by tsetse. The ideal situation is one in which the methods of land utilization adopted render the area untenable by tsetse. This has been successfully achieved in some places

[1] For further information on this subject readers are referred to papers presented at the 'East African Wildlife—Land Use Symposium' held at Nairobi in 1967 and to publications by Ledger (1964); Dasman (1964); Riney (1965); and Talbot and Payne (1965).

but it is an ideal which is singularly difficult to attain in many parts of Africa.

In West Africa, the use of land solely for seasonal pasturage has little effect on tsetse infestation. It has seldom proved possible to exploit agricultural practices to destroy the habitats of riverine tsetse or even to prevent the regrowth of vegetation which has been cleared as an anti-tsetse measure. In some places, however, the cultivator has been induced to destroy islands of riparian vegetation or to adopt farming methods which will restrain the regeneration of cleared vegetation as, for example, by the cultivation of sugar cane or rice.

An outstanding example of the great benefits which can be derived from tsetse reclamation combined with planned land utilization is provided by a major re-settlement scheme carried out in the Anchau area of northern Nigeria (often referred to as the Anchau Corridor) and described by Nash (1948). This area, which extends to about 700 square miles, was severely affected by sleeping sickness transmitted by tsetse of the *palpalis* group. The measures adopted to control the vectors included discriminative clearing of the local streams, the provision of barrier clearings to prevent wet season re-infestation from a larger river, and the creation of forest reserves along the latter so as to minimize human contact with tsetse. Other measures carried out concurrently included movement of the local inhabitants to the lightly forested watershed area, the planned siting and layout of villages, and the use of the land for the cultivation of staple grain crops, sugar cane, groundnuts and cotton, and, to some extent, for the maintenance of livestock. These combined measures were successful in converting an unhealthy and unproductive community into a healthy and prosperous one. There can be little doubt that, had they not been taken, the area would have been depopulated. The fact that the project area subsequently became engulfed and infiltrated by an advance of *G. morsitans* has prevented the full development of balanced agricultural practice and constant vigilance is required to prevent the regrowth of habitats liable to infestation by riverine tsetse.

In areas where tsetse control has been achieved by mechanical clearing of upland bush, failure to institute appropriate regimes for the management of pasture and agriculture may lead to uncontrolled regeneration followed by reinfestation. It may be difficult to persuade the cultivator to adopt land use practices which are strange to him but essential if regrowth is to be prevented. In some places, knowledge of suitable methods for the management of pasture and crop land is highly developed while in other areas this has yet to be obtained.

Uncontrolled cultivation by expanding tribes may result in the disappearance of tsetse of the *morsitans* group from thousands of square miles of infested country but riverine tsetse usually remain. The latter may constitute a serious threat to human health but the risk to livestock is often insufficiently great to preclude the seasonal exploitation of pasturage by Zebu stock. But unless the land resources in such areas are defined, mapped and allocated to the purposes for which they are best suited—cultivation, grazing, forestry, etc.—there will be a grave danger that valuable natural resources will be dissipated and possibly new tsetse habitats created.

In agricultural communities in which significant numbers of livestock are kept, it may be possible so to arrange the areas cultivated as to ensure that stock are kept at some distance from the 'fly front', and to reinforce this measure by bush clearance, the application of insecticides and the use of drugs to protect the stock. In some areas infested by tsetse of the *morsitans* group, this may be the most practical means of maintaining livestock, but if it is to be successful care must be taken to avoid overstocking and the development of drug resistance.

The greatest opportunities for proper land utilization are to be found in large areas in which the need and potential for development exist and in which it has been shown that all types of tsetse infestation can be eliminated by the application of appropriate techniques. In such circumstances a substantial proportion of the land resources may be uninhabited and therefore available for allocation to the type of land usage for which it is best suited. The optimal use of land resources calls for careful planning based on the combined efforts of surveyors, soil scientists, ecologists, specialists on pastoral, arable and forestry matters, and persons qualified to advise on human and animal health hazards. It is valuable also to have experimental evidence on the potential uses to which different types of land resources can be put. The skilled interpretation of aerial photographs may yield important information and, in all work of this kind, accurate maps are essential.

An example of this type of rational approach is provided by current projects in northern Nigeria involving two extensive areas of 22,600 and 36,900 square miles, respectively. The first phase of these projects involved an investigation of the feasibility of tsetse extermination. This was undertaken jointly by an ecologist and a tsetse control officer who, over a period of twenty months, studied the areas on the ground, sifted all available local data and assessed the experiences gained over a period of twelve years. On this basis, they concluded that tsetse extermination was feasible over the whole of the first area of 22,600 square miles and over 21,475 square miles of the second area (Glover & Aitcheson, 1966, 1967). The second phase, currently in progress, is to prepare a comprehensive land use plan and, in this work, technical experts from the Land Resources Division of the United Kingdom Directorate of Overseas Surveys are collaborating with the appropriate local authorities and their experts. The third and final stage of these projects will be the execution of plans evolved in this way. It may prove to be easier to eliminate tsetse than to ensure that the recommendations made for the use of the land are carried out but, at least, an opportunity for sound development will have been created.

Forest reserves merit special consideration since they may, and indeed have, become the means of perpetuating and extending areas of tsetse infestation. Policies for the reservation of forest should be formulated for each major vegetation zone with the object of meeting the forestry requirements of the community without, at the same time, maintaining or increasing areas of tsetse infestation. The policy to be adopted in a particular locality will vary according to local circumstances but, in formulating it, certain general principles should be observed. The size of the reserve is important. The needs of the community and the requirements for tsetse control or eradication would seem to be best served by the creation of small units in which, if necessary, tsetse control measures can be effectively applied. Large reserves are liable to prejudice the success of future tsetse eradication projects and if they are already, or should become, infested, tsetse extermination is difficult to achieve. When a reserve is not already infested but is liable to become so at some future date, care should be taken to isolate it within an area which is unsuitable for tsetse as, for example, an area of cultivation. The distances between reserves should be sufficiently great to prevent the spread of tsetse from one reserve to another. Proposals for the creation of forest reserves should always be referred to the medical and veterinary authorities for their comments. Some of these principles do not, of course, apply to those parts of Africa which are specifically set aside to maintain the natural heritage in its entirety as in National Parks and Game Reserves.

MEASURES FOR THE ELIMINATION OR LIMITATION OF TSETSE FLY POPULATIONS

The various methods available for the eradication or limitation of tsetse fly populations have been described in detail in Part II and it is only necessary here to consider the practical implications of applying them to the protection of livestock in the field.

The need to control trypanosomiasis is usually dictated by some pressing local human or animal health problem. It is necessary at the outset to decide upon the method or methods best suited to the attainment of the desired objective.

Methods of controlling trypanosomiasis involving a direct attack on the insect vector fall into two distinct categories: (1) measures designed to achieve complete elimination of the fly which, if successful, provide a permanent solution, and (2) those which do not achieve complete elimination and therefore involve continuing expenditure on their maintenance. The former will be referred to here as *extermination* and the latter as *control* measures.

Extermination measures may be directed against all species of tsetse present in the area or may be restricted to the species known to be responsible for the transmission of trypanosomiasis (Du Toit, 1954; MacLennan, 1967). Unless all contiguous areas can be included in the elimination operation, control measures will be required to prevent re-invasion since suitable tsetse habitats may persist, or be re-created, within the area from which the fly has been eliminated. Assuming that, in a given area, an effective and economic technique is available to ensure extermination of all tsetse, the ultimate success of the operation will depend on the ability to achieve complete elimination in the total area of infestation or, where this is unattainable, to prevent re-invasion by some economically justifiable method.

Destruction of Game Animals

In certain circumstances, it has been found possible to reclaim areas from tsetse infestation and to control the spread of tsetse by the destruction of game animals. A full account of the development and use of this method has been given in Chapter 28. In practice, the method, alone or combined with other measures, has been used with success against tsetse of the *morsitans* group in Uganda, Rhodesia and the southern Sudan.

Cattle Fences

Cattle fences, sometimes many hundreds of miles in length, are erected in some territories to prevent the movement of cattle into areas in which they would be exposed to greater risk of contracting trypanosomiasis, and from which they would be liable to bring back trypanosomes and tsetse flies into clean areas. Cattle fences are used in conjunction with game eviction and game fences to eliminate the favoured food sources of savanna tsetse populations and thereby limit the diffusion or actual advance of tsetse infestation.

Clearing of Vegetation

The clearing of vegetation—partial or complete—has been described in Chapter 27. These methods have been successfully applied in various parts of Africa to obtain more or less permanent elimination of tsetse but the extent to which they are currently used is determined by cost; for example, the cost of clearing heavy riverine vegetation in West Africa in 1967 was estimated to be of the order of £2,a00 per square mile. It is difficult to control the regeneration of woody vegetation which follows clearing and long-term surveillance is required. The most favourable results are obtained when, following clearing, the local population can be induced to adopt practices which prevent regeneration such as cultivation of the land and pasture management by controlled grazing and burning. This may be very difficult to achieve if the local population is not naturally inclined to follow them. Protection of large areas against fire, essential if late or postponed burning is to be relied upon to control woody regrowth, is exceedingly difficult to ensure in localities in which the dry season is pronounced and prolonged, and in which the traditional practice is to burn early.

Arboricides are not only expensive to buy but are surprisingly costly to apply. The time of their application in relation to the growth phase of the species to be treated is of critical significance and this no doubt accounts for the inconsistent results which have been reported. Species of tree vary greatly in susceptibility to aboricides; some common woodland species may be quite resistant. So far, no really effective arboricide has become available which is capable of dealing with all the important species which provide suitable habitats for tsetse. The powers of survival of African trees are remarkable; trees which have apparently been killed may spring into leaf even after the lapse of eighteen months. Arboricides are probably of greatest value for the control of regrowth after clearing.

Clearing measures are still practical and effective methods of dealing with local problems affecting village and urban communities and ranches where the use of insecticides would yield only transient results.

Insecticides

The insecticides which have been used for the control of tsetse populations have been described in detail in Chapters 23 and 24.

In field practice, insecticides have been employed in one of two main ways, namely, (a) the repeated and relatively non-selective dispersal of low-dosage, non-persistent aerosols, and (b) the restricted application to known tsetse resting places of a single or a limited number of treatments with a relatively heavy, persistent deposit.

One of the more significant achievements in tsetse extermination has been the elimination of *G. pallidipes* from 7,000 square miles of Zululand, using insecticides applied mainly as non-persistent aerosols (Du Toit, 1954). This was a prolonged operation; insecticidal applications of various kinds were made intermittently over a period of three years. The whole campaign including initial surveys and the search for effective extermination methods lasted for seven years. The insecticides employed were DDT and BHC. Methods of application ranged from aerial applications by fixed wing aircraft and helicopters to ground based methods such as thermal smoke generating canisters, dust dispersal, and application to cattle by dipping. The area included three well stocked game reserves. Surveys based on the collection of pupal cases were relied upon to define the most significant habitats utilized by *G. pallidipes* which were estimated to occupy only 3% of the total infested area. Furthermore, it was demonstrated in preliminary trials that, although the fly dispersed very widely from its concentrated breeding areas, the dispersed population collapsed if insecticidal applications were confined to these limited localities. In this campaign the considerable experimentation in the course of the search for extermination methods led ultimately to the conclusion that the eradication of *G. pallidipes* could be achieved by, at the most, ten applications of BHC in exhaust aerosol form (*see* Chapter 24), at three to four week intervals, to accurately defined breeding areas in favourable terrain. Areas with more numerous valleys may require additional applications by helicopters, and discriminative clearings may be required in mountainous country. The writer makes the point that the concentration of the principal breeding sites of *G. pallidipes* into 3% of the infested area enabled the discriminative and economical application of insecticides.

The use of persisting deposits entails much heavier local application rates of insecticide. The economic feasibility of this method is therefore dependent on a technique of restricted application to features of the tsetse environment used as perching places by tsetse. Stages in the process of restricted selection of sites of application have been described by Davies (1964) who defined two phases, 'discrimination' to indicate the choice of those vegetative communities within the infested area in which numbers of tsetse were observed to concentrate (e.g. thicket, riparian strips, ecotones) and 'selection' to indicate those places within such communities where the flies actually perch (e.g. on tree trunks to certain heights, certain types of branches). When selected to this degree, the places to which the insecticide is applied may occupy a minute proportion of the infested area, and if restricted to places adopted by the flies as a result of some environmental stress factor, the measures become increasingly effective and economical.

The degree to which the principles of selection and discrimination can be applied vary greatly with circumstances, particularly with the species of *Glossina* and environmental influences such as vegetation zone, vegetation type and climate. Success is more likely in places near the drier limits of distribution of the species concerned and is facilitated by the occurrence of any stress factor such as limitation in the extent of suitable vegetational environment, inhospitable climate or shortage of food sources. Success is dependent on a thorough knowledge of the bionomics of the species concerned. There is a danger that 'atypical' habitats may be overlooked and so lead to re-infestation.

Under favourable circumstances in northern Nigeria, for example in *Isoberlinia* woodland, the discriminative application of insecticide to vegetation in ecotones and other features of the environment such as paths frequented by *G. morsitans*, and the selective application to branch resting sites within these localities as described by MacLennan (1967) led to application rates of 0·09 to 0·15 lb. of DDT (active ingredient) per acre of overall infestation. In fact the degree of discrimination practised meant that attention was devoted to only 7 to 13% of the infested area, dependent on the prevalence of concentration habitat, to which the rate of application was 1·3 to 0·98 lb. per acre.

It has proved possible to prevent re-invasion of part of the project area by repeating the measures in a buffer zone on the infested portion of the project perimeter over a period of four years but these repetitive measures cost as much annually as an annual phase of work in the extermination area.

Any advantage in cost of the single application of a persistent deposit over repeated aerosol applications derives from the degree of discrimination and selection which is possible. Elsewhere in northern Nigeria, in the relatively dry Sudan savanna zones, *G. morsitans* and *G. tachinoides* have been eliminated from substantial areas by the single restricted application of DDT WP at the rate of 0·45 to 0·11 lb. actual DDT per acre of infested area. Near the northern limit of infestation success has been achieved by applications limited to a height of two feet above ground level.

The behaviour of the insecticide formulations on the substrate (usually bark, occasionally leaves) to which it is applied is of crucial significance and climatic factors appear to exert a great influence. It is often impossible to achieve the elimination of *G. palpalis* by a single application, even of the more potent dieldrin, because the activity of the deposit declines more rapidly in the moister habitat essential for this fly than in the drier parts which can be utilized by the savanna species and *G. tachinoides*, and *G. palpalis* may be inherently less susceptible to insecticides. In Kenya it is the normal practice to use four applications for the control of the *palpalis* group of tsetse. Workers in northern Nigeria have shown that deposits applied to bark in the dry state may show lethal activity through the ensuing rains, the following dry season and even, to some slight degree, to the commencement of the second rainy season, whereas insecticide applied to bark in a moister, though not wet, state after the rains have set in is very rapidly lost (MacLennan, 1967).

Most studies of biological persistence have used exposures of test *Glossina* of short (say one minute) duration. Lycklama (*in press*) has shown that such tests, which may be dependent on a lethal dose adhering to the tarsi of the fly may fail to reveal the potential activity of certain types of deposit of small amount and that exposures of much longer duration (two hours) will give much higher mortalities. For example, a dieldrin deposit of 10 mg./square foot will kill 80 to 100% of test flies, control corrected, and deposits of 50 mg./square foot DDT will kill 30%. The deposits were fourteen months old and gave negligible mortalities with the short exposure test. It is not known how long a fly will voluntarily remain in contact with a toxic deposit, or how many shorter exposures it would experience in nature, but such studies are essential to the formulation of effective insecticide preparations. This experiment indicates the much greater toxicity of weathered deposits of dieldrin relative to DDT.

One of the more important factors which determine the feasibility of the extermination of *Glossina* infestations is the quality of persistence of the deposit since, if adequate persistence can be secured, an extermination operation may advance in a series of annual phases using a single application, until the whole infestation is eliminated. Re-invasion of sprayed areas by *G. morsitans* may take place in some depth within twelve months, but field experiences suggest that self-sustaining colonies may not be able to establish themselves until the second rainy season after the insecticide was applied, in the type of infestation which is encountered in the *Isoberlinia* woodland savanna of northern Nigeria. Otherwise, the re-invasion problem threatening extermination projects which do not eliminate a complete tsetse infestation, can only be handled by the creation of cleared barriers, the required extent of which will vary greatly according to circumstances or, alternatively, by the siting of fly pickets, by the creation of an insecticidal buffer zone from which re-infestation is periodically eliminated, or by combinations of these methods. In some instances the tsetse environment in the extermination area can be so modified through settlement and development that re-infestation is no longer possible. The magnitude and cost of such measures, which must include repetitive resurveys, can sometimes render extermination projects economically unacceptable, though it is sometimes possible to select a feasible perimeter. The larger the extermination area the smaller, relatively speaking, will be the cost of perimeter control measures in relation to area reclaimed, and the greater the scope for selecting a sound perimeter.

A further point of practical significance is the development of reliable techniques for the detection of *Glossina* in low density. The demoralizing experience of searching for stray specimens of *Glossina* over hundreds of square miles of territory during a period of years, with repeated negative findings, militates against the efficiency of the searches. It has not proved possible to use existing types of traps effectively for this purpose in northern Nigeria though they have been used at other places. A really effective attractant would improve the efficiency of both traps and chemical control agents.

There is accordingly some difficulty in assessing the results of tsetse extermination operations in those instances in which the tsetse environment is not rendered unsuitable for infestation because of developments in the reclaimed area. A period of seven to ten years should probably elapse before success can be confidently claimed.

Problems of Control of *Glossina* to Protect Livestock

Some examples, by no means comprehensive, are quoted below to illustrate the way in which the variety of situations encountered may be categorized.

(1) Areas from which the vector has been exterminated. The Zululand campaign covering 7,000 square miles eliminated *G. pallidipes* which was only one, though the most significant for the health of livestock, of three species of

Glossina. An area of *G. brevipalpis* was incidentally eliminated but *G. austeni* remained untouched (Du Toit, 1954).

(2) Places in which large area extermination seems feasible and in which it is proceeding. Examples are the Nyanza project in Kenya against *G. fuscipes* and *G. pallidipes* the first phase of which covers 800 square miles, and the Ankole campaign against *G. morsitans* in Uganda in the initial phase of which game eviction methods were applied to 1,700 square miles, now being extended by a combination of insecticide and bush clearing methods to include a further 600 square miles. The Bunyoro campaign, also in Uganda, initially dealt with *G. morsitans submorsitans* and *G. pallidipes* infestations over an area of almost 3,000 square miles, to which a further 750 square miles have now been added after a re-invasion set-back. In northern Nigeria, extermination operations against *G.m. submorsitans* and *G. tachinoides* have been completed within an area of 12,541 square miles and are in progress in two other areas, with additional *G. palpalis* infestations which cover 28,089 and 21,177 square miles, respectively, consequent on feasibility studies carried out by Glover and Aitcheson (1965, 1967).

Though the final objective of the permanent extermination of *Glossina* from several of these places has yet to be achieved, this goal appears to have been attained in some and to be in the process of achievement in others.

(3) Areas in which *Glossina* is controlled but not permanently eradicated, either to halt a tsetse advance, to enable agricultural settlement within an enclave or salient in tsetse infested country (the settlement activity within the salient rendering the tsetse habitat unsuitable for primary infestation), or to break the cycle of transmission of sleeping sickness. Tsetse are controlled to allow agricultural development in parts of Tanzania where the projects have been usually less than 200 square miles in extent. A degree of risk to livestock from trypanosomiasis is inherent in this situation which may be countered by exploiting the premune response, or by the use of chemotherapy, or by a combination of both these measures. In a cleared enclave in southern Guinea savanna, at Mokwa in northern Nigeria, which has heavy *G. morsitans* infestations on the perimeter, infections of trypanosomiasis in susceptible cattle were reduced to a low level simply by not grazing cattle within half a mile of the uncleared perimeter, and treating all of the minimum number of shade trees retained on the ranch with persisting insecticide deposits. Tsetse flies are stated not to be able to see food sources at 200 yards (Bax, 1937). Those transported into the ranch area will settle on the shade trees which function as the bait of the insecticidal trap. The ability of *Glossina* to cross open spaces varies with the species and with response to climatic factors.

(4) The major part of the tsetse infested region of Africa where no tsetse reclamation activity is yet feasible. Reclamation operations are usually too costly to contemplate as an annual repetition simply to control *Glossina* species in enclaves within infested areas, except under circumstances indicated above. Although effective measures are feasible over extensive areas, it is unfortunately true that, over much of the infested area of Africa, the tsetse problem is too general, extensive and diffuse, or our knowledge of the ecology of the flies is still too limited, to enable an economic form of control or extermination to be

devised which could be justified by the productive capacity of the reclaimed area. Some infested areas have low production potential. The factors involved in the maintenance of stock in the presence of risk from *Glossina* have been dealt with in the chapters on epizootiology and chemotherapy and involve considerations such as the premune response (a breed characteristic), the degree of risk from *Glossina*, the level of husbandry practised, and the efficiency of the drugs available for the treatment or prevention of trypanosomiasis.

It is important to mention here that the relevance of tsetse infestation and the desirability of tsetse reclamation in relation to the rural economy is not uncontroversial. The Land Utilization Conference of 1949 resolved that 'reclamation of large tsetse infested areas for African-owned herds maintained on a primitive pastoral system of management would be uneconomic'. Though this was before the extensive use of insecticide, the view has also been taken that tsetse infestations are conserving land resources which would otherwise be dissipated. Hornby, at the Goma Soils Conference in 1948, said that whilst in the past he had taken the view that he would only remove tsetse where he was convinced that stock density on the reclaimed land would be controlled, he now concluded that 'tsetse have contributed to the conservation of large areas at the cost of more intense erosion of other large areas and their implement of conservation has been the death of man and animals' (Ford, 1958). The concept that disease in man and his animals can result in the conservation of land resources is neither new nor peculiar to trypanosomiasis. Though the issue with regard to man has a special significance, the mortality of livestock assumes less prominence but, even so, to hold this concept with regard to livestock is to abandon hope and to overlook some of the indirect results. The consequence of infestation is not simply one of mortality. The fact is that tsetse reclamation in some places can facilitate the development of improved husbandry methods, the utilization of improved breeds and of generally sounder agricultural practices, there being no doubt at all about the detrimental influence of trypanosomiasis over large tracts of Africa.

For example, agricultural economists have called attention to the fact that, over much of Northern Nigeria, the income of the peasant farmer and therefore his ability to improve his farm, is strictly limited by the amount of land he can cultivate manually. This also accounts in part for the relatively high cost of local staple foods. As a general rule the agricultural tractor is not economically acceptable in relation to returns obtainable and it cannot utilize farm by-products. Work oxen which provide motive power, and which are an important component of mixed farming practice in tsetse-free areas, cannot be used where there is risk of contracting trypanosomiasis. Furthermore, in quite substantial areas, the elimination of tsetse offers the only opportunity of making available substantial land resources for integration in a planned development of the rural economy which incorporates livestock more closely with agriculture and the forest estate.

It has been pointed out that, in the eastern portion of the areas, tsetse infestation may be associated with the absence of man and not that infestation is preventing man from occupying infested areas, or that the country is infested because it is not suited to human occupation. This is undoubtedly the case in some places but has not been so in parts of Uganda, the Congo and Nigeria. There have been spectacular epidemics, and even depopulations, in several areas resulting from Gambian sleeping sickness, and this has led to the abandonment of fertile country, followed in many instances by the extension of *G. morsitans* and other infestations. The combined result has been the complete abandonment of populous, exceptionally valuable land resources and a high incidence of disease in man and livestock in peripheral localities. It is important though that wider issues are kept fully in view and that major extermination operations are based on very comprehensive feasibility studies supported by land use surveys. Within the huge area infested by different species of *Glossina* under diverse ecological conditions it is impossible to generalize.

THE USE OF DRUGS FOR THE PREVENTION AND CURE OF TRYPANOSOME INFECTIONS OF LIVESTOCK

The chemotherapeutic and chemoprophylactic agents used against various forms of trypanosomiasis in livestock have been reviewed in detail in Chapter 7 and the care and treatment of individual animals have been described in Chapter 42. The practical aspects of the use of drugs for the prevention and cure of the trypanosomiasis of livestock in the field are considered here.

Curative Treatment in the Field

In practice, curative agents are administered to stock exposed to the risk of contracting trypanosomiasis, and also to stock no longer so exposed either because of seasonal cessation of transmission or because the animals have been withdrawn from the areas of risk. When curative agents are used whilst stock are still at risk it appears that it is only a question of time before a level of drug resistance can be detected. Nevertheless, curative treatment under conditions of light risk has been widely resorted to in Africa and although resistance to most of the modern anti-trypanosomal drugs has developed, the practice has been justified in most places by the numbers of livestock which have been saved. What is justifiable is largely a question of degree. Curative treatment should not be given to stock retained in areas of substantial risk and it is questionable whether these drugs should be made freely available in areas of risk which are overstocked or where livestock are not part of productive farming practice. The correct course of action may be difficult to determine in circumstances in which the loss of livestock, even though not productive, would lead to evacuation of a cultivated area with the consequent liability for tsetse infestation to extend. The use of prophylactic drugs is described later (pp. 816–818) and also the practical significance of drug resistance (pp. 819–820).

The drugs in current use belong to the quinaldine group (quinapyramine sulphate *B. vet. C.*),[1] the phenathridine group (homidium *B. vet. C.*,[2] and

[1] Antrycide (ICI).
[2] Ethidium (Boots), Novidium (M & B).

isometamidium chloride[1]), and the diamidine group (diminazene aceturate *B. vet. C.*[2] and suramin (*B. vet. C.*[3]). The precursors of these drugs have been superseded either because the newer compounds are less toxic or are more effective. Antimonial compounds are no longer in current use.

It has been observed in the field, using a variety of anti-trypanosomal drugs, that effectiveness and toxic side effects, local and general, vary significantly in different territories. Stress factors such as malnutrition, high ambient temperatures, thirst and arduous work may contribute to treatment accidents. Complications occurring after the use of some drugs include delayed liver or kidney damage and photosensitization. The history of past treatment may be of value in selecting the most appropriate drug to use.

Since drugs vary in their effectiveness for different species of trypanosomes, the infecting organism must be identified before an appropriate drug can be selected. This is comparatively straightforward for most types of livestock but presents some difficulty when the mass treatment of cattle is involved. In the latter case, random blood smears should be taken from a suitable proportion of animals at the time of treatment. It is essential to determine not only the prevailing rate of infection in stock presented for treatment but also the extent to which the infecting strains of trypanosomes are sensitive to the drug in use. This is particularly necessary when mass therapy has been given over a period of years. A method for the detection of drug-resistant strains, involving the inoculation of multiple samples into experimental calves and treating them during the pre-patent period, has been described by Jones-Davies and Folkers (1966). Such a method can be used to locate resistant strains and adapted to determine their frequency in smaller groups.

Animals presented for mass treatment are usually selected and brought to a central point by their owners. Cattle-owners are often shrewd observers and many readily recognize early symptoms of trypanosomiasis in their animals. Accurate diagnosis of infection cannot yet be made sufficiently reliably or rapidly to warrant disregard of the owners' views even though, because of the non-specific nature of some of the observed symptoms, this may involve the treatment of some uninfected animals. The reliability of methods of diagnosis is discussed on pp. 790–792 Cunningham and Van Hoeve (1965) have drawn attention to the shortcomings of different diagnostic techniques.

If the occurrence of drug resistance is to be minimized, and if appropriate action is to be taken when it develops, it is essential that the State Veterinary Service should retain control over the circumstances in which mass therapy is administered and over the type of drug used. Usually this means the inclusion of antitrypanosomal drugs in a pharmacy ordinance and legislation to ensure that treatment is always under professional surveillance. A close watch must be maintained on dosage rates and drug concentrations. Practice in the field varies considerably between territories. Lack of adequate control rapidly encourages the development of drug resistance; in such circumstances the veterinary profession may be unaware of the occurrence and extent of drug resistance and can do little to rectify it once it has developed.

[1] Samorin (M & B). [2] Berenil (Hoechst). [3] Antrypol (ICI), Naganol (Bayer).

Drugs used for Curative Treatment

Of the drugs in current use **quinapyramine sulphate** has been used very extensively. It is generally effective against *T. vivax*, *T. congolense*, *T. brucei* and *T. evansi* in all classes of stock. A mild reaction envinced by salivation and muscular tremors is often observed. In animals under physical stress, as when long journeys are undertaken immediately before or after treatment, fatalities may occasionally occur but can be avoided by rest and watering on the day before and the day after treatment. The colourless character of this drug sometimes enables stock owners to present cattle twice for treatment and this may lead to fatalities or the occurrence of severe general symptoms. If this is a significant problem it may be necessary to colour-mark treated animals. Severe and immediate general reactions resulting in collapse are of common occurrence when the drug is administered to horses; these symptoms usually subside after a short time but are sometimes fatal. It is advisable to have a suitable antidote at hand and to divide the amount of drug given into two or three equal doses administered at six-hourly intervals subcutaneously; if administered at different sites this will also reduce the tendency to abscess formation at the injection site. Quite severe and sometimes fatal general reactions may sometimes be seen in dogs with doses in excess of 4·5 mg./kg.

Strains of *T. congolense* and *T. vivax* may readily develop a level of resistance to quinapyramine sulphate and it has been recorded that such resistant strains may also be resistant to homidium and to iso-metamidium chloride. A degree of cross-resistance to diminazene aceturate after laboratory enhancement of puinapyramine resistance has been recorded but this was not a fixed characteristic (Whiteside, 1962). However, there is a tendency for quinapuramine-resistant strains of trypanosomes to be resistant also to other anti-trypanosomal compounds. *T. simiae* may develop resistance to this drug.

Of the phenanthridine group, **homidium** compounds (both chloride and bromide) have been in general field use in some territories for almost as long as quinapyramine. These drugs are effective against *T. vivax* and *T. congolense* in all classes of stock and are usually well tolerated. Severe general reactions have only occasionally been seen in horses. The drugs may cause local reactions and should be administered by deep intra-muscular injection taking care to avoid leakage into subcutaneous tissues. Muscle lesions resulting from deep injections may lead to down grading of quality joints but this can be avoided by using the musculature of the mid-neck or by subcutaneous administration into the dewlap. Local reactions in the horse may be reduced by dividing the dose between two sites.

After some years of mass field therapy of cattle, infections with *T. congolense* resistant to the normal curative dose of 1 mg./kg. may become widespread but resistant strains of *T. vivax*, though they may occur (Stephen, 1963c), are evidently much less frequent in northern Nigeria (Jones-Davies & Folkers, 1966; Williamson & Stephen, 1960).

Isometamidium chloride is a very active anti-trypanosomal compound against *T. vivax* and *T. congolense* infections and, at higher dosages, is a potent prophylactic. The drug is particularly effective against strains of trypanosomes which have not been repeatedly exposed to chemotherapeutic agents but some field strains of *T. congolense* which are resistant to homidium may also be resistant to isometamidium at a dosage of 0·8 mg./kg., whilst some remain sensitive to doses of 0·25 and 0·5 mg./kg. (Jones-Davies & Folkers, 1967; Na'isa, 1967). Field experience with this drug has only been obtained in cattle. Local reactions are more severe than with homidium but under Nigerian conditions are acceptable at doses up to 0·8 mg./kg. administered in the muscles of the neck. Doses of up to 2 mg./kg. have been employed in Kenya to eliminate drug-resistant strains. Caution is required if doses in excess of 1 mg./kg. are employed or if the drug is to be used on grade or exotic stock; it is wise to undertake a small scale preliminary trial.

Of the diamidine group, **diminazene aceturate** is generally effective against *T. vivax, T. congolense* and *T. brucei.* Although this is the least toxic of current anti-trypanosomal drugs and is well tolerated by some classes of stock, symptoms of general malaise may be observed after administration to horses but are usually of a mild and temporary nature. However, local reactions in the horse can sometimes be severe and may be accompanied by abscess formation, necrosis and sloughing. It is advisable to divide the dose and to treat the injection sites by fomentation and massage twice a day for two to three days. Camels are sensitive to this drug and doses of 7 mg./kg. may prove fatal.

Though it was earlier believed that diminazene aceturate was very promptly eliminated from the treated animal it has been shown recently that this is not the case. It was also believed, since it was impossible or difficult to induce drug resistance in laboratory animals, that resistance was unlikely to develop following field use. But recent studies have confirmed the occurrence of field strains of *T. vivax* and *T. congolense* in cattle which were resistant to twice the recommended curative dose of 3·5 mg./kg. (MacLennan & Jones-Davies, 1967; Na'isa, 1967; Jones-Davies, 1967). This resistance seems more marked and troublesome in respect of *T. vivax* than it is of *T. congolense. T. brucei* also shows variations in sensitivity to this drug.

Suramin is effective against *T. evansi, T. brucei* and *T. equiperdum.* Two or three treatments given at weekly intervals are required to effect a cure and the drug must be administered intravenously. Laminitis may supervene in horses during treatment and to minimize this risk treatment should be spread over a longer period.

It is often impracticable to institute curative treatment of ***T. simiae*** infections because of early fatality after the onset of parasitaemia, but it may be feasible to treat milder infections if detected in time. Stephen (1966a) has reviewed the available information on the chemotherapy of *T. simiae* infections. Homidium compounds and diminazene aceturate are not effective but iso-metamidium chloride at 3 mg./kg. may clear the parasitaemia for 7 to 21 days or at 6 mg./kg. for 15 to 32 days. Quinapyramine sulphate administered at 3 to 5 mg./kg. also fails to effect radical cure and relapses may occur at 37 to 49 days, a period which may be sufficient to bring some pigs in the affected herd to a suitable condition for economic slaughter. Drug resistance may readily develop. Quinapyramine chloride effects a cure at doses of 50 mg./kg. (Nigeria) or 25 mg./kg. (Kenya) but the drug is not commercially available and on account of its insolubility is slow to act in circumstances which may require prompt results.

Watson and Williamson (1958) cured *T. simiae* infections in Nigeria with doses of 11·7 mg./kg. of quinapyramine prophylactic but because of possible variations in strain sensitivity this may not be effective in other territories. Curative treatment of very acute *T. simiae* infections in camels is not usually successful though it has been recorded that quinapyramine sulphate may save one animal in three. As indicated above, curative treatment cannot be relied upon to eliminate losses in pigs exposed to risk of infection with *T. simiae*.

Prophylactic Treatment in the Field

The distinction between the use of drugs for curative and prophylactic purposes may be one of quantity of dose, as with iso-metamidium chloride, or of administering a relatively insoluble compound, as with quinapyramine. With some other drugs the mode of action is not clearly established. The manner in which different prophylactic drugs produce their prolonged activity is described in Chapter 7. It is worth mentioning here that diminazene aceturate was originally reported to be rapidly excreted from the treated animal (Bauer, 1959; MacOwan, Fairclough, Hutchinson & Watson quoted by Van Hoeve & Cunningham, 1964). The latter workers were able to demonstrate biological activity for at least 14 days by using the serum of treated animals in an inhibition test in mice against a known sensitive strain of *T. brucei*. Activity was also demonstrated by exposure of treated cattle to natural field risk for 8 days. Untreated controls and one treated animal showed parasitaemia by the tenth day but the remaining animals did not exhibit parasitaemia until after the lapse of 31 days (7) or 57 days (2). In these studies the drug was administered at a dose of 7 mg./kg. Lumsden, Herbert and Hardy (1965b) demonstrated a protection period of at least 42 days in mice which received a dose of 91 mg./kg. Thus, even preparations whose chief merit appeared to be their transient activity in the treated animal may be discovered to possess some residual activity.

In practice, the use of prophylactic drugs against trypanosomiasis in livestock is fraught with difficulty. It is frequently impossible to make stockowners understand that treatment must be resumed *before* parasitaemia becomes evident. For economic reasons the period between treatments should be as long as possible yet it must also be adjusted to correspond to the severity of risk and the sensitivity of the infecting strains to the drug in use. Both these factors vary with the passage of time. When prophylaxis is waning in animals at risk, infection may occur some time before it is detectable by blood-slide examination. This favours the development or selection and propagation of strains of trypanosomes with some degree of drug resistance. The prophylactic selected should be of a different type from the curative drug used for mass field therapy and should be a compound which will not encourage resistance to an alternative curative drug.

Drugs used for Prophylactic Treatment

Quinapyramine prophylactic *B. vet C.*, isometamidium chloride, and phenathridinium-pyrimidinium[1] (pyrithidium *B. vet C.*) have been used to protect

[1] Prothidium (Boots).

cattle in the field. **Quinapyramine prophylactic** can readily give rise to resistant strains of trypanosomes and, as with all prophylactics, it is exceedingly important to ensure that larger animals are not underdosed. Similar systemic reactions may be observed as with the use of the sulphate. Permanent fibrous encapsulations shrinking to the size of a tennis ball are usual at the site of subcutaneous injection. Protection, in the absence of resistant strains, may last for two to three months according to the severity of risk and the standard of husbandry.

Isometamidium chloride is an exceedingly potent anti-trypanosomal drug with prophylactic properties at doses of 0·5 to 1 mg.k/g. The use of this drug to protect slaughter cattle in transit has been described on page 765. However, local toxic reactions at doses in excess of 0·8 mg./kg. have been observed in northern Nigeria but can be minimized by dividing the dose between two sites. Deep injection into the muscles of the mid-neck may avoid damage to expensive cuts of meat or alternatively the dose may be administered subcutaneously in the dewlap. The drug should be administered with particular caution if used to protect grade or exotic stock. Effective prophylaxis of two to four months' duration has been reported from Kenya at a dose rate of 1 mg./kg. Folkers (1966) working in northern Nigeria exposed a group of cattle to moderate continuous field risk from *G. morsitans* and treated them with isometamidium chloride at a dose rate of 0·25 mg./kg. after they became parasitaemic. The object was to observe any tendency towards the development of drug resistance as evinced by shortening of the period between treatments or by the occurrence of relapses after removal of the treated animals from exposure to risk. Groups were removed from risk after one to six treatments and were maintained thereafter at a low nutritional level. Only one animal relapsed after removal from risk and this one belonged to the group removed after the first isometamidium treatment. Only one animal exhibited an infection in the field which failed to respond promptly to the treatment and this was at the fifth such treatment. This failure was attributed to poor absorption of the drug due to an inflammatory reaction at the site of administration; the infection responded when the drug was injected at a different site. The full significance of these findings was obscured to some extent by possible cumulative effects and by deaths caused by insecticide poisoning and malnutrition after removal from risk but the drug clearly performed well under severe test conditions. The breakthrough period at the dose rate (0·25 mg./kg.) given whilst the stock were exposed to continuous risk varied from 36 to 101 (average 77) days and after the second treatment the period showed no definite tendency to shorten. The cattle remained in good condition in the field even though the last group was not removed from risk until after fifteen months had elapsed. In the belief that diminazene aceturate exhibits only transient activity in the treated animals and that resistance to this drug does not develop, all the experimental cattle, including the control group, received a clearing dose of 3·5 mg./kg. at the commencement of the experiment. The control group became infected, as determined by blood film examination, after 13 to 41 (average 21) days. Under the conditions of the experiment the infecting strains of trypanosomes must have been derived from feral rather than domestic animals since there were no other stock in the vicinity. Later, Jones-Davies and Folkers (1966) showed that some field strains of *T. congolense* resistant to homidium at 1 mg./kg. in cattle may fail to be eliminated by doses of isomedamidium chloride of 0·8 mg./kg. whilst others will respond to doses of 0·25 mg./kg. In a comparative study of the prophylactic value of metamidium chloride, quinapyramine sulphate and quinapyramine prophylactic undertaken in an area of moderate risk from *G. morsitans*, Kirkby (1961) found that metamidium chloride afforded protection to cattle for an average period of 94 days at a dose level of 1 mg./kg. and for 125 days at 2 mg./kg., whereas at a dose level of 5 mg./kg. quinapyramine sulphate protected for 53 days and quinapyramine prophylactic for 60 days. The local reactions to metamidium chloride at these dosages were too severe to be generally acceptable. A later modification of this drug, isomethamidium chloride, produces less reaction and it has been found that, for the treatment of Zebu cattle in Nigeria, reactions are acceptable so long as doses of 0·8 mg./kg. or more are divided between two injection sites.

Phenanthridinium-pyrimidinium (pyrithidium) has not afforded longer protection at recommended dosages than quinapyramine prophylactic in northern Nigeria. High dosages can be associated with weight loss and delayed deaths, the causation of which has not been fully determined. However, in parts of East Africa the drug has been used in the field and has afforded adequate protection under certain conditions at doses of 2 mg./kg. It is advisable to administer the drug subcutaneously in the dewlap but a shoulder site may also be used. A bulky local reaction is usual which eventually resolves to a smaller fibrous nodule. This drug should only be used with caution in grade and exotic stock and is not suitable for use in sheep and goats.

Effective anti-trypanosomal agents have been evolved by compounding various curative drugs with suramin (*see* Chapter 7). The resultant, slightly toluble, **suramin complexes** are potent prophylactics but they cause rather severe tissue reactions at the injection site in most classes of livestock and the complexes themselves are not easy to handle. Attempts to circumvent these tissue reactions have not been sufficiently successful to justify taking these agents into general field use. Stephen and Gray (1960) and Gray (1961a) have, however, recorded that, in pigs, the reaction to quinapyramine-suramin complex does not produce swelling, that this drug does not interfere with normal weight gain, and that it may safely be used in sows at an advanced stage of pregnancy. A single injection of 40 mg./kg. administered deeply in the neck anterior to the shoulder will protect young actively growing pigs for at least twelve weeks, and adults for at least six months, against severe *T. simiae* risk. Stephen (1966a) advises the use of quinapyramine-suramin complex at a dose of 40 mg./kg. or quinapyramine chloride at 50 mg./kg., the latter administered some time before the pigs are exposed to risk, followed by quinapyramine-suramin complex 40 mg./kg. every six months. Newborn pigs, if exposed to risk, should be kept in screened accommodation until weaned and growing pigs should receive 40 mg./kg. of the complex at three-monthly intervals until the pig is nine months old after which the interval is extended to six months. The dose rate of the complex refers to the quantity of the basic drug, in this case quinapyramine. Extensive practical experience of this regimen has not yet been obtained.

It is evident from what is on record that the prophylactic or indeed the curative anti-trypanosomal drugs at present available have important limitations. Furthermore, practice in the usage of these agents must vary greatly according to circumstances.

Drug Resistance

The means by which drug resistance may be brought about have been discussed in Chapter 7. From the practical viewpoint the picture at present is not clear. In the past, distinctions have not always been clearly drawn between types of drug resistance nor between the different species of trypanosome involved. Species vary in their ability to produce strains which are resistant and cross-resistant to therapeutic doses of different curative drugs.

There are practical difficulties in meeting the resistance problem by simply increasing the dose. The limitations may be economic (cost of drug and cost of administration), physical (solubility and volume of dose), or toxic (local, general and delayed reactions). Furthermore, if the resistance is due to adaptation, increased dosage may prove to be only temporarily effective. But if the resistance has arisen as the result of the selection of type with a fixed characteristic it is possible that increased dosage might eliminate the resistant strain. It is clear that, after ten years' general field use, strains of *T. congolense* which are resistant to the normal therapeutic dose of homidium are widespread in northern Nigeria. Strains of *T. vivax* resistant to homidium are not prevalent. In cattle, resistance of *T. congolense* to homidium is readily enhanced by sub-curative treatment but with *T. vivax* in sheep Stephen (1963) failed to produce a significant degree of resistance by sub-curative treatment, alone or in combination with cyclical transmission through *G. palpalis*.

The only available means of circumventing *T. congolense* resistance is to use a drug to which cross-resistance is not expected, for example, diminazene aceturate. But it is now known that at least some strains of *T. congolense* are appearing which are resistant to twice the normal therapeutic dose of 3·5 mg./kg. of diminazene aceturate. It is not known whether these strains are capable of adapting to higher doses. Laboratory evidence suggests, however, that this is not likely; more extensive investigation is required. Following the field use of diminazene aceturate at 3·5 mg./kg. strains of *T. vivax* resistant to 7 mg./kg. have been noted. Whether this resistance is capable of enhancement, or whether other strains may be available for selection with yet higher levels of tolerance to the drug, is not known. So far, in northern Nigeria, *T. vivax* strains which are able to tolerate this dose of diminazene aceturate have proved susceptible to homidium at 1 mg./kg. (Jones-Davies, 1967). In Rhodesia, a degree of isometamidium resistance has been observed in a strain of *T. vivax* which, however, remained sensitive to diminazene aceturate 3·5 mg./kg. Much more factual information from the field and from the laboratory is required before the problems of drug resistance can be fully elucidated and methods devised to counter them.

It is important to know the extent to which drug-resistant strains of trypanosomes contribute to the field risk to which livestock may be exposed. It has been established that strains of *T. congolense* which have become resistant to homidium retain this resistance after transmission through *Glossina* (Gray &

Roberts, 1968) and in many other instances it has been shown that drug-resistance, once acquired, is not readily lost. In northern Nigeria, resistant strains can now be easily located by exposing calves to normal field risk from tsetse. The most serious situation arises when infection in tsetse is derived from cattle which have been under drug prophylaxis, rather than from wild animals. An explanation for the apparent success of certain drugs in protecting animals exposed to severe challenge in the field may be that the local tsetse have been infected from wild animals in areas not normally frequented by treated livestock. Wild animals and livestock which have become tolerant to trypanosome infection can, however, become reservoirs of drug-resistant trypanosomes. Resistant strains may remain highly pathogenic for newly infected, untreated animals although their pathogenicity in treated animals may be variable, presumably as a result of activation of the immune response. Slaughter cattle exposed to risk while under waning drug prophylaxis may show heavy parasitaemia but little evidence of clinical illness; on occasion such animals have been observed to thrive (*see* page 765). This is, perhaps, an extreme example. In other circumstances, field strains in cattle which have been ineffectively treated, or in which prophylaxis is waning, often cause well defined clinical illness.

The practical significance of drug resistance varies with circumstances. The advent of a significant degree of resistance may be deferred by careful usage of the drug concerned but, in the present state of knowledge, it cannot always be avoided. Grave difficulties have arisen on farms, ranches and settlement schemes which have been attributed to the depradations of drug-resistant trypanosomes. Much can be done to rectify such situations by sound professional guidance (Kirkby, 1963) but the necessary expert advice is not always immediately available in developing countries.

The stage to which the propagation of drug-resistant strains has developed must also be considered. In the case of livestock destined for slaughter where the chances of resistant strains infecting tsetse from the surrounding locality are minimal, the consequences are less grave than where such strains are liable to be actively transmitted between individuals within the group. An even more dangerous situation arises where resistant strains occur amongst breeding stock and are transmitted over wider areas to become part of the natural field risk, or where the infection spreads to tolerant cattle and wild animals.

Drugs and the Immune Response Factor

Active immunizing procedures are not yet available for practical exploitation and many difficulties have still to be resolved (*see* Chapter 6). The full significance of the host defence mechanism in the epizootiology of trypanosomiasis in Zebu cattle in parts of Africa is not always realized though it has long been recognized in tolerant stock. But for this phenomenon, losses of Zebu stock resulting from periodic exposure to risk of infection, a common occurrence in parts of Africa, would have been much more serious than was the case before the advent of modern drugs.

At present the only available means of exploiting the immune response is to expose animals to risk and, when necessary, to rely on the judicious use of drugs to assist recovery from the infection which is necessary to stimulate the host's defence mechanism; the possible occurrence, and consequences, of drug-resistance must be kept in mind.

If, in the future, a significant degree of drug resistance should develop and become widespread, it may well be that the best, and perhaps the only effective, means of combating trypanosomiasis in livestock will be to combine drug therapy with at least partial stimulation of the immune response.

REFERENCES

ABEDI, Z. H., and MILLER, M. J. (1963). 'Tsetse fly puparia: a new collecting technique,' *Science*, N.Y. **141,** 264.

ACS, G., REICH, E., and MORI, M. (1964). 'Biological and biochemical properties of the analogue antibiotic Tubercidin,' *Proc. Nat. Acad. Sci.*, **52,** 493.

ACTOR, P., WIND, S., and PAGANO, J. F. (1962). 'Potentiation of amphotericin B activity against *Trypanosoma congolense* in mice,' *Proc. Soc. exp. Biol.*, **110,** 409.

ADAMSON, JOY (1961). *Living Free: The Story of Elsa and her Cubs.* London, Collins and Harvill Press.

ADRIAENSSENS, K. (1960). 'Furaltadone in human Rhodesian sleeping sickness. Report of the first three cases,' *Ann. Soc. belge Méd. trop.*, **40,** 715.

ADRIAENSSENS, K. (1961). 'Nota over de toxiciteit van MEL B in *Trypanosoma rhodesiense* slaapziekte,' *Trop. Dis. Bull.*, **58,** 424.

ADRIAENSSENS, K. (1962). 'Furaltadone in the treatment of Rhodesian sleeping sickness,' *Trop. geogr. Med.*, **14,** 171.

ADRIAENSSENS, K. (1962a). 'Preliminary report of 3 cases of Rhodesian sleeping sickness treated with NF-902 (a levo-isomer of Furaltodone),' *Ann. Soc. belge Méd. trop.*, **42,** 31.

AKWEI, E. (1952). 'Planning the control of sleeping sickness: a sequel,' *Trans. R. Soc. trop. Med. Hyg.*, **46,** 437.

ALBERT, A. (1966). *The Acridines*, 2nd edition. London, E. Arnold & Co.

ALEXEIEFF, A. (1913). 'Introduction à la révision de la famille Herpétomonadidae (=Trypanosomidae Doflein, 1911),' *Arch. Protistenk.*, **29,** 313.

ALLISON, A. C. (1968). 'The role of lysosomes in the action of drugs and hormones,' *Adv. Chemotherapy*, **3,** 253.

ALLISON, A. C., and YOUNG, M. R. (1964). 'Uptake of dyes and drugs by living cells in culture,' *Life Sciences*, **3,** 1407.

AMREIN, Y. U. (1965). 'Genetic transfer in trypanosomes. 1. Syngamy in *Trypanosoma cruzi*,' *Exp. Parasit.*, **17,** 261.

AMREIN, Y. U. (1965a). 'Genetic transfer in trypanosomes. II. Genetic transformation in *Trypanosoma equiperdum*,' *Exp. Parasit.*, **17,** 264.

AMREIN, Y. U., and FULTON, J. D. (1959). 'Attempts to transfer drug-resistance of trypanosomes *in vivo*,' *J. Protozool.*, **6,** 120.

AMREIN, Y. U., GEIGY, R., and KAUFMANN, MARIANNE (1965). 'On the reacquisition of virulence in trypanosomes of the *brucei* group,' *Acta trop.*, **22,** 193.

ANDERSSON, C. J. (1856). *Lake Ngami, or Explorations and Discoveries, during four years' wanderings in the wilds of South Western Africa.* London.

ANDREWARTHA, H. G., and BIRCH, L. C. (1954). *The Distribution and Abundance of Animals.* Chicago, University of Chicago Press.

ANON. (1968). 'The Sengwa Research Project. A study of game–tsetse fly relationships (a communication from the Tsetse & Trypanosomiasis Control Branch of the Dept. of Vet. Services and the Dept. of National Parks and Wild Life Management, Rhodesia),' *Rhodes. Sci. News*, **2,** 11, p. 236.

APTED, F. I. C. (1953). 'The treatment of advanced cases of Rhodesian sleeping sickness by MEL B and Arsobal,' *Trans. R. Soc. trop. Med. Hyg.*, **47,** 387.

APTED, F. I. C. (1957). 'Four years' experience of melarsen oxide/BAL in the treatment of late stage Rhodesian sleeping sickness,' *Trans. R. Soc. trop. Med. Hyg.*, **51,** 75.

APTED, F. I. C. (1960). 'Nitrofurazone in the treatment of sleeping sickness due to *Trypanosoma rhodesiense*,' *Trans. R. Soc. trop. Med. Hyg.*, **54,** 225.

APTED, F. I. C. (1962). 'Sleeping sickness in Tanganyika, past, present and future,' *Trans. R. Soc. trop. Med. Hyg.*, **56,** 15.

APTED, F. I. C., ORMEROD, W. E., SMYLY, D. P., STRONACH, B. W., and SZLAMP, E. L. (1963). 'A comparative study of the epidemiology of endemic Rhodesian sleeping sickness in different parts of Africa,' *J. trop. Med. Hyg.*, **66,** 1.

ASCHER, K. R. S. (1964). 'A review of chemosterilants and oviposition-inhibitors in insects,' *World. Rev. Pest Control*, **3,** 7.

ASHCROFT, M. T. (1957). 'The polymorphism of *Trypanosoma brucei* and *T. rhodesiense*, its relation to relapses and remissions of infections in white rats, and the effect of cortisone,' *Ann. trop. Med. Parasit.*, **51,** 301.

ASHCROFT, M. T. (1959). 'The importance of African wild animals as reservoirs of trypanosomiasis,' *E. Afr. med. J.*, **36,** 289.

ASHCROFT, M. T. (1959a). 'The Tinde experiment: a further study of the long-term cyclical transmission of *T. rhodesiense*,' *Ann. trop. Med. Parasit.*, **53,** 137.

ASHCROFT, M. T. (1959b). 'A critical review of the epidemiology of human trypanosomiasis in Africa,' *Trop. Dis. Bull.*, **56,** 1073.

ASHCROFT, M. T. (1963). 'A comparative study of the epidemiology of endemic Rhodesian sleeping sickness in different parts of Africa,' *J. trop. Med. Hyg.*, **66,** 133.

ASHCROFT, M. T., BURTT, E., and FAIRBAIRN, H. (1959). 'The experimental infection of some African wild animals with *Trypanosoma rhodesiense*, *T. brucei* and *T. congolense*,' *Ann. trop. Med. Parasit.*, **53,** 147.

ASHLEY, J. N., BERG, S. S., and LUCAS, J. M. S. (1960). '3:3′-Diamidinocarbanilide: a new drug active against babesial infections,' *Nature*, Lond. **185,** 461.

AUSTEN, E. E. (1903). *A monograph of the tsetse flies (genus* Glossina, *Westwood) based on the collection in the British Museum.* London, British Museum (Natural History).

AUSTEN, E. E. (1911). *A Handbook of the Tsetse-flies (genus* Glossina). London, British Museum (Natural History). 110 pp.

AUSTEN, E. E. (1923). 'A new East African tsetse-fly (genus *Glossina* Wied.) which apparently disseminates sleeping sickness,' *Bull. ent. Res.*, **13,** 311.

AUSTEN, E. E., and HEGH, E. (1922). *Tsetse-flies, their Characteristics, Distribution and Bionomics with some account of possible methods for their Control.* London.

AZEVEDO, J. FRAGA DE, DA COSTA MOURAO, M., and DE CASTRO SALAZAR, J. M. (1962). 'L'involution biologique de la population de *Glossina palpalis palpalis* au cours de la campagne d'éradication dans l'Ile du Prince (1956–8),' *11th Int. Congr. Ent.*, **2,** 412.

AZEVEDO, J. F. DE, and PINHÃO, R. DA C. (1964). 'The maintenance of a laboratory colony of *Glossina morsitans* since 1959,' *Bull. Wld. Hlth. Org.*, **31,** 835.

AZEVEDO, J. F. DE, and PINHÃO, R. DA C. (1968). 'Prospects offered by the laboratory breeding of *Glossina morsitans* in Lisbon.' Paper presented in January 1967 to the Panel on Control of Livestock Insect Pests by the Sterile-male Technique. Joint FAO/IAEA, Vienna, *Panel Proceedings Series*, STI/PUB/184, 1968. 102 pp.

REFERENCES

BACH, H., PFEIL, E., PHILIPPAR, W., and REICH, M. (1963). 'Molekülbau und Haftung substantiver Farbstoffe auf Cellulose,' *Angew. Chem.*, **75,** 407.

BAGSHAWE, A. G. (1908). 'Experiments on flight of *Glossina palpalis*.' (Abstract from Dr Bagshawe's August [1906] Report), *Rep. Sleep. Sick. Comm. Roy. Soc.*, **9,** App, 45.

BAILEY, N. M. (1967). 'The trypanocidal activity of Berenil following oral administration and its application in the prophylaxis of human trypanosomiasis.' *See* ISCTR (1967), p. 159.

BAILEY, N. M. (1967a). 'The antitrypanosomal activity of drugs following oral administration to laboratory rats.' *See* EATRO (1967), p. 80.

BAILEY, N. M. (1968). 'Oral Berenil in the treatment and prophylaxis of human trypanosomiasis,' *Trans. R. Soc. trop. Med. Hyg.*, **62,** 122.

BAILEY, N. M., CUNNINGHAM, M. P., and KIMBER, C. D. (1967). 'The indirect fluorescent antibody technique applied to dried blood, for use as a screening test in the diagnosis of human trypanosomiasis in Africa,' *Trans. R. Soc. trop. Med. Hyg.*, **61,** 696.

BAKER, C. E. W. (1958). *Symposium on Animal Trypanosomiasis.* CCTA Publication No. 45, p. 29.

BAKER, J. R. (1960). 'The influence of the number of trypanosomes inoculated on the prepatent period of the subsequent trypanosomiasis in laboratory rodents,' *Ann. trop. Med. Parasit.*, **54,** 71.

BAKER, J. R. (1962). 'Infection of the chimpanzee (*Pan troglodytes verus*) with *Trypanosoma rhodesiense* and *T. brucei*,' *Ann. trop. Med. Parasit.*, **56,** 216.

BAKER, J. R. (1963). 'Speculations on the evolution of the family Trypanosomatidae Doflein, 1901,' *Exp. Parasit.*, **13,** 219.

BAKER, J. R. (1967). 'Trypanosome infections in wild African mammals,' *Trans. R. Soc. trop. Med. Hyg.*, **61,** 132.

BAKER, J. R. (1968). 'Experimental infections with *Trypanosoma brucei* and *T. rhoedsiense* in chimpanzees,' *Trans. R. Soc. trop. Med. Hyg.*, **62,** 138.

BAKER, J. R., SACHS, R., and LAUFER, I. (1967). 'Trypanosomes of wild mammals in an area north-west of the Serengeti National Park, Tanzania,' *Z. Tropenmed. Parasit.*, **18,** 280.

BALBIANI, G. (1888). 'Évolution des micro-organismes animaux et végétaux parasites. Les Mastigophores,' *J. Micrograph.*, **12,** 394.

BALDRY, D. A. T. (1963). 'An evaluation by bioassay of the persistence of DDT deposits on riverine vegetation in the North Guinea savannah vegetation zone of Nigeria, and observations on factors influencing the availability of deposits to *G. palpalis*,' *Bull. ent. Res.*, **54,** 497.

BALDRY, D. A. T. (1964). 'Observations on a close association between *Glossina tachinoides* and domestic pigs near Nsukka, Eastern Nigeria. II. Ecology and trypanosome infection rates in *G. tachinoides*,' *Ann. trop. Med. Parasit.*, **58,** 32.

BALDRY, D. A. T. (1964a). 'An assessment by bioassay of the comparative toxicity and persistence of dieldrin and isobenzan deposits on riverine vegetation in the Northern Guinea savannah zone of Nigeria in relation to the control of *G. palpalis* (*R.-D.*),' *Bull. ent. Res.*, **55,** 49.

BALDRY, D. A. T. (1965). The Nigerian Institute for Trypanosomiasis Research. *Annual Report 1964.*

BALDRY, D. A. T. (1967). 'On the distribution of *Glossina tachinoides* in West Africa. I. The distribution of *G. tachinoides* in Southern Nigeria. II. An assessment of the probable present distribution of *G. tachinoides* in West

Africa and of possible future extensions, based on existing records and recent observations in Southern Nigeria.' *See* ISCTR (1967), p. 103.

BALFOUR, A. (1906). 'Biting and noxious insects other than mosquitoes,' 2nd rep. *Wellcome Res. Lab.*, 29.

BALIS, J., and BERGEON, P. (1968). 'Étude de la répartition des glossines en Éthiopie,' *Bull. Wld. Hlth. Org.*, **38,** 809.

BARBER, H. J., and BERG, S. S. (1962). 'Structure and activity of antiprotozoal drugs,' in *Drugs, Parasites and Hosts* (ed. L. G. Goodwin and R. H. Nimmo-Smith). London, J. & A. Churchill Ltd., pp. 165–79.

BARDOS, T. J., DATTA-GUPTA, N., and HEBBORN, P. (1966). 'Synthesis, chemistry & preliminary pharmacology of arsenical nitrogen mustards and structurally related nonalkylating arsenicals,' *J. med. Chem.*, **9,** 221.

BAROTTE, J. (1925). 'Les trypanosomiases de l'Afrique du Nord,' *Mém. Soc. Sci. Nat. Maroc.*, **11,** 1.

BARRASS, R. (1960). 'The settling of tsetse flies *Glossina morsitans* Westwood (Diptera, Muscidae) on cloth screens,' *Entomologia exp. & appl.*, **3,** 59.

BARRETT, A. J., and DINGLE, J. T. (1967). 'A lysosomal component capable of binding cations and a carcinogen,' *Biochem. J.*, **105,** 20 P.

BAUER, F. (1958). 'Über den Wirkungsmechanismus des Berenil (4, 4'Diamidino-diazoaminobenzol), bei *Trypanosoma congolense*,' *Zentbl. Bakt. ParasitKde Abt.*, 1 Originale, **172,** 605.

BAUER, F. (1962). 'The development of drug-resistance to Berenil in *Trypanosoma congolense*,' *Vet. Rec.*, **74,** 265.

BAUER, F. (1963). 'Chemotherapeutische Untersuchungen bei experimentellen Infektionen durch *Trypanosoma evansi*,' *Zbl. Vet. Med.*, Ser. A, **10,** 21.

BAUER, F. (1964). 'The development of resistance to drugs and to antibodies by *Trypanosoma congolense*,' *Proc. 3rd Intern. Congr. Chemotherapy*, Stuttgart, 1963, **2,** 1548.

BAUER, F. (1966). 'Zur Behandlung der *Babesia canis*-Infektion mit Berenil.' *Z. Tropenmed. Parasit.*, **17,** 390.

BAUER, W., and VINOGRAD, J. (1968). 'The interaction of closed circular DNA with intercalative dyes,' *J. Mol. Biol.*, **33,** 141.

BAX, S. N. (1937). 'The senses of smell and sight in *Glossina swynnertoni*,' *Bull. ent. Res.*, **28,** 539.

BAX, S. N. (1943–4). 'A practical policy for tsetse reclamation and field experiment,' *E. Afr. agric. J.*, **9,** Nos. 1–3, pp. 2, 83, 157. Nairobi, 1943–4.

BEAUDIMENT, R., CANVIN, L., and LEPROUX, R. (1954). 'Accidents due to treatment with Lomidine in the French Cameroons. Their therapeutics and prevention (Experiments with 4·891 RP).' *See* ISCTR (1954), p. 130.

BEAUDOIN, A. R. (1964). 'The teratogenicity of Congo Red in rats,' *Proc. Soc. exp. Biol. Med.*, **117,** 176.

BEAUDOIN, A. R., and PICKERING M. J. (1960). 'Teratogenic activity of several synthetic compounds structurally related to Trypan Blue,' *Anat. Rec.*, **137,** 297.

BELDING, D. L. (1965). *Textbook of Parasitology*, 3rd edition. New York, Appleton-Century-Crofts.

BÉNAZET, F. (1962). 'Relations entre la fixation tissulaire et l'action tissulaire et la durée d'action des trypanocides,' *Rev. Élev. Méd. vét. Pays. trop.*, **15,** 11.

BENNETT, JR., L. L. (1965). 'Phthalanilides and some related dibasic and polybasic compounds: a review of biological activities and modes of action,' *Progr. exp. Tumor. Res.*, **7,** 259.

BENNETT, S. L. J. (1933). 'The control of camel trypanosomiasis,' *J. comp. Path. Ther.*, **46**, 67 and 174.

BENTZ, M., and DIALLO, I. (1963). 'Technique simplifiée pour la recherche systématique d'une bêta-2-macroglobulinémie pathologique en milieu tropical,' *Bull. Soc. Path. exot.*, **56**, 434.

BENTZ, M., and MACARIO, C. (1963). 'Le traitement systématique des individus porteurs d'hyper-bêta-2-macroglobulinémies (AIE qualitatives) en zone d'endémie trypanique,' *Bull. Soc. Path. exot.*, **56**, 416.

BERG, S. S. (1961). 'The search for new trypanocides. VI. Amidinophenyldiazoaminoquinolinium and -quinazolinium salts,' *J. chem. Soc.*, 4041.

BERG, S. S. (1962). 'The search for new trypanocides. VII. *m*-Amidinophenyldiazoaminostyryl quinolinium salts,' *J. chem. Soc.*, 677.

BERG, S. S. (1963). 'The search for new trypanocides. VIII. Coupling of *m*-amidinobenzenediazonium chloride with 3,8-diamino-5-ethyl-6-phenyl phenanthridinium chloride,' *J. chem. Soc.*, 3635.

BERG, S. S., BROWN, K. N., HILL, J., and WRAGG, W. R. (1961). 'A new prophylactic trypanocidal drug, 2,7-*bis* (*m*-amidinophenyldiazoamino)-10-ethyl-9-phenylphenanthridinium chloride dihydrochloride (M. & B. 4596),' *Nature*, Lond. **192**, 367.

BERG, S. S., BROWN, K. N., and LUCAS, J. M. S. (1961). 'The trypanocidal activity and local tolerance of sparingly soluble salts of metamidium,' *Ann. trop. Med. Parasit.*, **55**, 298.

BERG, S. S., and PARNELL, E. W. (1961). 'Bisquaternary salts related to quinapyramine (Antrycide). Replacement of the quinoline nucleus by other heterocycles,' *J. chem. Soc.*, 5275.

BERNFELD, P. (1963). 'Polyanionic inhibitors,' *Metabolic Inhibitors*, Vol. II. (ed. R. M. Hochster and J. H. Quastel). New York, Academic Press, p. 437.

BERTRAND, E., BAUDIN, L., VACHER, R., DUCASSE, B., SENTILHES, L., and VEYRET, V. (1967). 'Les signes cardio-vasculaires dans la trypanosomiase africaine à *Trypanosoma gambiense*,' *Méd. trop.*, **27**, 381.

BERTRAND, E., SENTILHES, L., DUCASSE, B., VACHER, P., and BAUDIN, L. (1965). 'L'atteinte du coeur dans la trypanosomiase africaine à *Trypanosoma gambiense* à propos notamment des constatations ECG chez 60 malades,' *Méd. trop.*, **25**, 603.

BEVAN, LL. E. W. (1928). 'A method of inoculating cattle against trypanosomiasis,' *Trans. R. Soc. trop. Med. Hyg.*, **22**, 147.

BEVAN, LL. E. W. (1936). 'Notes on immunity in trypanosomiasis,' *Trans. R. Soc. trop. Med. Hyg.*, **30**, 199.

BEZON, A., and DUCASSE, P. (1958). 'Caractères généraux et particuliers de la grippe asiatique en milieu d'endémie trypanosomienne (Abengourou, Côte d'Ivoire),' *Méd. trop.*, **18**, 806.

BINGGELI, M. (1963). *Radioisotopes and ionizing radiations in entomology*. IAEA Biblio. Series No. 9. 414 pp.

BINGGELI, M. (1965). *Radioisotopes and ionizing radiations in entomology, 1961–3*, IAEA. Biblio. Series No. 15. 564 pp.

BINGGELI, M. (1967). *Radioisotopes and ionizing radiations in entomology, 1964–5*. IAEA. Biblio. Series No. 24. 454 pp.

BINNS, H. R. (1938). 'Observations on the behaviour in laboratory animals of *T. congolense* Broden, 1904,' *Ann. trop. Med. Parasit.*, **32**, 425.

BIRCH, L. C. (1948). 'The intrinsic rate of natural increase of an insect population,' *J. anim. Ecol.*, **17**, 15.

BIRD, R. G., MOLLOY, J. O., and ORMEROD, W. E. (1966). 'Granules and tubules in the cytoplasm of the sleeping sickness trypanosome: an electron microscope study,' *Trans. R. Soc. trop. Med. Hyg.*, **60,** 753.

BIRKETT, J. D. (1958). *Symposium on Animal Trypanosomiasis.* CCTA Publication No. 45. p. 32.

BLACKLOCK, B., and YORKE, W. (1913). 'The trypanosome causing Dourine (Mal de Coit or Beschälseuche),' *Proc. Roy. Soc.*, B, **87,** 89.

BLAIR, D. M. (1939). 'Human trypanosomiasis in Southern Rhodesia 1911–38,' *Trans. R. Soc. trop. Med. Hyg.*, **32,** 729.

BLOCH, A., and NICHOL, C. A. (1965). 'Nucleoside antibiotics related to adenosine,' *Antimicrobial Agents and Chemotherapy*, 1964 (ed. J. C. Sylvester). Ann Arbor, Mich. American Society for Microbiology. p. 530.

BLOCH, A., LEONARD, R. J., and NICHOL, C. A. (1965). 'On the mode of action of the nucleoside antibiotic Tubercidin (7-deaza-adenosine),' *Fed. Proc.*, **25,** 454.

BOREHAM, P. F. L. (1966). 'Pharmacologically active peptides produced in the tissues of the host during trypanosome infections,' *Trans. R. Soc. trop. Med. Hyg.*, **60,** 124.

BOREHAM, P. F. L. (1968). 'Immune reactions and kinin formation in chronic trypanosomiasis,' *Br. J. Pharmacol. Chemother.*, **32,** 493.

BOREHAM, P. F. L., and GOODWIN, L. G. (1967). 'A pharmacological and pathological study of the vascular changes which occur in chronic trypanosomiasis of the rabbit.' *See* ISCTR (1967), p. 83.

BORSTEL, R. D. VON (1960). 'Population control by release of irradiated males,' *Science*, N.Y. **131,** 880.

BOUANCHAUD, D. H., SCAVIZZI, M. R., and CHABBERT, Y. A. (1969). 'Elimination by Ethidium bromide of antibiotic resistance in enterobacteria and staphylococci,' *J. gen. Microbiol.*, **54,** 417.

BOUET, G., and ROUBAUD, E. (1910). 'Expériences diverses de transmission des trypanosomes par les glossines. I, II, *Ann. Inst. Pasteur*, **24,** 658; III, IV, *Bull. Soc. Path. exot.*, **3,** 599 and 722.

BOWMAN, I. B. R., and FLYNN, I. W. (1968). 'The isolation and metabolic properties of polymorphic *brucei* subgroup trypanosomes,' *Trans. R. Soc. trop. Med. Hyg.*, **62,** 133.

BOYCOTT, A. E., and PRICE-JONES, C. (1913). 'Experimental trypanosome anaemia,' *J. Path. Bact.*, **17,** 347.

BOYDEN, S. V. (1951). 'The adsorption of proteins on erythrocytes treated with tannic acid and subsequent haemagglutination by antiprotein sera,' *J. exp. Med.*, **93,** 107.

BOYT, W. P., LOVEMORE, D. F., PILSON, R. D., and SMITH, I. D. (1963). 'A preliminary report on the maintenance of cattle by various drugs in a mixed *Glossina morsitans* and *G. pallidipes* fly-belt.' *See* ISCTR (1963), p. 71.

BRAND, T. VON (1956). 'Beziehungen zwischen Stoffwechsel und taxonomischer Einteilung der Saügetier-trypanosomen,' *Zool. Anz.*, **157,** 199.

BRAZZAVILLE CONFERENCE REPORT (1950). *Conférence africaine sur la tsétsé et la trypanosomiase*, Brazzaville, 2–8 février, 1948. Toulouse, 1950.

BRETSCHER, M. S., and MARCKER, K. A. (1966). 'Polypeptidyl-s-ribonucleic acid and amino acyl-s-ribonucleic acid binding sites on ribosomes,' *Nature*, Lond. **211,** 380.

BROCKMAN, R. W. (1961). 'Symposium on the experimental pharmacology and clinical use of antimetabolites.' Part VI. Mechanisms of resistance to metabolite analogues with anticancer activity,' *Clin. Pharmacol. Therap.*, **2,** 237.

BRODEN, A. (1904). 'Les infections à trypanosomes au Congo chez l'homme et les animaux,' *Bull. Soc. Études Colon.* (Brussels), February.

BRODIE, B. B. (1967). 'Physicochemical and biochemical aspects of pharmacology,' *J. Amer. med. Assn.*, **202,** 600.

BROOKER, B. E. (1965). 'Lysosome-like bodies in trypanosomatid flagellates,' *Progress in Protozoology*. Int. Congr. Series 91. Excerpta Medica Foundation, Amsterdam. p. 138.

BROOM, J. C., and BROWN, H. C. (1940). 'Studies in trypanosomiasis. IV. Notes on the serological character of *Trypanosoma brucei* after cyclical development in *Glossina morsitans*,' *Trans. R. Soc. trop. Med. Hyg.*, **34,** 53.

BROWN, H. C., and BROOM, J. C. (1938). 'Studies in Trypanosomiasis. II. Observations on the red cell adhesion test,' *Trans. R. Soc. trop. Med. Hyg.*, **32,** 209.

BROWN, K. N. (1963). 'The antigenic character of the *Brucei* trypanosomes,' in *Immunity to Protozoa* (ed. P. C. C. Garnham, A. E. Pierce, I. Roitt). Oxford, Blackwell Scientific Publications. p. 204.

BROWN, K. N., ARMSTRONG, J. A., and VALENTINE, R. C. (1965). 'The ingestion of protein molecules by blood forms of *Trypanosoma rhodesiense*,' *Experimental Cell Research*, **39,** 129.

BROWN, K. N., HILL, J., and HOLLAND, A. E. (1961). 'Antitrypanosomal activity of certain phenyldiazoamino- and phenylazoamino-phenanthridin iumcompounds,' *Brit. J. Pharmacol.*, **17,** 396.

BROWN, K. N., and WILLIAMSON, J. (1962). 'Antigens of *Brucei* trypanosomes,' *Nature*, Lond. **194,** 1253.

BROWN, K. N., and WILLIAMSON, J. (1964). 'The chemical composition of trypanosomes. IV. Location of antigens in subcellular fractions of *Trypanosoma rhodesiense*,' *Exp. Parasit.*, **15,** 69.

BROWNING, C. H., COHEN, J. B., GAUNT, R., and GULBRANSEN, R. (1922). 'Relationships between antiseptic action and chemical constitution with special reference to compounds of the pyridine, quinoline, acridine and phenazine series,' *Proc. Roy. Soc.*, B, **93,** 329.

BROWNING, C. H., COHEN, J. B., and GULBRANSEN, R. (1922). 'The antiseptic properties of cyanine dyes,' *Brit. med. J.*, 514.

BROWNING, C. H., and GULBRANSEN, R. (1934). 'Prophylaxis of experimental trypanosome infections by chemotherapeutic agents,' *J. Path. Bact.*, **39,** 75.

BRUCE, D. (1895). *Preliminary Report on the Tsetse Fly Disease or Nagana in Zululand.* Durban.

BRUCE, D. (1897). *Further Report on the Tsetse Fly Disease or Nagana in Zululand.* London.

BRUCE, D. (1909). 'A trypanosome from Zanzibar,' *Proc. Roy. Soc.*, B, **81,** 14.

BRUCE, D. (1914). 'Classification of the African trypanosomes pathogenic to man and domestic animals,' *Trans. Roy. Soc. trop. Med. Hyg.*, **8,** 1.

BRUCE, D. *et al.* (1909). 'The development of *Trypanosoma gambiense* in *Glossina palpalis*,' *Proc. Roy. Soc.*, B, **81,** 405; *Repts. Sleep. Sickn. Comm. Roy. Soc., 1910*, **10,** 46.

BRUCE, D., *et al.* (1910). 'Trypanosome diseases of domestic animals in Uganda. I. *Trypanosoma pecorum* sp. nov,' *Proc. Roy. Soc.*, B, **82,** 468; *Repts. Sleep. Sickn. Comm. Roy. Soc.*, **11,** 128.

BRUCE, D., *et al.* (1911). 'Further researches on the development of *Trypanosoma gambiense* in *Glossina palpalis*,' *Proc. Roy. Soc.*, B, **83,** 513; *Repts. Sleep. Sickn. Comm. Roy. Soc.*, **11,** 34.

BRUCE, D., *et al.* (1911a). 'The development of trypanosomes in tsetse flies,' *Repts. Sleep. Sickn. Comm. Roy. Soc.*, **11,** 12.

BRUCE, D., *et al.* (1911b). 'Further researches on the development of *Trypanosoma vivax* in laboratory-bred *Glossina palpalis*,' *Repts. Sleep. Sickn. Comm. Roy. Soc.*, **11,** 50.

BRUCE, D., *et al.* (1911c). 'Trypanosome diseases of domestic animals in Uganda. III. *Trypanosoma vivax* (Ziemann),' *Repts. Sleep. Sickn. Comm. Roy. Soc.*, **11,** 150.

BRUCE, D., *et al.* (1911d). 'Trypanosome diseases of domestic animals in Uganda. *Trypanosoma uniforme* sp. nov,' *Repts. Sleep. Sickn. Comm. Roy. Soc.*, **11,** 160.

BRUCE, D., *et al.* (1912). The morphology of *Trypanosome simiae* sp. nov. *Proc. Roy. Soc.*, B, **85,** 477; *Repts. Sleep. Sickn. Comm. Roy. Soc., 1914*, **15,** 11.

BRUCE, D., *et al.* (1913). 'Trypanosome diseases of domestic animals in Nyasaland.' II. *Trypanosoma caprae* (Kleine),' *Proc. Roy. Soc.*, B, **86,** 278.

BRUCE, D., *et al.* (1914). 'Trypanosome disease of domestic animals in Nyasaland. I. *Trypanosoma simiae* sp. nov. Parts II and III,' *Repts. Sleep. Sickn. Comm. Roy. Soc.*, **15,** 121 and 131.

BRUCE, D., *et al.* (1914a). 'The trypanosome causing disease in man in Nyasaland. Pt. III. Development in *Glossina morsitans*,' *Proc. Roy. Soc.*, B, **87,** 516; *Repts. Sleep. Sickn. Comm. Roy. Soc., 1915*, **16,** 135.

BRUCE, D., *et al.* (1914b). 'Description of a strain of *Trypanosoma brucei* from Zululand. Part III. Development in *Glossina morsitans*,' *Proc. Roy. Soc.*, B, **87,** 526; *Repts. Sleep. Sickn. Comm. Roy. Soc., 1915*, **16,** 145.

BRUCE, D., *et al.* (1914c). 'The trypanosome causing disease in man in Nyasaland. Pt. III. Development in *Glossina morsitans*,' *Proc. Roy. Soc.*, B, **88,** 213; *Repts. Sleep. Sickn. Comm. Roy. Soc., 1915*, **16,** 151.

BRUCE, D., *et al.* (1914d). '*Glossina brevipalpis* as a carrier of trypanosome disease in Nyasaland,' *Proc. Roy. Soc.*, B, **88,** 20; *Repts. Sleep. Sickn. Comm. Roy. Soc., 1915*, **16,** 157.

BRUCE, D., *et al.* (1915). 'Trypanosome diseases of domestic animals in Nyasaland. XXXV. *Trypanosoma pecorum*,' *Repts. Sleep. Sickn. Comm. Roy. Soc.*, **16,** 174.

BRUCE, D., *et al.* (1915a). '*Trypanosoma caprae* (Kleine),' *Repts. Sleep. Sickn. Comm. Roy. Soc.*, **16,** 182.

BRUCE, D., *et al.* (1915b). Trypanosome disease of man and domestic animals in Nyasaland. *Repts. Sleep. Sickn. Comm. Roy. Soc.*, **16,** 29.

BRUTSAERT, P., and HENRARD, C. (1938). 'L'hémoculture comme moyen auxiliaire de diagnostic de la maladie du sommeil,' *C. R. Séanc. Soc. Biol.*, **127,** 1469.

BUCHANAN, J. C. R., (1929). 'Some clinical aspects of Trypanosomiasis rhodesiensis,' *Trans. R. Soc. trop. Med. Hyg.*, **23,** 81.

BURCHARD, R. P., and BALDRY, D. A. T. (1970). 'Polytene chromosomes of *Glossina palpalis* Robineau-Desvoidy (Diptera: Muscidae) I. The preliminary demonstration,' *Proc. R. ent. Soc. Lond.*, (A) **45** (*in press*).

BURNETT, G. F. (1954). 'The effect of poison bait cattle on populations of *Glossina morsitans* and *G. swynnertoni*,' *Bull. ent. Res.*, **45,** 411.

BURNETT, G. F. (1955). 'Non-persistent insecticides and tsetse flies—the effect of variation in life-cycle, interval between applications and percentage kill,' Tropical Pesticides Research Institute, Tanzania, *Miscellaneous Report No. 136.* 16 pp.

BURNETT, G. F. (1961). 'Effect of age and pregnancy on the tolerance of tsetse flies to insecticides,' *Nature*, Lond. **192,** 188 (Corresp.).

BURNETT, G. F. (1961–3). 'The susceptibility of tsetse flies to topical applications of insecticides I–VI,' *Bull. ent. Res.*, **52,** 531–9; 763–8; **53,** 337–45; 347–54; 747–52; 753–61.

BURNETT, G. F., ROBINSON, J., and LEROUX, J. G. (1957). 'Comparative trials of DDT and Dieldrin for the control of the riverside tsetse *Glossina palpalis fuscipes*,' *E. Afr. agric. J.*, **22,** 142.

BURNETT, G. F., and THOMPSON, B. W. (1956). 'Aircraft applications of insecticides in East Africa. X. An investigation of the behaviour of coarse aerosol clouds in woodland,' *Bull. ent. Res.*, **47,** 495.

BURNETT, G. F., YEO, D., MILLER, A. W. D., and WHITE, P. J. (1961). 'Aircraft applications of insecticides in East Africa. XIII. An economical method for the control of *Glossina morsitans* Westw.,' *Bull. ent. Res.*, **52,** 305.

BURNETT, G. F., CHADWICK, P. E., MILLER, A. W. D., and BEESLEY, J. S. S. (1964). 'Aircraft applications of insecticides in East Africa. XIV. Very-low-volume aerosols of dieldrin and telodrin for the control of *Glossina morsitans.* West.,' *Bull. ent. Res.*, **55,** 527.

BURSELL, E. (1955). 'The polypneustic lobes of the tsetse larva (*Glossina*, Diptera),' *Proc. Roy. Soc.*, B, **144,** 275.

BURSELL, E. (1955a). 'Experiments in tsetse control in southern Tanganyika,' *Bull. ent. Res.*, **46,** 3, 589.

BURSELL, E. (1957). 'The effect of humidity on the activity of tsetse flies,' *J. exp. Biol.*, **34,** 42.

BURSELL, E. (1957a). 'Spiracular control of water loss in the tsetse fly,' *Proc. R. ent. Soc., Lond.* (A) **32,** 21.

BURSELL, E. (1958). 'The water balance of tsetse pupae,' *Phil. Trans. Roy. Soc. Lond., Ser. B.*, **241,** 179.

BURSELL, E. (1959). 'Determination of the age of tsetse puparia by dissection,' *Proc. R. ent. Soc. Lond.*, **34,** 23.

BURSELL, E. (1959a). 'The water balance of tsetse flies,' *Trans. R. ent. Soc. Lond.*, **111,** 205.

BURSELL, E. (1960). 'The measurement of size in tsetse flies,' *Bull. ent. Res.*, **51,** 33.

BURSELL, E. (1960a). 'The effect of humidity and temperature on the extent of abdominal pigmentation in *Glossina pallidipes* Austen,' *Bull. ent. Res.*, **51,** 39.

BURSELL, E. (1960b). 'The effect of temperature on the consumption of fat during pupal development in *Glossina*,' *Bull. ent. Res.*, **51,** 583.

BURSELL, E. (1960c). 'Loss of water by excretion and defaecation in the tsetse fly,' *J. exp. Biol.*, **37,** 689.

BURSELL, E. (1961). 'Starvation and desiccation in tsetse flies (*Glossina*),' *Entomologia exp. & app.*, **4,** 301.

BURSELL, E. (1961a). 'The behaviour of tsetse flies (*Glossina swynnertoni* Austen) in relation to problems of sampling,' *Proc. R. ent. Soc. Lond.*, (A) **36,** 9.

BURSELL, E. (1961b). 'Post-teneral development of the thoracic musculature in tsetse flies,' *Proc. R. ent. Soc. Lond.*, (A) **36,** 69.

BURSELL, E. (1963). 'Aspects of the metabolism of amino acids in the tsetse fly, *Glossina* (Diptera),' *Jour. Ins. Physiol.*, **9**, 439.

BURSELL, E. (1965). 'Oxaloacetic carboxylase in flight musculature of the tsetse fly,' *Comp. Biochem. Physiol.*, **16**, 259.

BURSELL, E. (1965a). 'Nitrogenous waste products of the tsetse fly *Glossina morsitans*,' *Jour. Ins. Physiol.*, **11**, 993.

BURSELL, E. (1966). 'Aspects of the flight metabolism of tsetse flies (*Glossina*),' *Comp. Biochem. Physiol.*, **19**, 809.

BURSELL, E. (1966a). 'The nutritional state of tsetse flies from different vegetation types in Rhodesia,' *Bull. ent. Res.*, **57**, 171.

BURSELL, E. (1968). *A Prospect of Tsetse Flies. An inaugural lecture given in the University College of Rhodesia.* Salisbury, University College of Rhodesia.

BURSELL, E., and GLASGOW, J. P. (1960). 'Further observations on lake-side and riverine communities of *G. palpalis fuscipes* Newstead,' *Bull. ent. Res.*, **51**, 47.

BURSELL, E., and the late JACKSON, C. H. N. (1957), 'Notes on the choriothete and milk gland of *Glossina* and *Hippobosca* (Diptera),' *Proc. R. ent. Soc. Lond.*, (A) **32**, 30.

BURSELL, E., and SLACK, E. (1968). 'Indications concerning the flight activity of tsetse flies (*Glossina morsitans*) in the field,' *Bull. ent. Res.*, **58**, 3, 575.

BURTT, B. D. (1942). 'Some East African Vegetation Communities,' *J. Ecol.*, **30**, 65. [Burtt Memorial Supplement.]

BURTT, E. (1946). 'Incubation of tsetse pupae: increased transmission rate of *Trypanosoma rhodesiense* in *Glossina morsitans*,' *Ann. trop. Med. Parasit.*, **40**, 18.

BURTT, E. (1946a). 'Salivation by *Glossina morsitans* on to glass slides: a technique for isolating infected flies,' *Ann. trop. Med. Parasit.*, **40**, 141.

BURTT, E. (1947). 'Incubation of tsetse pupae: the temperature range experienced by pupae kept under normal laboratory conditions at Tinde,' *Ann. trop. Med. Parasit.*, **41**, 50.

BURTT, E. (1952). 'The occurrence in nature of tsetse pupae (*Glossina swynnertoni* Austen),' *Acta tropica*, **9**, 304.

BURTT, E., and JACKSON, C. H. N. (1951). 'Illustrations of tsetse larvae,' *Bull. ent. Res.*, **41**, 523.

BURTT, E. T., and CATTON, W. T. (1956). 'Electrical responses to visual stimulation in the optic lobes of the locust and certain other insects,' *J. Physiol.*, **133**, 1, 68.

BUSVINE, J. R., ABDURRAHIM, U., and MOHAMMED, N. N. (1967). 'The relative potency of insecticides to tsetse flies assessed by two methods,' *Bull. ent. Res.*, **57**, 321.

BUTLER, G. C., DUGGAN, A. J., and HUTCHINSON, M. P. (1957). 'Melarsen in the treatment of *Trypanosoma gambiense* infection in man,' *Trans. R. Soc. trop. Med. Hyg.*, **51**, 69.

BUXTON, P. A. (1955). *The natural history of tsetse flies*, Mem. Lond. Sch. Hyg. Trop Med. No. 10. London, H. K. Lewis. xviii + 816 pp.

BUXTON, P. A. (1955a). 'Tsetse and climate: a consideration of the growth of knowledge,' *Proc. R. ent. Soc. Lond.*, (C. **19**), 11, p. 71.

BUXTON, P. A., and LEWIS, D. J. (1934). 'Climate and tsetse flies: Laboratory studies upon *Glossina submorsitans* and *tachinoides*,' *Phil. Trans. Roy. Soc. Lond.*, B, **224**, 175.

References

BUYCKX, E. J. (1965). 'Applications par voie aérienne de Telodrine dans la lutte contre *G. morsitans* au Bugesera (Rwanda).' *See* ISCTR (1965), p. 145.

CALVER, K. M. (1945). 'Chemotherapeutic studies on *T. congolense* infection,' *Trop. Dis. Bull.*, **42,** 704.

CAMERON, A. E. (1926). 'Bionomics of the Tabanidae (Diptera) of the Canadian prairie,' *Bull. ent. Res.*, **17,** 1.

CAMPION, D. G. (1965). 'The present status of research on chemosterilants in the United States and Central America for the control of insect pests,' *Pest Articles and News Summary*, Sec. A., **11,** 467.

CANTRELL, W. (1958). 'Mutation rate and antigenic variation in *Trypanosoma equiperdum*,' *J. infect. Dis.*, **103,** 263.

CAPPONI, M. (1953). 'Sur un cas de trypanosomiase congénitale à Douala,' *Bull. Soc. Path. exot.*, **46,** 667.

CARMICHAEL, J. (1933). 'The virus of rinderpest and its relation to *Glossina morsitans.* Westw.,' *Bull. ent. Res.*, **24,** 337.

CARMICHAEL, J. (1939). 'Turning sickness of cattle and *Trypanosoma theileri* (Laveran),' *Parasitology*, **31,** No. 4.

CARPANO, M. (1932). 'Localisations du *Trypanosoma theileri* dans les organes internes des bovins, son cycle évolutif,' *Ann. Parasit. hum. comp.*, **10,** 305.

CARPENTER, G. D. H. (1912). 'Progress report on investigations into the bionomics of *Glossina palpalis*, July 27, 1910, to August 5, 1911,' *Repts. Sleep. Sick. Comm. Roy. Soc.*, **12,** 79.

CARPENTER, G. D. H. (1919). '3rd, 4th and 5th Reports on the bionomics of *Glossina palpalis* on Lake Victoria,' *Repts. Sleep. Sick. Comm. Roy. Soc.*, **17.**

CARPENTER, G. D. H. (1920). *A Naturalist on Lake Victoria.* London, T. Fisher Unwin.

CARPENTER, G. D. H. (1923). 'Report on a test of a method of attacking *Glossina* by artificial breeding places,' *Bull. ent. Res.*, **13,** 443.

CARTER, R. M. (1906). 'Tsetse fly in Arabia,' *Brit. Med. J.*, ii, 1393.

CASTELLANI, A. (1903). '*Trypanosoma* in sleeping sickness,' *Brit. med. J.*, Pt. 1, 1218.

CASTILLO, A. M. (1962). 'Studies on surra. II. Treatment with Antrycide salts,' *Philipp. J. Anim. Ind.*, **20,** 97.

CASTRO, V. A., FINLAYSON, T. M., and ORMEROD, W. E. (1967). 'Reaction of the popliteal gland to infection with *Trypanosoma brucei* (laboratory demonstration),' *Trans. R. Soc. trop. Med. Hyg.*, **61,** 12.

CAWDERY, M. J. H. (1963). 'Investigations in Uganda on the chemotherapy of bovine trypanosomiasis with particular reference to the local reactions of prophylactic compounds.' *See* ISCTR (1963), p. 87.

CAWDERY, M. J. H., and KNIGHT, R. H. (1961). 'A new method for the administration of trypanocidal drugs to animals,' *Vet. Rec.*, **73,** 982.

CECCALDI, J. (1952). 'Du traitement des nouveaux trypanosomés par le 3·854 RP ou Arsobal,' *Bull. Soc. Path. exot.*, **45,** 652.

CECCALDI, J., TRINQUIER, E., ARNOULT, H., and MENU, P. (1950). 'Contribution au traitement de la trypanosomiase humaine par les arsénoxydes,' *Bull. Soc. Path. exot.*, **43,** 83.

CHADWICK, P. R. (1964). 'Effect of two chemosterilants on *G. morsitans*,' *Nature*, Lond. **204,** 299.

CHADWICK, P. R., BEESLEY, J. S. S., WHITE, P. J., and MATECHI, H. T. (1964). 'An experiment on the eradication of *G. swynnertoni* by insecticidal treatment of its resting sites,' *Bull. ent. Res.*, **55,** 411.

CHALLIER, A. (1963). 'Campagne de lutte contre *G. palpalis gambiensis* Vanderplank dans le foyer de Bamako.' *See* ISCTR (1963), p. 265.

CHALLIER, A. (1963a). 'Sensibilité de *Glossina palpalis gambiensis* au DDT et à la dieldrine determinée au moyen de la trousse standard OMS pour moustiques adultes,' *Bull. Soc. Path. exot.*, **56,** 519.

CHALLIER, A. (1964). 'Observations sur l'ovulation chez *Glossina palpalis gambiensis* Vanderplank, 1949,' *Bull. Soc. Path. exot.*, **57**, 985.

CHALLIER, A. (1965). 'Amélioration de la méthode de détermination de l'âge physiologique des glossines,' *Bull. Soc. Path. exot.*, **58,** 250.

CHALLIER, A., EYRAUD, M., and DEDEWANOU, B. (1965). 'Étude de l'effet de l'HCH nébulisé sur une population de *G. palpalis gambiensis* Vanderplank 1949 dans une galerie forestière (Kankalaba, République de Haute-Volta).' *See* ISCTR (1965), p. 133.

CHANDLER, R. L. (1952). 'Comparative tolerance of West African N'Dama cattle to trypanosomiasis,' *Ann. trop. Med. Parasit.*, **46**, 127.

CHANDLER, R. L. (1958). 'Studies on the tolerance of N'Dama cattle to trypanosomiasis,' *J. comp. Path.*, **68,** 253.

CHAPMAN, R. F. (1960). 'A note on *Glossina medicorum* Aust. (Diptera) in Ghana,' *Bull. ent. Res.*, **51,** 435.

CHAPMAN, R. F. (1961). 'Some experiments to determine the methods used in host-finding by the tsetse fly, *Glossina medicorum* Austen,' *Bull. ent. Res.*, **52,** 83.

CHARDOME, M., and PEEL, E. (1954). 'Étude expérimentale d'une souche appelée *T. congolense* var. *berghei* transmise par *Glossina brevipalpis* du Mosso (Urundi),' *Ann. Soc. belge Méd. trop.*, **34,** 311.

CHARDOME, M. and PEEL, E. (1967). *Les trypanosomes transmis par* Glossina morsitans *au Bugesera* (*Rwanda et Burundi*). Brussels: Goemaere.

CHARGAFF, E., BANCROFT, F. W., and STANLEY-BROWN, MARGARET (1936). 'Studies on the chemistry of blood coagulation. II. On the inhibition of blood clotting by substances of high molecular weight,' *J. biol. Chem.*, **115,** 155.

CHATERJI, A., and SEN GUPTA, P. C. (1962). 'Adrenals in *Trypanosoma evansi* infection in white rats,' *Nature*, Lond. **193,** 78.

CHESTERS, J. K. (1966). 'Protein synthesis by cell-free extracts of *Crithidia oncopelti*,' *Biochim. biophys. Acta*, 114, 385.

CHORLEY, C. W. (1933). Traps for tsetse-flies of the "Crinoline" and "Ventilator" forms. *Bull. ent. Res.*, **24,** 315.

CHORLEY, J. K. (1929). 'The bionomics of *Glossina morsitans* in the Umniati fly belt, Southern Rhodesia, 1922–3,' *Bull. ent. Res.*, **20,** 279.

CHORLEY, J. K. (1929a). 'Experiments in grass fires against *Glossina morsitans* in Southern Rhodesia,' *Bull. ent. Res.*, **20,** 377.

CHORLEY, J. K. (1954). 'Annual Report of the Director of Tsetse Fly Operations for the year October 1, 1951, to September 30, 1952,' *Rhod. Agric. J.*, **51,** 197.

CHORLEY, J. K. (1958). 'La lutte contre la mouche tsé-tsé en Rhodesie du Sud.' *See* ISCTR (1958), p. 123.

CHORLEY, T. W., and HOPKINS, G. H. E. (1942). 'Activity of *Glossina pallidipes* at night (Diptera),' *Proc. R. ent. Soc. Lond.*, (A) **17,** 93.

CHRISTY, C. (1903). 'The distribution of sleeping sickness, *filaria perstans*, etc., in East Equatorial Africa,' *Repts. Sleep. Sickn. Comm. Roy. Soc.*, **2,** 2.

CHRISTY, C. (1904). 'The cerebrospinal fluid in sleeping sickness (trypanosomiasis) 104 lumbar punctures. Second interim report of the expedition of the Liverpool School of Tropical Medicine to the Congo, 1903,' *Memoirs of the Liverpool School of Tropical Medicine*, **13,** 57.

CLAPIER, P. (1921). 'Constatation de *Trypanosoma gambiense* en grande abondance dans le liquide d'hydrocèle,' *Bull. Soc. Path. exot.*, **14,** 378.

CLARK, R. (1840). 'Observations on the disease Lethargus: with cases and pathology,' *Lond. Med. Gaz.*, Series II, 970.

CLARK, T. B. (1959). 'Comparative morphology for four genera of Trypanosomatidae,' *J. Protozool.*, **6,** 227.

CLARK, T. B., and WALLACE, F. G. (1960). 'A comparative study of kinetoplast ultrastructure in the Trypanosomatidae,' *J. Protozool.*, **7,** 115.

CLARKE, J. E. (1964). 'Game elimination as a means of tsetse control with special reference to host preferences,' *Puku*, **2,** 67.

CLARKSON, M. J., and AWAN, M. A. Q. (1967). 'Immunological studies on *Trypanosoma vivax* in the sheep,' *Trans. R. Soc. trop. Med. Hyg.*, **61,** 142.

CMELIK, S. H. W., BURSELL, E., and SLACK, E. (1969). 'Composition of the gut content of third-instar larvae (*Glossina morsitans* Westw.),' *Comp. Biochem. Physiol.*, **29,** 447.

COCKBILL, G. F. (1960). 'The control of tsetse and trypanosomiasis in Southern Rhodesia,' *Proc. & Trans. Rhod. Sci. Assoc.*, **47,** 1.

COCKBILL, G. F. (1964). 'Report of Tsetse and Trypanosomiasis Control Branch in Dept. of Veterinary Services, Federation of Rhodesia and Nyasaland,' *Annual Report, 1963*. Salisbury, Govt. Printer.

COCKBILL, G. F. (1965). *Report* of the Assistant Director of Veterinary Services (Tsetse and Trypanosomiasis Control) for year ended September 30, 1965. Salisbury, Govt. Printer.

COCKBILL, G. F. (1967). 'The history and significance of trypanosomiasis problems in Rhodesia,' *Proc. & Trans. Rhod. Sci. Assoc.,*, **52,** 7.

COCKBILL, G. F., LOVEMORE, D. F., and PHELPS, R. J. (1963). 'The control of tsetse flies (*Glossina*, Diptera, Muscidae) in a heavily infested area of Southern Rhodesia by means of insecticide discharged from air craft, followed by the settlement of indigenous people,' *Bull. ent. Res.*, **54,** 93.

COCKERELL, T. D. A. (1918). 'New species of North American fossil beetles, cockroaches, and tsetse flies,' *Proc. U.S. natn. Mus.*, **54,** 301.

COHEN, A., KING, H., and STRANGEWAYS, W. I. (1932). 'Trypanocidal action and chemical constitution. Part XIV. The relative velocity of oxidation of arylarsenoxides,' *J. chem. Soc.*, 2866.

COLLOMB, H. (1957). 'Encéphalite de la trypanosomiase humaine africaine. Synthèse anatomo-clinique,' *Gaz. méd. Fr.*, **64,** 1069.

COLLOMB, H., AYATS, H., and MARTINO, P. (1964). 'Les causes de déçès dans la trypanosomiase humaine africaine,' *Bull. Soc. méd. Afr. noire Lang. fr.*, **9,** 54.

COLLOMB, H., AYATS, H., MARTINO, P., and LARIVIÈRE, M. (1964a). 'Les incidents et accidents du traitement de la trypanosomiase par le Mel W. (Deuxieme note à propos de 40 nouvelles observations),' *Bull. Soc. méd. Afr. noire Lang. fr.*, **9,** 325.

COLLOMB, H., BERT, J., MATTERN, P., and HOCQUET, P. (1963). 'Étude clinique, biologique, électro-encéphalographique de la trypanosomiase expérimentale chez *Erythrocebus patas*,' *Bull. Soc. Path. exot.*, **56,** 971.

COLLOMB, H., GALLAIS, P., and PLANQUES, L. (1956). 'La trypanosomiase chez l'Africain transplanté,' *Bull. Soc. Path. exot.*, **49**, 900.

COLLOMB, H., LARIVIERE, M., AYATS, H., DIOP, M., and MARTINO, P. (1964b). 'Les échecs du traitement de la trypanosomiase par le Mel W,' *Bull. Mém. mixte méd. Pharm., Dakar*, **12**, 156.

COLLOMB, H., and MILETTO, G. (1957). 'Les séquelles de la trypanosomiase humaine africaine,' *Bull. Soc. Path. exot.*, **50**, 573.

COLLOMB, H., MILETTO, G., and LEVRON, M. (1956). 'Troubles de la glycorégulation et diamidines. (À propos de trois observations de diabète après traitement par la Lomidine),' *Méd. trop.*, **16**, 786.

COLLOMB, H., ZWINGELSTEIN, J., AYATS, H., and SECK, I. (1963). 'Les incidents et accidents du traitement de la trypanosomiase par le Mel W. À propos de 38 observations,' *Bull. Soc. méd. Afr. noire Lang. fr.*, **8**, 61.

CONRAN, P. (1921). 'Intermissions in trypanosomiasis,' *Brit. med. J.*, June 18, p. 916.

CONTENT, J., and COGNIAUX-LECLERC, J. (1968). 'Comparison of the *in vitro* action of Ethidium chloride on animal viruses with that of other photodyes,' *J. gen. Virol.*, **3**, 63.

COOKE, W. E., GREGG, A. L., and MANSON-BAHR, P. H. (1937). 'Recent experiences of mild or symptomless infections with *Trypanosoma gambiense* from the Gold Coast and Nigeria,' *Trans. R. Soc. trop. Med. Hyg.*, **30**, 461.

COONS, A. H. (1956). 'Histochemistry with labelled antibody,' *Int. Rev. Cytol.*, **5**, 1–23.

COONS, A. H., and KAPLAN, M. H. (1950). 'Localization of antigen in tissue cells. II. Improvements in a method for the detection of antigens by means of fluorescent antibody,' *J. exp. Med.*, **91**, 1.

CORSON, J. F. (1938). 'A third note on a strain of *T. gambiense* transmitted by *G. morsitans*,' *Ann. trop. Med. Parasit.*, **32**, 245.

COTTRELL, C. B. (1962). 'General observations on the imaginal ecdysis of blowflies,' *Trans. R. ent. Soc. Lond.*, **114**, 317.

COURTOIS, D., and BIDEAU, J. (1966). 'L'immunofluorescence appliqué au diagnostic de la trypanosomiase africaine. Valeur comparative avec le titrage de l'immunoglobulins IgM,' *Bull. Soc. Path. exot.*, **59**, 809.

CRAIG, C. F. (1948). *Laboratory diagnosis of protozoan diseases*, 2nd edition. London, Kimpton.

CRAWFORD, T. B. B., and LEVVY, G. A. (1947). 'Changes undergone by phenyl arsenious acid and phenyl arsonic acid in the animal body,' *Biochem. J.*, **41**, 333.

CROOKSHANK, E. M. (1886). 'Flagellated protozoa in the blood of diseased and apparently healthy animals,' *J. R. micro. Soc.*, **6**, 913.

CROSS, G. A. M. (1966). 'Protein synthesis in a cell-free system from *Crithidia oncopelti*,' *J. gen. Microbiol.*, **44**, iii.

CROSS, G. A. M. (1968). 'Physical properties of ribosomes from a protozoan,' *J. gen. Microbiol.*, **50**, ix.

CROWLE, A. J. (1961). *Immunodiffusion.* New York and London, Academic Press.

CULWICK, A. T., and FAIRBAIRN, H. (1947). 'Polymorphism in *Trypanosoma simiae* and the morphology of the metacyclic forms,' *Trans. R. Soc. trop. Med. Hyg.*, **41**, 415.

CUNNINGHAM, K. G., HUTCHINSON, S. A., MANSON, W., and SPRING, F. S. (1951). 'Cordycepin, a metabolic product from cultures of *Cordyceps militaris* (Linn.) Link. Part I. Isolation and characterisation,' *J. chem. Soc.*, 2299.

CUNNINGHAM, M. P. (1967). 'Vaccination of cattle against trypanosomes by infection and treatment.' *See* ISCTR (1967), p. 65.

CUNNINGHAM, M. P., BAILEY, N. M., and KIMBER, C. D. (1967). 'The estimation of IgM immunoglobulin in dried blood, for use as a screening test in the diagnosis of human trypanosomiasis in Africa,' *Trans. R. Soc. trop. Med. Hyg.*, **61,** 688.

CUNNINGHAM, M. P., KIMBER, C. D., BAILEY, N. M., and HARLEY, J. M. P. (1967). 'Seventh Seminar on Trypanosomiasis,' *Trans. R. Soc. trop. Med. Hyg.*, **61,** 146.

CUNNINGHAM, M. P., LUMSDEN, W. H. R., and WEBBER, W. A. F. (1963b). 'Preservation of viable trypanosomes in lymph tubes at low temperature,' *Exp. Parasit.*, **14,** 280.

CUNNINGHAM, M. P., and VAN HOEVE, K. (1965). 'Diagnosis of trypanosomiasis in cattle.' *See* ISCTR (1965), p. 51.

CUNNINGHAM, M. P., VAN HOEVE, K., and LUMSDEN, W. H. R. (1963a). 'Variable infectivity of organisms of the *T. brucei* subgroup during acute relapsing infections in rats.' *See* EATRO (1963a), p. 21.

CUNNINGHAM, M. P., and VICKERMAN, K. (1962). 'Antigenic analysis of the *Trypanosoma brucei* group, using the agglutination reaction,' *Trans. R. Soc. trop. Med. Hyg.*, **56,** 48.

CURASSON, G. (1925). '*Trypanosoma theileri* au Soudan Français,' *Bull. Soc. Path. exot.*, **18,** 823.

CURASSON, G. (1943). *Traité de protozoologie vétérinaire et comparée. Tome I: Trypanosomes.* Paris, Vigot-Frères.

CURTIS, C. F. (1968). 'Radiation sterilization and the effect of multiple mating of females in *Glossina austeni*,' *J. Insect. Physiol.*, **14,** 1365.

CURTIS, C. F. (1968a). 'A possible genetic method for the control of insect pests with special reference to tsetse flies (*Glossina* spp.),' *Bull. ent. Res.*, **57,** 509.

CURTIS, C. F. (1968b). 'Possible use of translocations to fix desirable genes in insect pest populations,' *Nature*, Lond., **218,** 368.

CURTIS, C. F., and HILL, W. B. (1968). 'Theoretical and practical studies on a possible genetic method for tsetse fly control,' *Isotopes and Radiations in Entomology*, p. 233. Vienna, International Atomic Agency.

CUTHBERT, A. W. (1967). 'Membrane lipids and drug action,' *Pharmacol. Rev.*, **19,** 59.

DA COSTA, B. F. B., SANT'ANNA, J. F., DOS SANTOS, A. C., and ALVARES, M. J. DE A. (1915). *Sleeping Sickness, a record of four years war against it in Principe, Portuguese West Africa.* Transl. by J. A. Wylie, 1916, London.

DAME, D. A. (1968). 'Chemosterilization, rearing and ecological studies of *Glossina*.' Paper presented in January 1967 to the Panel on Control of Livestock Insect Pests by the Sterile-male Technique. Joint FAO/IAEA, Vienna, *Panel Proceedings Series* STI/PUB/184, 1968, 102 pp.

DAME, D. A., BIRKENMEER, D. R. and BURSELL, E. (1969). 'Development of the thoracic muscle and flight behaviour of *Glossina morsitans orientalis* Vanderplank,' *Bull. ent. Res.*, **59** (1968), 345.

DAME, D. A., DEAN, G. J. W., and FORD, J. (1965). 'Investigations of the sterile male technique with *Glossina morsitans*.' *See* ISCTR (1965), p. 93.

DAME, D. A., and FORD, H. R. (1966). 'Effect of the chemosterilant Tepa on *Glossina morsitans* Westw,' *Bull. ent. Res.*, **56,** 649.

DAME, D. A., and FORD, H. R. (1968). 'Multiple mating of *G. morsitans* Westw. and its potential effect on the sterile male technique,' *Bull. ent. Res.*, **58,** 213.

DAME, D. A., and MACKENZIE, P. K. I. (1968). 'Transmission of *Trypanosoma congolense* by chemosterilised male *G. morsitans.*,' *Ann. trop. Med. Parasit.*, **62,** 372.

DAME, D. A., WOODARD, D. B., FORD, H. R., and WEIDHAAS, D. E. (1964). 'Field behaviour of sexually sterile *Anopheles quadrimaculatus*,' *Mosquito News*, **24,** 6.

DANFORTH, W. F. (1967). 'Respiratory metabolism,' in *Research in Protozoology*, Vol. 1 (ed. T. T. Chen), p. 201.

DANIELS, C. W. (1916). 'Eye lesions as a point of importance in directing suspicion to possible trypanosome infection,' *Trop. Dis. Bull.*, **8,** 265.

DARLING, F. F. (1941). *A Herd of Red Deer: A Study in Animal Behaviour*, 2nd edition. Oxford.

DARLING, F. F. (1947). *Natural History in the Highlands and Islands*, London.

DARRÉ, H., MOLLARET, P., TANGUY, Y., and MERCIER, P. (1937). 'Hydrocéphalie congénitale par trypanosomiase héréditaire. Démonstration de la possibilité du passage transplacentaire dans l'espèce humaine,' *Bull. Soc. Path. exot.*, **30,** 159.

DASMAN, F. (1964). *African Game Ranching*. Oxford, Pergamon Press.

DAVEY, J. B. (1936). 'Trypanosomiasis,' *Br. med. J.*, June 27, 1321.

DAVID, –. –., and PAPE, –. –. (1942). 'Deux cas d'hérédo-trypanosomiase,' *Rev. Sci. Méd. Pharm. et Vét. de l'Afrique Francaise libre*, Brazzaville, **1,** 92.

DAVIES, H. (1964). 'Eradication of tsetse in the Chad River System of Northern Nigeria,' *J. app. Ecol.*, **1,** 387.

DAVIES, H. (1967). *Tsetse Flies in Northern Nigeria, A handbook for Junior Control Staff*, 2nd edition. Ibadan University Press.

DAVIES, H., and BLASDALE, P. (1960). 'The eradication of *Glossina morsitans submorsitans* Newst. and *G. tachinoides* Westw. in part of a river flood plain in Northern Nigeria by chemical means. Part III,' *Bull. ent. Res.*, **51,** 265.

DAVIES, J. B. (1961). 'Dieldrin in the control of *Glossina palpalis* in the Southern Guinea Savannah of Northern Nigeria.' *See* ISCTR (1961) p. 277.

DAVIES, J. N. P. (1962). 'The cause of sleeping sickness, Pts. 1 and 2,' *East Afric. med. J.*, **39,** 81 and 145.

DAVIS, B. S. (1952). 'Studies on the trypanosomes of some California mammals,' *Univ. California Pub. Zool.*, **57,** 145.

DAVIS, N. T. (1964). 'Studies of the reproductive physiology of Cimicidae (Hemiptera). I. Fecundation and egg maturation,' *J. Insect Physiol.*, **10,** 947.

DEAN, G. J. W. and CLEMENTS, S. A. (1969). 'Effect of gamma-radiation on *Glossina pallidipes* Aust.' *Bull. ent. Res.*, **58,** 755.

DEAN, G. J. W., DAME, D. A., and BIRKENMEYER, D. R. (1969). 'Field cage evaluation of the competitiveness of male *Glossina morsitans orientalis* Vanderplank sterilised with tepa or gamma irradiation.' *Bull. ent. Res.*, **59,** (1968), 339.

DEAN, G. J. W., PAGE, J., and WILSON, F. (1969). 'Observations on the behaviour of tsetse flies (*Glossina morsitans orientalis* Vanderplank and *G. pallidipes* Aust.) during an attempt to concentrate breeding around cattle.' *J. appl. Ecol.*, **6,** 13.

DEAN, G. J. W., WILLIAMSON, B. R., and PHELPS, R. J. (1969). 'Behavioural studies of *Glossina morsitans* Westw. using tantalum-182.' *Bull. ent. Res.*, **58,** 763.

DEAN, G. J. W. and WORTHAM, S. M. (1969). 'Effect of gamma-radiation on the tsetse fly *Glossina moritans* Westw.' *Bull. ent. Res.*, **58,** 505.

DECKER, K., FRANZ, H. F., and FRANZ, M. (1964). 'Vergleichende Untersuchungen über die Wirkung von Puromycin und Aminonucleosid auf die Proteinsynthese,' *Klin. Wschr.*, **12,** 583.

DE DUVE, C., PRESSMAN, B. C., GIANETTO, R., WATTIAUX, R., and APPELMANS, F. (1955). 'Tissue fractionation studies. 6. Intracellular distribution patterns of enzymes in rat-liver tissue,' *Biochem. J.*, **60,** 604.

DE JONGH, R. T., and FRIEDHEIM, E. A. H. (1959). 'Le pentylthiarsphénylmélamine (Mel W) dans le traitement de trypanosomiase à *T. gambiense*,' *Bull. Soc. Path. exot.*, **52,** 769.

DELANÖE, P. (1912). 'L'importance de la phagocytose dans l'immunité de la souris à l'égard de quelques flagellés,' *Ann. Inst. Past.*, **26,** 172.

DE RAADT, P. (1967). 'Reactive encephalopathy occurring as a complication during treatment of *Trypanosoma rhodesiense* infections with non-arsenical drugs.' *See* EATRO (1967), p. 85.

DE RAADT, P., and KIMBER, C. E. (1966). 'A drug trial with Astiban.' *See* EATRO (1966), p. 59.

DESART, THE EARL OF (Chairman) (1914). *Report of the Inter-departmental Committee on Sleeping Sickness.* Cd. 7349 and *Minutes of Evidence*, Cd. 7350, London, HMSO 26 and 330 pp.

DESOWITZ, R. S. (1956). 'Effect of antibody on the respiratory rate of *Trypanosoma vivax*,' *Nature*, Lond., **177,** 132.

DESOWITZ, R. S. (1959). 'Studies on immunity and host-parasite relationships. I. The immunological response of resistant and susceptible breeds of cattle to trypanosomal challenge,' *Ann. trop. Med. Parasitol.*, **53,** 293.

DESOWITZ, R. S. (1959a). 'Paper electrophoresis of trypanosomal extracts,' *Nature*, Lond., **184,** 986.

DESOWITZ, R. S. (1960). 'Studies on the immunity and host-parasite relationships. II. The immune response of antelope to trypanosomal challenge,' *Ann. trop. Med. Parasit.*, **54,** 281.

DESOWITZ, R. S., and FAIRBAIRN, H. (1955). 'The influence of temperature on the length of the developmental cycle of *T. vivax* in *G. palpalis*,' *Ann. trop. Med. Parasitol.*, **49,** 161.

DESOWITZ, R. S., and WATSON, H. J. C. (1951). 'Studies on *Trypanosoma vivax*. I. Susceptibility of white rats to infection,' *Ann. trop. Med. Parasit.*, **45,** 207.

DESOWITZ, R. S., and WATSON, H. J. C. (1952). 'Studies on *Trypanosoma vivax*. III. Observations on maintenance of a strain in white rats,' *Ann. trop. Med. Parasit.*, **46,** 92.

DESOWITZ, R. S., and WATSON, H. J. C. (1953). 'Studies on *Trypanosoma vivax*. IV. The maintenance of a strain in white rats without sheep serum supplement,' *Ann. trop. Med. Parasit.*, **47,** 62.

DESOWITZ, R. S., and WATSON, H. J. C. (1953a). 'The maintenance of a strain of *Trypanosoma simiae* in rabbits,' *Ann. trop. Med. Parasit.*, **47,** 324.

DETHIER, V. G. (1954). 'Notes on the biting response of tsetse flies,' *Amer. Jour. trop. Med. & Hyg.*, **3,** 160.

DETINOVA, T. S. (1955). 'Age changes in the ovaries of *Hippobosca capensis*,' *Dokl. Acad. Sci. USSR*, **5**, 937.

DETINOVA, T. S. (1962). *Age grouping methods in Diptera of medical importance*. W. H. O. Monograph 47, Geneva.

DIALLO, J. (1951). 'Resultats de la chimioprophylaxie par les diamidines dans le secteur special No. 3 a Guekedou-Kissidougou (Guinée),' *Bull. Soc. Path. exot.*, **44**, 93.

DIAS, E., and FREITAS, L. DE (1943). 'Introdução ao estudo biometrico dos hemoflagelados do genero *Schizotrypanum*,' *Mem. Inst. O. Cruz.*, **38**, 427.

DIAS, J. A. TRAVASSOS DOS SANTOS (1961). 'Trypanosomes found in antelopes of a region infested by *Glossina austeni* Newstead, 1912, in Mozambique.' *See* ISCTR (1961), p. 175.

DIAS, J. A. TRAVASSOS DOS SANTOS (1961a). 'Resultado de um reconhecimento Glossinico em algumas circonscricaos do Distríto de Cabo Delgado,' *Anais Servs. Vet. Ind. anim. Moçamb.*, **7**, 167.

DIAS, J. A. TRAVASSOS DOS SANTOS (1962). 'The status of the tsetse fly in Mozambique before 1896,' *S. A. J. Sci.*, **58**, 243.

DIAS, V. A. S. (1946). 'Notulas parasitólogicas. III. Da existência em Angola do *Tr. uniforme* Bruce & Coll. 1911,' *An. Serviç. Veter. Industr. Anim.*, Angola, p. 94.

DICKINSON, L., CHANTRILL, D. H., INKLEY, G. W., and THOMPSON, M. J. (1953). 'The antiviral action of phenanthridinium compounds,' *Brit. J. Pharmacol.*, **8**, 139.

DIXON, H. (1966). 'Blood platelets as a source of enzyme activity in washed trypanosome suspensions,' *Nature*, Lond., **210**, 428.

DODIN, A., and FROMENTIN, H. (1962). 'Mise en évidence d'un antigène vaccinant dans le plasma de la souris expérimentalement infecté par *Trypanosoma gambiense* et par *T. congolense*,' *Bull. Soc. Path. exot.*, **55**, 128.

DODIN, A., and FROMENTIN, H. (1963). 'Réaction d'hémagglutination passive dans la trypanosomiase humaine.' *See* ISCTR (1963), p. 369.

DONNELLY, J. (1958). 'Methods for the study of Blowfly Populations. III. The fate and distribution of ^{32}P, in Blowflies labelled in the larval stage,' *Ann. appl. Biol.*, **46**, 2, 243.

DUGGAN, A. J. (1962). 'A survey of sleeping sickness in Northern Nigeria from the earliest times to the present day,' *Trans. R. Soc. trop. Med. Hyg.*, **56**, 439.

DUGGAN, A. J. (1962a). 'The occurrence of human trypanosomiasis among the Rukuba tribe of Northern Nigeria,' *J. trop. Med. Hyg.*, **65**, 151.

DUGGAN, A. J., and HUTCHINSON, M. P. (1966). 'Sleeping sickness in Europeans: A review of 109 cases,' *J. trop. Med. Hyg.*, **69**, 124.

DUKE, H. L. (1912). 'The transmission of *Trypanosoma nanum*,' *Repts. Sleep. Sickn. Comm. Roy. Soc.*, **12**, 111.

DUKE, H. L. (1913). 'A trypanosome from British East Africa showing posterior-nuclear forms,' *Repts. Sleep. Sickn. Comm. Roy. Soc.*, **13**, 67.

DUKE, H. L. (1919). 'An enquiry into the relations of *Glossina morsitans* and ungulate game, with special reference to rinderpest.' *Bull. ent. Res.*, **10**, 7.

DUKE, H. L. (1923). 'An enquiry into an outbreak of human trypanosomiasis in a *Glossina morsitans* belt to the east of Mwanza, Tanganyika Territory,' *Proc. R. Soc.*, B, **94**, 250.

DUKE, H. L. (1923a). 'Further enquiries into the zoological status of the polymorphic mammalian trypanosomes of Africa, and the means by which they are spread in nature,' *Parasitology*, **15**, 258.

DUKE, H. L. (1928). 'Studies on the bionomics of the polymorphic trypanosomes of man and ruminants,' *Final Rept. League of Nations Intern. Comm. on Hum. Trypanosomiasis* (Geneva), 21.

DUKE, H. L. (1930). 'On the occurrence in man of strains of *T. gambiense* non-transmissible cyclically by *G. palpalis*,' *Parasitology*, **22**, 490.

DUKE, H. L. (1933). 'Studies on the factors that may influence the transmission of the polymorphic trypanosomes by tsetse,' Parts IV and VI, *Ann. trop. Med. Parasit.*, **27**, 431 and 451.

DUKE, H. L. (1934). 'On the transmissibility by *Glossina* of *T. brucei*, *T. rhodesiense* and *T. gambiense* with special reference to old laboratory strains,' *Parasitology*, **26**, 153.

DUKE, H. L. (1935). 'Old "laboratory" strains of the polymorphic trypanosomes,' *Lancet*, **229**, 665.

DUKE, H. L. (1935a). 'Further studies on the behaviour of *T. rhodesiense* recently isolated from man, in antelope and other African game animals,' *Parasitology*, **27**, 68.

DUKE, H. L. (1936). 'On the prophylactic action of "Bayer 205" against the trypanosomes of man,' *Lancet*, **230**, 463.

DUKE, H. L. (1937). 'Studies on the effect on *T. gambiense* and *T. rhodesiense* of prolonged maintenance in mammals other than man. V. The effect of prolonged maintenance away from man of the infectivity of *T. rhodesiense* for man,' *Parasitology*, **29**, 12.

DUKE, H. L., METTAM, R. W. M., and WALLACE, J. M. (1934). 'Observations on the direct passage from vertebrate to vertebrate of recently isolated strains of *T. brucei* and *T. rhodesiense*,' *Trans. R. Soc. trop. Med. Hyg.*, **28**, 77.

DUKE, H. L., and WALLACE, J. M. (1930). 'Red cell adhesion in trypanosomiasis of man and animals,' *Parasitology*, **22**, 414.

DU TOIT, R. (1954). 'Trypanosomiasis in Zululand and the control of tsetse flies by chemical means,' *Onderstepoort Jnl. vet. Res.*, **26**, 317.

DU TOIT, R., KLUGE, E. B., and FIEDLER, D. G. H. (1954). 'The eradication of *G. pallidipes* from Zululand by chemical means.' *See* ISCTR (1954), p. 141.

DUTTON, J. E. (1902). 'Preliminary note upon a trypanosome occurring in the blood of man,' *Thomson Yates Lab. Repts.*, **4**, 455.

DUTTON, J. E., and TODD, J. L. (1903). 'First report of the trypanosomiasis expedition to Senegambia (1902),' *Liverpool School of Tropical Medicine Memoir XI.*

DYE, W. H. (1926). 'The serum-formalin reaction in *T. rhodesiense* infection,' *Trans. R. Soc. trop. Med. Hyg.*, **20**, 74.

DYE, W. H. (1927). 'The relative importance of man and beast in human trypanosomiasis,' *Trans. R. Soc. trop. Med. Hyg.*, **21**, 187.

DYLEFF, P. (1932). 'Quelques réflexions sur la disparition spontanée des trypanosomes chez trois Européens reconnus porteurs des trypanosomes,' *Bull. Soc. Path. exot.*, **25**, 956.

EATRO (1950). *Annual Report 1949.* EA Tsetse and Trypanosomiasis Research and Reclamation Organization. Nairobi, EA High Commission.

EATRO (1950a). *Annual Report 1950.* EA Tsetse and Trypanosomiasis Research and Reclamation Organization. Nairobi, EA High Commission.

EATRO (1952). *Annual Report 1951.* EA Tsetse and Trypanosomiasis Research and Reclamation Organization. Nairobi, EA High Commission.

EATRO (1953). *Annual Report 1952.* EA Tsetse and Trypanosomiasis Research and Reclamation Organization. Nairobi, EA High Commission.

EATRO (1954). *Annual Report 1953.* EA Tsetse and Trypanosomiasis Research and Reclamation Organization. Nairobi, EA High Commission.

EATRO (1955). *Notes for field studies of tsetse flies in East Africa.* EA Tsetse and Trypanosomiasis Research and Reclamation Organization. Nairobi, EA High Commission.

EATRO (1955a). *Annual Report 1954–5.* EA Tsetse and Trypanosomiasis Research and Reclamation Organization. Nairobi, EA High Commission.

EATRO (1956). *Annual Report 1955–6.* EA Trypanosomiasis Research Organization. Nairobi, EA High Commission.

EATRO (1958). *Annual Report 1956–7.* EA Trypanosomiasis Research Organization. Nairobi, EA High Commission.

EATRO (1959). *Annual Report 1958.* EA Trypanosomiasis Research Organization. Nairobi, EA High Commission.

EATRO (1960). *Annual Report 1959.* EA Trypanosomiasis Research Organization. Nairobi, EA High Commission.

EATRO (1961). *Annual Report 1960.* EA Trypanosomiasis Research Organization. Nairobi, EA High Commission.

EATRO (1963). *Annual Report 1961.* EA Trypanosomiasis Research Organization. Nairobi, EA High Commission.

EATRO (1963a). *Annual Report 1962–3.* EA Trypanosomiasis Research Organization. Nairobi, EA High Commission.

EATRO (1966). *Annual Report 1965.* EA Trypanosomiasis Research Organization. Entebbe, Govt. Printer.

EATRO (1967). *Annual Report 1966.* East African Trypanosomiasis Research Organization. Entebbe, Govt. Printer.

EDDY, G. W., ROTH, A. R., and ABRAHAMSEN, L. R. (1965). 'Sterilant effect of some materials on *Aedes aegypti* (L) feeding on treated mice,' *Mosquito News*, **25,** 169.

EDNEY, E. B., and BARRASS, R. (1962). 'The body temperature of the tsetse fly, *Glossina morsitans* Westwood (Diptera, Muscidae),' *J. Insect. Physiol.*, **8,** 469.

EDNEY, E. B., and BARRASS, R. (1962a). 'Transpiration and the body temperature of tsetse flies (*G. morsitans*),' *American Zoologist*, **2,** 406.

EDWARDS, E. E., JUDD, J. M., and SQUIRE, F. A. (1956). 'Observations on trypanosomes in domestic animals in West Africa. I.' *Ann. trop. Med. Parasit.*, **50,** 223.

EDWARDS, F. W., OLDROYD, H., and SMART, J. (1939). *British blood-sucking flies.* Lond., Brit. Mus. (Nat. Hist.).

EHRLICH, P. (1911). 'Über chemotherapie,' *Zbl. Bakt.*, I. Abt. Ref., **50,** Beiheft, 94.

EHRLICH, P., ROEHL, W., and GULBRANSEN, R. (1909). 'Über serumfeste Trypanosomenstämme. Bemerkungen zu der Arbeit von Levaditi und Mutermilch,' *Z. Immun.-Forsch.*, **3,** 296.

ELEK, S. D. (1949). 'The serological analysis of mixed flocculating systems by diffusion gradients,' *Brit. J. exp. Path.*, **30,** 484.

ELLIOTT, W. H. (1963). 'The effects of antimicrobial agents on deoxyribonucleic acid polymerase,' *Biochem. J.*, **86,** 562.

ENDERLEIN, G. (1936). 'Diptera,' in *Die Tierwelt Mitteleuropas*, **6,** T. 2, p. 259S. Leipzig.

ERCOLI, N. (1962). 'Drug sensitivity and serological variations in *Trypanosoma equiperdum* following nitrogen mustard treatment,' *J. Protozool.*, **9,** 474.

ERCOLI, N. (1967). 'Selective antagonism of arsenicals and antimonials,' *Nature*, Lond., **216,** 398.

ERCOLI, N. (1968). 'Chemotherapeutic and toxicological properties of antimonyl tartrate-dimethylcysteine chelates,' *Proc. Soc. exp. Biol. Med.*, **129,** 284.

EVANS, G. (1880). *Report on 'surra' disease in the Dera Ismail Khan district.* Punjab Govt. Milit. Dept. No. 493, 446.

EVENS, F., (1953). 'Dispersion géographique des glossines au Congo Belge,' *Mem. Inst. r. Sci. nat. Belg.*, 2nd Ser. Fasc., **48,** 70 pp.

EVENS, F. and NIEMEGEERS, C. J. E. J. (1954). 'Recherches sur l'élevage et la biologie de *Glossina palpalis martinii*,' *Mém. Inst. r. Sci. nat. Belg.*, **54,** 1.

EVENS, F., NIEMEGEERS, C., and CHARLES, P. (1963). 'Maladie du sommeil à *T. gambiense*. Étude de quelques réactions biochimiques du sérum humain,' *Acad. Roy. des Sci. d'Outre Mer. Classe des Sci. Naturelles et Méd.* (NS), **14,** 179.

EVENS, F., NIEMEGEERS, K., and PACKCHANIAN, A. (1957). 'Nitrofurazone therapy of *Trypanosoma gambiense* sleeping sickness in man,' *Am. J. trop. Med. Hyg.*, **6,** 665.

EVENS, F., SCHOENAERS, F., NEUJEAN, G., KAECKENBEEK, A., and STYNS, J. (1953). 'Valeur pratique de la réaction de fixation du complément dans la maladie du sommeil à *T. gambiense*. II. La réaction de fixation du complément lors d'une rechute après traitement médicamenteux,' *Ann. Soc. belge Méd. trop.*, **33,** 389.

FAIRBAIRN, H. (1948). 'Sleeping sickness in Tanganyika Territory, 1922–46,' *Trop. Dis. Bull.*, **45,** 1.

FAIRBAIRN, H. (1953). 'Studies on *T. vivax*. IX. Morphological differences in strains and their relation to pathogenicity,' *Ann. trop. Med. Parasit.*, **47,** 394.

FAIRBAIRN, H. (1954). 'The animal reservoirs of *T. rhodesiense* and *T. gambiense*,' *Ann. Soc. belge Méd. trop.*, **34,** 663.

FAIRBAIRN, H. (1956). 'The infectivity to man of syringe-passaged strains of *Trypanosoma rhodesiense* and *T. gambiense*,' *Ann. trop. Med. Parasit.*, **50,** 167.

FAIRBAIRN, H. (1958). 'The penetration of *T. rhodesiense* through the peritrophic membrane of *G. palpalis*,' *Ann. trop. Med. Parasit.*, **52,** 18.

FAIRBAIRN, H. (1962). 'Measurements of strains of *T. congolense*,' *Ann. trop. Med. Parasit.*, **56,** 218.

FAIRBAIRN, H., and BURTT, E. (1946). 'The infectivity to man of a strain of *Trypanosoma rhodesiense* transmitted cyclically by *Glossina morsitans* through sheep and antelope: evidence that man requires a minimum infective dose of metacyclic trypanosomes,' *Ann. trop. Med. Parasit.*, **40,** 270.

FAIRBAIRN, H., and CULWICK, A. T. (1950). 'The transmission of the polymorphic trypanosomes,' *Acta trop.*, **7,** 19.

FAIRBAIRN, H., and GODFREY, D. G. (1957). 'The local reaction in man at the site of infection with *Trypanosoma rhodesiense*,' *Ann. trop. Med. Parasit.*, **51,** 464.

FAIRBAIRN, H., and GODFREY, D. G. (1958). 'Sections cut through a chancre developing in a human volunteer previously exposed to the bite of an infected tsetse (laboratory demonstration),' *Trans. R. Soc. trop. Med. Hyg.*, **52,** 21.

FAIRBAIRN, H., and WILLIAMSON, J. (1956). 'The composition of tsetse fly saliva. I. Histochemical analysis,' *Ann. trop. Med. Parasit.*, **50,** 322.

FAIRCLOUGH, R. (1956). 'Insecticidal fogs against tsetse flies on trains,' *Bull. ent. Res.*, **47,** 193.

FAIRCLOUGH, R. (1963). 'A summary of the use of Berenil in Kenya.' *See* ISCTR (1963), p. 81.

FAIRCLOUGH, R. (1963a). 'Observations on the use of Berenil against trypanosomiasis of cattle in Kenya,' *Vet. Rec.*, **75,** 1107.

FALCONE, A. B., MAO, R. L., and SHRAGO, E. (1962). 'A study of the action of hypoglycaemia-producing biguanide and sulfonylurea compounds on oxidative phosphorylation,' *J. biol. Chem.*, **237,** 904.

FARNHAM, A. E., and DUBIN, D. T. (1967). 'Studies on the mechanism of action of Puromycin aminonucleoside in L cells,' *Biochim. biophys. Acta*, **138,** 35.

FARRELL, J. A. K. (1961). 'The control of a tsetse fly advance by use of residual insecticide.' *See* ISCTR (1961), p. 265.

FASTIER, F. N. (1962). 'Structure-activity relationships of amidine derivatives,' *Pharmacol. Rev.*, **14,** 37.

FAVIER, J. (1963). 'Prophylaxie et traitement de la dourine par l'Antrycide en Algérie.' Thesis, Paris (Alfort). *Vet. Bull.* 1964, **34,** Abstr. 2850.

FERGUSON, W. (1964). 'A survey of disease incidence in slaughter cattle in Northern Nigeria,' *Bull. epizoot. Dis. Afr.*, **12,** 331.

FERNANDEZ, D. B., RICO, F., and DUMAG, P. U. (1965). 'Observations on an outbreak of surra among cattle,' *Philipp. J. anim. Ind.*, **21,** 221.

FERNANDO, S. D. A., and JAYASINGHE, J. B. (1965). 'The use of Spirotrypan in the treatment of surra in dogs,' *Vet. Rec.*, **77,** 44.

FERONE, R., BURCHALL, J. J., and HITCHINGS, G. H. (1969). '*Plasmodium berghei* dihydrofolate reductase. Isolation, properties and inhibition by antifolates,' *Molec. Pharmacol.*, **5,** 49.

FERREIRA, F. S. DA CRUZ and DA COSTA, F. M. C. (1963). 'Resultados do tratamento da trypanosomíase humana Africana com o arsobal,' *Gaz. Méd. Portoguese*, **16,** 611.

FIEDLER, O. G. H., and KLUGE, E. B. (1954). 'The parasites of tsetse flies with special reference to the influence of the hosts on them,' *Onderstepoort, J. Vet. Res.*, **26,** 399.

FIEDLER, O. G. H., DU TOIT, R., and KLUGE, R. (1954). 'The influence of the tsetse fly eradication campaign on the breeding activity of Glossinae and their parasites in Zululand,' *Onderstepoort J. vet. Res.*, **26,** 389.

FIELD, M. J. (1968). 'Chronic psychosis in rural Ghana,' *Br. J. Psychiat.*, **114,** 31.

FIENNES, R. N. T-W- (1946). '*Trypanosoma congolense* (Broden) disease of cattle: the parenchymatous lesion and its relation to the cellular defences,' *J. comp. Path. Therap.*, **56,** 29.

FIENNES, R. N. T-W- (1950). 'The cattle trypanosomiases: some considerations of pathology and immunity,' *Ann. trop. Med. Parasit.*, **44,** 42.

FIENNES, R. N. T-W- (1950a). 'The cattle trypanosomiases: cryptic trypanosomiasis,' *Ann. trop. Med. Parasit.*, **44,** 222.

FIENNES, R. N. T-W- (1952). 'Pigment in trypanosomiasis of cattle,' *Trans. Roy. Soc. trop. Med. Hyg.*, **46,** 462.

FIENNES, R. N. T-W- (1952a). 'Trypanosome infections of cattle—diagnosis of blood infections of cattle when parasites are rare,' *Vet. Rec.*, **46,** 733.

FIENNES, R. N. T-W- (1952b). 'The cattle trypanosomiases; a cryptic focus of parasites in association with a secondary stage of disease,' *Brit. vet. J.*, **108,** 298.

FIENNES, R. N. T-W- (1953). 'The therapeutic and prophylactic properties of Antrycide in trypanosomiasis of cattle,' *Brit. vet. J.*, **109,** 280 and 330.

FIENNES, R. N. T-W- (1953a). 'The results of autopsies on trypanosome-infected cattle,' *Brit. vet. J.*, **109,** 511.

FIENNES, R. N. T-W- (1954). 'Haematological studies in trypanosomiasis of cattle,' *Vet. Rec.*, **66,** 423.

FIENNES, R. N. T-W-, JONES, E. R., and LAWS, S. G. (1946). 'The course and pathology of *Trypanosoma congolense* (Broden) disease of cattle,' *J. comp. Path. Therap.*, **56,** 1–27.

FINELLE, P. (1963). 'Rapport sur les progrès récents de la chimiothérapie des trypanosomiases animales.' *See* ISCTR (1963), p. 55.

FINELLE, P. (1965). 'Rapport sur les progrès récents de la chimiothérapie des trypanosomiases animales.' *See* ISCTR (1965), p. 35.

FINELLE, P. (1967). 'Nouvelle note sur un essai de lutte contre *Glossina fuscipes* en République Centrafricaine.' *See* ISCTR (1967), p. 139.

FINELLE, P., ITARD, J., YVORE, P., and LACOTTE, R. (1963). 'Répartition des Glossines en République Centrafricaine état actuel des connaissances,' *Revue Élev. Méd. vét. Pays trop.*, **16,** 337.

FINELLE, P., and LACOTTE, R. (1965). 'Essais des médicaments trypano-préventifs chez les ânes.' *See* ISCTR (1965), p. 31.

FINELLE, P., LAURENT, J. and RAYNAUD, J. B. (1963). 'Note complémentaire sur un essai de lutte contre *Glossina fuscipes* en République Centrafricaine.' *Revue Élev. Méd. vét. Pays trop.*, **15,** 403.

FINELLE, P., and YVORE, P. (1963). 'Possibilités d'utilisation du Metamidium par injection intraveineuse.' *See* ISCTR (1963), p. 69.

FINK, L. D., and WRIGHT, H. N. (1948). 'An investigation of the nature and extent of the binding of oxophenarsine (Mapharsen) by the red blood cell of the rabbit *in vitro*. I. Adsorption on the cell surface,' *J. Pharmacol.*, **94,** 455.

FINLAYSON, L. H. (1967). 'Behaviour and regulation of puparium formation in the larva of the tsetse fly *Glossina morsitans orientalis* Vanderplank in relation to humidity, light and mechanical stimuli,' *Bull. ent. Res.*, **57,** 301.

FISCHL, V., and SCHLOSSBERGER, H. (1932). *Handbuch der Chemotherapie, I. Metallfreie organische Verbindungen.* Leipzig, Fischers Medizinische Buchhandlung.

FISCHL, V., and SCHLOSSBERGER, H. (1934). *Handbuch der Chemotherapie, II. Metallderivate.* Leipzig, Fischers Medizinische Buchhandlung.

FISHER, J., BRUCE, J. I., BOURGEOIS, J. G., BUEDING, E., SADUN, E. H., WITHERSPOON, C., and PETERS, P. (1966). 'Effect of a subcurative dose of TWSb on the levels of phosphate esters in *Schistosoma mansoni*,' *Amer. J. trop. Med. Hyg.*, **15,** 507.

FISKE, W. F. (1920). 'Investigations into the bionomics of *Glossina palpalis*,' *Bull. ent. Res.*, **10,** 347.

FLORINI, J. R., BIRD, H. H., and BELL, P. H. (1966). 'Inhibition of protein synthesis *in vitro* and *in vivo* by Nucleocidin, an antitrypanosomal antibiotic,' *J. biol. Chem.*, **241,** 1091.

FLYNN, I. W., and BOWMAN, I. B. R. (1968). 'A comparative study of trypanosome and mammalian pyruvate kinase and the action of arsenical drugs,' *Trans. R. Soc. trop. Med. Hyg.*, **62,** 132.

FLYNN, I. W., and BOWMAN, I. B. R. (1969). 'Further studies on the mode of action of arsenicals on trypanosome pyruvate kinase,' *Trans. R. Soc. trop. Med. Hyg.*, **63,** 121.

FOLKERS, C. (1966). 'The effect of repeated use of isometamidium at low dosage on the development of drug-resistant strains of cattle trypanosomes,' *Bull. epizoot. Dis. Afr.*, **14,** 301.

FOLKERS, C., and JONES-DAVIES, W. J. (1966). 'The incidence of trypanosomes in blood smears of cattle presented for treatment in Northern Nigeria,' *Bull. epizoot. Dis. Afr.*, **14,** 409.

FOLKERS, C., and MOHAMMED, A. N. (1965). 'The importance of biting flies other than *Glossina* in the epidemiology of trypanosomiasis in cattle in Shika, Northern Nigeria,' *Bull. epizoot. Dis. Afr.*, **13,** 331.

FORD, J. (1940). 'The action of predators on tsetse pupae,' *Tsetse Research Report 1935–38*. Dar es Salaam, Govt. Printer, p. 53.

FORD, J. (1953). 'Aerial photography in tsetse survey.' *See* EATRO (1953), p. 28.

FORD, J. (1954). 'Discriminative treatment of bush against *G. morsitans*.' *See* ISCTR (1954), p. 90.

FORD, J. (1958). 'Tsetse fly reclamation and development in Eastern Africa,' *Proc. 6th International Congress on Tropical Medicine & Malaria*, **3,** 223.

FORD, J. (1960). 'A note on the location of *Glossina morsitans* Westw. on transect fly-rounds.' *See* ISCTR (1960), p. 237.

FORD, J. (1960a). 'The influence of tsetse flies on the distribution of African cattle,' *Proc. 1st. Fed. scient. Congr.*, Salisbury, p. 357.

FORD, J. (1961). 'The advance of *Glossina morsitans* and *Glossina pallidipes* into the Sabi and Lundi river basins, Southern Rhodesia.' *See* ISCTR (1961), p. 219.

FORD, J. (1963). 'Microclimates of tsetse fly resting sites in the Zambesi Valley, Southern Rhodesia.' *See* ISCTR (1963), p. 165.

FORD, J. (1963a). 'Game conservation and farming in relation to cattle farming and bovine trypanosomiasis.' *See* ISCTR (1963), p. 119.

FORD, J. (1963b). 'The distribution of the vectors of African pathogenic trypanosomes,' *Bull. World Hlth. Org.*, **28,** 653.

FORD, J. (1964). 'The geographical distribution of trypanosome infections in African cattle populations,' *Bull. epizoot. Dis. Afr.*, **12,** 307.

FORD, J. (1965). 'Distributions of *Glossina* and epidemiological patterns in the African trypanosomiases,' *J. trop. Med. Hyg.*, **68,** 211.

FORD, J. (1966). 'The role of elephants in controlling the distribution of tsetse-flies,' *Bull. Int. Un. Conserv. Nat., N.S.*, **19,** 6.

FORD, J. (1968). 'The control of populations through limitation of habitat distribution as exemplified by tsetse flies,' *Insect Abundance; R. ent. Soc. Symposium:* No. 4, 109 (ed. T. R. E. Southwood), Oxford.

FORD, J. (1969). 'Feeding and other responses of tsetse flies to man and ox and their epidemiological significance,' *Acta trop.*, **26,** 249.

FORD, J. (1970). 'The role of the trypanosomiases in African ecology.' Oxford, Clarendon Press.

FORD, J., GLASGOW, J. P., JOHNS, D. L., and WELCH, J. R. (1959). 'Transect fly rounds in field studies of *Glossina*,' *Bull. ent. Res.*, **50,** 275.

FORD, J., and LEGGATE, B. M. (1961). 'The geographical and climatic distribution of trypanosome infection rates in *G. morsitans* group of tsetse-flies,' *Trans. R. Soc. trop. Med. Hyg.*, **55,** 383.

FORÉAMI (1959). (Fonds Reine Élizabeth pour l'assistance Médicale aux Indigènes du Congo Belge) (1959). *Rapport sur l'activité durant l'année 1958*. Brussels.

FOSTER, R. (1957). 'Observations on laboratory colonies of the tsetse flies *Glossina morsitans* Westw. and *Glossina austeni* Newstead,' *Parasitology*, **47,** 361.

FOSTER, R. (1963). 'Infestation of *Glossina palpalis* R.-D. 1830 (Diptera) by larval Mermithidae Braun 1883 (Nematoda) in West Africa, with some comments on the parasitization of man by the worms,' *Ann. trop. Med. Parasit.*, **57,** 347.

FOSTER, R. (1963a). 'Contributions to the epidemiology of human sleeping sickness in Liberia,' *Trans. R. Soc. trop. Med. Hyg.*, **57,** 465.

FOSTER, R. (1964). 'Contributions to the epidemiology of human sleeping sickness in Liberia, bionomics of the vector *Glossina palpalis* (R.-D.) in a forest habitat,' *Bull. ent. Res.*, **54,** 4, p. 727.

FOSTER, R., WHITE, P. J., and YEO, D. (1961). 'Preliminary attempts to reduce the cost of controlling tsetse species *Glossina morsitans* Westw., *Glossina swynnertoni* Aust., and *G. pallidipes* Aust. in savanna woodland,' *Bull. ent. Res.*, **52,** 293.

FOX, J. J., WATANABE, K. A., and BLOCH, A. (1966). 'Nucleoside antibiotics,' in *Progress in Nucleic Acid Research and Molecular Biology* (ed. J. N. Davidson and W. E. Cohen). New York, Acad. Press, **5,** 251.

FRANCO, L. T. DE A. (1960). 'A velocidade de sedimentação dos eritrócitos na tripanossomíase humana (*T. gambiense*),' *Anais Inst. Med. trop. Lisboa*, **17,** 967.

FRASER, A. D., and DUKE, H. L. (1912). 'The development of trypanosomes in *Glossina palpalis*,' *Repts. Sleep. Sick. Comm. Roy. Soc.*, **12,** 36.

FRENCH, M. H. (1935). 'Nitrogen and mineral metabolism in *Trypanosoma congolense* disease,' *Rep. Dept. Vet. Sci., Tanganyika* (1934), p. 59.

FREY, J. R., DE WECK, A. L., and GELEICK, H. (1966). 'Sensitization, immunological tolerance and desensitization of guinea pigs to Neoarsphenamine,' *Int. Arch. Allergy*, **30,** 288.

FRIEDHEIM, E. A. H. (1941). 'L'acide triazine-arsénique dans le traitement de la maladie du sommeil africaine. Étude expérimentale et clinique,' *Schweiz. med. Wschr.*, **71,** 116.

FRIEDHEIM, E. A. H. (1949). 'Mel B in the treatment of human trypanosomiasis,' *Am. J. trop. Med.*, **29,** 173.

FRIEDHEIM, E. A. H. (1951). 'Mel B in the treatment of tryparsamide-resistant *T. gambiense* sleeping sickness: observations on drug resistance in the trypanosomes of the French Cameroun,' *Am. J. trop. Med.*, **31,** 218.

FRIEDHEIM, E. A. H. (1953). 'MSb and MSbB in the treatment of sleeping sickness due to infection with *Trypanosoma gambiense*,' *Ann. trop. Med. Parasit.*, **47,** 350.

FRIEDHEIM, E. A. H. (1959). 'Some approaches to the development of chemotherapeutic compounds,' *Ann. trop. Med. Parasit.*, **53,** 1.

FRIEDHEIM, E. A. H., DA SILVA, J. R., and MARTINS, A. V. (1954). 'Treatment of schistosomiasis *mansoni* with antimony α, α'-dimercapto-potassium succinate (TWSb),' *Amer. J. trop. Med. Hyg.*, **3,** 714.

FROST, D. V. (1967). 'Arsenicals in biology—retrospect and prospect,' *Fed. Proc.*, **26,** (1), 194.

FULLER, W., and WARING, M. J. (1964). 'A molecular model for the interaction of Ethidium bromide with DNA,' *Ber. Bunsenges. physik. Chem.*, **68,** 805.

FULTON, J. D., and SPOONER, D. F. (1959). 'Terminal respiration in certain mammalian trypanosomes,' *Exp. Parasit.*, **5,** 59.

FURON, R. (1962). *The Geology of Africa.* Edinburgh.

FUSSGÄNGER, R. (1951). 'Spirotrypan (Ein neues Arsenobenzolpräparat), *Der Hautarzt*, **9,** 413.

FUSSGÄNGER, R., and BAUER, F. (1960). 'Investigations on Berenil resistance of trypanosomes,' *Vet. Rec.*, **72,** 1118.

GADDUM, J. H. (1958). *Pharmacology*, 5th edition. London, Oxford University Press, p. 504.

GALE, E. F., and FOLKES, J. P. (1967). 'Actions of pentamidine on the metabolism of *Staphylococcus aureus*,' *Biochim. biophys. Acta*, **144,** 467.

GALL, D. (1954). 'The chemoprophylaxis of sleeping sickness with the diamidines,' *Ann. trop. Med. Parasit.*, **48,** 242.

GALL, D. (1956). 'Blood protein changes in sleeping sickness,' *J. West. Afric. Sci. Ass.*, **2,** No. 2, 152.

GALL, D., HUTCHINSON, M. P., and YATES, W. (1955). 'The estimation of cerebrospinal-fluid protein in sleeping sickness: Sicard and Cantaloube's method and a sulphosalicylic acid method,' *Ann. trop. Med. Parasit.*, **49,** 419.

GALL, D., HUTCHINSON, M. P., and YATES, W. (1957). 'The erythrocyte sedimentation rate in sleeping sickness,' *Ann. trop. Med. Parasit.*, **51,** 136.

GALLAIS, P., COLLOMB, H., MILETTO, G., DUTERTRE, J., and BÉRARD-BADIER (1956). 'L'apport de la pneumo-encéphalographie dans l'interprétation et le classement de l'encéphalite de la trypanosomiase humaine africaine. Intérêt doctrinal et thérapeutique,' *Méd. trop.*, **16,** 5.

GASCHEN, H. (1945). 'Les glossines de l'Afrique Occidentale Française,' *Acta trop.* supp. 2, Basle, 131 pp.

GEIGY, R. (1948). 'Élevage de *Glossina palpalis*,' *Acta trop.*, **5,** 201.

GEISLER, –. (1912). 'Trypanosomen beim ostafrikanischen Warzenschwein,' *Arch. Schiffs. Tropenhyg.*, **16,** 197.

GELFAND, M. (1947). 'Transitory neurological signs in sleeping sickness,' *Trans. R. Soc. trop. Med. Hyg.*, **41,** 255.

GELFAND, M. (1961). *Northern Rhodesia in the Days of the Charter.* Oxford. 291 pp.

GELFAND, M. (1966). 'The early clinical features of Rhodesian trypanosomiasis with special reference to the "chancre" (local reaction),' *Trans. R. Soc. trop. Med. Hyg.*, **60,** 376.

GELFAND, M., and FRIEDLANDER, J. (1963). 'Jaundice in Rhodesian sleeping sickness. Report on two European cases,' *Trans. R. Soc. trop. Med. Hyg.*, **57,** 290.

GILL, B. S. (1961). 'Studies on surra. I. Therapeutic activity of Antrycide, suramin, Berenil, pentamidine, propamidine, stilbamidine, Antimosan and tartar emetic against *Trypanosoma evansi* in albino rats,' *Ind. J. vet. Sci.*, **31,** 93.

GILL, B. S. (1962). 'Therapeutic activity of MSb, MSbB, Mel W, TWSb and Te 85 against *Trypanosoma evansi* in rats,' *Ind. J. Microbiol.*, **2,** 13.

GILL, B. S. (1962a). 'Prophylactic action of TWSb, MSb, Prothidium, Metamidium and its suraminate and quinapyramine against *Trypanosoma evansi* in mice and rats,' *Ind. J. Microbiol.*, **2,** 25.

GILL, B. S. (1963). 'Therapeutic activity of suramin complexes against *Trypanosoma evansi* in rats,' *Ind. J. Microbiol.*, **3,** 95.

GILL, B. S. (1964). 'A procedure for the indirect haemagglutination test for the study of experimental *Trypanosoma evansi* infections,' *Ann. trop. Med. Parasit.*, **58,** 473.

GILL, B. S. (1964a). 'Laboratory studies on the chemotherapy and chemoprophylaxis of *Trypanosoma evansi* infection,' *Trans. Roy. Soc. trop. Med. Hyg.*, **58,** 9.

GILL, B. S. (1965). 'Properties of soluble antigens of *Trypanosoma evansi*,' *J. gen. Microbiol.*, **38,** 361.

GILL, B. S. (1966). 'Indirect haemagglutination test using formolised cells for detecting *Trypanosoma evansi* antibody in experimental sera,' *Ann. trop. Med. Parasit.*, **60,** 276.

GILL, B. S., and MALHOTRA, M. N. (1963). 'Prophylactic activity of suramin complexes in "surra" (*Trypanosoma evansi*),' *Nature*, Lond., **200,** 285.

GILL, B. S., and MALHOTRA, M. N. (1963a). 'Prophylactic activity of Antrycide and MSb against repeated infections of *Trypanosoma evansi* in mice,' *Ind. J. Microbiol.*, **3,** 9.

GILL, B. S., MALHOTRA, M. N., SEN, D. K., and SAMADDAR, J. (1963). 'Chemotherapeutic effect of nitrofurazone in experimental *Trypanosoma evansi* infection of mice and rats,' *Indian J. Microbiol.*, **3,** 5.

GILLAIN, J. (1937). 'Quel est le trypanosome virulent des suidés au Congo Belge? Que penser de *T. montgomeryi* en tant qu'espèce,' *Ann. Soc. belge Méd. trop.*, **17,** 219.

GILLMAN, J., GILBERT, C., GILLMAN, T., and SPENCE, I. (1948). 'A preliminary report on hydrocephalus, spina bifida and other congenital anomalies in the rat produced by Trypan Blue,' *S. Afr. J. Med. Sci.*, **13,** 47.

GILMOUR, J. S. L., and HESLOP-HARRISON, J. (1954). 'The deme terminology and the units of micro-evolutionary change,' *Genetica*, **27,** 147.

GLASGOW, J. P. (1946). 'The seasonal abundance of blood-sucking flies in a grassed woodland area in central Tanganyika,' *J. anim. Ecol.*, **15,** 93.

GLASGOW, J. P. (1953). 'The extermination of animal populations by artificial predation and the estimation of populations,' *J. anim. Ecol.*, **22,** 32.

GLASGOW, J. P. (1954). '*Glossina palpalis fuscipes* Newstead in lake-side and in riverine forest,' *Bull. ent. Res.*, **45,** 563.

GLASGOW, J. P. (1956). '*Tsetse Research.*' *See* EATRO (1956), p. 9.

GLASGOW, J. P. (1960). 'Variations in the venation of *Glossina* Wiedemann (Diptera: Muscidae),' *Proc. R. ent. Soc. Lond.*, (A) **35,** 49.

GLASGOW, J. P. (1960a). 'Shinyanga: a review of the work of the Tsetse Research Laboratory,' *E. A. Agr. For. J.*, **26,** 22.

GLASGOW, J. P. (1961). 'The variability of fly-round catches in field studies of *Glossina*,' *Bull. ent. Res.*, **51,** 781.

GLASGOW, J. P. (1961a). 'The feeding habits of *Glossina swynnertoni* Austen,' *J. anim. Ecol.*, **30,** 77.

GLASGOW, J. P. (1961b). 'Seasonal changes in the breeding places of *Glossina morsitans morsitans* Westwood,' *Acta tropica*, **18,** 252.

GLASGOW, J. P. (1961c). 'Selection for size in tsetse flies,' *J. anim. Ecol.*, **30,** 87.

GLASGOW, J. P. (1961d). 'Seasonal variation in size and colour and daily changes in the distribution of *Glossina pallidipes* Aust., in the South Busoga forest, Uganda,' *Bull. ent. Res.*, **52,** 647.

GLASGOW, J. P. (1961e). 'Ecological effects of tsetse fly control in particular as a consequence of bush clearing,' *Int. Union for Conservation of Nature and National Resources.* Symposium Warszwa, July 1960. Leiden 1961. p. 85.

GLASGOW, J. P. (1963). *The Distribution and Abundance of Tsetse.* Oxford, Pergamon Press. 252 pp.

GLASGOW, J. P. (1967). 'Recent fundamental work on tsetse flies,' *Ann. Rev. Ent.*, **12,** 421.

GLASGOW, J. P., and BURSELL, E. (1961). 'Seasonal variations in the fat content and size of *Glossina swynnertoni* Austen,' *Bull. ent. Res.*, **51,** 705.

GLASGOW, J. P., and DUFFY, B. J. (1947). 'The extermination of *Glossina palpalis fuscipes* Newstead by hand-catching,' *Bull. ent. Res.*, **38,** 465.

GLASGOW, J. P., and DUFFY, B. J. (1949). 'Observations on lateral scour in the Kuja River, Kenya,' *E. Afr. Agric. J.*, **15,** 29.

GLASGOW, J. P., and DUFFY, B. J. (1951). 'Further observations on the extermination of *Glossina palpalis fuscipes* Newstead by hand-catching,' *Bull. ent. Res.*, **42,** 55.

GLASGOW, J. P., and DUFFY, B. J. (1961). 'Traps in field studies of *Glossina pallidipes* Austen,' *Bull. ent. Res.*, **52,** 795.

GLASGOW, J. P., and GLASGOW, S. (1962). 'Histology of the growth of flight muscles in *Glossina* (Diptera: Muscidae),' *Proc. R. ent. Soc. Lond.*, (A) **37,** 35.

GLASGOW, J. P., ISHERWOOD, F., LEE-JONES, F., and WEITZ, B. (1958). 'Factors influencing the staple food of tsetse flies,' *J. anim. Ecol.*, **27,** 59.

GLASGOW, J. P., and WELCH, J. R. (1962). 'Long-term fluctuations in numbers of the tsetse fly *Glossina swynnertoni* Austen,' *Bull. ent. Res.*, **53,** 129.

GLASGOW, J. P., and WILSON, F. (1953). 'A census of the tsetse fly *Glossina pallidipes* Austen and of its host animals,' *J. anim. Ecol.*, **22,** 47.

GLEDHILL, J. A., and CAUGHEY, W. (1963). 'Report on a field trial in the use of Dieldrin for the control of *G. morsitans* in the Zambesi Valley—1961.' *See* ISCTR (1963), p. 239.

GLOVER, P. E. (1961). *The Tsetse Problem in Northern Nigeria.* Nairobi, Patwa News Agency.

GLOVER, P. E. (1963). 'A further note on the extermination of *G. palpalis* in Nyanza Province of Kenya.' *See* ISCTR (1963), p. 253.

GLOVER, P. E. (1965). 'A review of recent knowledge on the relationship between the tsetse fly and its vertebrate hosts.' (Presented at the First International Congress of Parasitology, Rome, September 1964.) *I.U.C.N. Pubn.* New Series No. 6. (Published by the Fauna Preservation Society for Conservation of Nature and National Resources, London, 1965.)

GLOVER, P. E. (1967). 'The importance of ecological studies in the control of tsetse flies,' *Bull. Wld. Hlth. Org.*, **37,** 581.

GLOVER, P. E., and AITCHISON, P. (1966). *Tsetse control and land use in Northern Nigeria: a feasibility survey of Area I.* Mimeographed by Veterinary Tsetse and Trypanosomiasis Unit, Ministry of Animal and Forest Resources, Kaduna, Northern Nigeria.

GLOVER, P. E., JACKSON, C. H. N., ROBERTSON, A. G., and THOMSON, W. E. F. (1955). 'The extermination of the tsetse fly *Glossina morsitans*, Westw. at Abercorn, Northern Rhodesia,' *Bull. ent. Res.*, **46,** 57.

GLOVER, P. E., LE ROUX, J. G., and PARKER, D. F. (1960). 'The extermination of *Glossina palpalis* on the Kuja-Migori river systems with the use of insecticides.' *See* ISCTR (1960), p. 331.

REFERENCES

GLOVER, P. E., TRUMP, E. C., and WILLIAMS, R. (1959). 'A note on mechanical bush clearing,' *E. Afr. agric. J.*, **25**, 18.

GODFREY, D. G. (1960). 'Types of *Trypanosoma congolense*. I. Morphological differences,' *Ann. trop. Med. Parasit.*, **54**, 428.

GODFREY, D. G. (1961). 'Types of *Trypanosoma congolense*. II. Differences in the course of infection,' *Ann. trop. Med. Parasit.*, **55**, 154.

GODFREY, D. G., and KILLICK-KENDRICK, R. (1961). 'Bovine trypanosomiasis in Nigeria. I. The inoculation of blood into rats as a method of survey in the Donga Valley, Benue Province,' *Ann. trop. Med. Parasit.*, **55**, 287.

GODFREY, D. G., and KILLICK-KENDRICK, R. (1962). '*Trypanosoma evansi* in camels in Nigeria,' *Ann. trop. Med. Parasit.*, **56**, 1, 14.

GOLDSCHMIDT, R. (1938). *Physiological Genetics*. London, McGraw-Hill.

GOODIER, R. (1960). 'Some effects of bush clearing in Southern Rhodesia.' *See* ISCTR (1960), p. 241.

GOODIER, R. (1961). 'Discriminative bush-clearing against tsetse in the south-east of Southern Rhodesia.' *Bull. No. 2102 of the Federal Ministry of Agriculture*, 1961. (Reprinted from *Rhodesia Agric. J.*, **58**, 4, p. 262.)

GOODWIN, L. G. (1964). 'The chemotherapy of trypanosomiasis,' *Biochem. Physiol. Protozoa*, **3**, 495.

GOODWIN, L. G., and BOREHAM, P. F. L. (1966). 'Pharmacologically active peptides in trypanosome infections,' in *Hypotensive peptides* (ed. E. G. Erdös, N. Back, and F. Sicuteri). Springer-Verlag, New York Inc. pp. 545–50.

GOODWIN, L. G., and PAGE, J. E. (1943). 'A study of the excretion of organic antimonials using a polarographic procedure,' *Biochem. J.*, **37**, 198.

GOODWIN, L. G., and RICHARDS, W. H. G. (1960). 'Pharmacologically active peptides in the blood and urine of animals infected with *Babesia rodhaini* and other pathogenic organisms,' *Br. J. Pharmac. Chemother.*, **15**, 152.

GOODWIN, L. G., and THIEL, C. C. (1967). 'A portable slow-coding device,' *Trans. R. Soc. trop. Med. Hyg.*, **61**, 134.

GORDON, J., ROSE, B., and SEHON, A. H. (1958). 'Detection of "non-precipitating" antibodies in sera of individuals allergic to ragweed pollen by an *in vitro* method,' *J. exp. Med.*, **108**, 37.

GORDON, R. M. (1957). *Trypanosoma congolense* in its passage through the peritrophic membrane of *G. morsitans*,' *Trans. R. Soc. trop. Med. Hyg.*, **51**, 296.

GORDON, R. M., and CREWE, W. (1948). 'The mechanisms by which mosquitoes and tsetse-flies obtain their blood-meal, the histology of the lesions produced, and the subsequent reactions of the mammalian host; together with some observations on the feeding of *Chrysops* and *Cimex*,' *Ann. trop. Med. Parasit.*, **42**, 334.

GORDON, R. M., CREWE, W., and WILLETT, K. C. (1956). 'Studies on the deposition, migration and development to the blood forms of trypanosomes belonging to the *Trypanosoma brucei* group. I. An account of the process of feeding adopted by the tsetse fly when obtaining a blood meal from the mammalian host, with special reference to the ejection of saliva and the relationship of the feeding process to the deposition of the metacyclic trypanosomes,' *Ann. trop. Med. Parasit.*, **50**, 426.

GORDON, R. M., and WILLETT, K. C. (1956). 'A preliminary account of the deposition by the tsetse fly of the infective forms of *Trypanosoma rhodesiense*, their subsequent migration to the general circulation and their development to the blood forms,' *Ann. trop. Med. Parasit.*, **50**, 314.

GORDON, R. M., and WILLETT, K. C. (1958). 'Studies on the deposition, migration and development to the blood forms of trypanosomes belonging to the *T. brucei* group. III. The development of *T. rhodesiense* from the metacyclic forms, as observed in mammalian tissue and in culture,' *Ann. trop. Med. Parasit.*, **52**, 346.

GRABAR, P. (1964). 'Immuno-electrophoresis,' in *Immunological Technique*. (ed. J. F. Ackroyd). Oxford, Blackwell Scientific Publications. pp. 79–91.

GRABAR, P., and WILLIAMS, C. A. Jr. (1955). 'Méthode immuno-électrophorétique d'analyse de mélanges de substances antigéniques,' *Biochim. biophys. Acta*, **17**, 67.

GRABER, M. (1966). 'Chad Institute d'Élevage et de Médecine Vétérinaire des Pays Tropicaux,' *Rapport annuel 1965*. Fort Lamy, Chad, Laboratoire de Farcha.

GRAF, H. (1929). 'Report on 4 cases of trypanosomiasis occurring in Europeans of the British Cameroons,' *Trans. Roy. Soc. trop. Med. Hyg.*, **23**, 95.

GRAF, H. (1929a). 'Beitrag zur Pathologie des *Glossina palpalis*-Stichs und der Inkubationszeit bei Schlafkrankheit,' *Arch. Schiffs. Tropenhyg.*, **33**, 219.

GRAF, H. (1937). 'Über den Primäraffekt und die Inkubationszeit der Schlafkrankheit,' *Arch. Schiffs. Tropenhyg.*, **41**, 213.

GRANT, P. T. (1966). 'The selective inhibition of energy-yielding reactions,' *Symp. Soc. gen. Microbiol.*, **16**, 281.

GRANT, P. T., and SARGENT, J. R. (1960).' Properties of L-α-glycerophosphate and its role in the respiration of *Trypanosoma rhodesiense*,' *Biochem. J.*, **76**, 229.

GRANT, P. T., SARGENT, J. R., and RYLEY, J. F. (1961). 'Respiratory systems in the Trypanosomatidae,' *Biochem. J.*, **81**, 200.

GRASSÉ, P. P. (1952). 'Ordre des Trypanosomides,' *Traité de Zoologie* (Paris), **1** (1), 602.

GRASSÉ, P. P. (1961). 'La reproduction par induction du blépharoplaste et du flagelle de *Trypanosoma equiperdum* (Flagellé Protomonadine),' *C. R. Acad. Sci.*, **252**, 3917.

GRASSÉ, P. P., and PYNE, C. K. (1965). 'Sur l'origine et l'homologie du cinétoplaste,' in *Progress in Protozoology*, Int. Congr. Series 91, Excerpta Medica Foundation, Amsterdam, 131–2.

GRAY, A. R. (1961). 'Soluble antigens of *Trypanosoma vivax* and of other trypanosomes,' *Immunology*, **4**, 253.

GRAY, A. R. (1961a). 'Suramin complexes. VIII. A further trial of the prophylactic activity of Antrycide-suramin complex and Antrycide chloride against *Trypanosoma simiae* in pigs,' *Ann. trop. Med. Parasit.*, **55**, 432.

GRAY, A. R. (1962). 'The influence of antibody on the serological variation in *Trypanosoma brucei*,' *Ann. trop. Med. Parasit.*, **56**, 4.

GRAY, A. R. (1965). 'Antigenic variation in clones of *Trypanosoma brucei*. I. Immunological relationships of the clones,' *Ann. trop. Med. Parasit.*, **59**, 27.

GRAY, A. R. (1965a). 'Antigenic variation in a strain of *Trypanosoma brucei* transmitted by *Glossina morsitans* and *G. palpalis*,' *J. gen. Microbiol.*, **41**, 195.

References

GRAY, A. R. (1966). 'Antigenic variation in clones of *Trypanosoma brucei*. II. The drug sensitivities of variants of a clone and the antigenic relationships of trypanosomes before and after drug treatment,' *Ann. trop. Med. Parasit.*, **60,** 265.

GRAY, A. R., and ROBERTS, C. J. (1968). 'Experiments on the cyclical transmission of drug-resistant strains of trypanosomes,' *Trans. Roy. Soc. trop. Med. Hyg.*, **62,** 126.

GRAY, A. R., and STEPHEN, L. E. (1962). 'A comparative trial of the local toxicity and prophylactic activity against trypanosomiasis in West African zebu cattle of Metamidium chloride, suramin salt and embonate with Antrycide pro-salt,' *Vet. Rec.*, **74,** 696.

GREATHEAD, D. J. (1967). 'The Bombyliidae (Diptera) of northern Ethiopia,' *J. nat. Hist.*, **1,** 195.

GREWAL, M. S. (1960). 'On a new trypanosome, *Trypanosoma helogalei* Grewal 1956, from the blood of an African mongoose, *Helogale undulata rufula* Peters (Peters' pigmy mongoose),' *Ind. J. med. Res.*, **48,** 418.

GREWAL, M. S. (1961). 'A new trypanosome, *Trypanosoma ichneumoni* Grewal, 1961, from the blood of an Egyptian mongoose (ichneumon), *Herpestes ichneumon* Linnaeus,' *Res. Bull. (N.S.) Panjab Univ.*, **12,** 39.

GRIMSTONE, A. V. (1961). 'Fine structure and morphogenesis in protozoa,' *Biol. Rev.*, **36,** 97.

GROSSOWICZ, N., and RASOOLY, G. (1958). 'Evaluation of some trypanostatic agents by means of *Herpetomonas culicidarum*,' *J. Protozool.*, **5,** 249.

GROVES, M. J., and WILMSHURST, E. C. (1964). 'Preparation and biological activity of some complexes of trypanocidal phenanthridinium compounds,' *J. Pharm. Pharmacol. Suppl.*, **16,** 140.

GRUVEL, J. (1966). 'Les glossines vectrices des trypanosomiases au Tchad,' *Revue Élev. Méd. vét. Pays trop.*, **19,** 169.

GUTTERIDGE, W. E. (1966). 'Further investigations on the mode of action of pentamidine,' *Trans. R. Soc. trop. Med. Hyg.*, **60,** 120.

GUTTERIDGE, W. E. (1967). 'Further investigations of the mode of action of pentamidine,' *Trans. R. Soc. trop. Med. Hyg.*, **61,** 136.

GUTTERIDGE, W. E. (1969). 'Some effects of pentamidine di-isethionate on *Crithidia fasciculata*,' *J. Protozool.*, **16,** 306.

GUTTERIDGE, W. E., JAFFE, J. J., and MCCORMACK, J. J. (1968). 'Presence and properties of dihydrofolate reductases within the genus *Trypanosoma*,' *Brit. J. Pharmacol.*, **34,** 191 P.

GUTTMAN, H. N., and WALLACE, F. G. (1964). 'Nutrition and physiology of the Trypanosomatidae,' in *Biochemistry and Physiology of Protozoa* (ed. S. H. Hutner). New York, Academic Press. **3,** 460.

HAESELBARTH, E., SEGERMAN, J., and ZUMPT, F. (1966). 'The arthropod parasites of vertebrates in Africa south of the Sahara (Ethiopian Region) Vol. III (Insecta excl. Phthiraptera).' *Publ. S. Afr. Inst. Med. Res.* Johannesburg, **13,** No. 52.

HAGAN, H. R. (1951). *Embryology of the Viviparous Insects.* New York, Ronald Press Company.

HAIG, D. A., and LUND, A. S. (1948). 'Transmission of the South African strain of dourine to laboratory animals,' *Onderstepoort J.*, **23,** 59.

HANSSON, H. A. (1966). 'Selective effects of metabolic inhibitors on retinal cultures,' *Exp. Eye Res.*, **5,** 335.

HARDING, R. D. (1940). 'The influence of sleeping sickness on mortality in two districts of Northern Nigeria,' *Trans. R. Soc. trop. Med. Hyg.*, **33,** 483.

HARDING, R. D. (1945). 'Late results of treatment of sleeping sickness in Sierra Leone by Antrypol, tryparsamide, pentamidine and propamidine, singly and in various combinations,' *Trans. R. Soc. trop. Med. Hyg.*, **39,** 99.

HARDING, R. D., and HUTCHINSON, M. P. (1948). 'Sleeping sickness of an unusual type in Sierra Leone and its attempted control,' *Trans. R. Soc. trop. Med. Hyg.*, **41,** 481.

HARDY, G. H. (1944). 'The copulation and the terminal segments of Diptera,' *Proc. Roy. ent. Soc. Lond.*, (A) **19,** p. 37.

HARLEY, J. M. B. (1954). 'The breeding sites of the tsetse fly, *Glossina morsitans*,' *Acta tropica*, **11,** 379.

HARLEY, J. M. B. (1958). 'The availability of *Glossina morsitans* Westw. in Ankole, Uganda,' *Bull. ent. Res.*, **49,** 225.

HARLEY, J. M. B. (1959). 'The biting behaviour of *G. swynnertoni*.' *See* EATRO (1959), p. 38.

HARLEY, J. M. B. (1960). 'A review of entomological research carried out by the East African Trypanosomiasis Research Organization,' *Report of the 7th Commonwealth Entomological Conference 1960*. London, Commonwealth Institute of Entomology, p. 246.

HARLEY, J. M. B. (1965). 'Activity cycles of *Glossina pallidipes* Aust., *G. palpalis fuscipes* Newst. and *G. brevipalpis* Newst.,' *Bull. ent. Res.*, **56,** 141.

HARLEY, J. M. B. (1966). 'Seasonal and diurnal variations in physiological age and trypanosome infection rate of females of *Glossina pallidipes* Aust., *G. palpalis fuscipes* Newst. and *G. brevipalpis* Newst,' *Bull. ent. Res.*, **56,** 4, p. 595.

HARLEY, J. M. B. (1966a). 'Studies on age and trypanosome infection rate in females of *Glossina pallidipes* Aust., *G. palpalis fuscipes* Newst., and *G. brevipalpis* Newst. in Uganda,' *Bull. ent. Res.*, **57,** 23.

HARLEY, J. M. B. (1967). 'The influence of sampling method on the trypanosome infection rate of catches of *Glossina pallidipes* and *G. fuscipes*,' *Entomologia exp. appl.*, **10,** 240.

HARLEY, J. M. B. (1967a). 'Further studies on the age and trypanosome infection rates in *Glossina pallidipes* Aust., *G. palpalis fuscipes* Newst. and *G. brevipalpis* Newst. in Uganda,' *Bull. ent. Res.*, **57,** 3, p. 459.

HARLEY, J. M. B. (1968). 'The influence of temperatures on reproduction and development in four species of *Glossina* (Diptera: Muscidae),' *Proc. Roy. ent. Soc. Lond.*, (A) **43,** 170.

HARLEY, J. M. B., CUNNINGHAM, M. P., and VAN HOEVE, K. (1966). 'The numbers of infective *Trypanosoma rhodesiense* extruded by *Glossina morsitans* during feeding,' *Ann. trop. Med. Parasit.*, **60,** 455.

HARLEY, J. M. B., and PILSON, R. D. (1961). 'An experiment in the use of discriminative clearing for the control of *Glossina morsitans* Westw. in Ankole, Uganda,' *Bull. ent. Res.*, **52,** 561.

HARRIS, R. H. T. P. (1930). Report on the bionomics of the tsetse fly (*Glossina pallidipes* Aust)., and a preliminary report on a new method of control, presented to the Provincial Administration of Natal. Fol. 75 pp. Pietermaritzburg.

HARRISON, H. (1940). 'The game experiment,' *Tsetse Research Report 1935–8*. Dar es Salaam, Govt. Printer. p. 27.

REFERENCES

RT, P. D'A. (1968). '*Mycobacterium tuberculosis* in macrophages: effect of certain surfactants and other membrane-active compounds,' *Science*, N.Y., **162,** 686.

HARTMANN, M., and NÖLLER, W. (1918). 'Untersuchungen über die Cytologie von *Trypanosoma theileri*,' *Arch. Protistenk.*, **38,** 355.

HAWKING, F. (1937). 'Studies on chemotherapeutic action. I. The absorption of arsenical compounds and tartar emetic by normal and resistant trypanosomes and its relation to drug-resistance,' *J. Pharmacol.*, **59,** 123.

HAWKING, F. (1940). 'Three cases of trypanosomiasis relapsing during treatment with Bayer 205 (Germanin),' *Trans. R. Soc. trop. Med. Hyg.*, **34,** 217.

HAWKING, F. (1962). 'Trypanocidal action of *p*-biguanidoacetophenone amidinohydrazone,' *Brit. J. Pharmacol.*, **19,** 324.

HAWKING, F. (1962a). 'Estimation of the concentration of melarsoprol (Mel B) and Mel W in biological fluids by bioassay with trypanosomes *in vitro*,' *Trans. R. Soc. trop. Med. Hyg.*, **56,** 354.

HAWKING, F. (1963). 'Chemotherapy of trypanosomiasis,' in *Experimental Chemotherapy* Vol. 1 (ed. R. J. Schnitzer, and F. Hawking). New York, Academic Press. p. 129.

HAWKING, F. (1963a). 'Action of drugs upon *Trypanosoma congolense, T. vivax* and *T. rhodesiense* in tsetse flies and in culture,' *Ann. trop. Med. Parasit.*, **57,** 255.

HAWKING, F. (1963b). 'Drug resistance of *Trypanosoma congolense* and other trypanosomes to quinapyramine, phenanthridines, Berenil and other compounds in mice,' *Ann. trop. Med. Parasit.*, **57,** 262.

HAWKING, F. (1966). 'Chemotherapy of trypanosomiasis,' in *Experimental Chemotherapy* Vol. IV (ed. R. J. Schnitzer, and F. Hawking). New York, Academic Press. p. 398.

HAWKING, F. (1966a). 'Arsenical resistance and tartar emetic resistance,' *Trans. R. Soc. trop. Med. Hyg.*, **60,** 123.

HAWKING, F., and GREENFIELD, J. G. (1941). 'Two autopsies on *rhodesiense* sleeping sickness: visceral lesions and significance of changes in cerebrospinal fluid,' *Trans. Roy. Soc. trop. Med. Hyg.*, **35,** 155.

HAWKING, F., HENNELLY, T. J., and QUASTEL, J. H. (1937). 'Trypanocidal activity and arsenic content of the cerebrospinal fluid after administration of arsenic compounds,' *J. Pharmacol.*, **59,** 157.

HAWKING, F., and WALKER, P. J. (1966). 'Analysis of the development of arsenical resistance in trypanosomes *in vitro*,' *Exp. Parasit.*, **18,** 63.

HAZARD, E. I., LOFGREN, C. S., WOODARD, D. B., FORD, H. R., and GLANCEY, B. M. (1964). 'Selection of *Aedes aegypti* for resistance to the chemical sterilant apholate,' *Science*, N.Y., **145,** 500.

HEGH, E. (1929). *Les Tsé-tsés*, Tome 1er. Brussels, Ministère des Colonies. xiv + 742 pp.

HEISCH, R. B., KILLICK-KENDRICK, R., DORRELL, J., and MARSDEN, P. D. (1968). 'The behaviour of trypanosomes in testicles,' *Trans. R. Soc. trop. Med. Hyg.*, **62,** p. 5.

HEISCH, R. B., MCMAHON, J. P., and MANSON-BAHR, P. E. C. (1958). 'The isolation of *Trypanosoma rhodesiense* from a bushbuck,' *Brit. med. J.*, ii, 1203.

HENDERSON, J. F. (1963). 'Inhibition of purine metabolism in Ehrlich ascites carcinoma cells by phenanthridinium compounds related to Ethidium bromide,' *Cancer Res.*, **23,** 491.

HENDERSON, W. (1931). 'The relationship of pica in cattle to trypanosomiasis,' *Vet. J.*, **87,** 518.

HENDERSON-BEGG, A. (1946). 'Heterophile antibodies in trypanosomiasis,' *Trans. Roy. Soc. trop. Med. Hyg.*, **40,** 331.

HENNING, M. A. (1956). *Animal Diseases in South Africa*, 3rd edition. Central News Agency, South Africa.

HENRARD, C. (1952). 'Une tsé-tsé nouvelle du groupe "*fusca*", *Glossina van-hoofi*, sp. nov.,' *Rev. zool. Bot. Afr.*, **45,** 193.

HERBERT, I. V. (1964). '*Trypanosoma theileri* Laveran, 1902,' *Vet. Bull.*, **34,** 563.

HESSE, A. J. (1956). 'A revision of the Bombyliidae (Diptera) of Southern Africa, III,' *Ann. S. Afr. Mus.*, **35,** 465.

HILL, D. H. (1955). '*Trypanosoma brucei* in the cat.' *Brit. vet. J.*, **111,** 77.

HILL, D. H. (1956). *Inter-African Bureau Epizoot. Dis. Afr.*, Tec. Rep. 12/55.

HILL, J. (1962). 'Virulence of *Trypanosoma congolense* in mice treated with a prophylactic phenanthridinium drug (M. & B. 459–6B),' *Ann. trop. Med. Parasit.*, **56,** 426.

HILL, J., and MCFADZEAN, J. A. (1963). 'Studies on isometamidium. Depots of isometamidium in mice and rats and their importance for prophylaxis against *Trypanosoma congolense*,' *Trans. R. Soc. trop. Med. Hyg.*, **57,** 476.

HILL, K. R. (1948). 'The protein content of cerebrospinal fluid in trypanosomiasis,' *Trans. R. Soc. trop. Med. Hyg.*, **41,** 641.

HINTON, H. E. (1968). 'Spiracular gills,' *Adv. Insect. Physiol.*, **5,** 65.

HIRT, R., and BERCHTOLD, R. (1961). 'Biophysikalische Studien mit synthetischem Lecithin als Weg zu neuartigen Chemotherapeutika,' *Experientia*, **17,** 418.

HISSETTE, J. (1932). 'Considérations pratiques sur des accidents oculaires de la trypanosomiase ou de son traitement,' *Ann. Soc. belge Méd. trop.*, **12,** 531.

HOARE, C. A. (1931). 'Studies on *Trypanosoma grayi*. III. Life cycle in the tsetse fly and in the crocodile,' *Parasitology*, **23,** 449.

HOARE, C. A. (1936). Morphological and taxonomic studies on mammalian trypanosomes. II. *Trypanosoma simiae* and acute porcine trypanosomiasis in tropical Africa. *Trans. R. Soc. trop. Med. Hyg.*, **29,** 619.

HOARE, C. A. (1938). 'Morphological and taxonomic studies on mammalian trypanosomes. V. The diagnostic value of the kinetoplast,' *Trans. R. Soc. trop. Med. Hyg.*, **32,** 333.

HOARE, C. A. (1940). 'Studies on the behaviour of *Trypanosoma evansi* in tsetse flies, with special reference to its phylogeny,' *Parasitology*, **32,** 105.

HOARE, C. A. (1943). 'Biological races in parasitic protozoa,' *Biol. Rev.*, **18,** 137.

HOARE, C. A. (1947). 'Tsetse-borne trypanosomiases outside their natural boundaries,' *Ann. Soc. belge Méd. trop.* (Liber Jubilaris J. Rodhain), 267.

HOARE, C. A. (1948). 'The relationship of the haemoflagellates,' *Proc. IV. Intern. Congr. Trop. Med. Malaria*, Washington, **2,** 1110.

HOARE, C. A. (1949). *Handbook of Medical Protozoology*. London, Baillière, Tindall & Cox.

HOARE, C. A. (1955). 'Intraspecific biological groups in pathogenic protozoa,' *Refuah Veterinarith*, Tel-Aviv, **12,** 263.

HOARE, C. A. (1956). 'Morphological and taxonomic studies on mammalian trypanosomes. VIII. Revision of *Trypanosoma evansi*,' *Parasitology*, **46,** 130.

HOARE, C. A. (1957). 'The spread of African trypanosomes beyond their natural range,' *Ztschr. Tropenmed. Parasit.*, **8,** 157.

HOARE, C. A. (1957a). 'The classification of trypanosomes of veterinary and medical importance,' *Vet. Rev. Annot.*, **3,** 1.

HOARE, C. A. (1959). 'Morphological and taxonomic studies on mammalian trypanosomes. IX. Revision of *Trypanosoma dimorphon*,' *Parasitology*, **49,** 210.

HOARE, C. A. (1962). 'Reservoir hosts and natural foci of human protozoal infections,' *Acta tropica*, **19,** 281.

HOARE, C. A. (1964). 'Morphological and taxonomic studies on mammalian trypanosomes. X. Revision of the systematics,' *J. Protozool.*, **11,** 200.

HOARE, C. A. (1966). 'The classification of mammalian trypanosomes,' *Ergebn. Mikrobiol.*, **39,** 43.

HOARE, C. A. (1967). 'Evolutionary trends in mammalian trypanosomes,' *Advances in Parasitology*, **5,** 47.

HOARE, C. A., and BROOM, J. C. (1938). 'Morphological and taxonomic studies on mammalian trypanosomes. IV. Biometrical study of the relationship between *T. uniforme* and *T. vivax*,' *Trans. R. Soc. trop. Med. Hyg.*, **31,** 517.

HOARE, C. A., and WALLACE, F. G. (1966). 'Developmental stages of Trypanosomatid flagellates: a new terminology,' *Nature*, Lond., **212,** 1385.

HOCKING, K. S. (1961). 'Discriminative application of insecticide against *Glossina morsitans*,' *Bull. ent. Res.*, **52,** 17.

HOCKING, K. S. (1962). 'The population dynamics of tsetse flies with particular reference to their control by insecticides,' *XIth International Congress for Entomology, Vienna, 1960*, **2,** 409.

HOCKING, K. S. *et al.* (1962a). 'Expert Committee on Trypanosomiasis, First Report.' *W.H.O. techn. Rep. Ser.*, 1962 No. 247. 57 pp.

HOCKING, K. S., LAMERTON, J. F., and LEWIS, E. A. (1963). 'Tsetse fly control and eradication,' *Bull. Wld. Hlth. Org.*, **28,** 811.

HOCKING, K. S., LEE, C. W., BEESLEY, J. S. S., and MATECHI, H. T. (1966). 'Aircraft applications. XVI. Airspray experiment with endosulfan against *Glossina morsitans*, *G. swynnertoni* and *G. pallidipes*,' *Bull. ent. Res.*, **56,** 737.

HOCKING, K. S., PARR, H. C. M., YEO, D., and ANSTEY, D. (1953). 'Aircraft applications. IV. Application of coarse aerosols in savanna woodland containing the tsetse flies, *Glossina morsitans* and *G. swynnertoni*,' *Bull. ent. Res.*, **44,** 627.

HOCKING, K. S., and YEO, D. (1956). 'Aircraft applications. XI. Applications of a coarse aerosol to control *G. morsitans* Westw. at Urambo, Tanganyika and *G. morsitans* and *G. pallidipes* Aust. in Lango Country, Uganda,' *Bull. ent. Res.*, **47,** 631.

HOFFMANN, R. (1954). 'Zur Fortpflanzungensbiologie und zur intrauterinen Entwicklung von *Glossina palpalis*,' *Acta trop.*, **11,** 1.

HOLDSTOCK, D. J., MATHIAS, A. P., and SCHACHTER, M. (1957). 'A comparative study of kinin, kallidin and bradykinin,' *Br. J. Pharmac. Chemother.*, **12,** 149.

HOLLINS, C., and LEWIS-FANING, E. (1947). 'The sedimentation rate in the African peasant with special reference to trypanosomiasis,' *Trans. R. Soc. trop. Med. Hyg.*, **41,** 217.

HOLZ, J. (1965). 'Das Verhalten von *Trypanosoma evansi* unter Einfluss des Diacethyl-N^2-guanyl-N^2-(*p*-amidinophenyl)-dihydrazon-dihydrochlorid,' *Zbl. Vet. Med.*, **12B,** 67.

HOPE-GILL, C. W. (1938). 'A study of the reaction rate of the serum-formalin reaction in *Trypanosoma gambiense* sleeping sickness,' *Trans. R. Soc. trop. Med. Hyg.*, **31**, 507.

HORN, A. E. (1910). 'A report on sleeping sickness in the Volta River district of the Gold Coast with suggestions for dealing with it,' *Bull. Sleep. Sickn. Bur.*, **2**, 222.

HORNBY, H. E. (1941). 'Immunization against bovine trypanosomiasis,' *Trans. Roy. Soc. trop. Med. Hyg.*, **35**, 165.

HORNBY, H. E. (1952). *Animal trypanosomiasis in East Africa, 1949.* London, HMSO.

HORNBY, H. E. (1953). (*Trypanosomiasis*, unpublished MS.)

HORNBY, H. E., and BAILEY, H. W. (1929). 'Research on trypanosomiasis,' *Ann. Rep. Dept. Vet. Sci. Anim. Husbandry, Tanganyika* (1928), 19.

HORNBY, H. E., and BAILEY, H. W. (1932). 'Research on trypanosomiasis,' *Ann. Rep. Dept. Vet. Sci. Tanganyika* (1931), p. 10.

HOUBA, V., and ALLISON, A. C. (1966). 'M-antiglobulins (rheumatoid-factor-like globulins) and other gamma-globulins in relation to tropical parasitic infections,' *Lancet*, **i**, 848.

HUDSON, B., and VINOGRAD, J. (1967). 'Catenated circular DNA molecules in HeLa cell mitochondria,' *Nature*, Lond., **216**, 647.

HUGHES, D. E. (1951). 'A press for disrupting bacteria and other organisms,' *Brit. J. exp. Path.*, **32**, 97.

HUGHES, J. C. (1957). 'Olfactory stimulation of tsetse flies and blowflies,' *Bull. ent. Res.*, **48**, 561.

HULLEY, P. E. (1968). 'Mitotic chromosomes of *Glossina pallidipes* Aust.,' *Nature*, Lond., **217**, 977.

HURST, E. W. (1959). 'The lesions produced in the central nervous system by certain organic arsenical compounds,' *J. Path. Bact.*, **77**, 523.

HUTCHINSON, M. P. (1953). 'The epidemiology of human trypanosomiasis in British West Africa. I and II: The Gambia,' *Ann. trop. Med. Parasit.*, **47**, 156.

HUTCHINSON, M. P. (1954). 'The epidemiology of human trypanosomiasis in British West Africa. III. Sierra Leone,' *Ann. trop. Med. Parasit.*, **48**, 75.

HUTCHINSON, M. P., BARRY, A., and BRENGUES, J. R. J. (1964). 'Trypanosomiasis in Kissi.' *Report on CCTA Mission.* Mimeographed copies, OCCGE, Centre Muraz, Bobo Dioulasso.

HUTCHINSON, M. P., and WATSON, H. J. C. (1962). 'Berenil in the treatment of *Trypanosoma gambiense* infection in man,' *Trans. R. Soc. trop. Med. Hyg.*, **56**, 227.

HUXLEY, J. (1942). *Evolution, the Modern Synthesis.* London, Allen & Unwin. 645 pp.

IKEJIANI, O. (1947). 'The antigenic composition and the effect of various extracts of *Trypanosoma equiperdum* and *Trypanosoma lewisi* on the leucocyte picture in experimental trypanosomiasis,' *Amer. J. Hyg.*, **45**, 144.

IMMS, A. D. (1957). *A General Textbook of Entomology*, 9th edition, revised by O. W. Richards and R. G. Davies. London, Methuen.

INOKI, S. (1960). 'Studies on antigenic variation in the Wellcome strains of *Trypanosoma gambiense*. II. On the first relapse of mice treated with human plasma,' *Biken. J.*, **3**, 223.

INOKI, S., OSAKI, H., and NAKAPAYASHI, T. (1956). 'Studies on the immunological variation in *Trypanosoma gambiense*. II. Verifications of the new variation system by Ehrlich's and *in vitro* methods,' *Med. J. Osaka Univ.*, **7**, 165.

ISCTR (1954). 'International Scientific Committee for Trypanosomiasis Research. Fifth Meeting, Pretoria, 1954,' *Publ. perm. inter-afr. Bur. Tsetse Tryp.*, No. 206. Leopoldville, 1954.

ISCTR (1958). 'International Scientific Committee for Trypanosomiasis Research. Sixth Meeting, Salisbury, 1956,' *Comm. tech. Co-op. Afr. S. Sahara* [London], 1958.

ISCTR (1960). 'International Scientific Committee for Trypanosomiasis Research. Seventh Meeting, Brussels, 1958,' *Publ. Comm. tech. Co-op. Afr. S. Sahara*, No. 41, [London], 1960.

ISCTR (1961). 'International Scientific Committee for Trypanosomiasis Research. Eighth Meeting, Jos, 1960,' *Publ. Comm. tech. Co-op. Afr. S. Sahara*, No. 62. [London], 1961.

ISCTR (1963). 'International Scientific Committee for Trypanosomiasis Research. Ninth Meeting, Conakry, 1962,' *Publ. Comm. tech. Co-op. Afr.* No. 88. [London], 1963.

ISCTR (1965). 'International Scientific Committee for Trypanosomiasis Research. Tenth Meeting, Kampala, 1964,' *Publ. Comm. tech. Co-op. Afr.* No. 97. [London], 1965.

ISCTR (1967). 'International Scientific Council for Trypanosomiasis Research. Eleventh Meeting, Nairobi, 1966,' *Publ. scient. tech. Res. Commn, Org. Afr. Unity*, No. 100. Lagos, 1967.

ISHERWOOD, F. (1957). 'The resting sites of *Glossina swynnertoni* Aust. in the wet season,' *Bull. ent. Res.*, **48**, pt. 3, p. 601.

ITARD, J. (1966). 'Cycle de l'óogénese chez les femelles de *Glossina tachinoides* West. et détermination de l'âge physiologique,' *Rev. Élev. Méd. vét. Pays trop.*, **19**, 331.

ITARD, J. (1966a). 'Chromosomes de Glossines (Diptera: Muscidae) (Note presentée par M. Clémont Bressou, Séance du 24 Octobre, 1966),' *C. R. Acad. Sc. Paris*, **263**, 1395 (Ser. D).

ITARD, J. (1968). 'Premiers résultats d'essai d'irradiation gamma sur des pupes et des mâles adultes de *G. morsitans morsitans*.' Panel on Control of Livestock Insect Pests by the Sterile-male Technique (Joint FAO/IAEA, Vienna), *Panel Proc. Series* STI/PUB/184, 1968.

ITARD, J. (1968a). 'Résultats récents d'un élevage de *Glossina tachinoides* Westw. entrepris à Maisons-Alfort (France).' Paper presented in January, 1967 to the Panel on Control of Livestock Insect Pests by the Sterile-male Technique (Joint FAO/IAEA, Vienna), *Panel Proc. Series*, STI/PUB/184, 1968, 102 pp.

ITARD, J. (1969). *Les caryotypes de six espèces de Glossines*. First Symposium on the breeding of the tsetse fly in the laboratory and its practical application. April 22–3, 1969. Lisbon.

ITARD, J., and MAILLOT, L. (1966). 'Notes sur un élevage de Glossines (Diptera: Muscidae) entrepris, à partir de pupes expédiées d'Afrique, à Maisons-Alfort (France),' *Rev. Elev. Méd. vét. Pays trop.*, **19**, 29.

JACK, R. W. (1912). 'Observations on the breeding haunts of *Glossina morsitans*,' *Bull. ent. Res.*, **2**, 357.

JACK, R. W. (1914). 'Tsetse fly and big game in Southern Rhodesia,' *Bull. ent. Res.*, **5**, 97.

JACK, R. W. (1939). 'Studies in the physiology and behaviour of *Glossina morsitans* Westw.,' *Southern Rhodesia: Mem. Dept. Agr.*, **1**, pp. 1–203.

JACK, R. W. (1941). 'Notes on the behaviour of *Glossina pallidipes* and *G. brevipalpis* and some comparisons with *G. morsitans*,' *Bull. ent. Res.*, **31,** 407.

JACK, R. W. (1941a). 'Further studies in the physiology and behaviour of *Glossina morsitans* Westw.,' *Southern Rhodesia: Mem. Dept. Agric.* No. 3.

JACK, R. W., and WILLIAMS, W. L. (1937). 'The effect of temperature on the reaction of *Glossina morsitans* Westw. to light,' *Bull. ent. Res.*, **28,** 499.

JACKSON, C. H. N. (1930). 'Contributions to the bionomics of *Glossina morsitans*,' *Bull. ent. Res.*, **21,** 491.

JACKSON, C. H. N. (1933). 'On an advance of tsetse fly in central Tanganyika,' *Trans. R. ent. Soc. Lond.*, **81,** 205.

JACKSON, C. H. N. (1933a). 'The causes and implications of hunger in tsetse flies,' *Bull. ent. Res.*, **24,** 443.

JACKSON, C. H. N. (1933b). 'On a method of marking tsetse flies,' *J. anim. Ecol.*, **2,** 289.

JACKSON, C. H. N. (1937). 'Some new methods in the study of *G. morsitans*,' *Proc. zool. Soc. Lond.* 1936, p. 811. (London, January 20, 1937.)

JACKSON, C. H. N. (1940). 'An outline of experiments in Kakoma,' *Tsetse Research Reports 1935–8*, pp. 11–15. Dar-es-Salaam, Govt. Printer.

JACKSON, C. H. N. (1941). 'The economy of a tsetse population,' *Bull. ent. Res.*, **32,** 53.

JACKSON, C. H. N. (1941a). 'The anaylsis of a tsetse fly population,' *Ann. Eugen. Camb.*, **10** (1940), 332 [1941].

JACKSON, C. H. N. (1944). 'The analysis of a tsetse fly population. II.,' *Ann. Eugen. Camb.*, **12,** 176.

JACKSON, C. H. N. (1945). 'Pairing of *Glossina morsitans* Westwood with *G. swynnertoni* Austen (Diptera),' *Proc. R. ent. Soc. Lond.*, (A) **20,** 106.

JACKSON, C. H. N. (1945a). 'Comparative studies of the habitat requirements of tsetse fly species,' *J. anim. Ecol.*, **14,** p. 46.

JACKSON, C. H. N. (1946). 'An artificially isolated generation of tsetse flies (Diptera),' *Bull. ent. Res.*, **37,** 291.

JACKSON, C. H. N. (1948). 'The analysis of a tsetse fly population. III,' *Ann. Eugen. Camb.*, **14,** 91.

JACKSON, C. H. N. (1948a). 'Some further isolated generations of tsetse flies,' *Bull. ent. Res.*, **39,** 441.

JACKSON, C. H. N. (1948b). 'The eclosion of tsetse (*Glossina*) larvae (Diptera),' *Proc. R. ent. Soc. Lond.*, (A) **23,** 36.

JACKSON, C. H. N. (1949). 'The biology of tsetse flies,' *Biol. Rev.*, **24,** 174.

JACKSON, C. H. N. (1950). 'Wet season fraying of wings of tsetse flies, *Glossina morsitans*,' *Bull. ent. Res.*, **41,** p. 159.

JACKSON, C. H. N. (1950a). 'Some reflections on "Land Management" as the solution of the tsetse problem,' *Brazzaville Conference Report*, 1950, (q.v.), pp. 315–16.

JACKSON, C. H. N. (1950b). 'On two advances of tsetse fly in Central Tanganyika,' *Proc. R. ent. Soc. Lond.*, (A) **25,** 29.

JACKSON, C. H. N. (1952). '*Tsetse Research*.' *See* EATRO (1952), p. 9.

JACKSON, C. H. N. (1953). 'A mixed population of *Glossina morsitans* and *G. swynnertoni*,' *J. anim. Ecol.*, **22,** 78.

JACKSON, C. H. N. (1953a). 'Seasonal variations in the mean size of tsetse flies,' *Bull. ent. Res.*, **43,** 703.

JACKSON, C. H. N. (1954). 'The availability of tsetse flies.' *See* ISCTR (1954), p. 97.

JACKSON, C. H. N. (1954a). '*Tsetse research.*' *See* EATRO (1954), p. 20.

JACKSON, C. H. N. (1954b). 'The hunger cycles of *Glossina morsitans* and *G. swynnertoni* Austen,' *J. anim. Ecol.*, **23,** 368.

JACKSON, C. H. N. (1955). 'The pattern of *Glossina morsitans* communities,' *Bull. ent. Res.*, **46,** 517.

JACKSON, C. H. N. (1955a). '*Tsetse Research.*' *See* EATRO (1955a), p. 13.

JACKSON, C. H. N., and VANDERPLANK, F. L. (1941). 'Diameters of mammalian erythrocytes,' *Proc. zool. Soc. Lond.* (A) **112,** 57.

JACQUEMIN, P. (1956). 'Un dispositif pratique pour nourrir les arthropodes hématophages,' *Ann. Parasit. hum. comp.*, **31,** 476.

JAFFE, J. J. (1963). '*In vivo* activity of L-azaserine against *Trypanosoma equiperdum,*' *J. Protozool.*, **10,** 431.

JAFFE, J. J. (1965). 'Sensitivity of *Trypanosoma equiperdum* to the action of tumor-inhibitory antibiotics *in vitro,*' *Biochem. Pharmacol.*, **14,** 1867.

JAFFE, J. J. (1967). Sensitivity of *Trypanosoma equiperdum* to the action of tumour-inhibitory antibiotics *in vivo,*' *Nature*, Lond., **213,** 704.

JAFFE, J. J. (1967a). 'Sensitivity of trypanosomes to metabolic inhibitors,' *Trans. N.Y. Acad. Sci.*, Ser. II, **29,** 1057.

JANCSÓ, N., and JANCSÓ-GÁBOR, A. (1952). 'Suramin (Bayer 205) in animal tissues,' *Nature*, Lond. **170,** 567.

JANSSEN, P. G, VAN BOGAERT, L., and HAYMAKER, W. (1956). 'Pathology of the peripheral nervous system in African trypanosomiasis. A study of seven cases,' *J. Neuropath. and exper. Neurol.*, **15,** 269.

JANSSENS, P. G., VAN BOGAERT, L., MICHIELS, A., and VAN DE STEEN, R. (1960). 'Trypanosomiase africaine, affection virale, Mel B et encéphalite,' *Ann. Soc. belge Méd. trop.*, **40,** 759 and 769.

JANSSENS, P. G., KARCHER, D., VAN SANDE, M., LOWENTHAL, A., and GHYSELS, G. (1961). 'Étude enzyme-électrophorétique du LCR de patients atteints de trypanosomiase africaine *T. gambiense,*' *Bull. Soc. Path. exot.*, **54,** 322.

JEANNEL, R. (1942). 'La génése des faunes terrestres,' *Éléments de Biogéographie.* Paris.

JEANNEL, R. (1961). 'La Gondwanie et le peuplement de l'Afrique,' *Annls. Mus. r. Afr. cent.*, Ser. 8°. Tervuren.

JENKIN, P. M., and HINTON, H. E. (1969). 'Apolysis in arthropod moulting cycles,' *Nature*, Lond., **211,** 871.

JENKINS. A. R., and ROBERTSON, D. H. H. (1959). 'Hepatic dysfunction in human trypanosomiasis. II. Serum proteins in *Trypanosoma rhodesiense* infections and observations on the alterations found after treatment and during convalescence,' *Trans. R. Soc. trop. Med. Hyg.*, **53,** 524.

JENKINS, D. W. (1962). 'Radioisotopes in ecological and biological studies of agricultural insects,' *Radioisotopes and radiation in entomology sponsored by the International Atomic Energy Agency and held in Bombay*, 5–9 December, 1960, p. 3. Vienna, International Atomic Energy Agency.

JENKINS, D. W. (1964). 'Pathogens, parasites and predators of medically important arthropods. Annotated list and bibliography,' *Bull. Wld. Hlth. Org.*, **30** suppl., Geneva. 150 pp.

JEWELL, G. R. (1956). 'Marking of tsetse flies for their detection at night,' *Nature*, Lond., **178,** 750.

JEWELL, G. R. (1958). 'Detection of tsetse at night,' *Nature*, Lond., **181,** 1354.

JEWELL, G. R. (1958a). 'Quantitative studies of the breeding places of *G. morsitans*.' *See* EATRO (1958), p. 58.

JOBLING, B. (1933). 'A revision of the structure of the head, mouth-parts and salivary glands of *Glossina palpalis*.' *Parasitology*, **24**, 449.

JOHNS, D. L. (1958). 'Estimation of *Glossina* populations.' *See* EATRO (1958), p. 46.

JOHNS, D. L. (1958a). 'Antennal sense organs of *Glossina*.' *See* EATRO (1958), p. 48.

JOHNSON, H. M., BRENNER, K., and HALL, H. E. (1966). 'The use of a water-soluble carbodiimide as a coupling reagent in the passive hemagglutination test,' *J. Immunol.*, **97**, 791.

JOHNSON, P., NEAL, R. A., and GALL, D. (1963). 'Protective effect of killed trypanosome vaccines with incorporated adjuvants,' *Nature*, Lond., **200**, 83.

JOHNSON, W. B., and LLOYD, LL. (1923). 'First report of the tsetse fly investigation in the Northern Provinces of Nigeria,' *Bull. ent. Res.*, **13**, 373.

JOHNSTONE, R. M. (1963). 'Sulfydryl agents: arsenicals,' in *Metabolic Inhibitors*, Vol. II (ed. R. M. Hochster and J. H. Quastel). New York, Academic Press. pp. 99–118.

JOLLY, G. M. (1965). 'Explicit estimates from capture–recapture data with both death and immigration–stochastic model,' *Biometrika*, **52**, 225.

JONCHÈRE, H. (1951). 'Chimioprophylaxie de la trypanosomaise humaine en AOF,' *Bull. Soc. Path. exot.*, **44**, 83.

JONES-DAVIES, W. J. (1967). 'The discovery of Berenil-resistant *Trypanosoma vivax* in Northern Nigeria,' *Vet. Rec.*, **80**, 531.

JONES-DAVIES, W. J. (1967a). 'A Berenil-resistant strain of *Trypanosoma vivax* in cattle,' *Vet. Rec.*, **81**, 567.

JONES-DAVIES, W. J. (1967b). 'The protection of a small group of Nigerian trade cattle from trypanosomiasis using Samorin,' *Bull. epizoot. Dis. Afr.*, **15**, 323.

JONES-DAVIES, W. J. (1968). 'Diminazene aceturate and homidium chloride resistance in tsetse fly-transmitted trypanosomes of cattle in Northern Nigeria,' *Vet. Rec.*, **83**, 433.

JONES-DAVIES, W. J., and FOLKERS, C. (1966). 'The prevalence of homidium-resistant strains of trypanosomes in cattle in Northern Nigeria,' *Bull. epizoot. Dis. Afr.*, **14**, 65.

JONES-DAVIES, W. J., and FOLKERS, C. (1967). 'Some observations on cross-resistance to Samorin and Berenil of homidium-resistant field strains of *Trypanosoma congolense* in Northern Nigerian cattle.' *See* ISCTR (1967), p. 35.

JORDAN, A. M. (1958). 'The mating behaviour of females of *Glossina palpalis* (R.-D.) in captivity,' *Bull. ent. Res.*, **49**, 35.

JORDAN, A. M. (1961). 'An assessment of the economic importance of the tsetse species of southern Nigeria and the southern Cameroons based on their trypanosome infection rates and ecology,' *Bull. ent. Res.*, **52**, 431.

JORDAN, A. M. (1962). 'A redescription of the signum of *Glossina nashi* Potts,' *Ann. trop. Med. Parasit.*, **56**, 1, 70.

JORDAN, A. M. (1962a). 'The ecology of the *fusca* group of tsetse flies (*Glossina*) in southern Nigeria,' *Bull. ent. Res.*, **53**, 355.

JORDAN, A. M. (1962b). 'The pregnancy rate in *Glossina palpalis* (R.-D.) in Southern Nigeria,' *Bull. ent. Res.*, **53**, 387.

REFERENCES

JORDAN, A. M. (1964). 'Trypanosome infection rates in *Glossina morsitans submorsitans* Newst. in Northern Nigeria,' *Bull. ent. Res.*, **55,** 219.

JORDAN, A. M. (1965). 'The hosts of *Glossina* as the main factor affecting trypanosome infection rates of tsetse flies in Nigeria,' *Trans. R. Soc. trop. Med. Hyg.*, **59,** 423.

JORDAN, A. M. (1965a). 'The status of *Glossina fusca* Walker. (Diptera: Muscidae) in West Africa,' *Ann. trop. Med. Parasit.*, **59,** 2, 219.

JORDAN, A. M. (1965b). 'Long-term fluctuations in numbers of a population of *Glossina palpalis palpalis* (R.-D.).' *See* ISCTR (1965), p. 85.

JORDAN, A. M., LEE-JONES, F., and WEITZ, B. (1961). 'The natural hosts of tsetse flies in the forest belt of Nigeria and the southern Cameroons,' *Ann. trop. Med. Parasit.*, **55,** 167.

JORDAN, A. M., LEE-JONES, F., and WEITZ, B. (1962). 'The natural hosts of tsetse flies in Northern Nigeria,' *Ann. trop. Med. Parasit.*, **56,** 430.

JORDAN, A. M., NASH, T. A. M., and BOYLE, J. A. (1966). 'The large-scale rearing of *Glossina austeni* (Newst.) in the laboratory. II. The use of calves as hosts on seven days of the week,' *Ann. trop. Med. Parasit.*, **60,** 461.

JORDAN, A. M., NASH, T. A. M., and BOYLE, J. A. (1967). 'The rearing of *Glossina austeni* Newst. with lop-eared rabbits as hosts. I. Efficacy of the method,' *Ann. trop. Med. Parasit.*, **61,** 182.

JUNERT, H. (1939). 'Veranderungen im klinischen Bild der ostafrikanischen Schlafkrankheit,' *Arch. Schiffs. Tropenhyg.*, **43,** 205.

KAGWA, B. H. (1967). 'Endemic viral encephalitis in Uganda,' *E. Afr. med. J.*, **44,** 333.

KAHAN, D., ZAHALSKY, A. C., and HUTNER, S. H. (1968). 'Protein synthesis in cell-free preparations of *Crithidia fasciculata*,' *J. Protozool.*, **15,** 385.

KANDASWAMY, T. S., and HENDERSON, J. F. (1962). 'Intracellular differentiation of purine ribonucleotides derived from endogenous and exogenous sources,' *Biochim. biophys. Acta.*, **61,** 86.

KANDASWAMY, T. S., and HENDERSON, J. F. (1962a). 'Inhibition of ascites tumour growth with the trypanocide, Ethidium bromide, in combination with azaserine,' *Nature*, Lond. **195,** 85.

KANDASWAMY, T. S., and HENDERSON, J. F. (1963). 'Alteration of the biochemical effects of Ethidium bromide by exposure of the cells to hypotonic media,' *Nature*, Lond. **199,** 807.

KANDASWAMY, T. S., and HENDERSON, J. F. (1963a). 'The metabolism of Ethidium bromide in normal and neoplastic tissues,' *Cancer Res.*, **23,** 250.

KEAY, R. W. J. (1953). *An Outline of Nigerian Vegetation*, 2nd edition. Lagos, Govt. Printer.

KEAY, R. W. J. (1959). *Vegetation Map of Africa South of the Tropic of Cancer*, published on behalf of l'Association pour l'Étude Taxonomique de la Flore d'Afrique Tropicale, with the assistance of UNESCO. Oxford University Press.

KEEVILL, A. J. (1934). 'Subsequent histories of six cases of *Trypanosoma rhodesiense* infection treated with "Bayer 205" or "Fourneau 309",' *Trans. R. Soc. trop. Med. Hyg.*, **28,** 101.

KELLERSBERGER, E. R. (1933). 'African sleeping sickness. A review of 9,000 cases from a Central African clinic,' *Am. J. trop. Med.*, **13,** 211.

KENDREW, W. G. (1953). *The Climates of the Continents*, Oxford.

KERNAGHAN, R. J. (1961). 'Insecticidal control of vectors of human trypanosomiasis in N. Nigeria,' *J. trop. Med. Hyg.*, **64,** 303.

KERNAGHAN, R. J. (1962). 'An experiment in the control of *Glossina palpalis* over a limited area,' *J. trop. Med. Hyg.*, **65** (6), 146.

KERNAGHAN, R. J., and JOHNSTON, M. R. L. (1962). 'A method of determining insecticide persistence in tsetse fly control operations,' *Bull. Wld. Hlth. Org.*, **26**, 139.

KERNAGHAN, R. J., and NASH, T. A. M. (1964). 'A technique for the dispatch of pupae of *Glossina* and other insects by air from the tropics,' *Ann. trop. Med. Parasit.*, **58**, 355.

KERRICH, G. J. (1960). 'The forms of *Syntomosphyrum* Hym. (Eulophidae) parasitic on tsetse flies,' *Bull. ent. Res.*, **51**, 21.

KERRIDGE, D. (1958). 'The effect of actidione and other antifungal agents on nucleic acid and protein synthesis in *Saccharomyces carlsbergensis*,' *J. gen. Microbiol.*, **19**, 497.

KEYMER, I. F. (1967). '*Trypanosoma* (*Megatrypanum*) spp. Hoare, 1964 of ruminants,' *Vet. Rec.*, **80**, 286.

KEYMER, I. F. (1969). A survey of trypanosome infections in wild ungulates in the Luangwa valley, Northern Rhodesia (Zambia). *Ann. trop. Med. Parasit.*, **63**, 195.

KILGORE, W. W., and DOUTT, R. L. (1967). Editors. *Pest Control. Biological, Physical and Selected Chemical Methods*. New York, Academic Press. 477 pp.

KILLICK-KENDRICK, R. (1964). 'The apparent loss of the kinetoplast of *Trypanosoma evansi* after treatment of an experimentally infected horse with Berenil,' *Ann. trop. Med. Parasit.*, **58**, 481.

KILLICK-KENDRICK, R., and GODFREY, D. G. (1963). 'Observations on a close association between *Glossina tachinoides* and domestic pigs near Nsukka, Nigeria. I,' *Ann. trop. Med. Parasit.*, **57**, 225.

KING, H., LOURIE, E. M., and YORKE, W. (1937). 'New trypanocidal substances,' *Lancet*, **233**, 1360.

KINGHORN, A., and YORKE, W. (1912). 'Trypanosomes obtained by feeding wild *Glossina morsitans* on monkeys in Luangwa valley, Northern Rhodesia,' *Ann. trop. Med. Parasit.*, **6**, 317.

KINGHORN, A., and YORKE, W. (1912a). 'On the influence of meteorological conditions on the development of *Trypanosoma rhodesiense* in *Glossina morsitans*,' *Ann. trop. Med. Parasit.*, **6**, 405.

KINSKY, S. C. (1967). 'Polyene antibiotics,' in *Antibiotics* Vol. I (ed. D. Gottlieb and P. D. Shaw). New York, Springer-Verlag. 122–41.

KIRKBY, W. W. (1961). 'Therapeutic trial using M & B 4404, Homidium bromide and Antrycide methylsulphate.' *See* ISCTR (1961), p. 129.

KIRKBY, W. W. (1961a). 'Comparative prophylactic trial using Prothidium, Antrycide pro-salt and M & B 4404.' *See* ISCTR (1961), p. 135.

KIRKBY, W. W. (1961b). 'Prophylaxis under continuous exposure to the risk of natural infection with trypanosomiasis by tsetse flies. A comparative trial of metamidium chloride, Antrycide pro-salt and Antrycide methylsulphate,' *Vet. Rec.*, **73**, 1411.

KIRKBY, W. W. (1963). 'A review of the trypanosomiasis problem on the Shika stock farm, N. Nigeria, from 1929 to the present day,' *Bull. epizoot. Dis. Afr.*, **11**, 391.

KIRKBY, W. W., and BLASDALE, P. (1960). 'The eradication of *Glossina morsitans submorsitans* Newst. and *Glossina tachinoides* Westw., in part of a river flood plain in Northern Nigeria by chemical means. Part II,' *Bull. ent. Res.*, **51**, 253.

KLEINE, F. K. (1909). 'Positive Infektionsversuche mit *T. brucei* durch *G. palpalis*,' *Deutsch. Med. Wschr.*, **35,** 469.

KLEINE, F. K. (1909a). 'Weitere wissenschaftliche Beobachtungen über die Entwicklung von Trypanosomen in Glossinen,' *Deutsch. med. Wschr.*, **35,** 924.

KLEINE, F. K. (1910). 'Trypanosomenbefunde am Tanganjika und andere Beobachtungen,' *Deutsch. med. Wschr.*, **36,** 1400.

KLEINE, F. K. (1919). 'Die Schlafkrankeit in Kamerun,' *Arch. Schiffs. Tropenhyg.*, **23,** 315.

KLEINE, F. K., and TAUTE, M. (1911). 'Ergänzungen zu unseren Trypanosomenstudien,' *Arb. GesundhAmt.*, **31** (2), 321.

KLENOW, H. (1963). 'Formation of the mono-, di-, and triphosphate of Cordycepin in Ehrlich ascites-tumor cells *in vitro*,' *Biochim. biophys. Acta*, **76,** 347.

KLIGER, I. J., OLITZKI, L., and KLIGER, H. (1940). 'The antigenic composition and immunising properties of trypanosomes,' *J. Immunol.*, **38,** 317.

KNIGHT, R. H., and SOUTHON, H. A. W. (1963). 'A simple method for marking haematophagous insects during the act of feeding,' *Bull. ent. Res.*, **54,** 3, p. 379.

KNIPLING, E. F. (1960). 'The eradication of the screw-worm fly,' *Scientific American*, **203,** 54.

KNIPLING, E. F. (1963). *Potential role of the sterility principle for tsetse fly eradication.* WHO/Vector Control/27, 17 mimeo pages.

KNIPLING, E. F. (1964). 'The potential role of the sterility method for insect population control with special reference to combining this method with conventional methods,' *U.S. Dept. Agriculture, ARS. 33–98.* 54 pp.

KNIPLING, E. F. (1964a). 'The sterility principle of insect population control,' *Pest Articles and News Summary*, Sec. A, **10,** 587.

KNUTH, P., and DU TOIT, P. J. (1921). 'Tropenkrankheiten der Haustiere,' in Mense's *Handb. Tropen-Krankh.*, 2nd edition, v. **6.** Leipzig.

KOCH, H. (1914). 'Bericht über einen Versuch *Glossina palpalis* durch Fang zu beseitigen,' *Arch. Schiffs. Tropenhyg.*, **18,** (24), 807.

KOPP, I., and SOLOMON, H. C. (1940). 'The untoward reactions of tryparsamide,' *Am. J. Syph. Neurol.*, **24,** 265.

KOZMA, C. (1962). 'Über den Nachweis spezifischer Herz-Autoantikörper bei der Chagas-Myokarditis,' *Zeit. Tropenmed. u. Parasitol.*, **13,** 175.

KRANEVELD, F. C. (1931). 'Einzelne Uebertragungsversuche von *Trypanosoma theileri* Laveran, 1902, mit Tabaniden,' *Nederl.-Ind. Blad. Diergeneesk*, **43,** 132.

KUNERT, H. (1939). 'Veränderungen im klinischen Bild der ostafrikanischen Schlafkrankheit,' *Arch. Schiffs. Tropenhyg.*, **43,** 205.

KURZ, H. (1964). 'The permeation of drugs across the so-called blood-brain-barrier at low temperature,' *Experientia*, **20,** 96.

LA BRECQUE, G. C., and KELLER, J. C. (1965). Editors. 'Advances of insect population control by the sterile-male technique,' *IAEA Tech. Rept. Series*, No. 44. 79 pp.

LA BRECQUE, G. C., and SMITH, C. N. (1968). Editors. *Insect Chemosterilization.* Appelton-Century-Croft. 354 pp.

LA CROIX, E. A. S. (1961). 'Some entomological aspects of a series of outbreaks of human trypanosomiasis in northern Ghana in 1957–59.' *See* ISCTR (1961), p. 65.

LAGANE, L. (1913). 'Pouls lent dans la trypanosomiase humaine,' *Bull. Soc. Path. exot.*, **6**, 269.

LAMBORN, W. A. (1915). 'A preliminary report on the problem of controlling *Glossina* in Nyasaland.' *Bull. ent. Res.*, **6**, 59.

LAMBORN, W. A. (1915a). 'Second report on *Glossina* investigations in Nyasaland,' *Bull. ent. Res.*, **6**, 249.

LAMBORN, W. A. (1916). 'Third report on *Glossina* investigations in Nyasaland,' *Bull. ent. Res.*, **7**, 29.

LAMBORN, W. A. (1922). 'Report of the Medical Entomologist,' *Ann. Med. Rep. of the Nyasaland Prot. for the year ended 31 December, 1921.*

LAMBORN, W. A. (1925). 'An attempt to control *Glossina morsitans* by means of *Syntomosphyrum glossinae* Waterston,' *Bull. ent. Res.*, **15**, 303.

LAMBORN, W. A., and HOWAT, C. H. (1936). 'A possible reservoir host of *Trypanosoma rhodesiense*,' *Br. med. J.*, June 6, 1153.

LAMBRECHT, F. L. (1954). 'Note sur l'armature génitale mâle de *Glossina morsitans* Westw,' *Rev. Zool. Bot. Afr.*, **50**, 3–4, p. 189.

LAMBRECHT, F. L. (1964). 'Aspects of evolution and ecology of tsetse flies and trypanosomiasis in prehistoric African environment,' *J. Afric. History*, **5**, 1.

LAMERTON, J. F. (1962). 'Manda valleys in Tanganyika,' *J. Ecol.*, **50**, 771.

LAMPREY, H. F., GLASGOW, J. P., LEE-JONES, F., and WEITZ, B. (1962). 'A simultaneous census of the potential and actual food sources of the tsetse fly *Glossina swynnertoni* Austen,' *J. anim. Ecol.*, **31**, 151.

LANFRANCHI, A. (1915). 'Sur le passage des trypanosomes dans le lait,' *Bull. Soc. Path. exot.*, **8**, 438.

LANGLEY, P. A. (1965). 'The neuroendrocrine system and stomatogastric nervous system of the adult tsetse fly *Glossina morsitans*,' *Proc. zool. Soc. Lond.*, **144**, 415.

LANGLEY, P. A. (1966). 'The effect of environment and host type on the rate of digestion in the tsetse fly, *Glossina morsitans* Westw.,' *Bull. ent. Res.*, **57**, 39.

LANGLEY, P. A. (1966a). 'The control of digestion in the tsetse fly *Glossina morsitans:* enzyme activity in relation to the size and nature of the meal,' *Jour. Ins. Physiol.*, **12**, 439.

LANGLEY, P. A. (1967). 'The control of digestion in the tsetse fly *Glossina morsitans:* a comparison between field flies and flies reared in captivity,' *Jour. Ins. Physiol.*, **13**, 477.

LANGLEY, P. A. (1967a). 'Experimental evidence for a hormonal control of digestion in the tsetse fly, *Glossina morsitans* Westwood: a study of the larva, pupa and teneral adult fly,' *Jour. Ins. Physiol.*, **13**, 1921.

LANGLEY, P. A. (1967b). 'Digestion in the tsetse fly *Glossina morsitans* Westw.: the effect of feeding field-caught flies on guinea pigs in the laboratory,' *Bull. ent. Res.*, **57**, 447.

LANGLEY, P. A. (1967c). 'Effect of ligaturing on puparium formation in the larva of the tsetse fly, *Glossina morsitans* Westwood,' *Nature*. Lond. **214**, 389.

LANGRIDGE, W. P. (1961). 'Scent attractants for tsetse flies,' *See* ISCTR (1961), p. 235.

LANHAM, S. M. (1968). 'Separation of trypanosomes from the blood of infected rats and mice by anion-exchangers,' *Nature*, Lond. **218**, 1273.

LAPEYSSONNIE, L. (1960). 'Deuxième note concernant un cas exceptionnel de trypanosomiase. Parasitémie observée depuis 21 ans sans signes cliniques appréciables chez une malade traitée inefficacement pendant les dix premières années,' *Bull. Soc. Path. exot.*, **53**, 28.

LAUFER, I. (1955). 'Aspects of medical control of Rhodesian sleeping sickness in Tanganyika,' *E. Afr. med. J.*, **32,** 465.

LAUNOY, L., GUILLOT, M., and JONCHÈRE, H. (1960). 'Étude du stockage et de l'élimination de la pentamidine chez la souris et le rat blanc,' *Ann. Pharm. fr.*, **18,** 273 and 423.

LAUNOY, L., and LAGODSKY, H. (1940). 'Documents relatifs à l'activité trypanocide de quelques diamidines,' *Bull. Soc. Path. exot.*, **33,** 320.

LAVERAN, A. (1905). 'Note pour servir à l'histoire des trypanosomiases du Soudan Anglo-Egyptien,' *C. R. Soc. Biol.*, **57,** 292.

LAVERAN, A. (1906). 'Trypanosomiases du Haut-Niger: un nouveau trypanosome pathogène,' *C. R. Acad. Sci.*, **143,** 94.

LAVERAN, A. (1909). (In footnote to Montgomery, R. E. and Kinghorn, A. [1909], *q.v.*).

LAVERAN, A. (1911). 'Les trypanosomes ont-ils des formes latentes chez leurs hôtes vértebrés?' *C. R. Acad. Sci.*, **15,** 649.

LAVERAN, A., and BLANCHARD, R. (1895). 'Les hématozoaires de l'homme et des animaux,' *1e Part. Protozoaires du sang.* Paris.

LAVERAN, A., and MESNIL, F. (1904). 'Sur un trypanosome d'Afrique pathogène pour les Équidés, *Tr. dimorphon* Dutton et Todd,' *C. R. Acad. Sci.*, **138,** 732.

LAVERAN, A., and MESNIL, F. (1905). 'Sur le Surra et la différenciation des trypanosomiases,' *C. R. Acad. Sci.*, Paris, **140,** 831.

LAVERAN, A., and MESNIL, F. (1912). *Trypanosomes et trypanosomiases.* Paris, Masson et Cie.

LAVIER, G. (1927). 'The posterior-nuclear form,' *Interim Rept. League of Nations Comm. Hum. Trypanosomiasis*, Geneva. p. 118.

LAVIER, G. (1927a). 'On the existence of *T. vivax* in man,' *Interim Rept. League of Nations Internat. Comm. on Hum. Trypanosomiasis*, Geneva. p. 144.

LAVIER, G. (1933). 'Sur le polymorphisme réel de certains trypanosomes réputés monomorphes,' *Ann. Parasitol.*, **11,** 280.

LAVIER, G., and LEROUX, R. (1939). 'Lésions cardiaques dans la maladie du sommeil,' *Bull. Soc. Path. exot.*, **32,** 927.

LEACH, T. M. (1961). 'Observations on the treatment of *Trypanosoma evansi* infection in camels,' *J. comp. Path.*, **71,** 109.

LEACH, T. M. (1964). West African Institute for Trypanosomiasis Research *Annual Report 1963.*

LEACH, T. M. (1965). Nigerian Institute for Trypanosomiasis Research *Annual Report 1964.*

LE BERRE, R., and ITARD, J. (1960). 'Validité des sous-espèces *Glossina fusca fusca* Walker, 1879, et *G. fusca congolense* Newstead et Evans, 1921, Diptera, Muscidae,' *Bull. Soc. Path. exot.*, **53,** 542.

LEDGER, H. P. (1964). 'The role of wildlife in African agriculture,' *E. Afr. agric. For. J.*, **30,** 137.

LEE, C. W., and MILLER, A. W. D. (1966). 'Trials with devices for atomising by exhaust gases from a Cessna 182 aircraft engine,' *Agric. Aviation*, **8,** 19.

LEE-JONES, F. (1961). In 'Report of the first Seminar on fundamental research in trypanosomiasis,' *Ann. trop. Med. Parasit.*, **55,** 141.

LÉGER, L. (1904). 'Les affinités de l'*Herpetomonas subulata* et la phylogènie des trypanosomes,' *C. R. Soc. Biol.*, **57,** 615.

LEGGATE, B. M., and PILSON, R. D. (1961). 'The diurnal feeding activity of *Glossina pallidipes* Aust. in relation to trypanosome challenge,' *Bull. ent. Res.*, **51,** 697.

LEHMANN, D. L. (1964). 'The selective action in culture of some trypanocidal drugs on *Trypanosoma rhodesiense* and *T. brucei*,' *Ann. trop. Med. Parasit.*, **58,** 189.

LE PAGE, R. W. F. (1967). 'Studies on the variable antigens of *Trypanosoma brucei*,' *Trans. R. Soc. trop. Med. Hyg.*, **61,** 139.

LE PAGE, R. W. F. (1968). 'Further studies on the variable antigens of *Trypanosoma brucei*,' *Trans. R. Soc. trop. Med. Hyg.*, **62,** 131.

LE PECQ, J. B., and PAOLETTI, C. (1967). 'A fluorescent complex between Ethidium bromide and nucleic acids,' *J. mol. Biol.*, **27,** 87.

LE PORT, L.-R. (1935). 'Les plexo-choroidites rhomboidiennes au début de la maladie du sommeil,' *Bull. Méd. du Katanga*, **12,** 41.

LE ROUX, P. L. (1933). *Annual Report Animal Health, N. Rhodesia.* p. 43.

LE ROUZIC (1949). 'Chimio-prophylaxie en AOF,' *Bull. méd. AOF,* no. spéc., pp. 53–61.

LESTER, H. M. O. (1933). 'The characteristics of some Nigerian strains of the polymorphic trypanosomes,' *Ann. trop. Med. Parasit.*, **27,** 361.

LESTER, H. M. O. (1933a). 'Sleeping sickness in Northern Nigeria,' *W. Afr. med. J.*, **6,** 50.

LESTER, H. M. O. (1934). 'Report on the tsetse investigation,' *Rep. med. Hlth. Serv. Nigeria 1933*, 74–83.

LESTER, H. M. O. (1938). 'The progress of sleeping sickness work in Northern Nigeria,' *W. Afr. med. J.*, **10,** 2.

LESTER, H. M. O., and LLOYD, L. (1928). 'Notes on the process of digestion in tsetse flies,' *Bull. ent. Res.*, **19,** 39.

LEUPOLD, F. (1928). 'Untersuchungen über Rezidivstämme bei Trypanosomen mit Hilfe des Rieckenberg-Phänomens,' *Z. Hyg. InfektKr.*, **109,** 144.

LEVADITI, C., and MCINTOSH, J. (1910). 'Mécanisme de la création de races de trypanosomes résistantes aux anticorps,' *Bull. Soc. Path. exot.*, **3,** 368.

LEVADITI, C., and MUTERMILCH, S. (1910). 'Mécanisme de la phagocytose,' *C. R. Soc. Biol.*, **68,** 1079.

LEWIN, P. K., and MOSCARELLO, M. A. (1968). 'Nucleolar changes in HeLa cells grown in the presence of aminonucleoside,' *Lab. Invest.*, **19,** 265.

LEWIS, C. T. (1954). 'Studies concerning the uptake of contact insecticides. I. The anatomy of the tarsi of certain Diptera of medical importance,' *Bull. ent. Res.*, **45,** 711.

LEWIS, D. J. (1934). 'The behaviour of the larvae of tsetse flies before pupation,' *Bull. ent. Res.*, **25,** 195.

LEWIS, D. J. (1953). 'The Tabanidae of the Anglo Egyptian Sudan,' *Bull. ent. Res.*, **44,** 175.

LEWIS, E. A. (1939). 'Observations on *Glossina fuscipleuris* and other tsetses in the Oyani Valley, Kenya Colony,' *Bull. ent. Res.*, **30,** 345.

LEWIS, E. A. (1942). 'Notes on *Glossina longipennis* and its breeding-places,' *Bull. ent. Res.*, **32,** 303.

LEWIS, E. A. (1950). 'Tsetse flies carried by railway trains in Kenya Colony,' *Bull. ent. Res.*, **40,** 511.

LEWIS, E. A. (1953). 'Land use and tsetse control,' *E. A. Agric. J.*, **18,** 1.

LINGARD, A. (1904). 'The *Trypanosoma* of dourine and its life history,' *Cbl. Bakt., I. Abt. orig.*, **37,** 537.

LIVINGSTONE, D. (1857). *Missionary Travels in South Africa.* London. John Murray. p. 80.

LIVINGSTONE, D., and LIVINGSTONE, C. (1895). *Narrative of an expedition to the Zambesi and its tributaries: and of the discovery of the lakes Shirwa and Nyasa, 1859–64*. London, John Murray.

LLOYD, H. M. (1935). 'Notes on the bionomics of *Glossina swynnertoni* Austen,' *Bull. ent. Res.*, **26**, 439.

LLOYD, J. B., BECK, F., GRIFFITHS, A., and PARRY, L. M. (1968). 'The mechanism of action of acid bisazo dyes,' in *The Interaction of Drugs and Subcellular Components on Animal Cells* (ed. P. N. Campbell). London, J. & A. Churchill Ltd. p. 171.

LLOYD, LL. (1912). 'Notes on *Glossina morsitans* Westw. in the Luangwa Valley, Northern Rhodesia,' *Bull. ent. Res.*, **3**, 233.

LLOYD, LL. (1914). 'Further notes on the bionomics of *Glossina morsitans* in Northern Rhodesia,' *Bull. ent. Res.*, **5**, 49.

LLOYD, LL. and JOHNSON, W. B. (1924). 'The trypanosome infections of tsetse flies in Northern Nigeria and a new method of estimation,' *Bull. ent. Res.*, **14**, 265.

LLOYD, LL., JOHNSON, W. B., and RAWSON, P. H. (1927). 'Experiments in the control of tsetse fly,' *Bull. ent. Res.*, **17**, 423.

LLOYD, LL., JOHNSON, W. B., YOUNG, W. A., and MORRISON, H. (1924). 'Second report of the tsetse fly investigation in the Northern Provinces of Nigeria,' *Bull. ent. Res.*, **15**, 1.

LODHA, K. R., and SINGH, B. (1963). 'Surra in cattle in Rajasthan,' *Ceylon vet. J.*, **11**, 66.

LOEWE, H. (1964). 'Amidinophenoxy-pyrimidinium-Verbindungen, eine neue Klasse von Trypanociden,' *Proc. III Internat. Congr. Chemotherapy 1963* (Stuttgart), H9, p. 1552. G. Thieme Verlag.

LOEWE, H., and URBANIETZ, J. (1965). '6-Amidino-4-amino-chinaldine, ein neuer Typ aromatischer Amidine,' *Arzneim.-Forsch.*, **15**, 604.

LOEWE, H., URBANIETZ, J., and MIETH, H. (1967). 'Über neue Diamidine,' *Proc. V. Internat. Congr. Chemotherapy, 1967.* (Vienna). A.V1/16, p. 645.

LOTTE, A. (1951). 'Enseignements de quatre années de chimioprophylaxie en AEF,' *Méd. trop.*, **11**, 737.

LOTTE, A. (1951a). 'Enseignement de quatre années de chimioprophylaxie en AEF,' BPITT No. 146/0 in *Trop. Dis. Bull.*, **49**, 246.

LOTTE, A. (1954). 'The prophylaxis of sleeping sickness in aquatic regions.' *See* ISCTR (1954), p. 29.

LOURIE, E. M., and O'CONNOR, R. J. (1937). 'A study of *Trypanosoma rhodesiense* relapse strains *in vitro*,' *Ann. trop. Med. Parasit.*, **30**, 179.

LOURIE, E. M., and YORKE, W. (1939). 'The trypanocidal action of certain aromatic diamidines,' *Ann. trop. Med. Parasit.*, **33**, 298.

LOVEMORE, D. F. (1963). 'The effects of anti-tsetse shooting operations on the game populations as observed in the Sebungwe District, Southern Rhodesia,' *Rep. Symposium, Conservation of Nature and Natural Resources in modern African States*, Arusha, Tanganyika, September 1961. IUCN, Morges, Switzerland, 232–4.

LOW, G. C., and MOTT, F. W. (1904). 'The examination of the tissues of the case of sleeping sickness in a European,' *Brit. med. J.*, i, 1000.

LUCAS, J. M. S. (1955). 'Transmission of *Trypanosoma congolense* in cattle under field conditions in the absence of tsetse flies,' *Vet. Rec.*, **67**, 403.

LUCASSE, C. (1964). 'Fluorescent antibody test as applied to cerebrospinal fluid in human sleeping sickness,' *Bull. Soc. Path. exot.*, **57**, 283.

LUMSDEN, W. H. R. (1952). 'The crepuscular biting activity of insects in the forest canopy in Bwamba, Uganda,' *Bull. ent. Res.*, **42**, 721.

LUMSDEN, W. H. R. (1962). 'Trypanosomiasis in African wild life,' *1st. Int. Conf. on Wild Life Disease*, New York, Jan. 24–7, pp. 68–88.

LUMSDEN, W. H. R. (1965). 'The estimation of the concentration of the IgM class of immunoglobulins in the serum as an aid to the diagnosis of trypanosomiasis in man.' *See* ISCTR (1965), p. 203.

LUMSDEN, W. H. R., CUNNINGHAM, M. P., WEBBER, W. A. F., VAN HOEVE, K., and WALKER, P. J. (1963). 'A method for the measurement of infectivity of trypanosome suspensions,' *Exp. Parasit.*, **14**, 269.

LUMSDEN, W. H. R., CUNNINGHAM, M. P., WEBBER, W. A. F., VAN HOEVE, K., KNIGHT, R. H., and SIMMONS, V. (1965). 'Some effects of hydrogen ion concentration on trypanosome numbers and infectivity,' *Exp. Parasit.*, **16**, 8.

LUMSDEN, W. H. R., and HARDY, G. J. C. (1965a). 'Nomenclature of living parasite material,' *Nature*, Lond. **205**, 1032.

LUMSDEN, W. H. R., HERBERT, W. J., and HARDY, G. J. C. (1965b). '*In vivo* prophylactic activity of Berenil against trypanosomes in mice,' *Vet. Rec.*, **77**, 147.

LUMSDEN, W. H. R., HERBERT, W. J., and MCNEILLAGE, G. J. C. (1967). 'Nomenclature of antigenic types of trypanosomes,' *Vet. Rec.*, **81**, 237.

MAC's and MC's, *see* pp. 874–876.

MACARIO, C. (1963). 'La reviviscence d'un foyer de trypanosomiase africaine,' *Méd. trop.*, **23**, 493.

MACHADO, A. DE BARROS (1954). 'Museu do Dundo. Subsídios para o estudo da biologia na Lunda. Révision systématique des Glossines du groupe *palpalis* (Diptera),' *Publ. cult. Cia. Diamantes de Angola*, No. 22. Lisbon.

MACHADO, A. DE BARROS (1959). 'Museu do Dundo. Subsídios para o estudo da biologia na Lunda. Nouvelles contributions a l'étude systématique et biogéographique des Glossines (Diptera),' *Publ. cult. Cia. Diamantes de Angola*, No. 46. Lisbon.

MACHADO, A. DE BARROS (1964). 'Mission de Zoologie médicale au Maniema (Congo, Léopoldville). 13. Diptera – Glossinidae,' *Ann. Mus. r. Afr. Centr.*, Sér. 8° *Zool.*, **132**, 247.

MACHADO, A. DE BARROS (1965). 'Museu do Dundo. Subsídios para o estudo da biologia na Lunda. Réexamen des Glossines (Diptera) supposées avoir été rapportées du Zambèze par la deuxième expédition de Livingstone,' *Publ. cult. Cia Diamantes Angola*, No. 69, p. 117. Lisbon.

MACHADO, A. DE BARROS (1966). 'Remarques sur la systématique des Glossines du groupe *morsitans*,' *Proc. First Internat. Congr. Parasitology, Rome, 1964* (ed. A. Corradetti), p. 981, Rome.

MAEGRAITH, B. (1948). *Pathological Processes in Malaria and Blackwater Fever*. Oxford, Blackwell Scientific Publications.

MAEGRAITH, B. (1963). 'Unde venis?' *Lancet*, **284**, p. 401.

MAHOOD, A. R. (1961). 'An experiment on the control of *G. palpalis* in Southern Zaria Province, Northern Nigeria by chemical means.' *See* ISCTR (1961), p. 269.

MAHOOD, A. R. (1963). 'Control of *G. palpalis* (R.-D.) in the Guinea savannah zone of N. Nigeria,' *See* ISCTR (1963), p. 171.

MAHOOD, A. R. (1963a). 'A note on the ecology of *Glossina morsitans submorsitans* Newst. in the Guinea savannah zone of Northern Nigeria.' *See* ISCTR (1963), p. 181.

MALDONADO, –. (1910). (English abstract of Portuguese texts of 1906 and 1909), *Sleeping Sickness Bureau Bull.*, **2,** 26.

MANSELL-PROTHERO, R. (1965). *Migrants and Malaria.* London, Longmans.

MANSON-BAHR, P. E. C. (1959). (Laboratory demonstration), *Trans. R. Soc. trop. Med. Hyg.*, **53,** 310.

MANSON-BAHR, P. E. C., and CHARTERS, A. D. (1963). 'Myocarditis in African trypanosomiasis,' *Trans. R. Soc. trop. Med. Hyg.*, **57,** 119.

MANSON-BAHR, P. H. (1966). *Manson's Tropical Diseases,* 16th edition. London, Baillière, Tindall & Cassell.

MARNEFFE, J. (1955). 'Observation d'un foyer de *T. rhodesiense* en Urundi. Historique et aspect géographique—clinique—traitement—prophylaxie—1954–55,' *Ann. Soc. belge Méd. trop.*, **35,** 357.

MARTIN, L., and DARRÉ, H. (1908). 'Sur les symptômes nerveux du début de la maladie du sommeil,' *Bull. Soc. Path. exot.*, **1,** 15.

MASSEGUIN, A., CAUSSE, M., and RICOSSÉ, M. (1955). 'Note préliminaire sur l'association lomidine-moranyl dans la prévention de la maladie du sommeil,' *Bull. Soc. Path. exot.*, **48,** 36.

MASSEYEFF, R., and GOMBERT, J. (1962). 'Le diagnostic sérologique de la trypanosomiase africaine à *T. gambiense* par le test d'inhibition de la respiration des trypanosomes. Étude de 100 sérums,' *Bull. Mlm. Fac. mixte Méd. Pharm., Dakar,* **10,** 104.

MATTERN, P. (1962). 'β_2-macroglobulinorachie importante chez des malades atteints de trypanosomiase africaine,' *Ann. Inst. Pasteur,* **102,** 64.

MATTERN, P. (1962a). 'A propos de la présence de β_2-macroglobuline dans le liquide céphalo-rachidien,' *C. R. Soc. Biol.*, **156,** 158.

MATTERN, P. (1964). 'Techniques et intérêt épidémiologique du diagnostic de la trypanosomiase humaine africaine par la recherche de la β_2-macroglobulins dans le sang et dans le LCR,' *Ann. Inst. Pasteur,* **107,** 415.

MATTERN, P., DURET, J., and PAUTRIZEL, R. (1963). 'Hyper-β_2-macroglobulinémie au cours de la trypanosomiase expérimentale du lapin à *T. equiperdum,*' *C. r. Hebd. Séanc. Acad. Sci., Paris,* **256,** 820.

MATTERN, P., FROMENTIN, H., and PILO-MORON, E. (1963). 'Comportement de la β_2 macroglobulins sérique chez le singe experimentalement infecté par un trypanosome sp. souche Feo,' *Bull. Soc. Path. exot.*, **56,** 301.

MATTERN, P., MASSEYEFF, R., MICHEL, R., and PERETTI, P. (1961). 'Étude immunochimique de la β_2-macroglobuline des sérums de malades atteints de trypanosomiase africaine à *Trypanosoma gambiense,*' *Ann. Inst. Pasteur,* **101,** 382.

MATTERN, P., PILLOT, J., and BONNARDOT, R. (1965). 'Contribution à l'étude des immuno-globulines du liquide céphalo-rachidien responsables du phénomène d'immuno-fluorescence dans la neuro-syphilis at dans la trypanosomiase nerveuse,' *Méd. Afr. noire,* **12,** 219.

MAYER, M. (1912). ('Bemerkungen' to Geisler (1912) q.v.), *Arch. Schiffs. Tropenhyg.*, **16,** 197.

MAYR, E. (1942). *Systematics and the Origin of Species from the Viewpoint of a Zoologist.* New York, Colombia University Press. xiv + 334 pp.

MAYR, E., LINSLEY, E. G., and USINGER, R. L. (1953). *Methods and Principles of Systematic Zoology.* New York, Toronto, London, McGraw-Hill.

MELLANBY, H. (1937). 'Experimental work on reproduction in the tsetse fly, *Glossina palpalis,*' *Parasitology,* **29,** 131.

MELLANBY, H., and MELLANBY, K. (1937). 'Rearing tsetse flies in captivity,' *Proc. R. ent. Soc. Lond.*, (A) **12,** 1.

MELLANBY, K. (1936). 'Experimental work with the tsetse fly *Glossina palpalis* in Uganda,' *Bull. ent. Res.*, **27,** 611.

MELLANBY, K. (1939). 'Fertilization and egg production in the bedbug, *Cimex lectularius* L.,' *Parasitology*, **31,** 193.

MERRYMAN, H. T. (1966). In *Cryobiology* (ed. H. T. Merryman), New York, Academic Press. pp. 70–5.

MERRYMAN, H. T., and WEINMAN, D. (1968). In *Infectious Blood Diseases* (ed. D. Weinman and M. Ristic), New York, Academic Press. pp. 343–65.

MESNIL, F., and BRIMONT, E. (1909). 'Sur les propriétés protectrices du sérum des animaux trypanosomiés: Races résistantes à ces sérums,' *Ann. Inst. Pasteur*, **23,** 129.

MEYER, R. R., and SIMPSON, M. V. (1969). 'Differential inhibition of mitochondrial and nuclear DNA polymerases by the mutagenic dyes Ethidium bromide and acriflavin,' *Biochem. biophys. Res. Commun.*, **34,** 238.

MICHEL, R. (1964). 'Reflexmikroskopische und enzymatische Untersuchungen der zytoplasmatischen Granula von *Trypanosoma gambiense*,' *Z. Tropenmed. Parasit.*, **15,** 400.

MICHEL, R. (1966). 'Korrelation zwischen der Häufigkeitsverteilung cytoplasmatischer Ribonucleinsäure-und Sulfhydril-Granula einiger Trypanosomenarten und dem Infektionsverlauf im Wirbeltierwirt,' *Z. Tropenmed. Parasit*,, **17,** 68.

MILL, K. R. (1948). 'The protein content of cerebrospinal fluid in trypanosomiasis,' *Trans. R. Soc. trop. Med. Hyg.*, **41,** 641.

MILLER, A. W. D., and CHADWICK, P. R. (1963). 'Swathe marking in aerial spraying,' *Agric. Aviation*, **5,** 114.

MILLER, J. K. (1965). 'Variation of the soluble antigens of *Trypanosoma brucei*,' *Immunology*, **9,** 521.

MINCHIN, E. A. (1905). 'Report on the anatomy of the tsetse fly (*Glossina palpalis*),' *Proc. Roy. Soc.*, (B) **76,** No. B512, 531.

MINCHIN, E. A. (1908). 'Investigations on the development of trypanosomes in tsetse flies and other Diptera,' *Q. J. micro. Sci.*, **52,** 159.

MINCHIN, E. A. (1909). 'The structure of *T. lewisi* in relation to microscopical technique,' *Q. J. micro. Sci.*, **53,** 755.

MINCHIN, E. A., and THOMSON, J. D. (1915). 'The rat trypanosome, *T. lewisi*, in its relation to the rat-flea, *Ceratophyllus fasciatus*,' *Quart. J. micr. Sci.*, **60,** 463.

MITTENDORF, H. J., and WILSON, S. G. (1961). *Livestock and Meat Marketing in Africa.* Rome, FAO.

MOGGRIDGE, J. Y. (1936). 'Experiments on the crossing of open spaces by *Glossina swynnertoni*,' *Bull. ent. Res.*, **27,** 435.

MOGGRIDGE, J. Y. (1948). 'Night activity of tsetse (*Glossina*) on the Kenya coast,' *Proc. R. ent. Soc. Lond.*, (A) **23,** 87.

MOISER, B. (1912). 'Notes on the haunts and habits of *G. tachinoides* near Geidam, Bornu Province, Northern Nigeria,' *Bull. ent. Res.*, **3,** 195.

MOLLOY, J. O., and ORMEROD, W. E. (1965). 'Two types of cytoplasmic granule in *Trypanosoma rhodesiense*,' *Exp. Parasit.*, **17,** 57.

MONNET, A., and BAYLET, R. (1951). 'Étude de l'élimination urinaire du 3854 RP (Mel B Friedheim—Arsobal Spécia),' *Trop. Dis. Bull.*, **48,** 958.

MONNET, A., and BAYLET, R. (1951a). 'Contribution à l'étude du métabolisme du mélaminyl 4 phényl—arsénodithioglycerine en solution dans le propylene glycol: son passage dans le liquide céphalo-rachidien,' *Bull. Soc. Path. exot.*, **44,** 754.

MONTGOMERY, R. E., and KINGHORN, A. (1909). 'A further report on trypanosomiasis of domestic stock in Northern Rhodesia (North-Eastern Rhodesia),' *Ann. trop. Med. Parasit.*, **3,** 311.

MOODY, J. P., and WILLIAMS, R. T. (1962). 'The fate of arylarsonic acids in the hen,' *Biochem. J.*, 4P.

MOREAU, R. E. (1967). *The Bird Fauna of Africa and its Islands.* London.

MORRIS, K. R. S. (1934). 'The bionomics and importance of *Glossina longipalpis* Wied. in the Gold Coast,' *Bull. ent. Res.*, **25,** 309.

MORRIS, K. R. S. (1944). 'A large scale experiment in the eradication of tsetse (*G. palpalis* and *G. tachinoides*),' *Farm and For.*, **5,** 149.

MORRIS, K. R. S. (1946). 'The control of trypanosomiasis by entomological means,' *Bull. ent. Res.*, **37,** 201.

MORRIS, K. R. S. (1949). 'Planning the control of sleeping sickness,' *Trans. R. Soc. trop. Med. Hyg.*, **43,** 165.

MORRIS, K. R. S. (1951). 'The ecology of epidemic sleeping sickness. I. The significance of location,' *Bull. ent. Res.*, **42,** 427.

MORRIS, K. R. S. (1959). 'The epidemiology of sleeping sickness in East Africa. A sleeping sickness outbreak in Uganda in 1957,' *Trans. R. Soc. trop. Med. Hyg.*, **53,** 384.

MORRIS, K. R. S. (1960). 'Studies on the epidemiology of sleeping sickness in East Africa. II. Sleeping sickness in Kenya,' *Trans. R. Soc. trop. Med. Hyg.*, **54,** 71.

MORRIS, K. R. S. (1960a). 'Studies on the epidemiology of sleeping sickness in East Africa. III. The endemic area of Lakes Edward and George in Uganda,' *Trans. R. Soc. trop. Med. Hyg.*, **54,** 212.

MORRIS, K. R. S. (1960b). 'Trapping as a means of studying the game tsetse, *Glossina pallidipes* Aust.,' *Bull. ent. Res.*, **51,** p. 533.

MORRIS, K. R. S. (1961). 'Problems in the assessment of tsetse populations,' *Bull. ent. Res.*, **52,** p. 239.

MORRIS, K. R. S. (1961a). 'Effectiveness of traps in tsetse surveys in the Liberian rain forest,' *Amer. J. trop. Med. Hyg.*, **10,** 905.

MORRIS, K. R. S. (1962). 'The food of *Glossina palpalis* (R.-D.) and its bearing on the control of sleeping sickness in forest country,' *J. trop. Med. Hyg.*, **65,** p. 12.

MORRIS, K. R. S. (1962a). 'The epidemiology of sleeping sickness in East Africa. V. Epidemics on the Albert Nile,' *Trans. R. Soc. trop. Med. Hyg.*, **56,** 316.

MORRIS, K. R. S., and MORRIS, M. G. (1949). 'The use of traps against tsetse in West Africa,' *Bull. ent. Res.*, **39,** p. 491.

MORRIS, M. G. (1950). The persistence of toxicity in DDT-impregnated hessian and its use on tsetse traps,' *Bull. ent. Res.*, **41,** 259.

MORTON, G. O., LANCASTER, J. E., VAN LEAR, G. E., FULMAR, W., and MEYER, W. E. (1969). 'The structure of Nucleocidin. III. (A new structure),' *J. Amer. chem. Soc.*, **91,** 1535.

MOTT, F. W. (1899). 'The changes in the central nervous system of 2 cases of negro lethargy: sequel to Dr. Manson's clinical report,' *Brit. med. J.* **(ii).** 1666.

MOTT, F. W. (1906). 'Histological observations on sleeping sickness and other trypanosome infections,' *Reports of the Sleeping Sickness Commission of the Royal Society*, **7,** 3.

MOUCHET, J. (1963). 'L'éradication des Glossines aux confins du Nord-Cameroun et du Tchad.' *See* ISCTR (1963), p. 229.

MOUCHET, J., DELAS, A., and YVORE, P. (1961). 'La campagne expérimentale de lutte contre *G. tachinoides* à Logone-Birni (Cameroun et Tchad),' *Bull. Soc. Path. exot.*, **54,** 875.

MOUCHET, J., and GARIOU, J. (1966). 'Notice de la carte de répartition des Glossines au Cameroun,' Cahiers ORSTOM, *Ent. Med.*, 83.

MOUCHET, J., GARIOU, J., and RATEAU, J. (1958). 'Distribution géographique et écologique de *Glossina palpalis palpalis* Rob. Desv. et *Glossina fuscipes fuscipes* Newst. au Cameroun,' *Bull. Soc. Path. exot.*, **51,** 652.

MSHELBWALA, A. S. (1967). 'Infectivity of *Trypanosoma rhodesiense* to tsetse flies fed through animal membranes,' *Nature*, Lond. **215,** 441.

MÜHLPFORDT, H. (1963). 'Über die Bedeutung und Feinstruktur des Blepharoplasten bei parasitischen Flagellaten,' *Z. Tropenmed. Parasit.*, **14,** 357.

MÜHLPFORDT, H. (1964). 'Über den Kinetoplasten der Flagellaten,' *Z. Tropenmed. Parasit.*, **15,** 289.

MÜHLPFORDT, H., and BAYER, M. (1961). 'Elektronmikroskopische Untersuchungen an Protozoen (*Trypanosoma gambiense*),' *Z. Tropenmed. Parasit.*, **12,** 334.

MUIRHEAD THOMSON, R. C. (1968). *Ecology of Insect Vector Populations.* London, Academic Press Inc., pp. vii + 174.

MUTERMILCH, S., and SALAMON, E. (1928). 'Mechanism of the crisis in the trypanosome-infected guinea pig,' *C. R. Soc. Biol.*, **98,** 348.

MWAMBU, P. M. (1967). 'Cattle trypanosomiasis survey in the area adjoining the south Busoga fly belt.' *See* ISCTR (1967), p. 25.

MACADAM, R. F., and WILLIAMSON, J. (1964). 'The effect of some trypanosomicidal drugs on the fine structure of *Trypanosoma rhodesiense*,' *Trans. R. Soc. trop. Med. Hyg.*, **58,** 7.

MACADAM, R. F., and WILLIAMSON, J. (1967). 'The effect of drugs on the fine structure of trypanosomes,' *Parasitology*, **57,** 21P–22P.

MACADAM, R. F., and WILLIAMSON, J. (1969). 'Lesions in the fine structure of *Trypanosoma rhodesiense* specifically associated with drug treatment,' *Trans. R. Soc. trop. Med. Hyg.*, **63,** 421.

MACFIE, J. W. S. (1913). 'On the morphology of the trypanosome (*Trypanosoma nigeriense*, n. sp.) from a case of sleeping sickness from Eket, Southern Nigeria, *Ann. trop. Med. Parasit.*, **7,** 339.

MACFIE, J. W. S. (1917). 'Preliminary note on a monomorphic trypanosome found in the blood of a native of the Gold Coast,' *Brit. med. J.*, pt. 1, 12.

MACFIE, J. W. S., and GALLACHER, G. H. (1914). 'Sleeping sickness in the Eket district of Nigeria,' *Ann. trop. Med. Parasit.*, **8,** 379.

MACGREGOR, D. E. (1965). *Annual Report* on the Veterinary Division of the Ministry of Animal and Forest Resources, Northern Nigeria, 1962–3. Kaduna. Min. of Int. Affairs.

MACGREGOR, D. E. (1966). *Annual Report* of Animal Health Division, Northern Nigeria, 1963–4. Kaduna. Govt. Printer.

MACKICHAN, I. W. (1944). 'Rhodesian sleeping sickness in eastern Uganda,' *Trans. R. Soc. trop. Med. Hyg.*, **38,** 49.

MACKIE, F. P. (1935). 'The Jarisch-Herxheimer reaction in trypanosomiasis—with a note on the morular cells of Mott,' *Trans. Roy. Soc. trop. Med. Hyg.*, **28,** 377.

MACKIE, T. J., and MCCARTNEY, J. E. (1953). *Handbook of Practical Bacteriology*, 9th edition. Edinburgh and London, E. & S. Livingstone.

MACLEAN, G. (1926). 'History of an outbreak of Rhodesian sleeping sickness in the Ufipa District of Tanganyika Territory with short notes on cases and treatment,' *Ann. trop. Med. Parasit.*, **20,** 329.

MACLEAN, G. (1930). 'Sleeping sickness measures in Tanganyika Territory,' *Kenya and East African med. J.*, **7,** 120.

MACLENNAN, K. J. R. (1957). 'A staining technique for the identification of trypanosomes in thick blood films,' *Trans. R. Soc. trop. Med. Hyg.*, **51,** 301.

MACLENNAN, K. J. R. (1963). 'Cattle trypanosomiasis in Northern Nigeria. The problem in the field,' *Bull. epizoot. Dis. Afr.*, **11,** 381.

MACLENNAN, K. J. R. (1965). 'Report on results from insecticidal control projects for the eradication of *Glossina* in the Sudan vegetational zone of Northern Nigeria.' *See* ISCTR (1965), p. 125.

MACLENNAN, K. J. R. (1967). 'Recent advances in tsetse fly control with special reference to Northern Nigeria,' *Bull. Wld. Health Organisation*, **37,** 615.

MACLENNAN, K. J. R. (1968). 'Some recent findings concerning the use of Berenil for the treatment of bovine trypanosomiasis in Northern Nigeria,' *Trans. R. Soc. trop. Med. Hyg.*, **62,** 139.

MACLENNAN, K. J. R., and AITCHISON, P. J. (1963). 'Simultaneous control of three species of *Glossina* by the selective application of insecticides,' *Bull. ent. Res.*, **54,** 199.

MACLENNAN, K. J. R., and JONES-DAVIES, W. J. (1967). 'The occurrence of a Berenil-resistant *Trypanosoma congolense* strain in Northern Nigeria,' *Vet. Rec.*, **80,** 389.

MACLENNAN, K. J. R., and KIRKBY, W. W. (1958). 'Eradication of *Glossina morsitans submorsitans* and *G. tachinoides* in part of a river flood plain in Northern Nigeria by chemical means. I,' *Bull. ent. Res.*, **49,** 123.

MACLEOD, J., and DONNELLY, J. (1957). 'Individual and group marking methods for fly-population studies,' *Bull. ent. Res.*, **48,** 585.

MACOWAN, K. D. S. (1961). *Annual Report.* Veterinary Department, Kenya, 1960, 47–50.

MCCULLOCH, B. (1967). 'Trypanosomes of the sub-group *brucei* as a probable cause of disease in wild zebra (*Equus burchelli*),' *Ann. trop. Med. Parasit.*, **61,** 261.

MCDONALD, W. A. (1957). 'A Calliphorid host of *Thyridanthrax abruptus* Lw. in Nigeria (Diptera: Bombyliidae),' *Bull. ent. Res.*, **48,** 533.

MCDONALD, W. A. (1960). 'Nocturnal detection of tsetse flies in Nigeria with ultra-violet light,' *Nature*, Lond. **185,** No. 4176, p. 867.

MCDONALD, W. A. (1961). 'Insecticidal spraying against *Glossina palpalis* in Nigeria based on a study of its nocturnal resting sites with ultra-violet light.' *See* ISCTR (1961), p. 243.

MCDONALD, W. A. (1961a). 'The laboratory rearing of *Glossina morsitans submorsitans* Newst. in Northern Nigeria.' *See* ISCTR (1961), p. 247.

MCKELVEY, E. M., and FAHEY, J. L. (1965). 'Immunoglobulin changes in disease: quantitation on the basis of heavy polypeptide chains, IgG (γG), IgA (γA), and IgM (γM), and of light polypeptide chains, type K (I) and type L (II),' *J. clin. Invest.*, **44,** 1778.

MCLETCHIE, J. L. (1948). 'The control of sleeping sickness in Nigeria,' *Trans. R. Soc. trop. Med. Hyg.*, **41,** 445.

MCLETCHIE, J. L. (1953). 'Sleeping sickness activities in Nigeria 1931–52. Part II,' *W. Afr. med. J.*, New Series, **2,** 138.

MCQUEEN, J. D., and MEGO, J. L. (1964). 'Tissue-concentration ratios of arsenate-^{74}As and labeled organic conjugates,' *J. Neurosurg.*, **21** (8), 641.

NAIRN, R. C. (1964). *Fluorescent Protein Tracing*, 2nd edition. Edinburgh and London, E. & S. Livingstone, Ltd.

NA'ISA, B. K. (1967). 'Follow-up on a survey of the prevalence of Homidium-resistant strains of trypanosomes in cattle in Northern Nigeria and drug cross-resistance tests on the strains with Samorin and Berenil,' *Bull. epizoot. Dis. Afr.*, **15,** 231.

NAJARIAN, H. H. (1965). 'The effect of paromomycin on *Trypanosoma equiperdum* infection in mice,' *Texas Rep. Biol. Med.*, **23,** 481.

NASH, T. A. M. (1930). 'A contribution to our knowledge of the bionomics of *Glossina morsitans*,' *Bull. ent. Res.*, **21,** 201.

NASH, T. A. M. (1933). 'The ecology of *Glossina morsitans* Westw., and two possible methods for its destruction—Part I,' *Bull. ent. Res.*, **24,** 107.

NASH, T. A. M. (1933a). 'The ecology of *Glossina morsitans* Westw., and two possible methods for its destruction—Part II,' *Bull. ent. Res.*, **24,** 163.

NASH, T. A. M. (1935). 'The effect of high maximum temperatures upon the longevity of *Glossina submorsitans* Newst. and *G. tachinoides* Westw.,' *Bull. ent. Res.*, **26,** 103.

NASH, T. A. M. (1936). 'The relationship between the maximum temperature and the seasonal longevity of *Glossina submorsitans* Newst. and *G. tachinoides* Westw. in Northern Nigeria,' *Bull. ent. Res.*, **27,** 273.

NASH, T. A. M. (1936a). 'The part played by micro-climates in enabling *Glossina submorsitans* and *G. tachinoides* to withstand the high temperatures of a West African dry season,' *Bull. ent. Res.*, **27,** 339.

NASH, T. A. M. (1937). 'Climate, the vital factor in the ecology of *Glossina*,' *Bull. ent. Res.*, **28,** 75.

NASH, T. A. M. (1939). 'The ecology of the puparium of *Glossina* in Northern Nigeria,' *Bull. ent. Res.*, **30,** 259.

NASH, T. A. M. (1940). 'The effect upon *Glossina* of changing the climate of the true habitat by partial clearing of vegetation,' *Bull. ent. Res.*, **31,** 69.

NASH, T. A. M. (1942). 'A study of the causes leading to the seasonal evacuation of a tsetse breeding-ground,' *Bull. ent. Res.*, **32,** 327.

NASH, T. A. M. (1944). 'The control of sleeping sickness in the *Raphia* pole trade,' *Bull. ent. Res.*, **35,** 49.

NASH, T. A. M. (1944a). 'A low density of tsetse flies associated with a high incidence of sleeping sickness,' *Bull. ent. Res.*, **35,** 51.

NASH, T. A. M. (1947). 'A record of *Syntomosphyrum glossinae* from Nigeria,' *Bull. ent. Res.*, **38,** 525.

NASH, T. A. M. (1948) *The Anchau Rural Development and Settlement Scheme.* London, HMSO.

NASH, T. A. M. (1948a). *Tsetse Flies in British West Africa.* London, HMSO.

NASH, T. A. M. (1948b). 'A note on the effect of high temperature on the pupal stage of *Glossina* in relation to the transmission rate of trypanosomes,' *Ann. trop. Med. Parasit.*, **42,** 30.

NASH, T. A. M. (1952). 'Some observations on resting tsetse-fly populations and evidence that *Glossina medicorum* is a carrier of trypanosomes,' *Bull. ent. Res.*, **43,** 33.

NASH, T. A. M. (1955). 'The fertilisation of *Glossina palpalis* in captivity,' *Bull. ent. Res.*, **46,** 357.

NASH, T. A. M. (1960). 'The effect of different types of man–fly contact upon the distribution of *T. gambiense* sleeping sickness in Nigeria.' *See* ISCTR (1960), p. 191.

NASH, T. A. M. (1960a). 'A review of the African trypanosomiasis problem,' *Trop. Dis. Bull.*, **57,** 973.

NASH, T. A. M. (1969). *Africa's Bane: the Tsetse Fly.* London, Collins.

NASH, T. A. M., and DAVEY, J. T. (1950). 'The resting habits of *Glossina medicorum, G. fusca* and *G. longipalpis*,' *Bull. ent. Res.*, **41,** 153.

NASH, T. A. M., and JORDAN, A. M. (1959). 'A guide to the identification of the West African species of the *fusca* group of tsetse-flies, by dissection of the genitalia,' *Ann. trop. Med. Parasit.*, **53,** 72.

NASH, T. A. M., JORDAN, A. M., and BOYLE, J. A. (1966). 'Effect of host pregnancy on pupal production by the tsetse fly,' *Nature*, Lond. **212,** 1581.

NASH, T. A. M., JORDAN, A. M., and BOYLE, J. A. (1966a). 'A promising method for rearing *Glossina austeni* Newst. on a small scale, based on the use of rabbits' ears for feeding,' *Trans. Roy. Soc. trop. Med. Hyg.*, **60,** 183.

NASH, T. A. M., JORDAN, A. M., and BOYLE, J. A. (1966b). 'The large-scale rearing of *Glossina austeni* in the laboratory. III—Confirmation of the value of pregnant goats as hosts,' *Ann. trop. Med. Parasit.*, **60,** 469.

NASH, T. A. M., JORDAN, A. M., and BOYLE, J. A. (1967). 'A method of maintaining *Glossina austeni* Newst. singly, and a study of the feeding habits of the female in relation to larviposition and pupal weight,' *Bull. ent. Res.*, **57,** 327.

NASH, T. A. M., JORDAN, A. M., and BOYLE, J. A. (1967a). 'Retraction of the claim that host pregnancy affects pupal production by the tsetse fly,' *Nature*, Lond. **216,** 163.

NASH, T. A. M., JORDAN, A. M., and BOYLE, J. A. (1968). 'The large-scale rearing of *Glossina austeni* Newst. in the Laboratory. IV. The final technique,' *Ann. trop. Med. Parasit.*, **62,** 336.

NASH, T. A. M., and KERNAGHAN, R. J. (1964). 'The feeding of haemato-phagous insects on goats and sheep: techniques for host restraint and cage application,' *Ann. trop. Med. Parasit.*, **58,** 168.

NASH, T. A. M., and KERNAGHAN, R. J. (1965). 'The weight and viability of puparia of *Glossina austeni* in relation to the conditions provided for pupal development,' *Ann. trop. Med. Parasit.*, **59,** 226.

NASH, T. A. M., and KERNAGHAN, R. J. (1965a). 'The function of the sternal and anal plates of females of *Glossina austeni* Newst. (Diptera: Muscidae),' *Proc. R. ent. Soc. Lond.*, (A) **40,** 1–3, p. 35.

NASH, T. A. M., KERNAGHAN, R. J., and BOYLE, J. A. (1966). 'The large-scale rearing of *Glossina austeni* Newst. in the laboratory. I. The use of pregnant and non-pregnant goats as hosts,' *Ann. trop. Med. Parasit.*, **60,** 39.

NASH, T. A. M., KERNAGHAN, R. J., and WRIGHT, A. I. (1965). 'A method for the prevention of skin reactions in goats used for feeding tsetse flies, *Glossina* spp.,' *Ann. trop. Med. Parasit.*, **59,** 88.

NASH, T. A. M., and PAGE, W. A. (1953). 'The ecology of *Glossina palpalis* in Northern Nigeria,' *Trans. R. ent. Soc. Lond.*, **104,** 71.

NASH, T. A. M., PAGE, W. A., JORDAN, A. M., and PETANA, W. (1960). 'The rearing of *Glossina palpalis* in the laboratory for experimental work.' *See* ISCTR (1960), p. 343.

NASH, T. A. M., and STEINER, J. O. (1957). 'The effect of obstructive clearing on *Glossina palpalis*,' *Bull. ent. Res.*, **48,** 323.

NASS, M. M. K., NASS, S., and AFZELIUS, B. A. (1965). 'The general occurrence of mitochondrial DNA,' *Experimental Cell Research*, **37,** 516.

NEAVE, S. A. (1909). 'Some notes on the distribution of *Glossina palpalis* (Rob-Desv.),' *J. econ. Biol.*, **4,** 109.

NELSON, R. A. (1953). 'The immune-adherence phenomenon. An immunologically specific reaction between micro-organisms and erythrocytes leading to enhanced phagocytosis,' *Science*, N.Y. **118,** 733.

NELSON, R. A., and NELSON, D. S. (1959). 'On the mechanisms of immuno-adherence. II. Analogy to mixed aggregation of sensitized antigens in the presence of complement: Immuno-adherence with blood platelets,' *Yale J. Biol. Med.*, **31,** 201.

NEUJEAN, G. (1950). 'Contribution à l'étude des liquides rachidiens et céphaliques dans la maladie du sommeil à "*Trypanosoma gambiense*",' *Ann. Soc. belge Méd. trop.*, **30,** 1125.

NEUJEAN, G., and EVENS, F. (1958). 'Diagnostic et traitement de la maladie du sommeil à *T. gambiense*. Bilan de dix ans d'activité du centre de traitement de Léopoldville,' *Acad. r. Sci. col. Cl. Sci. nat. Méd.*, v. 7, Mém. No. 8, No. spéc., 175 pp.

NEUMANN, R. (1911). 'Zur Kenntnis der Immunität bei experimenteller Trypanosomeninfektion,' *Z. Hyg. InfektKr.*, **69,** 109.

NEWSTEAD, R. (1910). 'On three new species of the genus *Glossina*, together with a description of the hitherto unknown male of *Glossina grossa*, Bigot,' *Ann. trop. Med. Parasit.*, **4,** 369.

NEWSTEAD, R. (1911). 'A revision of the tsetse flies (*Glossina*) based on a study of the male genital armature,' *Bull. ent. Res.*, **2,** 9.

NEWSTEAD, R., and EVANS, A. M. (1921). 'New tsetse-flies (*Glossina*) from the Belgian Congo,' *Ann. trop. Med. Parasit.*, **15,** 95.

NEWSTEAD, R., EVANS, A. M., and POTTS, W. H. (1924). 'Guide to the study of tsetse-flies,' *Liverpool Sch. trop. Med., Mem.* (*New Series*) No. 1. Liverpool Univ. Press. xi + 382 pp.

NEWTON, B. A. (1962). 'The effect of quaternary ammonium trypanocides on cell division, nucleic acid and protein synthesis,' in *Drugs, Parasites and Hosts* (ed. L. G. Goodwin and R. H. Nimmo-Smith), London, J. & A. Churchill Ltd., p. 142.

NEWTON, B. A. (1963). 'Interaction of Antrycide with isolated ribosomes,' *Biochem. J.*, **89,** 93P–94P.

NEWTON, B. A. (1964). 'Mechanisms of action of phenanthridine and amino-quinaldine trypanocides,' *Adv. Chemotherapy*, **1,** 35.

NEWTON, B. A. (1965). In *Annual Report, 1965*, Nigerian Institute for Trypanosomiasis Research, p. 34.

NEWTON, B. A. (1966). 'Effects of antrycide on nucleic acid synthesis and function,' *Symp. Soc. gen. Microbiol.*, **16,** 213.

NEWTON, B. A. (1968). 'Biochemical peculiarities of trypanosomatid flagellates,' *Ann. Rev. Microbiol.*, **22,** 109.

NEWTON, B. A., and LE PAGE, R. W. F. (1967). 'Preferential inhibition of extranuclear deoxyribonucleic acid synthesis by the trypanocide Berenil,' *Biochem. J.*, **105,** 50P.

NEWTON, B. A., and LE PAGE, R. W. F. (1968). 'Interaction of Berenil with trypanosome DNA,' *Trans. R. Soc. trop. Med. Hyg.*, **62,** 131.

NIESCHULZ, O. (1930). 'Surrauebertragungsversuche auf Java und Sumatra,' *Veeartsenijk. Meded.*, Utrecht, **75.**

NITR (1964). Nigerian Institute for Trypanosomiasis Research. *Annual Report, 1964.*

NITR (1965). Nigerian Institute for Trypanosomiasis Research. *Annual Report, 1965.*

NJOGU, A. R. (1967). 'Histochemical demonstration of pyridine-nucleotide-linked dehydrogenases and diaphorases of *Brucei* subgroup trypanosomes after starch-gel electrophoresis,' *Trans. R. Soc. trop. Med. Hyg.*, **61,** 136.

NJOGU, A. R., and HUMPHRIES, K. C. (1967). 'Electrophoretic separation of the soluble proteins of *Brucei* subgroup trypanosomes,' *Nature*, Lond. **216,** 280.

NJOGU, A. R., and HUMPHRIES, K. C. (1967a). 'Distribution of the soluble dehydrogenases and diaphorases of *Brucei* subgroup trypanosomes in starch-gel electropherograms,' *Nature*, Lond. **216,** 1308.

NNOCHIRI, E. (1964). 'Observations on the treatment of onchocerciasis in an endemic area of Western Nigeria,' *Trans. R. Soc. trop. Med. Hyg.*, **58,** 413.

NOBLE, E. R. (1955). 'The morphology and life cycles of trypanosomes,' *Quart. Rev. Biol.*, **30,** 1.

NOBLE, E. R., MCRARY, W. L., and BEAVER, E. T. (1953). 'Cell division in trypanosomes,' *Trans. Amer. micro. Soc.*, **72,** 236.

NODENOT, L., RIDET, J., CHARTOL, A., and DESMOULINS, G. (1960). 'Un médicament nouveau contre la maladie du sommeil le Mel W,' *Méd. trop.*, **20,** 679.

NÖLLER, W. (1925). 'Der Nachweis des Uebertragers des gemeinen Rinder-trypanosomas, *T. theileri*, mit Hilfe des Kulturverfahrens,' *Cbl. Bakt.* (*I. Referate*), **79,** 133.

NORTHERN NIGERIA, MINISTRY OF HEALTH (1964). *Rural Health Report, 1963.* Kaduna, Govt. Printer.

NOSSAL, G. J. V. (1962). 'Cellular genetics of immune responses,' *Advances in Immunology*, **2,** 163.

NOVY, F. G., DE KRUIF, P. H., and NOVY, R. L. (1917). 'Anaphylatoxin and Anaphylaxis. I. Trypanosome anaphylatoxin,' *J. infect. Dis.*, **20,** 499.

NUTTALL, G. H. F. (1904). *Blood immunity and blood relationships.* Cambridge University Press.

OAKLEY, C. L., and FULTHORPE, A. J. (1953). 'Antigenic analysis by diffusion,' *J. Path. Bact.*, **65,** 49.

OCCGE (Organisation de Coordination et de Coopération pour la Lutte contre les Grandes Endémies) (1966). *Report of Sixth Technical Conference*, **2,** 384.

OCEAC (Organisation de Coordination pour la Lutte contre les Endémies en Afrique Centrale) (1967). *Report of the Second Technical Conference*, **1,** 225.

OCHMANN, R. (1905). 'Trypanosomiasis beim Schweine,' *Berl. tierärztl. Wschr.*, **19,** 337.

OLESON, J. J., BENNETT, P. L., HALLIDAY, S. L., and WILLIAMS, J. H. (1955). 'The effect of the hydrolysis products of puromycin in mouse mammary tumours,' *Acta Un. int. Cancer*, **11,** 161.

ONYANGO, R. J., DE RAADT, P., and MBWABI, D. (1967). 'A trial of isometamidium in a patient with a Mel B resistant *T. rhodesiense* infection.' *See* EATRO (1967), p. 88.

ONYANGO, R. J., HOEVE, K. VAN, and RAADT, P. DE (1966). 'The epidemiology of *T. rhodesiense* sleeping sickness in Alego Location, Central Nyanza, Kenya. I. Evidence that cattle may act as reservoir hosts of trypanosomes infective to man,' *Trans. R. Soc. trop. Med. Hyg.*, **60,** 175.

ORMEROD, W. E. (1958). 'A comparative study of cytoplasmic inclusions (volutin granules) in different species of trypanosomes,' *J. gen. Microbiol.*, **19,** 271.

ORMEROD, W. E. (1960). 'Cell inclusions and the epidemiology of Rhodesian sleeping sickness,' *Trans. R. Soc. trop. Med. Hyg.*, **54,** 299.

ORMEROD, W. E. (1961). 'The epidemic spread of Rhodesian sleeping sickness 1908–60,' *Trans. R. Soc. trop. Med. Hyg.*, **55,** 525.

ORMEROD, W. E. (1961a) 'The study of volutin granules in trypanosomes,' *Trans. R. Soc. trop. Med. Hyg.*, **55,** 313.

ORMEROD, W. E. (1962). 'The appearance of "volutin granules" in *Trypanosoma rhodesiense* studied by phase-contrast and electron microscopy,' *Parasitology*, **52,** 9P–10P.

ORMEROD, W. E. (1963). 'A comparative study of growth and morphology of strains of *Trypanosoma rhodesiense*,' *Exp. Parasit.*, **13,** 374.

ORMEROD, W. E. (1966). 'New evidence of the nature and significance of cytoplasmic granules in trypanosomes,' *Proc. I. Intern. Congr. Parasitology*, Rome, 1964, **1,** 322.

ORMEROD, W. E. (1966a). 'The trypanosome as a secretory cell. Sixth seminar on trypanosomiasis,' *Trans. R. Soc. trop. Med. Hyg.*, **60,** 117.

ORMEROD, W. E. (1967). 'Taxonomy of the sleeping sickness trypanosomes,' *J. Parasit.*, **53,** 824.

ORMEROD, W. E., and SHAW, J. J. (1963). 'A study of granules and other changes in phase-contrast appearance produced by chemotherapeutic agents in trypanosomes,' *Brit. J. Pharmacol.*, **21,** 259.

OSAKI, H. (1959). 'Studies on the immunological variation in *Trypanosoma gambiense* (Serotypes and mode of relapse),' *Biken J.*, **2,** 113.

OUCHTERLONY, O. (1948). '*In vitro* method for testing the toxin-producing capacity of diphtheria bacteria,' *Acta Path. Microbiol. Scand.*, **23,** 186.

OUCHTERLONY, O. (1964). 'Gel-Diffusion Techniques,' in *Immunological Methods* (ed. J. F. Ackroyd). Oxford, Blackwell. pp. 55–78.

OUDIN, J. (1946). 'Méthode d'analyse immunochimique par précipitation spécifique en milieu gélifié,' *C. R. Acad. Sci.*, Paris, **222,** 115.

OVAZZA, M. (1956). 'Contribution à l'étude des diptères vulnérants de l'Empire d'Éthiopie. IV. *Glossina*,' *Bull. Soc. Path. exot.*, **49,** 204.

OVERBY, L. R., and FREDERICKSON, R. L. (1963). 'Metabolic stability of radioactive arsanilic acid in chickens,' *J. Agr. Food. Chem.*, **11,** 378.

OVERBY, L. R., and FREDERICKSON, R. L. (1965). 'Metabolism of arsanilic acid. II. Localization and type of arsenic excreted and retained by chickens,' *Toxicol. Appl. Pharmacol.*, **7,** 855.

PAGE, W. A. (1959). 'The ecology of *Glossina palpalis* (R.-D.) in Southern Nigeria,' *Bull. ent. Res.*, **50,** 617.

PAGE, W. A., and MCDONALD, W. A. (1959). 'An assessment of the degree of man–fly contact exhibited by *Glossina palpalis* at water holes in northern and southern Nigeria,' *Ann. trop. Med. Parasit.*, **53,** 162.

PARKER, A. H. (1956). 'Laboratory studies on the selection of the breeding-site by *Glossina palpalis*,' *Ann. trop. Med. Parasit.*, **50,** 49.

PARKER, A. H. (1956a). 'Experiments on the behaviour of *G. palpalis* larvae, together with observations on the natural breeding-places of the species during the wet season,' *Ann. trop. Med. Parasit.*, **50,** 69.

PARKIN, B. S. (1948). 'The demonstration and transmission of the South African strain of *T. equiperdum* of horses,' *Onderstepoort J.*, **23,** 41.

PATRICK, J. B., and MEYER, W. E. (1968). 'The structure of Nucleocidin. II,' *Amer. chem. Soc. 156th Meeting*, Abstr. MEDI 024.

PATRICK, H., VOITLE, R. H., HYRE, H. M., and MARTIN, W. G. (1964). 'Incorporation of arsenic into cock sperm,' *Proc. Soc. exp. Biol.*, **117,** 365.

PATTON, W. S. (1934). 'Studies on the higher Diptera of medical and veterinary importance. A revision of the species of the genus *Glossina* Wiedemann, based on a comparative study of the male and female terminalia,' *Ann. trop. Med. Parasit.*, **28,** 315.

PATTON, W. S. (1936). 'Studies on the higher Diptera of medical and veterinary importance. A revision of the species of the genus *Glossina* Wiedemann based on a comparative study of the male and female terminalia,' *Ann. trop. Med. Parasit.*, **30,** 71.

PATTON, W. S. (1936a). 'Studies on the higher Diptera of medical and veterinary importance. A revision of the species of the genus *Glossina* Wiedemann based on a comparative study of the male and female terminalia,' *Ann. trop. Med. Parasit.*, **30,** 151.

PATTON, W. S. (1936b). 'Studies on the higher Diptera of medical and veterinary importance. A revision of the species of the genus *Glossina* Wiedemann based on a comparative study of the male and female terminalia,' *Ann. trop. Med. Parasit.*, **30,** 305.

PAUL, H. E., and PAUL, M. F. (1966). 'The nitrofurans-chemotherapeutic properties,' in *Experimental Chemotherapy*, Vol. IV (ed. R. J. Schnitzer and F. Hawking). New York, Academic Press, pp. 521.

PAUL, M. F., PAUL, H. E., BENDER, R. C., KOPKO, F., HARRINGTON, C. M., ELLS, V. R., and BUZARD, J. A. (1960). 'Studies on the distribution and excretion of certain nitrofurans,' *Antibiot. Chemotherapy*, **10,** 287.

PAUTRIZEL, R., LAFAYE, A., and DURET, J. (1959). 'Diagnostic sérologique de la maladie du sommeil. I. Amélioration de l'antigène préparé à partir de *Trypanosoma equiperdum*,' *Bull. Soc. Path. exot.*, **52,** 318.

PAUTRIZEL, R., MATTERN, P., and DURET, J. (1960). 'Diagnostic sérologique de la maladie du sommeil. II. Les anticorps fixant le complément au cours de l'infection,' *Bull. Soc. Path. exot.*, **53,** 878.

PEARCE, L., and BROWN, W. H. (1918). 'Experimental trypanosomiasis: its application in chemotherapeutic investigations,' *J. exp. Med.*, **28,** 109.

PEARSALL, W. H. (1959). 'Game protection as a form of land-use,' *Oryx*, V, 19.

PEEL, E., and CHARDOME, M. (1953). 'Note préliminaire sur *Trypanosoma suis*, évoluant dans les glandes salivaires de *Glossina brevipalpis*,' *Ann. Soc. belge Méd. trop.*, **33,** 457.

PEEL, E., and CHARDOME, M. (1954). '*Trypanosoma suis* Ochmann, 1905, trypanosome monomorphe pathogène de mammifères, évoluant dans les glandes salivaires de *G. brevipalpis* Newst., Mosso (Urundi),' *Ann. Soc. belge Méd. trop.*, **34,** 277.

PEEL, E., and CHARDOME, M. (1954a). 'Étude expérimentale d'une souche considerée comme *Trypanosoma congolense* Broden, 1904 et transmise par *Glossina brevipalpis* du Mosso (Urundi),' *Ann. Soc. belge Méd. trop.*, **34,** 297.

PEEL, E., and CHARDOME, M. (1954b). 'Étude expérimentale d'une souche appelée *Trypanosoma congolense* var. *urundiense* transmise par *Glossina brevipalpis* du Mosso (Urundi),' *Ann. Soc. belge Méd. trop.*, **34,** 303.

PEEL, E., and CHARDOME, M. (1954c). 'Étude expérimentale d'une souche appelée *Trypanosoma congolense* var. *mossoense* transmise par *Glossina brevipalpis* du Mosso (Urundi),' *Ann. Soc. belge Méd. trop.*, **34,** 321.

PEEL, E., and CHARDOME, M. (1954d). 'Étude expérimentale de souches de *Trypanosoma simiae* Bruce 1912, transmises par *G. brevipalpis* du Mosso (Urundi),' *Ann. Soc. belge Méd. trop.*, **34,** 345.

PEEL, E., and CHARDOME, M. (1954e). '*Trypanosoma suis* Ochmann, 1905, a porcine trypanosome from the Belgian Congo, with metacyclic development in the salivary glands of *Glossina*,' *Trans. R. Soc. trop. Med. Hyg.*, **48,** 288.

PELLEGRINI, D. (1948). '*Trypanosoma simiae* (Bruce) infection of the camel,' *E. Afr. agric. J.*, **13,** 207.

PENTSCHEW, A. (1958). 'Vergiftung durch organische Arsenverbindungen,' *Handbuch der speziellen pathologischen Anatomie und Histologie*, (ed. W. Scholz) 13ster Band, 2ter Teil: *Erkrankungen des zentralen Nervensystems II*, 2078–2102. Berlin, Springer.

PEOPLES, S. A. (1964). 'Arsenic toxicity in cattle,' *Ann. N.Y. Acad. Sci.*, **111,** 644.

PERCIVAL, A. BLAYNEY (1918). 'Game and Disease,' *J. E. Afr. Uganda Nat. Hist. Soc.*, **13,** 302.

PERSOONS, C. J. (1967). 'Trapping *G. pallidipes* and *G. palpalis fuscipes* in scented traps.' *See* ISCTR (1967), p. 127.

PERUZZI, M. (1928). 'Pathologico-anatomical and serological observations on the trypanosomiases,' *Final Report League of Nations International Commission on Human Trypanosomiasis*, Geneva. 245–324.

PETANA, W. B. (1963). 'A method for counting trypanosomes using Gram's iodine as diluent,' *Trans. R. Soc. trop. Med. Hyg.*, **57,** 382.

PETANA, W. B. (1964). 'The action of oxytetracycline upon African trypanosomes *in vitro*,' *Ann. trop. Med. Parasit.*, **58,** 13.

PHELPS, R. J. and BURROWS, P. M. (1969). 'Lethal temperatures for puparia of *Glossina morsitans orientalis* Vanderplank.' *Entomologia exp. appl.*, **12,** 23.

PHELPS, R. J., and BURROWS, P. M. (1969a). Puparial duration in *G. morsitans orientalis* Vanderplank under conditions of constant temperatures,' *Entomologia exp. appl.*, **12,** 33.

PHELPS, R. J., and BURROWS, P. M. (1969b). 'Prediction of pupal duration of *Glossina morsitans orientalis* Vanderplank under field conditions.' *J. appl. Ecol.*, **6,** 323.

PHELPS, R. J., SIMMONDS, A. M., and PARSONS, R. (1966). 'Pupal collection and respiratory physiology,' *Agricultural Research Council of Central Africa Annual Report, 1966*, 77.

PHILIPS, F. S., STERNBERG, S. S., CRONIN, A. P., SODERGREN, J. E., and VIDAL, P. M. (1967). 'Physiologic disposition and intracellular localization of Isometamidium,' *Cancer Res.*, **27,** 333.

PIERAERTS, G. (1952). 'Sur le fond d'oeil dans la trypanosomiase humaine,' *Bull. Soc. Path. exot.*, **45,** 357.

PILLE, G. (1953). 'Considérations pharmacologiques sur les diamidines et leur utilisation dans la trypanosomaise,' *Méd. trop.*, **13,** 859.

PILSON, R. D. (1967). 'Behaviour studies of the vector in relation to the control of trypanosomiasis,' *Proc. & Trans. Rhod. Sci. Assoc.*, **52,** 21.

PILSON, R. D., and HARLEY, J. M. B. (1959). 'The importance of cattle as a host of *Glossina morsitans* in Ankole,' *See* EATRO (1959), p. 45.

PILSON, R. D., and LEGGATE, B. M. (1962). 'A diurnal and seasonal study of the feeding activity of *Glossina pallidipes* Aust,' *Bull. ent. Res.*, **53,** 541.

PILSON, R. D., and LEGGATE, B. M. (1962a). 'A diurnal and seasonal study of the resting behaviour of *Glossina pallidipes* Aust.,' *Bull. ent. Res.*, **53,** 551.

PILSON, R. D., and PILSON, B. M. (1967). 'Behaviour studies of *Glossina morsitans* Westw. in the field,' *Bull. ent. Res.*, **57,** 227.

PINTO, A. C. DU R. (1960). 'Um caso de doença de sono congénita,' *Anai. Inst. Med. trop. Lisb.*, **17,** 1195.

PINTO, A. R., PARREIRA, F., and FRANCO, A. (1953). 'A mielocultura na doença do sono,' *Trop. Dis. Bull.*, **50,** 800.

PIRES, F. A. (1960). 'Uma nova espécie de *Glossino* do grupo *Morsitans* (Diptera, Muscidae) *Glossina borgesi* sp. nov.,' *Bol. Soc. Est. Moçambique*, **29,** No. 125, Section D, No. 4, 4 pp. text, 8 pp. figs.

PIRES, F. A., and DA SILVA, J. M. (1960). 'Subsídios para o estudo das *Glossinas* do Ultramar português. Sobre a morfologia da armadura genital da *G. pallidipes* Austen, 1903. (Diptera),' *Bol. Soc. Est. Moçambique*, V. **29,** No. 125, Section D, No. 3, 10 pp. text, 14 pp. figs.

PLIMMER, H. G., and BRADFORD, J. R. (1899). 'A preliminary note on the morphology and distribution of the organism found in the tsetse fly disease,' *Proc. Roy. Soc.*, B, **65,** 274.

POLGE, C., and SOLTYS, M. A. (1957). 'Preservation of trypanosomes in the frozen state,' *Trans. R. Soc. trop. Med. Hyg.*, **51,** 519.

POTTS, W. H. (1924). 'A new variety of *Glossina schwetzi* Newstead & Evans, from the Belgian Congo,' *Ann. trop. Med. Parasit.*, **18,** 205.

POTTS, W. H. (1930). 'A contribution to the study of numbers of tsetse fly (*Glossina morsitans* Westw.) by quantitative methods,' *S. Afr. J. Sci.*, **27,** 491.

POTTS, W. H. (1933). 'Observations on *Glossina morsitans* Westw. in East Africa,' *Bull. ent. Res.*, **24,** 293.

POTTS, W. H. (1937). 'The distribution of tsetse flies in Tanganyika Territory,' *Bull. ent. Res.*, **28,** 129.

POTTS, W. H. (1950). '*Tsetse Research.*' *See* EATRO (1950), p. 6.

POTTS, W. H. (1950a). '*Tsetse Research.*' *See* EATRO (1950a), p. 11.

POTTS, W. H. (1953–4). *Distribution of tsetse species in Africa, compiled from information collated by W. H. Potts.* London. Directorate of Colonial Surveys.

POTTS, W. H. (1955). 'A new tsetse-fly from the British Cameroons,' *Ann. trop. Med. Parasit.*, **49,** 218.

POTTS, W. H. (1956). 'Genitalia of *Glossina palpalis* collected on the Zambesi river by Sir John Kirk in 1864,' *Trans. R. Soc. trop. Med. Hyg.*, **50,** 303.

POTTS, W. H. (1958). 'Sterilization of tsetse flies (*Glossina*) by gamma irradiation,' *Ann. trop. Med. Parasit.*, **52,** 484.

POTTS, W. H. (1965). 'The gamma irradiation of *Glossina* puparial stages and control,' *Proc. XII Intern. Congr. Ent. Lond.*, 1964, 254. London. 1965.

POTTS, W. H., and JACKSON, C. H. N. (1952). 'The Shinyanga game destruction experiment,' *Bull. ent. Res.*, **43,** 365.

POWER, R. J. B. (1964). 'The activity pattern of *Glossina longipennis* Corti,' *Proc. R. ent. Soc. Lond.*, (A) **39,** 5.

PRATES, M. M. (1928). 'Report 7. Organisation of experimental work on Glossinae at the Entebbe laboratory,' *Final Report of the League of Nations International Commission on Human Trypanosomiasis*, Geneva. p. 233.

PRATT, D. J., GREENWAY, P. J., and GWYNNE, M. D. (1966). 'A classification of East African rangeland with an appendix on terminology,' *J. appl. Ecol.*, **3,** 369.

PRATT, H. S. (1899). 'The anatomy of the female genital tract of the Pupipara as observed in *Melophagus ovinus*,' *Z. wiss. Zool.*, **66,** 16.

PREER, J. R. (1956). 'A quantitative technique of double diffusion in agar,' *J. Immunol.*, **77,** 52.

RADERMECKER, J. (1954). 'Sur la précocité des modifications EEG dans la trypanosomiase humaine expérimentale,' *Bull. Soc. Path. exot.*, **47,** 397.

RAFFEL, S. (1934). 'Studies in immunity to trypanosomes. I. Acquired immunity in *Trypanosoma equiperdum* infected rats. The Rieckenberg reaction,' *Amer. J. Hyg.*, **19,** 416.

RAJAGOPAL, P. K., and BURSELL, E. (1965). 'The effect of temperature on the oxygen consumption of tsetse pupae,' *Bull. ent. Res.*, **56,** 219.

RAJAGOPAL, P. K., and BURSELL, E. (1966). 'The respiratory metabolism of resting tsetse flies,' *Jour. Ins. Physiol.*, **12,** 287.

RAY, H. N., DAS GUPTA, N. N., DE, M. L., and GUHA, A. (1955). 'A new structure observed in *Trypanosome evansi*,' *Nature*, Lond. **175,** 392.

RAY, H. N., and MALHOTRA, M. N. (1960). 'Akinetoplastic strain of *Trypanosoma evansi* produced by "Prothidium",' *Nature*, Lond. **188,** 870.

REES, R. J. W., and HART, P. D'A. (1956). 'The enhancement of experimental tuberculosis in the mouse by suramin,' *Tubercle*, **37,** 327.

REGENDANZ, P., and HOEPPLI, R. (1929). 'Die Einwanderung der Trypanosomen in das Gewebe und die dadurch bewirkten histopathologischen Veränderungen,' *Arch. Schiffs. Tropenhyg.*, **33,** 376.

REGIONAL ECONOMIC ATLAS (1965). 'Africa.' Oxford, Clarendon Press.

REICHENOW, E. (1921). 'Untersuchungen über das Verhalten von *Trypanosoma gambiense* im menschlichen Körper,' *Z. Hyg.*, **94,** 266.

REICHENOW, E. (1929). 'Über *Trypanosoma gambiense* im Liquor cerebrospinalis des Menschen,' *Berlin Klin. Woch.*, **58,** 251.

REICHENOW, E. (1937). 'Dauerkultur pathogener Trypanosomen,' *C. R. XII Congr. Intern. Zool.*, Lisbon 1935, p. 1955.

REICHENOW, E. (1940). 'Ostafrikanische Beobachtungen an Trypanosomiden,' *Arch. Protistenk.*, **94,** 267.

REICHENOW, E. (1940a). 'Zur Frage der Bedeutung des Blepharoplasts der Trypanosomen,' *Archos Inst. biol.*, San Paulo, **11,** 433.

RENNISON, B. D., LUMSDEN, W. H. R., and WEBB, C. J. (1958). 'Use of reflecting paints for detecting tsetse fly at night,' *Nature*, Lond. **181,** 1354.

RENNISON, B. D., and SMITH, I. M. (1961). 'Studies of the sampling of *Glossina pallidipes* Aust. IV. Some aspects of the use of Morris traps,' *Bull. ent. Res.*, **52,** 609.

REPORT (1964). *See* under Northern Nigeria.

RICH, N. A., MEYERS, P., WEINBAUM, G., CORY, J. G., and SUHADOLNIK, R. S. (1965). 'Inhibition of human tumour cells by Cordycepin,' *Biochim. biophys. Acta*, **95,** 194.

RICHARDS, W. H. G. (1965). 'Pharmacologically active substances in the blood, tissues and urine of mice infected with *Trypanosoma brucei*,' *Br. J. Pharmac. Chemother.*, **24,** 124.

RICHARDSON, U. F., and KENDALL, S. B. (1957). *Veterinary Protozoology.* 2nd ed. London and Edinburgh, Oliver & Boyd.

RICHET, P. (1954). 'Diverse considerations on the prophylaxis of human trypanosomiasis in French Equatorial Africa.' *See* ISCTR (1954), p. 72.

RICHET, P. (1965). 'L'histoire et l'oeuvre de l'OCCGE en Afrique Occidentale Francophone,' *Trans. R. Soc. trop. Med. Hyg.*, **59,** 234.

RICHET, LOTTE, and DUCASSE (1958). 'Gravité particulière de la grippe au cours de la récente épidémie chez des trypanosomes en basse Côte d'Ivoire,' *Bull. méd. AOF,* **3,** 91.

RICHET, P., LOTTE, M., and FOUCHER, G. (1959). 'Résultats des traitements de la trypanosomiase humaine à *T. gambiense* par le Mel B ou l'arsobal dans le secteur special No. 43 à Natitingou (Nord Dahomey),' *Méd. trop.*, **19,** 253.

RIDLEY, H. (1945). 'Ocular lesions in trypanosomiasis,' *Ann. trop. Med. Parasit.*, **39,** 66.

RIECKENBERG, H. (1917). 'Eine neue Immunitätsreaktion bei experimenteller Trypanosomen-Infektion: die Blutplättchenprobe,' *Z. Immun. Forsch.*, **26,** 53.

RINEY, T. (1965). *Freedom from Hunger*, **6,** 36.

RIORDAN, K. (1966). 'Measurement by two methods of susceptibility to DDT and Dieldrin of *Glossina palpalis* in Northern Nigeria,' *Bull. ent. Res.*, **57,** 49.

RIORDAN, K. (1968). 'Chromosomes of the tsetse fly, *Glossina palpalis*,' *Parasitology*, **58,** 835.

RIORDAN, K. (1970). 'Polytene chromosomes of *Glossina palpalis* Robineau-Desvoidy (Diptera: Muscidae) II. Their improved demonstration,' *Proc. R. ent. Soc. Lond.*, (A) **45** (*in press*).

RIOU, G. (1967). 'Induction d'une "dyskinétoplastie" par le bromure d'éthidium chez *Trypanosoma cruzi* cultivé *in vitro*,' *C. R. Acad. Sci., Paris*, **265,** 2004.

RIOU, G. (1968). 'Disparition de l'ADN du kinétoplaste de *Trypanosoma cruzi* cultivé en présence de Bromure d'Ethidium,' *C. R. Acad. Sci., Paris*, **266,** 250.

RITZ, H. (1914). 'On relapses in experimental trypanosomiasis,' *Deut. Med. Woch.*, **40,** 1355.

RITZ, H. (1916). 'On relapses in experimental trypanosomiasis: 2nd communication,' *Arch. Schiffs. Tropenhyg.*, **20,** 397.

ROBERTSON, A. G., and BERNACCA, J. P. (1958). 'Game elimination as a tsetse control measure in Uganda.' *See* ISCTR (1958), p. 103.

ROBERTSON, A. G., and KLUGE, E. B. (1968). 'The use of insecticide in arresting an advance of *Glossina morsitans* Westwood in the south east lowveld of Rhodesia,' *Proc. and Trans. Rhod. Sci. Ass.*, **53,** 17.

ROBERTSON, D. H. H. (1960). 'Nitrofurazone in *T. rhodesiense* sleeping sickness.' *See* EATRO (1960), p. 41.

ROBERTSON, D. H. H. (1961). 'Nitrofurazone-induced haemolytic anaemia in a refractory case of *T. rhodesiense* sleeping sickness: the haemolytic trait and self-limiting haemolytic anaemia,' *Ann. trop. Med. Parasit.*, **55,** 49.

ROBERTSON, D. H. H. (1961a). 'The haemolytic effect of primaquine and nitrofurazone in cases of sleeping sickness with the haemolytic trait,' *Ann. trop. Med. Parasit.*, **55,** 278.

ROBERTSON, D. H. H. (1962). 'Chemotherapy of African trypanosomiasis,' *Practitioner*, **188,** 80.

ROBERTSON, D. H. H. (1963). 'The treatment of sleeping sickness (mainly due to *T. rhodesiense*) with melarsoprol. I. Reactions observed during treatment,' *Trans. R. Soc. trop. Med. Hyg.*, **57,** 122.

ROBERTSON, D. H. H. (1963a). 'The treatment of sleeping sickness (mainly due to *T. rhodesiense*) with melarsoprol. II. An assessment of its curative value,' *Trans. R. Soc. trop. Med. Hyg.*, **57,** 176.

ROBERTSON, D. H. H. (1963b). 'A trial of Mel W in the treatment of *Trypanosoma rhodesiense* sleeping sickness,' *Trans. R. Soc. trop. Med. Hyg.*, **57,** 274.

ROBERTSON, D. H. H., and BAKER, J. R. (1958). 'Human trypanosomiasis in south-east Uganda. I. A study of the epidemiology and present virulence of the disease,' *Trans. R. Soc. trop. Med. Hyg.*, **52,** 337.

ROBERTSON, D. H. H., and JENKINS, A. R. (1959). 'Hepatic dysfunction in human trypanosomiasis. I. Abnormalities of excretory function, sero-flocculation phenomena and other tests of hepatic function with observations on the alterations of these tests during treatment and convalescence,' *Trans. R. Soc. trop. Med. Hyg.*, **53,** 511.

ROBERTSON, D. H. H., and KNIGHT, R. H. (1964). 'Observations on the polyneuropathy and the disordered pyruvate metabolism induced by nitrofurazone in cases of sleeping sickness due to *Trypanosoma rhodesiense*,' *Acta trop.*, **21,** 239.

ROBERTSON, D. H. H., MBWABI, D., and BAKARI, N. (1963). 'Laevo-furaltadone in *Trypanosoma rhodesiense* trypanosomiasis.' *See* EATRO (1963a), p. 40.

ROBERTSON, M. (1913). 'Notes on the life history of *Trypanosoma gambiense*,' *Repts. Sleep. Sickn. Comm. Roy. Soc.*, **13,** 119.

ROBINSON, E. M. (1926). 'Serological investigations into some diseases of domesticated animals in South Africa caused by trypanosomes,' *Rep. Dir. Vet. Educ. Res., Dept. Agric. S. Africa*, Nos. 11–12, 9.

ROBINSON, E. M. (1948). 'Notes on serological tests carried out on equine species infected with Dourine,' *Onderstepoort J.*, **23,** 33.

ROBINSON, E. M. (1948a). 'Dourine infection in young equines,' *Onderstepoort J.*, **23,** 39.

ROBINSON, G. G. (1964). 'Abnormality in tsetse fly,' *Trans. R. Soc. trop. Med. Hyg.*, **58,** 579.

ROBINSON, G. G. (1965). 'A note on nocturnal resting sites of *Glossina morsitans* Westw. in the Republic of Zambia,' *Bull. ent. Res.*, **56,** 351.

ROBSON, J. (1962). 'Prophylaxis against trypanosomiasis in zebu cattle. III. Potentiation trials and a trial of RD 2902 in an area of medium trypanosome risk,' *Vet. Rec.*, **74,** 481.

RODGER, F. C. (1958). 'Comparison of the effect upon onchocerciasis of five drugs and selection of the one best able to prevent ocular complications,' *Trans. R. Soc. trop. Med. Hyg.*, **52,** 462.

RODHAIN, J., VALCKE, G., and VAN GOIDSENHOVEN, C. (1941). 'Considérations sur le diagnostic et la thérapeutique de la méningo-encéphalite trypanosomique humaine d'apres l'observation de quatre Européens atteints de la maladie du sommeil. Existence dans le sang et liquide encéphalorachidies des malades des sensibilistarices fixant le complément,' *Ann. Soc. belge Méd. trop.*, **21,** 195.

RODHAIN, J., and VAN GOIDSENHOVEN, C. (1944). 'Persistance prolongée de sensibilisatrice fixant l'alexine après guérison de la trypanosomiase,' *Ann. Soc. belge Méd. trop.*, **24,** 235.

RODHAIN, J., and VAN HOOF, M. T. (1944). 'Au sujet d'un élevage de *Glossina palpalis* en Europe et de quelques essais d'évolution chez cette glossine des *Trypanosoma lewisi* et *cruzi*,' *Ann. Soc. belge Méd. trop.*, **24,** 54.

ROEHL, W. (1926). 'Über die Wirkungsweise von Stoffen aus der Reihe des "Bayer 205",' *Arch. Schiffs. Tropenhyg.*, **30** (Beiheft 1), 103.

ROLLO, I. M., and WILLIAMSON, J. (1951). 'Acquired resistance to "melarsen", tryparsamide and amidines in pathogenic trypanosomes after treatment with "Melarsen" alone,' *Nature*, Lond. Jan. 27, 147.

ROSENTHAL, F. (1913). 'Untersuchungen über die Genese des Rezidivs bei experimentellen Trypanosomen-Infektion,' *Z. Hyg. InfektKr.*, **74,** 489.

ROUBAUD, E. (1909). *La* Glossina palpalis *R.-Desv. sa biologie, son rôle dans l'étiologie des trypanosomiases*. Thesis No. 1344, Paris University.

ROUBAUD, E. (1913). 'Évolution comparée des trypanosomes pathogènes chez les glossines,' *Bull. Soc. Path. exot.*, **6,** 435.

ROUBAUD, E. (1917). 'Histoire d'un élevage de *Glossina morsitans* à l'Institut Pasteur de Paris,' *Bull. Soc. Path. exot.*, **10,** 629.

ROUBAUD, E. (1935). 'Les modalités atypiques de l'infection trypanosomienne cyclique chez les glossines,' *Ann. Inst. Pasteur*, **55,** 340.

ROUBAUD, E., and COLAS-BELCOUR, J. (1936). 'Observations biologiques sur les glossines (*Gl. palpalis, Gl. morsitans*),' *Bull. Soc. Path. exot.*, **29,** 691.

ROUBAUD, E., MAILLOT, L., and RAGEAU, J. (1951). 'Infection naturelle de *Glossina caliginea* Austen dans les gîtes à palétuviers de Douala (Cameroun Français),' *Bull. Soc. Path. exot.*, **44,** 309.

ROUBAUD, E., STEFANOPOULO, G. J., and DUVOLON, S. (1944). 'Étude chez le rat blanc d'une souche neurotrope de *Trypanosoma gambiense*,' *Bull. Soc. Path. exot.*, **37,** 292.

ROUBAUD, E., and TREILLARD, M. (1935). 'Un coccobacille pathogène pour les mouches tsétsés,' *C. R. Acad. Sci.*, **201,** 304.

ROUBAUD, E., and TREILLARD, M. (1936). 'Infection expérimentale de *Glossina palpalis* par un coccobacille pathogène pour les muscidés,' *Bull. Soc. Path. exot.*, **29,** 145.

RUDZINSKA, M. A. and VICKERMAN, K. (1968). 'The fine structure,' in *Infectious Blood Diseases of Man and Animals* (ed. D. Weinman and M. Ristic). Vol. 1, Part II, Chapter 4. New York and London, Academic Press.

RUSSELL, H. (1936). 'Observations on immunity in relapsing fever and trypanosomiasis,' *Trans. R. Soc. trop. Med. Hyg.*, **30,** 179.

RUTTER, T. E. G. (1967). 'Diseases of camels. Part 2. Protozoal diseases,' *Vet. Bull.*, **37,** 611.

RUTTLEDGE, W. (1928). 'Tsetse fly (*Glossina morsitans*) in the Koalib Hills, Nuba Mountains Province, Sudan,' *Bull. ent. Res.*, **19,** 309.

RYLEY, J. F. (1964). 'A chemoprophylactic approach to babesiasis,' *Res. in Vet. Sci.*, **5,** No. 4, 411.

RYLEY, J. F. (1966). 'Histochemical studies on blood and culture forms of *Trypanosoma rhodesiense*.' In *Proc. 1st Int. Congr. Parasitology*. Vol. I, p. 41.

SADUN, E. H., DUXBURY, R. E., WILLIAMS, J. S., and ANDERSON, R. I. (1963). 'Fluorescent antibody test for the serodiagnosis of African and American Trypanosomiasis in man,' *J. Parasit.*, **49,** 385.

SAUNDERS, D. S. (1960). 'The "white-clubbed" form of *Syntomosphyrum* (Hym., Eulophidae) parasitic on tsetse flies,' *Bull. ent. Res.*, **51,** 17.

SAUNDERS, D. S. (1960a). 'On the stages of development of *Syntomosphyrum albiclavus* Kerrich (Hym., Eulophidae) a parasite of tsetse flies,' *Bull. ent. Res.*, **51,** 25.

SAUNDERS, D. S. (1960b). 'The ovulation cycle in *Glossina morsitans* Westwood (Diptera: Muscidae) and a possible method of age determination for female tsetse flies by the examination of their ovaries,' *Trans. Roy. ent. Soc. Lond.*, **112,** 221.

SAUNDERS, D. S. (1961). 'Studies on ovarian development in tsetse flies (*Glossina*, Diptera),' *Parasitology*, **51,** 545.

SAUNDERS, D. S. (1962). 'Age determination for female tsetse flies and the age compositions of samples of *Glossina pallidipes* Aust., *G. palpalis fuscipes* Newst. and *G. brevipalpis* Newst.,' *Bull. ent. Res.*, **53,** 579.

SAUNDERS, D. S. (1964). 'Age changes in the ovaries in the sheep ked, *Melophagus ovinus* (L.) (Diptera: Hippoboscidae),' *Proc. R. ent. Soc. Lond.*, (A) **39,** 68.

SAUNDERS, D. S. (1967). 'Survival and reproduction in a natural population of the tsetse fly, *Glossina palpalis palpalis* (Robineau-Desvoidy),' *Proc. R. ent. Soc. Lond.*, (A) **42,** 129.

SAUVEL, R., THOMÉ, M., MAGIMEL, J., BALIS, J., and FINELLE, P. (1961). 'Recherches sur la toxicité et la valeur trypanopréventive du moranylate d'éthidium. I–IV,' *Rev. Élev. Méd. vét. Pays trop.*, **14,** 165.

SCANGA, F. (1959). *Atlante di microscopia elettronica.* Vol. 1. Roma, Pensiero Scientifico. p. 242–4.

SCHÄFER, G. (1963). 'Oligomycinähnlicher Effekt von Biguaniden,' *Biochem. Z.*, **339,** 46.

SCHANKER, L. S. (1962). 'Passage of drugs across body membranes,' *Pharmacol. Rev.*, **14,** 501.

SCHANKER, L. S. (1966). 'Passage of drugs into and out of the central nervous system,' in *Antimicrobial Agents and Chemotherapy* (ed. G. L. Hobby) Ann Arbor, Mich., American Society for Microbiology, 1965. p. 1044.

SCHILLING, C. (1902). 'Bericht über die Surra-Krankheit der Pferde und Rinder in Schutzgebiete Togo,' *Zbl. Bakt., I. Abt. orig.*, **31,** 452.

SCHILLING, C. (1935). 'Immunisation against trypanosomiasis,' *J. trop. Med. Hyg.*, **38,** 106.

SCHILLING, C. (1935a). 'Protective inoculation against tsetse fly disease and sleeping sickness,' *Tropenpflanzer*, **38,** 229.

SCHILLING, C. (1936). 'Immunization against trypanosomiasis,' *J. trop. Med. Hyg.*, **39,** 221.

SCHILLING, C. (1936a). 'Immunization against fly disease,' *Z. Immunforsch.*, **89,** 306.

SCHILLING, C. (1936b). 'Immunization against trypanosomiasis,' *Bull. Soc. Path. exot.*, **29,** 886.

SCHILLING, C., and NEUMANN, H. (1932). 'Zur Methodik der immunologischen Differenzierungsmethoden von Trypanosomenstämmen,' *Arch. Schiffs. Tropenhyg.*, **36,** 214.

SCHILLING, C., SCHRECK, H., NEUMANN, H., and KUMERT, H. (1933). 'Immunization against trypanosomal diseases,' *Deut. med. Woch.*, **59,** 1603.

SCHILLING, C., SCHRECK, H., NEUMANN, H., and KUMERT, H. (1933a). 'Immunization against trypanosomal diseases,' *Bull. Soc. Path. exot.*, **26,** 1004.

SCHILLING, C., SCHRECK, H., NEUMANN, H., and KUMERT, H. (1934). 'Immunization against trypanosomiasis,' *J. trop. Med. Hyg.*, **37,** 70.

SCHILLING, C., SCHRECK, H., NEUMANN, H., and KUMERT, H. (1934a). 'Research on protective inoculation against trypanosomiasis,' *Z. Immunforsch.*, **83,** 71.

SCHILLING, C., SCHRECK, H., NEUMANN, H., and KUMERT, H. (1935). 'Immunization against fly diseases,' *Z. Immunforsch.*, **85,** 513.

SCHILLING, C., SCHRECK, H., NEUMANN, H., and KUMERT, H. (1936). 'Immunization against fly diseases,' *Z. Immunforsch.*, **87,** 47.

SCHILLING, C., SCHRECK, H., NEUMANN, H., and KUMERT, H. (1936a). 'Immunization against fly diseases,' *Z. Immunforsch.*, **87,** 482.

SCHILLING, C., SCHRECK, H., NEUMANN, H., and KUMERT, H. (1936b). 'Experiments on protective inoculation against fly diseases,' *Z. Tschr. f. Immunitsf. u. Experim. Therap.*

SCHMIDT, G. (1965). 'Über die trypanocide Wirksamkeit von Terephthalaniliden,' *Experientia*, **21,** 276.

SCHNEIDER, J. (1963). 'Traitement de la trypanosomiase africaine humaine,' *Bull. Wld. Hlth. Org.*, **28** (5–6), 763.

SCHNEIDER, J., LEVEUF, J. J., and TANGARA, S. (1961). 'Traitement de la trypanosomiase africaine par le pentylthiarsphénylmélamine,' *Bull. Soc. Path. exot.*, **54,** 345.

SCHNITZER, R. J., and HAWKING, F. (1963). Editors. *Experimental Chemotherapy.* Vol. 1. New York and London, Academic Press. (Hawking, F. *Chemotherapy of Trypanosomiasis*, pp. 129–256.)

SCHOENAERS, F., NEUJEAN, G., and EVENS, F. (1953). 'Valeur pratique de la réaction de fixation du complément dans la maladie du sommeil à *T. gambiense.* I. Le diagnostic de la maladie,' *Ann. Soc. belge Méd. trop.*, **33,** 141.

SCHOENBACH, E. B., and GREENSPAN, E. M. (1948). 'The pharmacology, mode of action and therapeutic potentialities of stilbamidine, pentamidine, propamidine and other aromatic diamidines—a review,' *Medicine*, **27,** 327.

SCHUBERG, A., and BÖING, W. (1913). 'Über der Weg der Infektion bei Trypanosomen—und Spirochätenerkrankungen,' *Deut. med. Woch.*, **39,** 877.

SCHULZ, H., and MACCLURE, E. (1961). 'Elektronmikroskopische Untersuchung des *Trypanosoma cruzi* mit besonderer Berücksichtigung des Periplasten und des Blepharoplasten,' *Zeitschrift für Zellforschung*, **55,** 389.

SCHWETZ, J. (1928). 'A leishmanoid stage in the evolution of *Trypanosoma vivax* and *Trypanosoma congolense-dimorphon* in the vertebrate host (Bovine),' *Ann. Soc. belge Méd. trop.*, **8,** 315.

SCHWETZ, J. (1932). 'Sur la trypanosomiase virulente du porc,' *Bull. Soc. Path. exot.*, **25,** 906.

SCHWETZ, J. (1934). 'Contribution à l'étude des trypanosomes pathogènes des suidés,' *Bull. agric. Congo Belge.*, **25,** 313.

SCHWETZ, J. (1938). 'Quelques réflexions et suggestions pour une future classification des trypanosomes pathogènes,' *Ann. Soc. belge Méd. trop.*, **16,** 265.

SCHWETZ, J., and FORNARA, C. (1929). 'Developmental forms of trypanosomiasis in the vertebrate host,' *Bull. Soc. Path. exot.*, **22,** 862.

SCOTT, D. (1957). 'The epidemiology of human trypanosomiasis in Ashanti (Ghana),' *J. trop. Med. Hyg.*, **60,** 205.

SCOTT, D. (1959). 'Human trypanosomiasis in Northern Ghana, 1950–6. An epidemiological review,' *W. Afr. med. J.*, **8,** 165.

SCOTT, D. (1961). 'A recent series of outbreaks of human trypanosomiasis in Northern Ghana (1957–9),' *W. Afr. med. J.*, **10,** 122. *See* also ISCTR (1961), p. 45.

SCOTT, J. D. (1931). 'A practical method of marking insects in quantitative samples taken at regular intervals,' *S. Afr. J. Sci.*, **28,** 372.

SCOTT, J. D. (1934). 'Ecology of certain plant communities of the Central Province, Tanganyika Territory,' *J. Ecol.*, **22,** 177.

SCUDDER, S. H. (1892). '*U.S. Geological Survey, Bull. 93, 1892.* p. 19 [from Hegh, 1929, p. 71.]

SEBER, G. A. F. (1965). 'A note on multiple-recapture census,' *Biometrika*, **52,** 249.

SEED, J. R. (1963). 'The characterization of antigens isolated from *Trypanosoma rhodesiense*,' *J. Protozool.*, **10,** 380.

SEED, J. R., and BAQUERO, M. A. (1965). 'The characterization of hexokinase from *Trypanosoma rhodesiense* and *Trypanosoma gambiense*,' *J. Protozool.*, **12,** 427.

SEED, J. R., BYRAM, J., and GAM, A. A. (1967). 'Characterisation and localisation of acid phosphatase activity in *Trypanosoma gambiense*,' *J. Protozool*, **14,** 117.

SEED, J. R., and WEINMAN, D. (1963). 'Characterization of antigens isolated from *Trypanosoma rhodesiense*,' *Nature*, Lond. **198,** 197.

SEN, H. G., RAY, H. N., and DUTTA, B. N. (1954). 'Mode of action of Antrycide on *Trypanosoma evansi:* a preliminary note,' *Bull. Calcutta Sch. trop. Med.*, **2,** 18.

SERGENT, E., DONATIEN, A. L., PARROT, C. F., LESTOQUARD, F., PLANTUREUX, E., and BOUGEBIEF, N. (1924). 'Études expérimentales sur les piroplasmoses bovines d'Algérie,' *Ann. Inst. Pasteur*, **38,** 273.

SHINOZAWA, T., YAHARA, I., and IMAHORI, K. (1968). 'Interaction of polyvinyl sulfate with ribosomes,' *J. mol. Biol.*, **36,** 305.

SHIRCORE, J. O. (1914). 'Suggestions for the limitation and destruction of *Glossina morsitans*,' *Bull. ent. Res.*, **5,** 87.

SHIRCORE, J. O. (1916). 'A method for the trapping of *Glossina morsitans* suggested for trial,' *Trans. R. Soc. trop. Med. Hyg.*, **9,** No. 3, 101.

SHUTE, P. G., and MARYON, MARJORIE, E. (1966). *Laboratory Technique for the Study of Malaria.* 2nd edition. London, J. & A. Churchill.

SIEV, M., WEINBERG, R., and PENMAN, S. (1969). 'The selective interruption of nucleolar RNA synthesis in HeLa cells by Cordycepin,' *J. Cell. Biol.*, **41,** 510.

SILVA, M. A. DE A. (1957). 'The value of drugs commonly used in the treatment of *T. rhodesiense* sleeping sickness,' *An. Inst. Med. trop. Lisboa*, **14,** 159.

SILVA, M. A. DE A., and CASEIRO, A. (1957). 'Prophylactic action of diamidines against *T. rhodesiense* infection,' *An. Inst. Med. trop. Lisboa*, **14,** 171.

SILVA, M. A. DE A., and SILVA, J. M. DA (1960). 'On the incidence of trypanosomiasis in game.' *See* ISCTR (1960), p. 269.

SIMARD, R., and BERNHARD, W. (1966). 'Le phénomène de la ségrégation nucléolaire: spécificité d'action de certains antimétabolites,' *Int. J. Cancer*, **1,** 463.

References

SIMPSON, G. G. (1950). *The Meaning of Evolution*, London, Oxford University Press.

SIMPSON, H. R. (1958). 'The effect of sterilized males on a natural tsetse fly population,' *Biometrics*, **14**, 159.

SIMPSON, J. J. (1911). 'Entomological research in West Africa. I. Gambia,' *Bull. ent. Res.*, **2**, 187.

SIMPSON, J. J. (1918). 'Bionomics of tsetse and other parasitological notes in the Gold Coast,' *Bull. ent. Res.*, **8**, 193.

SLEEPING SICKNESS COMMITTEE (1914). *Report of the Departmental Committee on Sleeping Sickness.* London, HMSO, Cd. 7349.

SLEEPING SICKNESS COMMITTEE (1914a). *Minutes of Evidence taken by the Departmental Committee on Sleeping Sickness.* London, HMSO, Cd. 7350.

SMART, J. (1956). *A Handbook for the Identification of Insects of Medical Importance.* 3rd edition. London, Brit. Mus. (Nat. Hist.), 1956. xi + 303 pp.

SMEESTERS, C., and JACQUES, P. J. (1968). 'Influence of injected suramin on enzymic equipment of rat liver lysosomes *in vivo*,' *XII Int. Congress Cell. Biol.*, Brussels, 1968. *Excerpta Medica*, série intern. No. 166. Abstr. 143, p. 82.

SMITH, C. N., LA BRECQUE, G. C., and BORKOVEC, A. B. (1964). 'Insect chemosterilants,' *Ann. Rev. Ent.*, **9**, 269.

SMITH, G. W., and MILLER, J. M. (1955). 'Stilbamidine for tic douloureux,' *Lancet*, **269**, 723.

SMITH, I. M. (1958). 'The protection against trypanosomiasis conferred on cattle by repeated doses of Antrycide, along or with *Trypanosoma congolense*,' *Ann. trop. Med. Parasit.*, **52**, 391.

SMITH, I. M., and RENNISON, B. D. (1961). 'Studies on the sampling of *Glossina pallidipes* Aust. I. The numbers caught daily on cattle, in Morris traps and on a fly round,' *Bull. ent. Res.*, **52**, 165.

SMITH, I. M., and RENNISON, B. D. (1961a). 'Studies on the sampling of *Glossina pallidipes* Aust. II. The daily pattern of flies caught on cattle, in Morris traps and on a fly round,' *Bull. ent. Res.*, **52**, 183.

SMITH, I. M., and RENNISON, B. D. (1961b). 'Studies on the sampling of *Glossina pallidipes* Aust. III. The hunger stages of male flies caught on cattle and in Morris traps,' *Bull. ent. Res.*, **52**, 601.

SMITH, I. M., and SCOTT, W. N. (1961). 'Chemoprophylaxis against bovine trypanosomiasis. III. The cure of infected cattle removed from a high tsetse density,' *J. comp. Path.*, **71**, 325.

SMITH, K. G. V. (1967). 'The biology and taxonomy of the genus *Stylogaster* Macquart, 1835 (Diptera: Conopidae, Stylogasterinae) in the Ethiopian and Malagasy regions,' *Trans. R. ent. Soc. Lond.*, **119**, 47.

SNODGRASS, R. E. (1944). 'The feeding apparatus of biting and sucking insects affecting man and animals,' *Smithsonian Misc. Coll.*, **104**, No. 7.

SOCIÉTÉ DES USINES CHIMIQUES RHÔNE-POULENC (1961). 'Salt of suramin and chloroquine, an antimalarial agent,' *Patent Appl.*, July 27, 1960.

SOLTYS, M. A. (1955). 'Studies on resistance to *Trypanosoma congolense* developed by Zebu cattle treated prophylactically with Antrycide Pro-salt in an enzootic area of East Africa,' *Ann. trop. Med. Parasit.*, **49**, 1.

SOLTYS, M. A. (1957). 'Immunity in Trypanosomiasis. I. Neutralization reaction,' *Parasitology*, **47**, 375.

SOLTYS, M. A. (1957a). Immunity in Trypanosomiasis. II. Agglutination reaction with African trypanosomes. *Parasitology*, **47**, 390.

SOLTYS, M. A. (1958). 'Immunity in trypanosomiasis and its effect on chemotherapy,' *Vet. Rec.*, **70,** 657.

SOLTYS, M. A. (1964). 'Immunity in trypanosomiasis. V. Immunization of animals with dead trypanosomes,' *Parasitology*, **54,** 585.

SOUSA, A. E. DE (1961). 'The advance of *Glossina* in Southern Mozambique.' *See* ISCTR (1961), p. 203.

SOUTHON, H. A. W. (1959). 'The resting sites of *Glossina swynnertoni* at night.' *See* EATRO (1959), p. 55.

SOUTHON, H. A. W. (1959a). 'Studies in predation on *Glossina*.' *See* EATRO (1959), p. 56.

SOUTHON, H. A. W., and COCKINGS, K. L. (1963). 'Laboratory maintenance of *Glossina*.' *See* EATRO (1963), p. 30.

SOUTHON, H. A. W., and COCKINGS, K. L. (1963a). 'Fertilization of *G. morsitans* in the laboratory.' *See* EATRO (1963a), p. 33.

SOUTHON, H. A. W., and CUNNINGHAM, M. P. (1966). 'Infectivity of trypanosomes derived from individual *Glossina morsitans* Westw.,' *Nature*, Lond. **212,** 1477.

SOUTHON, H. A. W., and ROBERTSON, D. H. H. (1961). 'The isolation of *T. rhodesiense* from wild *G. palpalis*,' *Nature*, Lond. **189,** 411.

SOUTHWOOD, T. R. E. (1966). *Ecological Methods.* London, Methuen & Co. Ltd. xviii + 391 pp.

SPINKS, A. (1948). 'The persistence in the blood stream of some compounds related to suramin,' *Biochem. J.*, **42,** 109.

SQUIRE, F. A. (1950). 'Age-grouping of tsetse flies as an aid to the study of their bionomics,' *Nature*, Lond. **165,** 307.

SQUIRE, F. A. (1951). 'Seasonal variation in the incidence of *Trypanosoma vivax* in *Glossina palpalis* (R.-D.),' *Bull. ent. Res.*, **42,** 371.

SQUIRE, F. A. (1951a). 'Observations on mating scars in *Glossina palpalis* (R.-D.),' *Bull. ent. Res.*, **42,** 601.

SQUIRE, F. A. (1952). 'On the sex ratio in *Glossina*,' *Bull. ent. Res.*, **43,** 231.

SQUIRE, F. A. (1954). 'Observations on the incidence of trypanosomes in *Glossina palpalis* (R.-D.) in Sierra Leone,' *Bull. ent. Res.*, **45,** 745.

STEEL, J. H. (1885). 'Investigation into an obscure and fatal disease among transport mules in British Burma.'

STEEL, W. S., and GLEDHILL, J. A. (1960). 'The Broken Hill—Mulungushi Dam tsetse eradication scheme.' *See* ISCTR (1960), p. 247.

STEEL, W. S., GLEDHILL, J. A., and NORTON, L. B. (1960). 'Chingola tsetse control scheme.' *See* ISCTR (1960), p. 291.

STEELE, B. (1958). 'Report on the progress of a project to eradicate *Glossina brevipalpis* in the district of Karonga, Nyasaland.' *See* ISCTR (1958), p. 91.

STEFANOPOULO, G., CAUBET, P., and DUVOLON, S. (1945). 'Méningo-encéphalite a *Trypanosoma gambiense* (souche neurotrope) observée chez le lapin,' *Bull. Soc. Path. exot.*, **38,** 271.

STEINER, J. O. (1964). Tsetse control section of *Rural Health Report, 1963.* Min. of Health, Northern Nigeria. Govt. Printer, Kaduna.

STEINER, L. F., HARRIS, E. J., MITCHELL, W. C., FUJIMOTO, M. S., and CRISTENSON, L. D. (1965). 'Melon fly eradication by overflooding with sterile flies,' *J. econ. Ent.*, **58,** 519.

STEINERT, M. (1960). 'Mitochondria associated with the kinetonucleus of *T. mega*,' *Journal of Biophysical and Biochemical Cytology*, **8,** 542.

STEINERT, M. (1965). L'absence d'histone dans le kinétonucléus des trypanosomes,' *Exp. Cell Res.*, **39,** 69.

STEINERT, M., and VAN ASSEL, S. (1967). 'The loss of kinetoplastic DNA in two species of Trypanosomatidae treated with acriflavine,' *J. Cell. Biol.*, **34,** 489.

STEPHEN, L. E. (1962). 'Experimental *Trypanosoma congolense* infection in a horse,' *Vet. Rec.*, **74,** 853.

STEPHEN, L. E. (1962a). 'Suramin complexes. IX. An experiment to test the therapeutic activity of Antrycide-suramin complex against *T. simiae* in pigs,' *Ann. trop. Med. Parasit.*, **56,** 401.

STEPHEN, L. E. (1962b). 'Suramin complexes. X. Comparison of the prophylactic activity of Prothidium-suramin complex and Prothidium bromide in West African zebu cattle,' *Ann. trop. Med. Parasit.*, **56,** 406.

STEPHEN, L. E. (1962c). 'Some observations on the behaviour of trypanosomes occurring in cattle previously treated with prophylactic drugs,' *Ann. trop. Med. Parasit.*, **56,** 415.

STEPHEN, L. E. (1963). 'The chemotherapy and chemoprophylaxis of *Trypanosoma simiae* infections,' *Vet. Bull.*, **33,** 599.

STEPHEN, L. E. (1963a). 'On the validity of *Trypanosoma montgomeryi* Laveran, 1909,' *Ann. trop. Med. Parasit.*, **57,** 397.

STEPHEN, L. E. (1963b). 'A morphological and biometrical study of the blood forms of *Trypanosoma suis* Ochmann, 1905,' *Parasitology*, **53,** 217.

STEPHEN, L. E. (1963c). 'An attempt to produce resistance to homidium in a strain of *Trypanosoma vivax* transmitted by tsetse fly,' *Jour. comp. Path. Ther.*, **73,** No. 1, 76.

STEPHEN, L. E. (1966). 'Observations on the resistance of West African N'Dama and Zebu cattle to trypanosomiasis following challenge by wild *Glossina morsitans* from an early age,' *Ann. trop. Med. Parasit.*, **60,** 230.

STEPHEN, L. E. (1966a). *Pig Trypanosomiasis in Tropical Africa.* Commonwealth Bureau of Animal Health, Review Series No. 8. Farnham House, Farnham Royal, Bucks.

STEPHEN, L. E., and GRAY, A. R. (1960). 'Suramin complexes. VI. The prophylactic activity of Antrycide-suramin complex and Antrycide chloride against *Trypanosoma simiae* in pigs,' *Ann. trop. Med. Parasit.*, **54,** 493.

STEPHEN, L. E., and GRAY, A. R. (1961). 'Observations on the therapeutic activity of Metamidium, Tozocide and Nucleocidin against *Trypanosoma simiae* infections in pigs,' *Vet. Rec.*, **73,** 563.

STEPHEN, L. E., and MACKENZIE, C. P. (1959). 'Experimental *Trypanosoma vivax* infection in the horse,' *Vet. Rec.*, **71,** 527.

STEPHENS, J. W. W., and BLACKLOCK, B. (1913). 'On the non-identity of *Trypanosoma brucei* Plimmer and Bradford, 1899, with the trypanosome of the same name from the Uganda ox,' *Proc. Roy. Soc.*, (B) **86,** 187.

STEPHENS, J. W. W., and FANTHAM, H. B. (1910). 'On the peculiar morphology of a trypanosome from a case of sleeping sickness and the possibility of its being a new species (*Trypanosoma rhodesiense*),' *Proc. Roy. Soc.*, (B) **83,** 28.

STEWART, J. L. (1936). 'Porcine trypanosomiasis in the Gold Coast,' *Trans. R. Soc. trop. Med. Hyg.*, **30,** 313.

STEWART, J. L. (1937). *Report on the eradication of tsetse flies of the* palpalis *group, from the Pong Tamale area, Northern Territories.* Accra, Gold Coast Govt. Printer. No. 1 of 1937.

STEWART, J. L. (1951). 'The West African shorthorn cattle: their value to Africa as trypanosomiasis-resistant animals,' *Vet. Rec.*, **63,** 454.

STEYN, J. J. (1949). 'DDT field trials against *Glossina palpalis* on Nkusi Island, Lake Victoria,' *J. entom. Soc. Southern Africa*, **12,** 126.

STUHLMANN, F. (1907). 'Beiträge zur Kentniss der Tsetsefliege (*Glossina fusca* und *Gl. tachinoides*),' *Arb. Kaiserl. Gesundheits.*, **26,** 301.

SWYNNERTON, C. F. M. (1921). 'An examination of the tsetse problem in North Mossurisse, Portuguese East Africa,' *Bull. ent. Res.*, **11,** 315.

SWYNNERTON, C. F. M. (1923). 'The entomological aspects of an outbreak of sleeping sickness near Mwanza, Tanganyika Territory,' *Bull. ent. Res.*, **13,** 317.

SWYNNERTON, C. F. M. (1925). 'An experiment in the control of tsetse flies at Shinyanga, Tanganyika Territory,' *Bull. ent. Res.*, **15,** 313.

SWYNNERTON, C. F. M. (1933). 'Some traps for tsetse-flies,' *Bull. ent. Res.*, **24,** 69.

SWYNNERTON, C. F. M. (1936). 'The tsetse flies of East Africa. A first study of their ecology with a view to their control,' *Trans. R. ent. Soc. Lond.*, **84,** 1.

SYMES, C. B., HADAWAY, A. B., BARLOW, F., and GALLEY, W. (1948). 'Field experiments with DDT and Benzene Hexachloride against tsetse (*G. palpalis*),' *Bull. ent. Res.*, **38,** 591.

SYMES, C. B., and SOUTHBY, R. (1938). *The Reduction of* G. palpalis *in a Lake Shore Area by the 'Block' Method.* Nairobi, Govt. Printer.

SYMES, C. B., and VANE, R. T. (1937). *The eradication of* G. palpalis *from river areas by the 'block' method.* Nairobi, Govt. Printer. 61 pp.

TALBOT, L. M., and PAYNE, W. J. A. (1965). *The meat production potential of wild animals in Africa. A Review.* Commonwealth Agricultural Bureau, Farnham Royal.

TAVERNE, J. (1957). 'Immune-adherence of bacteriophage T_2,' *Brit. J. exp. Path.*, **38,** 377.

TAYLOR, A. E. R. (1966). 'The infectivity of *Trypanosoma vivax* (Desowitz strain) to mice,' *Trans. R. Soc. trop. Med. Hyg.*, **60,** 119.

TAYLOR, A. E. R., and BAKER, J. R. (1968). *The Cultivation of Parasites* in vitro. Oxford, Blackwell Scientific Publications.

TAYLOR, A. W. (1930). '*Glossina palpalis* and sleeping sickness at Ganawuri, Plateau Province, Northern Nigeria,' *Bull. ent. Res.*, **21,** 333.

TAYLOR, A. W. (1932). 'Pupal parasitism in *Glossina morsitans* and *G. tachinoides* at Gadau, Northern Nigeria,' *Bull. ent. Res.*, **23,** 463.

TAYLOR, A. W. (1932a). 'The development of West African strains of *Trypanosoma gambiense* in *Glossina tachinoides* under normal laboratory conditions and at raised temperatures,' *Parasitology*, **24,** 401.

TAYLOR, J. M., and STANNERS, C. P. (1968). 'The synthesis of RNA by mammalian cells treated with the aminonucleoside of Puromycin,' *Biochim. biophys. Acta*, **155,** 424.

TEESDALE, C. (1940). 'Fertilization in the tsetse fly *Glossina palpalis* in a population of low density,' *J. anim. Ecol.*, **9,** 24.

TEMPLETON, R. G. (1965). 'An attempt to eradicate *Glossina tachinoides* and *Glossina morsitans submorsitans* in an area of endemic sleeping sickness in Northern Nigeria by the use of residual insecticides.' *See* ISCTR (1965), p. 167.

TEMPLIS, C. H., and LOFY, M. F. (1963). 'A modified method for identification of mosquito blood meals,' *Am. J. trop. Med. Hyg.*, **12,** 825.

TERRY, R. J. (1957). 'Antibody against *Trypanosoma vivax* present in the cotton rat,' *Exp. Parasit.*, **6,** 404.

THEILER, A. (1903). 'A new *Trypanosoma* and the disease caused by it,' *J. comp. Path. Therap.*, **16,** 193.

THEILER, A. (1918). *Slapziekte in Horses in Griqualand West* (*Dourine*). Union of South Africa Dept. of Agriculture. Pretoria, Govt. Printing and Stationery Office.

THILLET, C. J., and CHANDLER, A. C. (1957). 'Immunization against *Trypanosoma lewisi* in rats by injection of metabolic products,' *Science*, N.Y. **125,** 346.

THOMAS, SIR W. E., DAVEY, T. H., and POTTS, W. H. (1955). 'Report of the Commission of Enquiry on human and animal trypanosomiasis in Southern Rhodesia,' *Federation of Rhodesia and Nyasaland, C. Fed.*, **24,** Salisbury. Govt. Printer. 115 pp.

THOMPSON, B. W. (1953). 'Aircraft applications of insecticides in East Africa III. Atmospheric turbulence in woodland,' *Bull. ent. Res.*, **44,** 611.

THOMPSON, P. E., OLSZEWSKI, B. J., ELSLAGER, E. F., and WORTH, D. F. (1963). 'Laboratory studies on 4,6-diamino-1-(*p*-chlorophenyl)-1,2-dihydro-2,2-dimethyl-*s*-triazine pamoate (C1–501) as a repository anti-malarial drug,' *Amer. J. trop. Med. Hyg.*, **12,** 481.

THOMSON, W. E. F., GLOVER, P. E., and TRUMP, E. C. (1961). 'The extermination of *G. pallidipes* from an isolated area on Lake Victoria with the use of insecticides.' *See* ISCTR (1961), p. 303.

THURSTON, J. P. (1958). 'The effect of immune sera on the respiration of *Trypanosoma brucei in vitro*,' *Parasitology*, **48,** 463.

TINLEY, K. L. (1964). 'Some observations on certain Tabanid flies in North-eastern Zululand,' *Proc. Roy. ent. Soc. Lond.*, (A) **39,** 73.

TOBIE, ELEANOR J. (1958). 'The cultivation of *Trypanosoma congolense in vitro*,' *J. Parasit.*, **44,** 241.

TOBIE, ELEANOR J., VON BRAND, T., and MEHLMAN, B. (1950). 'Cultural and physiological observations on *Trypanosoma rhodesiense* and *Trypanosoma gambiense*,' *J. Parasit.*, **36,** 48.

TODD, J. L. (1912). *Trans. XV Internat. Congress on Hyg., and Demography.* Washington, Sept. 25–28, 1912.

TOMCHICK, R., and MANDEL, H. G. (1964). 'Biochemical effects of Ethidium bromide in micro-organisms,' *J. gen. Microbiol.*, **36,** 225.

TOOTH, G. (1950). *Studies in mental illness on the Gold Coast.* Colonial Research Publication No. 6. London, HMSO.

TOTHILL, J. D. (1948). Editor. *Agriculture in the Sudan.* London, Oxford University Press.

TOULANT, M. (1950). 'Manifestations oculaires des trypanosomiases humaines,' *Maladie du sommeil—Fièvre de Rhodesie—Maladie de Chagas.* Paris, Masson et Cie. 103 pp.

TOURÉ, S. M. (1967). 'Répartition géographique et écologie spéciale des Glossines (Diptera, Muscidae) au Senegal.' FAO/IAEA Panel on control of Livestock Insect Pests by the Sterile-Male Technique, Vienna. (Typescript, 7 pp.)

TOUSSAINT, A. J., and ANDERSON, R. I. (1965). 'Soluble antigen fluorescent antibody technique,' *Appl. Microbiology*, **13,** 552.

TOUSSAINT, A. J., TARRANT, C. J., and ANDERSON, R. I. (1965a). 'An indirect fluorescent antibody technique using soluble antigens for serodiagnosis of *Trypanosoma cruzi* infection,' *Proc. Soc. exp. Biol., N.Y.*, **120,** 783.

TOWNSEND, C. H. T. (1923). 'The tsetse problem,' *S. A. J. nat. Hist.*, **4,** 36 and 139.

TRAGER, W. (1959). 'Tsetse fly tissue culture and the development of trypanosomes to the infective stage,' *Ann. trop. Med. Parasitol.*, **53,** 473.

TRÉFOUEL, J. (1962). 'Le rôle de Maurice Nicolle en chimiothérapie antitrypanosomes,' *Bull. Soc. Path. exot.*, **55,** 200.

TURK, J. L. (1958). 'Immune-adherence with stable antigens,' *Immunology*, **1,** 305.

TURK, J. L. (1964). 'The detection of antibodies by immune-adherence,' in *Immunological Methods*, (ed. J. F. Ackroyd) Oxford, Blackwell Scientific Publications. pp. 405–15.

TURNBULL, J. H. (1964). 'Enzymes, drugs and antibodies, some chemical factors,' *Experientia*, **20,** 113.

TURNER, E. C., and GERHARDT, R. R. (1965). 'A material for rapid marking of face flies for dispersal studies,' *J. econ. Ent.*, **58,** p. 584.

UNSWORTH, K. (1949). 'Trypanosomiasis researches,' *Nigerian Ann. Rep. Vet. Dept. 1948.*

UNSWORTH, K., and BIRKETT, J. D. (1952). 'The use of Antrycide prosalt in protecting cattle against trypanosomiasis when in transit through tsetse areas,' *Vet. Rec.*, **64,** 24, 351.

UNSWORTH, K., and NESBITT, P. E. (1952). 'Studies on *Trypanosoma vivax*. II. The maintenance of a strain in rabbits,' *Ann. trop. Med. Parasit.*, **46,** 85.

VAN BOGAERT, L. (1956). 'De quelques aspects neurologiques de la trypanosomiase africaine,' *Ann. Soc. belge Méd. trop.*, **36,** 645.

VAN BOGAERT, L. (1958). 'La trypanosomiase africaine,' *Handbuch der speziellen pathologischen Anatomie und Histologie*, (ed. W. Scholz) 13ster Band, 2ter Teil: *Erkrankungen des zentralen Nervensystems II*, 1089–1099. Berlin, Springer.

VAN BOGAERT, L., and DUBOIS, A. (1956). 'Sur l'encéphalite expérimentale à *Trypanosoma gambiense* chez le hamster de Syrie (*Mesocricetus auratus*),' *Rev. belge Path. et Méd. expér.*, **25,** 257.

VAN BOGAERT, L., and JANSSEN, P. (1957). 'Contribution a l'étude de la neurologie et neuropathologie de la trypanosomiase humaine,' *Ann. Soc. belge Méd. trop.*, **37,** 379.

VAN DEN BERGHE, L., and LAMBRECHT, F. L. (1954). 'Notes on the discovery and biology of *Glossina brevipalpis* Newst. in the Mosso Region, (Urundi),' *Bull. ent. Res.*, **45,** 501.

VAN DEN BERGHE, L., LAMBRECHT, F. L., and CHRISTIAENSEN, A. R. (1956). 'Étude biologique et écologique des glossines dans la région de Mutara (Ruanda),' *Mém. Acad. Royale Sci. Colon.* N.S., **4,** 2, 102 pp.

VAN DEN BERGHE, L., PEEL, E., and CHARDOME, M. (1963). 'Les trypanosomes transmis par *Glossina vanhoofi*,' *Ann. Soc. belge Méd. trop.*, **43,** 151.

VAN DEN BERGHE, L., and ZAGHI, A. J. (1963). 'Wild pigs as hosts of *Glossina vanhoofi* Henrard and *Trypanosoma suis* Ochmann in the Central African forest,' *Nature*, Lond. **197,** 1126.

VAN DEN BRANDEN, F. (1941). 'Considérations au sujet du sérodiagnostic de la trypanosomiase,' *Bull. Soc. Path. exot.*, **34,** 81.

VAN DEN BRANDEN, F., and APPELMANS, M. (1934). 'Les troubles visuels dans la trypanosomiase humaine,' *Ann. Soc. belge Méd. trop.*, **14,** 91.

VAN DYKE, K., and SZUSTKIEWICZ, C. (1968). 'Automated systems for the fluorometric determination of nucleic acids by the ethidium bromide technique,' *Anal. Biochem.*, **23,** 109.

VAN EMDEN, F. I. (1944). 'A new Sub-species of *Glossina* from Uganda (Diptera),' *Bull. ent. Res.*, **35,** 193.

VAN GOIDSENHOVEN, C., and SCHOENAERS, F. (1944). 'Sur la stabilisation des antigènes utilisés au sérodiagnostic des trypanosomiases,' *Ann. Soc. belge Méd. trop.*, **24,** 167.

VAN HOEVE, K., and CUNNINGHAM, M. P. (1964). 'Prophylactic activity of Berenil against trypanosomes in treated cattle,' *Vet. Rec.*, **76,** 260.

VAN HOEVE, K., CUNNINGHAM, M. P., and GRAINGE, E. B. (1965). 'Some observations on the treatment of cattle with Berenil.' *See* ISCTR (1965), p. 27.

VAN HOEVE, K., and GRAINGE, E. B. (1966). 'Berenil sensitivity *in vitro* of trypanosomes of the *T. brucei* subgroup and *T. congolense* group.' *See* EATRO (1966), p. 63.

VAN HOEVE, K., ONYANGO, R. J., HARLEY, J. M. B., and DE RAADT, P. (1967). 'The epidemiology of *Trypanosoma rhodesiense* sleeping sickness in Alego location, Central Nyanza, Kenya. II. The cyclical transmission of *Trypanosoma rhodesiense* isolated from cattle to a man, a cow and to sheep,' *Trans. R. Soc. trop. Med. Hyg.*, **61,** 684.

VAN HOOF, L. (1947). 'Observations on trypanosomiasis in the Belgian Congo,' *Trans. R. Soc. trop. Med. Hyg.*, **40,** 728.

VAN HOOF, L., and HENRARD, C. (1934). 'La transmission cyclique des races résistantes de "*Trypanosoma gambiense*" par "*Glossina palpalis*",' *Ann. Soc. belge Méd. trop.* (note complementaire), **14,** 109.

VAN HOOF, L., HENRARD, C., and PEEL, E. (1944). 'Pentamidine in the prevention and treatment of trypanosomiasis,' *Trans. R. Soc. trop. Med. Hyg.*, **37,** 271.

VAN HOOF, L., HENRARD, C., and PEEL, E. (1948). 'Quelques observations sur les trypanosomes des grands mammifères au Congo Belge,' *Acta tropica*, **5,** 327.

VAN HOOF, L., LEWILLON, R., HENRARD, C., PEEL, E., and RODJESTVENSKY, B. (1946). 'A field experiment on the prophylactic value of pentamidine in sleeping sickness,' *Trans. R. Soc. trop. Med. Hyg.*, **39,** 327.

VAN SACEGHEM, R. (1934). 'The immunization of cattle against trypanosomiasis,' *Bull. Soc. Path. exot.*, **27,** 170.

VAN SACEGHEM, R. (1936). 'The immunization of cattle against trypanosomiasis,' *Bull. agric. Congo belge*, **27,** 47.

VAN SACEGHEM, R. (1938). 'L'immunisation des bovidés contre la trypanosomiase,' *Bull. Soc. Path. exot.*, **31,** 296.

VAN ZINDEREN BAKKER, E. M., and CLARK, J. D. (1962). 'Pleistocene climates and cultures in North Eastern Angola,' *Nature*, Lond., **196,** 639.

VANDERPLANK, F. L. (1944). 'Hybridization between *Glossina* species and suggested new method for control of certain species of tsetse,' *Nature*, Lond. **154,** 607.

VANDERPLANK, F. L. (1947). 'Experiments in the hybridization of tsetse flies (*Glossina*, Diptera) and the possibility of a new method of control,' *Trans. R. ent. Soc. Lond.*, **98,** 1.

VANDERPLANK, F. L. (1947a). 'Experiments with DDT on various species of tsetse in field and laboratory,' *Trans. R. Soc. trop. Med. Hyg.*, **40,** 603.

VANDERPLANK, F. L. (1947b). 'Some observations on the hunger-cycle of the tsetse flies *Glossina swynnertoni* and *G. pallidipes* (Diptera) in the field,' *Bull. ent. Res.*, **38,** 431.

VANDERPLANK, F. L. (1948). 'Experiments in cross-breeding tsetse-flies (*Glossina* species),' *Ann. trop. Med. Parasit.*, **42,** 131.

VANDERPLANK, F. L. (1948a). 'Studies of behaviour of the tsetse fly, *Glossina pallidipes*, in the field; influence of climatic factors on activity,' *J. anim. Ecol.*, **17,** 245.

VANDERPLANK, F. L. (1949). 'The classification of *Glossina morsitans* Westwood (Diptera, Muscidae) including a description of a new subspecies, varieties and hybrids,' *Proc. R. ent. Soc. Lond.*, (B) **18,** 56.

VANDERPLANK, F. L. (1949a). 'Variation in the male genitalia of the tsetse fly *Glossina pallidipes* Austen and a note on *G. austeni* Newstead,' *Proc. R. ent. Soc. Lond.* (B) **18,** 65.

VANDERPLANK, F. L. (1949b). 'The classification of *Glossina palpalis* including the descriptions of new subspecies and hybrids,' *Proc. R. ent. Soc. Lond.*, (B) **18,** 69.

VANDERPLANK, F. L. (1950). 'Air-speed/wing-tip speed ratios of insect flight,' *Nature*, Lond., **165,** 806.

VATTIER, G. (1965). 'Étude de caractères morphologiques et anatomiques en relation avec l'âge physiologique des femelles de Glossines,' *Cah., Office de la Recherche Scientifique et Technique Outre-Mer* (Ent. Méd.), Paris, nom. 2 (1964), p. 21.

VAUCEL, M. (1943). 'Glossines du Cameroun Française,' *Rev. Sci. méd. Pharm. vét. Afr. franç. libre*, **2,** 97.

VAUCEL, M. (1952). *Médecine Tropicale*. Paris, Flammarion.

VAUCEL, M., DODIN, A., and FROMENTIN, H. (1964). 'Concentration des hémoparasites extracellulaires par une méthode nouvelle,' *Ann. Soc. belge Méd. trop.*, **44,** 353.

VAUCEL, M. A., WADDY, B. B., SILVA, M. A. DE A., and PONS, V. E. (1963). 'Répartition de la trypanosomiase africaine chez l'homme et les animaux,' *Bull. Wld. Hlth. Org.*, **28,** 545.

VICKERMAN, K. (1962). 'The mechanism of cyclical development in trypanosomes of the *Trypanosoma brucei* sub-group: an hypothesis based on ultrastructural observations,' *Trans. R. Soc. trop. Med. Hyg.*, **56,** 487.

VICKERMAN, K. (1965). 'Polymorphism and mitochondrial activity in sleeping sickness trypanosomes,' *Nature*, Lond. **208,** 762.

VICKERMAN, K. (1966). 'Genetic systems in unicellular animals,' *Science Progress*, Oxford, **54,** 13.

VICKERMAN, K. (1966a). 'Replication of the mitochondrion in trypanosomes,' *Proc. Sixth Int. Congress for Electron Microscopy*, Kyoto (1966), Vol. 2, 245.

VILAGINES, R., and ATANASIU, P. (1967). 'Action of Ethidium bromide on growth of Herpes virus in cell cultures,' *Nature*, Lond. **215,** 87.

VINCENT, V., and THOMAS, R. G. (n.d.). *An agricultural Survey of Southern Rhodesia. Part 1. Agro-ecological Survey*. Federation of Rhodesia and Nyasaland. Govt. Printer, Salisbury. 124 pp.

WADDY, B. B. (1956). 'Organisation and work of the Gold Coast Medical Field Units,' *Trans. R. Soc. trop. Med. Hyg.*, **50,** 313.

WAITR (1956). West African Institute for Trypanosomiasis Research. *Annual Report* 1955.

WAITR (1957). West African Institute for Trypanosomiasis Research. *Annual Report* 1956.

WAITR (1958). West African Institute for Trypanosomiasis Research. *Annual Report* 1957.

WAITR (1959). West African Institute for Trypanosomiasis Research. *Annual Report* 1958.

WAITR (1960). West African Institute for Trypanosomiasis Research. *Annual Report* 1959.

WAITR (1961). West African Institute for Trypanosomiasis Research. *Annual Report*, 1960.

WAITR (1963). West African Institute for Trypanosomiasis Research. *Annual Report*, 1963.

WALKER, P. J. (1964). 'Reproduction and heredity in trypanosomes. A critical review dealing mainly with the African species in the mammalian host,' *Int. Rev. Cytol.*, **17,** 51.

WALKER, P. J. (1966). 'Freeze preservation of parasitic protozoa,' *Lab. Pract.*, **15,** 423.

WALKER, P. J. (1968). In *Infectious blood diseases* (ed. D. Weinman and M. Ristic) New York, Academic Press. pp. 367–91.

WALKER, P. J., and ASHWOOD-SMITH, M. J. (1961). 'Dimethyl sulphoxide, an alternative to glycerol, for the low temperature preservation of trypanosomes,' *Ann. trop. Med. Parasit.*, **55,** 93.

WALKER, P. J., and WILÉN, M. J. (1967). 'A controlled rate liquid nitrogen cooling device suitable for freeze preservation of living cells,' *Lab. Pract.*, **16,** 480.

WALLACE, F. G. (1963). 'Criteria for the differentiation of genera among the Trypanosomatid parasites of insects,' *Proc. I. Intern. Conf. Protozool.*, Prague, 1961, p. 70.

WALLACE, F. G. (1966). 'The Trypanosomatid parasites of insects and arachnids,' *Exp. Parasit.*, **18,** 124.

WALLACE, J. M., and WORMALL, A. (1931). 'Red-cell adhesion in trypanosomiasis of man and other animals. II. Some experiments on the mechanism of the reaction,' *Parasitology*, **23,** 346.

WALLIS, O. C. (1966). 'The effect of pentamidine on ribosomes of the parasitic flagellate *Crithidia* (*Strigomonas*) *oncopelti*,' *J. Protozool.*, **13,** 234.

WALLS, L. P. (1947). 'The chemotherapy of phenanthridine compounds,' *J. Soc. chem. Ind.*, **66,** 182.

WALLS, L. P. (1963). 'The chemotherapy of trypanosomiasis,' *Progr. Med. Chem.*, **3,** 52.

WARING, M. J. (1964). 'Complex formation with DNA and inhibition of *Escherichia coli* RNA polymerase by ethidium bromide,' *Biochim. biophys. Acta*, **87,** 358.

WARING, M. J. (1965). 'The effects of antimicrobial agents on RNA polymerase,' *Molec. Pharmacol.*, **1,** 1.

WARING, M. J. (1965a). 'Complex formation between Ethidium bromide and nucleic acids,' *J. molec. Biol.*, **13,** 269.

WARING, M. J. (1966). 'Structural requirements for the binding of ethidium to nucleic acids,' *Biochim. biophys. Acta*, **114,** 234.

WARING, M. J. (1966a). 'Cross-linking and intercalation in nucleic acids,' in *Biochemical Studies of Antimicrobial Drugs* (ed. B. A. Newton and P. E. Reynolds) *16th Symp. Soc. gen. Microbiol.*, p. 235.

WARING, M. J. (1968). 'Drugs which affect the structure and function of DNA,' *Nature*, Lond. **219,** 1320.

WATKINS, J. F. (1964). 'Observations on antigenic variation in a strain of *Trypanosoma brucei* growing in mice,' *J. Hyg., Lond.*, **62,** 69.

WATSON, E. A. (1920). *Dourine in Canada 1904–20. History, Research and Suppression.* Dominion of Canada, Department of Agriculture. Ottawa, Thomas Mulvey.

WATSON, H. J. C. (1962). 'Mel W: a field trial in the treatment of *Trypanosoma gambiense* sleeping sickness,' *Trans. R. Soc. trop. Med. Hyg.*, **56,** 231.

WATSON, H. J. C. (1963). 'The domestic pig as a reservoir of *Trypanosoma gambiense*.' *See* ISCTR (1963), p. 327.

WATSON, H. J. C. (1965). 'Mel W. Final report on a field trial in the treatment of *T. gambiense* sleeping sickness,' *Trans. R. Soc. trop. Med. Hyg.*, **59,** 163.

WATSON, H. J. C., and WILLIAMSON, J. (1958). 'Suramin complexes. Part III. Preliminary experiments in *Trypanosoma simiae* infections in pigs,' *Ann. trop. Med. Parasit.*, **52,** 72.

WAUD, D. R. (1968). 'Pharmacological receptors,' *Pharmacol. Rev.*, **20,** 49.

WEBER, G. (1968). 'Carbohydrate metabolism in cancer cells and the molecular correlation concept,' *Naturwiss.*, **55,** 418.

WEINMAN, D. (1946). 'Cultivation of African sleeping sickness trypanosomes on improved, simple, cell-free medium,' *Proc. Soc. exp. Biol. Med.*, **63,** 456.

WEINMAN, D. (1960). 'Cultivation of the African sleeping sickness trypanosomes from the blood and cerebrospinal fluid of patients and suspects,' *Trans. R. Soc. trop. Med. Hyg.*, **54,** 180.

WEINMAN, D. (1963). 'Problems of diagnosis of trypanosomiasis,' *Bull. Wld. Hlth. Org.*, **28,** 731.

WEINMAN, D., and MCALLISTER, J. (1947). 'Prolonged storage of human pathogenic protozoa with conservation of virulence,' *Amer. J. Hyg.*, **45,** 102.

WEISSMANN, G., DAVIES, P., and KRAKAUER, K. (1969). 'Stabilization of lysosomes by stilbamidines,' *Fed. Proc.*, **28,** 265.

WEITZ, B. (1952). 'The antigenicity of sera of man and animals in relation to the preparation of specific precipitating antisera,' *J. Hyg., Camb.*, **50,** 275.

WEITZ, B. (1956). 'Identification of blood meals of blood-sucking arthropods,' *Bull. Wld. Hlth. Org.*, **15,** 473.

WEITZ, B. (1957). 'An automatic dispenser for multiple serological titrations,' *J. clin. Path.*, **10,** 200.

WEITZ, B. (1960). 'Feeding habits of blood-sucking arthropods,' *Parasitological Reviews Section, Exp. Parasit.*, **9,** 63.

WEITZ, B. (1960a). 'A soluble protective antigen of *Trypanosoma brucei*,' *Nature*, Lond. **185,** 788.

WEITZ, B. (1960b). 'The properties of some antigens of *Trypanosoma brucei*,' *J. gen. Microbiol.*, **23,** 589.

WEITZ, B. (1962). 'Immunity in Trypanosomiasis,' in *Drugs, Parasites and Hosts: Biological Council Symposium* (ed. L. G. Goodwin and R. H. Nimmo-Smith). London, J. & A. Churchill.

WEITZ, B. (1963). 'The feeding habits of *Glossina*,' *Bull. Wld. Hlth. Org.*, **28,** 711.

WEITZ, B. (1963a). 'The antigenicity of some African Trypanosomes,' in *Immunity to Protozoa.* Oxford, Blackwell.

WEITZ, B. (1963b). 'The specificity of trypanosomal antigens by immunofluorescence,' *J. gen. Microbiol.*, **32,** 145.

WEITZ, B. (1963c). 'Immunological relationships between the African trypanosomes and their hosts,' *Ann. N.Y. Acad. Sci.*, **113,** 400.

WEITZ, B. (1964). 'The reaction of trypanosomes to their environment,' in *Symposia of the Society of General Microbiology*, **14,** 'Microbial behaviour "*in vivo*" and "*in vitro*".' pp. 112–21.

WEITZ, B. (1967). 'Measurement of intensity of fluorescence,' *Trans. R. Soc. trop. Med. Hyg.*, **61,** 144.

WEITZ, B., and BUXTON, P. A. (1953). 'The rate of digestion of blood meals of various haematophagous arthropods as determined by the precipitin test,' *Bull. ent. Res.*, **44,** 445.

WEITZ, B., and GLASGOW, J. P. (1956). 'The natural hosts of *Glossina* in East Africa,' *Trans. R. Soc. trop. Med. Hyg.*, **50,** 593.

WEITZ, B., and JACKSON, C. H. N. (1955). 'The host-animals of *Glossina morsitans* at Daga-Iloi,' *Bull. ent. Res.*, **46,** 531.

WEITZ, B., LANGRIDGE, W. P., BAX, P. N., and LEE-JONES, F. (1960). 'The natural hosts of *Glossina longipennis* Corti and of some other tsetse flies in Kenya.' *See* ISCTR (1960), p. 303.

WELCH, J. R. (1960). 'Variations in the venation of *Glossina morsitans orientalis* Vanderplank (Diptera: Muscidae),' *Proc. R. ent. Soc. Lond.*, (A) **35,** 58.

WELCH, J. R. (1960a). 'Observations on deciduous woodland in the Eastern Province of Tanganyika,' *J. Ecol.*, **48,** 557.

WENYON, C. M. (1926). *Protozoology*. Vol. 1. London, Baillière, Tindall & Cox.

WERNER, R. (1954). 'Über die Frage der placentaren Trypanosomen-Infektioner und Übertragung von Trypanosomen und Antikörpern durch die Milch auf das Neugeborene,' *Z. Tropenmed. Parasit.*, **5,** 422.

WERNER, R., and KUNERT, R. (1958). 'Über die Ursache von congenitalen Protozoen-infektionen,' *Z. Tropenmed. Parasit.*, **9,** 17.

WESTWOOD, J. O. (1850). 'Observations on the destructive species of dipterous insects known in Africa under the names of Tsetse, Zimb and Tsaltsalya, and their supposed connexion with the fourth plague of Egypt,' *Proc. zool. Soc. Lond.*, part 18, p. 258.

WHARTON, R. H., SEOW, C. L., GANAPATHIPILLAI, A., and JABARATNAM, G. (1962). 'House fly populations and their dispersion in Malaya with particular reference to the fly problem in the Cameron Highlands,' *Med. J. Malaya*, **17,** 115.

WHITE, F. (1962). 'Geographic variation and speciation in Africa with particular reference to *Diospyros*,' in *Symposium on Taxonomy and Geography* (ed. D. Nichols). The Systematics Association Publ. No. 4, p. 71.

WHITE, P. J. (1963). 'Residual application of Dieldrin against tsetse in the Mara Valley,' *Trop. Pesticides Res. Inst. Arusha. Misc. Rep.*, No. 381, 6 pp.

WHITE, R. G. (1960). 'The relation of the cellular responses in germinal centres of lymph nodes to the production of antibody,' *Symposium on Mechanisms of Antibody Formation*. 1959. Czechoslovak Academy of Sciences, 25–9.

WHITESIDE, E. F. (1949). 'An experiment in control of tsetse with DDT-treated oxen,' *Bull. ent. Res.*, **40,** 123.

WHITESIDE, E. F. (1962). 'Interactions between drugs, trypanosomes and cattle in the field,' in *Drugs, Parasites and Hosts* (ed. L. G. Goodwin and R. H. Nimmo-Smith). London, J. & A. Churchill Ltd. p. 117.

WHITESIDE, E. F. (1962a). 'The control of cattle trypanosomiasis with drugs in Kenya: methods and costs,' *E. Afr. agric. J.*, **28,** 67.

WHITESIDE, E. F. (1963). 'A strain of *Trypanosoma congolense* directly resistant to Berenil,' *J. comp. Path.*, **73,** 167.

WHITTEN, J. M. (1957). 'The supposed pre-pupa in Cyclorrhaphous Diptera.' *Quart. J. Micr. Sci.*, **98,** 241.

WHITTEN, W. K. (1956). 'Physiological control of population growth,' *Nature*, Lond. **178,** 992.

WIGGLESWORTH, V. B. (1929). 'Digestion in the tsetse fly,' *Parasitology*, **21,** 288.

WIGGLESWORTH, V. B. (1965). *The Principles of Insect Physiology*, 6th edition. London, Methuen.

WIJERS, D. J. B. (1958). 'Factors that may influence the infection rate of *Glossina palpalis* with *Trypanosoma gambiense*. I. The age of the fly at the time of the infected feed,' *Ann. trop. Med. Parasit.*, **52,** 385.

WIJERS, D. J. B. (1959). 'Polymorphism in *Trypanosoma gambiense* and *T. rhodesiense* and the significance of the intermediate forms,' *Ann. trop. Med. Parasit.*, **53,** 59.

WIJERS, D. J. B., and WILLETT, K. C. (1960). 'Factors that may influence the infection rate of *Glossina palpalis* with *Trypanosoma gambiense*. II. The number and the morphology of the trypanosomes present in the blood of the host at the time of the infected feed,' *Ann. trop. Med. Parasit.*, **54,** 341.

WILDE, J. K. H., and FRENCH, M. H. (1945). 'An experimental study of *Trypanosoma rhodesiense* infection in zebu cattle,' *J. comp. Path.*, **55,** 206.

WILLETT, K. C. (1953). 'The laboratory maintenance of *Glossina*,' *Parasitology*, **43,** 110.

WILLETT, K. C. (1955). 'A special method for the dissection of *Glossina*,' *Ann. trop. Med. Parasit.*, **49,** 376.

WILLETT, K. C. (1956). 'An experiment on dosage in human trypanosomiasis,' *Ann. trop. Med. Parasit.*, **50,** 75.

WILLETT, K. C. (1963). 'Some principles of the epidemiology of human trypanosomiasis in Africa,' *Bull. Wld. Hlth. Org.*, **28,** 645.

WILLETT, K. C. (1965). 'Some observations on the recent epidemiology of sleeping sickness in Nyanza Region and its relation to the general epidemiology of Gambian and Rhodesian sleeping sickness in Africa,' *Trans. R. Soc. trop. Med. Hyg.*, **59,** 374.

WILLETT, K. C. (1966). 'Development of the peritrophic membrane in *Glossina* (tsetse flies) and its relation to infection with trypanosomes,' *Exp. Parasit.*, **18,** 290.

WILLETT, K. C. (1966a). 'The "trypanosome chancre" in Rhodesian sleeping sickness,' *Trans. R. Soc. trop. Med. Hyg.*, **60,** 689.

WILLETT, K. C., and GORDON, R. M. (1957). 'Studies on the deposition, migration, and development to the blood forms of trypanosomes belonging to the *T. brucei* group. II. An account of the migration of the trypanosomes from the site of their deposition in the rodent host to their appearance in the general circulation, with some observations on their probable routes of migration in the human host,' *Ann. trop. Med. Parasit.*, **51,** 471.

WILLETT, K. C., MCMAHON, J. P., ASHCROFT, M. T., and BAKER, J. R. (1964). 'Trypanosomes isolated from *Glossina palpalis* and *G. pallidipes* in Sakwa, Kenya,' *Trans. R. Soc. trop. Med. Hyg.*, **58,** 391.

WILLIAMS, J. S., DUXBURY, R. E., ANDERSON, R. I., and SADUN, E. H. (1963). 'Fluorescent antibody reactions in *Trypanosoma rhodesiense* and *T. gambiense* in experimental animals,' *J. Parasit.*, **49,** 380.

WILLIAMSON, J. (1956). 'The composition of tsetse fly saliva. II. Analysis of amino acids and sugars by paper partition chromatography,' *Ann. trop. Med. Parasit.*, **50,** 334.

WILLIAMSON, J. (1962). 'Chemotherapy and chemoprophylaxis of African trypanosomiasis,' *Exp. Parasit.*, **12,** 274.

WILLIAMSON, J. (1965). 'New aspects of trypanocidal drug action,' in *Progress in Protozoology.* Internat. Congr. Ser. No. 91. Excerpta Medica Foundation. Abstr. No. 77, p. 81.

WILLIAMSON, J. (1966). 'Cordycepin, an antitumour antibiotic with trypanocidal properties,' *Trans. R. Soc. trop. Med. Hyg.*, **60,** 8.

WILLIAMSON, J. (1966a). 'Trypanocidal drug action: some observations on synergism,' *Trans. R. Soc. trop. Med. Hyg.*, **60,** 121.

WILLIAMSON, J. (1969). 'The activity of drugs on *Trypanosoma congolense in vitro* at 37°C,' *Trans. R. Soc. trop. Med. Hyg.*, **63,** 422.

WILLIAMSON, J., and BROWN, K. N. (1964). 'The chemical composition of Trypanosomes. III. Antigenic constituents of *Brucei* trypanosomes,' *Exp. Parasit.*, **15,** 44.

WILLIAMSON, J., and COVER, B. (1966). 'Separation of blood-cell-free trypanosomes and malaria parasites on a sucrose gradient,' *Trans. R. Soc. trop. Med. Hyg.*, **60,** 425.

WILLIAMSON, J., and LOURIE, E. M. (1948). ' "Melarsen" and "Melarsen oxide",' *Nature*, Lond. Jan. 17, p. 103.

WILLIAMSON, J., and MACADAM, R. F. (1965). 'Effects of trypanocidal drugs on the fine structure of *Trypanosoma rhodesiense*,' *Trans. R. Soc. trop. Med. Hyg.*, **59,** 367.

WILLIAMSON, J., and STEPHEN, L. E. (1960). 'A test for drug-resistant trypanosomes in experimental tsetse-fly challenge of cattle,' *Ann. trop. Med. Parasit.*, **54,** 366.

WILSON, A. J., and GRAINGE, E. B. (1967). 'The effect of Berenil on *Trypanosoma theileri* Laveran infections in cattle.' *See* EATRO (1967), p. 79.

WILSON, S. G. (1948). 'The feeding of "Gammexane" and DDT to bovines,' *Bull. ent. Res.*, **39,** 423.

WILSON, S. G. (1949). '*Trypansosoma uniforme-Trypanosoma vivax* infections in bovines and *T. uniforme* infections in goats and sheep at Entebbe, Uganda,' *Parasitology*, **39,** 198.

WILSON, S. G. (1953). 'The control of *Glossina palpalis fuscipes* Newst. in Kenya colony,' *Bull. ent. Res.*, **44,** 711.

WINKLER, W. O. (1962). 'Identification of and estimation of the arsenic residue in livers of rats ingesting arsenicals,' *J. Ass. off. agric. Chem. Wash.*, **45,** 80.

WOLCOTT, G. B. (1952). 'Mitosis in *Trypanosoma lewisi*,' *J. Morph.*, **90,** 189.

WOODCOCK, K. E. (1949). 'Peripheral vegetation spraying on Ziribanje Island, Lake Victoria,' *Bureau Permanent Interafricaine de Tsetse et Trypanosomiase* No. 79. Brazzaville, 11 pp.

WOOFF, W. R. (1965). 'The eradication of *G. morsitans morsitans* in Ankole, western Uganda by Dieldrin application.' *See* ISCTR (1965), p. 157.

WOOFF, W. R. (1967). 'Consolidation in tsetse reclamation.' *See* ISCTR (1967), p. 141.

WORLD HEALTH ORGANISATION EXPERT COMMITTEE ON TRYPANOSOMIASIS (1962). *First Report.* Technical Report Series No. 247. Geneva and HMSO.

WORTHINGTON, E. B., and HARRIS, SIR DOUGLAS (1949). *A development plan for Uganda and the 1948 revision of the plan.* Entebbe, Govt. Printer.

YEO, D., and SIMPSON, H. R. (1960). 'The effect of repeated insecticidal applications on a natural tsetse population,' *Bull. ent. Res.*, **51,** 631.

YEO, D., and THOMPSON, B. W. (1954). 'Aircraft application of insecticides in East Africa. V. The deposition in open country of a coarse aerosol released from an aircraft,' *Bull. ent. Res.*, **45,** 79.

YORKE, W. (1921). 'Recent work on the treatment of sleeping sickness. A critical review,' *Trop. Dis. Bull.*, **18,** 155.

YORKE, W., MURGATROYD, F., and HAWKING, F. (1933). 'The relation of the polymorphic trypanosomes developing in the gut of *Glossina*, to the peritrophic membrane,' *Ann. trop. Med. Parasitol.*, **27,** 347.

YOSHIDA, T., YAMASHITA, F., and METCOFF, J. (1968). 'Metabolic basis of aminonucleoside nephrosis in rats. I. Inhibition of α-oxoglutarate oxidation by aminonucleoside,' *J. lab. clin. Med.*, **72,** 565.

YVORE, P., DESROTOUR, J., LAURENT, J., and FINELLE, P. (1963). 'Campagne d'éradication de *G. fuscipes fuscipes* par pulvérisation de Dieldrine en République Centrafricaine.' *See* ISCTR (1963), p. 187.

ZIEMANN, H. (1905). 'Beitrag zur Trypanosomenfrage,' *Cbl. Bakt.* (I. Abt.), **38,** 307, 429.

ZUMPT, F. (1936). '*Die Tsetsefliegen. Erkennungsmerkmale, Lebensweise und Bekämpfung*. Jena, G. Fischer.

Index

32